Clinical Ophthalmology
MEDICAL AND SURGICAL APPROACH

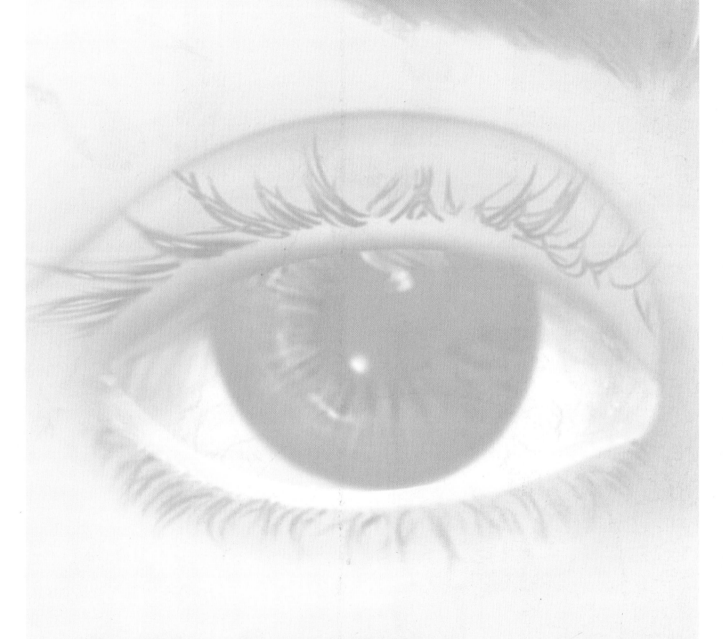

Clinical Ophthalmology
MEDICAL AND SURGICAL APPROACH

Second Edition

Editor

SANDEEP SAXENA MS MAMS

Member, National Academy of Medical Sciences, India
DAAD Visiting Professor, University of Bonn, Bonn, Germany
Visiting Professor, UNC-Chapel Hill, Chapel Hill, USA
Fellow, Barnes Retina Institute and Anheuser-Busch Eye Institute, St Louis, USA
Fellow, New York-Presbyterian Hospital, New York, USA

Professor, Department of Ophthalmology
CSM Medical University
(Erstwhile, King George's Medical University)
Lucknow, Uttar Pradesh, India

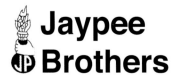

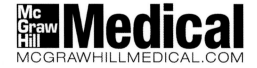

© 2012, Jaypee Brothers Medical Publishers
First published in India in 2011 by

Jaypee Brothers Medical Publishers (P) Ltd.

Corporate Office
4838/24 Ansari Road, Daryaganj, **New Delhi** - 110002, India, +91-11-43574357

Registered Office
B-3 EMCA House, 23/23B Ansari Road, Daryaganj,
New Delhi 110 002, India
Phones: +91-11-23272143, +91-11-23272703, +91-11-23282021,
+91-11-23245672, Rel: +91-11-32558559 Fax: +91-11-23276490,
+91-11-23245683
e-mail: jaypee@jaypeebrothers.com
Website: www.jaypeebrothers.com

First published in USA by The McGraw-Hill Companies, 2 Penn Plaza, New York, NY 10121. Exclusively worldwide distributor
except South Asia (India, Nepal, Sri Lanka, Bhutan, Pakistan, Bangladesh, Malaysia).

ISBN-13: 978-0-07-178129-9
ISBN-10: 0-07-178129-3

To

My parents
Dr R C Saxena and Mrs Madhu Saxena

&

My family
Sangeeta, Shreeya and Aishwarya

Contributors

Leonardo Akaishi, MD
Director
Hospital Oftalmólogico de Brasília
Modulo G, Brazil

Harmohina Bagga, MD
Formerly, Glaucoma Fellow
VST Center for Glaucoma Care
LV Prasad Eye Institute
Hyderabad, Andhra Pradesh, India

Samar K Basak, MD, DNB
Disha Eye Hospital and Research Center
Barrackpore, Kolkata, West Bengal, India

M Baskaran, DO, DNB
Consultant, Glaucoma Service
Sankara Nethralaya
Chennai, Tamil Nadu, India

Arnab Biswas, DOMS, FRCS
Consultant Oculoplastic and Orbital
Surgeon
Alo Eye Care
Kolkata, West Bengal, India

Jyotirmay Biswas, MS, FAMS
Head, Uveitis Service
Sankara Nethralaya
Chennai, Tamil Nadu, India

Gagandeep S Brar, MS
Formerly, Assistant Professor
Advanced Eye Center
Postgraduate Institute of Medical
Education and Research
Chandigarh, India

Arindam Chakravarti, MS
Vitreoretinal Consultant
Aditya Jyot Eye Hospital Private Limited
Mumbai, Maharashtra, India

Sunita Chaurasia, MS
Consultant, Cornea Service
LV Prasad Eye Institute
Hyderabad, Andhra Pradesh, India

Tanuj Dada, MD
Associate Professor
Dr Rajendra Prasad Center for
Ophthalmic Sciences
All India Institute of Medical Sciences
New Delhi, India

Taraprasad Das, MD, FRCS
Director
Head, Retina Service
LV Prasad Eye Institute
Bhubaneswar, Orissa, India

Sachi Devi, MS
Glaucoma Service
Sankara Nethralaya
Chennai, Tamil Nadu, India

Kumar Doctor, MS
Doctor Eye Institute
Mumbai, Maharashtra, India

Satpal Garg, MD
Professor
Dr Rajendra Prasad Center for
Ophthalmic Sciences
All India Institute of Medical Sciences
New Delhi, India

Ronnie George, MS, DO, DNB
Consultant, Glaucoma Service
Sankara Nethralaya
Chennai, Tamil Nadu, India

Lingam Gopal, MS, DNB, FRCS, FAMS
Director of Research
Medical and Vision Research Foundation
Sankara Nethralaya
Chennai, Tamil Nadu, India

Amod Gupta, MS, FAMS
Professor and Head
Advanced Eye Center
Postgraduate Institute of Medical
Education and Research
Chandigarh, India

Preeti Gupta, MS
Department of Ophthalmology
CSM Medical University
Lucknow, Uttar Pradesh, India

Vishali Gupta, MS
Associate Professor
Advanced Eye Center
Postgraduate Institute of Medical
Education and Research
Chandigarh, India

Albrecht Hennig, MD
Program Director
Sagarmatha Choudhary Eye Hospital
Lahan, Nepal

Santosh G Honavar, MD, FACS
Director, Ophthalmic Plastic Surgery
Orbital Diseases and Ocular Oncology
LV Prasad Eye Institute
Hyderabad, Andhra Pradesh, India

Chanda Hingorani, MS
Doctor Eye Institute
Mumbai, Maharashtra, India

Subhadra Jalali, MS
Head, Smt Kanuri Santhamma Retina
Vitreous Center
LV Prasad Eye Institute
Hyderabad, Andhra Pradesh, India

Apjit Kaur, MS
Professor
Department of Ophthalmology
CSM Medical University
Lucknow, Uttar Pradesh, India

Sushmita Kaushik, MS
Assistant Professor
Advanced Eye Center
Postgraduate Institute of Medical
Education and Research
Chandigarh, India

Mohit Khattri, MS
Department of Ophthalmology
CSM Medical University
Lucknow, Uttar Pradesh, India

Atul Kumar, MD, FAMS
Professor
Dr Rajendra Prasad Center for
Ophthalmic Sciences
All India Institute of Medical Sciences
New Delhi, India

Poonam Kishore, MS
Professor
Department of Ophthalmology
CSM Medical University
Lucknow, Uttar Pradesh, India

Ajit B Majji, MD
Consultant, Smt Kanuri Santhamma
Retina Vitreous Center
LV Prasad Eye Institute
Hyderabad, Andhra Pradesh, India

J Manju, B Opt
Electrodiagnostic Department
Sankara Nethralaya
Chennai, Tamil Nadu, India

Kanwar Mohan, MS
Formerly, Associate Professor
Department of Ophthalmology
Postgraduate Institute of Medical
Education and Research
Chandigarh, India

R Muralidhar, MS
Consultant, Cornea Service
LV Prasad Eye Institute
Hyderabad, Andhra Pradesh, India

Krishna R Murthy, MS
Vitreoretinal Department
Sankara Nethralaya
Chennai, Tamil Nadu, India

Praveen R Murthy, MS, DNB
Vitreoretinal Department
Sankara Nethralaya
Chennai, Tamil Nadu, India

Milind N Naik, MS
Consultant, Division of Ophthalmic
Plastic Surgery, Facial Aesthetic Surgery,
Orbit and Ocular Oncology
L V Prasad Eye Institute
Hyderabad, Andhra Pradesh, India

Arun Narayanaswamy, DNB
Consultant, Glaucoma Service
Sankara Nethralaya
Chennai, Tamil Nadu, India

S Natarajan, DO
Chairman and Managing Director
Aditya Jyot Eye Hospital Private Limited
Mumbai, Maharashtra, India

Aditya Neog, DO, DNB
Glaucoma Service
Sankara Nethralaya
Chennai, Tamil Nadu, India

Canrobert Oliveira, MD
Director, Refractive Surgery
Hospital Oftalmológico de Brasília
Modulo G, Brazil

Surinder S Pandav, MS
Additional Professor
Advanced Eye Center
Postgraduate Institute of Medical
Education and Research
Chandigarh, India

R Priya, M Phil (Opt)
Electrodiagnotic Department
Sankara Nethralaya
Chennai, Tamil Nadu, India

Jagat Ram, MS
Professor
Advanced Eye Center
Postgraduate Institute of Medical
Education and Research
Chandigarh, India

Kavita Rao, MS
Consultant
Aditya Jyot Eye Hospital Private Limited
Mumbai, Maharashtra, India

Srinivas K Rao DO, DNB, FRCS
Formerly, Consultant Cornea Service
Sankara Nethralaya
Chennai, Tamil Nadu, India

Ritika Sachdev, MS
Dr Rajendra Prasad Center for
Ophthalmic Sciences
All India Institute of Medical Sciences
New Delhi, India

Chinmaya Sahu, MS
Uveitis Service
Sankara Nethralaya
Chennai, Tamil Nadu, India

Virender Sangwan, MS
Associate Director
Director, Cornea and Uveitis Services
L V Prasad Eye Institute
Hyderabad, Andhra Pradesh, India

Puneet Saxena MS, MBA
Director, Industry Strategy
JDA
Dallas, USA

Sandeep Saxena MS MAMS
Professor
Department of Ophthalmology
CSM Medical University
Lucknow, Uttar Pradesh, India

G Chandra Sekhar, MD
Director
Head, VST Center for Glaucoma Care
LV Prasad Eye Institute
Hyderabad, Andhra Pradesh, India

Parveen Sen, MS
Consultant, Vitreoretinal Service
Sankara Nethralaya
Chennai, Tamil Nadu, India

Mahesh P Shanmugam, DO, DNB,
PhD, FRCS
Formerly, Consultant Vitreoretinal
Service
Sankara Nethralaya
Chennai, Tamil Nadu, India

Namrata Sharma, MD
Associate Professor
Dr Rajendra Prasad Center for
Ophthalmic Sciences
All India Institute of Medical Sciences
New Delhi, India

Rashmi Shetty, MBBS, FRSH
Consultant Cosmetic Physician
Revival Clinic
Mumbai, Maharashtra, India

Kirti Singh MD, DNB, FRCS
Professor, Glaucoma Division
Guru Nanak Eye Center
Maulana Azad Medical College
New Delhi, India

Vinita Singh, MS
Professor and Head
Department of Ophthalmology
CSM Medical University
Lucknow, Uttar Pradesh, India

Rajesh Sinha, MD, FRCS
Assistant Professor
Dr Rajendra Prasad Center for
Ophthalmic Sciences
All India Institute of Medical Sciences
New Delhi, India

Subijoy Sinha, MD
Dr Rajendra Prasad Center for
Ophthalmic Sciences
All India Institute of Medical Sciences
New Delhi, India

Late G Sitalakshmi, DO, FRCS
Consultant, Cornea Service
Sankara Nethralaya
Chennai, Tamil Nadu, India

Parul Sony, MD
Formerly, Senior Research Associate
Dr Rajendra Prasad Center for
Ophthalmic Sciences
All India Institute of Medical Sciences
New Delhi, India

S Sudharshan, DO
Consultant, Uveitis Service
Sankara Nethralaya
Chennai, Tamil Nadu, India

Radhika Tandon, MD
Professor
Dr Rajendra Prasad Center for
Ophthalmic Sciences
All India Institute of Medical Sciences
New Delhi, India

Mukesh Taneja, MS
Consultant, Cornea Service
L V Prasad Eye Institute
Hyderabad, Andhra Pradesh, India

Manoj K Tangri, MS
Senior Partner Manager
Hewlett-Packard Company
Fort-Collins, USA

Hem K Tewari, MD
Formerly, Professor and Chief
Dr Rajendra Prasad Center for
Ophthalmic Sciences
All India Institute of Medical Sciences
New Delhi, India

Jeewan S Titiyal, MD
Professor
Dr Rajendra Prasad Center for
Ophthalmic Sciences
All India Institute of Medical Sciences
New Delhi, India

Vasumathy Vedantham, MS, FRCS
Former Retina Fellow
Smt Kanuri Santhamma
Retina Vitreous Center
L V Prasad Eye Institute
Hyderabad, Andhra Pradesh, India

Geeta K Vemuganti, MD
Ophthalmic Pathology Division
L V Prasad Eye Institute
Hyderabad, Andhra Pradesh, India

Pradeep Venkatesh, MD
Associate Professor
Dr Rajendra Prasad Center for
Ophthalmic Sciences
All India Institute of Medical Sciences
New Delhi, India

Lalit Verma, MD
Formerly, Additional Professor
Dr Rajendra Prasad Center for
Ophthalmic Sciences
All India Institute of Medical Sciences
New Delhi, India

Lingam Vijaya, MS
Head, Glaucoma Service
Sankara Nethralaya
Chennai, Tamil Nadu, India

Foreword

The pace of change in ophthalmology is rapid and requires us to constantly update our skills and knowledge. We are subspecialized to a degree that demands that we must stay in close communication with our colleagues to be able to follow the advances occurring in the separate subdivisions of our specialty. In this challenging intellectual environment, a text bringing together respected authors from multiple disciplines is particularly welcome, and Dr Saxena has accomplished this task with great success. Twenty-one chapters cover new concepts and technological advances in the diagnosis and management of common ophthalmic disorders. Several chapters deal with advances in lens surgery, and several authorities cover new concepts in retinal disease including macular and submacular surgery. Modern concepts in corneal disease, glaucoma, oculoplastics, ocular oncology, infectious and inflammatory diseases, strabismus, trauma, and optic nerve 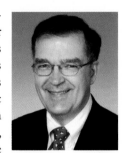 disorders are each presented by experts in ophthalmology. As ophthalmology has become more complex, we are driven to establish higher standards of scientific proof for our treatments and simultaneously to run our practices with greater efficiency to be able to bring the best of high technology to bear on our patients' problems while being mindful of cost. Thus, I was particularly pleased to see practice management and clinical trials covered in this text. Dr Saxena is an extraordinarily gifted and energetic physician and academician who, along with his fellow authors, has produced a book, which is an important contribution to contemporary ophthalmic education. Readers will benefit greatly from this accomplishment.

Travis A Meredith MD
Sterling A Barrett Distinguished Professor
Chairman, Department of Ophthalmology
University of North Carolina
Chapel Hill, USA

Preface to the Second Edition

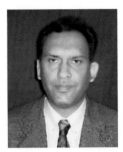

Ophthalmology is a continuously advancing field. As new technologies are being introduced at a rapid pace, the ophthalmologist must learn their intricacies as one begins to apply them to the treatment of ocular diseases. The adoption of new technology, in turn, brings with it the need to learn new skills and develop new treatment algorithms. Old concepts change and new ideas are plentiful. Everything is difficult before it becomes easy.

Clinical Ophthalmology: Medical and Surgical Approach is being launched as the second edition of *Clinical Practice in Ophthalmology*. This text attempts to update the state-of-the-art ophthalmology in a lucid, authoritative and well-illustrated manner. Ten sections encompassing forty-four chapters provide a new insight into the subject.

In this challenging intellectual environment *Clinical Ophthalmology: Medical and Surgical Approach* brings together a distinguished group of seventy-one experts and provides a comprehensive text combined with integrated visual reference, in the form of black and white and colored figures. The value of this book lays in the quality and expertise of the text chapter contributors. This book is intended for the experienced ophthalmologists, postgraduates as well as those in training. It is hoped that this book will be sufficiently comprehensive to aid the ophthalmologist in making diagnosis of common ophthalmic conditions as well as in performing competent surgeries. This pragmatic book provides an understanding of ophthalmology, important to the everyday practice. I hope this book will find a meaningful and valued place in the libraries of ophthalmologists, today and in future.

Sandeep Saxena

Preface to the First Edition

With the evolution of new diagnostic and therapeutic modalities, the ophthalmologist has become more involved in decision-making for patients. The challenge facing the ophthalmologist lies in maintaining an up-to-date practical knowledge. This thirst for knowledge is typical of those who are fascinated by the subject, but is also true of those who develop a great understanding of the subject.

Clinical Practice in Ophthalmology, a multi-authored text, was conceptualized in New York, USA. The publisher and the contributing authors were contacted on Internet to lay the groundwork. This book summarizes the present knowledge of clinical ophthalmology and practice management. The value of this book lies in the quality and expertise of the authors of the selected subjects. The authors have presented the material to provide the reader with a quick, but comprehensive review of the major ophthalmological issues. This pragmatic book provides an understanding of diseases so important to the everyday practice of ophthalmology. I hope this book will find a meaningful and valued place in the libraries of ophthalmologists, today and in future.

This book would not have been possible without the guidance of my mentors, cooperation of my family and help of Dr SK Bhasker.

Sandeep Saxena

Contents

Clinical Ophthalmology: Medical and Surgical Approach

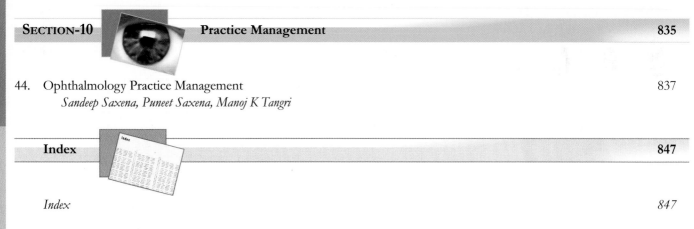

Clinical Ophthalmology: Medical and Surgical Approach

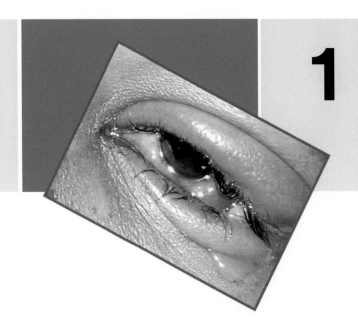

Corneal and External Diseases

1. **Investigations for Corneal and External Diseases**
2. **External Eye Diseases**
3. **Diseases of Cornea**
4. **Corneal Surgeries**
5. **Refractive Surgeries**

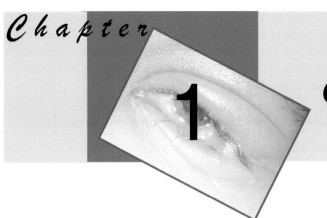

Chapter 1

Investigations for Corneal and External Diseases

Poonam Kishore, Preeti Gupta

INTRODUCTION

Conditions requiring investigations can be grouped as:
- Infectious keratitis
- Dry eye diseases
- Keratoplasty work-up

DIAGNOSIS IN INFECTIOUS KERATITIS

Corneal ulcer is an ocular emergency, which can lead to serious sight-threatening complications. Empirical treatment with broad spectrum antibiotic has to be started immediately after thorough clinical evaluation and after procuring the samples for microbiological evaluation. These microbiological investigations help in making accurate etiological diagnosis and in the modification of therapy in presence of non-improvement with the initial treatment.

Types of Samples

- Eyelid, corneal and conjunctival swabs
- Corneal scrapings
- Corneal biopsy
- Anterior chamber tap

Sample Collection Gadgets

The various sample collection gadgets, which are available and can be used are the platinum spatula, 26-gauge needle, Bard Parker blade no 57, hypodermic needle, surgical blade no 15 and calcium alginate swab.

Corneal Scraping

Corneal scraping is performed under topical anesthesia. The anesthetic agent, which is preferred is 0.5% proparacaine, as it is least bacteriostatic as compared to other anesthetic agents, such as tetracaine and xylocaine. General anesthesia and sedation may be required in children, uncooperative adults or mentally impaired patients. A lid speculum may be applied gently to separate the lids taking care not to cause undue pressure on the eyeball. Any mucous or debris on and around the ulcer is carefully cleaned with a sterile swab stick. After that the leading edges and base of the ulcer are scraped using a Kimura spatula or a Bard Parker knife. Multiple scrapings must be obtained to enhance the yield of the organisms. The material is gently transferred on to the glass slide. At least four slides are prepared. One for Gram staining, second for Giemsa staining, third for KOH wet preparation and fourth for viral antigen detection.

Transport of Sample

The single scraping sample obtained may either be transported in a liquid transport culture medium (indirect method) or inoculation of the multiple scrapes may be done directly onto the agar plates, which are preferred.

Corneal Biopsy

In certain cases of deep mycotic keratitis and intrastromal abscesses, a diagnostic superficial keratectomy or corneal biopsy may be necessary to harvest microbe-infested tissue to make an accurate microbiological diagnosis. The procedure is performed under an operating microscope under topical anesthesia. A dermatologic 2–3 mm trephine or a small Elliot microtrephine is advanced into the anterior corneal stroma, to incorporate both infected and clinically normal tissue. Subsequently a crescent blade or Bard Parker knife is used to undermine the tissue, which may then be cut with a surgical blade or microscissors.

Microbiological Investigations

Potassium Hydroxide Wet Mount Preparation

Ten percent KOH mount examined by conventional microscope is a useful test in helping identification of fungi and *acanthamoeba*. The test has high sensitivity (92%) and a high specificity (96%) and it can be performed in an outpatient area.

Gram Staining

Gram's stain identifies the organism correctly in up to 75% of the cases caused by a single organism and in 37% cases of polymicrobial keratitis. Overall, Gram's stain is accurate in approximately 61% of cases of bacterial keratitis.

Giemsa Staining

This stain differentiates bacteria from fungi, and also identifies chlamydia inclusion bodies and cysts and trophozoites of *acanthamoeba* species.

Special Stains

Ziehl-Neelsen acid-fast staining procedure identifies mycobacteria, actinomyces and nocardia.

Fluorochromatic Stains

Fluorochromatic stains, such as acridine-orange and calcofluor-white require the use of an epifluorescence microscope to visualize the organisms and the cells.

Culture Specimens

The corneal scrapings are routinely inoculated onto blood agar plate, chocolate agar plate, Sabouraud's dextrose agar plate (if fungus is suspected) and anaerobic media (if anaerobes are suspected). Routine culture media for various organisms are shown in Table 1.1.

Serological Investigations

These techniques (e.g. polymerase chain reaction) detect whether deoxyribonucleic acid (DNA) and ribonucleic acid (RNA) from a particular organism is present, but do not detect the viability of the organism. The advantages of polymerase chain reaction (PCR) include greater speed than culture methods (up to 4 hours) and the ability to analyze specimens far from where they are collected.

Role of Corneal Staining in Infectious Keratitis

Role of corneal staining is to determine the state of the corneal epithelium, the technique of corneal staining with a vital dye is employed, by which lesions often minute and invisible to the naked eye are dramatically accentuated in vivid colors. Three dyes are usually employed.

- Fluorescein is the most useful to delineate areas denuded of epithelium (abrasions, multiple erosions and ulcers), which stain a brilliant yellowish green, when examined with cobalt blue light.
- Rose bengal stains diseased and devitalized cells red.
- Alcian blue stains the mucus selectively and delineates excess mucus produced when there is a deficiency in tear formation.

DIAGNOSIS IN DRY EYE

Dry eye disease is a chronic inflammatory condition of the eye in which the precorneal film gets altered in function due to the dysfunction of tear volume or tear quality; alone or both leading to a complex symptomatology. The incidence varies from 8 to 30.5% in different countries. Various tests may be employed to help in the diagnosis of dry eye (Table 1.2).

Table 1.1: Routine culture media

Routine culture media	Growth	Incubation temperature
Soybean casein digest broth (trypticase soy broth)	Saturation of swabs	35°C
Blood agar plate	Aerobic bacteria, facultative anaerobic bacteria, fungi	35°C
Chocolate agar plate	Aerobic bacteria, facultative anaerobic bacteria, Neisseria, Hemophilus, Moraxella	35°C
Thioglycolate broth	Aerobic bacteria, anaerobic bacteria	35°C
Sabouraud's dextrose agar plate with antibiotic	Fungi	Room temperature
Brain heart infusion broth plate with antibiotic	Fungi	Room temperature
Special culture media		
Cooked meat broth	Anaerobic bacteria	35°C
Schaedler agar	Anaerobic bacteria	35°C
Thayer Martin blood agar plate	Neisseria	35°C
Brucella blood agar plate	Anaerobic bacteria	35°C
Lowenstein-Jensen media	Mycobacteria species	35°C with 3–10% CO_2
Middlebrook-Cohn agar	Mycobacteria, Nocardia	35°C with 3–10 % CO_2

Table 1.2: Tests for diagnosis of dry eye

Tear secretion	Schirmer's I test, Jone's test, Cotton-thread test, Dye clearance test, Fluorophotometry
Tear stability	Invasive BUT, Noninvasive BUT
Tear film integrity	Rose bengal staining
Physical features	Osmolarity, pH, Ferning, Evaporation rate
Chemistry	Electrolytes, Protein (Lysozyme, Lactoferrin)
Histology	Impression cytology, Lacrimal gland biopsy, Minor salivary gland biopsy

Tests of Tear Stability

Invasive Tear Break-up Time (Fluorescein Break-up Time)

This test requires observing the cornea using a slit-lamp biomicroscope, with a broad beam cobalt-blue light source set at, say, 10X magnification. To view the tear film, fluorescein dye is instilled. The patient is asked to refrain from blinking and in most cases within 60 seconds dark spots or streaks will form within the tear film. These discontinuities in fluorescence indicate breaks in the continuity of the tear film. The time elapsing between a complete blink and the appearance of the first 'dark spot or streak' is measured and taken to be the 'break-up time'. Five successive measures are routinely taken and the mean value is calculated (Fig. 1.1).

Disadvantages

*   There is a destabilizing effect of fluorescein on the tear film itself.
*   The volume of fluorescein added is uncontrolled and relatively large in comparison with the natural tear reservoir.
*   Contact with the ocular surface initiates some reflex lacrimation.

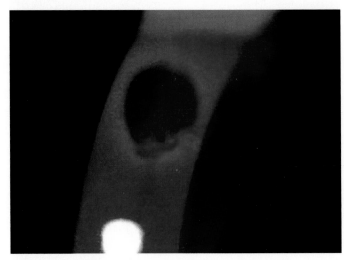

Fig. 1.1: Appearance of dark spot in tear break-up time
Normal = >10 seconds, Grade-1 =10 seconds
Grade-2 = 5–10 seconds, Grade-3 = 3–5 seconds
Grade-4 = < 3 seconds

Noninvasive Tests of Tear Film Stability

The fundamental principle common to these techniques are based on the reflective properties of smooth and stable tear film. As the tear film distorts (as it thins), its ability to reflect, undistorted, a regular optical array or pattern diminishes. Noninvasive tests of tear stability are based on observing the quality and stability of the first Purkinje image.

Corneal topographers based on the Placido disc can also be used to assess tear stability.

A device not reliant on the first Purkinje image is the Keeler Tearscope, an instrument which provides a wide field, specularly reflected view of the anterior surface, using a diffuse hemispheric light source. By measuring the time between a blink and the appearance of the first discontinuity in the lipid layer, the noninvasive break-up time can be measured.

Invasive Test for Tear Volume

It estimates for the volume of tears covering the ocular surface range from 2.74+–2.0 ml to 7 ml. The bulk of this volume is made up of fluid secreted by the main (primary) and secondary lacrimal glands.

Schirmer Test

Schirmer-1 test

This test is carried out with Whartmann-41 paper 5 mm × 35 mm whose end is bent to adjust on the lid. It is placed between inner 2/3rd and outer 1/3rd lid for 5 minutes. The room should have controlled humidity and temperature. In original test, the eye was kept open. However it can be kept closed. The inferences drawn from wetting of filter paper are:

*   If wetting < 3 mm = Very severe dry eyes
*   If wetting 3–5 mm = Severe dry eyes
*   If wetting 5–10 mm = Moderate dry eyes
*   If wetting is 10 mm = Mild dry eyes
*   If wetting is >10 mm = Normal

Schirmer-2 test

This test is carried out to note wetting of the filter paper after local anesthesia of conjunctival sac. This is carried out to note reading of basal tear function (Fig. 1.2).

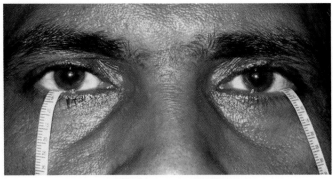

Fig.1.2: Schirmer test

Disadvantages

- Poor reproducibility.
- It is time consuming.
- It is irritating.
- It has poor diagnostic value especially when attempting to investigate the marginal dry eye.
- Type of paper and environmental factors affect the results.

Phenol Red Impregnated Cotton Thread Test

Cotton can soak up tear fluid by capillary action. The cotton thread is dyed with a pH sensitive phenol red, which changes from yellow-orange to red-orange on contact with tears. This is useful for quickly checking the length of wetted thread. The thread end is put in the lower fornix and readings are taken after two minutes (120 seconds). The wetting of thread is noted:
- Normal = >15 mm wetting (15–24 mm)
- Abnormal = <15 mm wetting: Aqueous deficiency.

The volume of tears taken up by the thread depends on the exact type of cotton and the duration of insertion.

The soft thin cotton is less irritating compared with the relatively stiffer Schirmer paper strip and more likely to infer basal tear volume.

Slit-lamp Fluorophotometry

Fluorophotometry is a laboratory-based system used to measure tear flow and turnover rates. A controlled measure of fluorescein is instilled in the eye and the fluorescence is gauged over time. The rate of decay in fluorescence indicates tear flow and turnover. By extrapolation, it is possible to predict the tear volume at the moment of fluorescein instillation.

Three microliter of 0.5% fluorescein solution was applied to cornea in untouched fashion. The ocular surface is washed after 10 minutes. After 20 minutes, corneal fluorescein is measured and converted into fluorescein concentration or is matched with standard fluorescein solution.

Interpretation

Grade-0 = No superficial punctum corneal stain.
Grade-1 = No severe superficial punctate keratitis at the center of cornea.
Grade-2 = Mild superficial punctate keratitis at the center of cornea.
Grade-3 = Severe superficial punctate keratitis at the center of cornea.
Fluorescein uptake: Normal = 22.4±16.9 ng/ml
Grade-1 = 96.4±51.2 ng/ml
Grade-2 = 318.6±146.0 ng/ml
Grade-3 = 1479.1±671.9 ng/ml

Noninvasive Test for Tear Volume

Tear Meniscus Height and Curvature

The tear meniscus is bound between the oculae surface, lid margin and the air. The surface exposed to air is concave and cylindrical. The distance from the lid margin to the boundary between the ocular surface and the edge of the tear rivulus is the tear meniscus height. It is claimed that 75 to 90% of the total fluid covering the ocular surface is contained within the upper and lower tear menisci. It follows that the height and curvature of either the lower or upper tear meniscus is proportional to the tear volume. In clinical practice tear meniscus height can be measured quickly and reliably at a magnification of 30 or more using a graduated eye piece (Table 1.3 and Fig. 1.3)

Ocular Protection Index

It is the tear break-up time in seconds divided by inter blink interval in seconds.

Inference: Ocular protection index <1 = Patient at risk
Ocular protection index >1 = Not at risk

The inter blink time can only be accurately measured with a camera interfaced with a computer. Furthermore, measurement of tear meniscus height is a useful noninvasive technique for investigating not only the dry eye, but also the patient complaining of occasional epiphora. If the tear meniscus height is constantly high there may be a partial blockage of the nasolacrimal drainage system that requires treatment.

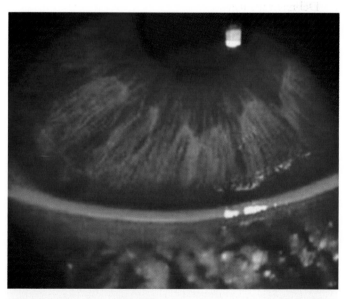

Fig. 1.3: Tear meniscus

Table 1.3: Tear meniscus curvature, height and width in dry eyes

	Tear meniscus curvature	Tear meniscus height	Tear meniscus width
Normal	0.54 ± 0.25 mm	0.46 ± 0.173 mm	0.017 ± 0.013 mm
Dry eyes	0.31 ± 0.16 mm	0.24 ± 0.089 mm	0.008 ± 0.0048 mm

Assessment of Tear Quality

Slit Lamp

I. The slit lamp is ideal tool to investigate ocular surface cellular damage using vital stains such as fluorescein, lissamine green or rose bengal.

Fluorescein stain test: The conjunctiva and cornea is examined for staining under blue filter.

No staining = Grade-0

          1/3 = Grade-1

          2/3 = Grade-2

          3/3 = Grade-3

Lissamine green stain or rose bengal test: It stains the cells, which are not covered by albumin or tears (Figs 1.4 and 1.5). A wet strip of filter paper dipped in Lissamine green stain is touched to the lower tarsal conjunctiva. The patients are asked to blink few times. The slit-lamp examination with 10x magnification using a yellow filter is carried out between 30 seconds to 2 minutes of the installation of dye and observation is noted. It is graded on the Oxford score. Each quadrant is graded from 0–4 and the total score is averaged.

    0= No stain;

    1= Mild staining dots;

    2=Staining dots multiple;

    3=Confined staining area;

    4=Very big patches of staining.

If cornea is stained, it is further graded into 0–4 scores as in conjunctiva.

i. Debris in the tears.

ii. Meibomian openings and oil droplets at the lid margins.

iii. Lashes for general state of hygiene, health and signs of inflammation.

iv. Contact lens, surface quality, movement and postlens debris.

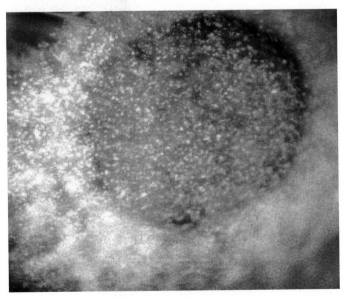

Fig 1.4: Lissamine green staining

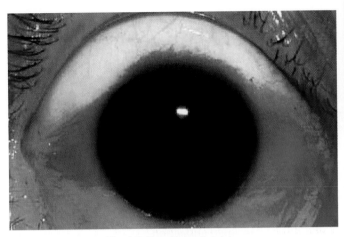

Fig. 1.5: Rose bengal staining

Nonroutine Tests in Dry Eye

Meibomiometry

The meibomian gland can be observed by appropriate lid eversion and retro-illumination using a suitable light source. This is a useful way of recording the overall quality and gross morphology of the glands. The meibomian oil droplets seen at the orifices of the gland can be harvested using thin strips of grease-proof paper and either the oil could be assayed or the area of the meibomian impressions could be measured. The area of the impression is an indication of lipid volume.

Lactoplate Test

The lysozyme and lactoferrin are the dominant proteins secreted by the lacrimal glands. These proteins protect the ocular surface by virtue of their antibacterial properties. In lacrimal gland dysfunction, the concentration of tear proteins is reduced. The Lactoplate test is a simple test for lactoferrin content.

Refractometry

Refractometry could prove to be a rapid objective indicator of lacrimal function by indicating protein concentration. Lactoferrin concentration in normal tear sample averages at 1.64 (S.D. $\pm$ 0.47) mg/ml and by exploration, it is estimated that tear refractive index reduces by 0.00095 units for 1 mg/ml fall in lactoferrin concentration.

Tear Ferning

When a tear sample is placed on a glass plate and allowed to dry out, the solid content of the sample precipitates forming an arborizing pattern. Dry eyes have tear ferning patterns different from normal because of reduced protein content. Monitoring tear ferning patterns could be useful in assessing the effects of treatment on dry eyes.

Osmolality

Osmolality can be determined by measuring the freezing point of minute (0.3 micro L) tear samples using a nanoliter osmometer. When lacrimal function is reduced, the osmolality of tear samples taken from the tear menisci increases from a normal level of <312 mOsm/kg to >320 mOsm/kg.

Laboratory Diagnosis

Impression Cytology

Impression cytology, a noninvasive or minimally invasive biopsy technique samples the superficial layers of the conjunctival and corneal epithelium. Impression cytology has become a useful research tool in both basic and clinical aspects for sampling ocular surface epithelium (Fig. 1.6).

Technique of Specimen Collection

Imprints from the surface of the bulbar and palpebral conjunctive are obtained using absorbent filter papers of different types. The widely accepted filter papers are those with pore size ranging from 0.025 μm and 0.45 μm, though 0.22 μm pore size renders the best results. They are pressed onto the ocular surface for 3–5 seconds with the aid of a solid rod and pealed off from the ocular surface. The back of the paper is marked before applying on to the surface for easy identification of the surface to be stained later.

Specimen Staining Technique

The commonly used stains for the routine histological staining of impression cytology specimens are the Papanicolaou or hematoxylin and periodic acid-Schiff (PAS) stains.

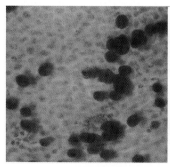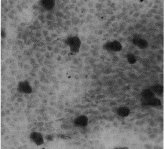

Fig. 1.6: Impression cytology in the normal eye

Applications of impression cytology

- Dry eye syndrome
- Ocular surface squamous neoplasia (OSSN)
- Vitamin A deficiency
- Diagnosis of limbal deficiency
- Detection of microorganism
- Monitoring effects of topical medication
- Other applications

Impression cytology technique has also demonstrated changes in the ocular surface in cases of chronic conjunctivitis or pterygium. In cases of systemic illnesses, such as diabetes, peripheral neuropathy, sick building syndrome, chronic renal failure, anorexia nervosa and radiation therapy, the utility of impression cytology has been reported in literature.

Corneal Aesthesiometer

It is concerned with the measuring of threshold of cornea to pressure stimuli with the help of a wire.

Nelson has done a cytological classification system of dry eye that is shown in Table 1.4.

DIAGNOSTIC MODALITIES IN KERATOPLASTY WORK-UP

Specular Microscopy

Optical Principles of Specular Microscopy

It is an epi-illuminated microscope that projects a slit of light onto the posterior corneal surface at nearly normal incidence. Most of this light is transmitted into aqueous humor. However, a small fraction of this light, 0.22% is reflected from the aqueous humor–endothelial cell interfaces back into cornea. The specularly reflected light is collected by the objective lens of photomicroscope and when the instrument is focused on posterior corneal surface, this light forms an image of corneal endothelium. The image may be viewed directly and photographed (Fig. 1.7).

According to Laing, if the beam is narrowed sufficiently four zones of reflection can be seen:

Zone 1 is the brightest region and is formed by the interfaces formed by the lens, coupling fluid and epithelium.

Table 1.4: Nelson's cytological classification system of dry eye

Grade					
				Properties	
	Epithelial cells	*Nucleus*	*N:c*	*Goblet cells*	*Stain pattern*
0	Small, round, eosinophilic cytoplasm	Large, basophilic	1:2	Abundant, plump, oval	Intense PAS positive cytoplasm
1	Slightly larger, more polygonal, eosinophilic staining cytoplasm	Smaller	1:3	Decreased in number, plump and oval	Intense PAS positive cytoplasm
2	Large and polygonal occasionally multinucleated, variably staining cytoplasm	Smaller	1:4–1:5	Markedly decreased in number and smaller in size	Poorly defined cellular border and less intensely PAS positive
3	Large and polygonal with basophilic staining cytoplasm	Small, pyknotic and absent in few cells	>1:6	Completely absent	–

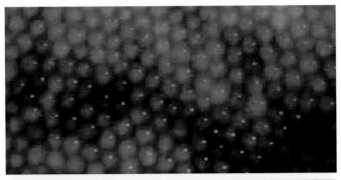

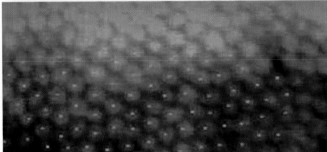

Fig. 1.7: Young normal corneal endothelial cells

Zone 2 is a larger region and represents light reflected from the stroma.

Zone 3 is the endothelial region.

Zone 4 represents light reflected from the aqueous humor.

Methods of Evaluation of Corneal Endothelium

Qualitative analysis: The normal specular micrograph should demonstrate a regular endothelia mosaic of hexagonal cells of approximately the same size. Cell boundaries should be well-defined.

Quantitative analysis: Quantitative analysis of a specular photomicrograph is the objective description of the attributes of a selected cluster of individual endothelial cells from a specular photomicrograph. Examples include cell density (measured as cells/mm^2) mean cell area (measured as mm^2/cell), and pleomorphism (usually measured as percentage of 3, 4, 5, 6, 7 or 8 sided cells).

Morphometric analysis: The variation in individual cell area (polymegathism) and cell shape, i.e. cells with a different number of sides (pleomorphism), may provide a better estimate of endothelial cell integrity and function.

Clinical Indications for Specular Microscopy

- Early diagnosis of Fuchs' endothelial dystrophy
- In certain eyes before cataract surgery
  - Previous trauma
  - Pseudoexfoliation
  - Recurrent uveitis
  - Corneal edema in contralateral eyes
  - Clear graft with operable cataract
  - Glaucomatous eye with cataract

- Subluxated lens or choosing the intraocular lens
  - Posterior polymorphous dystrophy
  - ICE syndrome, congenital glaucoma
  - Use of various types and designs of intraocular lenses
  - Effect of various irrigating solutions and intracameral products used during cataract on endothelium
  - Different techniques of cataract surgery, related instruments and endothelial response
- Evaluation of donor endothelium
- Various refractive surgical procedures like LASIK, LASEK and their term effect over corneal endothelium
- Contact lenses and phakic intraocular lenses

Advantages

- Operator independent
- Noninvasive
- Simultaneous measurement of cell count.

Disadvantages

- Time consuming
- Less reproducible than ultrasonic and ultrasound biomicroscopic pachymetric measurements.
- Impractical for use in operation rooms.
- Clinical use is limited to corneas that are free of edema, scarring, deposits or opacities that may distort light transmission.

Eye Bank Specular Microscopy

Evaluation of corneal tissue can be performed on whole globes as well as corneas stored in tissue culture media. Cell counts required for transplant surgery should be at least 2,000–2,500 cells/mm^2.

Eye bank specular microscope has a built-in high resolution camera that gives high quality images of donor cornea with a built-in cell analysis system. Instrument's XYZ and rocking platform mechanism makes tracking of the endothelial cell easy. It also has a built-in pachymeter.

Anterior Segment Optical Coherence Tomography and its Application in Corneal Diseases

Optical coherence tomography is a cross-sectional, three-dimensional and high resolution imaging modality that uses low coherence interferometry to achieve axial resolution in the range of 3–20 micrometers. It is a completely noninvasive technique. As it uses interferometry for depth resolution it can have a long working distance and a wide field of transverse scanning.

The primary limitation of optical coherence tomography imaging of the anterior segment is speed and penetration. The OCT systems used in commercial retinal scanner thus far have used 830 nm wavelength, with image acquisition time of 1 to 5 seconds. Recently ophthalmic optical coherence tomography system in 1310 nm wavelength with an acquisition time of 3.3 seconds have been introduced, which allowed deeper penetration. Cross-sectional imaging of the anterior chamber, including visualization of the angle is possible.

Applications in Cornea

1. Laser assisted in-situ keratomileusis and other refractive surgeries by directly measuring corneal flap thickness intra-operatively, provide the comprehensive pachymetry map of the entire cornea.
2. Anterior chamber width and other biometric parameters—Optical coherence tomography is a promising method for accurate anterior chamber depth owing to its high spatial resolution and can improve sulcus-supported phakic intraocular lens sizing also.
3. Anterior segment optical coherence tomography can also be of use in delineating the anterior segment anatomy in case of opaque corneas, failed grafts, adherent leucomas and help in the surgical planning prior to keratoplasty (Fig. 1.8).

Advantages

- Noncontact
- Rapid acquisition during the pachymetry scan ensures an accurate and repeatable pachymetry map
- High resolution
- Measures through corneal opacity.

Confocal Microscopy

The confocal microscope exploits the pinhole effect. Minsky carefully placed two pinholes, the first before the condenser, which focuses the light rays into the tissue, and the second before the eyepiece or camera, which focuses the reflected light rays into an image. Computer technology permitted three-dimensional reconstructions of the images. Overall, this new technology improved lateral and axial resolution to 1–6 and 4–15 mm, respectively, and increased magnification up to 600 times.

Indications of Confocal Microscopy

- Amiodarone, amyloid, chloroquine, ciprofloxacin, gold and iron-induced keratopathy

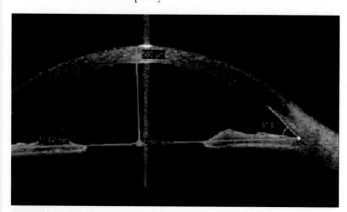

Fig. 1.8: Anterior segment analysis and pachymetry on optical coherence tomography

- Epithelial abnormalities like in Thygeson keratitis, Meesmann corneal dystrophy and Salzmann's nodular degeneration
- Dry eyes
- Stromal dystrophies-lattice dystrophy, Reis-Bücklers dystrophy, granular dystrophy, Schnyder crystalline corneal dystrophy and cornea farinata
- Keratoconus
- Cornea guttata or Fuchs endothelial dystrophy
- Primary congenital glaucoma with megalocornea.
- Role in corneal infections to visualize fungus, acanthamoeba, bacteria microsporidium and adenovirus
- Role in refractive surgeries to examine the LASIK flap interface.

Advantages

- It is noninvasive
- It allows observation of corneal structure at high magnification; and it allows visualization of keratocytes and corneal nerve fibers
- It offers moderate to good repeatability.

Disadvantages

- Poor agreement between confocal microscopy and ultrasound pachymetry; the latter apparently overestimating corneal thickness
- Slower data acquisition
- Poor penetration in corneal opacity.

Corneal Topography

Corneal topography or computerized videokeratography evolved from the need to measure corneal curvature and topography more comprehensively and accurately than keratometry. The purpose of computer-assisted corneal topography is to provide both qualitative and quantitative information about the corneal surface.

Projection Device Systems

Three types of projection device systems are currently used to measure corneal topography, and they are categorized as Placido based, elevation based, slit scanning and interferometric. All of them are capable of measuring and analyzing more than 8,000 points on the corneal surface.

Scanning Slit Imaging

The Orbscan uses a scanning slit-beam and direct stereotriangulation to measure the anterior corneal surface. During the 1.5 second examination, the patient fixes on a light source, whose reflex is aligned with the instrument axis. A "tracking system" (software image registration) attempts to minimize the influence of involuntary eye movement during the 1.5 second examination.

Formats for display of data: The interpretation of color contour maps is based on the recognition of the following regions:

Hot colors: Red, orange and yellow (steep zones of the cornea)

Intermediate colors: Green

Cool colors: Blue (flatter zones of the cornea)

Corneal power map (Axial/sagittal)

This is a 24 color representation of dioptric power at various points on the cornea. The radius of curvature is measured 360 times for each placido disc image, from center to vertex.

Numerical (Curvature) map: The corneal curvature of different areas on the cornea is shown in dioptric values.

Keratometric map: It depicts the two principal meridia (K_1 and K_2) of the cornea at 3 different zones, i.e. central 3 mm zone, intermediate 3 to 5 mm zone and the peripheral 5 to 7 mm zone.

Profile map: The profile map plots the steepest and flattest meridians of the cornea along with the difference in the two.

Tangential map: This gives a better geographical representation of the cornea.

Corneal topography in preoperative and postoperative cataract surgery through map is shown in Figures 1.9A and B.

Current Applications of Corneal Topography

- Screening patients before refractive surgery
- Diagnosis of irregular astigmatism and corneal warpage
- Diagnosis of early keratoconus.
- Evaluating postoperative changes in corneal shape after refractive surgery
- After cataract surgery, corneal topography has been used to understand the effect of cataract incision placement and size

- After penetrating keratoplasty
- An early application of corneal topography involved patients with high astigmatism who required relaxing incisions
- Surgical planning
- Corneal topography is used in planning astigmatic surgery. Symmetrical and asymmetrical bow tie pattern with against the rule and with the rule astigmatism can easily be picked up. Irregular astigmatism and asymmetric astigmatism can be identified.

Pachymetry

Pachymetry (Greek words: Pachos = thick + metry = to measure) is term used for the measurement of corneal thickness. It is an important indicator of health status of the cornea especially of corneal endothelial pump function. It also measures corneal rigidity and consequently has an impact on the accuracy of intraocular pressure measurement by applanation tonometry.

Corneal Thickness in Normal Eyes

The normal corneal thickness varies from central to peripheral limbus. It ranges from 0.7 to 0.9 mm at the limbus and varies between 0.49 mm and 0.56 mm at the center. The central corneal thickness (CCT) reading of 0.7 mm or more is indicative of endothelial decompensation. Peripheral corneal thickness is asymmetric so that temporal cornea is thinnest followed by the inferior cornea

Indications

- Glaucoma— for applying correction factor in actual intraocular pressure determination
- Congenital glaucoma— to assess the amount of corneal edema.

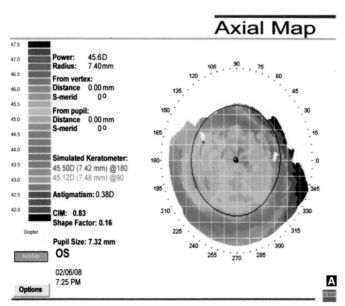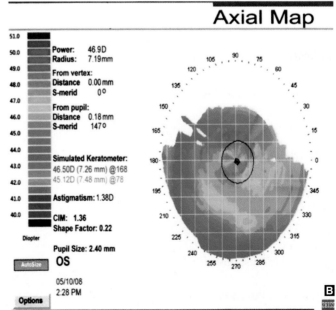

Figs 1.9A and B: Corneal topography in cataract surgery (A) Preoperative corneal topography (B) Postoperative corneal topography

- Refractive surgeries— (a) preoperative screening and (b) treatment plan of keratorefractive procedures like LASIK, astigmatic keratotomy, and previously even prior to radial keratotomy
- Postoperative follow-up of keratoplasty patients to determine endothelial cell function and its recovery and to become alert to early graft decompensation
- Contact lens—to assess corneal edema and in orthokeratology
- Assessing the thinness of the cornea as in corneal disorders like Terrien's and Pellucid marginal degenerations, keratoconus, keratoglobus and post LASIK ectasia
- Other cases if corneal decompensation— for monitoring and evaluating corneal edema and endothelial function as in herpetic endothelitis.

Correction Factor

To get a correct IOP reading, many correction factors have been reported by various researchers. It is recommended that in chronic eye diseases like glaucoma and glaucoma suspects for every increase in central corneal thickness of 50 μm, the correction done is to decrease the recorded IOP by 2.5 mm Hg.

Techniques of Pachymetric Measurements

There are two types of pachymetric techniques:

Spot measurements: These technologies include traditional optical pachymetry, specular and confocal microscopy, ultrasound pachymetry, and optical low-coherence reflectometry.

Wide area mapping: These provide the capability to map a wide area of the cornea. Pachymetric mapping technologies include slit-scanning optical pachymetry and very high–frequency ultrasound imaging.

Methods of Measurements

1. Ultrasonic techniques:
   a. Conventional ultrasonic pachymetry
   b. Ultrasound biomicroscopy
2. Optical techniques:
   a. Manual optical pachymetry
   b. Specular microscopy
   c. Scanning slit technology
   d. Optical coherence tomography
   e. Optical low coherence interferometry
   f. Confocal microscopy
   g. Laser Doppler interferometry
3. Alternative measurements:
   a. Pentacam
   b. Pachycam
   c. Ocular response analyzer

Ultrasonic Pachymetry

This is the most commonly used method these days and is regarded as the gold standard.

Principle

The ultrasonic pachymetry measurements depend on the reflection of ultrasonic waves from the anterior and posterior corneal surfaces. It is the measurement of the time difference (transit time) between echoes of ultrasonic signal pulses from the transducer of the probe and the reflected signal from the front and back surface of the cornea to the transducer.

Corneal thickness is calculated by following simple formula:
Corneal thickness = (Transit time × Propagation velocity) / 2
The sound velocity through normal cornea is taken as 1640 m/sec.

Disadvantages

- Contact method
- Accuracy is dependent on the perpendicularity of the probe's application to the cornea.
- Reproducibility relies on precise probe placement on the center of the cornea.
- Difficult to control the patients gaze during repeated measurements, so that the placement of the probe is difficult to reproduce. There is variable sound speed in wet and dry tissues.
- Low resolution
- Not accurate in edematous corneas.

Advantages

- Fast
- Simpler, therefore easier for paramedical staff to use
- Requires minimal observer judgment
- Portable
- Dry (no coupling medium required)
- Can be used intraoperatively.

Ultrasound Biomicroscopy

Ultrasound biomicroscopy is a high resolution ultrasound machine, which images the anterior segment of the eye. It has got a 12.5–50 MHz probe so that the depth of penetration is lesser (4 mm) than conventional ultrasound. It gives real-time images of anterior segment (Fig. 1.10).

Corneal thickness can be measured by the caliper incorporated in the machine or through the ultrasound biomicroscopy software after the acquisition of images.

Advantages

- Anterior segment examination (high resolution) can be carried out along with measurement of corneal thickness.
- Especially useful in cases where cornea is opaque.
- Various layers of cornea can be identified.

Disadvantages

- The main drawback of ultrasound biomicroscopy imaging is the inconvenient requirement of immersing the eye in a coupling fluid.
- Contact method

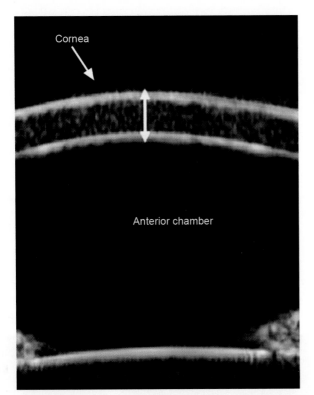

Fig. 1.10: Ultrasound biomicroscopy helps in the measurement of central corneal thickness

- Requirement for the patient to lie supine during the examination
- The device cannot be used intraoperatively
- Difficult to standardize.

Slit-Scanning Pachymetry

Principle

It measures anterior and posterior corneal elevations by comparing it to a best fit sphere. Pachymetry is done by calculating the difference between the elevation of anterior and posterior corneal surface.

Advantages

- It gives wide field pachymetry that is measurement across the entire cornea
- It also identifies the thinnest point in the cornea, both by value and location helping in the diagnosis of keratoconus.
- Corneal alignment is not required
- It can be used to calculate ablation depth and optical zones in corneal refractive surgeries.

Disadvantages

- It overestimates corneal thickness by 5%. The main drawback of Orbscan is the tendency to underestimate corneal thickness in Keratoconic, post-PRK and post-LASIK eyes

- This is not fast enough for pachymetric mapping because of motion artifacts in the measurements
- The Orbscan system shows decreased accuracy in measuring corneal thickness when clinically significant haze is present.

Pentacam

Pentacam analyses the complete anterior segment, corneal topography, the quantification of lens density, anterior chamber, angle measurements, and utility to monitor new therapeutic modalities like collagen crosslinking treatment for Keratoconus.

Principle

The Pentacam is also based on the true elevation measurement and images the anterior segment (cornea + lens) of the eye by a rotating Scheimpflug camera measurement, which supplies pictures in three dimensions.

Advantages

- Noninvasive, noncontact
- Even minute eye movements are captured and corrected simultaneously
- It gives precise representation and repeatability
- The high quality of the Scheimpflug image allows preoperative and postoperative monitoring as in the case of an intraocular contact lens.

Disadvantages

- It underestimates the corneal thickness in comparison to ultrasonic pachymetry.

Pachycam

The OCULUS Pachycam is compact and portable noncontact pachymeter with built-in keratometer. It can be mounted on slit lamp. It automatically corrects the intraocular pressure in accordance with various correction tables to obtain the "real" IOP. Image acquisition is done with the help of a 3-D alignment screen.

Principle

It is also based on Scheimpflug principle of the horizontal 4 mm cut image, which is evaluated and represented. It also gives central k-values as well as the local K-readings on the 4 mm cut.

Advantages

- Noncontact
- Portable and lightweight.

Chapter 2

External Eye Diseases

Samar K Basak

EYELIDS

DISORDERS OF EYELASHES

Trichiasis

Introduction

Trichiasis is the inward misdirection of eyelash, which irritates the cornea and/or the conjunctiva (Figs 2.1 and 2.2). Simple trichiasis involves only a few lashes and is relatively common. Diffuse trichiasis involves the entire lid margin and is much less common. It is seen primarily in countries where trachoma is endemic.

Trichiasis when associated with entropion is called pseudo-trichiasis (Fig. 2.3).

Diagnosis

Symptoms: Trichiasis is characterized by foreign body sensation, which may be present with watering and localized redness.

Signs: One or more misdirected eyelash may be turning towards the ocular surface and rubbing over it. This can cause punctate stain positive areas or corneal ulceration in chronic conditions.

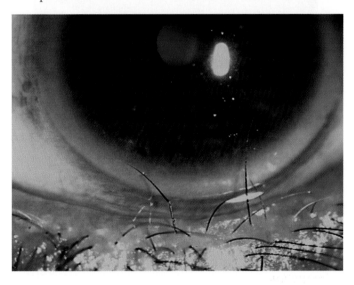

Fig. 2.2: Trichiasis—multiple eyelash

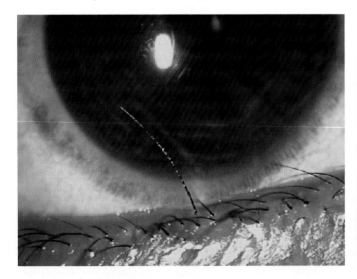

Fig. 2.1: Trichiasis—single eyelash

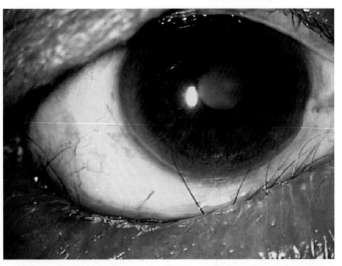

Fig. 2.3: Pseudotrichiasis in entropion

Treatment

Medical: The primary treatment of trichiasis is surgical. However, lubricants such as artificial tears and ointments, may decrease the irritant effect of lash rubbing. If a more serious disease is the cause then medical therapy should be directed towards that disease.

Surgical: Many procedures for trichiasis correction have been described. These procedures can be categorized as lash/follicle destroying or lash/follicle repositioning.

Trichiasis can be managed temporarily by epilation and permanently by electrolysis, cryotherapy or argon laser cilia ablation. If more cilia are involved, operative procedure for entropion correction is performed.

Madarosis

Introduction

Madarosis, refers to hair loss of the eyebrows (superciliary madarosis) or loss of eyelashes (ciliary madarosis). In addition to the obvious cosmetic blemish for which the patient usually presents to dermatologists or ophthalmologists, madarosis may be a sign of many systemic diseases.

Loss or scantiness of the eyelashes of one or both eyes can be found in the case of ulcerative blepharitis, Hansen's diseases, herpes zoster ophthalmicus, after radiation therapy, etc. (Figs 2.4 and 2.5).

Treatment

Identification of the cause and its treatment leads to reversal of madarosis in most cases. Surgical repair of the traumatic madarosis can be done, but good thickness of the eyelashes and ideal direction of their growth are difficult to achieve.

Poliosis

Introduction

Poliosis is the decrease or absence of melanin (or color) in eyebrows or eyelashes. This condition can cause white patches on the hair.

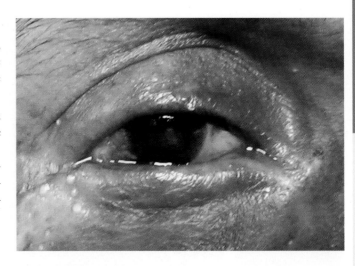

Fig. 2.5: Madarosis in herpes zoster ophthalmicus

Causes

Poliosis may occur in extreme old age, in Vogt-Koyanagi-Harada's syndrome or in oculocutaneous albinism (Figs 2.6 to 2.8).

Treatment

No treatment is required for this condition.

Blepharitis

Introduction

Blepharitis is an ocular disease characterized by subacute or chronic inflammation of the eyelid margins. It occurs mostly in children and is usually bilateral. It is often associated with seborrhea (dandruff) of the scalp.

Types

Anterior blepharitis
- *Squamous/seborrheic blepharitis:* This is the most common type of blepharitis and is usually one part of the spectrum of seborrhoeic dermatitis, which involves the scalp, lashes,

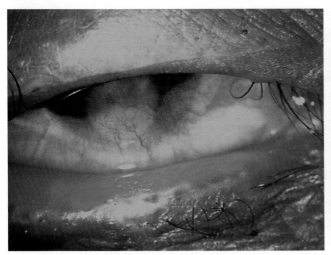

Fig. 2.4: Madarosis in blepharitis

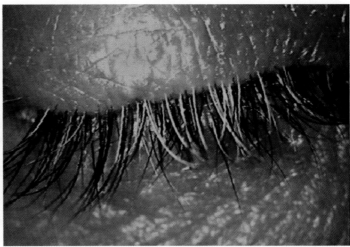

Fig. 2.6: Poliosis in aging

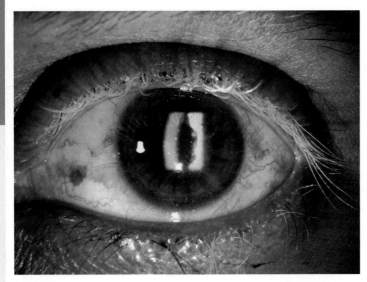

Fig. 2.7: Poliosis in Vogt-Koyanagi-Harada's syndrome

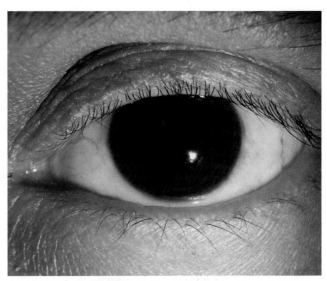

Fig. 2.9: Squamous blepharitis

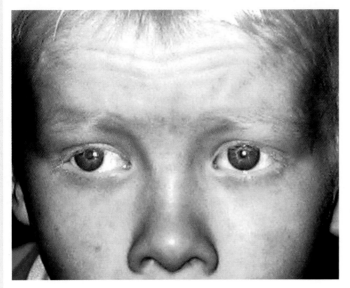

Fig. 2.8: Poliosis in oculocutaneous albinism

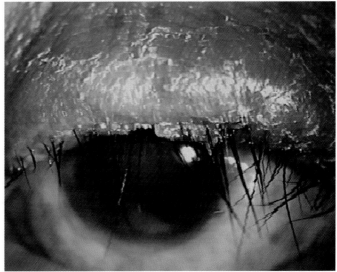

Fig. 2.10: Ulcerative blepharitis

eyebrows, nasolabial folds and ears. Hyperemia of the lid margins, white dandruff-like scales on the lid margins, falling of eyelashes (madarosis), and thickening of lid margins (tylosis) may occur. Treatment is best accomplished by a dermatologist (Fig. 2.9).

- *Ulcerative blepharitis:* Staphlycoccal blepharitis is caused by infection of the anterior portion of the eyelid by staphylococcal bacteria. As the infection progresses, foreign body sensation, matting of the lashes and burning may be noticed. The condition can sometimes lead to a chalazion or a stye, soreness of the lid margins, loss of eyelashes, and yellow crust at the root with matting and small ulcers at the base of crust. Marginal keratitis may also occur (Fig. 2.10).

- *Meibomianitis (Posterior blepharitis):* This is the chronic infection of the meibomian glands and occurs in the middle age. White, frothy secretion is present on the eyelid margins and at the canthi (seborrhea). Vertical yellowish streaks may be observed shining through the conjunctiva. Blocked meibomian ducts, thick secretion on expression ("toothpaste sign") are also observed (Figs 2.11 to 2.13).

Treatment

Anterior blepharitis: Lid hygiene (lid scrub), lid massage with steroid-antibiotic ointment, systemic tetracycline or doxycycline, and treatment of dandruff.

Meibomianitis (Posterior blepharitis): Hot compress, tarsal (vertical lid) massage, steroid-antibiotic ointment and systemic doxycycline.

Blepharoconjunctivitis

Introduction

Blepharoconjunctivitis can be acute or chronic. It may be infectious or inflammatory. *Staph. aureus* is the most common cause of infection. Other organisms are – *S. epidermidis, Propionibacterium*

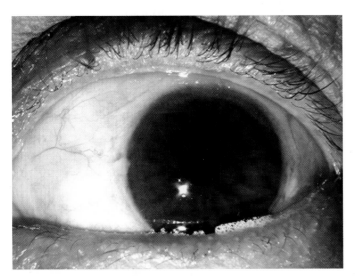

Fig. 2.11: Meibomian seborrhea

acnes, Corynebacterium Species or yeast *Pityrosporum*. It is often associated with ocular rosacea (Figs 2.14 and 2.15).

Diagnosis

Symptoms: Redness (acute or chronic), watering, swelling and crusting of the lids, and fall of eyelashes may occur.

Signs: Lid edema, erythema, matting of the eyelashes, tenderness and thickened lid margins may occur. Conjunctival congestion, mucopurulent discharge, tear film instability, corneal vascularization, marginal keratitis and other signs of meibomian gland dysfunction may also occur.

Treatment

Maintenance of lid hygiene, use of hot fomentation and topical broad spectrum antibiotic is advised. Tears substitutes, erythromycin/tetracycline eye ointment may be used at night. Systemic tetracycline (250 mg qid) or doxycycline (100 mg daily) may also

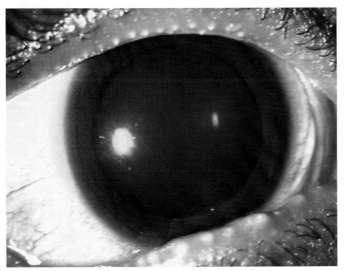

Fig. 2.12: Blocked ducts in meibomianitis

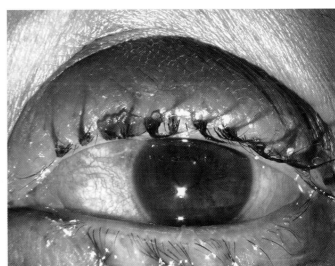

Fig. 2.14: Blepharoconjunctivitis

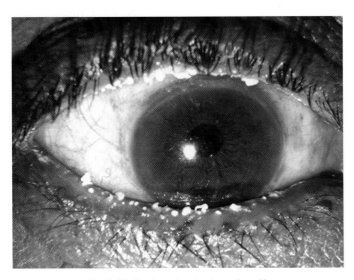

Fig. 2.13: Toothpaste sign in meibomitis

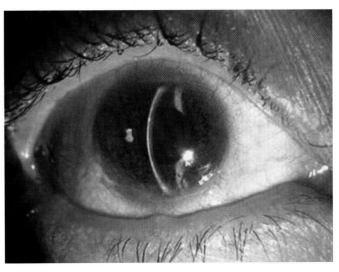

Fig. 2.15: Blepharoconjunctivitis—acne rosacea

be added for 4–6 weeks. Marginal keratitis may be treated with weak topical steroids along with other medication.

BENIGN NODULES

Chalazion

Introduction

Chalazion is a chronic nonspecific inflammatory granuloma of the meibomian gland. Chalazion also known as a meibomian gland lipogranuloma, is caused by inflammation of a blocked meibomian gland, usually on the upper eyelid.

Chalazia differ from styes (hordeolum) in that they are subacute, non-tender and usually painless nodules. Chalazion may become acutely inflamed, but unlike a stye, usually point inside the lid rather than on the lid margin. Chalazia are the most common inflammatory lesions of the eyelid.

Diagnosis

Symptoms: Painless nodular lid swelling always occurs away from the margin (Figs 2.16 and 2.17). Swelling on the eyelid, eyelid tenderness, sensitivity to light, increased tearing and heaviness of the eyelid may occur.

Signs: Tarsal conjunctiva is velvety red and slightly elevated. Chalazia may present as single or multiple nodules.

Treatment

Conservative management of chalazia includes lid hygiene and warm compresses. Topical antibiotic eye drops or ointment (e.g. chloramphenicol) is sometimes used for the initial acute infection.

If no evidence of infection is present, the chalazion can be injected with a steroid (e.g. triamcinolone, methylprednisolone) as they can frequently cause regression of the chalazion within a few weeks. 0.2–2 mL of 5 mg/mL triamcinolone can be injected directly into chalazion's center. A second injection may be necessary for larger chalazia. Complications of steroid injections include hypopigmentation, atrophy of the area, corneal

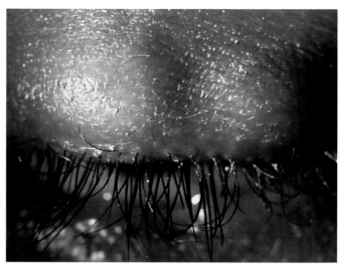
Fig. 2.17: Multiple chalazion

perforation and traumatic cataract, and potential exacerbation of bacterial or viral infection.

Incision and Curettage

Surgical steps: Surgical steps are performed under infiltrative anesthesia. Local anesthesia is not directly injected into the hordeolum; injection is done along the lid margins in a line above the upper tarsus or below the lower tarsus. Chalazion is fixed with a chalazion clamp; solid plate being towards skin surface. The eyelid is then everted and screw of the clamp is tightened. External incisions lead to scarring, so making external eyelid incisions or punctures is inadvisable, unless the hordeolum already is pointing externally. A large abscess may have multiple pockets and require multiple stabs. Internal incisions should be made vertically to minimize the area of cornea swept by a scar during blinking; external incisions should be made horizontally for optimal cosmesis (Fig. 2.18). When draining a lesion that points both externally and internally, make the incision internally and as far as possible from the site of external pointing. Combined overlying internal and external drainage

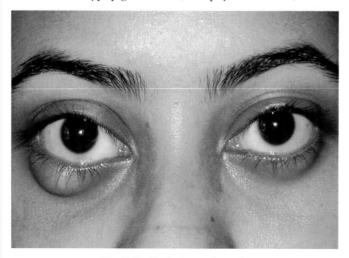
Fig. 2.16: Chalazion on lower lid

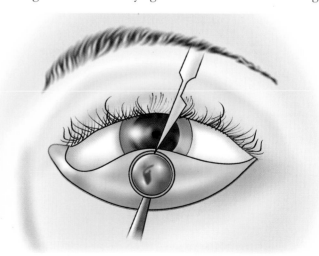
Fig. 2.18: Vertical incision for I and D in chalazion

increases the risk of later fistulae through the lid. To avoid disrupting normal growth of lashes, do not make incisions along eyelash margins. All contents (granulomatous materials with pus) are scooped out with a chalazion scoop. A thorough curettage is done by rotatory movement of the scoop. The clamp is removed and pressures are applied with a pellet inside and thumb outside for two minutes to secure hemostasis. Pad and pressure bandage is applied for 2–3 hours.

Internal Hordeolum (Infected Chalazion)

Introduction

An internal hordeolum (infected chalazion) is a secondary infection of meibomian glands in the tarsal plate. It is a unilateral acute infection of the meibomian gland. Tender, diffuse, inflamed swelling is present within the tarsal plate. The swelling is situated away from the lid margin. Pus-point is away from the eyelash root (Fig. 2.19). It may be associated with preseptal cellulitis.

Hordeola are found more frequently in persons who have the following: diabetes, other debilitating illnesses, chronic blepharitis, seborrhea and high serum lipids.

Treatment

Treatment of acute infection is done, which is followed by incision and curettage of the chalazion.

BACTERIAL INFECTIONS

External Hordeolum (Stye)

Introduction

Stye is acute suppurative inflammation of the eyelash follicle and the gland of Zeis and is caused by staphylococcus infection (Fig. 2.20).

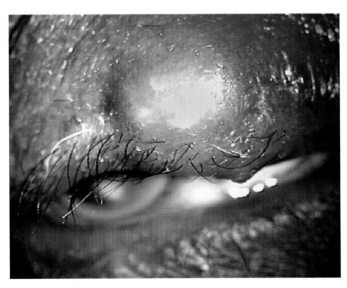

Fig. 2.19: Internal hordeolum

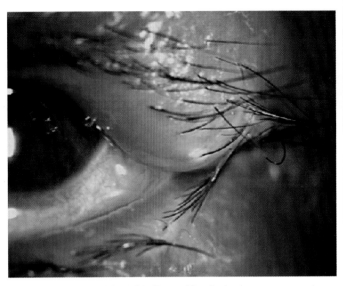

Fig. 2.20: External hordeolum

Diagnosis

Symptoms: Acute pain and swelling of the affected eyelid may occur.

Signs: Lid margin swelling may be associated with preseptal cellulitis. A whitish, round, raised pus point at the affected eyelash root may be present (Fig. 2.21).

Treatment

Hot compress, systemic analgesics, topical antibiotics and epilation of the affected eyelash are helpful.

VIRAL INFECTIONS

Herpes Zoster Ophthalmicus

Introduction

Herpes zoster ophthalmicus is caused by varicella-zoster virus affecting the elderly people. It occurs more common in immunocompromised hosts.

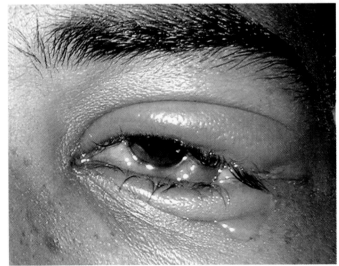

Fig. 2.21: External hordeolum with preseptal cellulitis

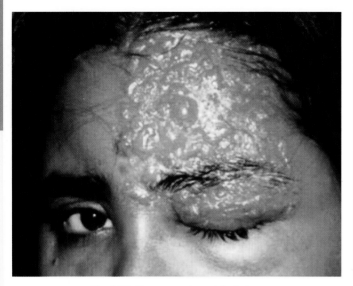

Fig. 2.22: Herpes zoster ophthalmicus

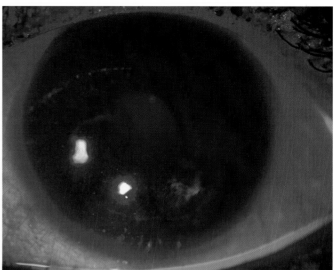

Fig. 2.24: Pseudodendritic lesion in herpes zoster ophthalmicus

Diagnosis

Symptoms: It is characterized by the presence of vesicular eruptions around the eye, forehead and scalp and severe pain along the ophthalmic division of fifth cranial nerve (Fig. 2.22).

Signs: Hutchinson's rule: When the tip of the nose is involved, the eye will also be involved, since both are supplied by the nasociliary nerve (Fig. 2.23).

The ocular lesions may be acute, chronic or recurrent:

Acute Ocular Lesions

1. *Lids:* Redness, edema and vesicular eruptions
2. *Cornea:* Punctuate epithelial keratitis.
   a. Microdendrites: small, fine, multiple dendritic or stellate lesions (Fig. 2.24).

   b. Nummular keratitis: multiple granular lesions surrounded by a halo of stromal haze (Fig. 2.25). Sensation may be diminished.
   c. Disciform keratitis.
3. *Iris:* Acute iridocyclitis with hyphema and patches of iris atrophy.
4. *Neuro-ophthalmological:* Optic neuritis and cranial nerve palsies affecting the third (commonest), fourth and sixth nerves.

Chronic Ocular Lesion

Ptosis occurs due to scarring of the lid. Trichiasis, entropion and lid notching; scleritis, nummular keratitis and ocular surface instability may be present.

Recurrent Ocular Lesion

They are associated with mucous plaque keratitis, neuroparalytic keratitis or secondary glaucoma.

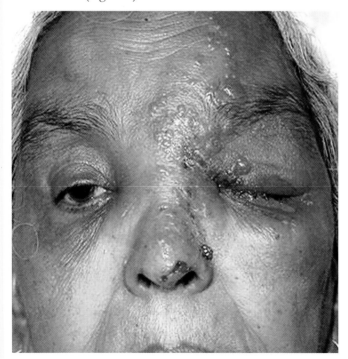

Fig. 2.23: Herpes zoster ophthalmicus—Hutchinson's rule

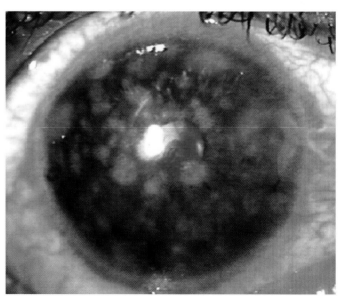

Fig. 2.25: Herpes zoster ophthalmicus—Nummular keratitis

Treatment

Oral acyclovir (800 mg) 5 times daily for 7–10 days is prescribed. Topical steroids are used in the presence of keratitis or iridocyclitis. Systemic corticosteroids are used in neuro-ophthalmologic problems.

Molluscum Contagiosum

Introduction

Molluscum contagiosum is a common skin infection in children caused by DNA poxvirus. It spreads by both sexual and non-sexual route like direct contact with infected skin or fomites. After an average incubation period of two to three months, flesh colored, dome-shaped, 3–5 mm sized papules with central umbilication appear on the face, trunk and exposed body parts. In patients with acquired immune disease syndrome, such lesions can occur on the eyelid, conjunctiva and can be large in size (10–15 mm) and number, resistant to therapy and more prone to secondary infection. Thus, all patients with the aforesaid presentation should be screened for HIV.

Increased number of lesions may also be seen in patients with atopic dermatitis, malignancies and, those on steroids and other immunosuppressive drugs. In immunodeficiency conditions (as in AIDS), it may be more severe and confluent, often in other parts of body. It may be associated with keratitis or follicular conjunctivitis.

Diagnosis

Symptoms: It is characterized by the presence of single or multiple small white lesions of the face, including the eyelids.

Signs: Single or multiple dome-shaped small yellowish-white umbilicated shiny nodules may be present (Figs 2.26 and 2.27). They may be associated with pannus, keratitis or follicular conjunctivitis (Fig. 2.28) and nevi.

Treatment

Investigations to find out immunodeficiency states should be performed. Chemical cautery or cryosurgery may be useful in some cases.

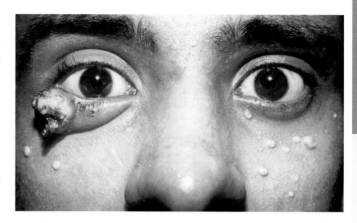

Fig. 2.27: Molluscum contagiosum in HIV positive patient

CONJUNCTIVA

Bacterial Conjunctivitis

Introduction

Bacterial conjunctivitis is mainly caused by *Staphylococcus aureus, Staphylococcus epidermidis, Streptococcus pneumoniae* and *Haemophilus influenzae* (in children). It may be associated with blepharitis.

Diagnosis

Symptoms: Redness in the white of the eye or inner eyelid, watering, and thick yellow discharge that crusts over the eyelashes, especially after sleep (in conjunctivitis caused by bacteria) is observed causing stickiness of eyelids. Itching and burning sensation, blurred vision, increased sensitivity to light and foreign body sensation is observed.

Signs: Clinically marked hyperemia, lid edema, matting of the eyelashes, conjunctival chemosis, petechial hemorrhages and mucopurulent discharge may be observed. Tarsal conjunctiva is a velvety red and not particularly follicular. Scarring of the tarsal conjunctiva may also occur (Figs 2.29A and B).

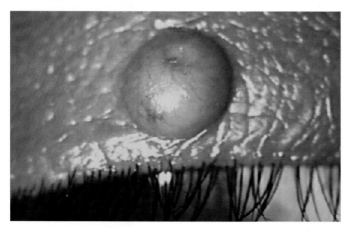

Fig. 2.26: Molluscum contagiosum

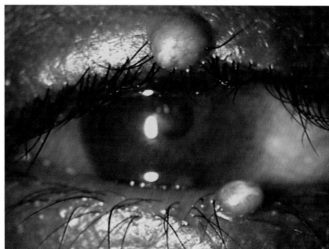

Fig. 2.28: Molluscum contagiosum with keratoconjunctivitis

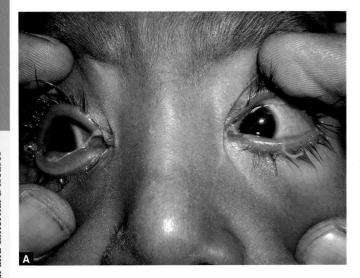

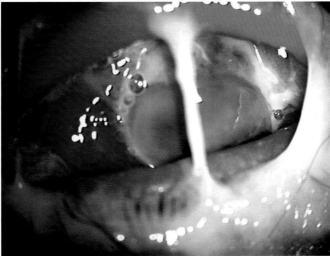

Fig. 2.30: Purulent conjunctivitis

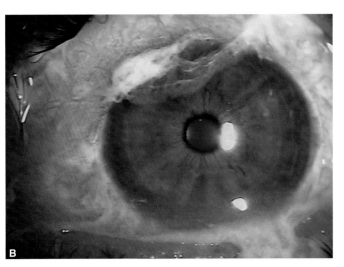

Figs 2.29A and B: Acute mucopurulent conjunctivitis

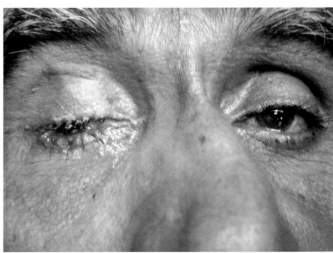

Fig. 2.31: Purulent conjunctivitis in the right eye

Treatment

Frequent eye wash with lukewarm water, broad-spectrum anti-biotic eye drops and antibiotic ointment at night is advised. Prevention of spread of the disease is also advised.

Gonococcal Keratoconjunctivitis

Introduction

Gonococcal keratoconjunctivitis is hyperacute conjunctivitis, resulting within 12–24 hours and is caused by *Neisseria gonorrhoeae*.

Diagnosis

Symptoms: It is characterized by sudden redness, swelling of the eyelids and pain with copious purulent discharge.

Signs: Copious purulent discharge, conjunctival chemosis, lid edema with crusting of eyelashes and preauricular lymphadenopathy may be present. Cornea may be involved in severe cases. Right eye is involved more frequently (Figs 2.30 and 2.31).

Treatment

Diagnosis is to be confirmed by bacterial culture. Isolation, frequent irrigation of eyes with lukewarm saline, systemic ciprofloxacin (500 mg bid for 5 days), penicillin (1:10,000 IU) or ciprofloxacin eye drop 2 hourly and ciprofloxacin eye ointment at night are advised.

Simultaneous treatment of sexual partner with oral antibiotics (Tab Ciprofloxacin) for gonorrhea is advised.

Ophthalmia Neonatorum

Introduction

Neonatal conjunctivitis by definition presents during the first month of life. It may be infectious or noninfectious.

Neonatal conjunctivitis, also known as ophthalmia neonatorum, is a form of bacterial conjunctivitis contracted by newborns during delivery. The baby's eyes are contaminated during passage through the birth canal from a mother infected with either *Neisseria gonorrhoeae* or *Chlamydia trachomatis*. In gonococcal

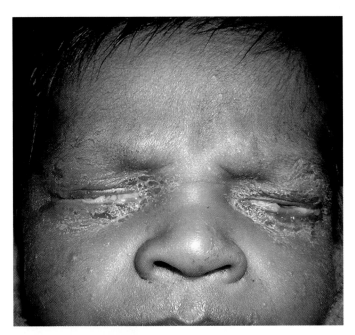

Fig. 2.32: Ophthalmia neonatorum

infection, hyperacute bilateral purulent conjunctivitis occurs within a week in neonates. In other cases, it is a catarrhal or mucopurulent conjunctivitis (Figs 2.32 and 2.33).

Types

Noninfectious: Chemical irritants, such as silver nitrate can cause chemical conjunctivitis, which usually lasts for 2–4 days.

Infectious: Many different bacteria and viruses can cause conjunctivitis in the neonate. The two most common ones being *N. gonorrhoeae* and *Chlamydia* acquired from the birth canal during delivery. Conjunctivitis secondary to infection with *Chlamydia trachomatis* produces conjunctivitis after 3 days of life, but may occur up to 2 weeks after delivery. The discharge is usually more

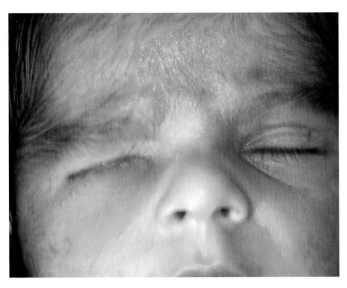

Fig. 2.33: Neonatal conjunctivitis—other cause

mucopurulent. Babies infected with *Chlamydia* may develop pneumonitis at a later stage. Infants with *Chlamydia pneumonitis* should be treated with oral erythromycin for 10–14 days.

Diagnosis

Symptoms: Acute onset redness is associated with purulent discharge, and swelling of the lids of a new born child. Maternal and antenatal history is important.

Signs: Tenderness in eyeball, swelling of lids, conjunctival discharge (purulent, mucoid or mucopurulent), conjunctival hyperemia and chemosis and observed. Corneal involvement, rarely, may occur in herpes simplex ophthalmia neonatorum.

Complications

Untreated cases may develop corneal ulceration, which may perforate resulting in corneal opacification and staphyloma formation.

Treatment

Prophylaxis needs antenatal, natal and postnatal care. Antenatal measures include thorough care of mother and treatment of genital infections. Natal measures include thorough cleaning of baby's closed eyelids. Postnatal measures include use of 1% tetracycline ointment or 0.5% erythromycin ointment or 1% silver nitrate solution into the eyes of babies immediately following birth. Single injection of ceftriaxone 50 mg/kg IM or IV should be given to new born of mothers with untreated gonococcal infection.

Neonates with gonococcal ophthalmia neonatorum should be treated for seven days with systemic antibiotic therapy.

Chlamydial Conjunctivitis

Introduction

Chlamydial conjunctivitis is a sexually transmitted disease, typically found in young adults. Associated history of leucorrhea, vaginitis or urethritis may be present. There may be history of bath in swimming pool.

Diagnosis

Symptoms: It is characterized by chronic red eye, watery or mucoid discharge, foreign body sensation, eyelids stickiness, etc.

Signs: Conjunctival follicles (inferior), superior pannus, preauricular lymphadenopathy is present (Fig. 2.34).

Treatment

Sulphacetamide (20%) eye drop qid for 4–6 weeks is prescribed. Alternately, erythromycin or tetracycline eye ointment bid for 4 weeks may be used. It is better to avoid bathing in swimming pool.

Oral azithromycin (1 gm) single dose or doxycycline 100 mg bid is advised for 7 days for patient and sexual partner.

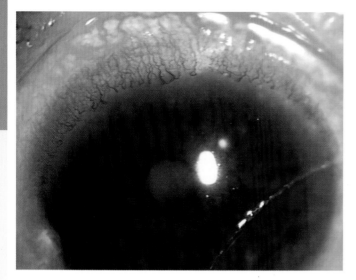

Fig. 2.34: Chlamydial conjunctivitis—pannus

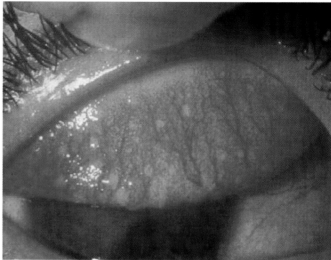

Fig. 2.35: Trachoma follicles

Trachoma

Introduction

Trachoma is chronic inflammation of the conjunctiva and the cornea. Trachoma is caused by *Chlamydia trachomatis*. It is characterized by follicles and papillary hypertrophy of the conjunctiva, with pannus formation over upper part of the cornea. Primarily, it occurs in developing countries (African and some Asian countries), in areas of poor sanitation and crowded condition. Trachoma has been included in *Vision 2020 program*. Although by the 1950s, trachoma had virtually disappeared from the industrialized world, it continues to plague the developing world. This potentially blinding disease remains endemic in the poorest regions of Africa, Asia, the Middle East, and in some parts of Latin America and Australia.

Globally, 84 million people suffer from active infection and nearly 8 million people are visually impaired as a result of this disease. In many of these communities, women are three times more likely than men to be blinded by the disease, due to their roles as caretakers in the family (Figs 2.35 and 2.36).

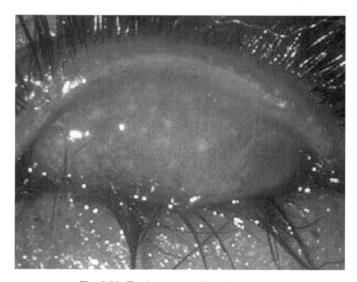

Fig. 2.36: Trachoma—papillary hypertrophy

Classification

WHO classification (FISTO)

- TF (**T**rachomatous inflammation: **F**ollicular): More than 5 follicles of > 0.5 mm in upper tarsus
- TI (**T**rachomatous inflammation: **I**ntense): Papillary hypertrophy and inflammation with thickening obscuring 50% of the tarsal blood vessels
- TS (**T**rachomatous **S**car): Cicatrization of tarsal conjunctiva with white fibrous band (Fig. 2.37)
- TT (**T**rachomatous **T**richiasis): Trichiasis of at least one eyelash or evidence of epilation (eyelash removal)
- CO (**T**rachomatous **C**orneal **O**pacity): CO involving at least part of the pupillary margin

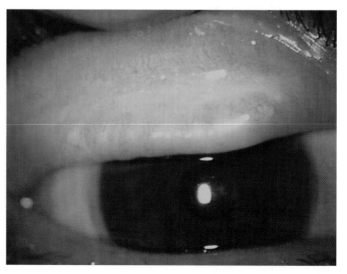

Fig. 2.37: Trachoma scar

McCallan's classification

McCallan in 1908, divided the clinical course of trachoma into 4 stages (Table 2.1).

Table 2.1: McCallan's classification

Stage 1 (Incipient trachoma)	Stage 2 (Established trachoma)	Stage 3 (Cicatrizing trachoma)	Stage 4 (Healed trachoma)
Hyperemia of palpebral conjunctiva	Appearance of mature follicle and papillae	Scarring of palpebral conjunctiva	Disease is cured or is not markable
Immature follicle	Progressive corneal pannus	Scars are easily visible as white bands	Sequelae to cicatrization cause symptoms

Diagnosis

Features

Bulbar conjunctival congestion with velvety papillary hypertrophy is present.

Follicles: Follicles are mostly seen in upper tarsal conjunctiva.

Pannus: Pannus is mainly seen at the upper limbus and upper part of cornea.

Herbert's pit: Pits are seen at the superior limbus. It is a pathognomonic sign (Fig. 2.38).

Scarring of upper tarsal conjunctiva is present.

Treatment

Sulphacetamide (20% or 30%) eye drops, qid; tetracycline eye ointment bid for 4–6 weeks; oral azithromycin—20 mg/kg as single dose; or oral doxycycline (100 mg) bid for 2 weeks is advised.

Prevention

SAFE strategy (by the WHO according to Vision 2020 program)

National governments in collaboration with numerous non-profit organizations are implementing trachoma control programs using the WHO recommended SAFE strategy, which includes:

S = Surgery to correct advanced stages of the disease for trichiasis and entropion

A = Antibiotics to treat active infection, using zithromax (azithromycin)

F = Facial cleanliness to reduce disease transmission

E = Environmental sanitation

Surgery

For individuals with trichiasis, a bilamellar tarsal rotation procedure (BTRP) is required to direct the lashes away from the globe. Early intervention is beneficial as the rate of recurrence is higher in more advanced disease.

Antibiotic Therapy

WHO guidelines recommend that a region should receive community-based, mass antibiotic treatment when the prevalence of active trachoma among one- to nine year-old children is greater than 10%. Subsequent annual treatment should be administered for three years, at which time the prevalence should be reassessed. Annual treatment should be continued until the prevalence drops below 5%. At lower prevalence, antibiotic treatment should be family based.

Antibiotic selection: (single oral dose of 20 mg/kg or topical tetracycline 1% eye ointment twice a day for six weeks). Azithromycin is preferred because it is used as a single oral dose. Although it is expensive, it is generally used as part of the international donation program organized by Pfizer through the International Trachoma Initiative. Azithromycin can be used in children from the age of six months and in pregnancy.

Cleanliness

Children with grossly visible nasal discharge, ocular discharge, or flies on their faces are at least twice as likely to have active trachoma as children with clean faces. Intensive community-based health education programs to promote face-washing can significantly reduce the prevalence of active trachoma, especially intense trachoma (TI). If somebody is already infected, washing one's face is strongly encouraged, especially a child, in order to prevent reinfection.

Environmental Improvement

Modifications in water use, fly control, latrine use, health education and proximity to domesticated animals have all been proposed to reduce transmission of *C. trachomatis*. These changes pose numerous challenges for implementation. It seems likely that these environmental changes ultimately impact on the transmission of ocular infection by the means of lack of facial cleanliness. Particular attention is required for environmental factors that limit clean faces.

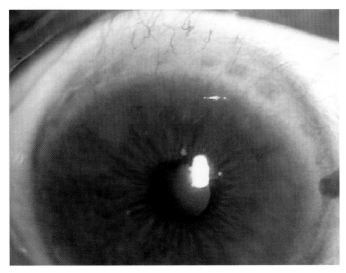

Fig. 2.38: Herbert's pit in trachoma

Viral Conjunctivitis

Adenoviral Keratoconjunctivitis

Introduction

Acute conjunctivitis is caused by adenoviral infection, which may be associated with keratitis after 2–3 weeks. It is responsible for epidemic keratoconjunctivitis.

Diagnosis

Symptoms: It is characterized by acute redness, watery discharge, photophobia and pain. It may be associated with recent upper respiratory tract infection.

Signs: Typical lesion is a keratoconjunctivitis with petechial hemorrhage and follicles (Figs 2.39 and 2.40). There is always a tendency for corneal involvement (superficial punctate keratitis) (Figs 2.41 and 2.42) and preauricular lymphadenopathy.

Treatment

Frequent hand washing, cold compress, astringents and antibiotic eye drops, preservative-free tear substitutes and judicious use of weak (soft) steroid drops in corneal involvement.

Prevention

Viral conjunctivitis is highly contagious. Patients should avoid touching their hands, hand shaking with others, and sharing towels and pillows, etc.

Acute Hemorrhagic Conjunctivitis

Introduction

Acute hemorrhagic conjunctivitis is associated with a large subconjunctival hemorrhage and is caused by *Picornavirus, Coxsackievirus* and *Enterovirus.*

Diagnosis

Symptoms: Acute hemorrhagic conjunctivitis begins with an initial period of catarrhal inflammation. The presentation becomes more dramatic with the appearance of conjunctival petechiae.

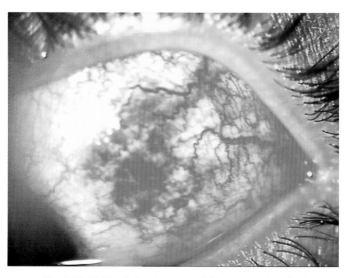

Fig. 2.40: Epidemic keratoconjunctivitis—subconjunctival petechial hemorrhage

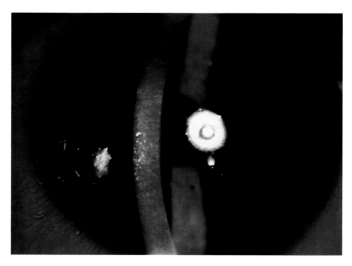

Fig. 2.41: Epidemic keratoconjunctivitis—fine superficial punctate keratitis

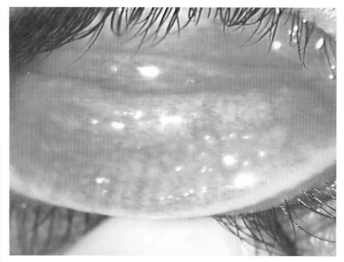

Fig. 2.39: Acute follicular conjunctivitis

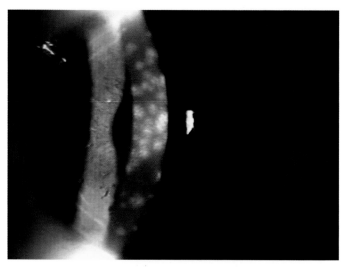

Fig. 2.42: Epidemic keratoconjunctivitis—coarse superficial punctate keratitis

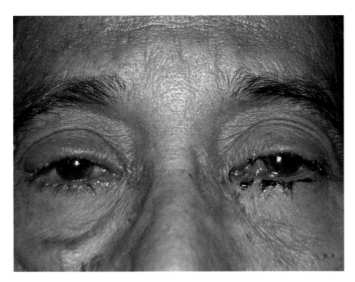

Fig. 2.43: Acute hemorrhagic conjunctivitis

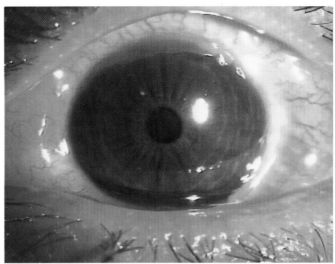

Fig. 2.44: Chemosis—allergic conjunctivitis

These conjunctival petechiae coalesce to form subconjunctival hemorrhages. These are associated with a painful, rapidly progressive follicular conjunctivitis. The lids often become swollen and indurated. The infection resolves within 5–7 days during which the symptoms of pain and irritation are present.

Punctate corneal epithelial defects have been noted and subepithelial corneal opacities have been described. Microbial corneal superinfection has occurred in cases receiving topical steroids. The infection resolves within 5–7 days without treatment. Sequelae in uncomplicated acute hemorrhagic conjunctivitis are rare.

Signs: There are large subconjunctival hemorrhages along with other signs of viral conjunctivitis (Fig. 2.43).

Treatment

The treatment is similar to adenoviral infection.

Allergic Conjunctivitis

Acute Allergic Conjunctivitis

Introduction

Acute allergic conjunctivitis results from acute allergic reaction of the conjunctiva to dust, pollens or other allergens.

Diagnosis

Symptoms: It is characterized by itching and watery discharge. A history of allergic diathesis is present.

Signs: Conjunctival chemosis, moderate to severe congestion, papillae and lid edema is present. No preauricular lymphadenopathy (Figs 2.44 and 2.45) may be present.

Treatment

Elimination of allergen; cold compress several times; frequent preservative-free tear substitutes; antihistaminic eye drops; olopatadine (0.1%), epinastine (0.05%) or ketotifen eye drops twice daily is advised. In severe cases, dilute (1/10th dilution

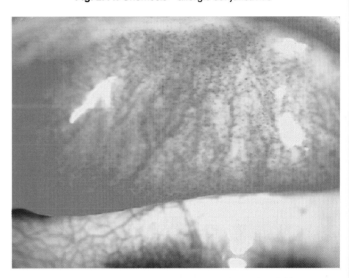

Fig. 2.45: Conjunctival papillae in allergic conjunctivitis

of dexamethasone) or soft steroid (fluorometholone or loteprednol) eye drops for 1–2 weeks and oral antihistaminics may be used.

Vernal Keratoconjunctivitis

Introduction

Vernal keratoconjunctivitis is a bilateral, recurrent, seasonal (spring) allergic conjunctivitis in children caused by exogenous allergens.

Types

The disease may be present in one of the three forms: palpebral, bulbar or mixed.

Palpebral: Cobblestone like papillary hypertrophy of the palpebral conjunctiva is present (Figs 2.46 and 2.47).

Bulbar: Multiple, small, nodule-like gelatinous thickening around the limbus, mostly at the upper limbus is present (Fig. 2.48).

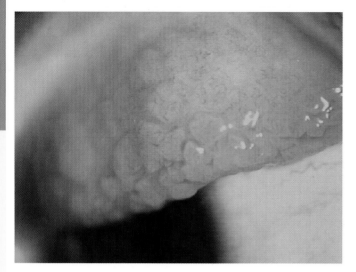

Fig. 2.46: Vernal conjunctivitis—palpebral type

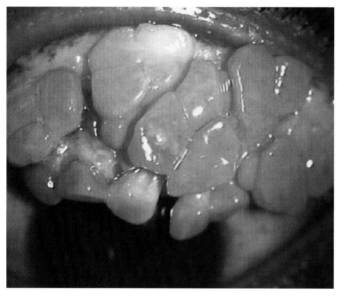

Fig. 2.47: Giant papillae in vernal keratoconjunctivitis

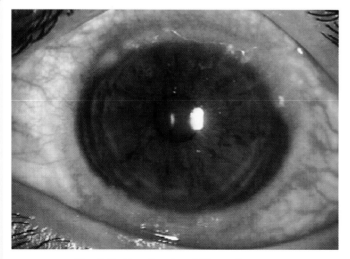

Fig. 2.48: Vernal conjunctivitis—bulbar type

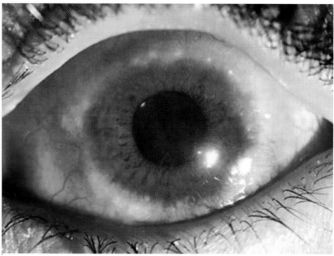

Fig. 2.49: Vernal keratoconjunctivitis—Horner-Trantas dots

Discrete superficial spots, called Horner-Trantas dots (Fig. 2.49) and micropannus around the upper limbus; epithelial microerosions leading to corneal ulceration (shield ulcer) (Fig. 2.50) are present.

Pseudogerontoxon: It resembles an arcus senilis with appearance of cupid's bow. Associated limbal deficiency, dry eye and keratoconus may be present.

Treatment

Cold compress, topical antihistaminics, frequent preservative-free tears substitutes, soft corticosteroids eye drops and mast-cell stabilizer eye drops are advised. Topical 2% cyclosporine has some role in severe cases.

Atopic Conjunctivitis

Introduction

Atopic keratoconjunctivitis is a type IV reaction, is seen in 30% of atopic dermatitis, especially with eczema. It is perennial in character with some seasonal exacerbation.

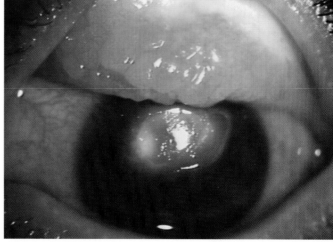

Fig. 2.50: Vernal keratoconjunctivitis—shield ulcer

Diagnosis

Symptoms: It is characterized by severe itching, watering, swelling of lids and photophobia (Fig. 2.51).

Signs: Thickened scaly dermatitis of the eyelids, conjunctival congestion, milky edema, papillary reaction of tarsal conjunctiva, superficial corneal vascularization and corneal opacity due to limbal stem cell dysfunction may be present. Associated skin lesions on face, neck, popliteal and antecubital areas are characteristic features. Hay fever, asthma and urticaria are often present.

Treatment

Tears substitutes, soft corticosteroid eye drops, tacrolimus (0.03%) ointment to treat lid condition and systemic immunosuppressants are advised.

Giant Papillary Conjunctivitis

Introduction

Giant papillary conjunctivitis is a foreign body (soft contact lenses, artificial eye and nylon sutures) associated allergic conjunctivitis with characteristic giant papillae (>1 mm).

Diagnosis

Symptoms: It is characterized by moderate itching, mucoid discharge and the heaviness of upper eyelids. History of using soft contact lens may be present.

Signs: Clinical picture is similar to palpebral type vernal conjunctivitis with the presence of giant papillae (Fig. 2.52).

Treatment

The treatment is similar as vernal keratoconjunctivitis. Avoidance of offending agents is advised for at least 6–8 weeks.

Stevens-Johnson Syndrome

Introduction

Erythema multiforme major is acute onset, mucocutaneous vesiculobullous disease caused by a hypersensitivity reaction

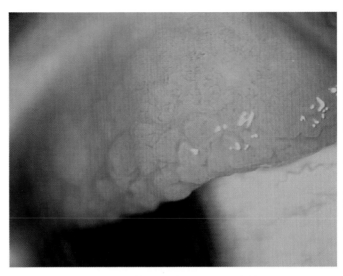

Fig. 2.52: Giant papillary conjunctivitis

to certain drugs like sulfa, penicillin, phenytoin, allopurinol or other drugs. It may also occur in some infection, like herpes simplex virus, mycoplasma pneumonia, or in malignancy. Conjunctiva is involved in 50% of cases.

Diagnosis

Symptoms: It is characterized by acute onset of fever, malaise, respiratory tract symptoms, and rash and redness of eyes. In late cases, there is dryness, foreign body sensation, dimness of vision and frequent blinking of eyes.

Signs: Mucopurulent conjunctivitis with pseudomembrane formation is present (Figs 2.53 and 2.54). Later on dry eye due to secondary scarring of the conjunctiva and lid margins with trichiasis and acquired distichiasis, symblepharon of various degrees, and obliteration of the fornices occurs (Fig. 2.55). There may be corneal ulceration, neovascularization, perforation

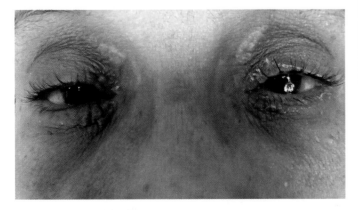

Fig. 2.51: Atopic keratoconjunctivitis

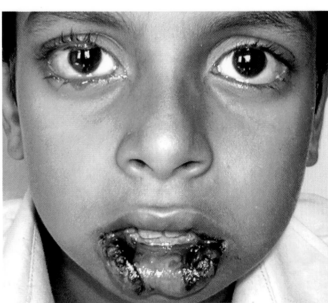

Fig. 2.53: Stevens-Johnson syndrome—conjunctival and oral lesion

or scarring (Fig. 2.56). Associated oral mucous membrane and cutaneous lesions are present (Figs 2.57 and 2.58).

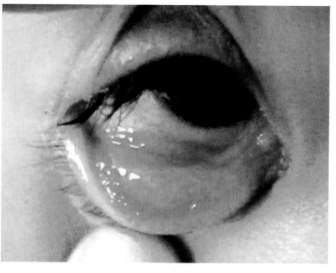

Fig. 2.54: Stevens-Johnson syndrome—pseudomembrane formation

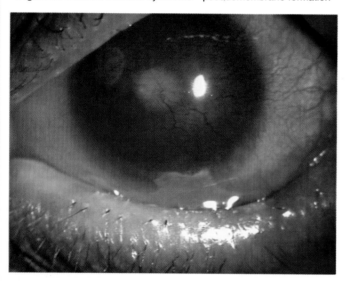

Fig. 2.55: Stevens-Johnson syndrome—symblepharon

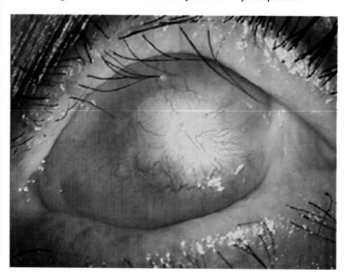

Fig. 2.56: Stevens-Johnson syndrome—symblepharon and vascularization

Treatment

Immediate hospitalization, remove or treat the offending cause and the supportive measures are suggested. Systemic methylprednisolone, cyclosporine or intravenous immunoglobulin (IVIG) are also important.

Preservative-free tear substitutes, antibiotic eye drops, soft steroid eye drops and amniotic membrane transplantation in large epithelial defects—for the initial phase. Later on treatment for symblepharon, trichiasis/distichiasis or other complications are required. Keratoprosthesis may be required in extreme situation.

Miscellaneous Conjunctivitis

Membranous Conjunctivitis

Membranous conjunctivitis is characterized by edema of the lids and mucopurulent or sanious discharge. Thick white or grayish-yellow membrane on the palpebral conjunctiva is

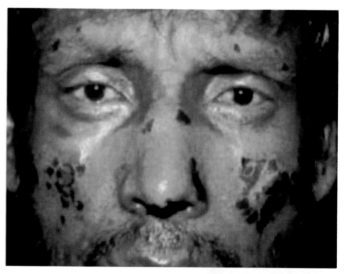

Fig. 2.57: Stevens-Johnson syndrome—skin involvement

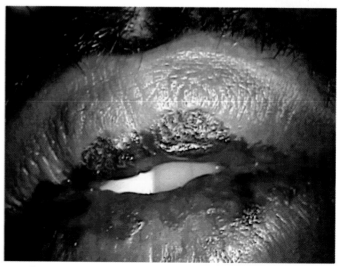

Fig. 2.58: Stevens-Johnson syndrome—oral lesion

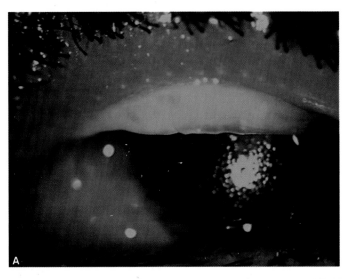

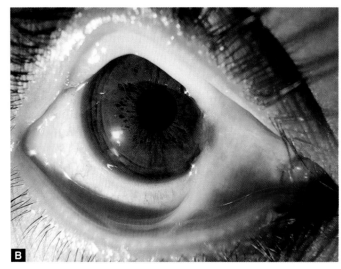

Figs 2.59 A and B: Membranous conjunctivitis

present. Bleeding is very common on removal of the membrane. Symblepharon may occur in late stage (Figs 2.59A and B).

Treatment

Isolation for the patient, crystalline penicillin, antidiphtheritic serum and erythromycin eye ointment is advised.

Angular Conjunctivitis

In angular conjunctivitis, conjunctival inflammation is limited to inner marginal strip, especially at the outer or inner canthi. Excoriation of the skin at the outer or inner canthi and congestion of adjacent bulbar conjunctiva (Fig. 2.60) are observed.

Treatment

Treatment includes oxytetracycline (1%) eye ointment and zinc oxide containing eye drops.

DEGENERATIONS

Pinguecula

Introduction

Pinguecula is due to hyaline infiltration and elastotic degeneration of the submucosal conjunctival tissue.

Diagnosis

Symptoms: Pinguecula is usually symptomless. Patient may complain for cosmetic reason or sometimes there may be localized redness.

Signs: There is yellowish, triangular deposit on the conjunctiva near the limbus at the palpebral aperture. The apex is towards the cornea. Pinguecula affects the nasal side first, then the temporal side (Figs 2.61 and 2.62).

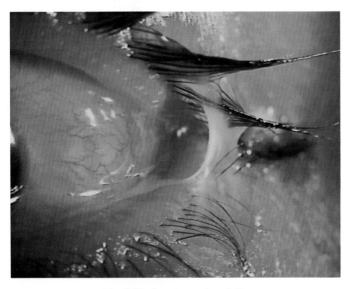

Fig. 2.60: Angular conjunctivitis

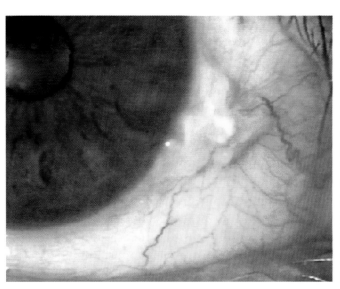

Fig. 2.61: Pinguecula

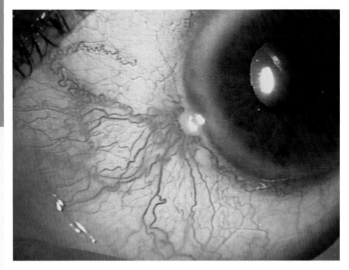

Fig. 2.62: Inflamed pinguecula

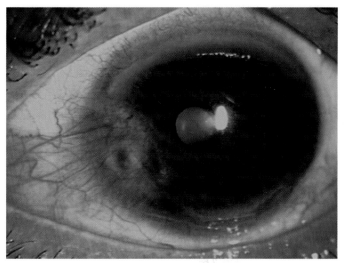

Fig. 2.63: Atrophic pterygium

Treatment

Pinguecula does not require any treatment. Sometimes, it may be inflamed and is then treated with dilute or soft corticosteroids eye drops qid for seven days.

Pterygium

Introduction

Pterygium results as the subconjunctival tissue proliferates as a triangular, wing-shaped tissue mass to invade the cornea to involve the Bowman's membrane and the superficial stroma.

Pterygium is usually bilateral. It may be asymmetrical and may occur among elderly individuals.

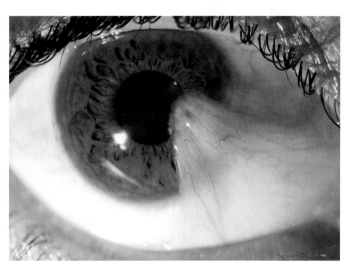

Fig. 2.64: Progressive pterygium

Types

Pterygium may occur as progressive (fleshy) and stationary (atrophic) types.

Atrophic (stationary) pterygium: Pterygium is thin and attenuated with poor vascularity. No opaque spot (cap) is seen (Fig. 2.63).

Progressive (fleshy) pterygium: Pterygium is thick, fleshy with prominent vascularity. It increases in size and encroaches towards the center of cornea. Opaque infiltrative spot (cap) with Stocker's line in the front of the apex is observed (Fig. 2.64).

Recurrent pterygium: Pterygium may recur with more scarring and wider area (Fig. 2.65).

Malignant pterygium: It is a recurrent pterygium with symblepharon formation, associated with the restriction of ocular movement on opposite side (Fig. 2.66).

Pseudopterygium: A pterygium is to be differentiated from a pseudopterygium (Fig. 2.67).

Treatment

Excision of pterygium (subconjunctival dissection) with conjunctival limbal autograft (CLAU) is the treatment of choice. Treatment of the bare sclera by mitomycin-C is another option.

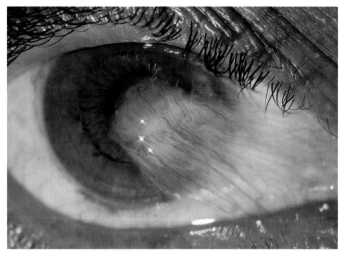

Fig. 2.65: Recurrent pterygium

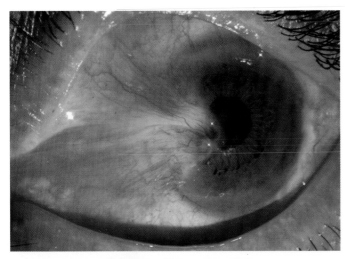

Fig. 2.66: Malignant pterygium

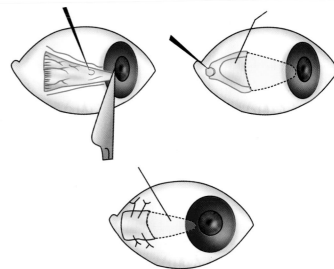

Fig. 2.68: Pterygium resection—bare sclera technique

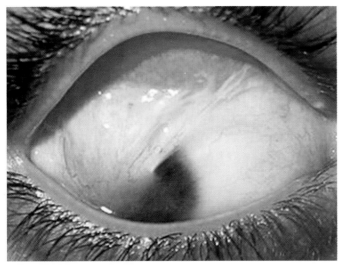

Fig. 2.67: Pseudopterygium

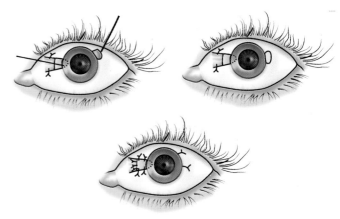

Fig. 2.69: Conjunctival limbal autograft

Surgical Steps of Pterygium Excision Surgery

Surgery is performed under topical anesthesia with local anesthetic infiltration within pterygium. Head of the pterygium is carefully resected from the cornea with fine blade. From the neck, two radial cuts are made on either side along the upper and lower border of the pterygium. The conjunctiva is undermined. Dissection of suncojunctival tissue is performed and is excised from deeper tissue. Conjunctiva is reposed and a triangular portion, which includes head and part of the body is removed, keeping 2–3 mm of bare sclera. A same-size rectangular piece of conjunctival tissue is dissected from the upper temporal limbus of the same eye and taken out as a limbal graft. The graft is oriented (matching the limbal edge) and placed over the bare sclera. This grafted tissue is sutured with 10-0 vicryl or monofilament nylon. Alternately tissue fibrin-glue can be used. Nylon sutures are removed after 2–3 weeks (Figs 2.68 and 2.69).

Benign Pigmented Lesions

Flat Superficial Pigmentation

These are common, congenital and small focal lesions (Fig. 2.70).

Causes

Conjunctival freckles, melanosis around Axenfeld loop (an intrascleral nerve loop 4 mm away from limbus) and melanosis around anterior ciliary artery.

No treatment is necessary.

Benign Epithelial Melanosis

It is a bilateral, yellowish-brown or brownish-black patches most prominent at the limbus. It is also present at the interpalpebral areas and gradually fades towards fornix. Lesions can be easily moved on the globe (Fig. 2.71).

No treatment is necessary.

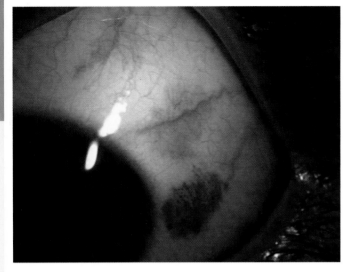

Fig. 2.70: Flat superficial pigmentation

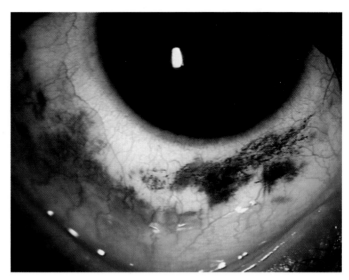

Fig. 2.72: Benign subepithelial melanocytosis

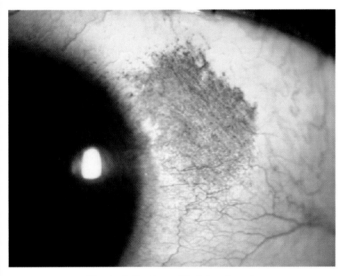

Fig. 2.71: Benign epithelial melanosis

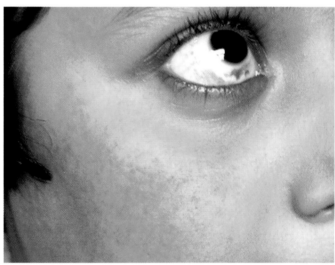

Fig. 2.73: Nevus of Ota

Benign Subepithelial Melanocytosis

It is a rare, unilateral congenital condition with a slate blue-gray discoloration. It affects the episcleral and scleral tissue and cannot be moved. It may affect the skin and mucous membrane in the distribution of fifth nerve (Fig. 2.72).

There may be isolated melanocytosis oculi or oculodermal melanocytosis (nevus of Ota), which involves both the skin and globe (Fig. 2.73).

No treatment is necessary.

Simple Nevus

This is a more common benign tumor. It is a single, sharply demarcated, flat or slightly elevated lesion and has predilection for the limbus, plica, caruncle or lid margin (Figs 2.74 to 2.76).

Most nevi have a tan or brown color, and 25% are nonpigmented, tends to enlarge or darken during puberty or pregnancy.

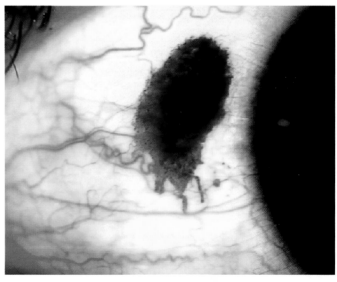

Fig. 2.74: Simple nevus

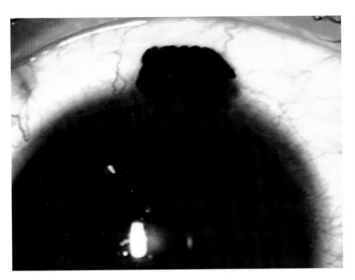

Fig. 2.75: Simple nevus—limbal

Treatment

Usually no treatment is necessary, but sometimes it may be excised for cosmetic reasons.

Melanocytoma

It is a very rare, congenital benign tumor. It is a black, slowly growing mass, which does not move freely over the globe and tends to enlarge during puberty (Fig. 2.77).

Treatment

Usually no treatment is necessary, but sometimes it may be excised for cosmetic reasons.

Malignant Lesions

Precancerous Melanosis

It is a small pigmented tumor, which spreads as a diffuse patch of pigmented lesion. It mostly occurs in elderly patients. In 20% cases, it proceeds to frank malignancy (Figs 2.78 and 2.79A and B).

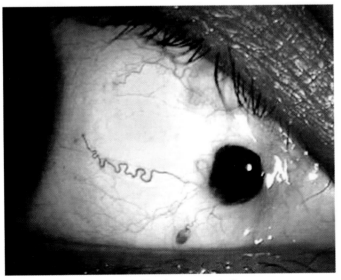

Fig. 2.76: Simple nevus—at plica

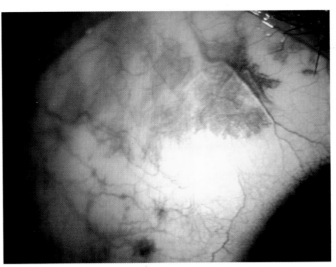

Fig. 2.77: Conjunctival melanocytoma

Treatment

Excision is performed in suspected cases.

Malignant Melanoma

It may be a pigmented or nonpigmented lesion, which affects elderly people.

Elevated lesion can occur in any part of conjunctiva, but has a predilection for limbus. Larger lesion may involve cornea, adjacent part of eyelid and orbit (Figs 2.80, 2.81A and B, and 2.83). Metastasis is common.

Treatment

Excision is performed in suspected cases.

DRY EYE

Introduction

Dry eye is a multifactorial disease of the tears and ocular surface that results in the symptoms of discomfort, visual disturbance,

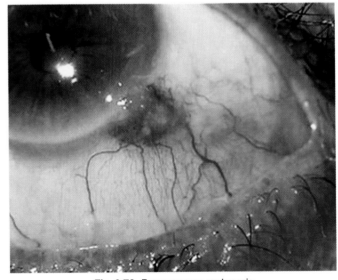

Fig. 2.78: Precancerous melanosis

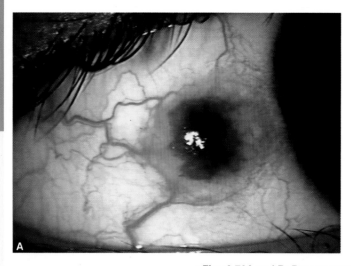

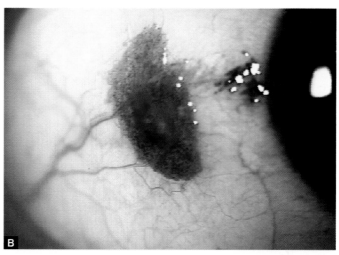

Figs 2.79A and B: Precancerous melanosis—malignant change

and tears film instability with potential damage to the ocular surface. It is accompanied by increased osmolarity of the tear film and inflammation of the ocular surface.

Definitions

Keratoconjunctivitis sicca: It is defined as deficiency of aqueous component of the tear film.
- *Primary keratoconjunctivitis sicca:* It is characterized by the involvement of the lacrimal gland alone without systemic involvement.
- *Secondary keratoconjunctivitis sicca:* It is associated with the additional feature of connective tissue disorders.

Xerosis: It is the dryness of the conjunctiva and presents as wrinkling, thickening, pigmentation and dryness of conjunctiva (Fig. 2.83).

Xerophthalmia: When the same xerotic process spreads over the cornea. It is mainly caused by vitamin-A deficiency (Fig. 2.84).

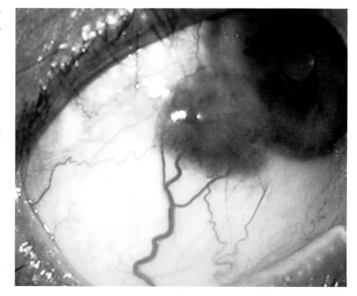

Fig. 2.80: Amelanotic melanoma

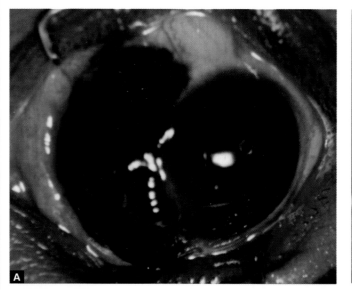

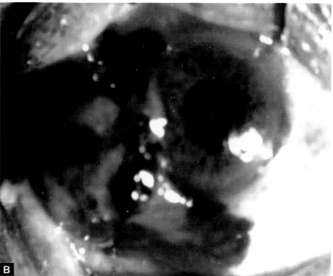

Figs 2.81A and B: Conjunctival melanoma

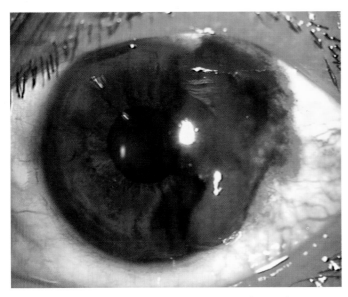

Fig. 2.82: Conjunctival melanoma—corneal extension

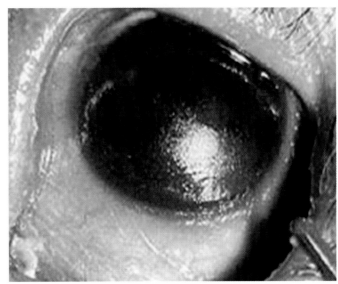

Fig. 2.84: Corneal xerophthalmia

Sjogren's syndrome: It is an autoimmune disease, characterized by dry eye and a dry mouth due to the involvement of both lacrimal and salivary glands.

- *Primary:* Involvement of both lacrimal and salivary glands without systemic problem.
- *Secondary:* Associated with problems of connective tissue disorders, as in rheumatoid arthritis, systemic lupus erythematosus, polymyositis and other disorders.

Diagnosis

Symptoms: It is characterized by burning, foreign body sensation, blurring of vision, discomfort and dry feeling.

Signs: It is characterized by low tear meniscus height, mucus debris on corneal surface, punctate staining of the cornea, filaments, Dellen and vascularization in severe cases (Figs 2.85 to 2.88).

Investigations

Level of dry eye:
- *Level 1:* Mild or episodic (under environmental stress) dry eye
- *Level 2:* Moderate or chronic dry eye
- *Level 3:* Severe dry eye
- *Level 4:* Most severe or disabling dry eye

Tear film break-up time: It is measured from one blink to the appearance of the tear film defect by using fluorescein stain under slit lamp. Normally it should be more than 10 seconds.

- *Schirmer's test:* After drying the eye of excess tears, Whitman filter paper is placed at lower fornix at the middle and lateral

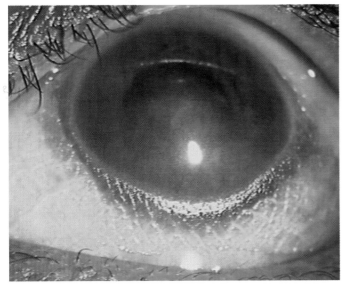

Fig. 2.83: Conjunctival xerosis

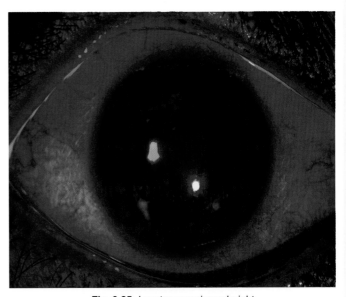

Fig. 2.85: Low tear meniscus height

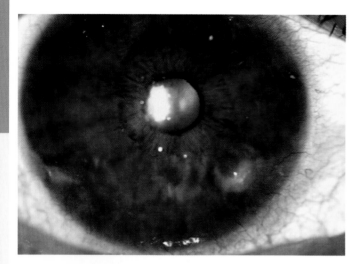

Fig. 2.86: Keratoconjunctivitis sicca—mucus debris

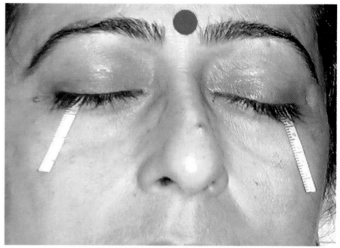

Fig. 2.89: Schirmer's test

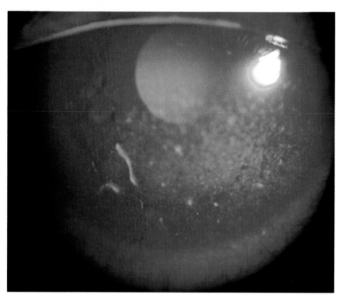

Fig. 2.87: Superficial punctate keratitis with filaments after fluorescein staining in dry eye

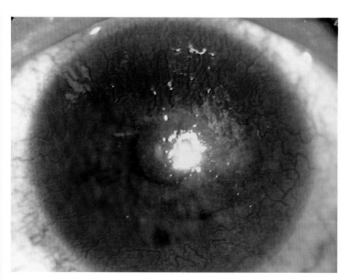

Fig. 2.88: Keratoconjunctivitis sicca—vascularization

third junction in each eye for five minutes. It is usually done without anesthesia (Schirmer I). Normal wetting is more than 10 mm (Fig. 2.89).

- *Staining of conjunctiva:* Staining is performed by rose bengal, fluorescein and lissamine green stain (Figs 2.90A and B and 2.91).
- *Other tests:* Tear osmolarity, tear ferning test, tear lysozyme assay, etc.

Treatment

- *Level 1 or mild dry eye:* Artificial tears four times daily and environmental education are most commonly used modes of therapy.
- *Level 2 or Moderate dry eye:* Preservative-free artificial tears on two hourly basis and gel at bed time. Cyclosporine (0.05%) eye drops or soft steroids eye drops two times daily. Tetracycline in case of meibomianitis.
- *Level 3 or Severe dry eye:* Along with it, autologous serum eye drops, mucolytic agents, punctal occlusion and contact lens are used.
- *Level 4 or disabling dry eye:* Additionally systemic anti-inflammatory agents, lid surgery, tarsorrhaphy, botulinum toxin and amniotic membrane transplant may be required.

EPISCLERA AND SCLERA

Episcleritis

Introduction

Episcleritis is a benign inflammation of the episcleral tissue and does not pose a serious problem.

Types

Simple: Sectoral redness involving the middle episcleral vessels is present (Fig. 2.92).

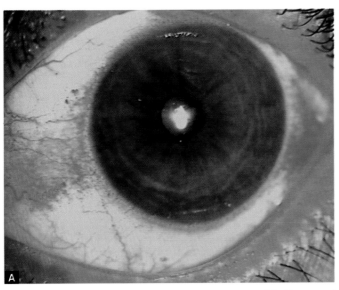

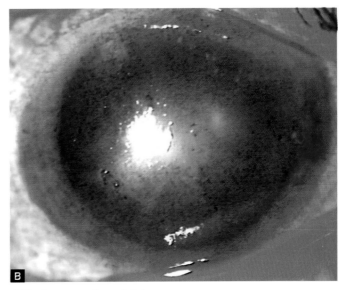

Figs 2.90A and B: Keratoconjunctivitis sicca—rose bengal stain

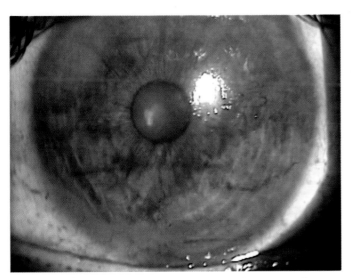

Fig. 2.91: Keratoconjunctivitis sicca—lissamine green stain

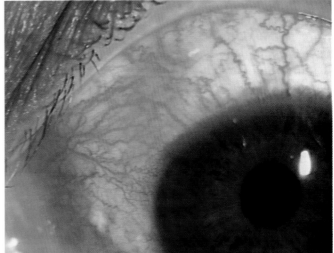

Fig. 2.92: Simple episcleritis

Nodular: Purple solitary nodule with surrounding injection, which can be moved over the sclera is present. It is situated 2–3 mm away from the limbus (Figs 2.93A and B).

Treatment

Oral anti-inflammatory agents, dilute topical corticosteroids or nonsteroidal anti-inflammatory eye drops are given.

Scleritis

Introduction

Scleritis is the inflammation of sclera and is associated with collagen disorders in 50% of the cases. Scleritis is associated with severe and boring pain in the affected eye.

Types

Scleritis may be diffuse, nodular or necrotizing:

Diffuse anterior scleritis: It involves either a segment or the entire anterior sclera. Diffuse redness and distortion of pattern of deep episcleral vascular plexus is present (Figs 2.94A and B).

Nodular scleritis (nonnecrotizing): It is extremely tender. Usually solitary or multiple firm immobile nodules are separated from the overlying congested episcleral tissue (Figs 2.95 and 2.96A and B).

Anterior necrotizing scleritis with inflammation: It is characterized by avascular patches with scleral necrosis and melting. Marked thinning of the sclera with increased visibility of underlying uvea is present (Figs 2.97 to 2.99).

Necrotizing scleritis without inflammation (scleromalacia perforans): It occurs in long-standing rheumatoid arthritis. It occurs as a painless, necrotic patch in normal sclera. Eventually, extreme scleral thinning with the exposure and bulging of underlying uvea occurs (Figs 2.100A and B).

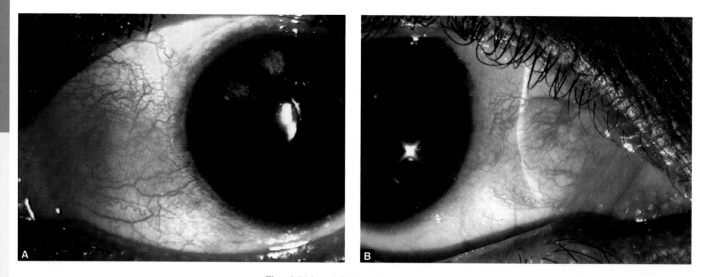

Figs 2.93A and B: Nodular episcleritis

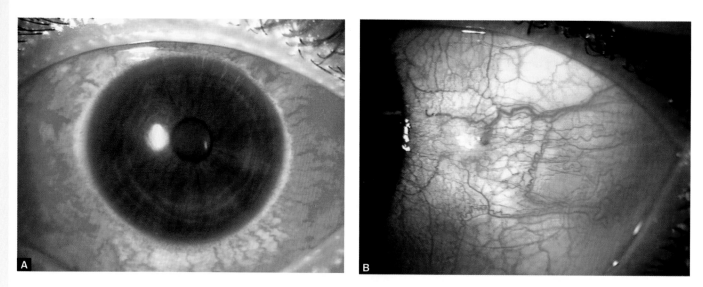

Figs 2.94A and B: Diffuse anterior scleritis

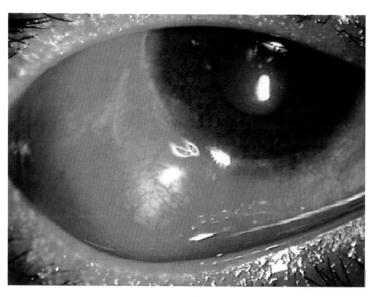

Fig. 2.95: Nodular scleritis—solitary

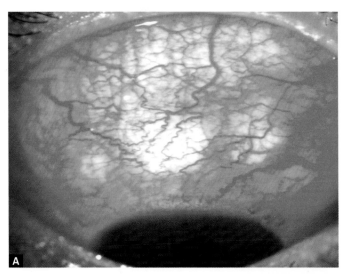
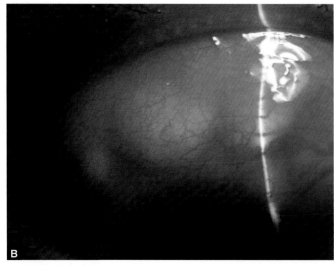

Figs 2.96A and B: Nodular scleritis—multiple

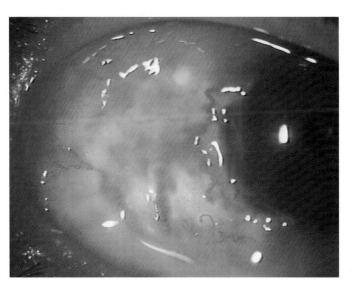

Fig. 2.97: Necrotizing scleritis with inflammation

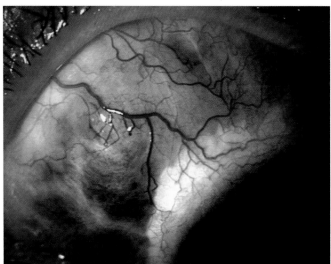

Fig. 2.98: Necrotizing scleritis—thinning

Treatment

Investigations for systemic collagen disorders may be required.

Systemic and topical corticosteroids as well as systemic and topical nonsteroidal anti-inflammatory drugs (like, indomethacin) are required. Systemic immunosuppressives may be required in severe and unresponsive cases.

Posterior Scleritis

Posterior scleritis may start as a posterior lesion or rarely be an extension of anterior scleritis. It may be associated with exudative retinal detachment, disc swelling, retinal hemorrhage, choroidal folds or detachment, and painful restricted motility or proptosis. It is usually unrelated to systemic collagen disorders (Fig. 2.101).

Treatment

Systemic aspirin, nonsteroidal anti-inflammatory drugs, corticosteroids or immunosuppressive therapy are given. Regular retinal consultation is required.

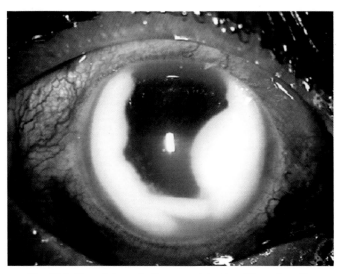

Fig. 2.99: Necrotizing scleritis—associated keratitis and uveitis

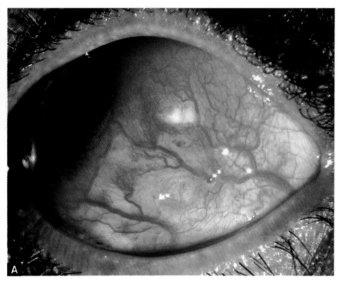

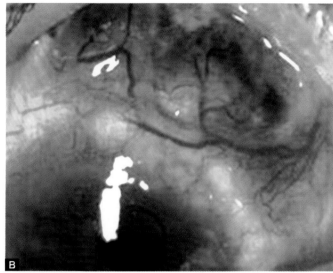

Figs 2.100A and B: Scleromalacia perforans

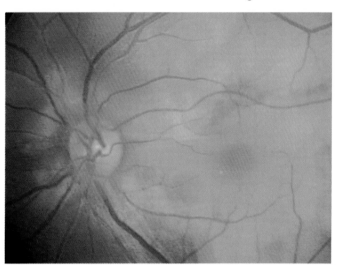

Fig. 2.101: Posterior scleritis

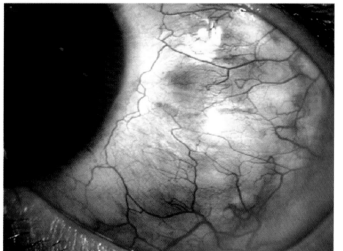

Fig. 2.102: Blue sclera

Scleral Discoloration

Blue Sclera

Sclera appears bluer than white, mainly due to increased visibility of the underlying uveal pigment through thin sclera (Fig. 2.102).

Causes

Osteogenesis imperfecta, buphthalmos, following diffuse scleritis, oculodermal melanocytosis and Marfan's syndrome (Figs 2.103 to 2.105).

Other Types of Discoloration

Localized blue or brown-black discoloration of the sclera may be seen in a variety of condition.

Causes

Healed focal scleritis, equatorial staphyloma, alkaptonuria, extreme old age, long-standing metallic foreign body (Figs 2.106 to 2.109).

Treatment

No treatment is required.

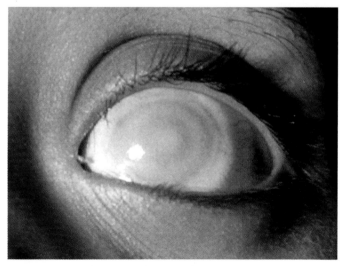

Fig. 2.103: Blue sclera—buphthalmos

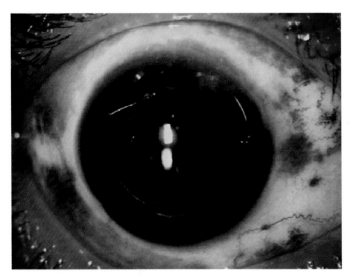

Fig. 2.104: Blue sclera—diffuse scleritis

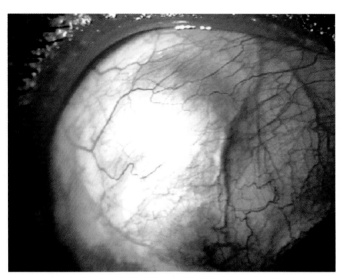

Fig. 2.107: Focal discoloration—equatorial staphyloma

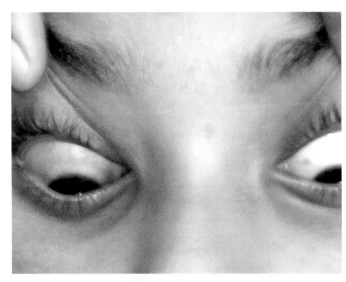

Fig. 2.105: Blue sclera—oculodermal melanocytosis

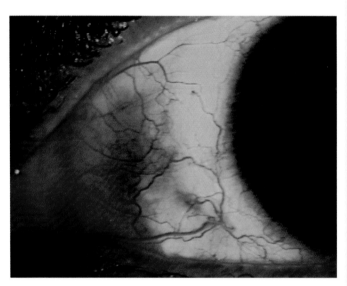

Fig. 2.108: Focal discoloration—alkaptonuria

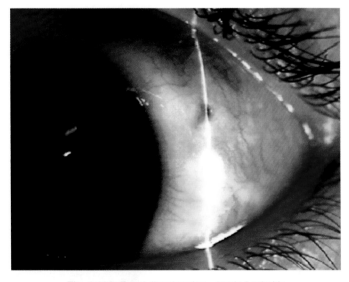

Fig. 2.106: Focal discoloration—healed scleritis

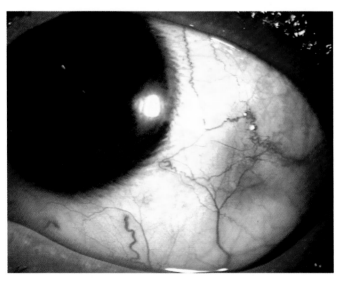

Fig. 2.109: Focal discoloration—old age

Diseases of Cornea

*Sunita Chaurasia, R Muralidhar,
Mukesh Taneja, Virender Sangwan*

BACTERIAL KERATITIS

Introduction

Bacterial keratitis is an ocular emergency that requires immediate and appropriate treatment to limit corneal morbidity and vision loss. Bacterial keratitis is the most prevalent type of serious ocular infection. The challenge for eye care providers is to distinguish bacterial keratitis from other infectious and noninfectious inflammatory conditions by assessing risk factors and evaluating clinical presentations.

Pathogens

The most common groups of bacteria responsible for bacterial keratitis are:

- Streptococcus
- Pseudomonas
- Enterobacteriaceae (including Klebsiella, Enterobacter Serratia, and Proteus), and
- Staphylococcus species.

Risk Factors

Several risk factors may lead to bacterial keratitis:

(a) Any factor that creates a breakdown of the corneal epithelium
(b) Exposure to some virulent bacteria that may penetrate intact epithelium (e.g. *Neisseria gonorrhoeae, Streptococcus pneumoniae*)
(c) Use of contact lenses, especially extended-wear contact lenses
(d) Contaminated ocular medications or contact lens solutions
(e) Decreased immunologic defenses secondary to malnutrition, alcoholism and diabetes
(f) Aqueous tear deficiencies
(g) Recent corneal disease (herpetic keratitis and secondary neurotrophic keratopathy)
(h) Structural alteration or malposition of the eyelids (entropion with trichiasis and lagophthalmos)
(i) Chronic dacryocystitis
(j) Use of topical corticosteroids

Pathophysiology

Interruption of an intact corneal epithelium permits the entrance of microorganisms into the corneal stroma, where they may proliferate and cause ulceration. Various virulence factors may initiate microbial invasion and effect or molecules may assist the infective process. Many bacteria display several adhesins on fimbriated and nonfimbriated structures that may aid in their adherence to host corneal cells. During the initial stages, the epithelium and stroma in the area of injury and infection swell and undergo necrosis. Acute inflammatory cells infiltrates base of the ulcer and cause necrosis of the stromal lamellae. Diffusion of inflammatory products (including cytokines) posteriorly elicits an outpouring of inflammatory cells into the anterior chamber and may create a hypopyon. Different bacterial toxins and enzymes (including elastase and alkaline protease) may be produced during corneal infection, contributing to the destruction of corneal substance.

History

Patients with bacterial keratitis are usually present with the rapid onset of pain, photophobia and decreased vision. It is important to document a complete systemic and ocular history in these patients to identify any potential risk factors that would have made them susceptible to develop this infection, including the following:

- Contact lens wear
- Trauma (including previous corneal surgery)
- Use of contaminated ocular medications
- Decreased immunologic defenses
- Aqueous tear deficiencies
- Recent corneal disease (herpetic keratitis, neurotrophic keratopathy)
- Structural alteration or malposition of the eyelids

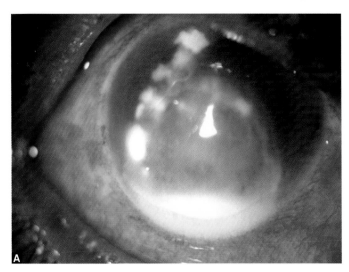

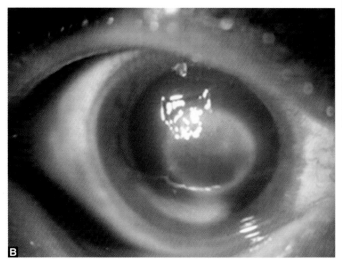

Figs 3.1A and B: Bacterial keratitis. *Pseudomonas* bacterial keratitis

Examination

On slit-lamp biomicroscopy, ulceration of the epithelium and corneal infiltration with no significant tissue loss may be observed. Dense, suppurative stromal inflammation with indistinct edges, stromal tissue loss and surrounding stromal edema may also be observed (Figs 3.1A and B and 3.2). There may be increased anterior chamber reaction with or without hypopyon, folds in the Descemet's membrane, upper eyelid edema, posterior synechiae and surrounding corneal inflammation may be observed which could be either focal or diffuse.. Conjunctival hyperemia and mucopurulent discharge is also observed. Endothelial inflammatory plaque/immune ring may also be present.

Microbiological Examination

A scraping of the corneal ulcer, including the edges, is obtained using a sterile Kimura's spatula or No. 15 Bard-Parker blade. Microscope slides are used for stained smears with Gram,

Giemsa, and acid-fast stain or KOH-calcofluor white (if fungi or acanthamoeba or microsporidia are suspected) (Figs 3.3 to 3.5).

Samples of the eyelids/conjunctiva, topical ocular medications, and contact lens cases and solutions also may be cultured. If the patient has been treated partially and the keratitis is mild or moderately severe, antibiotic therapy can be suspended for 12 to 24 hours before obtaining corneal samples for culture and sensitivity, to increase the yield of a positive culture. Cotton swabs contain fatty acids, which have an inhibitory effect on bacterial growth. On the other hand, calcium alginate moistened with trypticase soy broth can be used to obtain culture material to inoculate directly onto the culture media.

Topical anesthetic (proparacaine hydrochloride 0.5%) should be used to anesthetize the patient prior to culture scraping because it has the least inhibitory effect. Repeat cultures can be obtained if the original cultures were negative and the ulcer is not improving clinically.

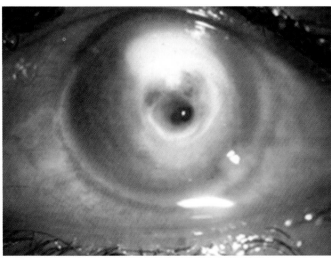

Fig. 3.2: Bacterial keratitis. *Pseudomonas* bacterial keratitis with the prolapse of iris

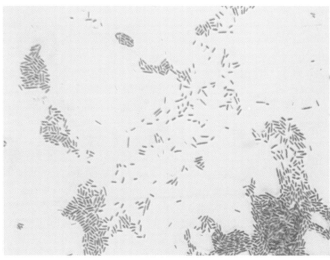

Fig. 3.3: Bacterial keratitis. Gram smears shows Gram-negative bacilli

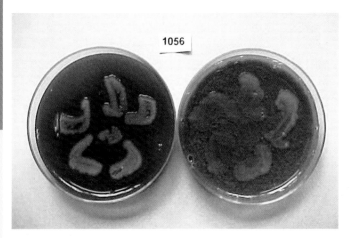

Fig. 3.4: Bacterial keratitis. Gray, moist colonies of *Pseudomonas*

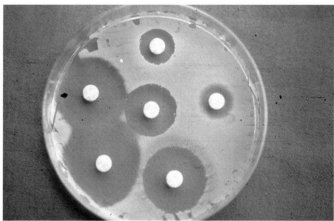

Fig. 3.5: Bacterial keratitis. Kirby Bauer disc diffusion method

Corneal biopsy using a small trephine or a corneal blade may be considered in the cases of deep stromal infiltrates, particularly if cultures are negative and the eye is not improving clinically.

Corneal Biopsy

A deep lamellar excision can be made using a disposable skin punch or a small Elliott corneal trephine. The superficial cornea is incised and deepened with a surgical blade to approximately 200 µm. Then, a lamellar dissection is performed and the material is plated directly onto the culture media. A portion also can be sent for histopathologic evaluation.

Histological Findings

During the initial stages, the epithelium and the stroma in the area of injury and infection swell and undergo necrosis. Acute inflammatory cells (mainly neutrophils) surround the beginning ulcer and cause necrosis of the stromal lamellae. In cases of severe inflammation, a deep ulcer and a deep stromal abscess may coalesce, resulting in thinning of the cornea and sloughing of the infected stroma.

As the natural host defense mechanisms overcome the infection, humoral and cellular immune defenses combine with antibacterial therapy to retard bacterial replication. Following this process, phagocytes of the organism and cellular debris take place, without further destruction of stromal collagen. During this stage, a distinct demarcation line may appear as the epithelial ulceration and stromal infiltration consolidate and the edges become rounded.

Vascularization of the cornea may follow if the keratitis becomes chronic. In the healing stage, the epithelium resurfaces the central area of ulceration and the necrotic stroma is replaced by scar tissue produced by fibroblasts. The reparative fibroblasts are derived from histiocytes and keratocytes that have undergone transformation. Areas of stromal thinning may be replaced partially by fibrous tissue. New blood vessel growth directed towards the area of ulceration occurs with the delivery of humoral and cellular components to promote further healing. The Bowman layer does not regenerate, but is replaced with fibrous tissue.

New epithelium slowly resurfaces the irregular base and vascularization gradually disappears. With severe bacterial keratitis, the progressive stage advances beyond the point in which the regressive stage can lead to the healing stage. In such severe ulcerations, stromal keratolysis may progress to corneal perforation. Uveal blood vessels may participate in sealing the perforation, resulting in an adherent vascularized leukoma.

Imaging

Slit-lamp photography can be useful to document the progression of the keratitis and in cases where the specific etiology is in doubt, it is used to obtain additional opinions, particularly in indolent and chronic cases not responding to antimicrobial therapy.

B-scan ultrasound can be obtained in eyes with severe corneal ulcers with no view of the posterior segment where endophthalmitis is being considered.

Management

Medical

If no organisms are identified on the slide smear, initiate broad-spectrum antibiotics with the following: Tobramycin/gentamicin (14 mg/mL) 1 drop every hour alternating with fortified cefazolin (50 mg/mL) 1 drop every hour. If the corneal ulcer is small, peripheral and no impending perforation is present, intensive monotherapy with fluoroquinolones is an alternative treatment. Other antimicrobials can be used, depending on the clinical progress and laboratory findings.

The fourth-generation ophthalmic fluoroquinolones include moxifloxacin and gatifloxacin and they are now being used for the treatment of bacterial conjunctivitis. Both antibiotics have better in vitro activity against gram-positive bacteria than ciprofloxacin or ofloxacin. Moxifloxacin penetrates better into ocular tissues than gatifloxacin and older fluoroquinolones; in vitro activity of moxifloxacin and gatifloxacin against gram-negative bacteria is similar to that of older fluoroquinolones. Moxifloxacin also has better mutant prevention characteristics than other fluoroquinolones. These findings support the use of the newer fluoroquinolones for the prevention and treatment of serious ophthalmic infections (e.g. keratitis, endophthalmitis) caused by susceptible bacteria.

In view of these findings, moxifloxacin or gatifloxacin may be a preferred alternative to ciprofloxacin as the first-line monotherapy in bacterial keratitis. Additionally, 0.5% moxifloxacin and, to a lesser extent, levofloxacin and ciprofloxacin have demonstrated significant effectiveness for reducing the number of mycobacterium abscesses in vivo, suggesting the potential use of these agents in the prevention of abscesses and keratitis. The frequency of antibiotic administration should be tapered off according to the clinical course using some of the following parameters:

Blunting of the perimeter of the stromal infiltrate; decreased density of the stromal infiltrate; decreased stromal edema and endothelial inflammatory plaque, decreased anterior chamber inflammation, reepithelialization of the corneal epithelial defect and improvement in symptoms and pain.

- • *Antibiotics*

Aminoglycosides: Aminoglycosides have a broad range of bactericidal activity against many bacterial species, particularly gram-negative rods. They have a selective affinity to bacterial 30S and 50S ribosomal subunits to produce a nonfunctional 70S initiation complex that results in the inhibition of bacterial cell protein synthesis. Unlike other antibiotics that impair protein synthesis, they are bactericidal. Their clinical activity is limited severely in anaerobic conditions. They have a low therapeutic/toxic ratio.

Cephalosporins: Cephalosporins have a broad spectrum of activity, including effective action against Haemophilus species. They contain a beta-lactam ring similar to penicillins, and a dihydrothiazine ring that makes them resistant to the action of penicillinases produced by staphylococci. They inhibit the third and final stage of bacterial cell wall formation by preferentially binding to one or more penicillin-binding proteins that are in the cytoplasmic membrane beneath the cell walls of susceptible bacteria. They are well tolerated topically.

Chloramphenicol: Chloramphenicol usually is reserved for specific infections, such as those associated with *H influenzae*. Its use has been limited by toxicity, including a dose-dependent bone marrow depression.

Macrolides: Macrolides are bacteriostatic agents (e.g. erythromycin, tetracycline) that can suppress the growth of susceptible gram-positive cocci. This class of drugs works by the inhibition of bacterial protein synthesis.

Glycopeptides: Glycopeptides have activity against gram-positive bacteria and methicillin- and penicillin-resistant staphylococci. They inhibit the biosynthesis of peptidoglycan polymers during the second stage of bacterial cell wall formation, at a different site of action from that of the beta-lactam antibiotics. They also have an excellent activity against a variety of gram-positive bacilli.

Sulfonamides: Sulfonamides have a structure similar to para-aminobenzoic acid, a precursor required by bacteria for folic acid synthesis. They competitively inhibit the synthesis of dihydropteroic acid, the immediate precursor of dihydrofolic acid from para-aminobenzoic acid pteridine. This inhibition does not affect mammalian cells because they lack the ability to synthesize folic acid and require preformed folic acid. They are active against gram-positive and gram-negative bacteria, and they are the preferred drugs against Nocardia keratitis.

Fluoroquinolones: Fluoroquinolones variably inhibit the action of bacterial DNA gyrase, an enzyme essential for bacterial DNA synthesis. They have activity against most aerobic gram-negative bacteria and some gram-positive bacteria. Concern has been generated regarding the emerging resistance to fluoroquinolones among staphylococci. Emerging resistance to these antimicrobials has been reported in nonocular and ocular isolates. They have limited efficacy against streptococci, enterococci, non-aeruginosa Pseudomonas and anaerobes. Two multicenter trials compared the efficacy of ciprofloxacin 0.3% and ofloxacin 0.3% solution versus fortified cefazolin and tobramycin, and reported favorable efficacy for a single agent fluoroquinolone therapy. They also have a record for low toxicity, good ocular surface penetration and prolonged tear film penetration. Monotherapy for bacterial keratitis using these classes of antibiotics has been proved to be effective in large clinical trials. However, emerging resistance to the fluoroquinolones is now being reported in nonocular and ocular isolates.

- • *Topical corticosteroids*

Anti-inflammatory agents that may impair host defenses and enhance microbial proliferation, but can reduce host inflammatory response that contributes to conjunctival or corneal scarring. Should not be used until specific antimicrobial therapy has controlled microbial proliferation and clear clinical improvement is evident. Judicious corticosteroid use entails dosage adjustment according to the severity of ocular inflammation and occurrence of side effects. Discontinuation should be gradual to minimize rebound of inflammation.

Surgical

The most common cause of corneal perforation is infection by bacteria, virus or fungus, accounting for 24 to 55% of all perforations, with bacterial infections being the most common.

Penetrating keratoplasty, sclerocorneal patch or application of cyanoacrylate tissue adhesive may be necessary in the cases of corneal perforation or imminent perforation.

Systemic intravenous antibiotics (alternatively ciprofloxacin 500 mg PO bid) should be started once an infected corneal ulcer has perforated and for three days following the penetrating keratoplasty. A clear plastic shield should be placed over the eye. The use of general anesthesia usually is preferred for keratoplasty surgery. Topical anesthesia can be used for the application of tissue adhesive. The size of the transplant should be the smallest trephine capable of incorporating the perforation site and any infected or ulcerated border. Donor generally is oversized by 0.5 mm. Cataract removal is left for a subsequent procedure because of the risk of expulsive hemorrhage and endophthalmitis. The anterior chamber should be irrigated to remove any necrotic or inflammatory debris. The donor cornea should be secured with 16 interrupted 10-0 nylon sutures. Subconjunctival injections of antibiotics can be given without depot steroid injection. The postoperative use of frequent topical fortified antibiotics is advocated. Corticosteroids, four times a day can be used immediately after surgery if it is believed that the infection was excised completely. Alternatively, steroids can be withheld for several days to monitor for infection. Once the acute postoperative period is over, long-term care is similar as that for uncomplicated penetrating keratoplasty. Topical antibiotics constitute the mainstay of treatment in the cases of bacterial keratitis, with subconjunctival antibiotics used only under unusual circumstances, and systemic antibiotics used only in the cases of perforation or specific organisms (e.g. *N. gonorrhoeae*). The use of topical corticosteroids remains controversial; however, when they are used, strict guidelines and close follow-up care are mandatory to ensure the best ultimate outcome of these patients.

Complications

The most feared complication of this condition is thinning of the cornea, secondary descemetocele and eventual perforation of the cornea that may result in endophthalmitis and loss of the eye.

Prognosis

The prognosis depends on several factors:
• Virulence of the organism
• Extent and location of the corneal ulcer
• Resulting vascularization and/or collagen deposition

FUNGAL KERATITIS

Introduction

Fungi are ubiquitous in the environment. Their spores can survive the extremes of temperature and desiccation. Fungi, particularly, Candida species are often a part of normal conjunctival flora. They have been isolated from the conjunctival sac in 3 to 28% of the healthy eyes. Fungi invade the ocular surface only when it is compromised, either from surface disease, topical steroid use or trauma. Ocular trauma, especially involving vegetable matter, is the most common risk factor for keratomycosis and accounts for 50% of the cases in most series. There has been an increase in the number of reported cases of fungal keratitis. The increasing use of broad-spectrum antibiotics may

provide a noncompetitive environment for fungi to grow. More recently, outbreaks of fungal keratitis due to contact lens solution (*Fusarium keratitis*) have also been reported.

Structural Characteristics of Fungi

Fungi are eukaryotes, have a membrane bound nucleus, a cell wall that contains chitin and a cell membrane that contains ergosterol. There are two broad categories of fungi, the yeasts or molds. Yeasts are usually unicellular and grow by budding. Molds, also called filamentous fungi, are composed of hyphae and are multicellular. Molds grow by the extension and branching of hyphae. Filamentous fungi may be septet or acetate. Septate hyphae have pores through which cytoplasm and nuclei pass to reach the growing tip.

Classification

A convenient method of classifying fungal isolates causing keratomycosis includes several diagnostic/laboratory groups, such as yeasts, moniliaceae and dematiaceae (Table 3.1).

Table 3.1: Fungal isolates causing keratomycosis

A	*Yeast*
	Candida species: Albicans, parapsilosis, krusei, tropicalis, guilliermondii
	Trichosporon beigelii
	Cryptococcus uniguttulans
B	*Filamentous septated*
	1. Nonpigmented hyphae (hyaline)
	Fusarium species: solani, oxysporum, moniliforme
	Aspergillus species: Fumigatus, flavus, terreus, glaucus, niger
	Acremonium species
	Cylindrocarpon species
	Paecilomyces species
	Scedosporium apiospermum
	2. Pigmented hyphae (dematiaceous)
	Alternaria species
	Curvularia species
	Cladosporium species
	Colleotricum species
	Phoma species

Clinical Features

The symptoms of fungal keratitis may not present as acutely as with other forms of microbial keratitis. Patients may report the initial symptom of foreign body sensation for several days associated with increasing pain. Presence of characteristic clinical features can be used as a diagnostic aid for suppurative keratitis caused by filamentous fungi. Serrated margins, raised slough, dry texture, satellite lesions and coloration other than yellow occur more frequently in the cases of filamentous fungal keratitis than bacterial keratitis. The probability of fungal infection if one clinical feature is present is 63%, increasing to 83% if all three features were present. Microbiological investigations should be performed whenever possible; however, where facilities are not available, a rapid presumptive diagnosis of suppurative keratitis may be possible by scoring clinical features. The appearance of macroscopic brown pigmentation is one specific sign seen in fungal keratitis due to dematiaceous fungus. The presence of intact epithelium with a deep stromal infiltrate may also be found in fungal keratitis (Figs 3.6 to 3.10).

Diagnosis

The Gram and Giemsa stains are the most common initial stains used for rapid diagnosis. Potassium hydroxide 10 to 20% wet mounts with calcofluor white is the best stain for fungi. Calcofluor white stains the chitin in the fungal cell wall and potassium hydroxide removes the non-fungal elements from the specimen.

In histopathology sections, hematoxylin and eosin, PAS stain and Gömöri methanamine silver stains are used. Culture media should include sheep blood agar, potato dextrose agar and Sabouraud's dextrose agar. Corneal biopsy may be necessary for deep keratomycosis. Anterior chamber tap may be useful in situations where organisms have penetrated the intact Descemet's membrane. Confocal microscopy is an important noninvasive tool in the cases of deep keratomycosis.

Management

Effective eradication of fungi is frequently difficult due to deeply invasive nature of the infectious process. Penetration of the fungus through the cornea into the anterior chamber may occur. Therefore, an effective agent for treating fungal keratitis should exhibit pharmacological properties that include excellent corneal and ocular penetration. Table 3.2 shows the effective drugs available for treating mycotic ocular infections.

Table 3.2: Classification of antifungal agents

Polyenes
- Amphotericin B
- Natamycin

Imidazoles
- Clotrimazole
- Miconazole
- Econazole
- Ketoconazole
- Fluconazole
- Itraconazole
- Voriconazole

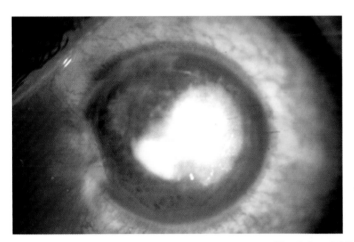
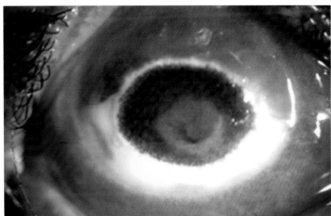

Figs 3.6 and 3.7: Fungal keratitis

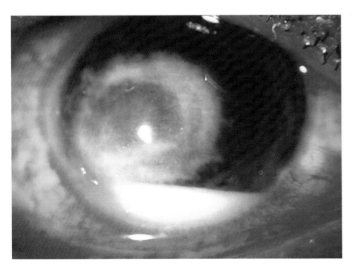

Fig. 3.8: Fungal keratitis. Hyphate edges

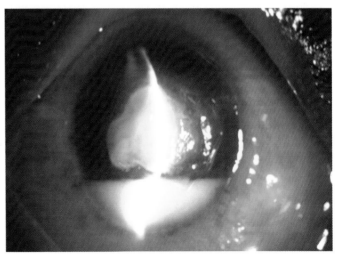

Fig. 3.9: Fungal keratitis. Dematiaceous fungus (pigmented plaque)

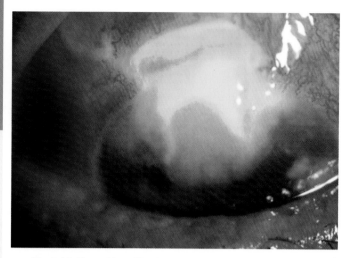

Fig. 3.10: Fungal keratitis. Postoperative tunnel infection due to filamentous fungus

Commercially available natamycin 5% suspension is the initial drug of choice for filamentous fungi. The corneal epithelium serves as a barrier to penetration in the view of high molecular mass of natamycin (665 kDa); hence debridement and superficial keratectomy are essential components in the management of fungal keratitis. If worsening is noted on topical natamycin treatment, amphotericin B 0.15% or azoles may be added as a second agent. Some of the newer antifungal agents have been tried topically. Voriconazole is one such medication, which may be promising in the management of keratitis.

Several clinical studies have reported favorable outcomes with the use of systemic antifungal agents, such as ketoconazole, fluconazole and itraconazole.

Intracameral injection of amphotericin B may have a role in the management of deep keratomycosis.

When progression of keratitis is noted, a therapeutic keratoplasty is indicated. The timing of penetrating keratoplasty is important. If the infectious agent were allowed to progress until it extends up to the limbus or sclera, outcomes of therapeutic keratoplasty would be unfavorable.

The use of corticosteroid in the postoperative period is controversial. Steroids should not be started before two weeks of penetrating keratoplasty. Majority of the recurrences occur during the initial postoperative period. Even if graft failure or rejection occurs, the patient can undergo a second penetrating keratoplasty subsequently.

Management

Treatment is influenced heavily by the interpretation of laboratory data. There is rarely a justification for empirical treatment with antifungal agents without corroborating evidence of a fungal etiology. Drug toxicity and necessity for prolonged treatment mitigate against the use of these agents empirically.

Signs of improvement include lessening of pain, decrease in the size of infiltrate, disappearance of satellite lesions and rounding out of feathery margins of the infiltrate.

HERPES SIMPLEX VIRUS KERATITIS

Introduction

Herpes simplex virus belongs to a family of viruses called Herpesviridae, which is a DNA virus that commonly affects humans.

There are two types of Herpes simplex virus, namely, type 1 and 2. In general, type 1 causes infection above, and type 2, below the waist. Therefore ocular herpes disease is usually caused by herpes simplex virus type 2 however, the rare neonatal herpes simplex virus infection, including herpetic keratitis and conjunctivitis is due to herpes simplex virus type 2 in a majority of cases as it is transmitted to neonates as they pass through the birth canal of a mother with genital herpes simplex virus type 2 infection.

Latency and Reactivation

Like other herpes viruses, herpes simplex virus has the ability to induce latent infection. After primary infection, that is, the host's first exposure at the peripheral site, the virus enters sensory nerve endings, which supply the site of peripheral epithelial infection, usually the oropharynx. Virus particles travel centripetally to the neuronal cell body by retrograde axoplasmic flow. Here, they can survive for decades, probably integrated into the host-cell nuclear DNA; yet they leave the cell morphologically, antigenically and functionally normal.

Primary Infection

Infection with herpes simplex virus for the first time can develop at any age although most cases occur within the first few years of life. Salivary contamination from a person with silent salivary shedding of herpes labialis is the most common source of infection. Aphthous stomatitis is the usual clinical picture, which can range from subclinical to very severe infection. However, primary herpes simplex virus infection can also occur in other mucous membranes, including the conjunctiva.

Primary ocular herpes simplex virus infection most commonly manifests as blepharoconjunctivitis, which is predominantly unilateral. The periorbital skin can develop intense blisters associated with conjunctivitis and blepharitis. Extensive spread on the facial skin can occur, particularly in eczematous individuals.

The conjunctivitis is usually follicular although severe cases may develop pseudo-membranous reaction. Preauricular lymphadenopathy often accompanies the conjunctivitis. Keratitis develops a few days after conjunctival involvement in 30 to 50% of cases. The morphology of the corneal lesions varies from superficial punctate keratitis, microdendrites or frank dendritic ulceration. Stromal involvement is rare. Interestingly, though subsequent recurrent disease is uncommon, it may occur as focal clusters of vesicles in the lids or as follicular conjunctivitis. In these cases corneal involvement is usually minimal or absent.

Recurrent Infection

The major factors which dictate the severity of recurrent herpes are: immune response of the host, the viral strain and treatment. Superficial corneal lesions (dendritic and geographic ulcers) are associated with the presence of replicating virus whilst deeper lesions (stromal and uveal) appear to be predominantly due to the immune response (Figs 3.11 to 3.13).

Corneal Epithelial Disease

The vast majority of the cases of herpes simplex virus keratitis are those which are present with a corneal epithelial lesion, usually a dendritic ulcer. Such individuals may experience this first episode in adulthood. This is due to the reactivation of a latent virus from a previously unrecognized primary ocular infection or from a virus, which has reached ophthalmic neurons in the trigeminal ganglion during primary infection of the oropharynx. It usually occurs as isolated lesion(s) without the involvement of conjunctiva and lids. The presenting symptoms include irritation, watering, photophobia, and occasionally, blurring of vision.

The morphology of the lesions is quite varied. They can appear as superficial punctate keratitis, stellate epithelial lesions, and dendritic or geographic ulcers. Ulcers are usually single, but may be several. The infected epithelial cells appear as opaque lesions, which form white plaques. Further enlargement results in the dendritic ulceration. The mechanism for dendrite formation is not known, but is thought to be related to the linear spread of virus from cell to cell in a contiguous manner. With further growth of the dendrite, the central epithelium is sloughed off and the lesion stains with fluorescein. The marginal infected cells take up rose bengal stain. The linear branches characteristically end in expansions called "terminal bulbs". The stroma under the ulcer may show a faint haze and there may be evidence of mild iritis. Corneal sensation is lost in

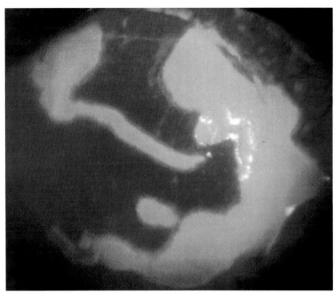

Fig. 3.12: Herpes simplex virus keratitis. Geographic ulcer

the areas where lesions are present. Repeated attacks may result in generalized corneal anesthesia.

Stromal Keratitis

Sight-threatening problems associated with herpes simplex virus type 1 infection appear to be largely due to an inflammatory response involving the corneal stroma. It is predominantly immune-mediated although in few cases direct invasion and active replication of the virus play a role. Secondary stromal inflammation can follow epithelial or endothelial involvement.

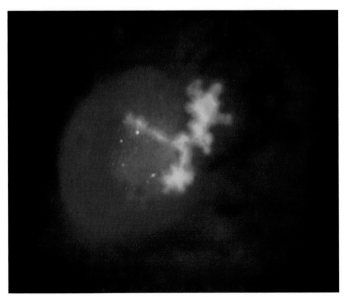

Fig. 3.11: Herpes simplex virus keratitis. Dendritic keratitis

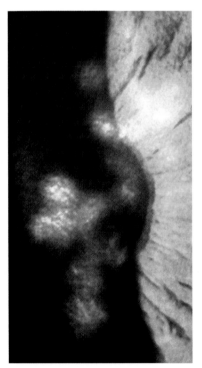

Fig. 3.13: Herpes simplex virus keratitis. Footprint scars

Immune-mediated stromal keratitis is the most common form of the stromal disease where an antibody response is mounted against the viral antigen present in the stroma expressed as a result of persistent infection. There is the deposition of antigen-antibody complement in the stroma. Animal studies show additional mechanisms involved in the stromal tissue destruction. It is proposed that CD4+ T cells play a significant role in the recognition of antigens presented by Langerhans cells, which migrate from limbus to central cornea after herpes simplex virus type 1 infection. The activated CD4+ T cells release cytokines, in particular interleukin 2 and gamma interferon. Both factors attract large numbers of polymorphonuclear leukocytes, which are responsible for corneal tissue destruction.

Clinically, there is a stromal infiltration without necrosis and ulceration. The size and the area involved may vary and include small infiltrates to large area of stromal haze. Some cases may be associated with dendritic lesions demonstrating the presence of the entire virus. The outcomes of these lesions vary. Progression or persistence of inflammation can occur. Neovascularization, secondary lipid keratopathy, thinning of the cornea and recurrent inflammation are well recognized. Another distinct form of stromal infiltrate is the immune ring of Wesley. This represents a circular deposit of antigen-antibody complexes with polymorphonuclear leukocyte infiltrate as a result of complement activation.

Necrotizing stromal keratitis is typically associated with ulceration (Fig. 3.14). It can follow epithelial disease, superficial stromal disease or disciform keratitis, and is believed to be due to active viral replication and intense immune stromal inflammation. It may be generalized or localized. These cases may have to be differentiated from the other forms of microbial keratitis and indeed secondary infection with bacteria and fungi can complicate herpes simplex virus stromal keratitis. Secondary complications include hypopyon, uveitis, posterior synechiae, glaucoma, retrocorneal membrane, cataract and rarely perforation.

Metaherpetic Ulcer

Development of persistent epithelial defects or recurrent epithelial erosions can be seen with herpes simplex virus epithelial infection. These are generally round or ovoid ulcers with a grey and thickened margin, which is due to piled up epithelial cells.

The mechanism appears to be due to damage to underlying basement membrane at the time of epithelial infection and denervation. Consequently the epithelium fails to adhere to the basement membrane resulting in persistent defect or recurrent erosion. Additional factors like the lack of trophic innervation, drug toxicity and stromal inflammation may play a role. Viral cultures are negative and the base of the ulcer stains with both rose bengal and fluorescein. Persistent ulcers have the potential to progress to corneal melt, perforation and super infection.

Metaherpetic ulcers (sometimes referred to as "neurotrophic") have to be differentiated from geographic ulcers, which are characteristically caused by inappropriate steroid use. The latter have flat edges and stain with rose bengal stain. They also change shape due to continued viral progression. Viral cultures will be positive (Fig. 3.15).

Herpes Simplex Virus Endotheliitis

Disciform keratitis is the most common form in which a disc-shaped area of stromal edema occurs without infiltration or vascularization. The area of involvement may be diffuse and central or eccentric. The presenting symptoms include watering, photophobia, discomfort or blurred vision. A history of herpetic eye disease is usually present. The involved cornea shows appreciable thickening of all layers sometimes with epithelial edema and often with folds in Descemet's membrane.

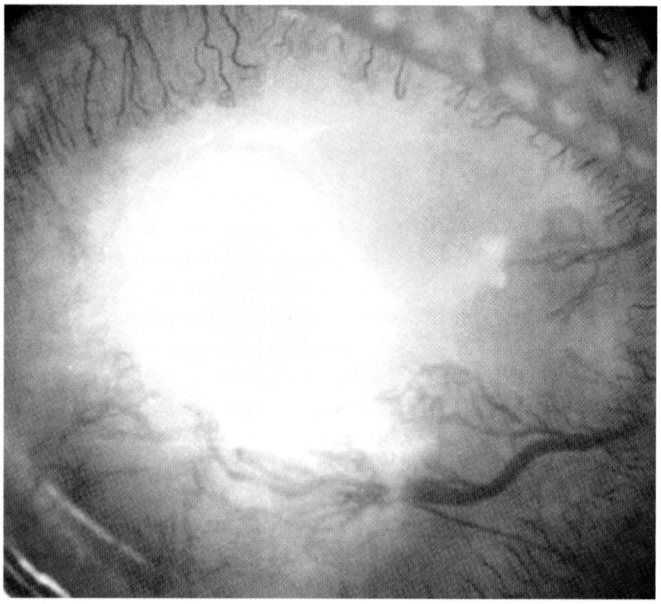

Fig. 3.14: Herpes simplex virus keratitis. Necrotizing keratitis

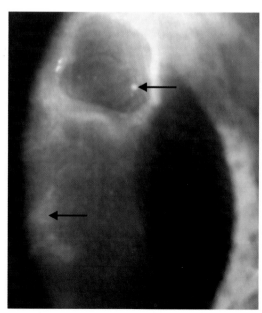

Fig. 3.15. Herpes simplex virus keratitis. Metaherpetic ulcer (←)

Careful examination usually reveals keratic precipitates in the affected area associated with mild anterior chamber activity (Fig. 3.16). Spontaneous clearing can follow although progression to necrotizing keratitis, vascularization, scarring and thinning is also possible. Delayed hypersensitivity mediated by T lymphocytes is probably important in the pathogenesis of disciform keratitis. The distribution of keratic precipitates strictly confined to the endothelium behind the swollen area suggests cell-mediated reaction directed at herpes simplex virus determinants on the surface of endothelial cells.

Rarely linear involvement of the endothelium can occur. In these cases stromal edema is seen associated with keratic precipitates separating the involved and uninvolved cornea similar to the Khodadoust line of corneal graft rejection. Slit-lamp examination may show dark areas in the endothelium, which appear as nonreflective black endothelial areas under a specular microscope. There may be progression of the endothelial line and the associated stromal edema. Immunological studies on the aqueous aspirates have revealed herpes simplex virus antigen in several of these cases.

Occasionally diffuse involvement of the endothelium can occur resulting in generalized corneal edema associated with scattered keratic precipitates.

Herpes Simplex Virus Iridocyclitis

All deeper forms of herpes simplex virus can be associated with uveitis. However, recurrent non-granulomatous anterior uveitis may be an isolated manifestation of herpes simplex virus ocular involvement, which can occur without a prior history of ocular herpes simplex virus infection. Immunological reaction was thought to be the cause in most of the cases although in some cases live viruses have been demonstrated in the anterior chamber and in iris tissue.

Clinically the severity can vary from mild to severe inflammation, which may result in fibrin formation, hypopyon, hyphema, posterior synechiae, segmental iris necrosis similar to the picture seen in zoster keratouveitis, and inflammatory membrane in the angle of the anterior chamber with secondary glaucoma (Fig. 3.17). The recent tendency to treat severe forms of anterior segment involvement with oral acyclovir is best reserved for those cases confirmed by laboratory diagnosis, as dosages and duration of treatment have not yet been defined.

Trabeculitis

Herpetic peripheral corneal involvement may extend to the trabecular meshwork resulting in trabeculitis. The resultant secondary glaucoma may be transient or lead to permanent damage.

Laboratory Diagnosis

Laboratory tests are not an absolute requisite for the diagnosis of herpes simplex virus infection as clinical features are often highly characteristic. However, we believe whenever possible they should be undertaken to establish a firm diagnosis. The chronic nature of the condition is such that a positive diagnosis once established, is invaluable in guiding management over what may be many years.

The available methods include virus culture, immunological tests and the histopathological examination of keratoplasty specimens.

The definitive method of diagnostic testing is isolating virus in tissue culture. The lesion is swabbed and placed in viral transport medium and sent to the laboratory. It is then inoculated onto cell monolayers and incubated at 37° C. A typical cytopathic effect is generally noticed in 2–4 days.

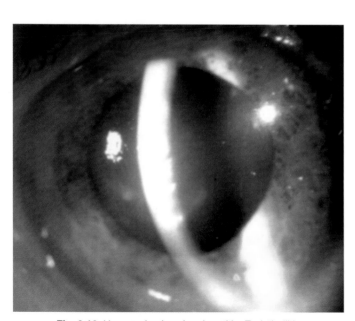

Fig. 3.16. Herpes simplex virus keratitis. Endotheliitis

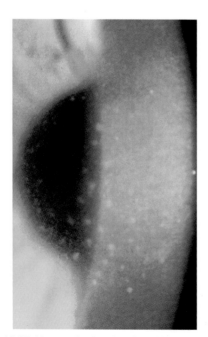

Fig.13.17: Herpes simplex virus keratitis. Iridocyclitis

A variety of immunological tests are available to detect herpes simplex virus antigens in specimens, namely, enzyme-linked immunosorbent assay (ELISA), immunofiltration test, latex agglutination and immunoperoxidase methods. In addition, an immunoaffinity membrane test has also been described. In this test a protein-binding affinity membrane used as a blotter is gently touched to the corneal lesion and processed with peroxidase-conjugated herpes simplex virus antibody. In few centers fluorescent antibody-staining technique is available for the rapid detection of herpetic antigen in cytoplasm or the nucleus of the cell.

Histopathological examination of keratectomy specimens may show granulomatous reaction in deep stroma and around Descemet's membrane. Immunocytochemistry may demonstrate herpes simplex virus antigens in stromal keratocytes, endothelial cells and epithelioid cells. These are more often seen with the necrotizing type of herpetic stromal keratitis.

Management

Management in these cases comprises of both medical and surgical procedures. The various medical agents which can be used are as follows:

Antiviral Agents

The following topical agents are currently available for use in herpes simplex virus keratitis:

Idoxuridine, a thymidine analogue was the first agent found to be effective in the treatment of herpes simplex virus keratitis. It is incorporated into the viral DNA, produces faulty DNA chain and also inhibits viral enzymes. It also incorporates into normal host cells, which accounts for its toxicity. Though idoxuridine is useful in treating epithelial infection, the problems of toxicity allergic reaction, clinical viral resistance, poor solubility and penetration, and rapid inactivation have led to the use of other antiviral drugs. Notable ocular side effects include contact dermatitis, punctate keratitis, epithelial opacification, chronic epithelial defects, lacrimal punctal stenosis, follicular conjunctivitis, corneal pannus and teratogenicity in rabbits.

Vidarabine, the second agent developed for human use, inhibits viral DNA polymerase and gets incorporated into both viral and host DNA. It is equally effective as idoxuridine in treating epithelial disease and being highly soluble, is available only as ointment. Although it is much less toxic, punctate keratopathy (similar to idoxuridine toxicity) can be a problem with topical use. Its use is generally restricted to viral strains resistant to other antiviral agents.

Trifluridine (trifluorothymidine) is a halogenated pyrimidine inhibiting thymidylate synthetase incorporated into viral DNA impairing transcription and translation. It is more potent than idoxuridine in healing dendritic ulcers. Also trifluorothymidine is superior to idoxuridine in the management of steroid-treated corneal ulcers. Although therapeutic levels of the drug can be achieved in the anterior chamber, its role in treating deep stromal diseases and uveitis is yet to be determined. Adverse effects include superficial punctate keratitis, follicular conjunctivitis, lacrimal punctal stenosis, corneal filaments, and contact dermatitis. Viral resistance to trifluorothymidine is rare.

Acyclovir is a purine analogue. It is specifically activated by virus-induced thymidine kinase, which initiates phosphorylation. Subsequently two additional phosphates are added by host-cell kinases to produce an active triphosphate form, which is inhibitorier to viral DNA polymerase than host-cell polymerase. Thus, acyclovir is specific to viral-infected cells with low toxicity. After topical application it achieves therapeutic concentration in the anterior chamber. Acyclovir is as equally effective as trifluorothymidine and ara–A in the treatment of herpes simplex keratitis. Acyclovir is less toxic to ocular surface than earlier generation antiviral agents and as such represents a major therapeutic advance. However, mutant virus strains with deficient thymidine kinase continue to replicate; therefore, the development of drug-resistant strain may post a problem.

Corticosteroids

Cautious use of steroids is recommended in the certain types of herpes simplex virus infection of the cornea. Corticosteroids suppress inflammation by interfering with the normal immunologic response to various stimuli and are an important management tool. Clinically they reduce infiltration, edema, inflammation and neovascularization. Generally their treatment is restricted to the management of stromal keratitis and herpetic uveitis. Steroids do not appear to increase the risk of acquiring herpes simplex virus infection, but certainly promote severity of the disease when present. Disadvantages include delayed epithelial and stromal healing, increased collagenolytic enzyme production, stimulation of viral replication, and risk of secondary infection, glaucoma and cataract. Infectious crystalline keratopathy is a recognized complication of steroid treatment for herpes simplex virus keratitis. The major problem with steroids is inappropriate use at the epithelial stage, particularly as it may improve the symptoms initially. Widespread over-the-counter treatment is undoubtedly responsible for converting what may have been relatively benign disease into irreversible corneal damage.

Systemic Treatment

Oral acyclovir appears to be as effective as topical acyclovir for herpes simplex virus epithelial keratitis, but cannot be recommended as it is much more expensive. However, oral acyclovir may be beneficial in reducing the ocular recurrence and may gain a place in deep corneal disease, keratouveitis and posttransplant management in proven cases.

Specific Treatment: Primary Infection

Antiviral treatment is generally advisable even though it is not absolutely indicated as primary blepharoconjunctivitis can resolve spontaneously. Acyclovir ointment is applied over the skin lesions and in the conjunctival sac up to five times a day.

Keratitis can be treated with antiviral alone or debridement and antiviral treatment. A shield to the eye may be necessary to prevent a child from rubbing the eye.

Specific Treatment: Recurrent Infection

Epithelial disease: Careful epithelial debridement is equally effective or even better than antiviral treatment alone. Epithelial keratitis is therefore treated with debridement, antiviral agent or a combination of both. Debridement involves removing the infected epithelial cells using a sterile cotton-tipped applicator after instillation of local anesthetic. The antiviral treatment is then initiated to improve viral clearance.

Acyclovir is the agent of choice (3% ointment, × 5 times a day). Treatment duration is usually for 10–14 days. It is to be noted that the epithelium often looks abnormal at the site of initial dendritic ulcer even resembling the original lesion, but without fluorescent staining. This may take several weeks to heal and treatment is not indicated. However, persistent epithelial lesions with the areas of fluorescent staining may indicate continued viral replication due to resistant strain or the development of metaherpetic disease. Presence of scalloped edges with progression indicates persistent infection and warrants a change of antiviral agent.

Epithelial indolent ulceration: Antiviral agents are not always needed as the underlying problem is damaged basement membrane and denervation. Generous use of lubricants, preferably unpreserved agents, often results in epithelial healing. Use of patch, bandage contact lens and occasionally a conjunctival flap, helps in resistant cases.

Stromal keratitis and immune keratitis: A combination of an antiviral agent and topical steroids is the preferred treatment. Topical steroids result in significantly reducing stromal inflammation and decrease the duration of stromal keratitis. The starting dose of topical steroids is adjusted to the level of inflammation, but it should always be a weak steroid. Once the inflammation is brought under control, gradually steroid drops are tapered and every attempt should be made to discontinue them. An individualized maintenance dose may be indicated for some patients who show frequent disease flare-up without steroid treatment. The use of oral acyclovir in addition to topical treatment does not appear to show any additional beneficial effect.

Necrotizing stromal keratitis: After culturing samples to exclude microbial secondary infection, antiviral treatment is started in suspected herpes simplex virus stromal keratitis. Topical steroids may be added cautiously if the overlying epithelium is intact. Continued stromal necrosis calls for surgical interventions, such as cyanoacrylate glue or penetrating keratoplasty.

Endotheliitis: A combination of topical steroids and antiviral agents is indicated to treat this form of herpes simplex virus infection. Additional treatment with oral acyclovir has also been found to be effective in the cases of linear endotheliitis.

Uveitis: Steroids are the treatment of choice. It is advisable to add topical antiviral treatment as some cases have been shown to be associated with live virus in the anterior chamber. Similarly oral acyclovir may be added if the response is not good or if live virus is isolated from the anterior chamber.

Trabeculitis: Antiglaucoma treatment should be initiated in addition to steroid and antiviral agents.

Surgical Procedures

Surgical procedures may sometimes be necessary to treat acute and/ or chronic complications of herpes simplex virus keratitis.

Penetrating keratoplasty: Penetrating keratoplasty is the procedure of choice to restore vision in those with significant corneal scarring due to recurrent herpes simplex virus keratitis. However, serious consideration must be given to the possibility of recurrence and rejection especially when the fellow eye may be normal. In parts of the world where donor corneas are in short supply penetrating keratoplasty for herpes simplex virus keratitis cannot be seen as a priority. Penetrating keratoplasty is also performed to re-establish the integrity of the globe after ulceration and perforation. This procedure also reduces the viral load in the cornea responsible for the repeated episodes of immune-mediated keratitis.

In patients with graft rejection, it is particularly difficult to differentiate it from the recurrence of herpetic uveitis. This is especially true in the cases of linear endotheliitis occurring in the grafted eye, which closely resembles a rejection episode with migrating line of KPs and stromal edema. However, linear endotheliitis crosses the graft host junction and responds well to oral acyclovir. It is therefore safe to treat any graft rejection with antiviral cover in such circumstances.

Other treatment modalities include the use of cyanoacrylate glue in small perforations as a temporary measure. Conjunctival flap, tarsorrhaphy and botulinum-induced ptosis may have a role in selected cases of nonhealing ulcers, particularly where access to corneal donor tissue and expert postoperative management is not available.

ACANTHAMOEBA KERATITIS

Introduction

Acanthamoeba spp. are ubiquitous organisms that can be isolated from a wide variety of environments, including water supplies, swimming pools, hot tubs, contact lenses, lens cases, and salt and bottled water. At least eight species of *Acanthamoeba* are known. *Acanthamoeba* exists in two forms, trophozoites and cysts. The trophozoite is motile and usually has one nucleolus, huge cytoplasmic vacuoles and feeds on bacteria. In unfavorable circumstances, trophozoites encyst. The cyst has a double wall containing cellulose and is 10–25 μm in diameter. The cystic form is extremely resistant to extreme conditions, such as desiccation, freezing, alterations in pH or chemical antimicrobial agents.

Predisposing Factors

Most patients who develop infection have at least three risk factors: corneal trauma, exposure to contaminated water, or contact lens solution and contact lens wear. It has been demonstrated in the animal experiments that corneal abrasion is necessary for the development of *Acanthamoeba* keratitis.

Clinical Features

One of the important symptoms is severe pain that is not commensurate with the clinical signs at least in the early phase of infection. The major clinical signs include: epithelial haze with elevated lines, epithelial defects, epithelial ridges, microcysts, pseudodendrite, stromal infiltrate, satellite lesions and ring infiltrate (Figs 3.18 and 3.19). Table 3.3 shows the major clinical signs and stages of *Acanthamoeba* keratitis.

Table 3.3: Clinical manifestations of *Acanthamoeba* keratitis

Early	Late	Advanced
Epithelial ridges	Epithelial defects	Ring infiltrate
Epithelial haze	Stromal infiltrate	Satellite lesions
Pseudodendrites	Nummular keratitis	Stromal abscess

Laboratory Diagnosis

It is important to establish the accuracy of diagnosis, as it requires prolonged treatment to eradicate the infection. Acanthamoeba trophozoites and cysts can be identified in smears by staining with Gram and Wright-Giemsa stains. Potassium hydroxide with calcofluor white is extremely useful for identification. Culturing the specimen on a confluent lawn of *E. coli*-plated on non-nutrient agar is a specific diagnostic technique. Confocal microscopy is another very sensitive and powerful technique for identifying *Acanthamoeba* cysts.

Management

Medical therapy has employed aminoglycosides, polymeric biguanides, diamidines and imidazoles in combinations. There is no reported standardization of treatment regimen. In vitro sensitivity testing has shown that few agents are effective in killing the trophozoites, but the cysts are resistant and a higher concentration of these drugs are necessary to kill them. The down side of such high concentration is toxicity to the corneal epithelium. Because of lower surface toxicity, polyhexamethylenebiguanide 0.02% and chlorhexidine 0.02% either alone or in combination have become the favored treatment modality. Propamidine isethionate 0.15% is another recommended drug, but usage is limited due to its availability. Oral administration of ketoconazole at a dose of 400 mg/day is also recommended.

Corticosteroids

The use of steroids is controversial. Corticosteroid reduces the sequelae of inflammation. However, they may exacerbate the infection by affecting the behavior of *Acanthamoeba spp.* Treatment with dexamethasone has been shown to induce rapid excystment, which was manifested in two to six fold increase in trophozoites. Moreover, it was shown to have stimulatory proliferation effect on trophozoites.

Keratoplasty

No clear guidelines are available about the appropriate timing for penetrating keratoplasty. Conventional strategy emphasizes on reserving keratoplasty for impending perforation or for visual rehabilitation once infection has cleared completely. However, recent management strategy is to plan for deep anterior lamellar keratoplasty in advanced cases less likely to improve on medical treatment, as the available literature suggests that the Descemet's acts as a barrier to these organisms.

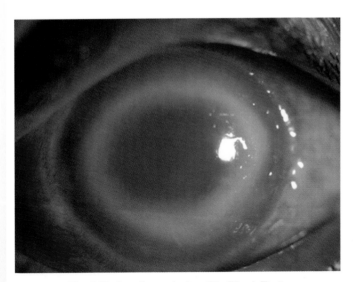

Fig. 3.18: Acanthamoeba keratitis. Ring infiltrate

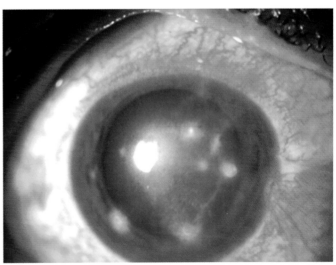

Fig. 3.19: Acanthamoeba keratitis. Contact lens related case of acanthamoeba keratitis

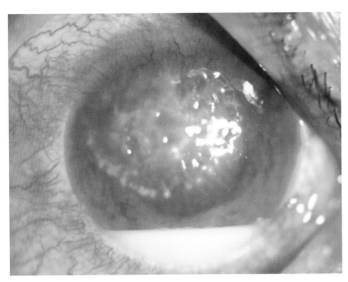

Fig. 3.20: Nocardia keratitis. Pinhead raised infiltrates and hypopyon is visible

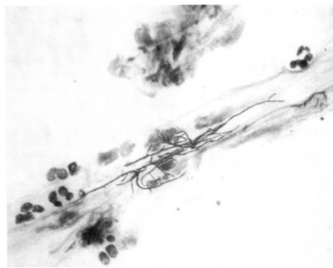

Fig. 3.22: Nocardia keratitis. Acid fast stain showing thin filaments

NOCARDIA KERATITIS

Introduction

The clinical diagnosis of Nocardia is often missed, as it is uncommon and picture may resemble mycotic keratitis. Nocardia are aerobic, gram-positive, thin branching filamentous bacteria (<1.5 μm in diameter). The filaments may be both acid fast and non-acid fast.

Predisposing Factors

Predisposing factors include trauma, contact lens use, postsurgical and corticosteroid use.

Clinical Features

Keratitis may be in the form of nonspecific punctate epitheliopathy or an ulcer with margins studded with yellow white discrete pinhead sized superficial infiltration (Figs 3.20 and 3.21 A and B). Patchy infiltrates, which are predominantly anterior stromal with the associated involvement of epithelial and subepithelial tissues are pathognomonic of Nocardia keratitis. The infiltrates may be arranged in a ring-like fashion, forming the characteristic wreath-like pattern. Satellite lesions may be noted.

Diagnosis

Corneal scraping smear that is positive for beaded gram-positive branching filaments and does not fluorescence with calcofluor white stain is suggestive of actinomycetes. It is an indication for extra smears for acid fast staining using 1% sulfuric acid (modified Kinyoun's method). Dry colonies, usually tiny and white, grow on blood agar and chocolate agar (Figs 3.22 and 3.23). Confocal microscopy is a useful noninvasive tool to diagnose Nocardia filaments.

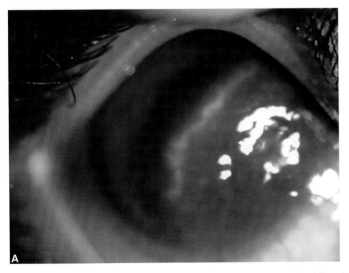

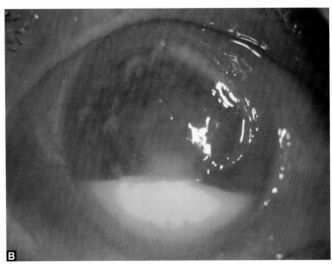

Figs 3.21A and B: Nocardia keratitis. Wreath-like pattern of infiltrates along with hypopyon

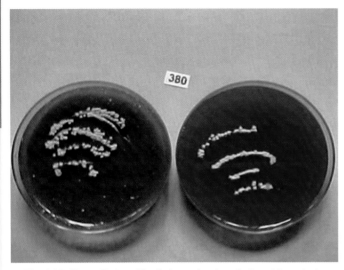

Fig. 3.23: Nocardia keratitis. Culture showing chalky white colonies

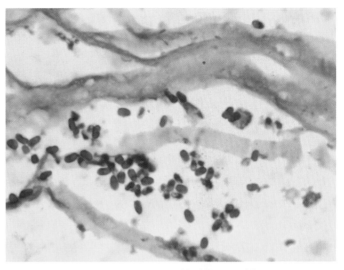

Fig. 3.25: Microsporidia keratitis. Microsporidia spores

Management

Topical Amikacin 2.5% or co-trimoxazole eyedrops (injectable preparation for topical use) are the drugs of choice.

MICROSPORIDIA KERATITIS

Introduction

Microsporidia are ubiquitous, obligate, intracellular, spore-forming obligate protozoan parasite. Five genera of Microsporidia are known to cause human diseases (*Nosema, Encephalitozoon, Enterocytozoon, Pleistophora* and *Septada*). Ocular infections more often occur by direct inoculation.

Clinical Features

Two clinical presentations have been described: Keratoconjunctivitis usually related to Encephalitozoon and stromal keratitis related to the *Nosema spp*. Ocular findings include conjunctival injection, mixed follicular-papillary tarsal conjunctival reaction and punctate epithelial keratopathy. The epitheliopathy is characterized by multiple coarse white to gray epithelial opacities. These infections rarely lead to corneal ulcerations. Stromal involvement may extend to deeper layers, taking disciform appearance similar to herpetic keratitis. The earlier belief that keratoconjunctivitis form occurs in immuno-deficient and stromal form in immunocompetent individuals is not universally true (Figs 3.24A and B).

Laboratory Diagnosis

Microsporidia is difficult to recover in culture, and the diagnosis is usually made by direct observation of the organism. Spores stain gram-positive, but staining is variable with routine methods, such as Giemsa, Gömöri silver or acid-fast staining (Figs 3.25 and 3.26). Potassium hydroxide calcofluor white staining is better for light microscopic diagnosis.

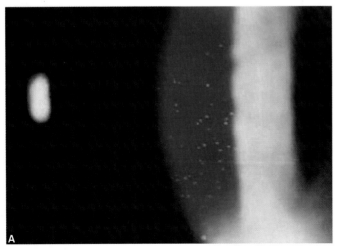

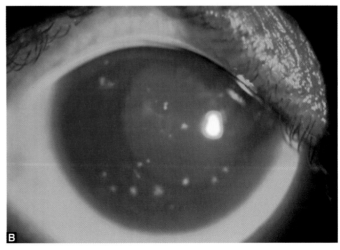

Figs 3.24A and B: Microsporidial keratoconjunctivitis

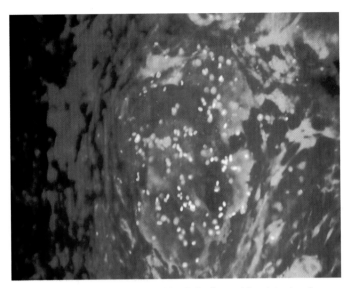

Fig. 3.26: Microsporidia keratitis. Calcofluor-white stain showing Microsporidia spores

Management

Superficial punctate keratopathy has a self-limiting course and treatment is supportive in the form of debridement and topical lubricants and prophylactic antibiotics. Medical treatments with topical antibiotics have demonstrated poor results in the stromal form. Itraconazole, polyhexamethylene biguanide and propamidine have been tried, but have resulted in the inconsistent clearance of microsporidia. Surgical treatment for the significant stromal involvement consists of penetrating keratoplasty as no effective topical drugs are available.

NEUROTROPHIC KERATITIS

Introduction

Neurotrophic keratitis is a degenerative disease of the corneal epithelium characterized by impaired healing. Absence of corneal sensitivity is the hallmark of the condition. The causes of decreased corneal sensations are myriad.

Pathogenesis

Reduced corneal sensations render the corneal surface vulnerable to occult injury and decreases reflex tearing. It also appears to the decrease healing rates of epithelial injury resulting in nonhealing epithelial defects. Normally a bidirectional interaction occurs between epithelial cells and nerve endings. Disruption of sensory and sympathetic pathways is thought to lead to decreased cell division.

Causes of corneal hypesthesia

- Infections: Herpes, leprosy
- Fifth nerve palsy: Surgery, neoplasia (acoustic neuroma), facial trauma, congenital
- Topical medications: Anesthetics, timolol, nonsteroidal anti-inflammatory drugs

- Corneal dystrophies: Lattice
- Systemic diseases: Diabetes
- Iatrogenic: Contact lens wear, LASIK, corneal incisions
- Toxic: Chemical injury.

Clinical Features

Corneal anesthesia triggers a variety of ocular surface abnormalities that produce ulcerations (Figs 3.27 to 3.29). Reflex tearing and blink rates are decreased secondary to the lack of afferent limb. Mackie characterized three stages of neurotrophic keratitis:

- Stage I includes subtle irregular corneal surface, which later develops into punctate erosions.
- Stage II is characterized by epithelial defects, associated with anterior stromal inflammation. The epithelium at the edges tends to be heaped up with grayish swollen epithelium. The ulcer is typically found in lower, exposed paracentral cornea and is generally oval in shape.
- Stage III involves stromal melting and occasional perforation.

Management

Stage I findings require topical lubricants, preferably preservative free solutions. Eyelid dysfunction must be carefully assessed to prevent exposure keratitis and progression to Stage II. For persistent epithelial defects and stromal lyses, soft contact lens may be tried, but patients respond best to lateral or medial tarsorrhaphy. Stage III disease may require cyanoacrylate application. More recent approaches using multilayered amniotic membrane transplantation have shown promising results in arresting the progression of stromal lysis.

PHLYCTENULAR KERATOCONJUNCTIVITIS

Introduction

It is an inflammatory disorder leading to conjunctival or corneal nodules, most commonly at the limbus. Phlyctenular keratoconjunctivitis is thought to be a delayed hypersensitivity (T cell-mediated type IV) to an antigen. The tuberculoprotein has been a common culprit. Other antigens implicated are *Staphylococcus, Candida, Chlamydia* and nematodes.

Clinical Features

Conjunctival phlyctenules are usually near the limbus, but can occur anywhere on the bulbar conjunctiva. They are initially seen as raised, amorphous, light grayish nodules that are 1–2 mm in diameter (Fig. 3.28). Corneal phlyctenules typically appear first at the limbus and may migrate either to the clear cornea or to the conjunctiva. When the phlyctenule migrates onto the cornea, strands of superficial blood vessels may arise

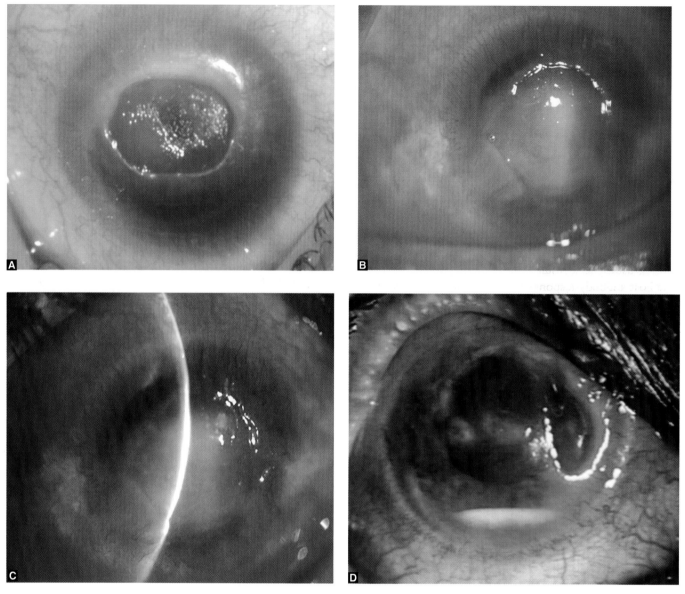

Figs 3.27A to D: Neurotrophic keratitis

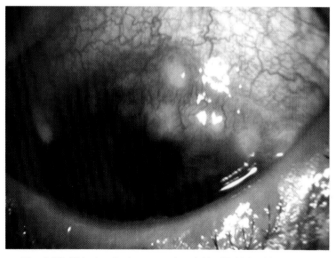

Fig. 3.28: Phlyctenular keratoconjunctivitis. Multiple phlyctenules

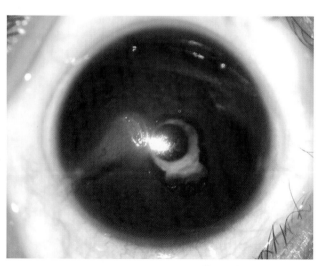

Fig. 3.29: Phlyctenular keratitis

from the limbus and follow the course of the phlyctenule (Fig. 3.29). Healing occurs leaving a vascularized, superficial scar.

Treatment

Treatment is determined by the etiology of phlyctenulosis. Treatment consists of topical corticosteroids. Attention should be paid to eyelid hygiene if necessary.

STAPHYLOCOCCAL MARGINAL KERATITIS

Introduction

Staphylococcal marginal keratitis is also called marginal catarrhal or catarrhal ulcers. It is most commonly caused by *Staphylococcus* species, usually as a result of chronic blepharoconjunctivitis. The host antibody response is responsible for corneal, which represents polymorphonuclear leukocytes resulting from antigen interaction.

Clinical Features

The disease usually begins with localized peripheral stromal infiltrates, which tend to occur at 2, 4, 8 and 10 o'clock positions. There is a clear lucid interval between the infiltrate and the limbus. With prolonged inflammation, the epithelium overlying the stromal infiltrates breaks down leading to ulceration and thinning (Fig. 3.30). Occasionally the thinning may result in perforation.

Management

Topical corticosteroids are the mainstay in the treatment. Management of the accompanying blepharoconjunctivitis is also necessary to decrease the frequency of recurrences.

PERIPHERAL ULCERATIVE KERATITIS

Introduction

Peripheral ulcerative keratitis is often a diagnostic challenge due to its multiple and varied etiology. The differential diagnosis is expansive and includes infectious and noninfectious disorders. It is important to ascertain the etiology as each has its own course of management. In most cases, a detailed history, appropriate investigations, and careful ocular and systemic examination would help to establish the diagnosis.

Pathogenesis

The peripheral cornea is immunologically different from the central cornea in the following aspects:

- This region being closest to conjunctiva is exposed to the immunologic machinery necessary to generate immune response.
- Peripheral cornea has more Langerhans cells compared to central cornea.
- Complement activation is more effective in this region.
- Immune complexes deposited in limbal vessels result in immune-mediated vasculitis.

Mooren's Ulcer

Mooren's ulcer is an idiopathic, painful, progressive ulceration of the peripheral cornea (Figs 3.31 and 3.32). It is a clinical diagnosis. It is not necessary to perform the entire battery of investigations, if Watson's criteria are fulfilled:

Watson's criteria

- Crescent-shaped peripheral corneal ulcer
- Extensive undermining of the central edge of the ulcer
- Corneal infiltrations along the leading edge

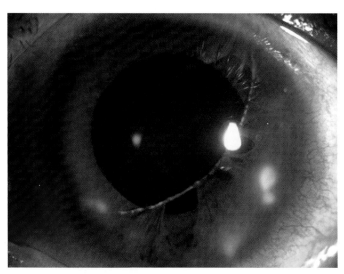

Fig. 3.30: Staphylococcal marginal keratitis

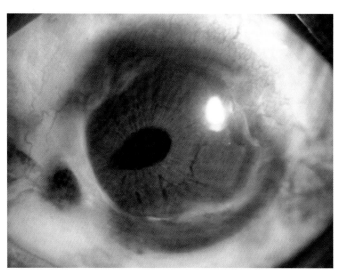

Fig. 3.31: Mooren's ulcer

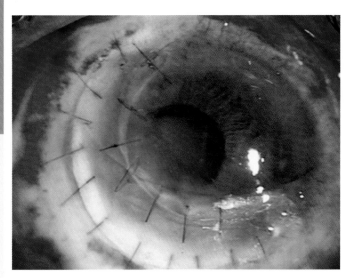

Fig. 3.32: Mooren's ulcer. A case of Mooren's ulcer managed with crescentric patch graft

- Absence of scleritis
- Absence of detectable systemic disease.

Pathogenesis

The pathogenesis is not clearly understood, but appears to involve an autoimmune reaction against a specific target molecule in the corneal stroma (corneal stromal protein, CO-Ag), which may occur in genetically susceptible individuals.

Three distinct types of presentation are described below:

1. Unilateral progressive
2. Bilateral aggressive
3. Bilateral indolent.

Management

The goals of therapy are to arrest the destructive process and to promote healing and reepithelialization. A stepladder approach for the management has been described below:

Topical steroids: Initial therapy should include intensive topical steroids on an hourly basis.

Conjunctival resection: Conjunctival resection along with tissue adhesive and bandage contact lens application in all active cases. Conjunctival excision should extend at least 2 o'clock hours on either side of the peripheral ulcer and approximately 4 mm beyond the corneoscleral limbus parallel to the ulcer.

Superficial keratectomy: The overhanging lip of the active edge of the ulcer should be debrided.

Systemic immunotherapy: Those cases of bilateral or progressive disease that fail to stabilize with the preceding therapeutic attempts will require systemic immunosuppressives. Initially systemic steroids should be started and tapered off based on clinical response. Among the immunomodulatory agents, the most commonly used are cyclophosphamide (2 mg /kg/body weight) and azathioprine (2 mg/kg body weight).

Collagen Vascular Disease-Related Peripheral Ulcerative Keratitis

Rheumatoid arthritis is the most common cause of collagen vascular disease related peripheral ulcerative keratitis. Frequently, there may be an associated scleritis. Other associated findings include keratoconjunctivitis sicca, episcleritis and sclerosing keratitis. Rheumatoid arthritis is clinically diagnosed on the basis of the criteria established by the American Rheumatism Association. The patients' clinical profile and positive serological indices will help in establishing diagnosis.

Other collagen vascular diseases associated with the peripheral ulcerative keratitis are:

Wegener's granulomatosis, polyarteritis nodosa, systemic lupus erythematosus and giant cell arteritis.

Management

It is important to perform certain serological tests where an underlying necrotizing vasculitides are suspected as these diseases may have lethal consequences if not managed appropriately. A complete blood counts, erythrocyte sedimentation rate, C-reactive protein, rheumatoid factor, c-ANCA and p-ANCA are recommended.

Topical steroids should be used with caution in these patients as these drugs inhibit collagen that increases the likelihood of perforation. Immunosuppressive therapy should be started.

Other causes of peripheral ulcerative keratitis include:

- Staphylococcal marginal keratitis
- Infections
- Ocular rosacea
- Contact lens-induced peripheral ulcer

INFECTIOUS CRYSTALLINE KERATOPATHY

Introduction

Infectious crystalline keratopathy is a unique pauci-inflammatory infection of the cornea characterized by minimal stromal inflammation with fine needle like extensions in the corneal stroma. Most common organism implicated is an alpha-hemolytic streptococcus. Other organisms include Streptococcus pneumoniae, *Staphylococcus epidermidis, Haemophilus, Pseudomonas,* Acinetobacter, Enterobacter, *Candida albicans* and *Mycobacterium fortuitum*. Characteristic clinical features include an indolent course, slow response to antimicrobial therapy, and frequent association with conditions leading to local immune compromise, such as previous keratoplasty and topical corticosteroid therapy.

Pathogenesis

Factors intrinsic to both the host and the infective organism have been proposed to contribute to the apparent abrogation of the host immune response. The clinicopathological features are partially explained by the formation of the biofilm. Mild pathogenic organisms invade the cornea and replicate, but incite little host response.

Management

A corneal biopsy may help to identify the causative organism. Aggressive therapy with antimicrobial agents for prolonged duration is needed in most cases. If unsuccessful, YAG laser or penetrating keratoplasty may be warranted.

FILAMENTARY KERATITIS

Introduction

It is a chronic disorder of the cornea characterized by one or more filaments that hang from the surface of cornea (Figs 3.33 A and B). Filamentary keratitis occurs secondary to various diseases or conditions, but in some cases no associated disease can be identified. Filaments appear as short tails, variable in length, but usually less than 2 mm long, being connected to the cornea. Beneath the attachment to the epithelium, there may be gray subepithelial granular opacity.

Histologically, filaments are composed of central mucin core with the scattered groups of inflammatory cells at the base of the filaments.

Theory of Filament Formation

As a normal epithelial surface degenerates due to dessication, some cells die and fall off, leaving a defect. Mucin may adhere to this defect and eventually epithelium grows down over mucin to form a filament.

Causes

- Dry eye disease, especially the tear deficient type
- Superior limbic keratoconjunctivitis
- Epidemic keratoconjunctivitis
- Eye surgery (penetrating keratoplasty, cataract surgery)
- Recurrent erosions
- Systemic diseases, such as sarcoidosis, diabetes, atopic dermatitis
- Medications.

Treatment

The underlying cause should be identified and managed to prevent recurrences. Intensive lubricants help in epithelialization. A bandage contact lens may be used to promote rapid healing and symptomatic relief.

METABOLIC KERATOPATHY

These diseases, while relatively rare, are of importance since the corneal findings may represent either the sole involvement or the earliest manifestation of the metabolic abnormality.

Systemic Mucopolysaccharidosis

These are lysosomal storage diseases that result from deficiency of enzymes involved in degradation of the glycosaminoglycans dermatan sulfate, heparin sulphate and keratan sulfate (Figs 3.34 to 3.38). Since the corneal stroma comprises ~ 4% of glycosaminoglycan, the accumulation of excessive dermatan and keratan sulfate is clinically apparent as stromal clouding. Heparan sulfate deposits in the retina and central nervous system account for the retinal pigmentary degeneration, papilledema and optic nerve atrophy. Ten different syndromes have been described to date. All are autosomal in inheritance, except Hunter syndrome, which is X-linked recessive. The main ocular features of various mucopolysaccharidosis types are summarized in the Table 3.4. The ocular and systemic variations of each major mucopolysaccharidosis disorder follow.

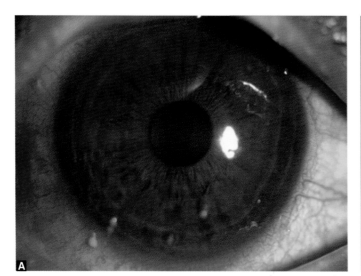
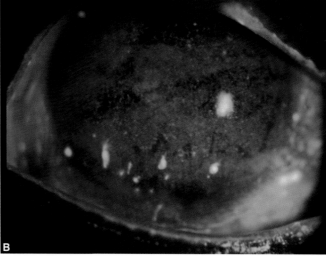

Figs 3.33A and B: Filamentary keratitis

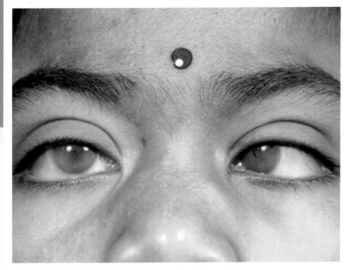

Fig. 3.34: Mucopolysaccharidosis

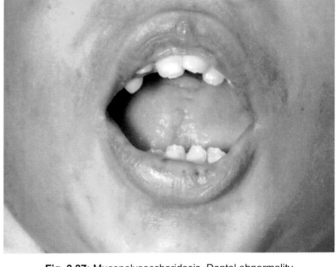

Fig. 3.37: Mucopolysaccharidosis. Dental abnormality

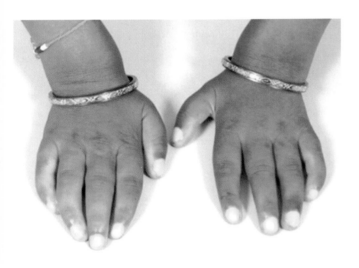

Fig. 3.35: Mucopolysaccharidosis. Short, stubby hands

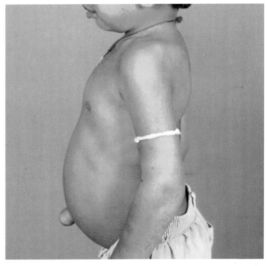

Fig. 3.38: Mucopolysaccharidosis. Umbilical hernia

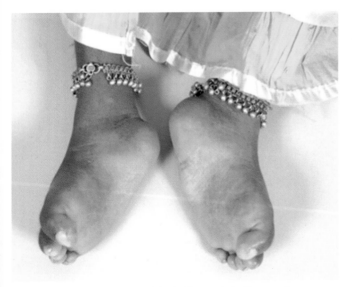

Fig. 3.36: Mucopolysaccharidosis. Congenital talipes equinovarus

Table 3.4: Ocular findings in mucopolysaccharidosis

Disease	Cornea	Retina	Optic nerve
MPS I-H (Hurler)	+	+	+
MPS I-S (Scheie)	+	+	+
MPS-II (Hunter)	-	+	+
MPS-III (Sanfilippo)	-	+	+
MPS-IV(Morquio)	+	-	+
MPS-VI (Maroteaux-Lamy)	+	-	+
MPS-VII (Sly)	+	-	-

MPS: Mucopolysaccharidosis

Hurler Syndrome

In this propotype of all MPS disorders, activity of lysosomal hydrolase A-1 iduronidase is absent. Although normal in infancy, dwarfism and coarse facial features become progressively manifest by the age of 2 or 3 years. Other findings include psychomotor retardation, deafness, stiff joints, hepatosplenomegaly, umbilical hernia. Corneal clouding is typically diffuse, with fine punctate opacities throughout the stroma. Other ocular findings are retinitis pigmentosa like picture, open-angle glaucoma, optic atrophy and/or papilledema. Death typically occurs by the age of 10 years secondary to respiratory infection or heart failure.

Scheie Syndrome

In marked contrast to MPS I-H, however, patients with MPS I-S have normal intelligence, stature and lifespan. Peripheral corneal clouding, progressing centrally is the predominant ocular finding.

Hunter Syndrome

Affected individuals appear normal in childhood. Later, the typical clinical features of coarse facies, stiff joints, heart disease and typical nodular skin develop. Ocular features include biomicroscopically subtle corneal haze without visual consequence, papilledema and retinal pigmentary degeneration.

Sanfilippo Syndrome

The corneas are clinically clear though subtle stromal opacities are biomicroscopically visible.

Morquio Syndrome

Corneal clouding with diffuse ground glass stromal opacification of variable intensity is common. Since no pigmentary degeneration occurs, corneal transplantation may be both anatomically and visually successful. Hypoplasia of odontoid process may predispose to atlantoaxial dislocation and spinal cord compression, so extreme care must be undertaken in performing general anesthesia.

Maroteaux-Lamy Syndrome

Ocular manifestations include mild corneal clouding, papilledema and optic atrophy. As with Morquio syndrome, hypolplasia of odontoid process may cause spinal cord compression.

Sly Syndrome

Corneal clouding is minimal. Corneal transplantation has been reported to be a valuable treatment option for visual rehabilitation despite shortened life span.

Cystinosis

This rare autosomal recessive disorder results in the accumulation of the amino acid cystine within lysosomes. Three variants are recognized based on the age of onset: infantile, intermediate and adult. Although the corneal findings are identical in the three disorders, the range of systemic manifestations extends from absent in the adult form to lethal in infantile cystinosis. In the cornea, crystals are preferentially located in the anterior stroma and are iridescent and polychromatic varying from needle like to rectangular. In mild cases only periphery may be involved, but with time the distribution extends deeper into the cornea. The crystals are not present at birth, but have been detected as early as 6 months of age. Corneal changes are usually present before nephropathy. The diagnosis can be made by conjunctival biopsy by either extracted free cystine or by electron microscopic detection of the characteristic crystals.

Dietary restriction has not been successful since cystine is synthesized from the essential amino acid methionine. Cysteamine eyedrops may prevent deposition of crystals in the cornea.

Wilson's Disease

It is an autosomal recessive disorder characterized by generalized accumulation of copper essentially in the liver, brain, kidneys and cornea. A sunflower cataract is also characteristic. The Kayser-Fleischer ring is a valuable diagnostic sign and management indicator, since its intensity is well correlated with the severity of disease, being invariably present in cases with neurologic manifestations. Equally important, regression of corneal copper deposition has been correlated with the success of treatment. The ring is brown to blue green, with characteristic progression first superiorly and inferiorly, then extending the full circumference of the cornea. As in the milder forms, the ring may be only detectable on gonioscopic visualization of Descemet's membrane.

DRUG-INDUCED KERATOPATHIES

Introduction

Lysosomal dysfunction may be caused by abnormal inclusions from exogenous sources. Drug usage is the most common precipitating cause. Cationic amphiphilic drugs are able to penetrate freely into the lysozymes, where they are protonated and complexed with polar lipids. Progressive accumulation of these complexes renders the lysosomal cells incompetent to perform its necessary functions.

Chloroquine

Ocular manifestations include a reversible keratopathy and an irreversible retinopathy. The bilateral keratopathy develops after the months of drug use and strongly resembles the verticillata keratopathy of Fabry's disease. Although the corneal changes do not usually produce symptoms, patients occasionally complain of halos or blurry vision in the absence of detectable retinopathy. The presence of this keratopathy is not an indication for cessation of therapy in contrast with retinopathy which warrants discontinuation of the drug.

Amiodarone

Long-term administration results in bilateral verticillate keratopathy clinically indistinguishable from chloroquine keratopathy. As the deposits do not hamper vision, the presence is no contraindication for continued amiodarone treatment.

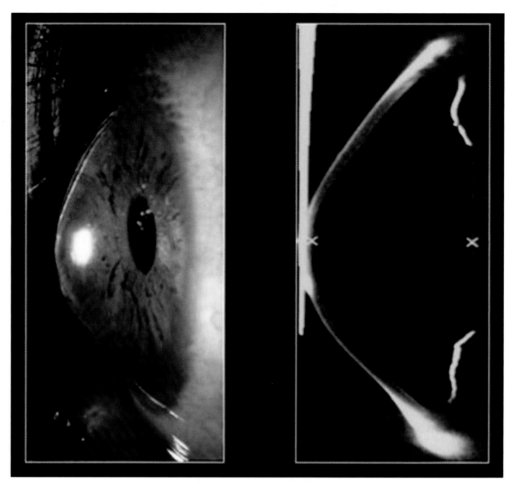

Fig. 3.39: Keratoconus

Other Agents

Chlorpromazine and related phenothiazines, clofazimine and tilorone are additional agents capable of producing lipidoses.

KERATOCONUS

Introduction

Keratoconus is a noninflammatory, bilateral (but usually asymmetrical) disease of the cornea, characterized by paracentral corneal thinning and ectasia so that the cornea takes the shape of a cone (Fig. 3.39). Visual loss occurs primarily from myopia and irregular astigmatism and secondarily from corneal scarring.

Reported prevalence in the general population varies (50–200 per 100,000), because of differences in diagnostic criteria. Keratoconus occurs in all ethnic groups with no male or female preponderance. It is commonly an isolated ocular condition, but sometimes coexists with other ocular and systemic diseases.

Commonly recognized ocular associations include vernal keratoconjunctivitis, retinitis pigmentosa and Leber congenital amaurosis; many of the connective tissue disorders (e.g. Ehlers-Danlos and Marfan syndromes), mitral valve prolapse, atopic dermatitis and Down syndrome.

Particular risk factors include atopic history, especially ocular allergies, rigid contact lens wear and vigorous eye rubbing. Most kertoconus cases appear spontaneously, although approximately 14% of them are present with the evidence of genetic transmission.

Keratoconus, generally manifests at puberty and is progressive until the third to fourth decade of life, when it usually arrests. Sometimes, however, it may commence later in life and progress or arrest at any age.

Pathophysiology

All layers of the cornea are believed to be affected by kertoconus, although the most notable features are the thinning of the corneal stroma, the fragmentation of the Bowman layer and the deposition of iron in the basal epithelial cells, forming the Fleischer ring. Folds and breaks in the Descemet's membrane result in acute hydrops and striae, respectively which results in variable amounts of diffuse scarring.

Clinical Features

Symptoms are highly variable and, in part, depend on the stage of the progression of the disorder. Early in the disease there may be no symptoms, and keratoconus may be noted by the ophthalmologist simply because the patient cannot be refracted to a clear 20/20 corrected vision. In advanced disease, there is significant distortion of vision accompanied by profound visual loss. Patients with keratoconus fortunately never become totally blind from their disease.

Clinical signs also differ depending on the severity of the disease. In moderate to advanced disease any one or combination of the following signs may be detectable by slit-lamp examination of the cornea: stromal thinning (centrally or paracentrally, most commonly inferiorly or inferotemporally); conical protrusion; an iron line partially or completely surrounding the cone (Fleischer's ring); and fine vertical lines in the deep stroma and Descemet's membrane that parallel the axis of the cone and disappear transiently on gentle digital pressure (Vogt's striae). Other accompanying signs might include epithelial nebulae, anterior stromal scars, enlarged corneal nerves, and increased intensity of the corneal endothelial reflex and subepithelial fibrillary lines.

Munson's sign and Rizzuti's sign are also useful adjunctive external signs associated with keratoconus. Munson's sign is a V-shaped conformation of the lower lid produced by the ectatic cornea in downgaze. Rizzuti's sign is a sharply focused beam of light near the nasal limbus, produced by lateral illumination of the cornea in patients with advanced keratoconus. Patients with advanced disease may occasionally be present with a sudden onset of visual loss accompanied by pain. On slit-lamp examination, the conjunctiva may be injected and a diffuse stromal opacity is noted in the cornea. This condition, referred to as "hydrops", is caused by breaks in Descemet's membrane with the stromal imbibition of aqueous through these breaks. The edema may persist for weeks or months, usually diminishing gradually, with relief of pain and resolution of the redness and corneal edema ultimately being replaced by scarring.

Early in the disease process the cornea may appear normal on slit-lamp biomicroscopy; however, there may be slight distortion or steepening of keratometry mires centrally or inferiorly. In such instances it is useful to dilate the pupil. Retroillumination techniques and scissoring of the retinoscopic reflex or the "Charleux" oil droplet sign are useful clinical signs to confirm the diagnosis in suspicious cases.

Diagnosis

Careful refraction, keratometry, corneal topography and slit-lamp biomicroscopy allow the clinician to observe evidence of keratoconus.

Imaging Studies

- *Keratometry*: Images of the keratometry mires commonly will be steep, highly astigmatic, irregular, and often appear egg-shaped rather than circular or oval in keratoconus.

A value of 47.2 D or greater is suggestive of keratoconus. Some patients with keratoconus will not show these signs.

- Corneal topography is helpful in reaching a diagnosis, especially when the typical biomicroscopy signs of Vogt striae and Fleischer ring are absent. Several quantitative indices are available using corneal topography information to screen for keratoconic corneal shape factors. The two most commonly known indices are those of Rabinowitz and Maeda and Klyce.

The Rabinowitz diagnostic criteria consist of three corneal topography derived indices, which, when abnormal in value, should alert the clinician to consider a diagnosis of keratoconus. These indices are as follows:

- K value quantifies the central steepening of the cornea that occurs in keratoconus. A value of 47.20 D or greater is suggestive of keratoconus.
- I-S value quantifies the inferior versus superior corneal dioptric asymmetry that occurs in keratoconus. A value of 1.4 D or greater is suggestive of keratoconus.
- KISA% incorporates the K and I-S values with a measure quantifying regular and irregular astigmatism into one index. This index is highly sensitive and specific in separating normal from keratoconic corneas. A value of greater than 100% is highly suggestive of frank keratoconus, and the range from 60 to 100% represents keratoconus suspects.

On the other hand, Maeda and Klyce designed an alternative computer expert program, based on linear discriminant analysis of 8 indices drawn from the corneal map and a binary decision tree. The program assigns the topographical map a quantitative percentage score of the severity of keratoconus called the KCI%. A value of greater than zero is believed to be suggestive of keratoconus.

Ultrasonic pachymetry may be useful to confirm corneal thinning in patients with suspected keratoconus on slit-lamp examination or videokeratography; however, it cannot be solely relied on to the diagnosis because of the large range and variation of pachymetry readings both centrally and paracentrally in the normal population. Modalities like Orbscan and Pentacam which provides both topography and pachymetry maps are particularly useful in making a diagnosis.

Histologic Findings

All layers of the cornea are affected by keratoconus. Superficial epithelial cells located at the nodule are elongated and arranged in a whorl-like fashion. Iron deposition in the basal corneal epithelial cells form the characteristic Fleischer ring. Localized breaks are present in the basement membrane. A decrease in the number of stromal collagen lamellae is present, as well as a loss of the fibular arrangement within the lamellae. Folds and ruptures occur in the Descemet's membrane. Some studies have reported endothelial cell loss in association with the rupture of the Descemet's membrane.

Management

Rigid gas permeable contact lenses are the mainstay of treatment.

- Patients with early keratoconus successfully may use spectacles or spherical/toric soft contact lenses. They may even rarely find that spectacle vision is superior to rigid contact lenses.
- Patients with modest-to-advanced keratoconus almost always require rigid contact lenses. When rigid contact lenses are no longer tolerated, some patients can maintain contact lens wear and usable visions with hydrogel contact lenses, piggyback contact lenses or scleral (haptic) contact lenses, but usually at a physiological or visual cost.
- Contact lens wear often is complicated by episodes of intolerance, allergic reactions (e.g. giant papillary conjunctivitis), corneal abrasions, neovascularization, and other problems, sometimes leading to total intolerance.

Certain surgical procedures which may prove useful in some cases are described below:

Although still controversial, intrastromal corneal rings (Intacs) have been implanted in the eyes of patients who have become intolerant to contact lenses. More traditionally, these patients (including those whose vision is not correctable to better than 20/40) are referred for corneal transplants (penetrating keratoplasty or deep anterior lamellar keratoplasty).

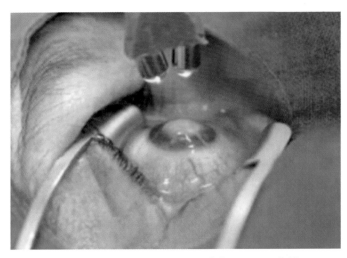

Fig. 3.40: Surgery for keratoconus. Collagen cross-linking

Corneal transplants are very successful in the treatment of keratoconus, resulting in clear visual axes in greater than 90% of all cases. Contact lenses are often still required post graft for optimum vision. Corneal grafts require continuing professional care to watch for rejection, suture-related problems, wound dehiscence and other difficulties. Although extremely rare, keratoconus can recur in a graft.

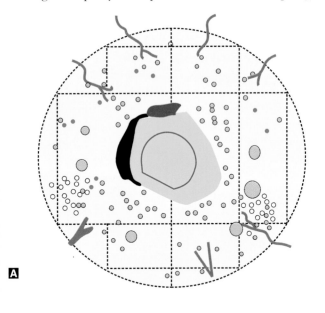

A

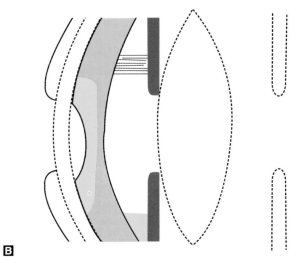

B

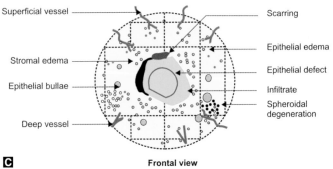

Superficial vessel

Stromal edema

Epithelial bullae

Deep vessel

Scarring

Epithelial edema

Epithelial defect

Infiltrate

Spheroidal degeneration

C   **Frontal view**

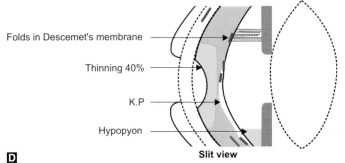

Folds in Descemet's membrane

Thinning 40%

K.P

Hypopyon

D   **Slit view**

Figs 3.41A to D

Color code used in corneal drawing

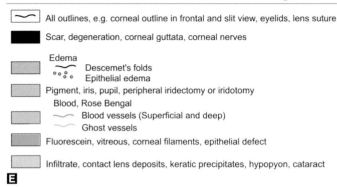

All outlines, e.g. corneal outline in frontal and slit view, eyelids, lens suture

Scar, degeneration, corneal guttata, corneal nerves

Edema
Descemet's folds
Epithelial edema
Pigment, iris, pupil, peripheral iridectomy or iridotomy
Blood, Rose Bengal
Blood vessels (Superficial and deep)
Ghost vessels
Fluorescein, vitreous, corneal filaments, epithelial defect

Infiltrate, contact lens deposits, keratic precipitates, hypopyon, cataract

E

Figs 3.41A to E: Documentation of clinical signs

A surgical treatment, involving riboflavin and ultraviolet light has been proposed (Fig. 3.40). With this treatment, the corneal epithelium is first removed, and the corneal stroma is subjected to riboflavin and exposed to ultraviolet light. The cornea is then allowed to reepithelialize. This treatment is an effort to induce increased collagen cross-linking to enhance corneal rigidity and to decrease keratoconic corneal steepening. While some act as advocates for this treatment, others have

significant concerns that it may be harmful rather than beneficial. Additional studies are in progress.

DOCUMENTATION OF CLINICAL SIGNS THROUGH CLINICAL DIAGRAMS

A clinical diagram is useful to document the type and position of corneal pathologies. The dimension of epithelial opacities and stromal ulceration and depth of new vessels and opacities should be documented. Color coding is extremely helpful (Figs 3.41A to E).

Opacities such as scars and degenerations are drawn in black.

Epithelial edema is drawn as fine blue circles; stromal edema is blue shading and folds in Descemet's membrane as wavy blue lines.

Hypopyon is shown in yellow.

Blood vessels are depicted in red. Superficial vessels are wavy lines that begin outside the limbus. Deep vessels are straight lines that begin at the limbus.

Pigments, such as iron rings and Krukenberg spindle are drawn in brown.

Chapter 4

Corneal Surgeries

Srinivas K Rao, Late G Sitalakshmi

CORNEAL TRAUMA

The cornea is prone to a variety of injuries by virtue of its exposed location as the window of the eye. These can range from relatively minor events, such as dust entering the eye to more serious injuries resulting from chemical or thermal insults. The management of these latter injuries is often medical at the time of presentation. The late sequelae in such injuries often result in cicatricial changes in the ocular surface.

This section deals with the principles of the management of lacerating and blunt injuries of the cornea that result in disruption of the stromal structure—at the time of presentation and later when visual rehabilitation is required. Corneal injuries of this nature can occur in two distinct populations—in young children from play-related activities and in young adults from their work environment. Although the general principles of management are not different, special consideration must be given to the timing of appropriate surgical interventions in the pediatric population, as the developing visual system in children is prone to amblyopic visual loss.

Such injuries can be caused by large blunt objects, which can result in irregular corneal tears and often ruptures of other parts of the ocular coats as well. On the other hand, sharp projectiles cause more limited corneal trauma and are in general associated with better outcomes than injuries caused by blunt trauma. With projectile injury, the nature and velocity of the injuring missile determines whether it lodges within the cornea or passes into the eye, damaging other structures as well. These factors also determine if the injuring agent is retained within the coats or intraocular structures. Apart from the physical damage to the ocular structures from the injuring agent, it is important to remember that these objects are quite frequently contaminated with infective agents and infection of the cornea and other structures may contribute significantly to the morbidity arising from such injuries. Medicolegal implications will also have to be considered, when managing patients who have suffered such injuries.

Assessment of the Eye

One of the most important determinations when examining a patient with corneal trauma is to distinguish between penetrating injuries (Fig. 4.1), which have breached the corneal integrity, but are contained within the corneal tissues, and perforating injuries (Fig. 4.2), which have caused full-thickness corneal damage. The classification of ocular trauma has been well described by numerous systems, including the Ocular Trauma Classification Group. For the context of this discussion, however, since only the management of corneal injuries is described, the distinction is based on whether the injury involves a partial – or full-thickness violation of the corneal structure—since the principles of management of these two groups are quite different.

The importance of this determination stems from the fact that in the latter injuries, there is a potential for infection to enter the eye (in 2 to 30% of eyes that have penetrating eye

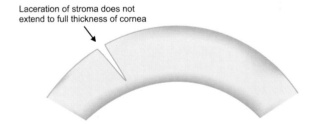

Laceration of stroma does not extend to full thickness of cornea

Fig. 4.1: Penetrating corneal injury

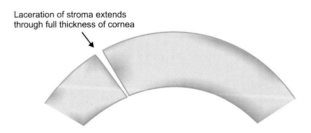

Laceration of stroma extends through full thickness of cornea

Fig. 4.2: Perforating corneal injury

trauma) and all such eyes must be treated as potential endophthalmitis until proven otherwise. Similarly, these eyes are also at risk of having a retained intraocular foreign body and investigations for the same are mandatory, and in the event of such a complication being present, the care of the eye may require the assistance of a vitreoretinal colleague. Finally, penetrating corneal injuries often do not require early or immediate surgical intervention, whereas perforating injuries often do.

In assessing patients with corneal trauma, it is important to first look for the coexistence of life-threatening systemic injuries, which if present should take precedence in management. A brief history as to the nature of the injuring agent and the circumstances of the injury are relevant as they help determine the possibility of a retained foreign body and its nature, the occurrence of infection, and possible medicolegal issues in work-related injuries and road traffic accidents. An assessment of the visual acuity of the injured eye must be performed before commencing the eye examination. In ocular trauma, the often-rapid occurrence of an anterior or posterior hemorrhage may preclude assessment of the visual potential of the eye and the state of the intraocular structures during subsequent examinations. Documentation in the records of very poor visual acuity at presentation will also serve to protect the examiner in the event of subsequent medicolegal litigation. Of particular relevance in corneal injuries is whether the location of such damage involves the visual axis of the eye, as this will help guide discussions regarding the visual consequences of the injury and the need, nature and timing of subsequent surgical interventions.

Isolated corneal injuries that are smaller than 8 mm in size tend to be associated with a better prognosis, especially if there is no vitreous, iris prolapse or vitreous hemorrhage. The presence of foreign bodies located within the cornea in penetrating corneal trauma and within the tissues of the eye in perforating trauma should be looked for. The presence of and potential for infection must be determined. The status of tetanus prophylaxis of the individual must be ascertained; and in the event of surgical repair being considered, the timing and nature of the last meal of the patient must be recorded. The patient should also be instructed to remain on nil oral diet since general anesthesia may have to be used during the surgical repair. Since one of the important goals in the management of these patients is the prevention of further damage to the injured eye, it is important that a rigid eye shield protects the injured eye until definitive care can be provided. Using a plastic rather than a metal shield is advantageous since this would allow the shield to remain in place during most radiographic imaging studies.

In addition to the above considerations, perforating injuries of the cornea are often associated with iris prolapse, lens damage, and retinal and choroidal injuries and these must be looked for, assessing also if there is evidence of endophthalmitis at presentation. Classic signs of associated scleral rupture are poor visual acuity, the presence of a boggy chemosis of the conjunctiva—often with hyphema and distortion of the pupil,

an afferent pupillary defect, a soft eye, and in severe cases, distorted globe contour. These often occur in the superonasal quadrant or at the site of insertion of the rectus muscles. Hidden occult perforations may also be present and the detection of these requires a higher index of suspicion. They should be suspected when lacerating injuries of the lids and brows are present. If the posterior segment of the eye cannot be visualized well, appropriate investigations, such as B-scan ultrasonography and radiologic imaging studies may be required for a complete assessment of the ocular status. In the succeeding sections, the surgical principles of corneal injury management are described.

Surgical Principles

It is best to have a soft eye with no vitreous upthrust when performing the surgical repair of the corneal tear. Thus, a deep plane of general anesthesia is desirable, and while the speculum chosen should provide a good exposure of the cornea, it is important to avoid pressure on the globe from the speculum. Bridle sutures of the rectus muscles are best avoided and povidone-iodine irrigation of the ocular surface should not be performed because of the exposure of intraocular contents in perforating injuries of the eye wall.

The ocular surface should be irrigated well with sterile balanced salt solution (BSS) to provide a good douche of the wound and remove all debris and contaminants from the surgical field. In eyes with a suspicion of corneal infection, a swab from the edges of the wound would help in better management of infections that develop in the postoperative period. A better inspection of the damage is possible in the operating room and the morphology of the tear, scleral or limbal involvement and loss of corneal tissue are determined.

Generally, 8-0 nylon for sclera, 9-0 nylon for limbus, 10-0 nylon for cornea and 11-0 nylon for complex corneal tears are the preferred suture materials. If iris is incarcerated in the wound and has not actually exited onto the surface of the eye, the use of intracameral pilocarpine (peripheral incarceration) or 1:10,000 adrenaline (central incarceration) may be tried to see if the movement of the iris is able to retract the incarcerated tissues into the anterior chamber. If, however, the iris has prolapsed onto the corneal surface and has been exposed for longer than 24 hours, there is a risk of introducing surface epithelium into the eye if the tissue is reposited. In this situation, it is important to abscise the prolapsed iris, by gently tugging on it and amputating it, flush with the corneal surface. The presence of a minimal ooze of blood from the cut end is a sign that all devitalized iris has been excised and only viable tissue is retained. In the presence of a shallow, but formed anterior chamber, a diamond knife is used to create a paracentesis, before the manipulations of the wound result in a total loss of the anterior chamber. This provides a port of access into the anterior chamber for use during subsequent maneuvers, such as introduction of viscoelastic to protect the endothelium, injection of air to maintain the chamber during suturing, and the use of a spatula to release iris adhesions to the wound. Excessive manipulations through the corneal tear should be avoided.

When repairing corneal tears, it is best to initiate suturing at the limbus, since the presence of the limbal palisades provides visual clues of the anatomic landmarks and allows precise apposition of the tear edges. Once the limbus has been reconstituted, sutures are placed to divide the tear into equal halves and the process is continued until the entire length of the tear has been sutured. Another important principle is to ensure that suture placement is perpendicular to the orientation of the tear at the point of the suture (Fig. 4.3). In long tears, a temporary suture may be applied in the middle of the wound to provide apposition of the wound edges and prevent excessive lateral displacement of the wound during suturing.

When dealing with curvilinear tears that extend to the center of the cornea, in addition to paying attention to the above issues, it is important to use the sutures to try and restore the shape of the corneal vault. Since deep, long and tight sutures tend to flatten the cornea curvature, these are used in the corneal periphery. As the corneal center is approached, shorter, more superficial and less tight sutures are employed. The use of viscoelastic or air to keep the anterior chamber formed during these maneuvers will help in the restoration of a more physiological corneal contour. In curved tears, continuous sutures are best avoided as they tend to straighten the suture line when tightened, which results in corneal distortion. Since each suture supports the wound for a distance equal to its length, it is possible to determine the number of sutures that is ideal for a given length of tear (Fig. 4.4).

It is important to ensure that the sutures produce good apposition of the edges of the corneal tear as this would help in reducing the occurrence of irregular astigmatism. To achieve this goal, the corneal bites should be of equal depth in both margins of the tear. In corneal tears complicated by extensive edema of the stromal edges, it is necessary to use long bites that are anchored in the normal corneal stroma, as this allows better judgment of the extent of suture tightening that is required. In very shelving corneal tears, it is important to use the posterior edge of the tear as the guide when determining the length of the suture bite in the two margins of the tear (Fig. 4.5).

Knots of 10-0 nylon sutures, which are used for corneal tear repair, are best buried in the corneal stroma as they can cause a significant discomfort and corneal problems if left exposed on the surface. It is better to bury the knot away from the side of the visual axis as maximal corneal scarring tends to occur in the corneal stroma around the knot. After burying the knot, a sharp pull in the reverse direction will reverse the orientation of the suture ends within the stroma, resulting in an arrowhead configuration that points to the surface, and facilitates easy removal later (Fig. 4.6). In shelving corneal tears, it is preferable to bury the knot on the side of the shorter anterior bite as the direction of the force applied during suture removal will support the wound and reduce the chance of wound dehiscence (Fig. 4.7).

Complex tears with a stellate configuration are harder to manage. It is best to suture the individual limbs of the tear first and tackle the stellate apex last. Since this is often composed of thin slivers of corneal tissue, a finer suture like 11-0 nylon may be preferable. A purse-string suture is effective in closing such wounds, but may lead to pursing and fish mouthing of the apex of the tear (Fig. 4.8). In tripartite tears, to avoid this problem, a variant of the purse-string suture, called the "star" suture, may be used. The bridging sutures crossing the apex help prevent fish mouthing of the apical tissues (Fig. 4.9).

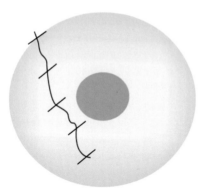

Fig. 4.3: Suturing a radial corneal tear

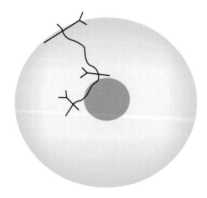

Fig. 4.4: Suturing a curvilinear corneal tear

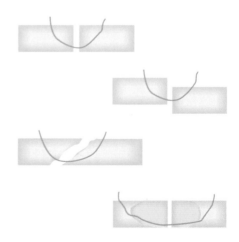

Fig. 4.5: Principles of suturing a corneal tear

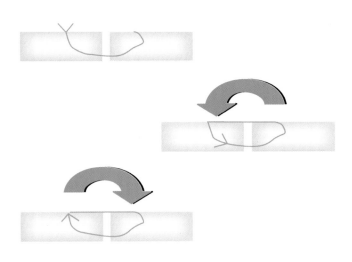

Fig. 4.6: Burying a corneal suture knot

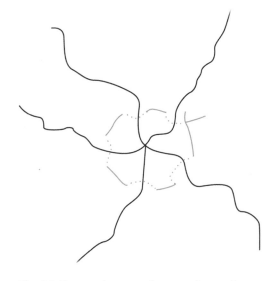

Fig. 4.8: Purse-string suture for apex of corneal tears

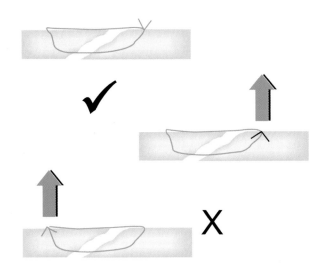

Fig. 4.7: Burying the suture knot in a shelving corneal tear

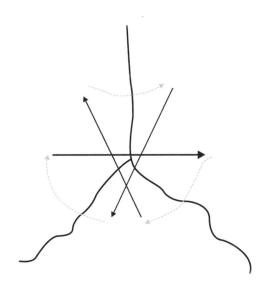

Fig. 4.9: Modified "'star'" suture for apex of stellate corneal tears

A leaking wound at the conclusion of the procedure is sometimes seen, especially when there has been some degree of tissue loss. If the leak is minimal, it can often be managed by the use of air in the anterior chamber and support with a bandage contact lens. When the leak is due to tissue loss, if this is minimal, the use of n-butyl cyanoacrylate glue or fibrin glue may be used to seal the leak, till corneal healing occurs. If, however, there has been more extensive tissue loss, corneal tissue transfer may be required to restore corneal integrity. A very challenging situation is in eyes with keratoglobus that have suffered corneal rupture, and these thin corneas are prone to corneal tears following relatively minor trauma. The extremely thin cornea in such eyes often does not support suturing well, and multiple leaks from the suture tracks may be seen. In cases of severe trauma in these eyes, primary corneal replacement may have to be considered, as globe saving maneuver. It is important that such patients are properly counseled regarding the risks and are encouraged to constantly wear protective polycarbonate spectacles, to prevent a future recurrence of a similar problem.

Another situation, where the extent of corneal damage is more extensive than would be expected from the nature of the injury, is in eyes that have had past incisional corneal surgical procedures, such as radial keratotomy or a corneal transplant. In these eyes, apparently well-healed scars after the incisional procedures tend to rupture, resulting in fairly extensive trauma. In eyes that have undergone radial keratotomy, the multiple petalloid pieces of interincisional corneal tissues are difficult to appose with interrupted sutures, as suturing one incision closed, results in further wound gape of the two adjacent incisions. In this situation, the Grene lasso suture is useful in tackling the problem. Originally described to counter excessive hyperopic shifts following radial keratotomy, this suture passes through adjacent incisions, in a circumferential manner at the periphery

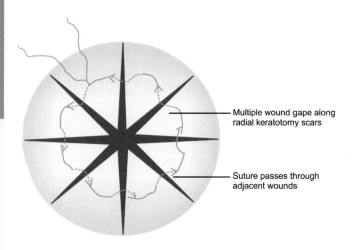

Fig. 4.10: Lasso suture for closing ruptured radial keratotomy incisions

Multiple wound gape along radial keratotomy scars

Suture passes through adjacent wounds

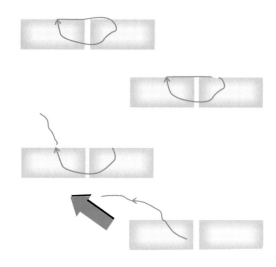

Fig. 4.11: Principles of corneal suture removal

of the cornea and tends to hold the individual corneal pieces together and provides stability (Fig. 4.10). Further interrupted sutures may then be applied as required. More than one lasso suture may also be applied.

Another peculiar situation that may sometimes occur in postoperative corneas is the traumatic displacement of the flap created during LASIK. When subjected to shearing forces, these apparently well-healed flaps tend to be disrupted and may sometimes be lost, or they may furl up in the interface—and this can result in severe astigmatism, and anatomical derangement due to the occurrence of an epithelial ingrowth. If the flap is lost, the surface will usually re-epithelialize and management would depend on the residual scarring and refractive error. Creating a flap from a donor eye and suturing it in place may be considered, if appropriate. If the flap is inturned, the interface is reopened, the flap unfolded, epithelium in the interface is removed, and the striae in the flap are removed by stretching the flap. After repositioning the flap, sutures may be required to ensure that the edge heals well and also to reduce the risk of recurrence of flap striae.

Suture removal should be performed at the appropriate time, when adequate wound healing has occurred, using a technique that reduces the risk of tracking epithelium and debris into the suture track. The corneal surface is first flushed with sterile solution to remove any debris on the suture. Antibiotics are applied prior to the procedure or topical povidone-iodine can be used. The suture is cut flush with the surface of the cornea at the end away from the suture knot, by introducing the tip of a blade or sterile disposable needle under the loop of suture. The instrument is again inserted under the loop of suture on the corneal surface at the knot end and the cut length of the surface suture is retracted onto the surface, without disturbing the corneal epithelium overlying the suture length. The exteriorized suture is then aligned with the knot and gradually increasing force used to pull out the entire suture (Fig. 4.11).

Penetrating Trauma—Management

When examining the cornea, the length (Fig. 4.12), depth (Fig. 4.13), and morphology of the corneal tear (Fig. 4.14), the presence of limbal involvement (Fig. 4.15), the extent of corneal edema (Fig. 4.16), and the presence of tissue loss, if any, must be determined.

General principles of penetrating corneal trauma management include the use of tetanus prophylaxis if required, antibiotic cover, the use of lubricants and a protective shield. Specific therapy is determined based on the characteristics of the wound. In the simplest situation, when the wound is less than 2 mm in length less than 25% of the corneal thickness, is away from the visual axis and has no associated edema, treatment consists of careful observation with the use of prophylactic topical antibiotics, lubricants and assessing if there are any changes in refraction after wound healing (Fig. 4.17).

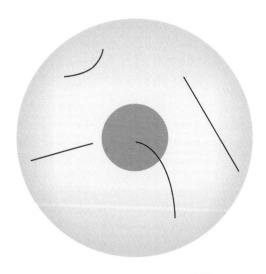

Fig. 4.12: Corneal tear assessment—length of tear

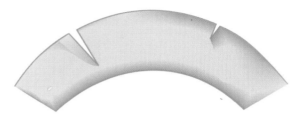

Fig. 4.13: Corneal tear assessment—depth of stromal damage

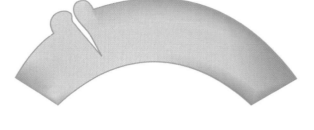

Fig. 4.16: Corneal tear assessment—edema of wound margins

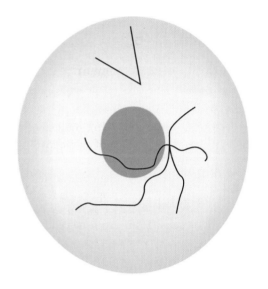

Fig. 4.14: Corneal tear assessment—morphology of tear

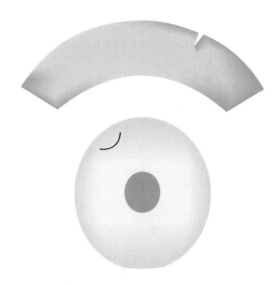

Fig. 4.17: Minimal penetrating corneal trauma

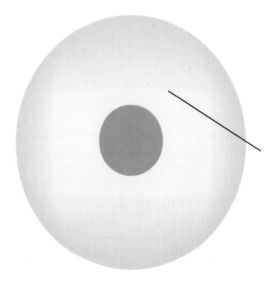

Fig. 4.15: Corneal tear assessment—involvement of limbus

In a larger tear that extends 5 to 6 mm in length, and involves 50% of corneal thickness, but does not involve the visual axis and has a shelving configuration, it should be possible to splint the tear with a stiff bandage contact lens that supports wound healing (such as the Bausch & Lomb Plano T). Topical antibiotics and lubricants can be used; and once the corneal edema resolves and scar progression is completed, any changes in refraction are addressed (Fig. 4.18).

If large tears extend longer than 6 mm and involve a corneal depth greater than 50%, involve the visual axis, or have a complex morphology—often stellate, it is necessary to suture the wound appropriately (Fig. 4.19). In the postoperative period, after confirming the clinical absence of corneal infection, the careful introduction of topical steroids concomitant with the use of topical antibiotics, may help reduce the extent and severity of corneal inflammation and resultant scarring. Sutures should be removed at the appropriate time to lessen the chances of complications from loosening, vascularization

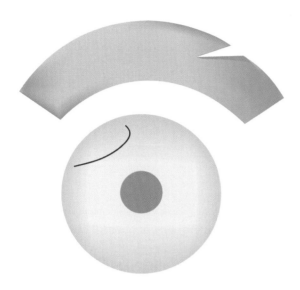

Fig. 4.18: Moderate penetrating corneal trauma

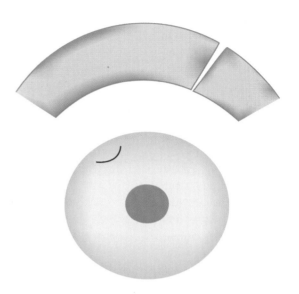

Fig. 4.20: Minimal perforating corneal trauma

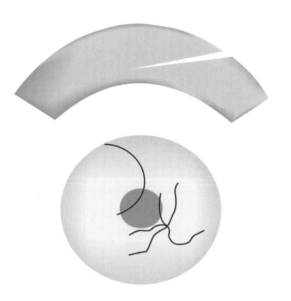

Fig. 4.19: Severe penetrating corneal trauma

and infection. The involvement of the visual axis will require further intervention to restore vision. If such complex corneal tears are not sutured, healing often occurs by secondary intention, with the tissues in the everted and unopposed position, which can result in large areas of scarring, severe distortion of the corneal surface contour and poor visual outcomes.

Perforating Trauma—Management

As with penetrating trauma, the treatment plan is decided after a detailed assessment, and is often surgical. However, in contrast to penetrating corneal trauma, topical medications especially ointments are best avoided as the injury track provides a pathway into the eye. In the mildest form of such an injury, a small track that is less than 2 mm in size, is self-sealed and Seidel test

negative, with no iris prolapse or infection—can be splinted with a bandage contact lens, and managed as in the case of a penetrating injury (Fig. 4.20). However, the portal of entry into the eye increases the risk of possible endophthalmitis, which must be watched for, and treatment with intravenous antibiotics considered, even though these are of unproven value.

In eyes with larger tears, that are Seidel test positive (the surface is painted with fluorescein strips treated with artificial tears and the presence of a leak is identified by the gradual change of the fluorescein from green to yellow due to dilution by the leaking aqueous), or have an active leak with a flat anterior chamber, iris prolapse, and or tissue loss, it would be best to suture the wound closed. The goals of surgery are to reconstruct the integrity of the damaged cornea and reform the anterior chamber, remove any disrupted lens material and unhealthy iris tissue, and remove intraocular foreign bodies that may be present. General anesthesia is preferred, although very small, uncomplicated tears can be repaired using preservative-free topical anesthetics. In any event, the eye should be protected with a pad and rigid shield till surgery; and if general anesthesia is considered, it would be necessary to avoid the use of a depolarizing muscle relaxant like succinylcholine, and to remove the supportive eye pad and shield only after anesthesia induction is completed.

In the event of the trauma also resulting in damage to the crystalline lens, the surgeon must evolve a plan for the management of the lens structures as well. A good view of the lens structures during surgery will help formulate an appropriate management strategy. In eyes with extensive corneal trauma, and fibrin formation in the anterior chamber precluding a good view of the lens structures despite attempting to shift the iris using a spatula and/or the use of micro hooks to retract the iris, it may be best to close the corneal wound and tackle the lens at a later stage when visualization improves. Tiny punctures of the anterior capsule often self-seal and result in limited opacities in the lens and are best observed. A tear in the anterior capsule with flocculent lens matter in the anterior chamber can be managed by trying to convert the anterior capsular tear into a rhexis and then extracting the lens nucleus and aspirating the cortex. Careful maneuvers are required as there may be coexisting zonular damage, in which case, the surgeon must be prepared for alternative approaches to extract the lens. Diligent efforts are made to retain the posterior capsular support for intraocular lens (IOL) implantation. If, however, there is extensive admixture of the vitreous and disrupted lens structures in the anterior chamber, a vitreous cutter may be required to remove the structures, provided an adequate view is possible through the cornea. Recent reports describe the use of an endoilluminator as a second instrument and intracameral triamcinolone to help visualize vitreous in the anterior chamber and facilitate its removal.

Common to both penetrating and perforating corneal trauma, injuries involving the visual axis will compromise visual function to varying extents after wound healing, depending on the location and density of the corneal scar. In minimal scarring, a change of spectacles may suffice; but with increasing irregularity of the corneal surface, the use of a rigid contact lens may have to be considered. If the density of the scar precludes good visual function, corneal replacement would have to be considered, and the techniques of lamellar and full-thickness corneal replacement have been discussed in other sections.

Outcomes of Corneal Trauma Management

Although corneal trauma is not unusual, provided it is recognized promptly and attended to, the resulting morbidity can be minimized. Paying attention to the principles described in this section can help restore useful visual function in many of these eyes. It must, however, be remembered that the prognosis for penetrating corneal trauma remains guarded, and it may also be dependent on the associated ocular damage. Thus, despite the numerous advances in instrumentation and surgical techniques, prevention remains better than cure. In this context, future attention to the epidemiology of such injuries, education of the public regarding the importance of protective measures, and the implementation of regulations and practices to enforce work safety is of paramount importance.

PTERYGIUM SURGERY

Indications for Surgery

A pterygium is a fibrovascular and wing-shaped encroachment of the conjunctiva onto the cornea. Ultraviolet light-induced damage to the limbal stem cell barrier with subsequent conjunctivalization of the cornea is the currently accepted etiopathogenesis of this condition. Indications for surgery include visual impairment, cosmetic disfigurement, motility restriction, recurrent inflammation, interference with contact lens wear, and rarely, changes suggestive of neoplasia. The main histopathologic change in primary pterygium is elastotic degeneration of the conjunctival collagen.

Problems with Assessment of Surgical Outcomes after Pterygium Surgery

There are numerous surgical procedures that have been advocated for the surgical management of pterygia, and each of these techniques has advantages and disadvantages. The ideal surgical procedure for this condition should be simple to perform, fast, with an acceptable complication rate, and have a very low recurrence rate and good cosmesis. Unfortunately, none of the currently available techniques fulfils all these criteria.

Some of the difficulty in evaluating the results of studies dealing with pterygium surgery include the lack of a standardized method of reporting for pterygium morphology or stage prior to surgery, variations in the indications for surgery and patient population, whether surgery was for a primary or recurrent pterygium, the exact surgical technique adopted, the postoperative medication(s) used, the duration of follow-up in the study and the definition of a recurrence. There is also the problem that some of the techniques used in pterygium surgery, such as the use of antimetabolites and beta-irradiation may have long-term sequelae, which are often not addressed in these studies.

Bare Sclera Excision

While there is no unanimity about the procedure of choice, accumulated evidence from a number of past studies clearly indicates that there is one established procedure, which should probably be discontinued. This is the bare sclera method of pterygium excision (Fig. 4.21). In this procedure, often performed using topical or subconjunctival anesthesia as an office procedure, the head of the pterygium is avulsed or shaved off the corneal surface and the body of the pterygium, including the overlying conjunctiva is excised. The resulting bare scleral surface is left exposed (Fig. 4.22), and the conjunctival margins may be sutured in place to the episcleral tissues (Fig. 4.23). Although considered a quick and easy method, the recurrence rates are very high and can approach 80%. This is unacceptably high and hence this method is best avoided.

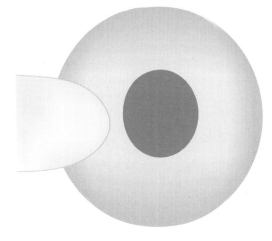

Fig. 4.21: Pterygium—localized loss of limbal barrier function

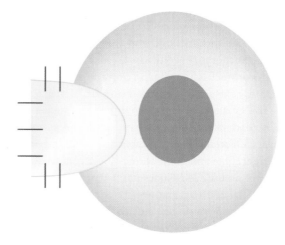

Fig. 4.22: Bare sclera excision with conjunctival sutures

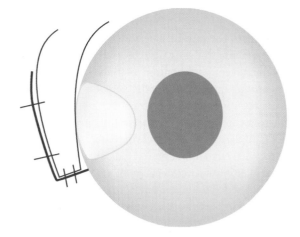

Fig. 4.24: Sliding conjunctival flap to close defect

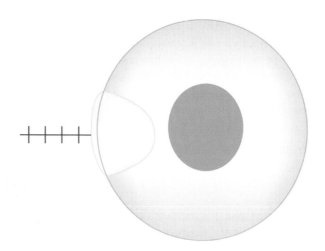

Fig. 4.23: Primary conjunctival closure after excision

Adjuncts to Bare Sclera Excision

In an effort to retain the simplicity of the bare sclera approach, but improve the recurrence rates, several intraoperative and postoperative adjuncts have been tried. These include the use of conjunctival closure techniques to cover the exposed scleral bed. In general, the conjunctiva over the pterygium is preserved; and after excision of the pterygial tissue, the conjunctiva is closed using sutures. With this approach, most studies report a recurrence rate of more than 50%; although in one study, the rate was as low as 2%. In some other instances, sliding flaps of conjunctiva are prepared from the superior or inferior conjunctiva (Fig. 4.24). Although two recent reports using the sliding flap technique describe a recurrence rate of 1.6% to 5.6%, loss to follow-up and study design issues indicate the need for further validation of this technique.

Another approach that has been popular in recent times is the use of the antimetabolites mitomycin-C or 5-fluorouracil. These medications attempt to reduce conjunctival fibroblast proliferation and thus, prevent a recurrence of pterygium after surgery. The optimal dose for intraoperative mitomycin-C use is still unclear, although the most commonly used dose appears to be 0.2 mg/ml applied for 3 minutes during the surgery. The recurrence rate with this technique is reported to be about 10%, but complications, such as severe pain, scleral necrosis and scleral perforation have been described—sometimes only on long-term follow-up. To overcome these complications, it has been suggested that the use of mitomycin-C be combined with a conjunctival graft or conjunctival closure, but long-term outcomes with this approach are still unavailable. Since there is potential for toxicity with mitomycin-C, the use of this medication as postoperative drops is discouraged, to avoid a potential for misuse by patients. The use of 5-fluorouracil intraoperatively at a dose of 25 mg/ml for 3 minutes has been described in a recent report. The authors also injected the medication into the pterygium when a recurrence was noted. Patients had pain and corneal surface toxicity with the use of this medication, and the 25% recurrence rate in this small series indicates the need for further evaluation of this approach.

The use of beta-irradiation in the dosage of 15 Gy in either single or divided doses, and the use of 1:2,000 thiotepa drops given every 3 hours for approximately 6 weeks has also been described. Despite reasonable outcomes, the potential for ocular tissue toxicity exists and therefore, these adjuncts should be used with caution. Since the use of these agents can result in toxicity, other approaches attempt to eliminate the need for such adjuvants by covering the area left bare by pterygium excision.

Conjunctival and Amniotic Membrane Grafting

This approach uses limbal-conjunctival autografting from the unaffected superotemporal quadrant of the bulbar conjunctiva (Fig. 4.25).

The surgical steps are described in detail below:
1. A wire speculum is used to separate the lids. A superior rectus bridle suture is inserted using 4-0 black silk. The suture is used to abduct the eye maximally (assume nasal pterygium), by clipping it to the drapes adjacent to the lateral canthus, after passing it under the arm of the wire speculum.

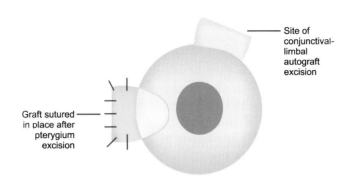

Graft sutured in place after pterygium excision

Site of conjunctival-limbal autograft excision

Fig. 4.25: Conjunctival-limbal autograft

2. A small incision is made in the conjunctiva just medial to the head of the pterygium avoiding the obviously altered conjunctiva on the head of the pterygium. Beginning here, the conjunctiva is progressively dissected from the body of the pterygium, towards the caruncle, using Westcott scissors. Care is taken to release only the conjunctiva and this is achieved by tenting up the dissected conjunctiva and snipping the taut adhesions to the subconjunctival tissue. The process is completed towards the upper fornix, caruncle and lower fornix in the shape of a triangle with its apex at the limbus, avoiding any conjunctival buttonholing. The head of the pterygium is left attached to the cornea and serves as a third hand for the surgeon, enabling easier dissection of the conjunctiva.

3. The corneal epithelium 1 mm ahead of the head of the pterygium is scraped off with a hockey-stick knife (Grieshaber). This exposes the altered epithelium just adjacent to the head of the pterygium, which is thickened and more firmly attached to the underlying cornea. The hockey-stick knife is used to elevate this thickened epithelium off the underlying cornea. Once this plane is defined, the pterygium head is easily avulsed using a combination of blunt dissection and traction. Residual fibrous tissue on the cornea is removed using sharp dissection with a no. 15 Bard-Parker blade.

4. In primary pterygia, a cotton bud can be used to elevate the body of the pterygium off the sclera. In recurrent pterygia, a combination of blunt and sharp dissection is used to remove the adherent fibrovascular tissue from the scleral surface. Especially in recurrent pterygia, extreme care is taken to avoid damage to the medial rectus muscle. In these lesions, extreme medial dissection is avoided as the vascular caruncular tissue is often dragged towards the cornea by the cicatricial tissue and damage to this tissue results in extensive bleeding.

5. The body of the pterygium with the involved Tenon's capsule and cicatrix is then excised, taking care to ensure the safety of the underlying medial rectus muscle and the overlying conjunctiva. In recurrent pterygia with extensive scarring, it may be prudent to tag and isolate the medial rectus muscle to ensure its safety. The abnormal tissue at the limbal end of the pterygium is aggressively resected often extending about 2 to 3 mm beyond the visible extent of the pterygium to avoid leaving behind any scaffold for a later recurrence and to have a good bed for placement of the graft.

6. The size of the conjunctival graft required to resurface the exposed scleral surface is determined using Castroviejo calipers in 3 directions—extent across the limbus, maximum circumferential extent of the bed, and maximum distance from the limbus. This allows the harvested graft to fit precisely in the bed.

7. Careful hemostasis of the exposed scleral surface is obtained using wet-field cautery. Extensive blanching of the scleral surface is avoided. The limbus is smoothed using a stroking motion with the edge of the hockey-stick knife held perpendicular to the limbal surface.

8. The bridle suture is used to rotate the globe downwards exposing the superior limbus and conjunctival surface. The measured dimensions are marked onto the superotemporal conjunctiva using several cautery spots. Using a Pierce-Hoskins forceps and Westcott scissors, the graft is excised starting at the forniceal end. Care is taken to obtain as thin a graft as possible without buttonholing. Once the limbus is reached, the graft is flipped over onto the cornea and the Tenon's attachments at the limbus are meticulously dissected. The flap is then excised using a Vannas scissors, taking care to include the limbal tissue.

9. After excision, the conjunctival-limbal graft is slid onto the cornea. Without lifting the tissue off the cornea, it is rotated and moved into its scleral bed with fine non-toothed forceps. A limbus-limbus orientation is maintained. This maneuver avoids inadvertent scrolling of the graft and possible inversion of the epithelial surface. The graft is smoothed out in its bed taking care to avoid any folding of the edges.

10. The eye is again abducted and the graft secured in position using interrupted 10-0 nylon sutures. The 4 corners of the graft are anchored with episcleral bites to maintain the graft in its position. The medial edge of the graft is sutured with 2 to 4 additional sutures, preferably including episclera. No sutures are placed on the limbal side of the graft.

11. The superior rectus bridle suture is removed and pulling the forniceal conjunctiva forwards covers the donor area and anchoring it to the limbal episcleral tissue with 2 interrupted 10-0 nylon sutures. No undermining of the superior conjunctiva is performed.

12. A dose of 0.5 cc dexamethasone is injected subconjunctivally at the conclusion of the procedure and the eye is patched firmly with antibiotic eye ointment.

Postoperatively, topical steroid eyedrops are used 2 hourly for the first postoperative week and then tapered over the next 5 to 6 weeks. Antibiotic ointment is used 3 times daily for the first 2 weeks. Retained sutures are removed at 6 weeks. The importance of using adequate steroid therapy in the postoperative management of these patients has been highlighted in a recent article.

Although considered technically more difficult than the standard resection procedures described earlier, requiring injection anesthesia and longer duration of surgery, this procedure has produced acceptable outcomes with excellent cosmesis. The rationale for the use of this procedure was the need to reconstruct the area of localized limbal insufficiency that has been described to occur in these eyes. However, other studies using a free conjunctival graft that does not contain limbal tissue have also resulted in low recurrence rates and this suggests that the barrier effect of the graft may also be important. Since there is some concern about creating extensive disturbances in the superior bulbar conjunctiva, in case such patients develop glaucoma later, it has been suggested that the inferior bulbar conjunctiva be used as a donor to cover the bare scleral bed after pterygium excision. In patients with double-headed pterygia, the use of a rotational autograft—wherein the conjunctiva is dissected off the body of the pterygium and replaced with the limbal side facing the canthus, has been described to produce acceptable recurrence rates, although the procedure has poorer cosmesis. In those with very extensive pterygia, the use of an annular graft to cover the bare area has been proposed.

The recurrence rate with the use of a conjunctival autograft technique, while generally acceptable, can vary from study to study. This variability is probably a result of individual variations in surgical technique, as this is a technically exacting procedure. Few serious complications result from this technique, and are usually related to hemorrhage under the graft or the inversion of the graft, in which instance the graft fails to be incorporated on the ocular surface.

Another option to resurface the scleral bed after pterygium excision is the use of an amniotic membrane graft. However, after initial enthusiasm regarding its use, recent papers indicate that the recurrence rates following the use of this technique are unacceptably high. Combining the use of amniotic membrane with limbal-conjunctival grafting may be an option in eyes with extensive lesions that result in symblepharon formation.

Apart from these techniques, there are some others, which are much less prevalent and not in common use—such as the use of lamellar corneal grafts, splitting and burying the head of the pterygium, etc. These are not well documented in the literature and their exact role in the surgical management of a pterygium is still not clear.

Although pterygium surgery is often considered a "simple" operation and is performed as an outpatient office procedure, the first surgery has the best chance of success with recurrent pterygia known to have a more aggressive behavior. Care is also required, since intraoperative complications like perforations during anesthetic injection, pterygium excision and sutures, disinsertion of recti, hemorrhage under the conjunctival graft, inverse placement of graft, and postoperative problems like infection, scarring, ocular movement disorders, scleral or corneal melting and recurrence can occur.

There are still many unanswered questions about pterygium pathogenesis and the optimal surgical solution. The ideal timing of surgical intervention and the effect of pterygium removal on corneal topography and final refractive error are still being studied. Based on current knowledge, until further improvements in surgical technique are available, the use of a conjunctival autograft appears to offer the best chance of success. Equivalent success can also be achieved using mitomycin-C, although the long-term consequences of such an approach are still unclear.

PENETRATING KERATOPLASTY

Indications and Patient Assessment

A corneal transplant is performed in eyes, which have visual potential that is not attained due to the corneal disease interfering with clarity, refractive ability, or integrity of the cornea. Other indications may be to relieve pain, or to treat infectious keratitis refractory to medical therapy, and rarely for cosmetic purposes. This procedure was first performed by Zirm in 1905; and with improvement in eye banking techniques, increasing numbers of procedures have been performed in the past decades, although there have been a very few changes in the underlying principles. However, with the advent and increasing popularity of the lamellar replacement techniques, the indications for a full-thickness corneal replacement procedure have decreased, but this is still the gold standard in corneal conditions that are not amenable to the lamellar procedures—as in full-thickness scars (Fig. 4.26). Careful assessment of the ocular status and the patient is important for successful corneal transplantation.

When assessing the eye, the existing vision and the potential improvement after surgery, the contribution of the corneal pathology to the visual deficit must be determined. It is important to rule out foci of infection in the ocular and periocular tissues, including the lids and nasolacrimal system. The presence of healthy, normal lids that can surface the cornea adequately during

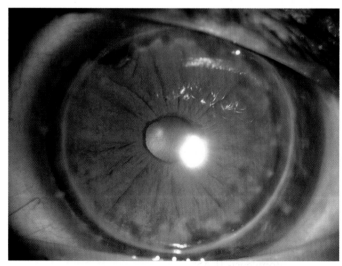

Fig. 4.26: Successful penetrating keratoplasty

blinking must be ensured. The presence of conditions like entropion, ectropion, trichiasis, distichiasis and lagophthalmos must be recognized and managed before performing the surgical procedure. A healthy tear film is essential for good anatomical and functional success after corneal grafting. The presence of a functional limbus and normal corneal innervation is important for adequate corneal healing after surgery. Corneal vascularization, scars, and previous corneal surgery, especially corneal grafting, increase the risk of failure. Evidence of past or present inflammation in the anterior chamber must be noted, as also the status of the crystalline lens. The intraocular pressure (IOP) and functional potential of the optic nerve and retina must be recorded. Factors known to be associated with worse outcomes include corneal vascularization, active inflammation at the time of transplantation or in the past, increased IOP, prior pregnancy or blood transfusion, trephine size < 7.0 mm or > 8.5 mm, and poor patient compliance.

The systemic health of the patient is evaluated with particular attention to diabetes, coagulation disorders, foci of sepsis, and other parameters that may affect the choice of anesthesia. The mental health of the patient, his or her expectations from the surgical procedure and the presence of a support system for postoperative care must be ensured. Apart from these considerations, it is also important for the surgeon to have a detailed discussion with the patient regarding the pros and cons of the procedure and the possible benefits of the procedure must be decided based on a realistic assessment of the chances of anatomical and functional success of the corneal graft, the vision in the other eye, the visual needs of the patient, and the possible need for and side effects of postoperative treatment regimens, such as systemic immunosuppression.

Contraindications

The *Eye Bank Association of America* has developed a set of criteria for donor corneas. Contraindications for the use of donor tissue for penetrating keratoplasty include:

- Death of unknown cause;
- Central nervous system diseases, such as Creutzfeldt-Jakob disease, subacute sclerosing panencephalitis, rubella, Reye's syndrome, rabies and infectious encephalitis;
- Infections such as human immunodeficiency virus, hepatitis, septicemia, syphilis and endocarditis;
- Eye diseases such as retinoblastoma, malignant tumor of anterior segment, and active ocular inflammation (e.g. uveitis, scleritis, retinitis and choroiditis);
- Prior ocular surgery (although pseudophakic eyes may be used if the endothelial cell density is good);
- Congenital or acquired anterior segment abnormalities, such as keratoconus and Fuchs endothelial dystrophy.

To this list must now be added the prior performance of corneal refractive surgical procedures, as the use of such eyes can result in unpredictable refractive outcomes and the laser in-situ keratomileusis (LASIK) flap is unlikely to withstand the surgical manipulations.

Surgical Technique

Preoperative antibiotics—one of the newer fluoroquinolones, is used topically preferably 2 hours before surgery, once every 30 minutes. Appropriate anesthesia is administered, which ensures that the patient is comfortably positioned, with no increase in orbital pressure and the eye in primary position. While some surgeons prefer general anesthesia routinely, the surgery can also be performed using orbital infiltration anesthesia. It is, however, important to use a long-acting agent (a 50:50 mixture of 2% lidocaine and 0.75% bupivacaine) and to use a Honan balloon or similar device to ensure a low orbital and IOP before commencing surgery. The patient should also understand that he should lie comfortably still without head movement and straining for the duration of the surgery—if local anesthesia is to be used. Routine asepsis and draping are performed ensuring that the lid margins are draped with sterile plastic to avoid the contamination of the operative field by meibomian gland secretions and the lashes.

A speculum is used to achieve good exposure of the cornea and care is taken when choosing the speculum to ensure that there is no untoward pressure on the globe. It is preferable to support the sclera with a Flieringa ring or similar device to reduce the risk of a severe scleral collapse when the eye is opened. This is particularly important in very young children, adults with keratoconus, high myopes and in aphakic eyes. Usually 4 to 6 interrupted sutures are used to anchor the ring to the episcleral tissues. A suture with sufficient tensile strength is used for this purpose, e.g. 8-0 nylon—and it is important to ensure that the sutures are placed equidistant from the limbus and from each other and tied with equal tension to reduce distortion of the host opening by the ring. Bridle sutures, to ensure horizontal placement of the eye and prevent torsion when trephination is performed, may be taken through the ring if it is used, or through the superior and inferior rectus muscles.

After ensuring proper tension on the bridle sutures, the corneal center is marked. In most instances of optical corneal grafting, it is preferable to center the trephine cut on this mark. Rare exceptions when a slight decentration is permitted are in eccentric cones seen in keratoconus and some corneal scars with localized thinning in the paracentral or peripheral cornea. However, it should be remembered that extensive decentration of the graft results in poor visual function. It is also important that the pupillary area is located behind the apex of the graft. Most optical corneal grafts use trephine sizes between 7 and 8.5 mm. Smaller sizes result in excessive astigmatism, suture placement close to the visual axis, and inadequate endothelial transfer. Larger grafts approach the limbal vasculature, increasing the risk of graft vascularization and immunological reactions, and may result in angle compromise and compression. It is ideal if the graft margin is central to the limbus by at least 1.5 mm all around as this will ensure that the corneal sutures do not engage limbal vessels—since this can promote the risk of such vessels crossing the graft-host junction and promoting an immune reaction. After ensuring proper graft size, a radial keratotomy marker is used to ink the corneal surface with radial marks that will serve as guides for the placement of sutures. The presence of the marks ensures more equitable distribution of the sutures around the circumference of the graft.

A variety of trephine systems are used to create the recipient opening and donor button. A free hand trephine can be used, but care is required during usage to avoid tilting of the trephine, which can result in irregularities in the edge profile and the shape of the corneal opening. Making sure of the vertical position of the trephine on the cornea before starting the cut can help achieve vertical walls. Rotating the trephine in one direction and making large (180°) rotations, rather than small side-to-side twisting motions, are also helpful. It is important to watch the central cornea through the barrel of the trephine; and if a localized wrinkling of the cut edges is seen, it indicates that the trephine is cutting deeper in that meridian and this will often result in a shelving corneal cut. To correct this, it is important to use more pressure on the trephine cut in the meridian opposite to where the wrinkles manifest. In eyes with advanced keratoconus, the steep cone may interfere with proper placement of the trephine. In such eyes, the application of cautery to the apex of the cone will result in shrinkage of the collagen and flattening of the cone—which will allow better placement of the trephine. It has been suggested that such cauterization may also improve the postoperative refractive outcomes of penetrating keratoplasty in these eyes. The vacuum-based systems, such as the Hessburg-Barron trephine, tend to perform better, since the vacuum in the barrel of the trephine holds the cornea against the cutting blade. The mechanized trephines like the Hanna system tend to provide excellent cuts in the recipient and have the advantage that they can also be used to prepare the donor button from the epithelial side, thus ensuring that the cuts are better matched. More recently, the use of a template and excimer laser corneal ablation has been described to achieve very precise cuts in the recipient and the donor. The use of a template also allows the creation of small teeth in the donor edge and matching notches in the recipient that allow the graft to fit securely in the bed. The use of the latter two systems, however, is associated with a significant increase in the cost of the procedure. With a good trephine cut, at the time of entry into the anterior chamber, most of the posterior surface should be cut and the walls of the cut should be vertical.

The cut can be completed with corneoscleral scissors taking care to maintain the plane of the trephine cut. To protect the iris and lens if present, the use of miotics and viscoelastics may be considered, but are not essential. Some surgeons prefer to leave a small posterior ledge of tissue in the recipient wound margin believing that this provides support during the placement of the donor button and increases the security of the closure. A situation where this modification is of particular help is in aphakic keratoplasty in which the performance of the anterior vitrectomy can sometimes result in a scleral collapse and distortion of the recipient opening despite the presence of a Flieringa ring. In such situations, the presence of a ledge in the recipient opening is helpful. In eyes with long-standing bullous keratopathy, the Descemet's membrane is often easily detached from the stroma. Failure to recognize and excise this diaphanous membrane during recipient corneal excision can result in the retention of this membrane and the formation of a double anterior chamber, which is noted in the postoperative period. This is sometimes compatible with graft endothelial function, although in some eyes the retained membrane can result in gradual clouding of the graft due to compromised endothelial function. Dealing with this retained membrane requires surgical excision or in the event of graft failure, a repeat keratoplasty. However, in some instances, the neodymium:yttrium-aluminum-garnet (Nd:YAG) laser can be used to make an opening in the retained membrane to allow the flow of aqueous into the second chamber, which may allow survival of the transplanted endothelium. After the graft is excised, any intraocular procedures that may be required are completed, such as, anterior vitrectomy, synechiolysis, pupilloplasty, cataract extraction, etc. In aphakic keratoplasty, particular attention is paid to in dealing with vitreous remnants in the anterior chamber, existing peripheral anterior synechiae, and the iris diaphragm itself, since the occurrence of peripheral anterior synechiae in these eyes in the postoperative period can result in serious problems like glaucoma, shallowing of the anterior chamber, endothelial loss and graft rejection. It is important to ensure complete removal of vitreous, if present, from the anterior chamber, especially from the angles. When vitreous bulges into the anterior chamber, using the vitrector positioned at the pupil may result in leaving behind residual small islands of gel in the angle recess. In time, these tend to contract and result in the formation of peripheral anterior synechiae, which can gradually progress in a zipper-like fashion around the circumference of the angle. The use of intracameral triamcinolone to help identify the vitreous may help in more thorough removal of the gel. Existing anterior synechiae of the peripheral iris to the cornea must be released. Tenuous adhesions are easily lysed with a blunt spatula or iris spatula. However, some of these adhesions tend to be more tenacious and in these eyes holding the host margin with forceps and using small dry Weck-Cel sponge bit held in a forceps to gently strip the adhesion from the center to the periphery can be a useful technique. If however, there are fibrous adhesions, then sharp dissection with scissors and/or a knife may be necessary. To ensure a thorough separation of the adhesions, the use of a small dental mirror to image the angle intraoperatively has been described. To ensure that these synechiae do not reform in the postoperative period, it is important to create a taut iris diaphragm. This is particular of importance in eyes that have received a sector iridectomy and have lax iris pillars that can move forward in the postoperative period (Fig. 4.27). Such a procedure may also have cosmetic benefits for the patient and in some eyes can result in a more central pupillary position and improved visual function. A peripheral iridectomy may be performed in phakic eyes or if increased anterior chamber reaction is anticipated in the postoperative period.

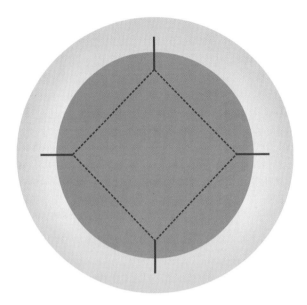

Fig. 4.27: Tension lines forming a square after 4 cardinal sutures

Cataract surgery is often combined with corneal transplantation. In eyes that have a relatively transparent cornea and a lens, which is not very dense, this can be achieved using phacoemulsification. If this is not possible due to poor visualization of the anterior chamber structures, then a partial-thickness trephination and removal of a 90% thickness anterior lamellar button within the trephination can be tried. If the thin posterior layers are sufficiently clear, the procedure may now be completed, especially if methylcellulose is placed over the corneal stroma. Even if complete phacoemulsification is not possible, an attempt is made to create an anterior capsulorhexis through the recipient cornea. If this can be achieved, the central corneal opening is then created and the rest of the cataract surgery is completed in an open-sky fashion. The presence of an anterior capsulorhexis allows secure in-the-bag placement of the IOL and this results in minimal optic iris contact and this can be of significant advantage in the context of a penetrating keratoplasty in which iritis can predispose to greater graft endothelial damage. The creation of a capsulorhexis in an open-sky approach is possible only if there is a very soft eye, with no upthrust, since these factors can result in a loss of the rhexis with the tear running peripherally. The determination of the appropriate intraocular lens power can prove to be a problem in such eyes, since the recipient cornea at the time of surgery has a very irregular surface (keratometry may not be possible) and the curvature of the postoperative corneal graft may be considerably different. Methods suggested to overcome this problem include—the use of an average postoperative keratometry value retrospectively calculated from the surgeon's series of patients; using keratometry data from the fellow eye; a standard value of 44 D; and using data from the cadaver donor eye. While an in-the-bag IOL would be ideal, anterior chamber lenses, iris, sulcus and scleral fixation have also been used.

After completion of the intraocular maneuvers, viscoelastic is used to cover the surface of the iris and lens and is also placed in the angle. Although mentioned after recipient bed preparation in this discussion, the surgeon must remember that during surgery, the donor graft is always prepared first—prior to recipient eye manipulations in penetrating keratoplasty. In the event of inadvertent damage to the donor button, surgery can be aborted without any recipient eye damage. For the same reason, it is also important that the assistant retains the excised recipient corneal button in the sterile surgical tray until the donor button has been safely transferred from the holding medium onto the recipient eye and has been anchored in place using sutures. In the event of the donor tissue becoming contaminated during transfer (if it is dropped, for instance), even if there is no other tissue available, the recipient button can be replaced and sutured and surgery repeated with good donor tissue at a subsequent time. The donor button is prepared by punching from the endothelial side with a free hand punch trephine after positioning the corneoscleral rim in a Teflon block. When using this system, it is important to ensure that a clean cut has been created all around with the trephine before it is lifted off the corneoscleral rim. This can be ensured by gently lifting the edges of the corneoscleral rim and ensuring that the rim rides up on the barrel of the trephine before lifting the trephine. In the event of an incomplete cut, the rim is shifted to the microscope and corneoscleral scissors are used to carefully complete the cut, and free the central disc of donor tissue. Occasionally, the cut button tends to remain within the barrel of the trephine, in which case BSS can be gently trickled onto the inner wall of the trephine to dislodge the button onto the underlying Teflon block.

In some systems, as mentioned earlier, an artificial anterior chamber allows the trephination of the donor from the epithelial surface. A Paton Spatula is used to transfer the donor button to the recipient eye. The graft is gently tipped into the recipient bed and rotated to ensure a proper fit. In general, the donor button is oversized by 0.25 to 0.50 mm to reduce the chances of angle compression and increased IOP in the postoperative period. A two-toothed Polack forceps is helpful in anchoring the donor button to enable easy passage of the first donor graft suture. The preferred suture material in corneal transplantation is 10-0 nylon. Although the first suture is technically the hardest to place because of the excessive movement of the free graft, it is the second suture, which is placed at 6 o'clock, which is the more important, since it determines the distribution of the graft tissue on the two sides of the meridian between 6 and 12 o'clock. The uses of marks in the recipient cornea facilitate the placement of the suture on the host margin. With the suture engaging the 6 o'clock position of the graft, the needle is positioned in the host; and before it is drawn through the tissue, an inspection of the tissue distribution on either side of the proposed suture is made to ensure that this is equitable. If there is too much overlap of the graft margin over the recipient rim on one side, then the needle is withdrawn from the host and repositioned away from the side of the overlap till good distribution is seen. After these two sutures, two others are placed at 3 and 9 o'clock and these four are termed the cardinal sutures. Since these serve as guides for the placement of the subsequent sutures, it is important to take time to ensure that these are well placed. The appearance of a furrow in the donor button, in the form of a square, connecting the edges of the 4 cardinal sutures indicates appropriate placement of these sutures (Fig. 4.28). Subsequent suture placement is relatively simpler—because the graft is now secured and tends to shift less, the needle needs to pass between each pair of cardinal sutures, and the position of the corneal furrow indicates the position of the bite in the donor corneal button.

Suturing is an important part of the procedure and care is taken to adhere to all the surgical tenets, as discussed in the section on corneal trauma. Briefly, interrupted sutures are passed radial to the graft-host junction, and are placed equidistant from the wound margin in both the donor and the recipient. The depth of the suture is ideally 90% in both tissues to ensure that there is good apposition of both the anterior and the posterior surfaces of the donor and the recipient. Care is taken to avoid excessive handling of the graft epithelium and margins by the forceps, and also to avoid excessive bending of the graft as this can result in increased endothelial damage. Although full-thickness suturing has been described, it is generally avoided as there can be increased leakage from the suture track, and there is also a risk of endophthalmitis when suture removal is required at a later date. The sutures are tied with equal tension to reduce the occurrence of high postoperative astigmatism. The knots are buried—usually in the recipient stroma—at the conclusion of the procedure, and rotated such that the arrowhead formed by the knot and the free ends point towards the surface. The knot is placed just beneath the surface as this facilitates easy and atraumatic removal later. Interrupted sutures are preferred in young children since wound healing can be very rapid in these eyes (Fig. 4.29). For the same reason, an interrupted suture technique is preferred in eyes, which have a

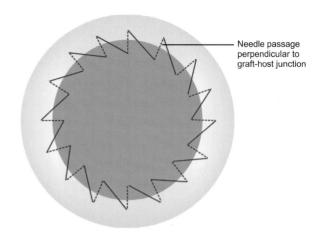

Fig. 4.29: Continuous running torque sutures

host rim that is irregular in thickness and vascularization. In the event of uneven healing in these eyes, some sutures may require removal at an early date because of loosening and in this context; a continuous suture is undesirable, as the loose loop would compromise the integrity of the suture in the other areas, which may have inadequate healing.

A continuous suture, however, offers greater security of closure and is faster to apply and, therefore, a good option in elderly patients with edematous corneas, in whom healing may be slower. A 24-bite continuous suture is usually preferred and can be applied using either the torque or anti-torque technique. In the former method, the bites of the needle across the graft-host junction are placed in a radial fashion (Fig. 4.30). Sometimes, two continuous sutures are employed, one with 10-0 and the other with 11-0 nylon, the rationale being, that in the event of high postoperative astigmatism, the 11-0 suture can be removed to modulate the astigmatism while the other suture continues to secure the wound. However, the preferred technique of astigmatism modulation with a continuous suture is suture adjustment. After determining the steep and flat axes of the graft in the early postoperative period, the patient can be treated either at the slit lamp or under the operating microscope, usually at 4 weeks after surgery, if astigmatism is > 3 D. The suture loops in the flat meridian are pulled into the

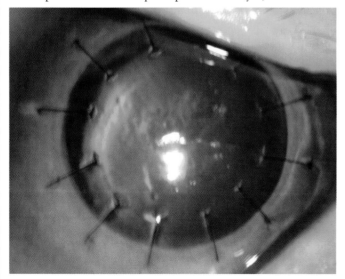

Fig. 4.28: Interrupted corneal graft sutures

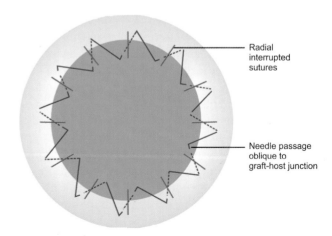

Fig. 4.30: Continuous running anti-torque sutures

steeper meridians to steepen the flat meridian and vice versa. This maneuver is performed with a pair of jeweler forceps or specially designed smooth rods that reduce the risk of suture breakage. As is obvious, the disadvantage of suture manipulation in the early postoperative period—apart from the risk of infection, is that suture breakage will require resuturing as the wound is still poorly healed.

Another approach uses a combination of interrupted and continuous sutures to secure the wound. After 12 deeply placed interrupted sutures have been placed to secure the graft and provide watertight closure, a 12-bite continuous anti-torque suture is passed. With this suture technique, the passage of the needle across the wound is in an oblique manner and the resultant suture looks like an equilateral triangle (Fig. 4.31). With this approach, the interrupted sutures can be removed as early as one month after surgery, based on the astigmatism, since the continuous suture ensures the safety of wound closure. At the conclusion of suturing, the use of a Troutman handheld qualitative keratometer helps determine if excessive astigmatism has been induced by the sutures. The room lights are dimmed and the keratometer is held close to the corneal surface. The epithelial surface of the graft is irrigated with BSS and the reflection of the keratometer mires from the central graft is noted. Circular mires indicate that the astigmatism is likely to be less than 3 D, while an oval pattern indicates astigmatism greater than this value with the steeper axis in the shorter meridian of the oval. The surgeon can then adjust the continuous suture or replace interrupted sutures to achieve a more regular corneal surface. The disadvantage of this approach, however, is that even if an ideal curvature is achieved at the end of the suturing process, the wound healing process is likely to resulting alterations in this endpoint.

After adequate suturing, it is important to ensure that a deep anterior chamber is formed by injecting BSS through the graft-host junction. At the conclusion of surgery, a subconjunctival injection of antibiotic and steroid is used as the graft is relatively unsterile (despite the presence of antibiotic in the corneal storage solution), and the steroid helps reduce inflammation.

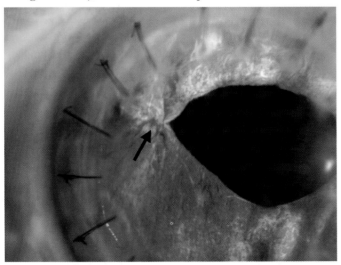

Fig. 4.31: Pupilloplasty to tighten lax iris diaphragm

Postoperative Care

Steroids still remain the mainstay of postpenetrating kerato-plasty treatment and are used frequently in the initial weeks after surgery—depending on the level of inflammation in the anterior chamber; a potent steroid, such as dexamethasone or prednisolone may be used hourly or 6 times a day. As the inflammation subsides, the dosage is rapidly reduced, and it is customary to use the medication 4 times a day by 6 weeks after surgery. Further tapering to once daily is usually possible by the fourth postoperative month; and thereafter, in uncomplicated surgeries, a less potent steroid like fluorometholone may be used at daily or alternate day dosage for longer periods. While there is no general consensus, some surgeons prefer to continue this low dose of medication for the life of the graft, in the absence of complications in the lens and IOP. Apart from steroids, a cycloplegic is usually used for the first 2 weeks, in the presence of anterior chamber inflammation. In keratoconus, this may be avoided if the Urrets-Zavalia syndrome is considered a risk. Intraocular pressure monitoring and management in the initial postoperative period is important to ensure adequate wound healing. In high-risk corneal transplants, it may be necessary to institute systemic immunosuppression and this is best done in consultation with an internist. Systemic steroids may be considered in eyes that have severe inflammation postoperatively. Topical tear substitutes in the initial postoperative period help in promoting epithelial health. Other medications may be needed in individual instances, such as oral acyclovir in a patient undergoing penetrating grafts for sequelae of herpes simplex keratitis, to reduce the risk of a viral recurrence in the postoperative period, especially during intensive steroid therapy.

Care of the post-transplant eye is important, especially in the early postoperative period when the following are monitored—signs of infection, poor graft-host wound apposition with leakage of aqueous, graft clarity and endothelial function, status of the corneal epithelium, depth and reaction in the anterior chamber, IOP, iris synechiae and pupillary block. Later, in the postoperative period, epithelial problems like superficial punctuate keratitis either due to sicca, irregular graft-host junction, trichiasis, exposure, or due to medication toxicity, epithelial defects, filaments, and suture loosening with or without infection, and sterile suture infiltrates may occur and need attention (Fig. 4.32). In the late postoperative period, important problems include astigmatism, immunological graft rejection, graft failure and glaucoma.

Graft rejection remains the most common cause of graft failure. Distinct types of rejection have been described and include—epithelial rejection (Figs. 4.33A and B), subepithelial infiltrates (Fig. 4.34), stromal rejection, endothelial rejection (Fig. 4.35), and mixed types. Of these, the most important is the endothelial rejection. Management of graft rejection is with steroids—depending on the severity and type of rejection, these may be used topically, orally, and as subconjunctival injections. The use of 500 mg intravenous methylprednisolone as a slow infusion in patients who present early in the rejection process has been

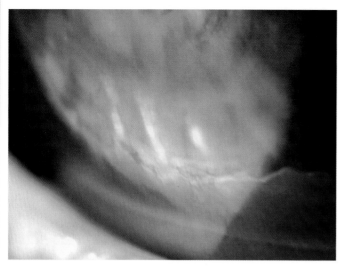

Fig. 4.32: Suture vascularization and multiple sterile infiltrates

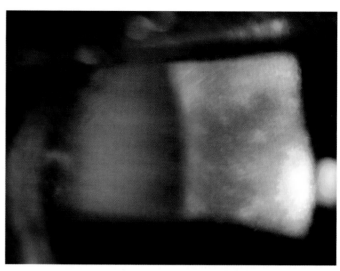

Fig. 4.34: Corneal graft rejection—subepithelial infiltrates

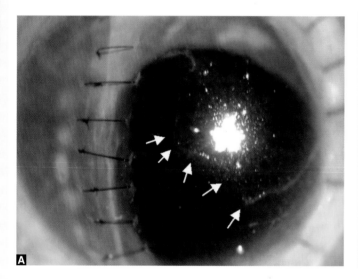

Figs 4.33A and B: Corneal graft rejection—epithelial (A) Epithelial rejection line, (B) Fluorescein staining

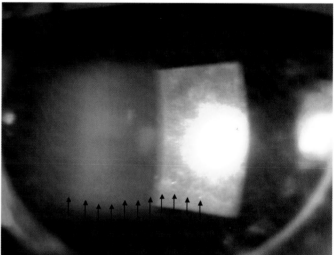

Fig. 4.35: Corneal graft rejection—Khodadoust line

shown to have a beneficial effect in reversing the rejection and may also confer some immunity against a subsequent recurrence. However, these infusions can be associated with significant electrolyte shifts and require the patient to be admitted and monitored during the infusion, as sudden death has been rarely reported. In addition, a more recent study reported no additional benefit with the use of pulse methylprednisolone therapy when compared with topical steroid therapy.

Therapeutic Penetrating Keratoplasty

This is a special indication for full-thickness penetrating keratoplasty in an eye with corneal infection that does not respond to medical therapy and requires surgical removal of the infiltrated tissue to preserve ocular integrity; and in some instances, to prevent further spread of the infection (Figs. 4.36A and B). In some of these eyes, a pre-existent corneal perforation may be present at the time of surgery. Apart from the general principles

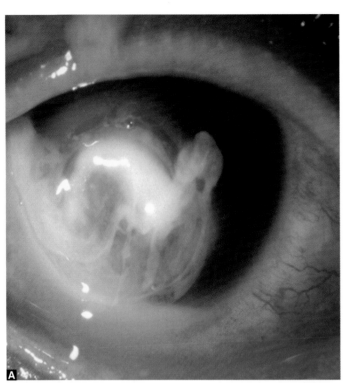
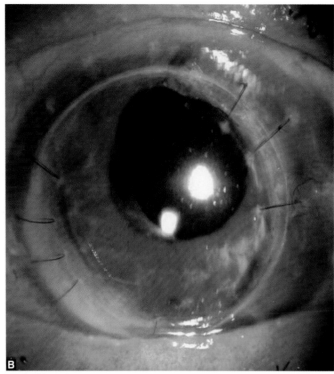

Figs 4.36A and B: Therapeutic penetrating keratoplasty—*Pseudomonas* keratitis (A) Corneal infection with hypopyon. (B) Post-therapeutic penetrating keratoplasty

described earlier, it is important to try and perform the surgery under general anesthesia when possible, especially if there is a corneal perforation. The use of intravenous mannitol prior to surgery may help reduce the vitreous pressure in these inflamed eyes. If there is a perforation, then attempts to trephine the recipient cornea of the soft eye are best avoided. After a mark with the appropriate sized trephine is made, it is preferable to introduce the scissors through the perforation and perform a radial cut to the trephine mark and then excise the cornea along the mark. It is important to ensure that all the infected corneal tissues are included in the excised corneal button, which is sent for microbiological evaluation. A hypopyon is usually present and must be cleared, and uveal tissue inflammation can result in the formation of extensive fibrin during the surgical procedure. Where possible, the lens is retained, even if cataractous, since it will serve as a barrier to the posterior migration of the infection. Suturing of the graft is usually performed with interrupted sutures. Since there is often choroidal swelling and sometimes detachment in these inflamed eyes, reforming the anterior chamber at the conclusion of suturing can be a challenge, and may sometimes require the retention of viscoelastic in the anterior chamber. If the pathogen is identified, it may be prudent to inject the appropriate antimicrobial subconjunctivally and intracamerally. In the case of fungal keratitis, steroid use is absolutely contraindicated intraoperatively, and in the first 2 weeks postoperatively, till it is clinically evident that infection has been eradicated (Figs 4.37 and 4.38). In the case of bacterial and acanthameba keratitis, if satisfactory excision of the infected tissues has been achieved and the initial postoperative period is uneventful, steroids can be initiated earlier (Fig. 4.39).

Total Corneoscleral Transplantation

In some eyes with advanced total corneal infections, in the end-stage of Mooren's ulcer, or with extensive immune-mediated corneal melting, it may be difficult to obtain a recipient corneal rim into which the donor cornea can be sutured. In these difficult situations, total corneoscleral transfer may offer the chance of salvaging the eye.

After a 360° peritomy in the recipient eye, a 50% partial thickness scleral incision is made circumferentially about 1 mm posterior to the limbus. A scleral flap is then dissected till the limbus using a crescent knife. Once this is completed all around the limbus, the anterior chamber is entered at the limbus, under the scleral frill. Corneoscleral scissors are used to complete the limbal cut and the entire cornea with the scleral frill is excised. A similar graft is fashioned from a whole donor globe, with the scleral frill 1.5 mm wide. This graft is then transferred to the recipient after placing viscoelastic on the iris. Interrupted sutures of 9-0 nylon are used to secure the scleral frill of the donor to the recipient scleral bed. At 12, 3, 6 and 9 o'clock, angle forming sutures are passed to ensure that some portions of the angle of the recipient eye remain functional. These are placed using 10-0 nylon double-armed sutures. At each of these sites, the suture needle is passed through the inner lip of the limbal-scleral rim in the host tissue and then passed out through the full thickness of the limbus in the donor graft in an *ab interno* fashion. The mattress suture is then tied on the surface of the donor limbus and the knot buried. At the conclusion of surgery, the conjunctiva is positioned over the donor scleral frill and sutured in place. Postoperatively, apart from the routine

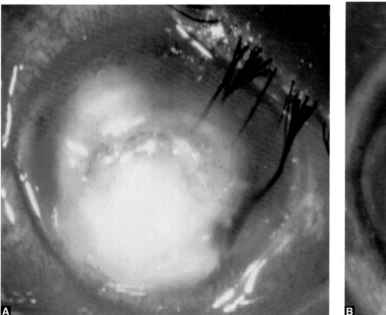

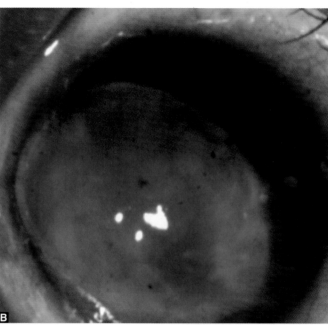

Figs 4.37A and B: Therapeutic penetrating keratoplasty—fungal keratitis. (A) Extensive fungal keratitis, (B) Anatomic success with opaque graft

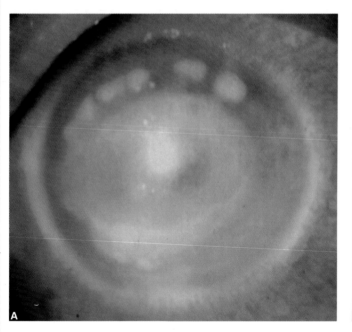

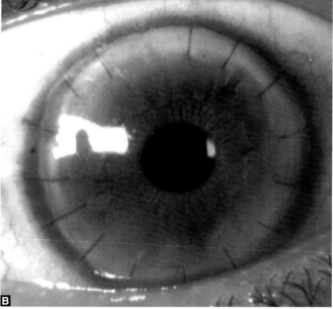

Figs 4.38A and B: Therapeutic penetrating keratoplasty—*Acanthamoeba* keratitis. (A) Acanthamoeba keratitis, (B) Anatomic success with clear graft

medications, immunosuppressive therapy is required and since glaucoma is a possibility, the IOP must be monitored periodically. Although technically more complicated than the other procedures described earlier, in some eyes where standard penetrating keratoplasty is considered impossible, this procedure offers an option for salvaging the eye (Figs 4.40 A and B).

Future Directions

The advent of newer immunosuppressive medications has improved the anatomical outcomes of corneal transplant procedures in high-risk eyes. Improved methods of trephination and an increased ability to modulate astigmatism in the postoperative period offer an opportunity to increase the functional success rates of penetrating keratoplasty. Better understanding of the potential of wavefront and topography modulated excimer ablations may also increase the functional success of these procedures, in eyes with clear grafts, but poor visual outcomes due to astigmatism and surface irregularities. Further advances in our knowledge of transplant immunology, specifically the issue of HLA matching may also offer new

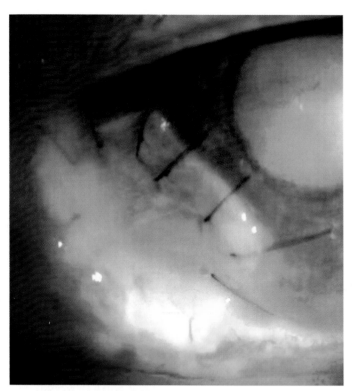

Fig. 4.39: Modified therapeutic penetrating keratoplasty. Full-thickness graft for peripheral perforated fungal ulcer

insights and improved success with penetrating keratoplasty in the coming years.

ANTERIOR LAMELLAR CORNEAL REPLACEMENT

Rationale

Although the technique of lamellar replacement of the anterior corneal layers has been in use for quite some time and was first described in 1830 by von Walther, initial success rates were less encouraging, largely due to the presence of interface scarring. With an improved understanding of corneal anatomy and the evolution of surgical techniques and instrumentation, an increased interest in such techniques in the recent past has resulted in the increasing popularity of this approach.

The idea of retaining the healthy host endothelium and limiting the surgical replacement of cornea to the diseased anterior stromal layers is obviously attractive—since most of the immunological consequences of the host immunological response affect the endothelium of the graft. While epithelial rejection is possible, it is seldom of serious import, and the occurrence of stromal rejection is quite rare. Achieving a regular stromal bed while ensuring the removal of all diseased stromal tissue and maintaining the transparency of the interface in the postoperative period, however, is technically demanding and it is possible that the presence of this interface may result in a quality of vision that is slightly less than that achieved by penetrating keratoplasty.

To ensure successful lamellar corneal surgery, it is important to pay attention to the surgical tenets described by Jose Barraquer. He proposed that it was important to achieve the deepest possible interface, with a uniform posterior stromal surface, and smooth sectioning of both the recipient and the donor interfaces, and to ensure that the interface remained free of deposits. In addition, it is important to ensure that the donor is of appropriate thickness, the edges coapt well, and appropriate suturing techniques are used to ensure a good refractive outcome. Improvements in surgical instrumentation and surgical techniques have allowed the present-day corneal surgeons to achieve many of these endpoints.

A major advance has been the understanding that the deeper the dissection in the cornea, the less the interface scarring. This is made possible by the differential structure of the

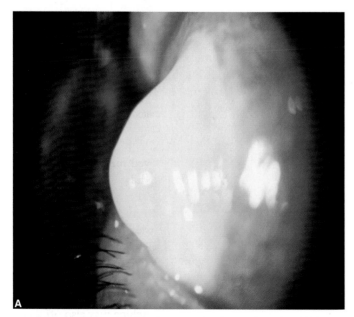
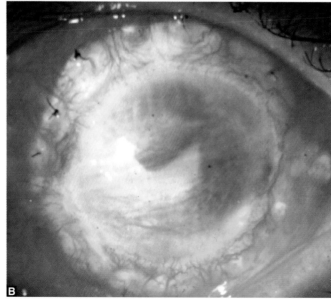

Figs 4.40A and B: Total corneoscleral transplantation. (A) Total corneal abscess, (B) Corneoscleral graft—early postoperative period

posterior corneal layers which course across the entire width of the cornea without a break. In general, the posterior stroma is more ordered, more hydrated, more easily swollen, and has a lower refractive index than the anterior stroma. The posterior lamellae are also wider and thicker (100–200 µm wide and 1.0–2.5 µm thick) than the anterior (0.5–30 µm wide and 0.2–1.2 µm thick). There are also differences in keratocyte morphology. These include a more regular arrangement of the collagen layers and a lesser keratocyte density.

Extending this concept of deep corneal dissection is the recognition that a potential plane of cleavage exists between the posterior stroma and the Descemet's membrane. Identification of this plane facilitates the removal of essentially the entire stroma leaving only the Descemet's membrane *in-situ*. However, a recent study indicates that this separation may occur within the banded and nonbanded portions of the Descemet's membrane in some eyes. Despite this, it is now clear that achieving this plane of dissection ensures an optimum quality to the interface, and most of the recent advances in anterior lamellar corneal surgery have focused on the development of techniques that permit the safe and reproducible creation of this plane during surgery.

Direct Surgical Dissection

With this approach, the goal is often to remove the bulk of the anterior corneal stroma by manual dissection using direct visualization, and this was initially described by Anwar. Of course, it is important to ensure that the residual stromal bed does not contain any of the opacified, scarred corneal tissue. In the event that the residual stroma contains opacified tissue, further dissection is performed in layers, until clear stroma is reached. An attempt to reach the plane of the Descemet's membrane is made only in the case of very deep opacities, since the risk of perforation increases greatly as the dissection is carried into the deeper layers. Normally, about 90% of the stromal tissue is removed as this provides the advantages of working in the posterior stromal layers, highlighted previously, and also produces a bed in which the donor tissue can be easily fitted (Fig. 4.41).

The surgical procedure can be performed using orbital local anesthetic infiltration and begins with marking of the corneal center. An appropriately sized trephine is then used to mark the area of corneal excision, centered on the corneal mark. Prior pachymetric mapping of the corneal surface will provide an idea of the thinnest corneal measurement and the trephine is set to cut to about 80% of this measurement. Alternatively, after the trephine makes the initial cut, the incision is deepened using a sharp knife in a freehand fashion. This allows the creation of a circular, vertical cut in the cornea following the mark of the trephine. Once a satisfactory depth has been reached, the cut central edge is held with corneal forceps and dissection is started in a horizontal plane at the base of the groove. This can be performed using a Grieshaber blade (No. 681.01), a crescent knife or the no. 15 Bard-Parker blade. When performing the dissection, it is important to ensure that the plane of

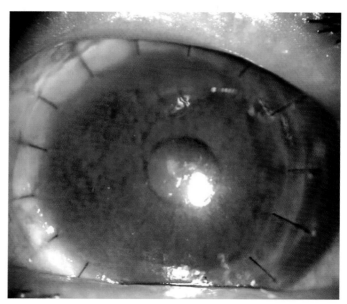

Fig. 4.41: Deep anterior lamellar keratoplasty—manual dissection. Post-deep anterior lamellar keratoplasty for extensive pseudopterygium

the dissection remains uniform, to achieve a smooth bed. In order to do this, the corneal stroma is retracted with a corneal forceps and the stretched corneal fibers are gently stroked with the blade held parallel to the posterior stromal surface. In this manner, the dissection is advanced across the corneal surface until the peripheral trephine dissected groove is reached in the opposite meridian, and the central disc of tissue can then be removed.

Several layers of tissue can be removed in succession using the same technique in order to ensure the two goals of removing all the opacified stroma and achieving a stromal bed that is only about 10% thick. When working close to the Descemet's membrane, a high IOP can predispose to perforation of the thin posterior layers. Thus, as the dissection proceeds posteriorly, it may be necessary to make a paracentesis to achieve a low IOP. Since the central corneal clarity is most critical for achieving a good visual outcome, once the initial dissection of the entire bed is completed, further attempts to remove tissue may be limited to the central part. Initiating the dissection can be performed by gently scratching on the exposed stromal surface using a sharp needle or knife. As the stromal fibers part, a new plane is created that can then be developed. A technique using the knife as described above can be used or a thin, smooth spatula can be inserted into the opening created and advanced in a sweeping maneuver to further separate the stromal layers prior to excision. Deroofing a 3 to 4 mm central window of Descemet's membrane or further thinning of the stroma in this region may suffice. A modification of this approach is the "divide and conquer" technique described by Tsubota et al. In this approach, after the initial partial-thickness trephination in the cornea, the disc is divided into 4 quadrants by two incisions at 90° to each other. This facilitates the dissection and removal of each of the 4 quadrants in turn.

Injection to Separate Descemet's Membrane

As mentioned earlier, it is preferable to achieve a plane of cleavage between the posterior stroma and the Descemet's membrane as this results in minimal interface scarring (Fig. 4.42). A variety of techniques have been described to help achieve this endpoint in a safe and reproducible manner. Variations and refinements have been described by Archila, Rostron, Sugita, Melles and Anwar. Briefly, the technique requires the use of air, viscoelastic or fluid injection into the corneal stroma and depends on the ability of the injected material to enter the pre-Descemet's space cleaving the stroma from the membrane. This separation allows the safe removal of the stroma, while retaining the Descemet's membrane.

Anwar described what he termed the "big bubble" technique, using air injection. Stromal trephination is first performed and between 60% and 80% of the stromal thickness is cut using a suction trephine. A 27 or 30-gauge needle is attached to an air filled syringe and bent at 60° with the bevel facing down. The needle is introduced into the trephined groove and advanced into the paracentral corneal stroma with the bevel facing down. This helps avoid inadvertent penetration of the Descemet's membrane and also facilitates the ability of the injected air to find the pre-Descemet's plane. When the needle tip is in the desired position, air is injected and an immediate whitening of the corneal stroma is noted due to the entry of air into the stromal lamellae. In an ideal situation a large bubble with a circular outline is noted, between the Descemet's membrane and the deep stroma and this is the desired endpoint. If, however, there is only a diffuse whitening of the stroma with no clear bubble formation, the process may be repeated at a second and third site.

The injection of air often results in an increase in IOP, due to the entry of air into the anterior chamber through the trabecular meshwork. A paracentesis is performed after air injection, to release some of the aqueous and reduce the IOP.

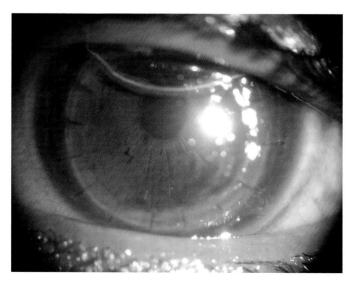

Fig. 4.42: Deep anterior lamellar keratoplasty—air injection. Post-deep anterior lamellar keratoplasty for advanced keratoconus

It is important, however, to avoid performing the paracentesis before air injection, since the entry of air through the cut in the Descemet's membrane may result in the enlargement of the tear. The anterior stroma is excised as described previously, exposing the roof of the "big bubble". A sharp knife is then used to enter the bubble tangentially, and the opening is carefully enlarged to permit the introduction of a spatula or cannula. The air usually escapes during this maneuver resulting in a collapse of the bubble. At this time, a low IOP is desirable and the paracentesis is used to release more aqueous. Using the entry created by the knife, a spatula is introduced to achieve further separation of the stroma from the Descemet's membrane, after which the anterior stromal layers are excised using scissors. Alternatively, viscoelastic can be used to achieve the same effect, and this also helps by coating the surface of the Descemet's membrane and prevents the scissors from dragging on the surface of the dry membrane.

During excision, it is important to avoid excessive traction on the corneal stroma as the attached fibers transmit the force to the delicate Descemet's membrane and can result in perforation. Making radial cuts in the roof of the bubble and removing the stroma in segments can also help. At the periphery of the stromal bed, a shelving cut is used to allow the retention of some stroma—as this allows safe suturing of the graft-host junction.

The use of fluid and viscoelastic injection is based on similar principles, but is less efficient and increases the risk of Descemet's rupture, as compared to the air injection technique. An excellent review of these techniques is available in an article by Anwar and Teichmann.

Closed Dissection Using Spatulated Dissectors

In an alternative approach that attempts to produce a defined depth of dissection in the corneal stroma, Melles used a closed approach and semi-sharp spatulas to produce a smooth plane in the dissected bed. The essence of this technique is to determine accurately the initial depth of entry into the corneal stroma as this determines the plane of subsequent dissection as well. In order to determine this depth, Melles has described a few signs. After creating an initial scleral incision at about 80% depth, a specially designed blunt spatula (DORC) is used to dissect into the peripheral corneal stroma. A paracentesis is made and the aqueous is completely replaced by air. The depth of dissection is checked by looking for the reflection of the instrument from the optical interface between the air and cornea. Two reflections are seen—one each from the anterior and posterior corneal surfaces and the position of the posterior corneal surface is halfway between these two reflections. As the spatula is advanced into the corneal stroma, it can be used to indent the air bubble, and this results in a semicircular specular reflex. The tip of the blade is separated from the reflex by the uncut posterior stroma, which appears as a dark band. The thinner the band, the deeper the position of the dissector in the corneal stroma and when this band is a thin dark line, the depth is approximately 90%. This is probably the most useful sign in determining the depth of the dissection, and can also be to periodically check the position of the instrument during the subsequent dissection as well. With the spatula in this position, a sweeping movement is performed in a side-to-side manner to create a pocket and using specially designed semi-sharp spatulated dissectors (DORC) the dissection is progressively increased to create a lamellar dissection of the entire corneal stroma from limbus to limbus at the same plane.

After this has been satisfactorily completed, viscoelastic is injected into the dissected pocket and a trephine used to cut through the anterior corneal layers. The viscoelastic protects the posterior layer from damage. After excision of the anterior stroma, surgery proceeds as with other techniques. With this approach, however, no attempt is made to reach the Descemet's membrane.

Donor Preparation

Since the accent in anterior lamellar keratoplasty today is to perform deep excision of the recipient stroma—be it to Descemet's or 90% depth, preparation of the donor button is relatively easy as the entire thickness of the button can be fitted into the stromal bed. Early attempts to use the donor button with the Descemet's membrane intact resulted in wrinkling of the membrane and possibly a greater potential for scarring and inflammation at the interface. Histopathologic evidence also indicates that retention of the Descemet's membrane can result in weaker graft-host bonding and could contribute to the formation of a pseudoanterior chamber at the interface. It is, therefore, preferable to remove the Descemet's membrane and endothelium from the donor button. This can be accomplished by staining the endothelium with trypan blue and using a dry Weck-Cel spear to detach the Schwalbe's line at the periphery and then rub off the entire membrane. Alternatively, after punching the appropriate size of corneal donor tissue, a fine forceps can be used to hold the cut edge of the Descemet's membrane and peel the entire circular disc as one continuous sheet. In an eye in which only a partial-thickness stromal removal has been performed, a dissection at a similar plane must be achieved in the donor—using either a whole donor globe, or the corneoscleral rim in an artificial anterior chamber in order to facilitate an appropriate recipient bed and donor tissue match. Such dissection is, however, technically more demanding and may result in greater potential for interface scarring.

It is also important to use talc-free gloves during the procedure and also ensure that the interface is free of lint or other debris. After thorough flushing of the stromal bed to remove residual viscoelastic, the donor button is placed in the bed and 10-0 nylon sutures are used to secure it in position. Care must be taken to ensure that the sutures achieve an even distribution of tension and that no perforation of the Descemet's membrane occurs. The use of air in the anterior chamber is helpful in promoting adhesion of the two layers, especially when the Descemet's membrane has been bared.

Anterior lamellar keratoplasty has improved significantly in the past few decades and is now a viable option in the management of corneal opacities that do not involve the Descemet's membrane and endothelium. Improvements in our knowledge of corneal surgical anatomy, wound healing, and surgical instruments and techniques now allows the safe and reproducible use of this technique in selected patients. The major complications are intraoperative and result from inability to remove the opaque corneal stroma in its entirety, failure to create a smooth interface, and perforation of the posterior stromal layer in the recipient eye. Although immunological reactions are rare, since the host endothelium is retained, they can occur in the transplanted stroma. A study has shown that in deep anterior lamellar keratoplasty, the recipient corneal endothelium has a small initial drop in endothelial cell density followed by a physiologic rate of cell loss. The authors indicate that they expect cell survival after lamellar keratoplasty to be better than after penetrating corneal grafting. Best corrected visual acuity (BCVA), refractive results, and complication rates also appear to be similar in the two procedures.

DEEP LAMELLAR ENDOTHELIAL KERATOPLASTY

Although full-thickness corneal transplantation has been the gold standard procedure for the management of corneal diseases affecting clarity and visual function, there are some problems associated with the procedure. These include the need to use sutures to secure the transplanted disc of donor cornea, which results in astigmatism, which can often be irregular. This can delay visual rehabilitation of the patient despite the presence of a clear-corneal graft. The use of sutures can sometimes also result in problems, such as early loosening with graft ectasia, late loosening with infiltrates, vascularization and rejection. The graft-host junction remains an area of potential weakness in the cornea that can rupture with trauma several years after the surgical procedure. The unpredictability of the postoperative corneal shape can also result in inaccurate estimation of the required IOL power in eyes undergoing combined cataract and corneal transplant surgery.

The recent improvements in techniques for lamellar replacement of the anterior corneal layers have aided the development of a similar technique for the selective replacement of the diseased corneal endothelium. Since the anterior layers remain undisturbed, surface corneal sutures as used in traditional corneal transplantation are not required. This provides early visual rehabilitation and reduced postoperative astigmatism. The corneal curvature remains more stable over time and large shifts in refraction do not occur. Late suture-related complications are not seen and the absence of a full-thickness vertical interface in the cornea increases the safety of the procedure—both during and after the surgical procedure. Finally, the minimal alteration in the contour of the cornea after surgery means that the predictability of IOL power calculations is enhanced.

Thus, in patients with corneal edema due to endothelial dysfunction, in whom there is no significant scarring, opacification or vascularization of the anterior layers, limited replacement of the posterior corneal layers appears to have many advantages over conventional full-thickness penetrating keratoplasty. These outcomes can be achieved by a number of techniques and this section briefly outlines the various ways in which these are achieved.

Microkeratome Flap-Assisted Deep Lamellar Endothelial Keratoplasty

This technique has been reported by Jones and Culbertson and Busin, Arffa and Sebastiani. A microkeratome is used to prepare a large diameter, thick (480 μm) hinged flap. After retracting the flap, a central disc of the posterior stromal bed is trephined. A donor disc that is about 250 μm thick is sutured into place in the bed created in the posterior stroma. The flap is then replaced and sutured into place as well. Encouraging results were obtained in the initial series, despite the occurrence of complications, such as epithelial ingrowth and corneal melt in the flap. The use of sutures, however, obviated some of the advantages of this approach. Since then other approaches have attempted to reduce the need for sutures in the cornea, and these are described below.

Large Incision Deep Lamellar Endothelial Keratoplasty

After the initial description of the technique of posterior lamellar corneal replacement in rabbits by Ko in 1993, it was the pioneering efforts of Melles that resulted in the first human surgical procedure using this approach. In his early procedures, Melles described the use of a 9.0 mm partial thickness superior scleral incision. Following a paracentesis, the anterior chamber was filled with air and the techniques described in the section on anterior lamellar corneal transplantation were used to reach 80% depth in the peripheral corneal stroma. Using the semi-sharp spatulated dissectors described earlier, the plane of dissection was carried across the entire cornea splitting the stroma from limbus to limbus. Into this space, a specially designed low-profile trephine was introduced and using the external handle, was rotated from side-to-side to effect a circular cut in the posterior stromal layer. After the initial trephine cut, specially designed microscissors were used to complete the cut and the disc of tissue was removed from the eye.

A whole donor eye was used in the initial series, but subsequently, a similar procedure was also performed on donor corneoscleral rims using an artificial anterior chamber. A similar plane of corneal dissection was achieved in the donor cornea, after which a same size corneal button was punched from the endothelial side using a punch trephine. The posterior layer of the donor cornea was then removed and placed endothelial side down on a specially designed spoon-shaped glide (DORC) coated with viscoelastic to protect the endothelium.

In the recipient eye, the glide carrying the disc of donor tissue was introduced into the anterior chamber and the disc was gently placed in the recipient bed that had been created in the posterior stroma. An air bubble was placed to assist in the attachment of the donor disc to the recipient stroma. After suturing the scleral incision, the air bubble was partially removed. The procedure resulted in clear recipient corneas, and the suture-induced astigmatism could be countered by suture removal, 3 months after the surgery. The desire to further reduce the size of the incision created in the sclera, however, led to the further modifications and the present refinement of the procedure.

Small Incision Deep Lamellar Endothelial Keratoplasty

The main reason for the large scleral incision required in the previous approach was the need to introduce the trephine into the stromal pocket created by the dissection. Despite a low profile, a significant separation of the wound lips is required to achieve proper central positioning of the trephine over the posterior corneal stroma, thereby requiring a relatively large scleral incision. The current evolution of the technique described by Melles and Terry does not require the use of an intrastromal trephine. Excision of the posterior stromal disc is achieved using specially designed highly curved scissors and hence, a 5 mm scleral incision is sufficient.

The procedure begins with a mark on the corneal surface using an appropriately sized trephine. The mark in inked over using a marker pen and serves as a guide during subsequent maneuvers to excise the posterior disc of stroma. The corneal dissection proceeds as with the previous technique. When a complete dissection of the corneal stroma has been achieved, the anterior chamber is entered using a keratome that perforates the posterior stromal layer in line with the surface marking, close to the superior or temporal scleral incision. Special scissors are then introduced through the scleral wound and positioned with one jaw in the anterior chamber and the other in the stromal pocket, to cut the posterior layer—following the outline of the mark made on the anterior surface. After the disc is removed, a similar technique is followed in the donor tissue, to separate the corneal stroma into thicker anterior and thinner posterior layers. A freehand trephine is used to punch a 0.5 mm oversized corneal button from the endothelial side. The posterior disc is carefully folded into a "taco" that is two-thirds in one portion and one-third in the other, over a thin tube of viscoelastic placed on the endothelium. The "taco" is held much like a foldable IOL, with a forceps that is designed to avoid crushing the tissue, prior to insertion. All viscoelastic is removed from the anterior chamber after which the "taco" is carried into the eye and unfolded so that the stromal surface hinges against the recipient bed. Air is then injected through a paracentesis to force the folded disc of donor corneal tissue to unfold completely. A 0.5 mm oversized disc of donor corneal tissue is used and the edges of the donor tissue are tucked into the recipient stromal bed at the periphery. The scleral incision is closed with 3 interrupted sutures and the air is partially removed (Fig. 4.43).

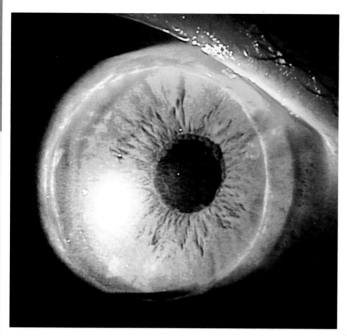

Fig. 4.43: Deep lamellar endothelial keratoplasty. Post-deep lamellar endothelial keratoplasty for bullous keratopathy

Results

Subsequent to the initial case series operated and presented by Melles, a larger number of patients have been operated using these techniques by Terry who has extensively published his results. Short and intermediate term follow-up of these patients, has shown encouraging results with regards the initial astigmatism, alteration in corneal contour, stability of the refraction, visual acuity, and endothelial cell counts. These appear to compare favorably with standard full-thickness penetrating keratoplasty results, and studies comparing the two procedures are currently underway.

Disadvantages with the deep lamellar endothelial keratoplasty approach include the need for specific instrumentation, a rather long learning curve and the need for excellent surgical technique. With the newer refinements using a small incision, the need to fold the corneal donor button results in some endothelial damage and care must be taken during surgery to minimize this complication. Postoperatively, dislocation of the transplanted disc of donor cornea can sometimes occur and may require surgical repositioning. The presence of the interface in the cornea can result in a marginal reduction in the quality of vision compared to the excellent vision afforded by successful full-thickness corneal transplantation. However, considering the other advantages of the deep lamellar endothelial keratoplasty approach, this may be an acceptable price to pay although longer-term results of the deep lamellar endothelial keratoplasty procedure are required.

Component corneal replacement is rapidly coming of age and the concepts of anterior and posterior lamellar corneal replacements are probably the beginning of an exciting new era in corneal transplant surgery. Future refinements could include the use of a femtosecond laser to perform the corneostromal

dissection and this would reduce the skill requirements for this procedure. To avoid the need to perform the recipient dissection, a newer approach attempts to remove only the Descemet's membrane—a procedure termed "descemetorhexis". However, current techniques do not permit the transfer of a similar piece of donor tissue and hence surgical technique is limited by the need to replace the recipient bed with a standard disc of posterior corneal stroma and endothelium from the donor eye. There is, therefore, a mismatch between the depth of the bed and the thickness of the donor tissue and preliminary experience indicates a higher dislocation rate of the donor disc with this approach, compared to the standard deep lamellar endothelial keratoplasty techniques. Recent approaches have attempted to detach the Descemet's membrane and endothelium from donor corneas and a search for a suitable system that allows implantation of these thin sheets is currently on. Endothelial culture techniques are being investigated and these may be suitably combined with deep lamellar endothelial keratoplasty techniques in the future.

CORNEAL TRANSPLANTATION—AUTOGRAFTS

Rationale

Although conventional penetrating keratoplasty enjoys a high degree of success today, immunological rejection remains a challenge. This is particularly important in young patients, eyes that have suffered trauma or previous inflammation, and in those that have corneal vascularization or prior attempts at surgery. Although various attempts have been made to overcome this important limitation, the ideal solution is still lacking. The benefits of HLA matching in these eyes are still debated with various reports providing conflicting evidence. The ideal way to avoid this serious problem would be to use tissue, which is immunologically identical to the recipient and thus, is tolerated by the immune defenses. The use of an autograft would solve the problem of immunologically mediated damage in corneal transplantation. This approach was first described by Plange in 1908, when he used a lamellar graft from one eye of a patient to replace a cornea opaque from lime burns in the fellow eye. Apart from the obvious advantages of using such a procedure in an eye unsuitable for conventional transplantation, there would also be a reduced need for prolonged, intensive steroid therapy in the postoperative period.

Types

Corneal autografts can be performed in a variety of ways depending on the situation that is present in a patient (Fig. 4.44). Tissue can be transferred in the same eye—the transfer can be full-thickness or partial and is performed for differing indications. A full-thickness trephination of the central cornea is performed to allow access to the intraocular contents—as in open-sky surgery for retinopathy of prematurity and rarely to provide a route for extracapsular cataract surgery in eyes with

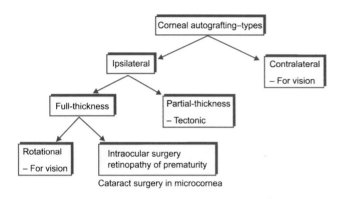

Fig. 4.44: Corneal autografting—options

small corneas. In eyes with a central opacity in the cornea and clear peripheral tissue, a rotational maneuver can help in bringing the clear peripheral cornea into the visual axis, helping the patient to see. In eyes with a small peripheral perforation, the use of a partial-thickness patch from the peripheral cornea has been described to restore the tectonic integrity of the cornea (Fig. 4.45). Corneal tissue can also be transferred between fellow eyes, using the clear cornea from a blind eye to reconstruct the anterior segment in the eye with visual potential, but an opaque cornea.

Ipsilateral Nonrotational Autografts

As mentioned previously, the use of such an approach has two indications. In eyes with complicated retinal detachments due to retinopathy of prematurity, the extreme contraction of fibrous tissue results in a relatively anterior position of the retina. In such eyes, a sclerotomy can result in unwanted complications, and in this context, using an open-sky approach for the removal of fibrous tissue is advantageous and removal of the cornea facilitates this. At the conclusion of surgery, the cornea

is replaced and sutured in place. A similar approach has been described to provide access for cataract surgery in eyes with micro cornea, although this surgery can possibly be performed by other approaches as well.

During surgery, a Flieringa ring is used to support the sclera and after marking the surface of the cornea with radial marks, an appropriate size of cornea is trephined and removed. Since the same tissue is to be replaced at the conclusion of intraocular maneuvers, it is important that undercutting of the tissue is avoided and vertical walls are obtained. This is facilitated by the use of a sharp vacuum trephine. During removal of the trephined cornea, it is important to ensure that the tissue is not excessively bent and chafing against the intraocular structures is avoided, as this helps preserve the endothelium. The use of good quality viscoelastics in the anterior chamber after entry into the eye can also help protect the endothelium. The excised cornea is temporarily stored in sterile corneal storage medium and at the end of surgery is replaced and sutured in place using standard techniques.

In eyes that have small peripheral perforations, the use of a disc of lamellar corneal tissue from the periphery can be used to restore the tectonic integrity of the eye. The use of a 50% thickness lamellar button from the thicker corneal periphery does not compromise corneal integrity at the donor site and this is a useful technique in an emergency when replacement tissue is unavailable.

Ipsilateral Rotational Autografts

This is a technique that works best in eyes that have a central corneal opacity and clear peripheral cornea. Often, these opacities result from penetrating central corneal trauma, while localized central corneal infections can also sometimes result in such a situation. An eccentric trephination is performed that allows the removal of a disc of cornea containing the central opacity. Intraocular maneuvers can then be performed if

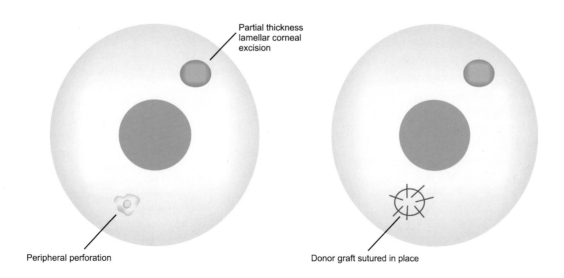

Fig. 4.45: Ipsilateral corneal autograft

desired, while the excised corneal button is temporarily stored in sterile corneal storage medium. After this is done, the disc of cornea is replaced and rotated to ensure that the opacity is now in the periphery and does not intrude into the visual axis. Interrupted sutures are then used to secure the graft.

It is important to be able to assess preoperatively, whether such a rotation is possible. In addition, evaluation of the endothelial counts in the clear-corneal periphery is important to ensure that there is adequate healthy endothelium to make the procedure viable. During excision of the corneal button, it is important to try and prevent excessive endothelial damage, and to have good vertical cuts in the trephined margins to avoid problems with wound apposition. During graft suturing, the use of interrupted sutures is preferred as the host and graft margins are of differing thickness and this technique offers greater scope for precise suture adjustment.

Measuring the appropriate size of the corneal button to be rotated and proper placement of the trephine are vital to ensure the success of this procedure. Various methods have been described for these calculations. It has been suggested that the diameter of the trephine to be used can be calculated as: 3/4 diameter of the cornea—1/2 the preoperative distance between the corneal center and the nearest edge of the opacity to the center (Fig. 4.46).
Various other methods have been described by other authors to determine the size of the trephine to be used; and with the advent of corneal imaging techniques, a recent approach describes the acquisition of a digitized image of the cornea to facilitate these calculations.

A simple approach that the author has been using with good success is described here. On the operating table, the geometrical center of the cornea is determined and marked [A] (assuming that the pupillary position matches this—in eyes with corectopia, surgical maneuvers are performed to achieve a central pupillary opening). Next, a mark is made 2.5 mm from the corneal center in the meridian where the opacity is largest [B]. This is to ensure that after rotation, there is at least 2 mm

of clear cornea in the visual axis—since the suture will require a 0.5 mm bite. In the meridian opposite to AB, at least 2 mm of clear cornea will be required (since the pupillary diameter is 3 to 4 mm), shown in the figure as AC. Thus, it is important to ensure that there is at least 4.5 mm of clear cornea in the periphery, as measured from C [CD]. The addition of AB + BC + CD provides the diameter of the required trephine. The trephine is placed with one edge passing through B, and the other preferably 0.5 to 1.0 mm within the limbus, at the peripheral mark D. Rotation of the excised corneal button ensures that CD is now placed centrally ensuring a 4 mm clear area in the corneal center and the sutures do not interfere with this zone (Fig. 4.47).

Despite the obvious advantages of this approach in avoiding immunological complications in this subset of high-risk eyes, it must be remembered that surgery increases the possibility of endothelial cell loss in these traumatized eyes. Studies have, however, shown that the rate of endothelial loss with this approach tends to be less than that seen after homologous corneal allografting (Fig. 4.48). Further, the mismatch between the thickness of the graft and recipient corneal margins can result in significant corneal astigmatism, which can limit the visual benefits of a clear central cornea. However, studies have shown that gratifying visual results can be obtained in such eyes.

Contralateral Autografts

As mentioned previously, the rationale of this approach is to achieve the transfer of healthy corneal tissue from a blind eye to the fellow eye, which has a corneal opacity, but good visual potential (Fig. 4.49). The donor eye in corneal autografting can be managed in one of the two ways. If retaining the donor globe is not important, the globe can either be enucleated, after which the corneal button can be excised, or the button can first

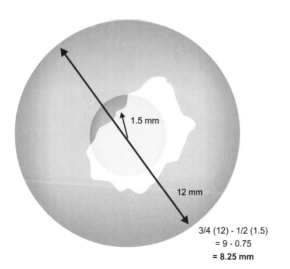

3/4 (12) - 1/2 (1.5)
= 9 - 0.75
= 8.25 mm

Fig. 4.46: Rotational corneal autograft—measuring graft size

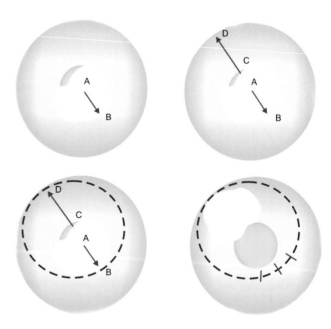

Fig. 4.47: Rotational corneal autograft—intraoperative measurements

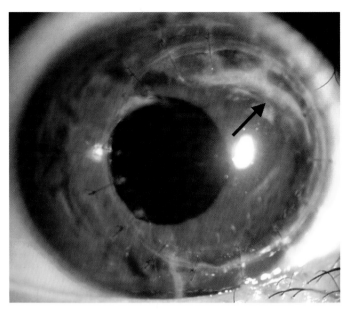

Fig. 4.48: Ipsilateral rotational corneal autograft. Arrow indicates peripheral location of scar and clear visual axis after surgery

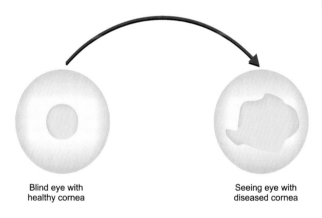

Blind eye with   Seeing eye with
healthy cornea   diseased cornea

Fig. 4.49: Contralateral corneal autograft

be removed after which the eye can be eviscerated. Advantages of this type of surgery would be a possible shorter duration of surgery, lesser risk of postoperative infection, and a reduced need for prolonged, postoperative medication and care in the blind eye. A major disadvantage of this approach would be the loss of one eye, which though blind, may have serious psychological implications for the patient. The other approach of retaining the donor eye can also be tackled in one of the two ways. Either the corneas can be switched with the blind eye receiving corneal tissue from the eye with visual potential and vice versa, or a donor allograft can be used.

Since it is preferable to oversize the graft in the healthy eye by 0.25 to 0.50 mm, if one switches the tissues between the two eyes, the use of an undersized graft in the blind eye can cause a period of increased IOP in this eye. To help reduce the chances of this complication, if the blind eye is phakic, it may be rendered aphakic by extracapsular cataract extraction (ECCE).

Since it is ideal to complete the procedure without the use of an allograft in the blind eye—to retain the immunological advantages—it may be ideal to temporarily close the corneal defect in the blind eye using a keratoprosthesis after excising the corneal button. Following surgery in the healthy eye is completed; the transfer of corneal tissue can be completed in the blind eye after removing the keratoprosthesis.

Corneal autografting is a valuable option in some patients with suitable conditions. Although the need for a more exacting surgical technique makes this a demanding surgical procedure, when performed well, it offers tremendous immunological advantages and should be considered whenever possible, especially in developing countries where quality corneal tissue is often scarce.

LIMBAL STEM CELL TRANSPLANTATION

Limbal Stem Cell

The limbus occupies a strategic location in the ocular surface and separates two distinct epithelial compartments—the corneal and conjunctival (Fig. 4.50). The epithelia in these two regions are structurally and functionally evolved for specialized functions and intermixing the two could have significant impact on ocular function. The barrier effect of the limbus is, therefore, considered quite important. The limbus is also the watershed region separating the corneal and scleral components of the ocular coat. Here again, despite the fact that both of these are composed of collagen, their organizational structure is quite different, as is their function in the eye.

Apart from the importance of its anatomic location, the limbus is important for another reason—current evidence indicates that the limbus is probably the seat of the stem cells of the corneal epithelium. The corneal epithelium, like that in other parts of the body is in a state of constant renewal. This process is best exemplified by what has been termed the XYZ hypothesis—it is proposed that there is a constant inflow of cells onto the corneal surface from the limbus in a centripetal

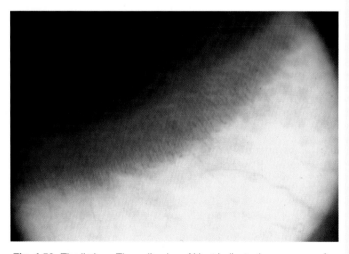

Fig. 4.50: The limbus. The palisades of Vogt indicate the presence of a healthy limbus

manner. In the cornea there is a vertical growth component with cells renewed at the basal layer and exerting a pressure towards the corneal surface. At the same time, there is cell loss from the surface cells, and to maintain the health of the epithelium, it is important that $X + Y = Z$.

The stem cell is believed to be capable of asymmetric cell division. The stem cell niche hypothesis was proposed by Schofield, and proposes that the limbal microenvironment maintains the stem cell in an undifferentiated state. When required, these slow cycling cells undergo cell division, and it is proposed that one of the daughter cells returns to the limbal niche to sustain the stem cell pool. The other daughter cell—termed the transient amplifying cell, is capable of a limited number of mitotic cycles, and resides in the corneal periphery. The products of the cell division cycle of these latter cells are termed postmitotic and terminally differentiated cells, and these constitute the specialized cells of the corneal epithelium. When there is a loss of some of the corneal epithelium, these processes are accelerated and the increased cell output reconstructs the corneal-epithelial barrier.

Stem Cell Dysfunction

In a normal eye, the above-mentioned process occurs at a constant rate on the corneal surface to ensure the maintenance of a normal corneal-epithelial barrier. It is believed that the constant growth pressure that is maintained by the corneal-epithelial pool may also be responsible for the conjunctival epithelium not encroaching on the cornea. In the event of stem cell dysfunction at the limbus, the normal homeostasis is disturbed. This can occur in two situations—either an external insult or an acquired condition damages the stem cell population at the limbus, as in chemical and thermal injury, Stevens-Johnson syndrome, badly fitted contact lenses, chronic limbitis, and repeated limbal surgeries. There are also a group of primary conditions that are associated with possible limbal dysfunction that adversely affect limbal stem cell health and function—as in aniridia.

In these conditions, if the limbal stem damage is minimal and focal; often, there is no obvious alteration in the corneal surface as there is sufficient reserve in the system to sustain function. However, if the extent of limbal damage exceeds this critical reserve, although the exact critical limit is still unclear, then the signs of limbal deficiency manifest themselves on the corneal surface. These have been described as a triad of ocular surface inflammation, recurrent epithelial breakdown, corneal vascularization, and eventually conjunctivalization—an invasion of conjunctiva onto the corneal surface. These changes often also result in patient discomfort, corneal opacity and poor visual function.

If the damage is gradual, as in aniridia or contact lens-induced changes, the limbal stem cell dysfunction and the resulting compensatory changes occur slowly and the surface integrity is often maintained although there is progressive loss of function. However, if the initial insult has been sudden and extensive as with chemical injury, there can also be damage to the underlying stroma, which further compromises corneal healing efforts. In this situation, a persistent epithelial defect can result and this leads to serious consequences (Fig. 4.51). Exposure of the stroma to the tear film neutrophils can result in stromal collagenolysis and ulceration, which can further slow down the process of re-epithelialization of the cornea. This situation of a compromised corneal surface can also result in corneal infection.

Correction of Limbal Stem Cell Dysfunction

In treating a corneal persistent epithelial defect, it is important to first ascertain the events that are taking place on the corneal surface—so that they can be addressed satisfactorily. The presence of an infection must be ascertained, as this would need to be tackled. If there is adequate limbal function, but excessive loss of epithelium occurs from the corneal surface due to lid or lash problems, these must be corrected to ensure a stable corneal surface. This can be an obvious defect as with trichiatic lashes or lagophthalmos. Sometimes, it can be subtler, as in the case of keratinization of the inner lid margin of the lids, in which case the act of blinking can result in constant scouring of the corneal surface and the resultant accelerated epithelial loss can result in increased proliferative stress on the corneal stem cell. Even if there is no increased loss of epithelium, the presence of an unhealthy stromal surface can cause epithelial problems, since the cells migrating into the corneal center from the limbus must be able to firmly adhere to the central corneal surface. In this situation, improving stromal health is vital. This can be attempted by the use of tear, substitutes, punctal

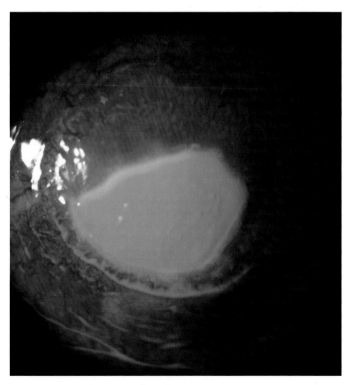

Fig. 4.51: Persistent epithelial defect. Fluorescein stain

occlusion, lubricating gel and dilute surface steroids to reduce inflammation. Oral tetracycline and vitamin C may alter collagenolytic processes and help in stromal healing. If these have been attempted, but there is still no satisfactory response, the use of a soft contact lens or autoserum tears can be considered. The latter are believed to help by providing the ocular surface with as yet unidentified biotrophic factors, which are not present in artificial tear substitutes.

If these measures do not result in rapid healing of the epithelial defect, then surgical intervention is planned. A superficial keratectomy may be considered to remove the unhealthy, spongy surface stroma, exposing the healthy underlying layers to support epithelial migration and attachment. This process helps also to remove heaped up, unhealthy epithelium at the edges of the persistent epithelial defect. Amniotic membrane can also be considered as an adjunct to the above procedure. The use of amniotic membrane is helpful as it serves as a good basement membrane for the epithelium, and has anti-inflammatory properties. It is also believed to promote epithelial health and reduce cell apoptosis. If these measures fail to help, the use of cyanoacrylate glue may be considered as this will seal the stromal surface and prevent ingress of the tear polymorphonuclear leukocytes. A tarsorrhaphy may be considered in desperate situations, as can a conjunctival flap.

However, if the reason for the occurrence of a persistent epithelial defect is the lack of support from the limbus, which is unable to output the required epithelial cell mass, a more logical approach would be to replenish the limbal stem cell reservoir so that healing can proceed. Such a procedure can be performed by transferring limbal tissue from a healthy fellow eye—a process called limbal autografting, or from the limbus of a healthy, living relative who has been HLA-matched with the recipient—a procedure termed live-related limbal allograft. If neither of these sources is available, then limbal tissue from a cadaveric eye can be considered—and this is termed cadaveric limbal allografting. Of these approaches, the best results are obtained with the limbal autograft, which is not surprising, since there is no immunological disturbance induced by the surgical process. Although initial results with HLA-matched live-related limbal allografting are encouraging, in the absence of systemic immunosuppression there is gradual deterioration of the corneal surface in these eyes. The use of systemic immunosuppression appears to prolong the survival of the transplanted limbal stem cells in intermediate-term follow-up. Similarly, with cadaver limbal transplantation, it appears that the ability to maintain corneal epithelial stem cell survival in the long-term in the recipient eyes is limited by the hostile environment of the ocular surface, the immunological mismatch, gradual attrition of transferred cell function, or possibly all of the above.

Surgical Procedures

Limbal Autografting

The surgical process begins in the recipient eye. A peritomy is made 1 to 2 mm from the limbus and extended for 360° around the limbus. The subconjunctival tissues are dissected till the scleral surface adjoining the limbus is exposed. The plane of the fibrovascular pannus at the limbus is identified, after which the entire sheet of pannus is peeled off the corneal surface using a combination of sharp and blunt dissection. The bleeding at the limbus is controlled using minimal cauterization, since it would be appropriate to preserve the vasculature for the success of the limbal graft. If there is a significant symblepharon formation, then more extensive dissection is required on the scleral surface to release these adhesions. After preparing the corneal surface of the recipient eye, the tissue removal from the fellow healthy eye is performed (Figs 4.52A and B).

In performing this procedure, it is important to ensure that the eye serving as the donor has not suffered an injury and that there is no limbal compromise. This is extremely important,

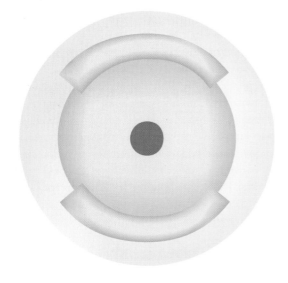

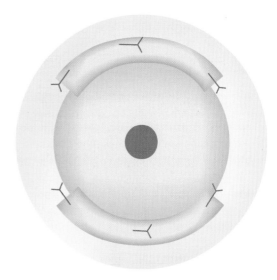

A

B

Figs 4.52A and B: Schematic diagrams of limbal autograft surgery. (A) Donor sites in healthy eye, (B) Grafts in-situ peritomy and pannus removal

since harvesting limbal tissue from a damaged eye would result in suboptimal surgical outcome in the recipient eye, and the loss of limbal tissue may also have serious consequences on the donor eye. After appropriate exposure, a marking pen is used to mark 2 clock hours at the superior and 2 clock hours at the inferior limbus. The conjunctiva 2 mm away from the limbus is also marked in a similar fashion. The conjunctiva at the site of the mark is tented up and incised using sharp Westcott scissors. The dissection then proceeds towards the limbus, avoiding the inclusion of Tenon's tissue in the graft. When the limbus is reached, a firmer attachment of the epithelium to the underlying tissue is noted.

With the conjunctiva held up firmly, the junction between the conjunctival attachment and the underlying stroma is stretched, and using a no. 15 Bard-Parker knife, the exposed adhesions can be lyzed gently. Care is taken to ensure that the knife is held parallel to the stromal surface, so that the surface is not incised. Instead the epithelium is gradually shaved off the surface. This process continues till the dissection ensures that the pigmented limbal palisades are included in the piece of conjunctiva that has been dissected. Once this endpoint is achieved, Vannas scissors are used to cut the attachment of the dissected tissue to the cornea, and the graft is placed in a bowl containing BSS. A similar procedure is carried out at the second site as well.

In the recipient eye, the conjunctival-limbal autograft is placed at the superior limbus. It is important to maintain the epithelial orientation of the tissue, using the marks made previously, and not invert it. It is also important to maintain the orientation of the limbal side of the graft and ensure that this margin of the graft is placed facing the recipient eye limbus. After this is ensured, interrupted 10-0 nylon sutures are placed at the 4 corners of the graft, passing through the episcleral tissue to ensure firm anchorage of the graft tissue. A similar procedure is followed at the inferior limbus.

Postoperatively, the eye can be patched with antibiotic-steroid ointment and reviewed daily until complete epithelialization or a soft contact lens can be applied. Frequent lubrication with unpreserved tears is helpful, and antibiotic eyedrops can be used till corneal surface healing is completed. The donor eye is treated with antibiotic ointment till the graft sites epithelialize.

Live-related Limbal Allograft

After appropriate HLA-matching, a similar surgical approach is followed in the recipient and donor eyes. The surgeries have to be performed in one session to ensure minimal delay in transfer of the limbal grafts to the recipient eye. Although the exact amount of limbal reserve in a normal eye is as yet unknown, it is generally considered safe to excise up to 5 clock hours of limbus from a healthy donor eye.

Cadaver Limbal Allografting

In this approach, one of the two techniques can be used to harvest the donor limbus. When the recipient cornea has a normal thickness, then in order to avoid a stepped corneal surface, it may be important to fashion a thin donor limbal graft. After the central corneal button has been punched from the endothelial side of a donor corneoscleral rim, the rest of the donor rim is placed on a sterile plastic sheet with the endothelial side facing up, on a cushion of viscoelastic to protect the epithelium. The undersurface of the limbus is held with a 0.12 mm forceps, and using sharp Vannas scissors a cut is made into the stroma of this tissue. This is gradually extended in a circumferential manner to systematically remove posterior stromal tissue. When the remaining anterior stromal tissue is judged to be sufficiently thin, the dissection is stopped. The entire ring of dissected anterior stroma and epithelium is transferred to the recipient surface which has been prepared as described previously, and sutured into place using interrupted 10-0 nylon sutures that suture the scleral portion of the rim to the recipient episcleral tissues.

However, if the disease process has left the recipient stroma thinner than normal, and this will be addressed using a lamellar or penetrating corneal transplant, the donor limbal tissue will need to be thicker, to try and maintain parity between the central donor cornea and the peripheral host rim thickness. To achieve this, the donor corneoscleral rim can be sutured onto a holder—the fashioning of which has been published earlier. Using a sharp crescent knife, dissection is initiated on the cut corneal edge at an appropriate depth and carried into the limbal and scleral portions of the corneoscleral rim. When this process has been completed all 360°, the sutures are cut and the anterior lamella of the donor rim, containing the epithelium and requisite thickness of the anterior stroma is taken for transplantation. If a combined penetrating keratoplasty is also to be performed in the recipient eye, then the central trephination is first performed. The donor corneal button is anchored in place using 4 interrupted sutures of 10-0 nylon. After this, the donor limbal ring is placed around the corneal graft, and interrupted sutures of 10-0 nylon are taken that encompass the donor corneal button, the peripheral host cornea, and the donor limbal ring. After 4 of these sutures, the first 4 sutures are replaced, and the process is completed using a total of 16 sutures. Finally, the scleral rim is sutured to the episcleral bulbar surface of the recipient eye, using three 10-0 nylon interrupted sutures in each quadrant to secure the limbal ring securely to the surface of the recipient eye. Amniotic membrane transplantation is then performed to cover the limbal and corneal allografts.

When limbal allografting is performed, systemic immunosuppression should be used to prevent immunological rejection of the vascularized, antigenic limbal grafts. These can be done using cyclosporine A, tacrolimus (FK 506), or mycophenolate mofetil. However, when using such medications, it may be better to co-manage the patient with an internist.

Experience With Ex Vivo Stem Cell Cultivation

The use of amniotic membrane in conjunction with stem cell grafting has helped with surface reconstruction, and also to promote the function of the transplanted stem cells. Since the use of large amounts of limbal tissue from a donor eye may compromise function in this eye in the long-term, there have been recent efforts to cultivate stem cells in the laboratory, from a small limbal biopsy, using amniotic membrane as a substrate. The expanded sheet of cultivated cells can then be used to reconstruct the corneal surface in the recipient. Obviously, the limbal biopsy can be performed from three different sources—the fellow eye of the patient, the eye of an HLA-match live relative or a cadaver eye. Although the technical feasibility of this approach has been shown in recent studies, the long-term results of this approach are still awaited. The surgical technique requires the preparation of the recipient eye as described, and placement of the epithelial cell containing amniotic membrane sheet over the corneal surface with the epithelial side facing up. The membrane is sutured to the limbal area using 10-0 nylon mattress sutures and a soft contact lens is placed to protect the epithelium. Encouraging results have been described using this approach—with the corneal surface reconstruction surviving well in the short and intermediate term. When combined limbal reconstruction and corneal transplants are performed, there is some evidence that it is better to perform these in a staged manner.

Future Directions

Current techniques of surgery are able to offer satisfactory reconstruction of the corneal surface in eyes with limbal deficiency. When combined with surface reconstruction, such procedures result in substantial anatomic and functional improvement in the eye. However, maintaining such outcomes beyond the short and intermediate term has proven to be difficult, even when experienced ophthalmologists perform such surgery. Part of the difficulty may stem from the fact that as yet, there are no unique markers that identify the limbal stem cell. Those that are available are only capable of identifying the differentiated and undifferentiated cells of the corneal epithelium. Identifying the stem cell would help us better understand the behavior of the transplanted cells in the recipient eye. This would be especially important in the case of the cultivated cell transplants as the amount of stem cells transferred may influence long-term outcomes. The ability to locate these specific cells would also help recognize their viability and ability to maintain an undifferentiated state in locations outside the limbal region.

The exact role of a natural tear film in these patients is also unclear, although it is apparent that such procedures fail to work in eyes with severe tear deficiency, especially if there is keratinization of the ocular surface structures. The nature of the biotrophic substances present in natural tears and their possible supplementation may prolong the survival of these transplanted cells. Similarly, the worse prognosis noted in eyes that have had limbal allografts as apposed to autografts suggests that immune-mediated damage may be responsible, at least partly for the damage. Existing immunosuppressive regimens may need to be modified to address these issues.

In conclusion, patients with limbal deficiency were until recently, considered to have an extremely poor prognosis, since the older surgical techniques failed to address the problems seen in such eyes. The recent explosion of knowledge regarding the limbal stem cell and its pivotal role in the management of such patients has led to improved techniques and a better outlook for such patients. However, further improvements are needed to ensure that the gains obtained are consolidated and lead to a more permanent solution in such eyes.

AMNIOTIC MEMBRANE TRANSPLANTATION

History of Amniotic Membrane Use

Although amniotic membrane is being increasingly used in ocular surgery today, it was first used in patients with extensive burns of the skin. In these patients, the use of this fetal membrane was associated with decrease in pain, reduced infection rates and accelerated wound healing. Subsequently, it was used in a wide variety of non-ocular surgical procedures, and was first used in the eye for conjunctival surface reconstruction by De Rotth in 1940. The technique used "live" fetal membranes, which included the use of the epithelium as well as the chorion, probably because of which, there was limited success. Sorsby and Symons were the first to use amniotic membrane alone in the treatment of ocular chemical injuries, and they reported encouraging results in 30 patients. However, there is little mention of amniotic membrane in ocular surgery in the ophthalmic literature of the next 50 years. Resurgence of interest occurred after the paper by Kim and Tseng in 1995, in which they described ocular surface rescue using preserved human amniotic membrane in a rabbit model of partial limbal deficiency. After this landmark paper, there has been a burgeoning use of this adjunct in ocular surgery and the list of indications has been expanding rapidly.

Properties of the Membrane

The structure of the membrane consists of a single layer of cuboidal, nucleated epithelial cells, with an underlying basement membrane and stroma. The stroma has been further categorized as a compact layer next to the basement membrane, a fibroblast layer, and a spongy layer, thus, making the amniotic membrane a 5-layered structure. The thickness of this membrane can vary from 0.02 to 0.50 mm, although tissue processing can alter this as noted in a subsequent paragraph. It is generally believed that the membrane is composed of type I and V collagen. In the placenta, the membrane functions as a protective layer, as a secretory epithelium, and helps support intercellular transport.

When used in the eye, it offers a variety of advantageous functions, which are fairly well described, although the exact mechanism of action is still unclear. It is able to facilitate epithelialization of the ocular surface, by acting as a basement membrane for cell adhesion, migration and proliferation. It also has an antiapoptotic effect and is believed to maintain the clonogenicity of epithelial progenitor cells. When used on the cornea, it promotes the differentiation of non-goblet cells; but when used in conjunctival reconstruction, it is believed to promote the differentiation of goblet cells, making it a very useful adjunct in eyes requiring ocular surface reconstruction. It reduces inflammation on the ocular surface, by excluding inflammatory cells with antiprotease activities, and is also thought to cause apoptosis of these cells. By suppressing the TGF-beta – signaling system, it is able to decrease myofibroblast differentiation from normal fibroblasts and hence, reduces scarring. Similarly, it also has antiangiogenic properties and decreases inflammatory vascularization of the ocular surface. Recently, it has been proposed that this membrane is able to maintain stem cell populations of the corneal epithelium, and the goblet cell precursors in conjunctival epithelium, when these tissues are cultured in vitro using amniotic membrane as a substrate.

Preparation and Storage

Although fresh amniotic membrane use has been described from centers where facilities for preservation do not exist, most centers today use preserved tissue. Some of the disadvantages of using nonpreserved tissue include the emergent nature of the ocular surgery when the amniotic membrane is available, the wastage that ensues unless a number of surgeries can be scheduled, and the lack of a "window period" to observe the donor. The latter refers to the protocol of screening the donor of the amniotic membrane for hepatitis B and C, syphilis and HIV-AIDS. Ideally such tests are repeated after 6 months, to ensure that the donor has not seroconverted in this period, before releasing the stored membrane for use—which is not possible if fresh tissue is used. The technique of preparation requires separation of the amnion, and washing in a solution of saline to which antibiotics have been added to remove all blood clots. Then, it is placed either in a vial of saline for use within 24 hours, or it can be flattened onto nitrocellulose paper with the epithelium facing up and stored in Dulbecco's modified Eagle medium and Glycerol (1:1) containing penicillin, streptomycin, neomycin and amphotericin B at –80°C. A more recent method of storage uses a low-heat drying dehydration method and the amniotic membrane resembles parchment paper. It is stored as a freestanding membrane without need for a carrier sheet and is rehydrated prior to use in the operation theater. This can be stored at room temperature.

Depending on the method of storage, the morphology of the membrane can vary. The freeze-dried membrane is 20 um in thickness, whereas the fresh fixed membrane is 65 um, and the preserved frozen is the thickest, at 463 um. These differences in characteristics may prove helpful during surgical use, and it has been suggested that the thinner membrane may be more suitable when used as a basement membrane, while the thicker membrane is more ideally suited for use in ocular surface reconstruction procedures. Although it was initially believed

that cryopreservation resulted in loss of some of the properties of the membrane, probably due to a loss of various biological growth factors, recent evidence indicates otherwise.

Surgical Technique

When using amniotic membrane on the cornea, it is preferable to use nonabsorbable sutures like 10-0 or 11-0 nylon. This is because the membrane tends to remain on the surface for variable lengths of time and it is preferable that premature suture dissolution does not occur. In the conjunctival surface on the other hand, since there is often more rapid incorporation of the membrane in the ocular tissues, absorbable sutures like 10-0 vicryl are preferred. On the corneal surface, the suture knots may be left exposed, as this facilitates easy removal. A bandage contact lens may be used to protect the lids from suture irritation.

Orientation of the membrane is generally with the basement membrane facing up. This allows the basement membrane to serve as a scaffold for the migrating epithelium to grow over, and also allows the stromal wound modulating properties to act on the corneal or scleral surface, on which the membrane is placed. The membrane is placed on the nitrocellulose paper with the stromal side adhering to the membrane. Even if this orientation is lost, it is relatively easy to discern the stromal surface. Touching this surface with a Weck-Cel sponge will result in the appearance of a strand of gel, much like vitreous (Fig. 4.53). On the other hand, touching the smooth basement membrane surface of the membrane does not result in this characteristic appearance.

It, however, does not seem to matter in clinical use which side of the membrane is placed on the stromal surface of the ocular tissues. It has been noted that placement of the membrane with the basement membrane facing up results in greater likelihood of the epithelium growing over the surface of the membrane, in which case the membrane is incorporated into the ocular surface and stays in place for varying periods of time. In some studies, the replacement of this membrane with a layer of fibrosis has been noted. If, however, the epithelium migrates under the membrane, then it is likely that the membrane will loosen and dislodge from the surface earlier.

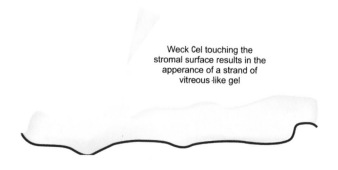

Weck Cel touching the stromal surface results in the apperance of a strand of vitreous-like gel

Fig. 4.53: Amniotic membrane—identifying the stromal surface

The amniotic membrane can be tailored to fit into the bed of a corneal epithelial defect if it is expected to promote epithelialization, as in a persistent epithelial defect. In this situation, it is termed an "inlay" graft. It has also been used to fill tissue defects or actual perforations in the cornea, and also in patients with a descemetocele. In some of these instances, it has been used in conjunction with fibrin glue. When used to fill up a stromal crater, either in the sclera or in the cornea, it has been used as multiple bits, or as one larger piece that has been folded upon itself (Fig. 4.54). When the membrane is sutured into the area of the persistent epithelial defect, the size of the membrane is cut to be about 1 mm larger than the defect (Figs. 4.55 and 4.56). Multiple mattress sutures are then taken to anchor the graft in place.

The amniotic membrane can also be used to cover the surface of the cornea, as in the above instances, to protect the "onlay" graft. It, therefore, serves the role of a biological contact lens and allows corneal healing to proceed undisturbed under the protective cover (Fig. 4.57). When used in this manner, it is termed an "onlay" graft. In this situation, multiple, circumferential, mattress sutures are used at the limbus to keep the tissue in place.

Yet another important role for amniotic membrane in ocular surface reconstruction is to serve as a "separator" to keep raw, granulating surfaces apart till they epithelialize (Figs 4.58 A to C). This property is used when repairing symblepharon of the ocular surface.

While these are standard uses for the amniotic membrane, it can be used following the same principles in other parts of the eye, for other surgical procedures. In recent times, it has gained popularity as the substrate for *ex vivo* cultivation of corneal and conjunctival epithelial sheets in the lab—both for research purposes, and also for transplantation onto the human eye—either as an autograft or in some instances, as an allograft. A composite graft of both corneal and conjunctival epithelium on amniotic membrane has also been used. Despite these expanded indications, it is most often used in ocular surgery for ocular surface reconstruction procedures.

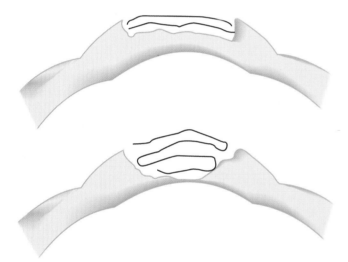

Fig. 4.54: Corneal ulceration—multilayer amniotic membrane transplantation

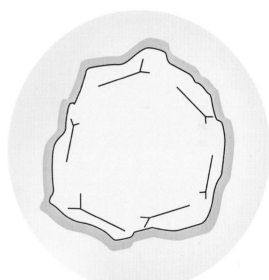

Fig. 4.56: Amniotic membrane transplant. Eye with larger persistent epithelial defect and limbal insufficiency

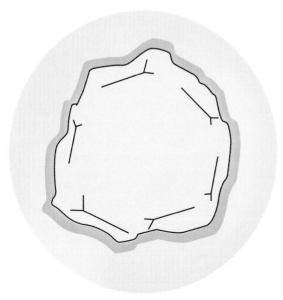

Fig. 4.55: Inlay amniotic graft for corneal epithelial defect

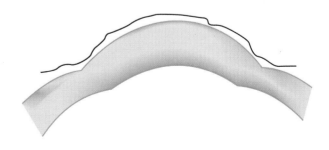

Fig. 4.57: Onlay amniotic graft for corneal surface protection

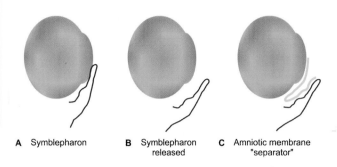

A Symblepharon   **B** Symblepharon released   **C** Amniotic membrane "separator"

Figs 4.58A to C: Amniotic membrane use in symblepharon repair

Review of Current Indications

Cornea

In the cornea, it has been used for the management of persistent epithelial defects, stromal ulceration and perforations, for treating patients with partial or complete limbal stem cell deficiency—often in conjunction with stem cell grafts, in acute chemical and thermal burns, in patients in the acute stage of toxic epidermal necrolysis or Stevens-Johnson syndrome, in the treatment of bullous keratopathy for pain relief, and for miscellaneous uses as in the treatment of band-shaped keratopathy after removal of the calcium, and to try and reduce scarring after excimer laser procedures.

Conjunctiva

It has been used fairly extensively in the management of both primary and recurrent pterygia, in reconstructing the surface after excision of limbal and other conjunctival tumors, in the management of conjunctivochalasis, leaking glaucoma blebs, in primary filtering surgery to reduce scarring in the scleral bed, in symblepharon release, and in recurrent retinal detachment surgery when it is used to decrease the chance of inflammatory fibrosis resulting in restricted motility of the extraocular muscles.

Sclera

As in the cornea, it has been used in the treatment of scleral ulceration.

Eyelid

Its use has been described also in the management of lid skin loss, and margin reconstruction, resurfacing the palpebral surface, and in entropion surgery.

As a substrate for the culture of corneal and conjunctival epithelium.

Although multiple uses have been described for amniotic membrane use in ocular surgery, very few of these have been validated in randomized comparisons with established procedures. Recent reports indicate that it may be less effective in pterygium surgery compared to conjunctival grafting, in glaucoma bleb revision compared to conjunctival advancement;

and in the management of significant limbal deficiency, amniotic membrane transplantation should be accompanied by stem cell transfer, since the membrane is only a substrate. While its use is safe with only minimal inflammatory reactions in the eye, it has been reported that *Staphylococcus* may adhere to the membrane and can cause infections, although this is uncommon.

However, despite its limitations, it has proved to be a very useful tool in the armamentarium of the corneal surgeon and has definitely played an important role in the improved management of ocular surface diseases in the last decade, since its reintroduction. Further refinement of processing techniques, and a better understanding of its exact mechanisms of action may facilitate a more rational approach to its use in the future, with hopefully better outcomes in more ocular conditions.

OCULAR SURFACE RECONSTRUCTION

Ocular Surface

The term ocular surface refers to a complex unit that is comprised of many structures acting in an integrated and coordinated fashion to achieve comfort and excellent vision for the patient. The lids form an important part of this functional complex as they serve to lubricate and protect the delicate structures of the eye. A healthy lid and blink mechanism helps to facilitate the proper spread of tears and also in maintaining the drainage dynamics. The lashes serve as sensors that initiate the protective blink reflex, and the meibomian glands in the lids are responsible for secreting the oily meibum, which serves as an important component of the tear complex. Diseases that interfere with the structure and function of the lids will result in damage to the ocular structures as well. A healthy tear film is vital for a healthy ocular surface. It provides lubrication, nutrition, trophic health factors, mechanical drainage conduits to remove trapped debris, and contains antimicrobial defense systems. Many conditions can affect tear quality and quantity and will have an adverse impact on the health of the other structures of the ocular surface. The conjunctival and corneal epithelial compartments constitute the physical ocular surface and their distinctness is supported and maintained by the presence of a healthy limbus. Since many diseases can affect one or more or sometimes all of these structures, the commonest example being chemical burns of the ocular surface; the reconstruction of these damaged eyes is a complex process and requires attention to the many alterations that are present. This holistic approach to restoring the health of the eye in these conditions is termed ocular surface reconstruction and often requires a staged approach by a team of specialists. In eyes with end-stage disease, resulting in a skin-like appearance of the ocular surface with extensive disorganization of the lid-eye relationships, a keratoprosthesis offers hope of visual rehabilitation (Fig. 4.59). The principles of surgery in such eyes are outlined in this chapter.

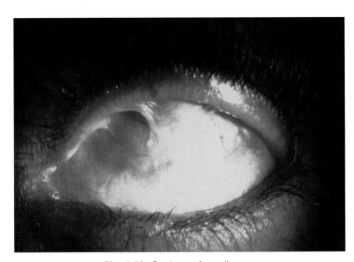

Fig. 4.59: Ocular surface disease

Lid and Tear Function

Structural disorders of the lids and adnexa, such as entropion, ectropion, trichiasis, distichiasis and lagophthalmos must be addressed prior to attempting surgery on the ocular surface. Appropriate oculoplastic consultation can be sought to help address these changes in the lids. An often-unrecognized cause of ocular surface damage in these eyes is the presence of a keratinized inner lid margin—during the blink reflex, these roughened surfaces tend to abrade the ocular surface repeatedly and this can result in increased corneal epithelial cellular loss. The increased demand on the limbal stem cells in this situation can then potentiate any exisiting limbal insufficiency. The XYZ hypothesis proposed by Richard Thoft postulates that the health of the corneal epithelial surface is maintained if the relationship $X + Y = Z$ is present. The term X refers to the centripetal migration of epithelial cells from the limbus into the corneal epithelial pool, while Y represents the upward epithelial migration from the basal layers of the epithelium. The combination of these two should match the factor Z that represents loss from the surface. Any imbalance in this relationship can affect the health and integrity of the corneal epithelial surface. Surgery to correct the keratinized lid margin can help in restoring the equilibrium in these eyes.

Along with the presence of healthy lids, normal tear function is also important, and current attempts to restore tear function focus on the use of newer tear substitutes that are either unpreserved or contain preservatives that are less toxic to the surface. Tear preservation is the next step in the management of tear insufficiency and can be achieved either by using punctal plugs or by using the surgical options described in another section. Restoring tear secretion by transfer of the parotid duct or transplantation of the submandibular salivary gland is yet to achieve widespread use and is technically demanding. The use of secretagogues like oral pilocarpine has shown some promise in early trials, despite the presence of significant side effects. Optimizing lid and tear function is vital for subsequent surgery of the ocular surface to achieve success.

Conjunctiva and Sclera

Cicatrization of the conjunctiva can result in tethering of the lids to the globe and can result in restriction of movement of both the lids and the globe. Apart from the visual consequences, failure of the lid to replenish the tear film on the surface of the globe during the blink reflex can result in deleterious changes in the ocular surface. Conjunctival cicatrization commonly results as a sequel to chemical or thermal burns, past trachoma or other cicatricial conjunctivitis, large ulcers causing extensive destruction of the conjunctiva, repeated ocular surface surgery, or ocular cicatricial pemphigoid. It is important to recognize the cause of conjunctival shrinkage, especially pemphigoid, as surgery in this condition in the absence of good control of the disease can further aggravate the ocular changes. In such patients, appropriate immunosuppressive therapy to achieve disease remission must first be used prior to conjunctival surgery.

The principles of surgery include the thorough release of all adhesions between the conjunctiva and the globe and excision of fibrotic scar tissues, thereby restoring the normal anatomy in the region. In order to prevent a recurrence of the condition, it is important that sufficient regenerative potential is present in the conjunctival tissues. In this context, it is important during surgery to use a substrate that will serve to separate the raw tissues of the globe and the lids and will also promote conjunctival epithelial healing, while at the same time reducing the scarring response of the ocular tissues. The ideal material that provides these functions is amniotic membrane and its use in this situation has been detailed in another section. In very extensive cicatrization, it may be necessary to first remove all adhesions and expose the entire bulbar scleral surface. Isolation and tagging of the four rectus muscles will aid in the performance of these steps. After hemostasis, amniotic membrane is draped over the exposed surface of the globe and mattress sutures are placed in each quadrant of the sclera between and at the level of the muscle insertions. Care is taken to ensure that the amniotic membrane adequately covers the insertion of the rectus muscles to help avoid their involvement in any subsequent scarring. The remainder of the amniotic membrane beyond the scleral anchor sutures is draped over the raw palpebral surfaces of the lids and a conformer is inserted to maintain the separation between the lids and the globe and reestablish the forniceal contour.

If, however, it appears that the extensive conjunctival loss has resulted in little potential for regeneration, it may be important to use a conjunctival substitute to reconstruct the surface. Traditionally, oral mucosa has been used and provides acceptable results, despite the anatomical differences compared to the normal conjunctiva. Currently described techniques of culturing conjunctival and oral mucosal epithelium in the laboratory offer new hope for such patients, although the initial results need to be substantiated in longer term studies, and greater number of patients. Defects in the underlying sclera can be reconstructed using preserved sclera, or lyophilized pericardium, and amniotic membrane transplantation has also been used in selected cases (Figs 4.60A and B).

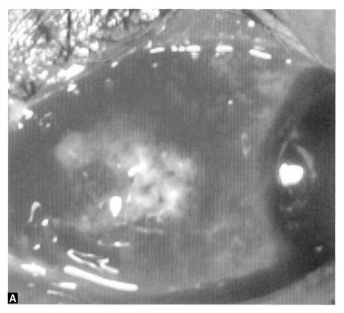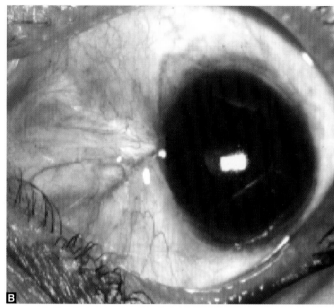

Figs 4.60A and B: Scleral patch graft. (A) Nocardia scleritis, (B) After scleral patch graft

Corneal Surface

While the preceding maneuvers are important for restoring normal anatomy, it is corneal surface reconstruction that restores the function of the eye and enables the patient to see. The concepts of limbal deficiency and the principles of repair of a damaged limbus have been discussed in a previous section. In the context of corneal surface reconstruction, one of the important problems that often confront a surgeon is the presence of a persistent epithelial defect. By definition, this is a corneal ulcer that has persisted for 2 weeks despite adequate therapy. Such a persistent breach in the corneal epithelium has the potential to progress, often rapidly, to serious complications, such as corneal infection, vascularization, thinning and even perforation. For the purpose of this discussion, it is assumed that the persistent ulcer is not due to corneal infection—as the treatment approach of this entity is beyond the scope of this chapter. If an infection has been ruled out, it may then be necessary to identify the actual cause of the persistent epithelial defect to allow a systematic approach to the diagnosis and management. The concept of the XYZ hypothesis is useful in addressing this problem.

If the problem is with the factor X—meaning that adequate corneal epithelial cells are not being produced by the limbus, it is necessary to pay attention to restoring the limbal stem cell population in these eyes. This has been described earlier. On the other hand, the problem may be with the factor Y—the cells produced at the limbus may have difficulty in migrating across the corneal surface, in adhering to the underlying structures; and therefore, unable to further multiply and provide the upward growth phase. If this is identified as a factor, then efforts to resolve the underlying issues can be undertaken. Depending on the underlying condition, one or more of the following options may be considered:

- Pressure patching/contact lens
- Diluted topical steroids
- Debridement/superficial keratectomy
- Corneal glue
- Anterior stromal puncture
- Amniotic membrane patch graft.

The issue of excessive cell loss or the factor Z has been dealt with earlier in this section.

Apart from the above there may be other aggravating factors such as:
- High IOP
- Uncontrolled diabetes mellitus
- Severe corneal edema
- Giant papillary conjunctivitis
- Floppy eyelid syndrome
- Neurotrophy
- Anesthetic abuse.

And the above mentioned factors must be identified and appropriately managed. In the context of neurotrophic keratitis, since it is possible that the absence of trophic factors can result in poor epithelial health, attempts have been made to use factors, such as fibronectin and epithelial growth factor to promote healing in such eyes. Since such factors are not commonly available, another option that can be considered is the use of autoserum tears, proposed by Tsubota. The rationale for their use is that the serum is likely to contain many of the trophic factors that are present in normal tears and the use of these factors as topical drops can help epithelial healing in such eyes. The method of preparation of these drops, their storage, use and precautions required are well-summarized recently. Lastly, the possibility that an underlying immune-mediated disorder is responsible for or aggravating the persistent epithelial defect must be considered, and appropriate investigations must be performed.

Similarly, these conditions, though rare, must also be considered:

- Mooren's ulcer
- Shield ulcer
- Conjunctival foreign body
- Severe dellen
- Factitious corneal ulcer.

Thus, ocular surface problems have many manifestations and causes and careful attention must be paid to the examination of such eyes, in order to determine the causative factors. A planned, often staged surgical approach must then be considered to ensure that these factors are tackled appropriately. When such an approach is followed, adequate restoration of ocular surface function is possible in most instances. However, in a subset of eyes with end-stage disease, where the surface appears keratinized, the hostile surface environment and total lack of an ocular surface defense, results in very poor survival of any transplanted biological tissues. In such eyes, the only hope for the restoration of visual function is the use of prosthetic devices and the basics of this approach are discussed in the next section.

Keratoprosthesis

Over the past decades, there have been many attempts to integrate a variety of prosthetic devices with the ocular structures using a number of different devices and approaches. Each of these has its merits and demerits and in this section one of the approaches will be described—the osteo-odonto-keratoprosthesis. Although originally described by Strampelli, it was Giancarlo Falcinelli who modified the technique to its presently used form. A description of the technique has been published by others. This technique uses a composite bone-tooth lamina to help anchor a polymethylmethacrylate (PMMA) cylinder to the cornea. The complex surgical procedure is performed in two stages.

In the first stage, a canine tooth is harvested from the mouth of the patient after X-ray screening has determined that the tooth has a healthy and viable root structure. A surgical motorized saw is used to excise the canine root encased in alveolar bone from the jaw. The lamina is fashioned by sawing through the root of the tooth in a longitudinal fashion to expose the dentine and the root canal. The pulp in the root canal is scraped off and a hole is drilled in the widest part of the root—to a size of 3 to 4 mm depending on the width of the root at that point. An appropriately sized plastic cylinder of suitable power (determined from the axial length of the eye) is then glued to the hole using dental cement. A subcutaneous pocket is created in the tissues of the cheek and the lamina-cylinder complex is placed in it and the pocket is sutured closed after instilling antibiotic powder. In the eye, the symblepharon are released, and scar tissue is excised as described earlier. A superficial keratectomy, including the Bowman's layer is performed to expose the bare corneal stroma after which a full-thickness circular piece of cheek mucosa about 4 cm in diameter is placed over the cornea

and sutured to sclera, also covering the muscle insertions (Figs 4.61A to D and 4.62A to D).

Stage II surgery is performed 2 to 3 months later to allow time for a connective tissue cover to develop around the lamina implanted in the cheek. If required, the integrity of the lamina can be checked by performing a spiral computed tomographic evaluation. During the second stage surgery, the lamina is retrieved from the subcutaneous location and excess connective tissue is removed from the two ends of the optic cylinder, and carefully trimmed over the rest of the lamina. The mucosal graft on the ocular surface is incised superiorly and reflected from the superior sclera and cornea, in a downward direction. The inferior attachment of the mucosal graft is left undisturbed to ensure that the blood supply is retained (Figs 4.63A to D and 4.64A to D).

A Flieringa ring is sutured in place and a 3 mm opening is created in the center of the cornea. Three radial incisions are made in the cornea extending till the limbus. The iris is disinserted at the root and removed by gently pulling on the tissue and hypotensive anesthesia is used to control the ooze. Constant irrigation with BSS also helps wash the blood away and prevents a large clot forming in the anterior chamber. The lens is then cryoextracted and the radial-corneal cuts are suture closed. A limited anterior vitrectomy is performed and the lamina is then placed over the cornea, such that the posterior part of the optic cylinder is in the anterior chamber—entering through the central corneal opening. The lamina is sutured into position using the connective tissue covering and episcleral bites. Air injection through the pars plana using a 30-gauge needle is used to maintain the IOP and avoid severe hypotony. At the conclusion of suturing, indirect ophthalmoscopy is performed to ensure that there is a good view of the disc and posterior pole, with the eye in the primary position. If this is not seen, a cylinder tilt may be responsible and the sutures are adjusted to straighten the cylinder position. Any bleeding into the vitreous cavity can also interfere with the visualization. After the cylinder and lamina are in satisfactory position, the mucosal flap is replaced and a small opening is created over the optic cylinder to allow the anterior portion of the cylinder to protrude through the mucosa. The superior edge of the mucosal flap is sutured in place and this completes the operation.

Since bleeding can occur during the ocular and oral surgical dissections, it is important that the patient is not on antiplatelet aggregators or anticoagulants. Infection is a major concern since oral tissues are used and extensive ocular surgery is performed. Intravenous antibiotics are used for the first week after surgery and oral antibiotics are continued for another week. This is more of a concern with stage I surgery. Treatment of the ocular surface mucosal graft is with antibiotic ointment and regular cleaning. Periodic follow-up is required to ensure early detection of problems with IOP and the stability of the graft. The presence of the lamina and the large mucosal graft preclude measurement of IOP using the current instrumentation.

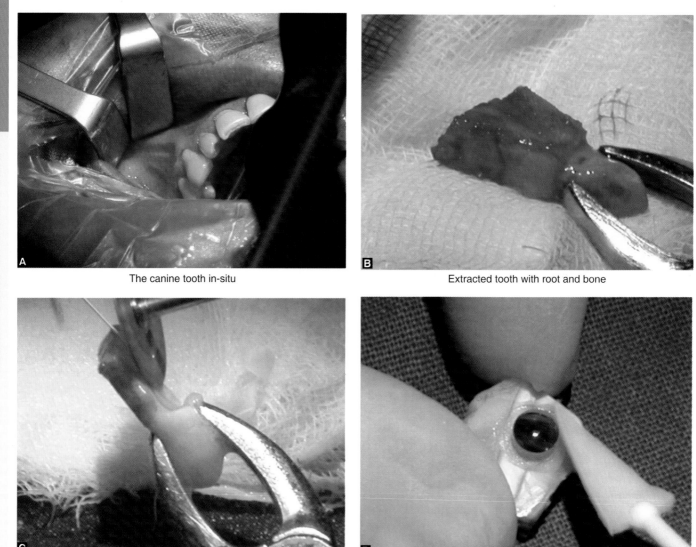

The canine tooth in-situ

Extracted tooth with root and bone

Fashioning the lamina

Cementing the optic cylinder

Figs 4.61A to D: Osteo-odonto-keratoprosthesis–Stage I surgery

IOP is estimated digitally and the health of the optic nerve is monitored using regular automated field measurements and visualization of the optic disc. The visual field provided by current cylinder designs is about 30 to 35°, but this allows good ambulant vision to the patient. With the technique of osteo-odonto-keratoprosthesis described in the previous paragraphs, prolonged retention times can be achieved with good visual function.

Future Prospects

Although the surgical approach to ocular surface reconstruction has improved considerably in the past decade, the ultimate goal of a truly artificial cornea is still a dream. An ideal keratoprosthesis—simple, cheap, fast and effective, is still elusive although many designs exist currently. Although the osteo-odonto-keratoprosthesis design, that the author is familiar with, is discussed here—alternative designs of keratoprostheses exist and have been used clinically. A detailed review of this subject,

however, is beyond the scope of this section. Other attempts at generating an artificial cornea include the creation of tissue engineered, transparent, collagen-based implants with inherent porosity that allow stromal cell ingrowth, epithelial overgrowth and rapid regeneration of a functional nerve complex. These, however, still require extensive clinical testing before they become a realistic option for corneal replacement.

PUNCTAL OCCLUSION

Tear Function and Drainage

Ocular comfort and function are closely related to the normal level and function of the tears in the eye. The integration of tears with the ocular surface is being increasingly recognized, and it is now believed that they function as one integrated unit. Similarly, although the earlier concept of the tear film was that of a tri-layered structure, it is now considered to resemble that

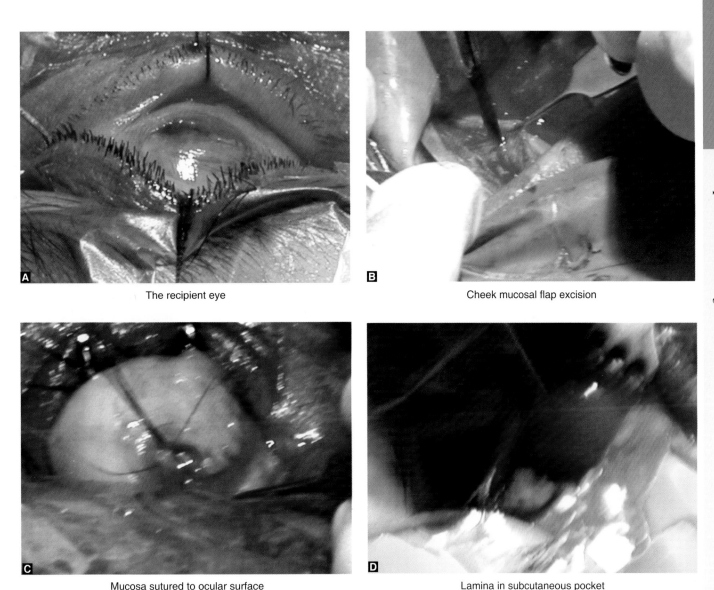

A The recipient eye	**B** Cheek mucosal flap excision
C Mucosa sutured to ocular surface	**D** Lamina in subcutaneous pocket

Figs 4.62A to D: Osteo-odonto-keratoprosthesis–Stage I surgery

of a gel, in which the mucus component is dispersed throughout the thickness of the tear film. The importance of the lipid layer in the structure and function of the normal tear film is also being increasingly stressed.

The advent of newer techniques and improvements in photographic methods now allows us to better understand the tear flow patterns in the eye. It appears that the punctal openings elevate themselves from the lid margin at the start of the closing phase of the blink, allowing their forceful meeting and occlusion by the time the closing lid is halfway down. Completion of lid closure then compresses the lacrimal canaliculi and sac, forcing contained fluid through the drainage system. The elastic expansion of the channels during the opening phase of the blink produces a suction effect, holding the lid margins at the punctal region together as the lids open. During the latter part of this opening, the punctal areas are seen to "pop" apart

suddenly as the vacuum is broken, and tear fluid from the marginal tear strips is drawn into the puncta in the first few seconds following the blink.

Indications

The improvements in our understanding of tear composition and function have been accompanied by many changes in the medical approaches to the management of tear insufficiency. Newer tear formulations are available, that mimic the natural tear composition more closely. These tears contain newer preservatives like purite and perborate, which are less toxic to the ocular surface compared to the earlier medications like benzalkonium chloride. They exist as preservatives while in solution; but when the drops come into contact with the ocular structures, they decompose into harmless physiological substances

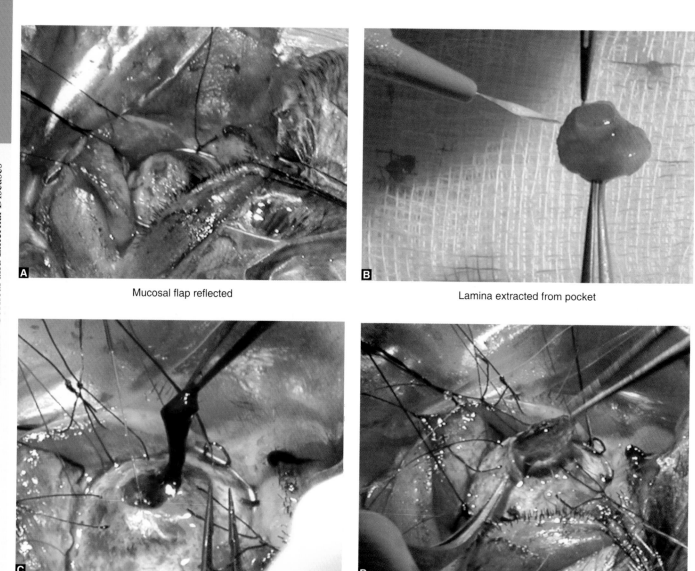

Mucosal flap reflected	Lamina extracted from pocket
Iris removal in recipient eye	Intracapsular lens extraction

Figs 4.63A to D: Osteo-odonto-keratoprosthesis–Stage II surgery

due to the action of ultraviolet light or the ocular surface enzymes.

Despite these advances, however, there are two fundamental issues that the artificial tears are unable to address. In a normal eye, tear supply is based on a demand-and-supply system regulated by a complex neurohumoral arc and this is difficult to replicate with artificial tear substitutes. Secondly, in addition to the electrolytes, normal tears are a complex mixture of other vital ingredients, many of which are yet to be identified, and these may be vital for the maintenance of the health of the normal ocular surface. Artificial tears do not replenish these biological substances. Thus, there is often a degree of severity of dry eye, in which tear replacement alone is insufficient to preserve the health of the ocular surface and provide comfort to the patient. In such a situation, interventional strategies can be employed to provide the desired outcomes.

Current understanding indicates that tear drainage is unequal through the upper and lower canalicular systems—with lower lid drainage being predominant. In a recent study, the authors used the "drop test" to study the relative contributions of the two drainage channels in normal subjects. They reported that in the supine position, up to 60% of the drainage occurs through the lower lid system. In the upright position, this may increase making the lower canaliculus the major cause of tear outflow from the ocular surface, apart from evaporation. Other studies have, however, shown that when normal physiology is altered by punctal occlusion, compensatory systems set in, which reduce tear production in the face of a reduced tear clearance rate.

Despite these limitations, recent studies have shown improvements in subjective patient symptoms, vital surface stain scores, and visual acuity in patients with Stevens-Johnson

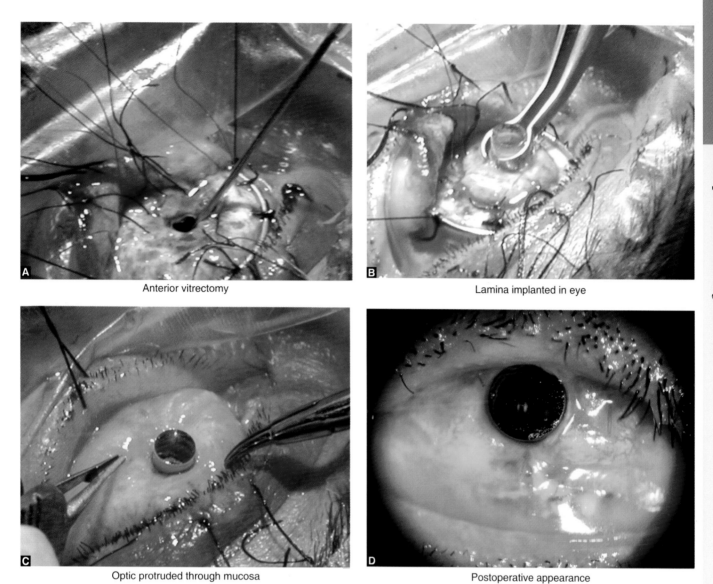

Figs 4.64A to D: Osteo-odonto-keratoprosthesis–Stage II surgery

syndrome and severe dry eye, after punctal occlusion. There has also been a recommendation for selective punctal occlusion in some diseases. In patients with superior limbic keratoconjunctivitis, the benefits of occluding only the superior lacrimal canaliculus has been described, and the authors indicate that the improvement results from the increase in local tear concentration in the region of the upper lid.

Approaches

Broadly, lacrimal punctal occlusion can be classified as temporary or permanent. In the former approach, a variety of materials, including hydroxypropyl methylcellulose, gelatin, collagen or catgut are used to block punctal drainage for a variable period of time ranging from a day to 2 weeks, to assess the effects of punctal occlusion. They are mostly used to assess for the occurrence of troublesome epiphora, prior to performing permanent occlusion. Improvement in patient symptoms and ocular surface scores can also be studied. If sufficient benefit is

noted with this approach, consideration is given to performing permanent occlusion. However, it is now apparent that these approaches only reduce tear flow through the canaliculus partially, by 60% to 80% and some patients can experience epiphora after punctal occlusion despite being asymptomatic after temporary occlusion.

Permanent occlusion is again subdivided into reversible and nonreversible methods. The former include approaches, such as the use of silicone, hydroxyethyl methacrylate or Teflon plugs that are placed in the punctum or canaliculus to obstruct drainage. The use of n-butyl cyanoacrylate would also be categorized here, although this is most often a temporary measure, with the glue falling out in time. Using a piece of autologous conjunctiva to create a mucosal patch that occludes the opening of the punctum is effective but reversible, because a cautery can be used to burn a hole in the mucosal patch when reopening of the drainage system is desired.

Irreversible methods include the destructive techniques using thermal—cautery or diathermy, and laser ablation to cause closure of the drainage channels. However, there is often breakdown of the scar created and recanalization results in renewed patency of the canaliculus in a large number of eyes treated with such techniques. Surgical excision of the lining epithelium and suturing of the canaliculus is a more permanent solution to this problem.

Surgical Technique

Since the occlusion procedure is designed to occlude the entrance into the lacrimal drainage system, for it to be effective, patency of the system should first be ensured. This will not only help decide if the procedure is necessary, but will also help prevent the occurrence of complications, such as dacryocystitis, which has been reported in patients who did not have a patent nasolacrimal duct.

Reversible punctal occlusion is a simple, office procedure—best performed with the patient seated at a slit lamp. Topical anesthesia is optional. The chosen temporary implant is held with a fine forceps and with the patient looking up, the medial aspect of the lower lid is gently retracted down, making the punctal opening more prominent. Under visualization, the implant is gently inserted into the vertical part of the lower canaliculus; and when in place, the closed tips of the forceps are used to gently advance the implant into the horizontal part of the canaliculus, so that it does not protrude and irritate the ocular surface. A similar procedure is performed for the upper lid with the lid retracted as the patient looks down. A similar technique is performed with the permanent plugs as well. While a wide variety of such devices are now available, they are generally designed to sit on the lid margin, partly protruding into the punctum and canaliculus, or are placed entirely within the horizontal portion of the canaliculus. With the former design, punctal dilatation is sometimes required to ensure proper placement of the device and topical anesthesia is then required, although this is still an office procedure. With plugs that sit within the canaliculus, often no anesthesia is required.

Thermal destruction requires that the lining of the mucosa of the canaliculus and punctum is destroyed and the healing process creates a scar that occludes drainage. The cautery or diathermy probe is inserted deep into the canaliculus and is then switched on for tissue destruction. While the procedure can be performed under topical anesthesia in some patients, the use of infiltration techniques may provide better pain relief. This can also be performed as an office procedure. The use of an argon laser to achieve these goals is a more elegant approach, but studies indicate that the recanalization rate is highest with this technique, which has, therefore, fallen out of favor in the face of more effective procedures.

The use of a conjunctival mucosal patch graft is technically more challenging and the procedure is performed in the operation theater using topical and infiltration anesthesia. A chalazion clamp is used to hold and evert the medial portion of the lid, so that the punctum is centered in the middle of the ring. The use of this clamp helps provide a bloodless operating field during excision of the conjunctiva around the punctum. A sharp knife is used to create a square mucosal incision that is centered on the punctum. Using the knife and 0.12 mm forceps, the mucosa outlined by the incision is excised. Bleeding is usually controlled by the presence of the chalazion clamp. A similar sized piece of free conjunctiva is excised from the inferior bulbar conjunctiva. The tissue is positioned in the raw area of the bed around the punctum, with the epithelial side facing up. The edges are sutured using 10-0 vicryl sutures (Figs 4.65A and B). After removing the clamp, a firm patch is applied with antibiotic ointment and is continued for a week. When reversal of effect is desired in the postoperative period, a cautery tip is used to make a hole in the center of the patch, which results in the reestablishment of patency of the canalicular system.

Surgical occlusion of the canalicular system requires a linear incision in the proximal part of the canaliculus, and this is facilitated by the insertion of a probe in the canal. Once the canalicular track is laid open, the epithelium lining the walls is scraped and 10-0 nylon sutures are used to approximate the walls. The resulting healing process causes obliteration of the canaliculus.

Complications

As with other surgical procedures, the above-mentioned techniques can also be associated with problems. These include extrusion of the plugs, damage to the punctal ring during dilatation, irritation or damage to the ocular surface from the presence of the plugs in the puncta, infective canaliculitis, migration of the plugs into the soft tissues surrounding the canaliculus, creation of false tracks and fistulae during the insertion procedure, dacryocystitis, canalicular stenosis, and pyogenic granuloma formation. Despite these problems, however, the use of punctal plugs remains an effective procedure in the surgical management of patients with tear insufficiency that is controlled poorly with medications.

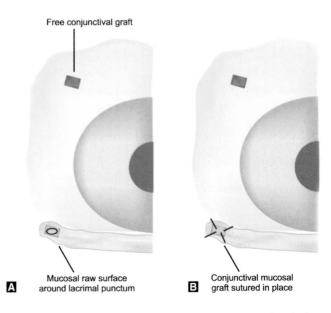

Free conjunctival graft

Mucosal raw surface around lacrimal punctum

Conjunctival mucosal graft sutured in place

Figs 4.65A and B: Conjunctival patch graft for punctal occlusion

There are other approaches that can be used to help such patients, if tear drainage blocking does not relieve symptoms. These include the addition of a lateral tarsorrhaphy to maintain the tear volume-surface area ratio, and the option of a free submandibular gland transplant—although the long-term efficacy of this complex surgical procedure is still unclear. Apart from these measures, the use of immunomodulators like topical cyclosporine A, autologous serum as eyedrops to supplement the biological trophic factors on the ocular surface, and the availability of oral secretagogues like pilocarpine may permit improved efficacy in the management of severe dry eye syndromes.

TECTONIC CORNEAL SURGERY

Limbal Fistula and Bleb Repair

With the increasing use of phacoemulsification for the surgical management of cataracts, the incidence of limbal fistulae and inadvertent fistula at the cataract wound is decreasing. However, in places where extracapsular cataract surgery is routinely performed, this entity continues to persist. A poorly constructed and sutured limbal wound, the use of excessive cauterization resulting in extensive tissue shrinkage, a patient predisposed to poor wound healing, and wound dehiscence in the early postoperative period are important predisposing factors. A communication exists between the anterior chamber and the external ocular surface; and if the area of wound dehiscence is unprotected, a fistula or cicatrix results. If the area of weakness in the wound is under an area covered by conjunctiva, an inadvertent bleb results. While the former is an area of direct communication with the interior of the eye and an important risk factor for endophthalmitis requiring early repair, the latter is not always an indication for surgery. If the patient has a non-leaking bleb, stable vision which does not fluctuate, normal IOP, has not developed past episodes of blebitis or endophthalmitis, and the bleb does not result in excessive irritation, dellen formation or astigmatism, observation would be acceptable. If the bleb violates one or more of the above conditions, surgical repair is probably indicated (Figs 4.66A and B).

The surgical procedure for both entities conforms to similar principles. Since there is an epithelium lined track communicating with the surface, simple suturing of the wound is unlikely to result in a good result, and a reestablishment of the communication is a virtual certainty. Over a period of time, there is sclerosis of the track with tissue scarring and contraction, and this combined with the possible initial tissue loss that resulted in this complication, also precludes simple wound resuturing. There is likely to be excessive compression of the wound when the retracted tissues are apposed and this will result in significant contour changes and unacceptable astigmatism. Thus, while an attempt is made to excise or destroy the epithelial lining, it is also important to reinforce the closure using a patch graft to close the communication.

The area of leak is identified (Fig. 4.67). If not obvious, the use of fluorescein and a Seidel test will be helpful. A paracentesis is made in the upper temporal quadrant to provide access to the anterior chamber during subsequent maneuvers. Since

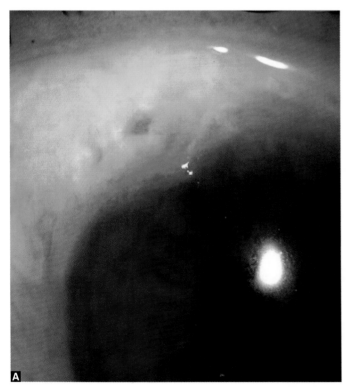
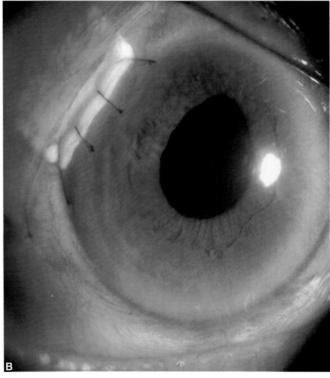

Figs 4.66A and B: Limbal fistula repair (A) Limbal inadvertent fistula, (B) Post-scleral patch graft

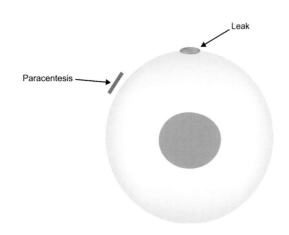

Fig. 4.67: Limbal fistula—paracentesis during surgery

the closure of the fistula is often associated with high spikes of IOP in the early postoperative period (till the dysfunctional trabecular meshwork begins functioning), this paracentesis can also serve to release some aqueous humor in the early postoperative period for control of the IOP, with the patient seated at the slit lamp.

The procedure starts with a peritomy at the site of the fistula or bleb to adequately expose the area of pathology (Fig. 4.68). Gentle cautery is performed to obtain adequate hemostasis without aggravating the existing tissue shrinkage. If a conjunctival bleb is present, a Beaver blade is used to shave the bleb from its attachments to the episclera, but care is taken to avoid opening the bleb as this can result in loss of the anterior chamber and a soft eye, making further dissection difficult. A partial-thickness incision is made in the sclera and cornea outlining a rectangle that is about 2 mm away from the margins of

the fistulous opening or bleb (Fig. 4.69). A dissection is initiated at the depth of the incision to create a bed in the sclera and cornea surrounding the fistula. This is performed using a Beaver blade, a no. 15 Bard-Parker blade or a crescent knife. A centripetal approach is used to encircle the fistula or bleb, working towards the area of pathology. It is important to ensure a good bed, particularly at the corners of the rectangle to enable the patch graft to fit well. The bleb is opened finally after the bed has been dissected satisfactorily.

The track of the fistula is scraped gently with a sharp knife or the bevel of a fine disposable needle to remove the epithelial lining. If there is a significant gape of the margins, a suture may be used to hold them together loosely, without creating any corneal distortion. Since the anterior chamber is likely to collapse at this stage, air or viscoelastic may be injected through the paracentesis to protect the endothelium and maintain the corneal contour when the graft is sutured. The dimensions of the rectangular bed are measured, and a similar sized graft is prepared either from preserved donor sclera or from the residual corneoscleral rim of a donor cornea that has been used for corneal transplantation. If the latter is used, the endothelium on the corneal portion is scraped off. While both are satisfactory, the use of a corneoscleral rim will result in better cosmesis, since the presence of a white, opaque scleral graft over the peripheral cornea can be avoided. The graft is sutured using 10-0 nylon sutures and the conjunctiva reposited over the scleral portion of the graft (Fig. 4.70).

In the event of a patch graft not being available, it is also possible to perform the same procedure using a rotational autograft. The initial steps remain the same. After adequate exposure of the fistula, a 50% scleral flap with the hinge at least 1.5 mm from the margin of the fistula is created (Fig. 4.71). This allows the folded flap to provide adequate compression and closure of the fistula. The area around the fistula is de-epithelialized and the superior flap is flipped over and sutured in place with the sutures passing through a groove created in the

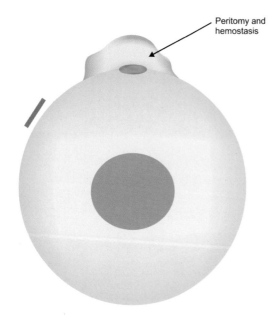

Fig. 4.68: Limbal fistula—exposure of leak site

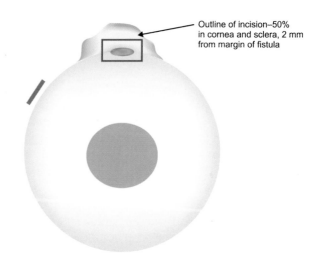

Fig. 4.69: Limbal fistula—incision for outline of patch graft

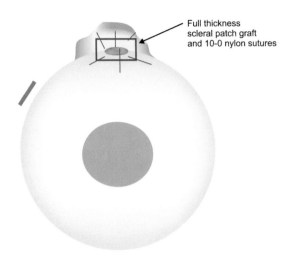

Fig. 4.70: Limbal fistula—scleral patch graft

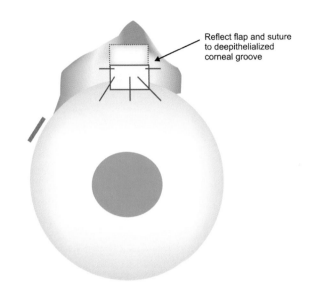

Fig. 4.72: Limbal fistula—suturing rotational scleral autograft

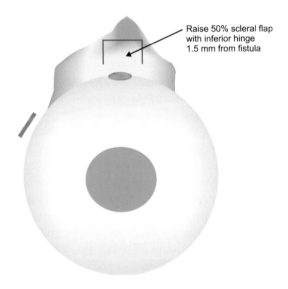

Fig. 4.71: Limbal fistula—fashioning rotational scleral autograft

cornea (Fig. 4.72). The conjunctiva is reposited over the scleral donor bed.

Corneal Perforations

Corneal perforations can result from trauma, infections and immunological melts of the corneal stroma. Those occurring from trauma often tend to be fairly large and their management has been dealt with in the section on corneal trauma. Those resulting from tissue necrosis or dissolution due to infective or immunological processes tend to be smaller, and need surgical repair to restore the integrity of the cornea. This would hopefully allow medical treatment of the underlying problem to resolve the infection or immunological disturbance (Fig. 4.73).

If the perforation is smaller than 1 mm, n-butyl cyanoacrylate glue remains a useful option (Figs 4.74A and B). The glue serves as a seal that protects the underlying corneal stroma

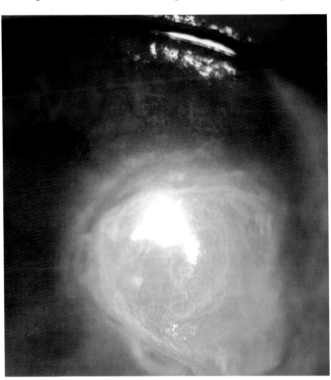

Fig. 4.73: Cyanoacrylate glue for peripheral perforation

from the deleterious effects of the tear film polymorphonuclear leukocytes, which are no longer able to accumulate and produce collagenolysis. Since the inflammatory component is excluded, stromal healing is able to proceed, allowing scarring and closure of the perforation.

Since the glue does not form a stable attachment to the corneal epithelium, it is important to perform a debridement of the epithelium and loose necrotic stroma surrounding the corneal perforation. The cyanoacrylate material tends to polymerize fairly quickly when it comes into contact with ocular fluids or the ocular surface; and therefore, it is important to achieve good drying of the surface before applying the

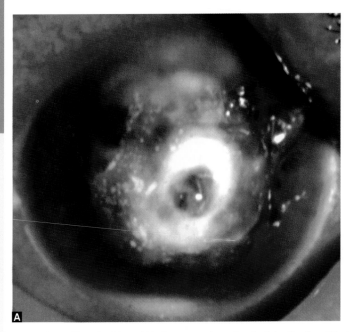 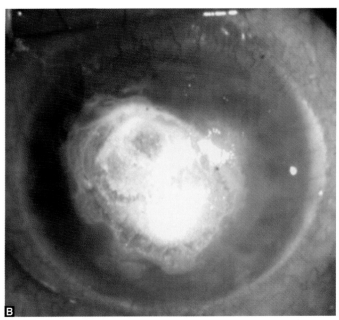

Figs 4.74A and B: Cyanoacrylate glue for infective keratitis (A) Keratitis with descemetocele, (B) Post-cyanoacrylate glue

glue. This prevents premature polymerization, which can result in an unsatisfactory seal. In eyes with a descemetocele and an impending perforation, the drying is easily achieved. However, if a perforation is actually present, the aqueous leak tends to pose problems. This can be countered by the injection of air into the anterior chamber. With the patient lying down, the air floats up and seals the leak due to its surface tension. In a larger perforation, very high-density viscoelastic may be used.

Applying the glue can be performed using one of the two techniques. A cotton swab can be cut in half and to the cut end of the stick, some sterile ointment is applied. Over this, a disc of sterile plastic is placed and the ointment serves to retain the disc in place. A drop of glue is placed over the plastic and this prevents premature polymerization (Fig. 4.75). The surgeon positions the stick over the site of the perforation and quickly inverts the whole complex such that the glue contacts the perforation and pressure is applied till polymerization occurs. Although a good technique, it is fairly cumbersome to use, with the main drawback being that the stick and plastic disc obscure a view of the actual site of application.

Another method to apply the glue would be to attach a fresh 30-gauge needle to a dry disposable tuberculin syringe in which some glue is taken. The glue is gradually expressed till a tiny bead appears at the tip of the needle (Fig. 4.76). This is then applied to the desired area under direct visualization and the surface tension of the drop is used to maintain contact with the corneal surface as the needle is slowly moved over the entire area where the glue is to be applied. Gentle pressure on the plunger provides more glue; and in this manner, the glue is "painted" over the entire area of application. The polymerized surface of the glue tends to have a craggy, rough surface, and it is important to place a bandage contact lens to protect the palpebral conjunctiva and also to reduce the disturbing effect of the lid on the glue.

Although there have been recent reports of the use of amniotic membrane pieces stuffed into the perforation to help close the defect, with further such pieces sewn to the corneal surface, further experience is probably required to assess the efficacy of this approach in the management of corneal perforations.

In eyes with perforations larger than 2 mm, glue does not work and a patch graft is required to ensure secure closure

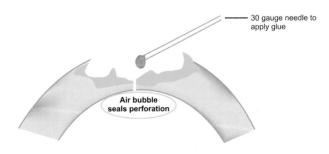

Fig. 4.75: Glue application in corneal perforation

Fig. 4.76: Glue application through a 30-gauge needle in corneal perforation

(Figs 4.77A and B). The caveats of the surgical procedure in these situations are described in this section. Assessment of the eye should be performed to determine the size of the perforation, and the presence of infection. The type of anesthesia to be used should be determined, and the surgical plan including the type of tissue to be used, as a patch graft should be determined, and the prognosis ascertained.

In the recipient eye, adequate exposure should be obtained during surgery, and the area for the surgical bed surrounding the perforation(s) should be outlined with appropriate sized trephines to provide a regular margin. However, a freehand marking in a rectangular shape should also be possible. The marks are deepened to 90% depth incisions using a diamond knife. A bed is then dissected in the area outlined, as mentioned in the procedure for fistula repair. Prolapsed iris serves to plug the opening and should be abscised after a paracentesis is created, to prevent premature loss of the anterior chamber, which makes subsequent dissection difficult.

Although a whole donor globe is best for fashioning the lamellar corneal patch graft, a corneoscleral rim can also be used for this purpose. Gauze wrapped around an appropriately sized acrylic ball implant can serve as a holder, onto which the corneoscleral rim can be sutured using 6-0 silk sutures. Since only an anterior lamellar patch is required, the endothelial damage that this maneuver creates is unimportant. The appropriate markings from the recipient bed are transferred onto the donor corneal surface and a similar 90% depth dissection is performed providing a patch of appropriate dimensions.

The graft is transferred to the recipient bed and the margins are matched. Cardinal sutures of 10-0 nylon are used to anchor the graft in place after which further interrupted sutures are used to achieve a secure watertight closure, ensuring good edge apposition. Sometimes, further trimming of the margins of the graft may be required to ensure a better fit in the bed. At the conclusion of the procedure, the knots of the interrupted sutures are buried in the corneal stroma and the anterior chamber is formed with BSS (Figs 4.78A and B).

Band-Shaped Keratopathy

In this condition, there is an accumulation of calcium in the interpalpebral subepithelial zone of the cornea. There are numerous causes, including chronic uveitis, especially in children, silicone oil in the eye, a familial variety, systemic disturbances in calcium metabolism and an idiopathic variety. The condition results in reduced visual function and also irritative symptoms due to the irregular and roughened corneal surface.

Management of the underlying condition may prevent recurrences of the corneal condition, but medical therapy of the condition is unsatisfactory. Removal of the calcium deposits can be easily performed using chelation with freshly prepared 1.5% to 3.0% disodium ethylenediaminetetraacetic acid (EDTA). The procedure can be performed either by using topical anesthesia with the patient seated at a slit lamp or by using an operating microscope, with the patient lying supine. A speculum is used to expose the cornea and the epithelium is removed from the area containing calcium, by scraping using a Beaver blade. Cotton swabs soaked in the EDTA solution are gently, but firmly rubbed against the exposed corneal deposits till satisfactory clearing is achieved. The eye is padded with atropine eyedrops and antibiotic eye ointment till epithelial integrity is re-established, followed by treatment with tear substitutes.

The removal of these deposits using the excimer laser has also been described. However, since calcium is vaporized rather slowly, it may be faster to physically remove larger plaques using a Beaver blade, and use the laser to achieve removal of the residual deposits and produce a smoother corneal surface.

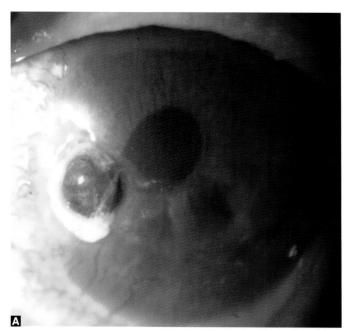

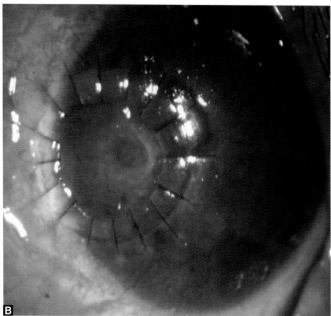

Figs 4.77A and B: Corneal patch graft for small perforation (A) Peripheral perforation, (B) Lamellar keratoplasty

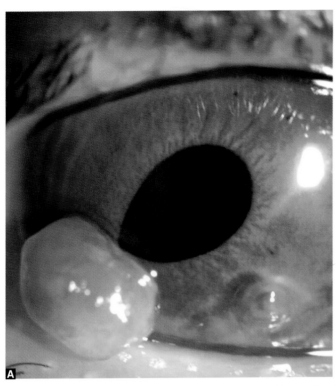
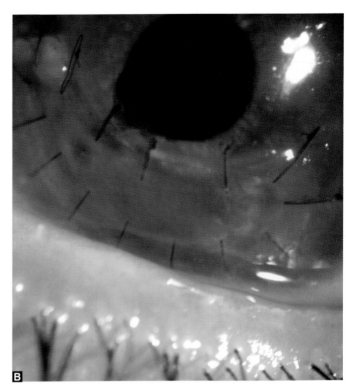

Figs 4.78A and B: Corneal patch graft for multiple perforation (A) Two peripheral perforations, (B) Lamellar keratoplasty

Anterior Stromal Puncture

Recurrent corneal erosions are caused following trauma to the corneal surface by sharp objects like a fingernail or the edge of a piece of paper. The resulting damage to the basement membrane of the corneal epithelium results in improper adhesion of the basal epithelium with the result that the epithelium in this area is prone to detachment—often when the patient wakes up at night or in the morning. Recent evidence also indicates that these eyes tend to have increased levels of matrix metalloproteinases in the tears and this may result in dissolution of the newly formed complexes, preventing a stable adhesion. In eyes, which do not respond to medical therapy including intense lubrication with eyedrops during the day and ointment at night, hypertonic saline, weak steroid eyedrops, and oral tetracyclines, a bandage contact lens may be tried. If even this fails, more invasive methods can be used, including anterior stromal puncture and excimer phototherapeutic keratectomy. Other options described in the management of this condition include—the use of a diamond burr to create a superficial keratectomy, botulinum toxin and autologous serum.

The purpose of the anterior stromal puncture is to create microtrauma to the Bowman's layer in the region of the epithelial erosion, thereby promoting scarring which firmly fixes the epithelium in place. It is performed using topical anesthesia with the patient seated at the slit lamp for better perception of corneal depth. After identifying the area of the erosion, the unhealthy epithelium is gently removed using a blunt Beaver blade. A 26 or 27-gauge needle with its tip bent is then used to make multiple punctures in the exposed Bowman's membrane.

A needle prefashioned for this purpose is also available commercially. The eye is then patched with atropine drops and antibiotic ointment to promote epithelial healing after which lubrication with tear substitutes and ointment is continued. It must be remembered, however, that the healing response in the Bowman's layer, which provides small microfingers of fibrosis anchoring the regenerated epithelium, also results in small corneal opacities in the area of treatment. Hence, this procedure should be reserved for small erosions that do not involve the visual axis. Also, this may not be the ideal solution for patients with corneal dystrophies involving a large area of the cornea.

Conjunctival Hooding

With the advent of newer options for the management of corneal disorders, this is a procedure that is seldom performed today. However, when indicated, as in a blind painful eye due to severe bullous keratopathy, this procedure provides satisfactory cosmesis and relief from symptoms. The procedure is also performed to cover a limited area of the cornea in some eyes with recurrent stromal inflammation and ulceration due to viral keratitis, if conservative treatment fails to satisfactorily resolve the condition.

The procedure of using the conjunctiva to cover the entire cornea—Gundersen's flap, can be performed using orbital infiltration anesthesia. A corneal suture is used to pull the globe in an inferior direction. A superior rectus bridle suture is avoided to prevent tears in the superior conjunctiva. Once the superior bulbar conjunctiva is exposed, a circumferential incision parallel to the superior limbus is made 12 mm from the limbus. Care is taken to avoid including the Tenon's tissue when dissecting

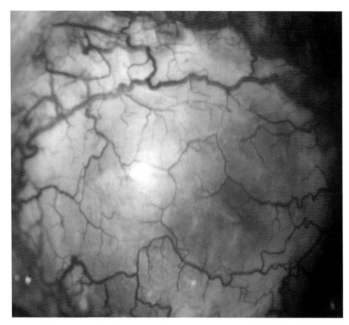

Fig. 4.79: Total conjunctival hooding

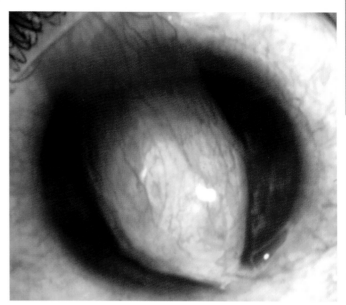

Fig. 4.80: Partial conjunctival flap

the conjunctival flap inferiorly to the superior limbus. When the dissection reaches the superior limbus, a perforation is made in the attachment of the conjunctiva to the limbus at 12 o'clock. This incision is then continued all around the limbus for 360° keeping the peritomy flush with the limbus. Attention is then paid to removing the corneal and limbal epithelium completely. Retention of this epithelium can result in cysts under the conjunctival flap. Once this has been accomplished, the superiorly dissected conjunctival flap is brought down and stretched over the denuded corneal surface, taking care to avoid buttonholing the flap. Relaxing incisions in the two "handles" of the flap may be required, to allow the flap to lie over the corneal surface without tension. The flap is then sutured to the limbal zone using interrupted 10-0 nylon sutures. The knots are not buried and can be removed between 4 and 6 weeks (Fig. 4.79).

Other alternatives that have been described for this condition include the use of extensive anterior stromal punctures over the entire corneal surface after removing the epithelium, and the use of amniotic membrane to patch the entire corneal surface after removing the edematous epithelium.

A similar approach, as described in the earlier paragraphs, is used for partial conjunctival hooding, but a superficial keratectomy is created to produce a bed for the conjunctival flap as the edge of a partial flap lying on the surface of the cornea is likely to be constantly contacted by the edge of the lid during blinking (Fig. 4.80).

Chapter 5

Refractive Surgeries

Ritika Sachdev, Namrata Sharma,
Rajesh Sinha, Jeewan S Titiyal

INTRODUCTION

Refractive surgery is one of the most rapidly developing aspects of ophthalmology. Prior to a detailed discussion of the refractive surgical procedures, it is imperative to understand the basic sciences and diagnostic tests, which are a critical to the practice of refractive surgery.

Relevant Anatomy and Corneal Biomechanics

The anterior corneal surface contributes to around two-third (approximately +48D) of the refractive power of the eye. The overall corneal power decreases (approximately +43D) due to the negative power of the posterior corneal surface.

Keratorefractive surgeries aim to alter the shape of the cornea in order to change the refractive status of the eye. Flattening the central cornea for myopic correction changes its shape from the natural prolate aspheric shape (steeper in the center) to an oblate profile (steeper in the periphery).

Corneal Topography

Placido-Disc Topography Systems

The Placido-disc topography systems are based on the reflection principle. A Placido disc is projected onto the cornea and the images of the Placido disc reflected off the corneal surface are captured. Information regarding the position of the Placido-disc rings is used to reconstruct the corneal shape.

These devices have excellent accuracy and reproducibility in anterior corneal curvature measurement. Limitations of these systems include the following:

- Data at the central zone have to be interpolated (although this unmeasured central zone is very small in some devices).
- The quality of tear film is critical since the images are obtained from light rays reflected off the tear film.
- Data is less accurate when mapping aspherical or irregular surfaces due to the assumption of sufficient smoothness in the radial direction used by some devices.

A normal cornea will have smooth contours, centrally uniform power and flattening toward the periphery—particularly toward the nasal side. Sim-K readings should be ~42.75 ± 1.6 D (standard deviation); a good rule of thumb would be to consider K readings less than 38 or greater than 47.5 D abnormal (± 3 standard deviations from the mean). Normal corneas may also present topography with a symmetrical bow tie pattern that represents cylinder.

Always perform corneal topography on both eyes, as pathology in one eye often forecasts the potential for pathology in the other eye (e.g. keratoconus).

Slit-Imaging Systems

The Orbscan system (Bausch & Lomb, Rochester, NY, USA) introduced in 1995 was based on the innovative principle of measuring the dimensions of a slit-scanning beam projected on the cornea.

Using slit or parallelepiped methodology, the curvature of the anterior surface of the cornea can be assessed along with the posterior surface and the anterior surface of the lens and iris. The Orbscan II incorporates a Placido-disc attachment to obtain curvature measurements directly and so attain the benefits of both approaches to cornea topography. During the acquisition, the Placido-disc is illuminated and the mire's reflection from the anterior corneal surface is stored. Subsequently, 40 slits, 20 from the right and 20 from the left, each 12.50 mm high and 0.30 mm wide, are projected on the cornea at an angle of 45 degrees to the instrument axis. As the light from these slits passes through the cornea, it is scattered in all directions, but, crucially, it is backscattered toward the digital video camera of the device, which records the appearance in 2-dimensional images. These data points are then used to create an elevation topographic representation of the anterior surface of the cornea. The triangulation of internal ocular surfaces is not as precise as that of the anterior surface because in addition to hardware and acquisition variables, it is also dependent on the precision of the anterior surface maps.

General guidelines for screening for "forme fruste conus" in LASIK using the Orbscan data

Posterior Elevation over Best Fit Sphere > 0.04 mm (Fig. 5.1)

Pachymetry

- Minimum pachymetry < 470 μm
- Difference of > 100 μm from 7 mm optical zone to thinnest point

The normal band scale setting depicts values within the normative range as green and highlights any gross abnormalities. It may be used for screening purpose (Figs 5.2A and B).

Scheimpflug Imaging: The Oculus Pentacam

The Pentacam (Oculus, Germany) and the Pentacam HR are Scheimpflug imaging devices, which utilize two cameras. The central camera monitors fixation while the second rotating Scheimpflug camera provides 25 or 50 cross-sectional corneal images during a scan of less than two seconds duration. Each image contains 500 elevation points with the standard Pentacam and 2,760 elevation points for the Pentacam HR, yielding a total of 25,000 or 138,000 total data points respectively. The Scheimpflug images are used to reconstruct the anterior and the posterior corneal surface. Other details obtained include corneal pachymetry, anterior chamber depth measurement (central and peripheral) as well as images of the iris, angle and the lens. Elevation data from the anterior and posterior corneal surface are depicted with respect to a reference shape (commonly a sphere) to produce elevation subtraction maps (Fig. 5.3). This aids in eliminating the "background noise" and highlights any abnormality. This system is perhaps the best tool for mapping the cornea prior to refractive surgery as it provides an accurate assessment of the posterior corneal surface, which is critical to the diagnosis of "forme fruste keratoconus".

General guidelines suggested by Belin and associates when screening patients for refractive surgery are as follows:

- Elevation values **>+10** μm for the anterior surface and >15 μm for the posterior surface for central or paracentral "islands" are considered abnormal.
- Abnormal islands in the pachymetry maps are typically associated with the displacement of the thinnest region in the pachymetry map towards the island.

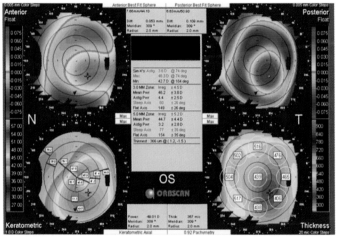

Fig. 5.1: Orbscan. Quad map (Orbscan) of a patient with keratoconus: Its four components include the anterior elevation map, the posterior elevation map, the keratometric map and the corneal pachymetry map

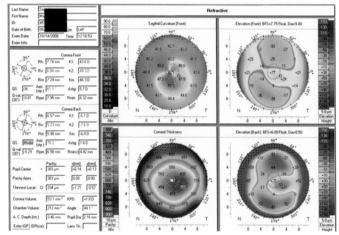

Fig. 5.3: Pentacam. The Pentacam map of a patient with keratoconus

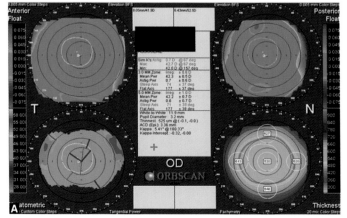

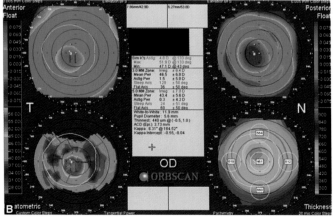

Figs 5.2A and B: Orbscan. Normal band scale quad map of a normal case (A) and a case with keratoconus (B)

Corneal Biomechanics

A recently introduced instrument, the Ocular Respose Analyzer (ORA, Riechert Ophthalmic Instruments, New York, USA) measures corneal biomechanical properties. It has been seen that in keratoconic corneas, the corneal hysteresis and corneal resistance factor were significantly lower than in the normal eyes. These parameters may be potentially useful in predicting whether a candidate seeking refractive surgery is at risk of developing post-LASIK ectasia.

Wavefront Analysis

Wavefront analysis allows a mathematical depiction of the irregularities in the cornea. The Hartmann-Shack wavefront sensor is the most commonly used instrument to measure wavefront aberrations clinically. These are then specified in terms of Zernike polynomials, much like a mathematical formula. Lower order aberrations (spherical errors are first order; regular astigmatism and defocus are second order) are commonly corrected with conventional LASIK. Higher order aberrations, such as coma and trefoil (third order) and secondary astigmatism or tetrafoil (fourth order) may increase after conventional LASIK surgery. Customized LASIK or wavefront-guided LASIK seeks to minimize these higher order aberrations in addition to elimination of the refractive error, so as to optimize the quality of vision.

What is Fourier Analysis?

The use of Fourier transformation to analyze a wavefront represents an alternative approach to Zernike polynomials. Despite potential advantages to either method, the increased resolution of complex shapes with Fourier transformation suggests that it may prove to be a useful modality in treating patients.

The VISX Star S4 system is the only laser with the advanced wavefront system, Fourier analysis.

KERATOREFRACTIVE PROCEDURES

These procedures aim to reshape the cornea in order to eliminate the refractive error.

Incisional Corneal Surgery

Incisional surgery for myopia and hyperopia has largely been replaced by excimer laser procedures. Astigmatic keratotomy still, however, retains its role in the treatment of astigmatism in patients undergoing cataract surgery and in correction of astigmatism after keratoplasty.

Radial Keratotomy for Myopia

Fyodorov is accredited with the development of modern radial keratotomy (RK). He devised basic instrumentation for the procedure and established that the diameter of the central clear optical zone was inversely proportional to the amount of myopic correction induced.

The procedure and its instruments were further refined by researchers in the United States.

Patient Selection

Radial keratotomy is suitable for patients with up to moderate myopia (1 to –4D). Treatment of higher degree of myopia often requires more than 8 incisions and longer incisions with smaller optical zones and may subsequently be fraught with complications.

Surgical Technique

Radial incisions produce a wound gape, increasing the radius of curvature of the central cornea and subsequently flattening it.

Radial incisions, centered on the pupil are performed with a diamond blade. The Russian technique advocated placement of centripetal (periphery to center) cuts while the American approach involves placement of centrifugal cuts (center to periphery). The Russian technique produces deeper cuts while the American technique minimizes the risk of extension of these cuts into the visual axis.

The incisions should ideally extend up to 85 to 95% of the corneal thickness. Deeper incisions produce more refractive correction, but are fraught with greater instability of the refractive outcome. Smaller optical zones produce greater myopic correction. The flattening produced by the incision also varies with the age of the patient, increasing by up to 1 D per decade of the patient's age.

Nomograms based on the degree of myopic correction desired and the age of the patient are used to guide the optimal sizing of the clear optical zone and estimate the number of incisions required.

Prospective Evaluation of Radial Keratotomy (PERK)

The PERK study conducted in 1982–83, evaluated the role of RK in patients with myopia ranging from – 2 D to – 8.75 D (diopters). All patients were treated with eight radial incisions with variable clear optical zones corresponding to the amount of myopic correction desired. Enhancement surgery was performed if required with an additional eight incisions. At ten years follow-up, the 53% of the patients were found to have best corrected visual acuity of 20/20 or better. Almost 85% of the patients achieved a BCVA of 20/40 or better. Loss of BCVA was noted in 3% of the patients, attributable to corneal scarring, irregular astigmatism and delayed onset bacterial keratitis.

A significant revelation in this trial was the documentation of the inherent instability of this procedure. A hyperopic shift of greater than 1 D was seen in 43% of the operated eyes. This shift did not regress even up to 10 years after the procedure and was noted to be associated with the length of the incision.

These findings led to the development of the mini-RK procedure with the use of shorter incisions.

Complications

- Diurnal fluctuations: The cornea gradually steepens during the waking hours. The PERK study demonstrated a difference of 0.31 D±0.58 D during the morning and evening spherical equivalents obtained after performing the refraction of patients who had undergone RK.
- Under correction and overcorrection
- Increased astigmatism
- Instability of refractive correction with hyperopic shift
- Starburst pattern and glare: Occurs due to scattering of light from the radial incisions or scars. Seen more commonly in patients with smaller clear optical zones (Figs 5.4A and B)
- Rare but blinding complications, such as perforation of the cornea, traumatic globe rupture and bacterial keratitis.

Hexagonal Keratotomy for Hyperopia

This procedure involved the placement of paracentral incisions in a hexagonal pattern in order to produce steepening of the central cornea. Significant problems like glare and irregular astigmatism plagued this procedure, which has now been largely abandoned.

Incisional Correction of Astigmatism

Transverse keratotomy consists of two linear incisions placed diametrically opposite each other along the steep axis of the cornea. These result in flattening along the steep meridian and associated steepening of the orthogonal meridian due to the phenomenon of "coupling". This procedure has, however, been largely replaced by the laser photoablative procedures, such as LASIK and photorefractive keratectomy (PRK).

Arcuate keratotomy (AK) and limbal relaxing incisions (LRI) are arcuate incisions centered on the steep axis placed in the in the midperipheral cornea and just anterior to the limbus respectively. "Coupling" causes the steepening of the orthogonal meridian, thereby keeping the spherical equivalent largely unchanged.

LASER-based Photoablative Procedures

Laser refractive surgery is based on the principle of modifying the refractive power of the cornea by ablating the stromal tissue. Laser procedures performed using excimer lasers to correct refractive errors are of two types:

- Surface treatment techniques or surface ablation procedures:
  - PRK
  - LASEK (laser-subepithelial keratomileusis)
  - Epi-LASIK
  - Surface ablation
- Lamellar treatment techniques:
  - Creation of a stromal flap
  - LASIK using the microkeratome
  - LASIK using the femtosecond laser

Surface Ablation Procedures

In the surface treatment techniques, corneal tissue is ablated with an excimer laser just below the corneal epithelium. The various techniques refer to how the corneal epithelium is removed.

- PRK epithelium is removed using a laser
- In LASEK an alcohol solution is used to abrade the epithelium
- In epi-LASIK, a microkeratome is used to remove a uniform sheet of epithelium
- In surface ablation, a mechanical instrument is used to scrape off the epithelium

The excimer laser procedure is performed and a bandage contact lens is placed. The corneal epithelium usually grows back in a couple of days (Figs 5.5 and 5.6).

In lamellar laser techniques, a microkeratome or a femtosecond laser is used to create a flap. The flap is everted on its hinge and the stroma is exposed for laser ablation. After ablation, the flap is reflected back in its original place where adhesions form within a few hours.

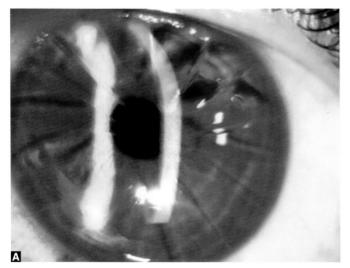
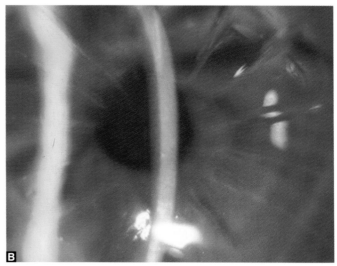

Figs 5.4A and B: Radial keratotomy (A) Radial incisions for the correction of myopia, (B) High magnification view. Note the small clear optical zone. The patient complains of "starburst" pattern

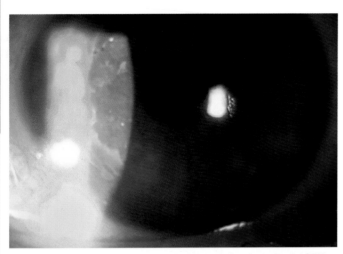

Fig. 5.5: LASEK. Postoperative appearance of patient after LASEK. Note the epithelial defect

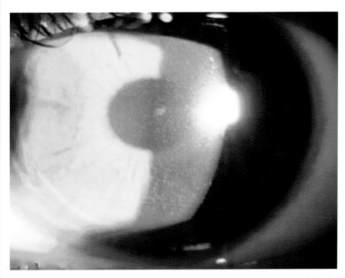

Fig. 5.6: LASEK. Postoperative appearance at 1 week. The epithelial defect has healed

In both the techniques refractive correction is achieved by photoablation of the corneal stroma by the excimer laser. The excimer laser system works on the principle of ablative photodecomposition using Argon Fluoride as the essential gas mixture. It is a Class IV laser with a wavelength of 193 nm. At this wavelength it causes selective ablation of corneal tissue according to preset parameters. For myopia greater ablation is done in the center of the cornea to flatten the corneal shape while in hyperopia, the peripheral tissue is ablated to cause the steepening of the cornea. The ablation protocol is determined specifically for each individual patient's refractive error and calculated accordingly by a software program in the laser system. The lasers may be delivered through an either large beam diameters of 5–7 mm or using the scanning technique to deliver a small spot or slit in a controlled manner on the stromal bed.

The depth of tissue ablation is calculated by Munnerlyn's equation, which in a simplified way states that

$$\text{Depth of ablation } (\mu m) = [\text{diameter of optical zone (mm)}]^2 \times 1/3 \text{ power (D)}$$

Hence, the amount of tissue that must be removed depends not only on the amount of refractive error, but also on the optical zone. Both the diameter and depth of ablation need to be optimized to attain best results. Smaller optical zones cause greater degree of regression and haloes while larger zones are beneficial in reducing night vision problems.

All laser systems come with their recommended list of safety precautions. All operating room personnel should avoid direct exposure to skin or eye with the primary laser beam. The area of potential hazard for the production of photochemical keratitis is less than 40 cm. Safety glasses should be worn within this range. Odors and fumes interfere with laser function and should not be allowed inside the laser room. The gas cylinders used in the laser have fluorine, argon, helium and neon. Fluorine is a highly toxic gas with a sharp odor that causes irritation to nose, eyes and throat at extremely low concentrations. Excimer lasers use < 0.25% concentration of fluroine. Argon, helium and neon are inert nontoxic gases with no color, odor or taste.

Strict environmental conditions need to be maintained in the laser suite for proper functioning of the laser system. Temperature range should not fluctuate beyond 60°–80° F and relative humidity should be between 35% and 65 %.

Indications of surface ablation procedures:
- Flat cornea
- LASIK complications in the contralateral eye
- Predisposition to trauma (flap), e.g. in contact sports
- Orbital anatomy precluding the use of microkeratome safely and effectively
- Irregular astigmatism (corneal topographical abnormalities not qualifying as keratoconus)
- Glaucoma and operated glaucoma with filtering bleb
- Deep set eye
- Small palpebral fissure

Contraindications
- Patient concerned about postoperative pain
- Keratoconus
- Pregnancy
- Diabetes (relative contraindication)
- Keloid

In higher amplitudes of refractive error, surface ablation can cause corneal haze and hence should be used along with mito-mycin-C intraoperatively (Fig. 5.7).

LASIK or Laser-Assisted in-situ Keratomileusis was origi-nally conceived by Barraquer in Colombia in 1949 where he created a free corneal cap, froze it, sculpted the undersurface on a cryolathe and sutured it back on the cornea. This was followed by automated lamellar keratoplasty in which after making a corneal flap, a microkeratome was used to excise a disc of stromal tissue and the flap was replaced without sutures. Burrato and Pallikaris first combined excimer laser with micro-keratome technology. Subsequent modification in technique

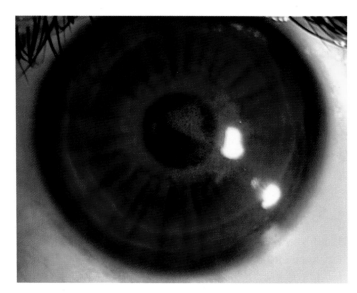

Fig. 5.7: Epi-LASIK. Epithelial haze after Epi-LASIK surgery in a case of refractive error with – 8 D of myopia

led to the current form of LASIK wherein an excimer laser is used to ablate the stromal bed after creating a hinged corneal flap with a very fine microkeratome blade, followed by accurate placement of the flap on the ablated stromal surface making it an extremely safe, precise and predictable procedure.

LASIK has become increasingly popular since 1995 and is now the most commonly performed refractive procedure to correct myopia, hyperopia and astigmatism. Errors ranging from – 0.5 to – 12 D of myopia, +0.5 to +4 D of hyperopia and up to 8 D of astigmatism can be treated. LASIK can also be used to treat residual refractive errors after PRK, RK, after cataract surgery with IOL implantation and penetrating kerato-plasty and combined with other refractive surgery (bioptics and trioptics), etc.

The basic instruments required for a LASIK procedure are the microkeratome and the excimer laser unit. A wide variety of microkeratomes are available, including the conventional mechanical keratome, disposable keratome, laser keratomes and water jets.

A microkeratome essentially consists of a fine oscillating blade, which can penetrate the cornea at predetermined depths to slice a smooth layer of corneal tissue. The adjustable param-eters allow the surgeon to decide the depth and diameter of the corneal flap with an accuracy of 5–10 μm. The assembly, opera-tion and maintenance of the microkeratome system are crucial to ensure the accurate and predictable resections of corneal tissue.

The microkeratome set-up includes a pneumatic suction ring, which fixates the globe and elevates the intraocular pres-sure up to 65 mm Hg to create an even and smooth corneal flap. On the surface of the suction ring, there are dove-tailed grooves over which the microkeratome head is placed and the motor allows the blade to advance to create a hinged corneal flap. A surgeon-controlled foot pedal ensures movement of the blade forward till the hinge is reached after which it is reversed

and the microkeratome is removed from the eye. The corneal flap is then gently lifted and everted to allow laser ablation on the stromal bed. The interface is irrigated, and the flap is replaced on the stromal bed after ensuring accurate placement. Visual recovery is almost immediate with a stable and precise refractive outcome.

Femtosecond Laser: A Breakthrough in Creation of the Stromal Flap for LASIK

A femtosecond laser represents a breakthrough in ultrafast laser science. The laser uses an infrared beam of light to pre-cisely separate tissue through a process called photo-disrup-tion by generating pulses as short as one-quadrillionth of a second (10-15 = femto-second). The IntraLase femtosecond laser (AMO, Santa Ana, CA, USA) is a 60 KHz diode pumped Nd:glass oscillator with a wavelength of 1053 nm based upon the technology whereby focused laser pulses divide material at the molecular level without transfer of heat or impact to the surrounding tissue.

The IntraLase femtosecond laser is used to create the cor-neal flap in a LASIK procedure eliminating the use and risk of a microkeratome and blade and increasing the overall safety, precision and accuracy (Fig. 5.8). The laser beam is focused on a pre-programmed depth and position within the cornea with each pulse forming a microscopic bubble. As the Intralase laser moves painlessly back and forth, the bubbles connect to form a flap with no trauma to adjacent tissue, the entire process taking around 20 seconds. The surgeon then lifts the flap to allow treatment by excimer laser. Laser specifications which can be modified to meet individual patient's needs include flap diam-eter, depth, hinge location and width and side-cut architecture.

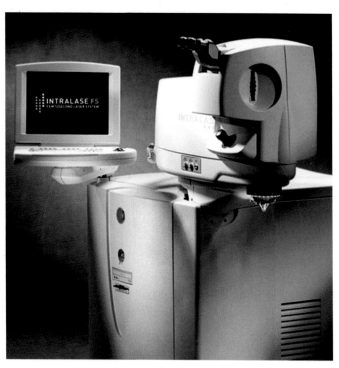

Fig. 5.8: IntraLase femtosecond laser system

The Intralase laser also creates a distinctive beveled edge flap which allows for precise re-positioning and alignment after Lasik is completed.

Intralase laser creates a corneal flap of precise size, shape and depth to micron-level accuracy 100% greater than that of blade-keratome and markedly reduces the risk of blade-related flap complications such as free caps, buttonholes, incomplete or decentered flaps. Unlike the meniscus shaped flap produced by the microkeratome, the flap created by the femtosecond laser is of uniform thickness (planar). It also creates fewer high and low-order aberrations which may cause glare and haloes at night. The precision of the flap also reduces the incidence of induced postoperative astigmatism as compared with microkeratome created flap.

Continued innovation in the femtosecond laser technology has led to the introduction of the next generation Intra Lase at 120 KHz which has now been commercially launched, signifying further advancements in refractive surgery.

LASIK in Myopia

LASIK is most commonly performed the world over for the correction of myopia. The prerequisites for LASIK include a minimum age of 18 years and refractive stability (no more than a ±0.5 D change in refraction in the last 6 months).

Preoperative Examination

Screening for LASIK must be done to eliminate patients who are unfit for the procedure. Contact lenses must be removed prior to the preoperative examination for a minimum of 7–14 days for soft contact lenses and 3 weeks for rigid gas permeable lenses. Systemic contraindications for LASIK include autoimmune disorders, collagen vascular disorders, diabetes mellitus and immunocompromised states. Pregnant and nursing women should also defer surgery due to fluctuation of refractive error during pregnancy, unstable tear film status and avoiding exposure of the fetus or neonate to medicines that may be required after the LASIK procedure. Patients on medications, such as amiodarone, isotretinoin and sumatriptan should be treated with caution as these medications may interfere with the wound healing response.

Ophthalmic contraindications include active ocular disease or inflammation as in conjunctivitis, scleritis, iritis or corneal ulcer. Severe dry eye associated with kerato-conjunctivitis sicca or exposure keratitis is an absolute contraindication. Herpes zoster ophthalmicus or herpetic keratitis especially if active in the previous 6 months is at risk for reactivation after exposure to ultraviolet radiation. Corneal ectasias seen in keratoconus, pellucid marginal degeneration and keratoglobus also preclude Lasik surgery. Glaucoma, diabetic retinopathy and progressive retinal disease make the patient unsuitable for a refractive procedure.

Ophthalmic Examination

A complete and detailed ophthalmic examination is mandatory before a patient is taken up for LASIK surgery. After a thorough history to rule out any contraindications, the patient undergoes measurement of unaided and best corrected visual acuity. A dry and cycloplegic refraction is performed. The patient is examined on the slit lamp to look for any lid abnormalities, corneal scarring or opacities or conjunctival disease. Any blepharitis or meibomitis must be treated to improve tear function and prevent trapping of any secretions at the flap interface.

A corneal topography and WaveScan measurement is performed. The corneal curvature, thickness, anterior and posterior floats are measured. Any corneal thinning or ectasia or early keratoconus (keratoconus forme fruste) is ruled out.

Performing the Laser Procedure

Based on the refraction, corneal topography and WaveScan measurements, the laser treatment plan is made. The information is complied together and the ablation profile is created keeping a residual bed of at least 250 μm. The laser technique is adopted depending on the amount of refractive error, the corneal thickness and the ablation depth required while maintaining the minimum bed thickness.

The ablation profile of an excimer laser corrects the spherical and cylindrical portions of the refractive error with lasers for myopia removing tissue from the center of the cornea to make the cornea flatter while hyperopic ablations are performed in the corneal periphery to make the central cornea steeper. Aspheric and wavefront-guided ablation profiles treat higher-order aberrations (HOA) of the eye and thus improve the patient's quality of vision.

Eye trackers monitor the center of the pupil and the iris pattern to prevent de-centered ablations and compensate for normal saccadic eye movements. The ablation procedure stops if the eye tracker cannot locate the pupil so that incorrect or poorly centered ablations are not performed.

Standard LASIK ablation parameters are available, like the Maloney's tables. These charts have the ablation depths calculated based on the refractive error and treat the spherical and cylindrical components. However, they do not treat the higher order aberrations (HOAs) and may even induce them especially during correction of high refractive errors. To avoid this, customized LASIK or C-Lasik is performed, which integrates wavefront technology with the laser treatment.

Lasik in Hyperopia

In contrast to the central ablation performed in myopia, in hyperopic refractive correction, the central area is steepened by ablation of a doughnut shaped area in the mid periphery.

Enhancement Procedures

Patients suffering from under and over corrections can undergo enhancements months to years later after their primary LASIK procedure. Flaps can usually be lifted with ease after delineating the flap edge carefully and reflecting it back gently. It is important to correctly identify the plane of the previous cut and keep the position of the hinge in mind to avoid tearing of the flap.

Anterior segment optical coherence tomography may be helpful in identifying the plane of the corneal flap.

The earliest an enhancement procedure should be performed should be after at least 3–6 months after the first refractive surgery to allow the refractive correction to stabilize. It is important to ensure that a residual bed thickness of 250 μm is maintained after the enhancement laser. Surface ablation or PRK may be considered for enhancement in patients with inadequate residual bed thickness or inability to lift the previous flap. Complications such as epithelial in growth are more common after enhancement procedures due to irregularity of the re-lifted flap edge.

Flap-Related Complications

The creation of a regular lamellar flap of uniform thickness is the most important step in the LASIK surgical procedure. The "ESP" approach to LASIK emphasizes the important safety aspects of this surgery, which stands for adequate Exposure, sufficient Suction and Precision and patience. Various flap-related complications include the following:

Interface debris

Etiology: Interface debris may be derived from various origins, which include metal fragments from blade shattering during the insertion of the flap, oil material from the microkeratome, meibomian gland secretions, powder from gloves, sponge debris, fibers and lint, or even eyelashes. Although small amount of debris is visually insignificant, larger debris may be associated with fibrosis and may cause diffuse lamellar keratitis.

Management: Interface debris, if significant, is treated by lifting the flap and cleaning of the interface by copious irrigation. We examine patients routinely at 30 minutes after the procedure and undertake early flap lifting and irrigation if significant axial debris or fibers are noted. This is not necessary with small amounts of non-axial interface debris, which is usually insignificant.

Prevention: The eyelids should be cleaned preoperatively and any blepharitis or anterior segment inflammation addressed prior to surgery. The measures include the use of lint – and powder-free gloves, gowns, draping the lashes and applying a draining sponge around the limbus, which prevents the regurgitation of surrounding secretions. An aspirating speculum may be used when irrigating the interface.

Epithelial Defect

The incidence of epithelial defects with LASIK is around 5%. It may vary from mild punctate epithelial changes to total dehiscence of the epithelial surface. The development of non-compression heads (Hansatome, Bausch & Lomb, Rochester, NY, USA) and dual motors to drive oscillation and translation have resulted in the reduced incidence of epithelial defects. Larger epithelial defects are more dangerous, especially, those with connection to the flap edge. There are increased chances of epithelial ingrowth and diffuse lamellar keratitis with the presence of epithelial defects.

Etiology: Epithelial toxicity subsequent to topical medications may predispose to intraoperative or postoperative epithelial defects. Anesthetic drops preoperatively should be limited.

Prevention: A thorough slit-lamp examination is mandatory preoperatively to rule to anterior basement membrane dystrophy. Limiting eyedrops preoperatively is essential in reducing the incidence of epithelial defects.

Treatment: With minor epithelial defects the epithelium can be repositioned and a contact lens placed in-situ. Pain relief may be required for 24 hours until the epithelium has healed. Epithelial defect increases the risk of epithelial ingrowth, and this needs to be monitored very closely in the postoperative period.

Incomplete Cap

Etiology: An incomplete cap is caused by the failure of traverse of the microkeratome. This may occur if the microkeratome is caught on the eyelid, lashes, speculum, loose epithelium or precipitated salts from irrigating solutions or there is a malfunction of the motor or gears. The incidence of this complication ranges from 0.3% to 1.2%.

Prevention: Exposure is the key to preventing an incomplete flap. The use of various specula to accommodate different eye shapes is essential. With good suction it is also possible to elevate the eye, or manipulate the eye to obtain clearance of the eyelids. A check of intraocular pressure is mandatory to rule out inadvertent loss of suction pressure when lifting the globe. Microkeratome jamming should be minimized by meticulous cleaning of its components and by inspection of its electrical connections.

Treatment: If there is inadequate stroma exposed to accommodate the ablation, the case should be aborted. The cap is then repositioned accurately and further surgery can be performed in three months' time, and will invariably do well. Any attempt to deliver the ablation where there is inadequate stroma will result in irregular astigmatism. In cases where retreatment is planned after 3 months, a deeper and a more peripheral cut should be planned to encompass the original area.

Buttonhole/Partial/Thin Cap

The incidence of thin flaps after LASIK varies from 0.3 to 0.75%. A flap which is <60 μm is suspicious as the thickness of the corneal epithelium is 50 μm (Figs 5.9A and B). Buttonholes may be partial thickness if they transect the Bowman's layer or full thickness if they exit through the epithelium. The incidence of buttonholes varies from 0.2 to 0.56%. A buttonhole is one of the most feared complications of LASIK surgery because it can result in irregular astigmatism, epithelial ingrowth and significant visual loss.

Etiology: Buttonholes are associated with steeper corneas, and it has been postulated that this occurs because of the buckling

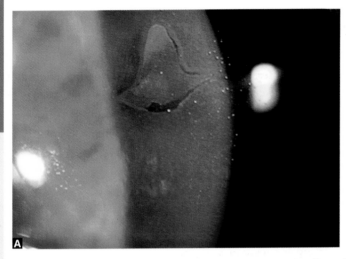
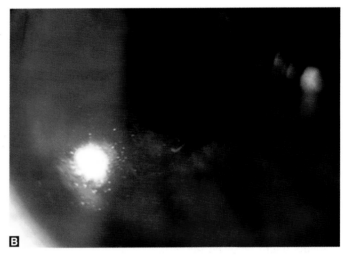

Figs 5.9A and B: Flap related complication. Buttonhole flap (A) Epithelial in growth in buttonhole flap (B)

of the cornea due to increased keratometric steepness. Leung and associates postulate that a lack of synchronization between the translational flap keratome movement and oscillatory blade movement results in the forward displacement of the tissue and hence may cause stepped, thin or button-holed caps.

Irregular caps may also result from damaged microkeratome blades, irregular oscillation speeds or poor suction. The poor suction is likely to be present in deep set eyes or small diameter corneas with less than optimal suction ring placement or conjunctival incarceration in the suction port generating a pseudosuction. The integrity of the blade is crucial to the occurrence of irregular flaps and the blade damage may occur either during manufacture or handling. The occurrence of previous ocular surgery is also a possible risk factor for occurrence of buttonholes.

Prevention: It is essential that the keratome chosen has in good working order. Extra care is taken with patients with steep corneas. It is imperative to ensure adequate suction by checking the intraocular pressure, which should be >65 mm Hg in order to create optimal flaps. Conjunctival incarceration due to repeated suction ring application may lead to a disparity between the intraocular pressure and the actual suction pressure.

Treatment: In cases of buttonhole, the complication should be recognized early, and excess manipulation of the cap is avoided. Sufficient time is given for corneal drying and a contact lens is placed in-situ. This may need to be left for 24 to 48 hours. No attempt is made to perform laser treatment. The patient is then followed closely over a three-month period to ensure that irregular astigmatism, haze or epithelial ingrowth does not occur. Three months later repeat surgery can be performed, planning a larger and a deeper cut. Alternatively, some surgeons advocate photorefractive keratectomy especially if the refractive error permits.

Free Cap

A free cap occurs when there is unintended complete dissection of the flap. This occurs more commonly in flat corneas and

was more common with the earlier microkeratomes (4.9%) as compared to the newer models (0.01 to 1%).

Etiology: The factors responsible for free cap are similar to those of thin flaps. Failure of microkeratome reversal coupled with an inadvertent or intended release of suction may cause the occurrence of a free cap.

Prevention: Same measures as for thin flaps should be taken.

Management: If the cap cannot be retrieved, the laser ablation is aborted and the epithelium is allowed to regenerate to cover the denuded area. If the cap is retrievable, pre-placed corneal markings should be used as a guide to correctly orient and place the flap/cap in position. Laser ablation may continue while the free cap is placed in the anti-desiccation chamber. A bandage contact lens should be placed after the procedure and alternatively, some surgeons have also applied sutures.

Dislodged Flap

A dislodged flap is an emergency (Fig. 5.10). It should be repositioned as soon as possible to prevent fixed folds, infection and epithelial ingrowth. The incidence varies between 1.1 to 2.0%.

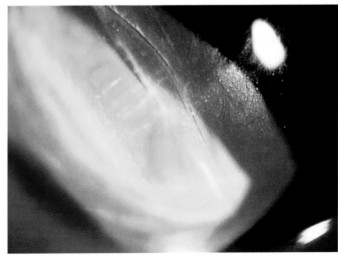

Fig. 5.10: Flap-related complication. Dislodged flap

Etiology: Mechanical movement by the lid action can result in flap displacement, especially if the ocular surface is dry. Larger diameter, thinner flaps and flaps with smaller hinge are more to get likely dislodged. Trauma, removal of contact lens and vitrectomy surgery may also cause the flap to be dislodged.

Management: The flap should be lifted and the surfaces should be inspected for any debris or epithelial ingrowth. A contact lens can then applied after scraping the surfaces to remove epithelial ingrowth.

Prevention: A contact lens may be applied after the LASIK surgery. Patients involved in contact sports should be counseled about the risk of late flap dislocation with LASIK and such patients might be given the option of PRK especially in low refractive errors.

Striae

Striae can either be minor and visually inconsequential, or severe or cause significant irregular astigmatism and loss of best corrected visual acuity, especially if visual axis is involved.

The flap striae or folds are of two types:

- Macrofolds: Macrofolds are easily visualized on slit lamp and are full thickness flap tenting in a linear manner.
- Microfolds: Microfolds on the other hand are within the flap itself and are in the form of wrinkles in the Bowman's layer or in epithelial basement membrane. These folds are best visualized on retro-illumination in the slit lamp.

  All folds/striae in the cap/flap do not require surgical intervention as the patients may not be symptomatic. The incidence of folds requiring reflotation of the flap varies from 0.2 to 1.5%.

Etiology: The causes of striae include malposition of the cap at the end of the LASIK surgery, or dislodgement due to excessive rubbing or blinking of the eyes postoperatively. There is an increased incidence of striae with thin flaps and with a small hinge. There are more chances of striae/folds in cases of high myopes and hyperopes, as due to a greater ablation and peripheral ablation respectively, more redundant hydrated flap has to cover the corneal convexity.

Prevention: Ensuring that the cap is well positioned at the end of the surgery is essential in the prevention of striae. The gutter should be checked to ensure that it is equal throughout the circumference of the cap, and excess hydration of the corneal flap should be avoided. This can result in fine microstriae.

Treatment: Striae are easy to manage if detected early. Ideally they are detected at the postoperative examination on the slit lamp, at which time the patient can be taken back to operation theater and the flap is refloated.

Perforation

The most ominous intraoperative complication in LASIK surgery is anterior chamber penetration.

Etiology: Anterior chamber penetration is totally microkeratome dependent. It may occur if assembly is incorrect. This may very rarely occur during laser ablation.

Prevention: There is a low risk of intraocular penetration with the newer microkeratomes. It is essential to ensure that the microkeratome is put together correctly and checked by the surgeon.

Treatment: The management of anterior chamber penetration involves immediate primary repair, and may involve cataract extraction, lens implant, iris restructuring, vitrectomy and even retinal detachment repair if it occurs.

Epithelial Ingrowth

Implantation of the epithelial cells in the interface occurs during surgery or migration of the epithelial cells under the flap.

Etiology: Most isolated nests of epithelial cells disappear without any consequences. The epithelial cells in connection with the flap edge have a bad prognosis as this may lead to irregular astigmatism with flap melting.

Management: Epithelial cells under the LASIK flap should be managed aggressively to prevent flap melting. The flap is lifted, the stromal bed as well as the flap surface is thoroughly irrigated and scraped and the flap is repositioned. Epithelial scraping may be done with a Bard-Parker knife, dedicated instruments or even with phototherapeutic keratectomy.

Prevention: Dedicated instruments for interface manipulation should be used, which do not come in contact with the surrounding epithelium. Meticulous attention should be given to avoid flap folds. Caution is mandatory especially when enhancement procedures are being undertaken.

Diffuse Lamellar Keratitis

Etiology: Also known as Sands of Sahara, diffuse lamellar keratitis is a sterile inflammatory reaction with a reported incidence of around 1.8%. The exact etiology is unknown, but is believed to be caused by foreign cells introduced at the time of surgery. These include gram negative bacterial endotoxins, residue from the microkeratome head, glove powder, etc. It is characterized by pain, blurred vision, foreign body sensation and light sensitivity and occurs usually 1–6 days after surgery, but can occur months to years later as well.

Grade I : This is a mild keratitis, which is localized at the periphery with minimal to no symptoms. Frequent topical steroids (prednisolone 1–2 hourly) should be started and patient should be reviewed in 1–2 days.

Grade II : Moderate infiltrates extending to the central cornea causing decreased vision and photophobia occur. Treatment includes frequent topical steroids along with oral steroids to control the inflammation.

Grade III : Clumping of inflammatory cells, which obscure the iris details and central infiltrates with a significant decrease in vision is seen. Along with topical and oral steroids, lifting the flap to brush the stromal bed and the flap underface and irrigation to remove all the inflammatory cells and debris is important to prevent permanent damage (Fig. 5.11).

Grade IV : Dense white central infiltrates maybe associated with corneal melting and loss of vision. The flap should be immediately lifted to scrape and remove all the interface debris and irrigated thoroughly. The infiltrate should be cultured to rule out an infective agent. A drop of steroid may be placed on the stromal bed to prevent further inflammation along with topical and oral steroids.

Management: Frequent topical steroids in hourly dosage along with topical antibiotics are given. Systemic corticosteroids have also been tried by some surgeons with a variable response.

In severe cases, flap relifting and irrigation may be indicated along with the topical steroids.

Laser-Related Complications

These include decentration and irregular astigmatism. Patients with high refractive error may find it difficult to fixate on the fixation light leading to decentered ablations. Switching off external light sources helps the patient to fixate on the target light. Lasers using iris registration to recognize and match the eye position relative to the preoperative WaveScan have lesser incidence of decentrations. Postoperative patients with decentered ablations complain of glare, haloes and ghosting of images due to light scattering at the edge of the ablation zone. Irregular astigmatism may occur due to decentered ablations and uneven flap healing. Central islands may occur when specific tissue areas are not ablated resulting in central elevated areas. Patients complain of poor vision and undercorrection. Customized lasers prevent such complications and provide better quality vision.

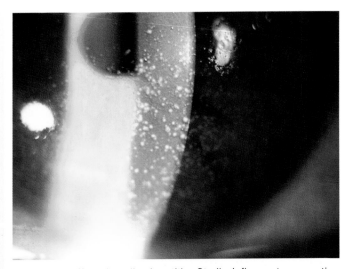

Fig. 5.11: Diffuse lamellar keratitis. Sterile inflammatory reaction Surface ablation procedures like PRK, LASEK and epi-LASEK do not require the creation of a stromal flap and thereby circumvent these potential flap-related complications. With the advent of femtosecond laser, however, flap creation has become more precise and safe even with the LASIK procedure

Infectious Keratitis

Though infectious keratitis after laser surgery is rare, it can be caused by *Streptococcus pneumoniae*, *Staphylococcus aureus*, *Mycobacterium chelonae* and *Nocardia asteroids*. Atypical mycobacteria have a predilection for the anoxic environment at the flap interface and may present 2–4 weeks after surgery with multiple dense infiltrates with feathery margins. Patients will complain of pain, redness and decreased vision. Early diagnosis and prompt intervention with aggressive antibiotics should be started. Fourth generation fluoroquinolones and cephalosporins are recommended. Cultures should be performed and flap amputation or penetrating keraoplasty may be needed in unresponsive cases.

Ectasia

Thinning and bulging of the cornea may occur due to biomechanical weakening of the corneal tissue following laser ablation. Patients with preoperative abnormal topography; keratoconus forme fruste cases which are missed but which may progress; thin corneas and high refractive errors; residual corneal bed thickness <250 μm are the risk factors. Patients will complain of decrease vision while topography will demonstrate irregular astigmatism with a myopic shift. Corneal cross linking with riboflavin 0.1% and ultraviolet radiation helps to increase the tissue rigidity and improve the biomechanical strength. Advanced cases may need corneal transplantation.

Dry Eye

Photorefractive keratectomy and laser in-situ keratomileusis can induce or exacerbate dry eye after surgery. This manifests as an increase in the degree and frequency of symptoms; corneal findings, such as superficial punctate keratopathy; and abnormal results of dry eye tests, such as the Schirmer test and tear break-up time. Corneal denervation is mainly implicated in its causation. Decreased corneal sensation results in decreased feedback to the lacrimal gland and reduced tear production. Dry eye is transient, lasting from a few weeks up to one year. Patients should be warned about this distressing complication. During a period of dry eye, artificial tears and punctal plugs are helpful in preventing or alleviating patient discomfort.

Corneal Haze

Different definitions of haze include: (1) a decrease in tissue transparency, (2) a marginal loss of corneal clarity and (3) a subepithelial stromal opacity.

Haze may be completely asymptomatic. It can also lead to starbursts and visual loss or, more seriously, to a stromal reaction that induces refractive regression, increases corneal surface irregularity, and leads to irregular astigmatism.

It is seen more commonly after PRK and surface ablation procedures. The surgically trauma induces a disruption of the basement membrane. Cascades of responses follow leading to keratocyte activation and transformation into fibroblasts with the subsequent deposition of extracellular matrix.

Clinically insignificant corneal haze is present in most eyes after PRK and may last for 1–2 years after surgery. Clinically significant haze only occurs in a small percentage of eyes, usually less than 0.5 to 4%, depending on the level of correction and other factors. A classification system described by Fantes is useful for grading the severity of corneal haze (Table 5.1).

Table 5.1: Fantes grading of corneal haze

Stage	Slit-lamp examination
0	Clear; no haze
0.5	Trace haze; seen with careful oblique examination
1	Haze not interfering with visibility of iris details
2	Mild obscuration of iris details
3	Moderate obscuration of iris and lens details
4	Complete opacification of the stroma obscuring anterior chamber

Significant corneal haze is usually associated with the correction of higher degrees of refractive error and smaller optical zones. Topical mitomycin-C (0.02%) is being increasingly used in surface ablation procedures to minimize the risk of developing significant corneal haze.

Thermokeratoplasty

Based on the application of heat to produce shrinkage of the corneal collagen fibers and subsequent alteration of the corneal surface.

Laser Thermokeratoplasty

The Holmium:ytterium-aluminium-garnet laser with a wavelength of 2100 nm was used to place circumferential spots in the corneal periphery in order to treat hyperopia up to 2.5 D. Visual fluctuations and refractive regression plagued the procedure and it has now largely been replaced by conductive keratoplasty.

Conductive Keratoplasty

It is based on the delivery of radiofrequency energy through a conducting tip inserted into the corneal stroma. As the current flows into the cornea, resistance to the current generates heat, which causes shrinkage of the collagen fibers. This procedure is FDA approved for the temporary treatment of hyperopia up to +3.0 D and presbyopic correction of the nondominant eye. It entails placement of one or more peripheral ring of spots with a fine conducting tip inserted into the cornea to deliver radiofrequency energy. Increasing number of spots or rings are used to correct higher degrees of hyperopia.

The "loss of effect" following this procedure is possibly a combination of regression and age-related hyperopic drift.

INTACS (Intrastromal Corneal Ring Segments)

INTACS are corneal implants which are used to change the shape of the cornea and correct the refractive error in patients with myopia and keratoconus (Fig. 5.12). Approved by the USFDA, they consist of two tiny clear crescent-shaped pieces of PMMA, which can be inserted into the cornea. For myopia, *INTACS* work by flattening the cornea to refocus light rays and improve vision while in keratoconus patients *INTACS* flatten the steep part of the cone and reduce vision distortions. *INTACS* are available in various sizes, which are chosen according to the refractive error and the corneal thickness of the patient.

A clear central cornea with a minimum corneal thickness of 450 μm at the incision site and a mesopic pupil size of less than 6 mm are preferred. After performing the corneal topography and the refraction, the size of the INTACS and placement is planned. The incision may be made mechanically with a diamond knife and a tunnel created by a dissector into which the ring segments are placed. Alternatively, the femtosecond laser can be used for the same using preprogrammed parameters.

INTACS offer the advantages of leaving the central cornea undisturbed. The results are rapid and predictable and if required, the INTACS can be removed or exchanged. The corneal asphericity is maintained with minimal adverse effects. Possible complications include epithelial defects, channel haze, under/over correction, sterile infiltrates/epithelial cysts, infectious keratitis and ring extrusion.

Newer Innovations

Femtosecond Lenticule Extraction

Femtosecond lenticule extraction (FLEx/FLE) consists of creation of a corneal lenticule with a femtosecond laser. A flap is subsequently created with the same laser and the lenticule is removed. The cornea is thus reshaped in order to correct the existing refractive error. At present the Zeiss femtosecond laser system (VisuMax) is equipped with the appropriate technology to perform this procedure for myopic correction.

Corneal Inlays for Correction of Presbyopia

A novel corneal implant technology may offer a new approach for improving near vision in emmetropic presbyopic patients.

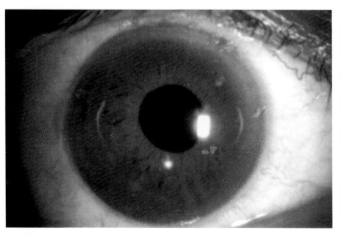

Fig. 5.12 : Intrastromal corneal ring segments. INTACS in myopia

Implantation of corneal inlays is a minimally invasive procedure, reversible and adjustable and which gives patients the ability to read without glasses.

Currently, three different corneal inlays are being developed: the AcuFocus/Bausch & Lomb ACI 7000, the Invue intracorneal microlens (Biovision, Brugges, Switzerland) and the PresbyLens (ReVision Optics, Lake Forest, CA, USA).

The ACI 7000 is a small diameter aperture optic and increases the depth of focus by using a pinhole optic. The inlay has a 1.6 mm center with a 3.6 mm surround. Peripheral rays are obscured and the central rays pass unaffected.

It generates improved near vision of about 1.5 D add, and does it with no measurable loss of distance vision. Placed on the nondominant eye, a corneal flap is cut as in standard LASIK, the inlay is placed on the stromal bed, and the flap is then replaced. The ACI 7000 doesn't change corneal power, but the depth of focus.

The Invue corneal inlay is a small hydrophilic acrylic lens that measures about 3 mm in diameter and is 15 μm to 20 μm thick. The device is implanted about 200 μm into the cornea of the patient's nondominant eye to create monovision.

The PresbyLens corneal inlay measures 1.5 mm and it is designed to change only a small central area of the cornea to increase near focusing power with little decrease in intermediate and distance focusing.

LENTICULAR REFRACTIVE SURGERY

Phakic Intraocular Lenses

Patients who have high refractive errors and/or thin corneas are unsuitable for corneal refractive surgery. For such patients lenticular refractive surgery is an option. This is available in the form of phakic intraocular lenses, which are implanted between the cornea and lens. Also termed "duophakia" or "artiphakia", the normal crystalline lens is retained and an additional intraocular lens is placed to correct the refractive error.

Selection of patients for phakic intraocular lenses:
1. Age above 18 years
2. Moderate to high myopes (>-9.0 D) and hyperopes (> 4.5 D)
3. Also indicated in lesser degrees of ametropias if LASIK is contraindicated such as
   • Corneas thinner than 500 μm
   • Steep or flat corneas
   • Topographic change suggestive of keratoconus
4. Endothelial cell density at least 2250–2500 mm^2.
5. Pupil smaller than 6 mm in scotopic luminance
6. Stable refraction for at least 1 year
7. Anterior chamber depth (excluding corneal thickness) at least 2.8 mm
8. Angle width at least 30 degrees
9. No eye pathology except refractive error
10. No systemic pathology, such as diabetes, collagen diseases, etc

The advantages of phakic intraocular lenses are the following:
• Allow the crystalline lens to retain its function
• Predictable
• Immediately stable, because the refractive outcome depends less on healing processes
• Excellent vision even in dim light conditions
• Removable and exchangeable
• Easily adjustable with complementary fine-tuning corneal surgeries.

Types of Phakic IOL

There are three types of phakic intraocular lenses. These include:
1. Anterior chamber angle-fixated intraocular lens, e.g. ZB M5, NuVita MA20 and Phakic 6.
2. Anterior chamber iris-fixated IOL, e.g. VeriSyse Phakic IOL (Artisan lens).
3. Posterior chamber sulcus fixated IOL, e.g. STAAR implantable contact lens and phakic refractive lens (PRL).

Angle-supported Phakic Intraocular Lenses

First generation angle-supported IOLs were developed by Baikoff and Joly in 1997. The first model (ZB-Domilens) was a modified Kelman type lens with a 4.0 mm optic and 2 haptics with a 4-point fixation in the angle. However, this lens had a high vault and was so close to the endothelium that it had to be explanted in 50% of the eyes due to endothelial damage.

In the line of Kelman type angle supported anterior chamber phakic IOL, the only available at present is PHAKIC 6 (Fig. 5.13), which is made of PMMA, has a 6.0 mm optic and 2 haptics with four-point fixation in the angle.

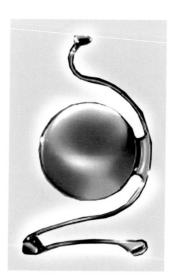

Fig. 5.13: Angle-supported phakic intraocular lenses. PHAKIC 6 IOL

Two types of foldable intraocular lenses in this group include:
1. Vivarte (Ciba Switzerland) and the Duet (Tekia, USA)
2. ICARE (Corneal, France) and AcrySof (Alcon, USA)

Vivarte (Fig. 5.14) and Duet have a foldable optic (acrylic) of 5.5 mm and 2 haptics made of PMMA with 3 points for angle fixation. The difference between these two intraocular lenses is that in the Duet the haptic and optic are implanted separately in the bag and the lens is assembled in the eye whereas in the ICARE and Acrysof the folding occurs outside the eye.

Iris-fixated Phakic Intraocular Lens

The prototype iris-fixated lens is the Artisan lens (Verisyse), which is a one-piece PMMA intraocular lens (Fig. 5.15). Available in two meniscus-shaped optic diameters of 5.0 and 6.0 mm, it has a fixed overall diameter of 8.5 mm and an average vaulting of 0.9 mm. Potential complications include progressive endothelial cell loss, chronic uveal inflammation, chafing of the iris stroma at the sites of enclavement, lens displacement/decentration, pigmentary dispersion syndrome and irregular pupil. The other phakic intraocular lenses include the Artiflex and Veriflex foldable iris supported lenses with a polysiloxane optic and rigid PMMA haptics and the Nikai lens, which is a one-piece silicone lens with a 3.2 mm concave optic and a frontal surface that projected anteriorly through the pupil. It is fixated behind the iris plane by two haptics and has a total length of 8.0 mm.

As regards sizing "one size fits all" as these implants are not dependent on the eye dimensions.

Surgical Technique

The steps of the surgery are as follows:
- Preoperative miosis is done
- Two side ports are made (2 mm away from each extremity of main incision)
- Main incision is made as a corneal or corneoscleral incision
- The anterior chamber is filled with a standard viscoelastic
- The intraocular lens is introduced
- The iris tissue is grasped into the claws
- The viscoelastic is washed out
- Iridectomy/Iridotomy is recommended.

Posterior Chamber Phakic Intraocular Lenses

In the years between 1990–1998, a new material came into vogue known as the Collamer. This was a hybrid of silicone and collagen and the lens was called as the implantable contact lens or ICL.

The PRL or the phakic refractive lens is another posterior chamber phakic IOL available with CIBA VISION. It is made of new generation ultra thin hydrophobic silicon. It has no anatomical fixation sites and floats on the layer of aqueous humor inside the posterior chamber exerting no traction on the ciliary structures and without coming in contact with the anterior capsule of the crystalline lens.

The StickLens (IOLTech, La Rochelle, France) made up of hydrophilic acrylic material is available. It sticks firmly to the anterior surface of the crystalline lens.

Implantable contact lens is indicated for placement in the posterior chamber of the phakic eye for the correction of moderate to high myopia ranging from –3.0 D to – 20.0 D. TORIC ICL (TICL) can correct up to – 3 to – 23D of sphere and + 1.0 to +6.0 D of cylinder. The TORIC ICL has the same overall design as the spherical ICL with the addition of a toric optic. The toricity is manufactured in the plus cylinder axis, within 22 degrees. The STAAR Visian ICL is made from a combination of copolymer and collagen called Collamer. This Collamer implantable contact lens reduces reflections and glare, and the collagen makes it extremely biocompatible. It is made up of 60% polyHEMA, water (36%), benzophenone (3.8%)

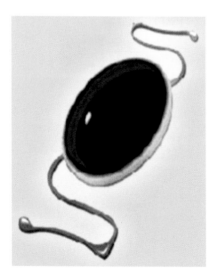

Fig. 5.14: Angle-supported phakic intraocular lenses. Vivarte

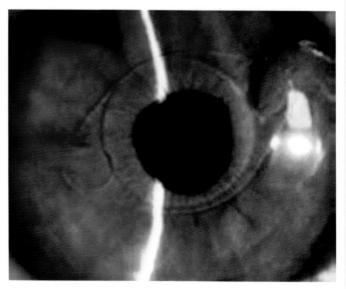

Fig. 5.15: Phakic intraocular lens. Artisan lens in-situ

and collagen (0.2%), it attracts the deposition of fibronectin on the lens surface, inhibits aqueous protein binding and makes the lens invisible to the immune system. We routinely use this phakic IOL in our clinical practice and shall be describing this in detail.

Calculation of power: ICL/TICL calculation and implantation software (Fig. 5.16) allows calculation of spherical and cylindrical power, length and generates the ICL/TICL implantation diagram (Fig. 5.17).

Measurement of white to white diameter: In the preoperative planning, the critical parameter in sizing the ICL is the white-to-white (WW) measurement, which can be measured with a Pentacam, OrbScan, ultrasound biomicroscopy or using calipers (Fig. 5.18). In myopic eyes, to determine the overall length (in mm) of the ICL, add 0.5 mm to the horizontal WW measurement. If the ICL is too short for the sulcus, the lens vault may be insufficient to clear the crystalline lens, exposing it to the risk of an anterior capsular cataract. If it is too long, the lens will vault excessively, crowding the angle and possibly causing closed-angle glaucoma.

Vault: Ideal ICL vault is approximately 500 μm, which is roughly one corneal thickness. There are concerns about high vault (1000 μm) leading to angle crowding and resulting in angle closure or synechiae formation. High vault may also increase iris chaffing and pigment dispersion, resulting in pigmentary glaucoma. Furthermore, low vault (125 μm) may also cause ICL contact with the crystalline lens and increase the risk of cataract formation over time.

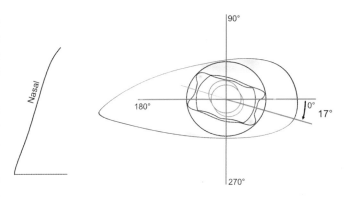

Rotate lens clockwise 17° after horizontal implantation

Fig 5.17: Posterior chamber phakic intraocular lens. TICL implantation diagram

Peripheral iridotomy: A peripheral iridotomy is performed 1–2 weeks before the surgery to provide an outlet for the aqueous flow around the lens. Alternatively it may be performed intraoperatively after ICL implantation with a Vannas scissors or a vitrectomy cutter. It should be sufficiently wide (at least 500 μm), positioned superiorly (from 11 to 1 o'clock) and well away from the haptics placement.

Procedure: The procedure is performed under topical anesthesia or a peribulbar block. After making a 0.6 mm side port, a 3.2 mm clear corneal incision is made on the steep meridian. The lens is introduced with angled-suture forceps or through the injector and positioned behind the iris on a horizontal axis with a cyclodialysis spatula (Figs 5.19A to C). To control for potential cyclotorsion in a supine position, the zero horizontal axis is marked preoperatively on the slit lamp. The lens is implanted temporally and gently rotated to align the axis with the cylindrical axis of the patient. Complete removal of viscoelastic material is essential. Presence of residual viscoelastic material behind the implant may cause opacification of the crystalline

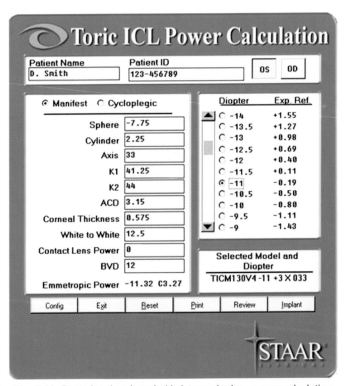

Fig. 5.16: Posterior chamber phakic intraocular lens power calculation. TICL calculation software

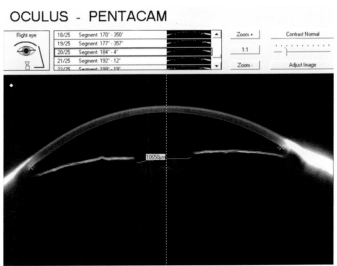

Fig. 5.18: Schiempflug image. Measurement of the white-to-white diameter with pentacam is shown

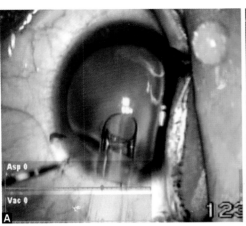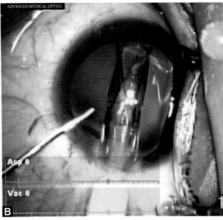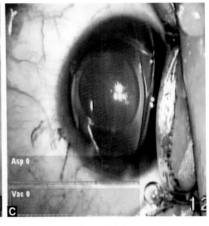

Figs 5.19A to C: Procedure of implantable contact lens implantation. Insertion of implantable contact lens with the STAAR injector system

lens. A miotic agent is injected and the aspiration is completed. The incision is closed by hydrating it.

Various studies have reported that phakic TICL implantation is a good option for the correction of moderate to high myopia, hyperopia, high myopic astigmatism, in eyes with keratoconus, correction of hyperopia post-radial keratotomy and post-penetrating keratoplasty.

Kamiya and associates studied long-term clinical outcomes of implantation of Visian implantable lens for moderate to high myopia in myopic refractive errors of − 4.00 to − 15.25 D. They concluded that implantation of ICLs is safe and effective and provides predictable and stable refractive results in the treatment of moderate to high myopia during a 4-year observation period.

Pesando and associates evaluated ICL in hyperopic eyes. Preoperatively, the spherical equivalent (SE) was between +2.75 D and +11.75 D and astigmatism was between +0.50 D and +1.00 D. The mean postoperative SE of the manifest refraction was +0.07 ± 0.54 D; refraction stabilized quickly and remained stable throughout the follow-up period. The results confirmed the long-term safety, efficacy, accuracy, and predictability of ICL for hyperopia.

Alfonso and associates evaluated the efficacy, predictability and safety of myopic phakic posterior chamber ICL to correct myopia associated with keratoconus. They showed that spherical equivalent refraction was within ±1.00 D of the desired refraction in all cases and 84% of cases were within ±0.50 D.

Alfonso and associates suggested that phakic intraocular lens implantation is a viable treatment for myopia and astigmatism after PKP in patients for whom glasses, contact lenses, or corneal refractive surgery is contraindicated.

Studies comparing ICL implantation with wavefront guided LASIK by Igarashi and associates have shown that ICL implantation induces significantly fewer ocular HOAs than wavefront-guided LASIK. Kamiya and associates compared Collamer toric ICL implantation and wavefront-guided laser in-situ keratomileusis for high myopic astigmatism and found that all eyes in the ICL group and 71% of eyes in the LASIK group were within ±1.00 D of the targeted SE correction at 6 months. They suggested that TORIC ICL implantation was better than wavefront-guided LASIK in eyes with high myopic astigmatism in almost all measures of safety, efficacy, predictability and stability.

The overall complication rate with ICL is low and most patients have a good visual recovery. The incidence of glare, haloes and night driving problems is also minimal.

Sanders and associates studied incidence of anterior subcapsular opacities and cataracts 5 years after surgery in the Visian implantable collamer lens FDA trial. Approximately 6 to 7% of eyes developed anterior subcapsular opacities at 7+ years following ICL implantation, but only 1 to 2% progressed to clinically significant cataract during the same period, especially very high myopes and older patients. Visual outcome following cataract extraction was good. Other reported complications of ICL are pigment dispersion and lens deposits, acute angle-closure glaucoma, late subluxation of ICL, endophthalmitis and retinal detachment.

Implantable contact lens is a safe and effective modality for correction of high myopia and for patients with thin corneas with excellent and stable postoperative results (Fig. 5.20). Advancements in anterior segment imaging and measurement technologies, such as ultrasonic biomicroscopy, optical coherence tomography and Scheimpflug imaging are now providing valuable information about anterior segment anatomy for custom-designed phakic intraocular lenses for the correction of moderate to high refractive errors.

Clear Lens Extraction

Refractive lensectomy with intraocular lens implantation is usually considered if alternative refractive procedures are not feasible. It is important to note that refractive lensectomy in a young patient will lead to the loss of accommodation and subsequent loss of near vision. Monovision, multifocal IOLs or accommodative IOLs may be used in order to minimize loss of near vision and maximize chances of spectacle independence.

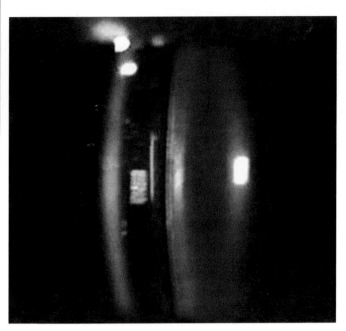

Fig. 5.20: Implantable contact lens. Postoperative slit lamp view of the implantable contact lens

Limbal relaxing incisions may be used to correct preexisting corneal astigmatism. Toric IOLs may also be implanted for the same.

Accurate calculation of intraocular lens power remains crucial to the outcome of this surgery. SRK/T formula is considerably accurate in patients with moderate to high myopia (axial); Hoffer Q is usually adopted in patients with moderate to high hyperopia.

Sequential rather than simultaneous surgery is preferred in order to minimize risk of bilateral endophthalmitis.

Bioptics

For eyes with large refractive errors, one procedure alone may not be sufficient to correct the entire refractive error. Combining two or three procedures together is called bioptics or trioptics respectively. Lenticular options are available in the form of phakic IOLs, toric IOLs and piggy back IOLs while corneal options for bioptics include corneal relaxing incisions (CRIs), anterior limbal relaxing incisions (ALRI), laser-assisted epithelial keratomileusis (LASEK), photorefractive keratectomy (PRK), conductive keratoplasty (CK) and intrastromal ring implants. Combinations for bioptics or trioptics include:

- Clear lens extraction with a monofocal or multifocal implant combined with limbal relaxing incisions to correct concomitant astigmatism
- Phakic IOL followed by LASIK to fine tune the residual refractive error if any
- Toric IOL in the bag, multifocal IOL in the sulcus followed by LASIK can be used for trioptics

Refractive surgery is one of the most evolved aspects of ophthalmic science and is undergoing rapid advancements each day in an endeavor to provide crystal clear vision without the aid of glasses and contact lenses. Sophisticated equipments and technological breakthroughs have greatly contributed, but at the base of all these innovations is the restless human mind searching for perfection. As this spirit continues, so will the quality of vision that we can provide to our patients with minimal complications.

Section

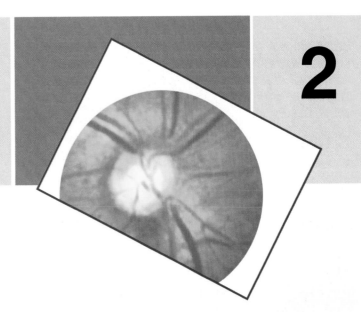

2

Glaucoma

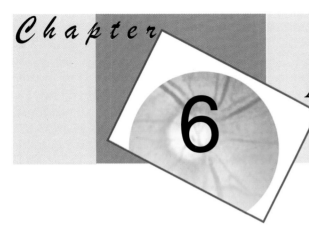

Chapter 6

Automated Visual Field Assessment, Optic Nerve and Nerve Fiber Layer Imaging

M Baskaran, Arun Narayanaswamy, Lingam Vijaya

AUTOMATED VISUAL FIELD ASSESSMENT

Introduction

A visual field is one of the principal components in the diagnosis of glaucoma. Documenting it has had a rapid evolution from manual to semiautomatic and now completely automated quantitative plotting of a field. The sound concepts introduced by Goldmann still forms the basis of automated perimetry though technology has made things faster, more detailed and statistically comparable. Software in these new generation machines has detailed data regarding the threshold sensitivity for each point for normal as well as glaucomatous patients. This data is compared with the patient data giving us a statistical probability and helps identify an abnormal field with a certain degree of accuracy. The complicated data that the computer generates can at the same time be prone to erratic interpretation and outcome if one is not careful in critically assessing the same.

This section would aim at broadly familiarizing oneself with the parameters of an automated visual field and a systematic evaluation to help differentiate between a normal and an abnormal field. Description would be limited to Humphrey field analyzer (HFA-II, Humphrey Systems, Dublin, CA, USA) results since it is the most widely used automated perimeter and programs (Table 6.1) of which we are most familiar with. It is very essential that a field report be always interpreted along with clinical data and never in isolation.

Test Algorithms

The following test algorithms are available in most of the 700 series of Humphrey perimeters.
- Full threshold
- Fastpac
- SITA* STANDARD
- SITA* FAST
- SWAP**

Table 6.1: Important test programs and their applications on the Humphrey perimeter (HFA II)

Screening programs*		
Test program	**Area and points tested**	**Application**
Central 76	30° 76 points	Glaucoma Neurological assessment
Full Field 120	60° 120 points	General Glaucoma Neurological assessment

Threshold programs**		
Central 30-2	30°/76 points 6° spacing	Glaucoma Neurological
Central 24-2	24°/ 54 points 6° spacing	Glaucoma Neurological
10-2	10°/68 points 2° spacing	Advanced glaucoma
Macula	5°/16 points 2° spacing	Macular assessment

* Screening programs are commonly used in situations of mass screening or as a prelude to actual full thresholding. Screening programs are effective to delineate hemianopic losses and glaucomatous patients who are unable to handle the stress of the longer duration threshold tests.

** The commonly used test point patterns are the central 30-2 and central 24-2. The 10-2 and macular programs are used to evaluate advanced glaucomas.

* Swedish Interactive Thresholding Algorithm

** Short Wavelength Automated Perimetry.

Full Threshold Program

This test is the gold standard and most commonly used algorithm for quantitative assessment of a visual field. Most discussion in the chapter would pertain to this strategy of testing. Sensitivity of a particular point is measured in decibels (dB) by convention. The perimeter is designed to project stimuli ranging from 0 dB (brightest) to 50 dB (dimmest) in a graded fashion to determine the threshold of a particular point and the same

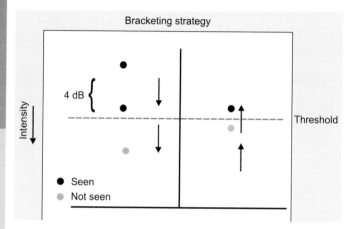

Fig. 6.1: Visual field. The bracketing strategy used by Humphrey perimeters starts with a particular decibel value and changes in 4 dB steps till threshold is crossed and the direction is then reversed with changes in 2 dB steps until second crossover. Crossovers may be from "not seen" to "seen" or vice versa

is referred to as the "bracketing" or "staircase strategy" (Fig. 6.1). This strategy involves stimulus presentation that is done in 4 decibel (dB) increments till "perception" from initial presentation and then reduced by 2 dB steps till a point when it is not perceived. The process involves a double-crossing of each point and tries to attain maximum accuracy in grading threshold of a particular point. Though a time consuming process, it has proved its validity with respect to accuracy. The "SITA standard" algorithm has evolved as a reliable and quicker alternative to full threshold and most practitioners have switched over to this mode of testing.

Evaluation of a Single Test

The standard Humphrey 30-2 full threshold printout contains a large amount of data with statistical analysis and systematic approach of evaluating each test report is always an ideal way of minimizing errors. The 30-2 and 24-2 programs are most commonly used test point patterns for glaucoma evaluation. A print out can be divided into seven sections (Fig. 6.2).

1. General information
2. Reliability indices
3. Raw data and gray scale
4. Total deviation
5. Pattern deviation
6. Global indices
7. Glaucoma hemifield test

The newer test reports of the 740 series perimeters include a "Gaze tracking" display at the bottom.

General Information

Section 1 displays this and it contains important data about the patients name, date of birth, test strategy, stimulus size and color, pupil size, background intensity, optical correction, age in years and visual acuity. These variables can significantly

affect raw and calculated data and to ensure their correct entry is important. Miotic pupils and incorrect refraction can reduce threshold estimation while a wrong date of birth will lead to incorrect age compared deviations and statistical abnormalities misleading the observer about a defect that may not exist. The fixation target used through the duration of test is usually central, unless the patient has a macular pathology for which larger targets like the small and large diamonds are used to ensure stable fixation and the same along with the method of fixation monitoring is printed in this area.

Reliability Indices

These parameters (section 2) determine the reliability of patient responses and patients concentration during the test. Fixation losses greater than 20% and false negative or positives greater than 33% are usually flagged (xx) to draw attention to unreliability of the test report. Test duration is another important parameter depicted here, automated perimetry is a demanding psychophysical test and long durations do create fatigue related defects allowing scope for the misinterpretation of test reports. This block also has the foveal threshold documented and this value should corelate to the best-corrected visual acuity.

Raw Data and Gray Scale

This (section 3) is a prominent portion of the printout representing both numeric and gray tone display of the actual threshold. Interpretation of the visual field entirely on the basis of it is difficult because it is an inferential representation that includes untested areas between points tested in a field by the software and is also influenced by artifacts. An overall impression of the field can be gauged in a reliable printout and it serves as a quick guide to defective areas so that one can study it in more detail on the total and pattern deviation plots. The raw data gives us actual threshold values of each point and bracketed values represent retested points.

Total Deviation

This area (section 4) represents the deviation of threshold from age-matched normal and is presented both numerically and with probability symbols. The numerical data depicts a point-to-point deviation in threshold values compared to a normal in the database. The probability symbols highlight points that are significantly less sensitive than normal and are graded from 5% to 0.5%. Cataract, refractive errors, corneal opacities and miosis contribute to this deviation and it represents an overall or generalized depression of visual field in comparison to age-related normal (Fig. 6.3). In the absence of secondary contributing factors mentioned above, a significant depression in this plot could be due to early glaucoma and one should view the same carefully and reassess the patient clinically.

Pattern Deviation

This (section 5) represents true focal depressions or scotomas and is frequently diagnostic. The statistical package provides

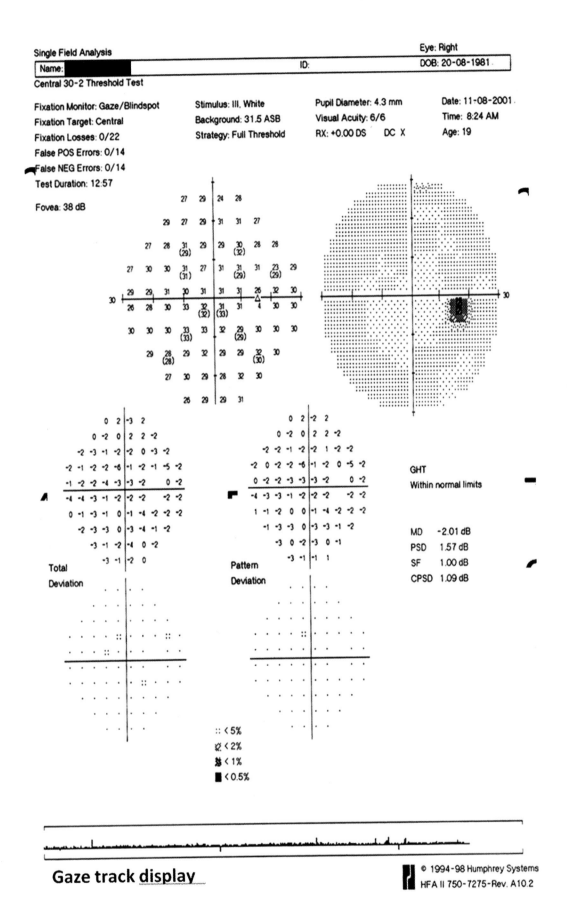

Fig. 6.2: Visual field. The printout is a typical Humphrey single field analysis. They have been bordered to divide them sequentially into seven sections for convenience

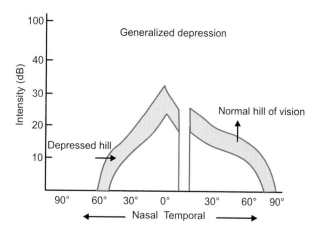

Fig. 6.3: Visual field. Depiction of the normal hill of vision compared to a patients hill of vision. A uniform and symmetric depression is noted when sensitivity is reduced by secondary contributing factors like cataract and refractive errors. The total deviation is a representation of the same in numerical values and probability plots

this information by correcting the deviation of the seventh highest threshold location within the program to zero deviation and adjusts the whole field by that value thereby eliminating effect of factors causing generalized depression and highlighting true scotomas (Fig. 6.4). The deviation is represented numerically and is complimented by a probability plot below it. A cluster of 3 contiguous non-edge points on the same side of horizontal with two points having a probability value <5% and one point <1% is considered as a significant defect.

Global Indices

There are four parameters in section 6, which are derived values calculated by the software from total deviation and pattern deviation. The deviations obtained are condensed to a single value and statistically analyzed. Any significance is complimented by probability percentages.

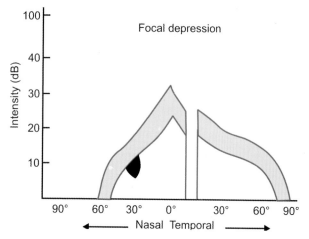

Fig. 6.4: Visual field. The pattern deviation extrapolates persistent areas of depressed sensitivity even after correction for factors contributing to generalized loss in the hill of vision and highlights the same. The focal area of depression marked black would be depicted as a nasal step in pattern deviation plot

Mean Deviation (MD)

It is a value representing the average height of hill of vision calculated from total deviation plot. Negative values indicate depression and are mainly due to cataract, refractive errors, etc., but significant glaucomatous damage does produce a more negative value.

Pattern Standard Deviation (PSD)

This value represents unevenness of the hill of vision and is also extrapolated from the total deviation plot. It is strongly influenced by localized defects.

Short-term Fluctuation (SF)

This parameter accounts for intra-test variability. It is the standard deviation of 10 points, thresholded twice, denoted by double bracketing in the raw data (section 3). The assessment of this is an effort by the software to calculate the error in threshold estimation during the test. An increase in the short-term index value usually represents poor patient reliability. The index can also be abnormal when there is a true field loss in and around the same areas where the 10 points are located. Poor reliability is confirmed when areas surrounding the points are normal.

Corrected Pattern Standard Deviation (CPSD)

An increased short-term fluctuation will cause enough deviation from normal to be represented in the pattern deviation plot leading us to assume the presence of a focal depression. The CPSD parameter represents PSD index corrected for short-term fluctuation in an attempt to eliminate the defects or depressions created by normal fluctuation. This will avoid attributing these defects to disease process. An increased short-term fluctuation index will create an abnormal PSD index, but a normal CPSD index when the same is due to poor patient reliability, true defects on the other hand will have an abnormal CPSD index with complimented probability values. The role of short-term fluctuation and CPSD in differentiating a normal and abnormal field is debated and newer algorithms like SITA have eliminated their use.

Glaucoma Hemifield Test

This analysis (section 7) is a representation of five zones in the superior half that are typically areas of glaucomatous loss compared to its counterpart in the inferior half (Fig. 6.5). Statistical differences between the matched zones are compared and test outcomes read in one of the five messages given below. Most observers regard this as an important diagnostic parameter for glaucoma.

- *Within normal limits:* Score difference between matched zones is statistically insignificant.
- *Outside normal limits:* Score difference between the matched zones has a probability value of <1%.

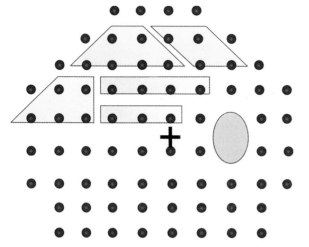

Fig. 6.5: Visual field. Glaucoma Hemifield Test message is analyzed by STATPAC software in Humphrey perimeters by comparing points shown above to their exact counterparts in the inferior hemifield and to a database of normals

- *Borderline:* Score difference between the matched zones has a probability value of <3%.
- *General reduction of sensitivity:* Associated with depressions that are equal on both sides of horizontal mid line and can also be seen in cases of advanced cataract or advanced glaucoma.
- *Abnormally high sensitivity:* This is seen in unreliable patients with high false positives.

The GHT parameter helps to label an abnormal field. This, along with a significant cluster of defects in the pattern deviation plot in a reliable test is definitely diagnostic.

The "Gaze track" display (Fig. 6.2) depicted in the lower most part of the printout provides accurate record of fixation throughout the test using the reflection of an infrared source over the cornea. Reliability of fixation cannot be concluded upon and the role of catch trials to monitor fixation continues to be important. The upward deflection reflects loss of fixation while downward deflection corresponds to a blink.

The assessment of the visual field should be done by a routine habitual evaluation (Tables 6.2 and 6.3) of each section mentioned above and conclusions regarding a pathological defect should be based on at least two reliable test reports with equal reproducibility and the same will serve as a baseline for comparison of future tests of the same patient. A few examples of early and late glaucomatous defects have been discussed in Figs 6.6 and 6.7A and B.

Table 6.2: Habitual approach for single field analysis

1. Ensure patient data is correct and test strategy used is what you recommended.
2. Establish that the field is reliable.
3. Assess total deviation plot and pattern deviation plot.
4. Look at global indices, GHT message.
5. Overview the grey scale.
6. Apply criteria for abnormality.

Table 6.3: Minimal criteria for abnormality on a visual field (Anderson's criteria)

A cluster of 3 or more non-edge points* in a location typical for glaucoma all of which are depressed on the pattern deviation plot at p < 5% level and one of which is at p < 1% level on 2 consecutive fields

or

A CPSD or PSD (in SITA) that occurs in less than 5% of normal fields on 2 consecutive fields

or

A GHT outside normal limits on 2 consecutive fields

*(Edge points valid in case of 24-2 program)

Common Factors Influencing Automated Perimetry

Automation in perimetry has been a big leap in terms of making perimetric evaluation more accurate, quantitative and quick and in eliminating technician bias. However, a human interaction is necessary to orient the patient with the machine, make him or her comfortable, encourage and monitor the test process to allow greater accuracy in performance. Below here are few examples of common artifactual errors that can produce erroneous results and mislead the observer. This can however be easily detected and corrected if one is systematic and pays attention to a few simple data or patient-related errors.

Cataract: The visual field generally shows a diffuse loss of sensitivity due to cataract. This leads to a depression on the total deviation plot while the pattern deviation, PSD and CPSD remain normal (Fig. 6.8). The GHT may also indicate generalized reduction of sensitivity. Depression associated with cataract can also be in the form of peripheral constriction or arcuate in nature, these depressions are more common with dense posterior subcapsular cataracts and generally disappear with larger targets (Size V).

Miotic pupil: An ideal pupil size for perimetry would be 3 mm and above. Pupils below this size should be dilated prior to testing because they can produce artifacts especially in the presence of associated cataractous changes as noted in Figure 6.9. It is important that the examiner and technician note pupil size before subjecting a patient to the test. It is also ideal to maintain similar size and test condition for every test to ensure stable output.

Edge artifacts: These artifacts (Fig. 6.10) are also known as lens rim artifacts and present as typical, sharply demarcated absolute defects (0 dB) in the periphery. The defects tend to be temporally skewed and broader towards the blind spot unlike typical arcuate scotomas that are broader nasally. Ptosis and prominent brow can produce similar superior depressions. A repeat test with careful head positioning and lens centration or use of contact lens will usually eliminate these defects.

Fatigue Related Artifacts

Automated perimetry is a demanding psychophysical test. Longer test durations do induce progressive deterioration in response pattern leading to increase in false negatives and

Single Field Analysis   Eye: Left

| Name: | ID: 310499 | DOB: 31-10-1959 |

Central 24-2 Threshold Test

Fixation Monitor: Gaze/Blindspot   Stimulus: III, White   Pupil Diameter: 6.8 mm   Date: 16-08-2001

Fixation Target: Central   Background: 31.5 ASB   Visual Acuity: 6/6   Time: 2:50 PM

Fixation Losses: 1/20   Strategy: Full Threshold   RX: +1.00 DS   DC X   Age: 41

False POS Errors: 1/13

False NEG Errors: 0/12

Test Duration: 11:32

Fovea: 30 dB ■

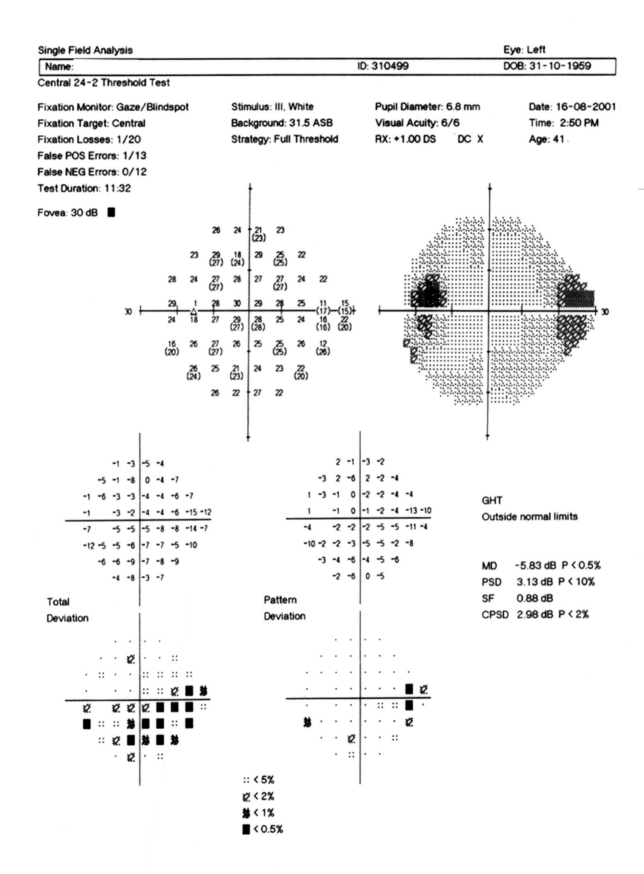

GHT

Outside normal limits

MD   -5.83 dB   P < 0.5%

PSD   3.13 dB   P < 10%

SF   0.88 dB

CPSD   2.98 dB   P < 2%

Total Deviation

Pattern Deviation

:: < 5%

🗴 < 2%

🗱 < 1%

■ < 0.5%

Fig. 6.6: Visual field. Early defect: Analyzing the above printout as per protocol, test strategy is 24-2 full threshold; General information is complete and normal; Reliability indices good; Total deviation reveals generalized depression; Pattern deviation reveals depression nasally on either side of horizontal; Global indices reveal CPSD < 2% and GHT is abnormal. Gray scale corresponds and points satisfy Anderson's criteria. The bottomline however is repeatability and clinical correlation

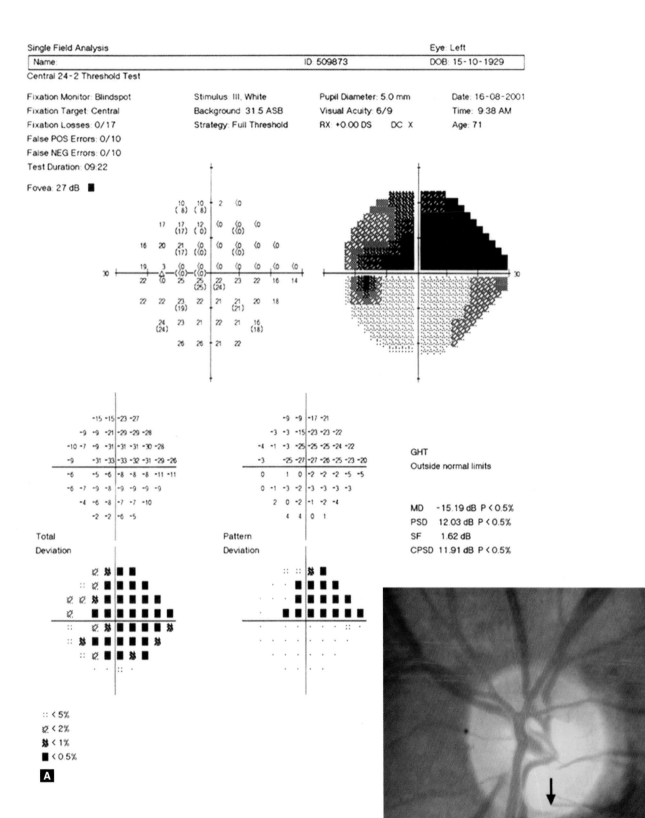

Single Field Analysis   Eye: Left

Name: ID: 509873   DOB: 15-10-1929

Central 24-2 Threshold Test

Fixation Monitor: Blindspot   Stimulus: III, White   Pupil Diameter: 5.0 mm   Date: 16-08-2001
Fixation Target: Central   Background: 31.5 ASB   Visual Acuity: 6/9   Time: 9:38 AM
Fixation Losses: 0/17   Strategy: Full Threshold   RX: +0.00 DS   DC X   Age: 71
False POS Errors: 0/10
False NEG Errors: 0/10
Test Duration: 09:22

Fovea: 27 dB ■

Total
Deviation

Pattern
Deviation

GHT
Outside normal limits

MD   -15.19 dB P < 0.5%
PSD   12.03 dB P < 0.5%
SF   1.62 dB
CPSD 11.91 dB P < 0.5%

:: < 5%
∅ < 2%
⊠ < 1%
■ < 0.5%

A

Figs 6.7A and B: Visual field. The visual field shows a dense superior arcuate scotoma (A) and all parameters are reliable and satisfy all components of Anderson's criteria, more importantly the disc corresponds (B)

B

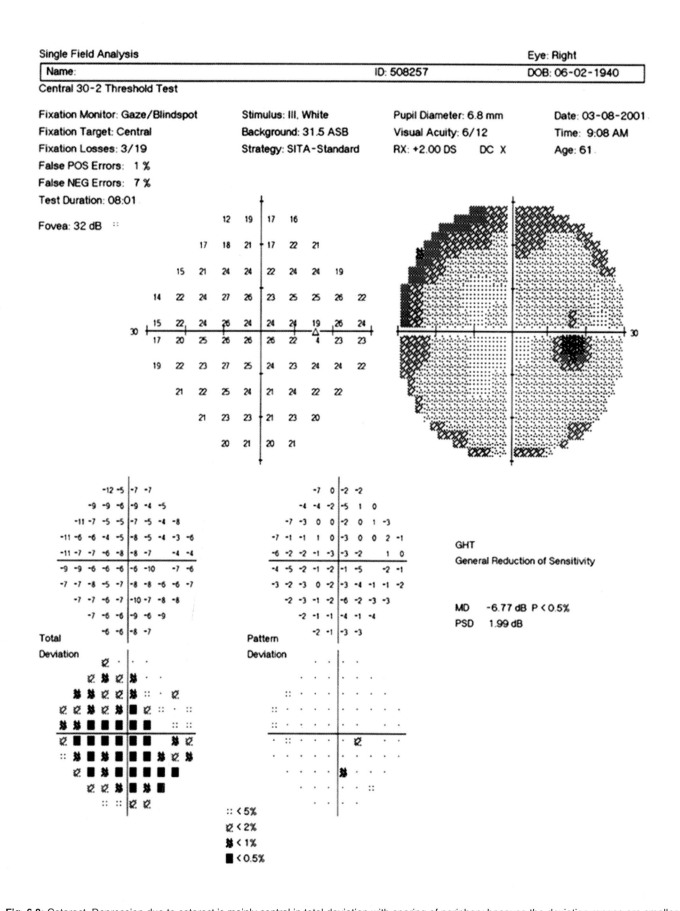

Eye: Right

Name: ID: 508257   DOB: 06-02-1940

Central 30-2 Threshold Test

Fixation Monitor: Gaze/Blindspot   Stimulus: III, White   Pupil Diameter: 6.8 mm   Date: 03-08-2001

Fixation Target: Central   Background: 31.5 ASB   Visual Acuity: 6/12   Time: 9:08 AM

Fixation Losses: 3/19   Strategy: SITA-Standard   RX: +2.00 DS   DC X   Age: 61

False POS Errors: 1 %

False NEG Errors: 7 %

Test Duration: 08:01

Fovea: 32 dB

Total Deviation

Pattern Deviation

GHT

General Reduction of Sensitivity

MD   -6.77 dB P < 0.5%

PSD   1.99 dB

:: < 5%

< 2%

< 1%

■ < 0.5%

Fig. 6.8: Cataract. Depression due to cataract is mainly central in total deviation with sparing of periphery because the deviation ranges are smaller for central points. The pattern deviation is clear, while GHT reads generalized reduction and PSD is insignficant. Important to note here that SITA strategy has been used—average test durations are shorter, reliability parameters are directly read in percentages, SF and CPSD are not tested for

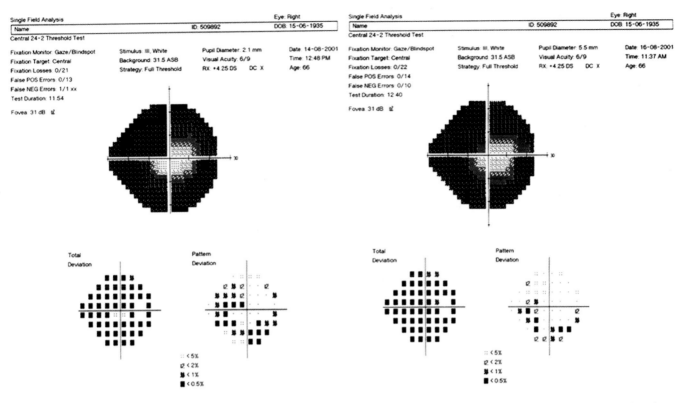

Fig. 6.9: Miotic pupil. Note pupil diameter in test one (2 mm), which shows significant loss both in gray scale as well as pattern deviation plot; a repeat test after dilatation (6 mm) clears up both areas significantly

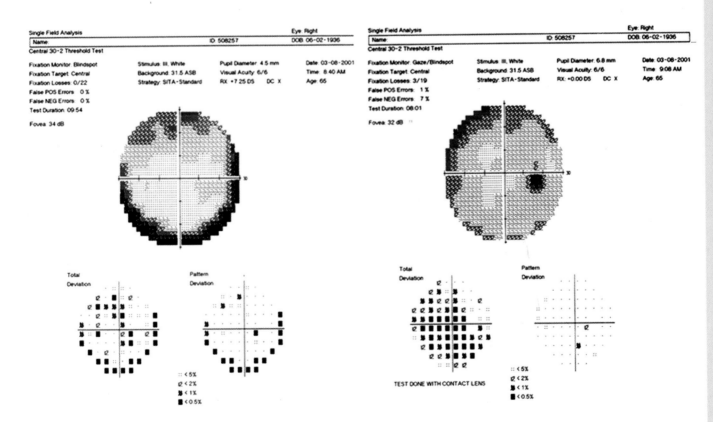

Fig. 6.10: Rim artifact. Visual field of a patient with peripheral artifact using a + 7.25 D sph lens, defects are sharply demarcated and absolute (0 dB on gray scale). This was corrected repeating the test with contact lenses

peripheral depressions resulting in typical clover leaf patterns (Fig. 6.11). This can be overcome by providing ideal test room conditions with comfortable seating for patients. An alert technician can always coax the patient and pause the test to give adequate rest. Faster strategies would be the alternative in old and easily fatigable patients.

Patient Behavior—Moderate and Extreme

The patient does have a challenge of living up to the expectations of a highly automated machine. It is fairly demanding to keep the momentum and coordination of pressing the button, which most patients vary in response during the initial testing phases leading to what's referred to as the "learning effect". Typically, they demonstrate decreased overall sensitivity and peripheral depression, which gradually improves with subsequent tests (Fig. 6.12). The extreme group of patients are either hyperactive or "trigger happy" causing abnormally high thresholds (40 dB) to be documented and cause typical "white scotomas" (Fig. 6.13) in the gray scale.

Criteria for Progression of Visual Field

A series of reliable visual fields need to be evaluated before we decide on the progression of glaucomatous loss. Ideally one should establish a set of baseline fields as discussed earlier with which all further tests are compared to comment on deterioration or progression. It is important to consider and rule out artifacts or role of cataract and refractive errors that can

influence test reports with time. A simple guideline to assess progression is outlined below, the software however has more detailed methods to analyze and detect progression.

Progression is suspected if:

* *New defect is noted in a previously normal area:* Cluster of 3 points worsened by 5 dB each, 1 of which has worsened by 10 dB.
* *Previously abnormal region has deepened if:* Three or more points have worsened by 10 dB.
* *Previously abnormal region has widened if:* Two or more new contiguous points are involved.

Advanced Analysis

The detection of progression in visual field loss is a complex issue because of various factors involved in the long-term fluctuation of test results. The software however has been designed to display serial visual field data to assist detection of progression. Three programs namely the "Overview" printout, "Change analysis" printout and "Glaucoma change probability" printout are available with current softwares.

The overview printout displays gray scale, measured threshold, total deviation and pattern deviation on a single sheet of paper. This allows only trends to be viewed over time in an easy format and up to 16 serial prints can be quickly reviewed. The change analysis printout displays serial data as a set of frequency distributions of actual threshold in the form of a box plot, which can be compared to a normal distribution also represented by a box plot. The print also displays changes in global

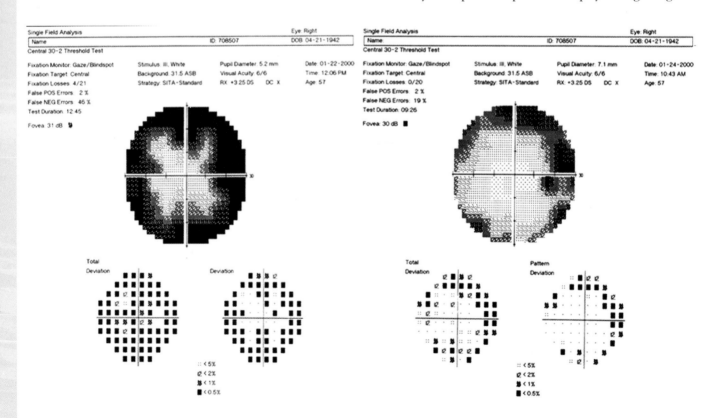

Fig. 6.11: Fatigue. Test shows a typical clover leaf pattern with increased false negatives. On a brighter morning, the same patient responded quicker (test duration shorter) and better

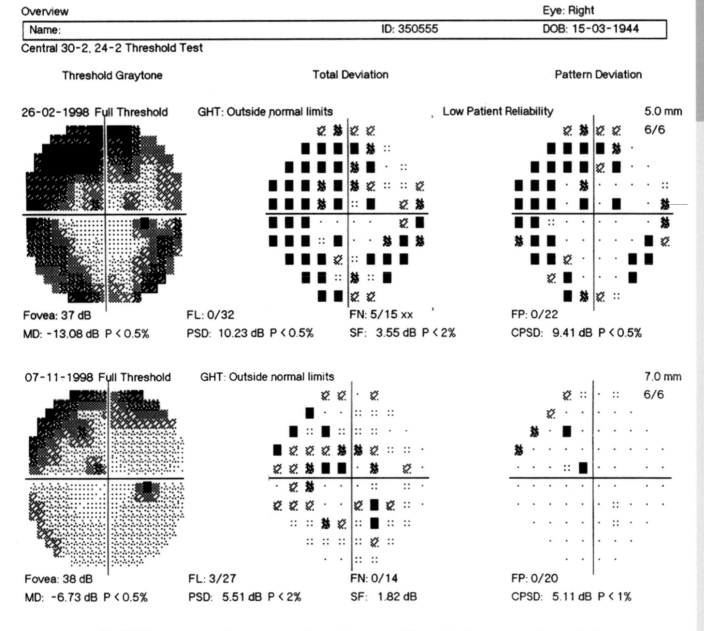

Fig. 6.12: Learning curve. An overview showing peripheral constriction, which disappears on subsequent tests

indices overtime in a graphical format. The glaucoma change probability analysis printout depicts and analyzes thresholds over a series of fields (at least 6) and is represented in the form of clear triangles (improved points) and black triangles (deteriorated points) allowing the clinician to detect progression.

Alternative Strategies and New Programs

Fastpac: This strategy was an attempt to quicken up prolonged full threshold test process. The presentation of stimulus is done in 3 dB steps compared to the 4-2 dB pattern of full threshold. Testing is stopped after one crossover from seeing to non-seeing area or vice versa unless there is a gross deviation from normal value, re-thresholding is done under such circumstances. The program reduced test time to 70% of full threshold, but had

its drawbacks in terms of increased short-term fluctuation and vulnerability to errors in patient's response. This strategy, at present, is considered ideal for screening. This is also useful in performing follow-up of largely normal fields and observing ocular hypertensive patients.

Swedish Interactive Thresholding Algorithms (SITA)

The full threshold was a well-accepted and durable program, but constant research aimed at developing a faster strategy yielded results after 10 years leading to the evolution of "SITA standard" and "SITA fast" algorithms. SITA standard has evolved into an accurate and intelligent alternative to full thresholding program and practitioners are switching over to this faster strategy for glaucoma evaluation. The strategy helped

Section 2 ■ Glaucoma

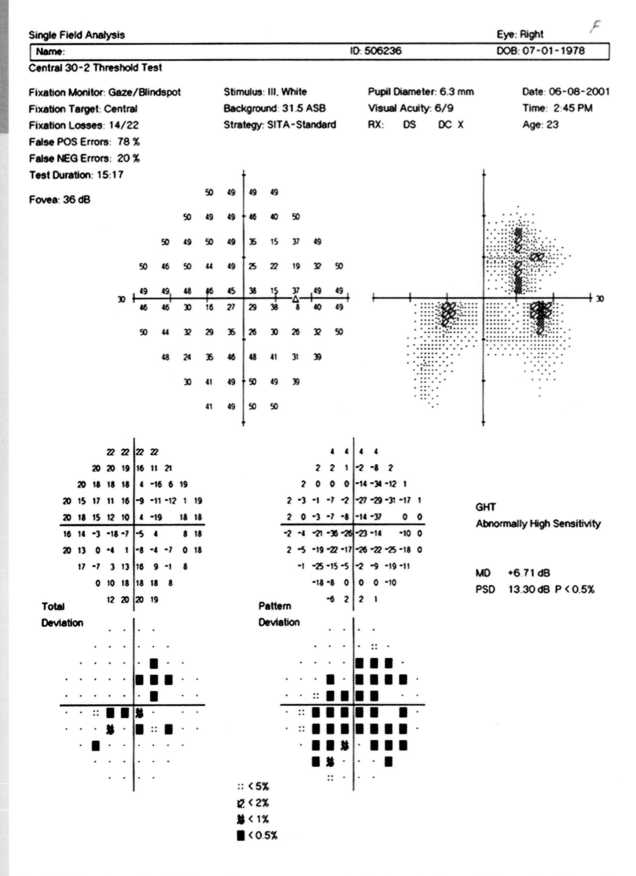

Fig. 6.13: Trigger happy. Visual field shows white scotomas on gray scale with abnormal values > 40 dB in raw data. False positives are high and GHT reads abnormally high sensitvity—typical of a trigger happy patient

in reducing test time by 50% retaining the same accuracy and reliability as the standard full threshold. This was possible as a result of a large database of visual field models from normal and glaucomatous patients. The testing pacing was modified based on patient's behavior and time-consuming catch trials were eliminated, but the program continued to retain its accuracy and reliability. SITA begins with prior probability models of normal and abnormal visual fields. The model is based on a large database of age-corrected values in normal and glaucomatous populations and correlation between adjacent test points. SITA is able to guess with ease the approximate threshold at each point based on the models in its data. This gives it a jump-start ahead of the full threshold strategy in estimating a particular point. The information index also adds to speed up by quickly approaching the selected levels based on responses of surrounding points. Testing is stopped if a particular point reaches a pre-selected threshold level. The program uses the standard deviation of patient's response time to determine the time interval during which to wait for a response before moving to next. The pacing is thus comfortably tuned to patient's speed and capacity. The full threshold algorithm does adjust pace based on reaction time, but there is an overall slowing up of the process even for fast responders. The SITA does have a capacity to precisely recompute all thresholds determined and re-evaluate validity of each response based on reaction time. This method of post-processing helps determine false positive responses thereby reducing the need for special catch trials to estimate reliability. The SITA ensures that threshold estimates are as reliable as full threshold by making sure that at least two crossovers are conducted at a point that does not match up to the pre-selected confidence limit, which otherwise is reduced to one crossover. The assessment of short-term fluctuation also was eliminated in SITA due to vastly improved estimation of false negative and false positive errors.

"SITA fast" runs in half the time of a fastpac test. Faster testing is achieved by stopping test once stimulus falls within the confidence limit unlike SITA standard where at least one crossover is necessary and two is required when deviation is grossly abnormal. Current practices recommend SITA fast in elderly or easily fatigued patients and as an alternative to less reliable supra threshold-screening strategies.

Short Wavelength Automated Perimetry

This is also known as blue-on-yellow perimetry evolved in the 1980's and is currently under clinical application for early detection of glaucoma. Developed by Davis and Berkeley labs, University of California, the principal basis of SWAP (Fig. 6.14) is to isolate the blue cone, which seems more susceptible to early glaucomatous damage. The other proposed basis is the low population of these ganglion cells (5%) that allows early detection in case of any damage. White-on-white perimetry stimulates all the cone systems while the wavelength of 440 nm is nearest to the peak response of blue cones. The intense yellow light serves to bleach the red and green systems reducing their sensitivities and the blue stimulus enhances the isolation of blue cone system. The blue cones have a much lower visual acuity (approximately 20/200) hence the "SWAP" stimuli are of size V and appear fuzzy and indistinct. Apart from the longer duration, the test parameters and color backgrounds make the test quite stressful in comparison to a standard white-on-white perimetry. Lenticular density affects blue transmission and it does produce a depression that could be profound and difficult to interpret and isolate from glaucomatous loss. Mild and moderate cataracts however do permit a reasonable test outcome with adequate specificity and reliable statistical data. It is important to remember "SWAP" results are only a part of the diagnostic picture. A clinical corelation of intraocular pressure and disc status is necessary to label a defect glaucomatous. SWAP can be resorted to when conventional tests have not been diagnostic in the evaluation of a suspicious patient.

Automated perimetry has been the cornerstone in terms of glaucoma diagnosis and management during the past three decades. Glaucoma as a disease process has become more complex in definition with intraocular pressure no longer being the only risk factor and quantitative perimetry has allowed deeper insights and is possibly the only simple diagnostic aid in such cases. Technology has provided an amazing finesse to this complex process of visual field analysis, but as always can be prone to errors that could be disastrous to the patient. The issue is challenging to the clinician and his role to understand the test process carefully and analyze the corresponding clinical picture to give an integrated judgment continues to be invaluable.

Frequency Doubling Technology Perimetry

Frequency doubling technology perimetry (FDT) is a new perimetry technique available for early glaucoma detection. The technology is based on the proposed evidence of loss in contrast sensitivity for frequency-doubled stimuli in glaucoma. The frequency doubling effect is mediated by the My-type (Magnocellular) subset of large ganglion cells, which have a propensity for early damage in glaucoma. The frequency doubling technology perimeter is a compact and portable machine (Fig. 6.15), which produces a frequency doubling illusion by causing a low spatial frequency sinusoidal grating to undergo high temporal frequency to produce an illusion of twice as many light and darks bars than actually present (Fig. 6.16).

The FDT can work on the screening mode as well as threshold mode. Two suprathreshold screening programs: C-20-1 and C-20-5 that test 17 locations over central 20° are available on the current perimeters. The area tested is divided into central circle of 5° diameter surrounded by sixteen 10° diameter squares. The C-20-1 program presents stimuli at 1% probability level (i.e. a contrast that is perceived by 99% of normal population) while the C-20-5 (Fig. 6.17) presents stimuli at 5% probability level and subsequently increases contrast level if response is negative. The C-20-1 is highly specific and appropriate for the mass screening and rapid evaluation of large population while

Single Field Analysis - BLUE-YELLOW   Eye: Right

| Name: | ID: 815143 | DOB: 07-06-1952 |

Central 24-2 Threshold Test

Fixation Monitor: Blindspot   Stimulus: V, Blue   Pupil Diameter: 3.0 mm   Date: 14-06-2001
Fixation Target: Central   Background: Yellow   Visual Acuity: 6/6   Time: 10:22 AM
Fixation Losses: 0/27   Strategy: Full Threshold   RX: +3.00 DS   DC X   Age: 49
False POS Errors: 0/18
False NEG Errors: 3/17
Test Duration: 16:05

Fovea: 19 dB

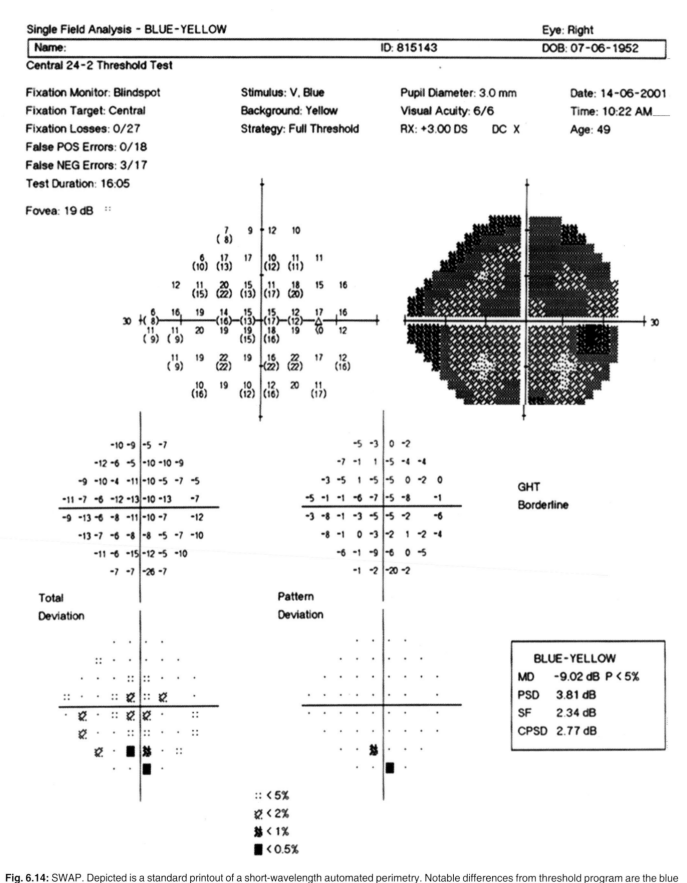

Total Deviation

Pattern Deviation

GHT
Borderline

BLUE-YELLOW
MD   -9.02 dB P < 5%
PSD   3.81 dB
SF   2.34 dB
CPSD 2.77 dB

:: < 5%
⌀ < 2%
▒ < 1%
■ < 0.5%

Fig. 6.14: SWAP. Depicted is a standard printout of a short-wavelength automated perimetry. Notable differences from threshold program are the blue on yellow stimulus presentation, stimulus size used is V and presentation is formatted on full threshold mode. Average test duration is longer and gray scale generally shows a diffuse depression depending on lenticular density. Global indices and GHT is calculated by the software

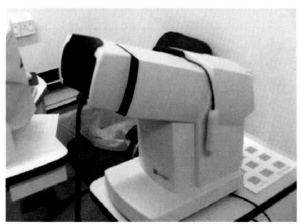

Fig. 6.15: The Humphrey-Welch Allyn FDT perimeter

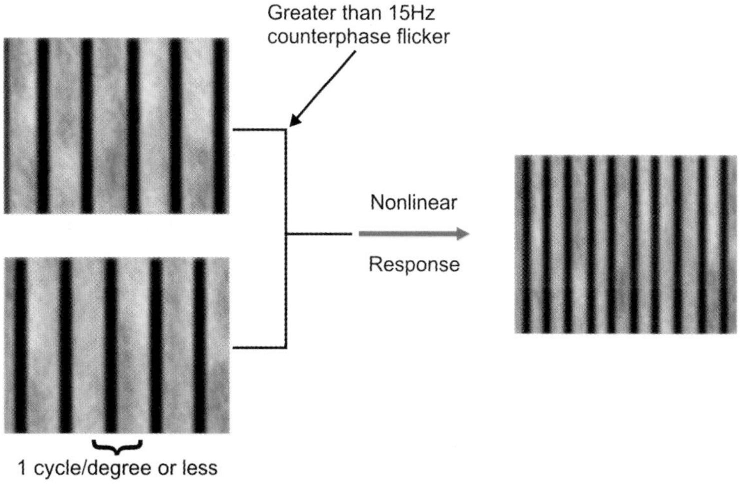

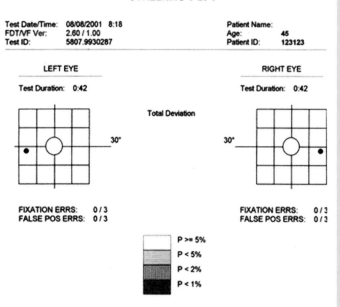

Fig. 6.16: Frequency doubling. A schematic representation of frequency doubling effect, which shows a low frequency sinusoidal grating that undergoes high temporal frequency counterphase flicker to create an illusion of doubling of the dark and light bands

C-20-5 program has a higher sensitivity and is ideal in a clinical setting and screening at risk patients.

The FDT in threshold mode tests central 20° with the C-20 program, the N-30 program (Fig. 6.18A) tests an additional two locations along the nasal step area on either side of the horizontal. The programs also run catch trials to assess reliability in terms of false positives, false negatives and fixation loss. The test printouts are fairly informative with actual threshold data along with a total deviation probability plot. Mean deviation (MD) and pattern standard deviation (PSD) are also represented and calculated by comparison to age-related normal data like in the Humphrey field analyzers. The newer versions of FDT have additional software that allows permanent data storage and more detailed printouts with total and pattern deviation plots depicted separately. The screening programs last about one minute per eye while threshold tests can take up to 5 minutes. The perimeter is much more patient friendly and test results are unaffected by room illumination and refractive errors of up to ± 7.00 D sph.

The FDT is being widely accepted as a useful screening tool for glaucoma and neurological cases. Correlation of defects in comparison to Humphrey programs has been well demonstrated (Fig. 6.18B). The instrument still has to prove its role in progression and monitoring disease process.

OPTIC NERVE AND NERVE FIBER LAYER IMAGING

Over the past decade computerized imaging technologies have evolved and been extensively refined for clinical assessment of the optic nerve and retinal nerve fiber layer (RNFL). These technologies have the ability to provide objective and quantitative measurements of the optic nerve and retinal nerve fiber layer. The quantitative measurements have been shown to have good correlation with the status of optic nerve structure and function thereby facilitating glaucoma diagnosis and monitoring. It is very important to remember that all these technologies can

Fig. 6.17: A sample of the C-20-5 screening test. The central circle is 5 degrees while the remaining test squares are 10 degrees each

only serve as adjuncts and data generated by these are best used with comprehensive information derived from clinical evaluation of the patient. The following technologies are currently the mainstay of optic nerve and nerve fiber layer imaging:

- Confocal scanning laser ophthalmoscopy (Heidelberg Retinal Tomograph [HRT]; Heidelberg Engineering, Heidelberg, Germany)
- Scanning laser polarimetry (GDx VCC; Carl Zeiss Meditec, Dublin, CA, USA)
- Optical coherence tomography (OCT; Carl Zeiss Meditec, Dublin, CA, USA).

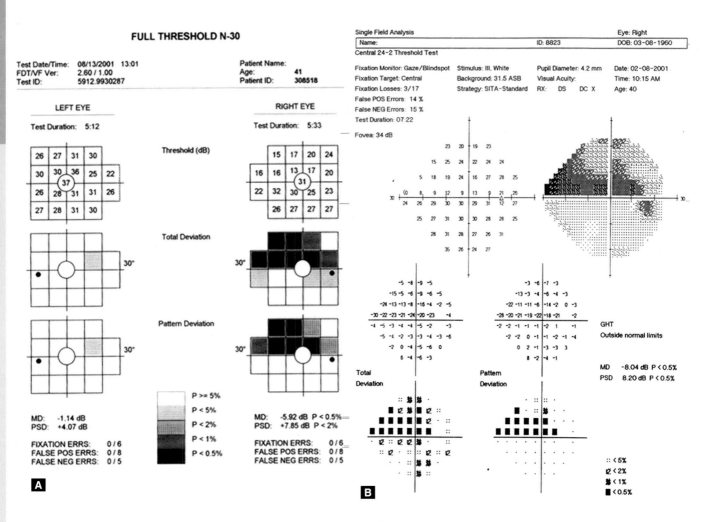

Figs 6.18A and B: The N-30 full threshold printout. The printout shows an addition of two squares in the nasal area (A). Printout is in typical format of Humphrey program and this depicts a superior arcuate scotoma. Good corelation is noted with tests of the same patient on HFA (B)

Heidelberg Retinal Tomograph

Introduction

The Heidelberg Retinal Tomograph (HRT) is a confocal scanning diode laser ophthalmoscope that analyzes three-dimensional images of the optic disc and peripapillary retina. Glaucoma is associated with loss of nerve fibers and this causes changes in the three-dimensional topography of the optic disc. The HRT allows a quantitative assessment of the optic disc topography and quantification of these changes at baseline as well as over a period of time.

Definition

The HRT uses a fixed 15 degree view centered on the optic disc with a resolution of 384 × 384 pixels per image plane. The instrument uses a 670 nm diode laser sharply focused at different depths within the eye to scan a series of 15 by 15 degree areas. Scans can be done in the undilated state of pupil following which images are generated along the x-y plane and standard scan depth is 2 mm resulting in 32 cross sectional images of the optic nerve. The scan depth gets automatically

adjusted depending on the depth of cupping. As cupping progresses, the resolution remains constant and therefore data can be compared over time. Once the images are captured, the next step involves marking the optic disc margin manually on the reflectance image provided by the computer. Marking can be refined by using the disc photograph as a guide. The subsequent analysis results in a color-coded topographic map (Figs 6.19A and B) and a printout with a long list of stereometric disc parameters like disc area, cup area, rim area, rim volume, cup shape measure, height variation contour, mean RNFL thickness and the Moorfields regression analysis.

Analysis of normality and abnormality is facilitated by the normative database of both stereometric disc parameters and Moorfields regression analysis database that is incorporated in the software. Moorfields regression analysis divides the optic disc into six sectors and the rim area (adjusted for cup area) is compared to normative database to asses for abnormality. Each sector is color coded either with a green check (normal), yellow exclamation (suspect) or a red cross (abnormal). The software also helps detect change in topography in subsequent follow-up reports when sessions of three or more are available. The current software version (HRT 3) is available with an enhanced normative database, glaucoma probability score and improved image scaling and alignment algorithm. In summary, HRT is a promising tool for diagnosis and monitoring patients with or at risk of glaucoma and can serve as a useful adjunct in the management of a glaucoma patient.

Scanning Laser Polarimetry

Introduction

The scanning laser polarimeter (GDx VCC) is based on the principle that birefringent retinal nerve fiber layer (RNFL) induces a change in the retardation of polarized light depending on its thickness. This change in retardation can be measured by an integrated retinal polarimeter and is an indirect estimate of RNFL thickness. RNFL thickness reduces significantly in glaucoma.

Definition

The GDx VCC has the ability to discriminate between healthy and glaucomatous eyes based on RNFL measurements and analyzing them against an age-based normative database.

The variable corneal compensator (VCC) allows eye specific compensation of anterior segment birefringence. GDx VCC uses a 780 nm polarization modulated diode laser with a field of view of 40 × 20 degrees, a resolution of 256 × 128 pixels and image reproducibility greater than 15 μm. The GDX VCC scans are done over the peripapillary NFL along a circular band that is centered around the optic disc. The band is 0.4 mm wide, and has an outer diameter of 3.2 mm and an inner diameter of 2.4 mm. The scanning generates deviation maps (Fig. 6.20) where in quantitative RNFL evaluation is provided through four key elements of the printout:

- Thickness map
- Deviation map
- TSNIT graph
- Parameter table.

The thickness map is color coded wherein thick RNFL values are colored yellow, orange and red while thin RNFL values are colored dark blue, light blue and green. The deviation map reveals the location and magnitude of RNFL defects over the entire thickness map. The deviation map uses a grayscale fundus image of the eye as a background, and displays abnormal grid values determined by a statistical comparison to normative database as colored squares over this image. TSNIT stands for temporal-superior-nasal-inferior-temporal and displays the RNFL thickness values along the calculation circle starting temporally and moving superiorly, nasally, inferiorly, and ending temporally. In a normal eye, the TSNIT plot follows the typical "double hump" pattern, with thick RNFL measures

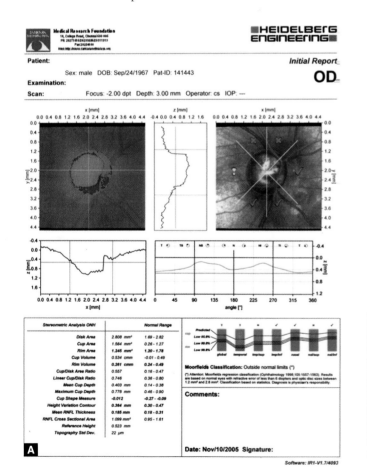

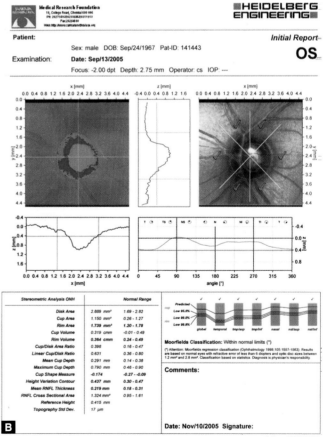

Figs 6.19A and B: Heidelberg retinal tomography. This instrument analyzes three dimensional images of the optic disc and peripapillary retina

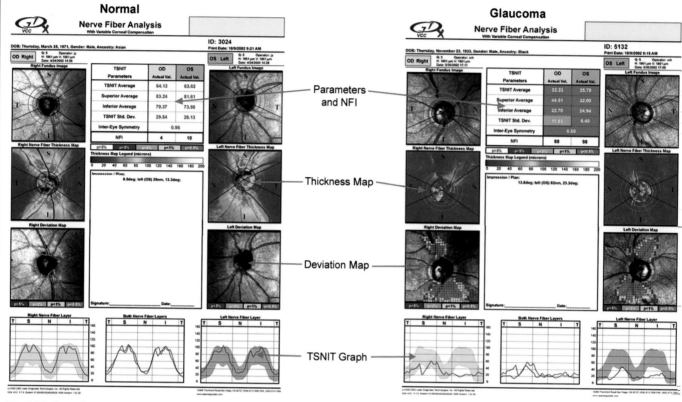

Fig. 6.20: Scanning laser polarimeter. This instrument diseriminates between healthy and glaucomatous eyes based retinal nerve fiber layer thickness

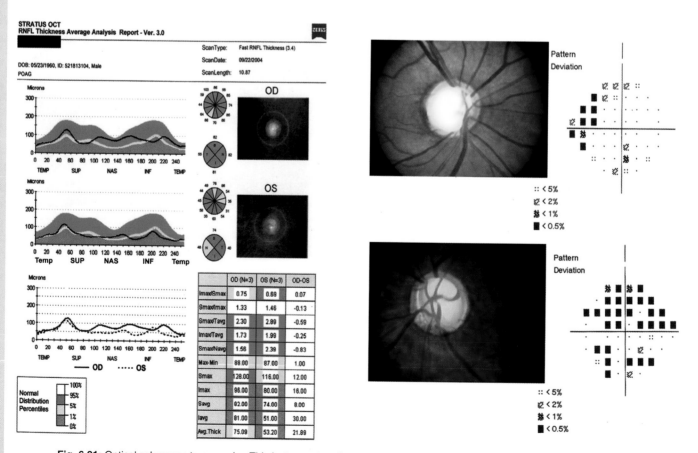

Fig. 6.21: Optical coherence tomography. This instrument analyzes retinal nerve fiber layer thickness and optic disc morphology

superiorly and inferiorly and thin RNFL values nasally and temporally. This pattern is disturbed when RNFL is lost due to glaucoma.

Parameter table depicts parameters that are automatically compared to the normative database and are quantified in terms of probability of normality. Normal parameter values are displayed in green, abnormal values are color coded based on their probability of normality with red having highest probability of being abnormal ($p < 0.5\%$), followed by yellow ($p < 1\%$), light blue ($p < 2\%$) and dark blue ($p < 5\%$). The parameter table includes the important parameter of nerve fiber indicator (NFI), which is a global measure based on the entire RNFL thickness map. It is calculated using an advanced form of neural network and utilizes information from the entire RNFL thickness map to optimize the discrimination between healthy and glaucomatous eyes. NFI output values range from 1–100, with classification based on the ranges: 1–30 is *Normal;* 31–50 is *Borderline;* 51 and above is *Abnormal*. Clinical research has shown that the NFI is the best parameter for discriminating normal from glaucoma. In summary, the GDX VCC is a useful adjunctive tool in the diagnosis of glaucoma and future improvements like the enhanced corneal compensation and progression algorithms will enhance its clinical applications.

Optical Coherence Tomography

Introduction

Optical coherence tomography (OCT) is a noninvasive, high-resolution imaging technique based on low coherence interferometry. It is analogous to an ultrasound with the primary difference being the usage of a coherent source of near infrared frequency light instead of sound waves. Changes in coherence are detected to an extent where the retinal layers can be resolved to 5 μm.

Definition

The ability of the OCT to achieve this resolution helps in a direct measurement of the thickness of RNFL and thereby behaves as an useful objective tool in the diagnosis of glaucoma. The imaging source is a diode laser with a wavelength of 840 nm and RNFL analysis is achieved by a circular scan line at 3.4 mm around the optic disc. RNFL thickness measurement is graphed in a TSNIT orientation and compared to age-matched normative data (Fig. 6.21).

Normality and abnormality is color coded as white (super normal), green (normal), yellow (borderline) and red (abnormal). Of the many parameters RNFL average and inferior RNFL thickness have been reported to have the best discriminating value in differentiating normal from glaucoma. The instrument also has abilities to analyze disc morphology. Radial line scans through optic disc provide cross-sectional information on cupping and neuroretinal rim area disc margins are objectively identified using signal from end of RPE. Key parameters include cup-to-disc ratio and horizontal integrated rim volume. Currently the third generation device Stratus OCT is available with an updated normative database is available for clinical use and it does appear to be a promising adjunctive objective tool in the evaluation of a glaucoma patient.

Chapter 7

Optic Disc Assessment

Harmohina Bagga, G Chandra Sekhar

INTRODUCTION

In the year 2000, approximately 67 million people throughout the world had glaucoma. This disease does not have any symptoms and that is why almost 50% patients are unaware that they are suffering from glaucoma. Rapid advances in imaging technologies, such as confocal scanning laser ophthalmoscopy; scanning laser polarimetry and optical coherence tomography allow detection of early glaucomatous damage with high sensitivity and specificity. New psychophysical procedures, such as short wavelength automated perimetry, frequency doubling perimetry and motion automated perimetry which are targeted at specific visual functions have been shown to be more sensitive and specific than standard automated perimetry for identifying glaucomatous damage. However, these may not be available to all clinicians and optic disc evaluation is usually performed at the slit lamp. Several studies have shown that abnormalities in the appearance of the optic disc may precede visual field defects.

Conventional stereoscopic clinical evaluation and imaging of the optic disc with fundus photographs is still the most frequently used and sensitive means of diagnosing glaucoma. Comparison of normal subjects with glaucoma patients with early to moderate visual field defects showed that qualitative optic disc evaluation and Heidelberg retinal tomography measurements had the highest sensitivity, specificity and area under the receiver operator characteristic (ROC) curves. With some training, it is possible to clinically evaluate optic nerve head and retinal nerve fiber layer stereoscopically and detect early glaucomatous damage. The aim of this communication is to describe the morphological changes of the optic nerve in glaucoma and highlight the techniques of clinical evaluation of the optic disc.

Methods of Optic Disc Examination

Traditionally, the direct ophthalmoscope has been used for the evaluation of the optic nerve head. Though it has the advantage of providing a magnified view, of being faster and easy to use, the lack of stereopsis can result in missing of subtle changes. Therefore, the use of the direct ophthalmoscope is to be strongly discouraged.

A variety of contact and noncontact lenses are available, which allow stereoscopic viewing of the fundus through the slit lamp. Contact lenses, such as Goldmann lenses are relatively uncomfortable for the patient, take longer time and the coupling fluid can cause transient blurring and difficulty in obtaining good quality fundus photographs. Noncontact lenses include +60 D, +78 D, +90 D and Volk SuperField lenses. These provide excellent stereoscopic and magnified view of the optic disc.

It is important to draw the appearance of the optic nerve head based on these methods. Though drawing of the optic disc suffers from the disadvantage of being subjective in nature, they offer a quick and inexpensive method of following the optic nerve head in the patients of glaucoma. In addition, photographs may not be possible in all cases, e.g. patients with rigid miotic pupils and those with significant media opacities. However, wherever possible, photographs are an indispensable adjunct to clinical evaluation.

Features of Glaucomatous Optic Disc Damage

Cup Disc Ratio

Early studies have reported that the vertical and horizontal cup-disc diameter ratios are useful for the quantification of glaucomatous optic neuropathy and for early detection of glaucoma. However, the ratio has limited value in the identification of glaucomatous damage, because of the wide variability in the size of the optic cup in the normal population. A high cup-disc ratio can be normal if the optic disc is large and a low cup-disc ratio may be glaucomatous if the optic disc is small. The problem with estimating cup-disc ratio as a measure of glaucomatous damage is that it is difficult to decide if the cup is physiological in a large disc or pathological in a small or normal sized disc. Vertical cup-disc diameter ratio corrected for the optic disc size has been found to be the best variable to separate between normal subjects and patients of ocular hypertension with retinal nerve fiber layer defect.

So in the clinical description of the optic nerve head, it is important to state the vertical cup-disc diameter ratio in combination with the estimated disc size. The disc diameter can be easily measured by adjusting the slit-lamp beam height to the edges of the disc while viewing the disc through a 60 D lens. The measurement by this method is roughly equal to the measurement obtained by the planimetry of disc photos by Litmann's correction. Measurements can also be made with other lenses by multiplying the measured value with the appropriate magnification factor–Goldmann contact lens (1.26) and Volk SuperField lens (1.5).

It is important to differentiate contour cupping from color cupping. The margin of the cup should be determined by the bend of the small vessels across the disc rim and not by the central area of disc pallor.

Asymmetry of Optic Disc Cupping

Asymmetry of cupping is seldom seen in normal eyes and until proven otherwise, must be taken as an indication of early glaucomatous damage. However, while assessing asymmetry, it is important to rule out asymmetry of the disc size, which may be due to anisometropia. This can result in difference in the cup-disc ratio between the eyes.

Neuroretinal Rim Evaluation

Glaucomatous damage can be diffuse, focal or a combination of both. Diffuse damage results in symmetrical enlargement of the cup. Focal damage usually involves a particular area of the rim. Normally, according to the ISNT rule, the inferior rim is the thickest followed by the superior, nasal and then the temporal. During optic nerve head evaluation, one must look carefully for any areas of thinning of the neuroretinal rim or for notching or in other words extension of the cup into the rim tissue. If the cup is especially deep in the notch, it is known as a pseudo-pit. Notching and pseudo-pits are usually seen at the superior or inferior poles. The width of the notch tends to correspond to the extent of the visual field defect (Figs 7.1A and B and 7.2). Optic rim pallor is another important indicator of glaucomatous disc damage. In the glaucomatous optic disc, the pale and translucent atrophic tissue may replace the normal pink color of the neuroretinal rim, this can result in a field defect in the corresponding opposite hemisphere (Fig. 7.3).

Vascular Changes

Splinter hemorrhages on the optic disc are a common finding in glaucoma patients (Fig. 7.4). Various studies have shown that disc hemorrhages in association with localized nerve fiber layer defects and notches of the neuroretinal rim are more common among patients of normal tension glaucoma. A possible explanation for the difference in frequency has been suggested. The amount of blood leaking out of a vessel into the surrounding tissue depends on the intraocular pressure when the bleeding occurs. The higher transmural pressure gradient in normal pressure glaucoma leads to larger disc hemorrhages. Also, since the absorption rate of disc hemorrhages depends on the size of the disc bleed, the hemorrhages in patients of normal pressure glaucoma may take a longer time to disappear and thus have a higher chance to be detected than the disc hemorrhages in patients of high pressure glaucoma. Disc hemorrhages in glaucoma usually appear as splinter or flame shaped hemorrhages on the disc surface. They usually precede neuroretinal changes and visual field defects corresponding to the location of the hemorrhage may be expected to appear weeks to years later.

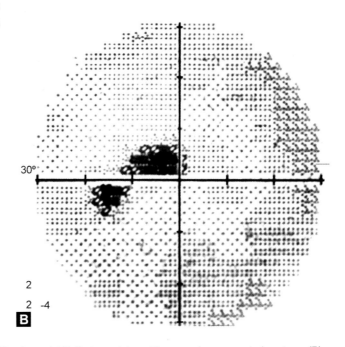

Figs 7.1A and B: Small disc with a localized notch at 6 o'clock position (arrow) (A), that correlates with a superior paracentral scotoma (B)

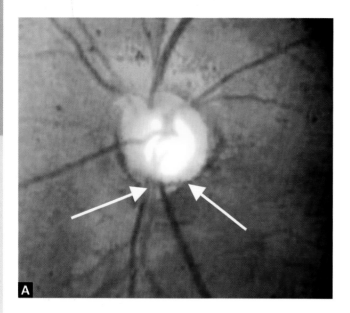

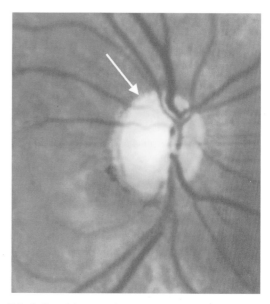

Fig. 7.3: Pallor of the superior neuroretinal rim (↓) that correlates with an inferior nasal step

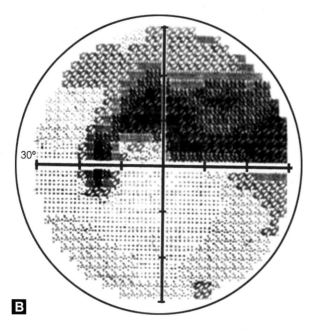

Figs 7.2A and B: A relatively wider inferior notch (↑) (A) that results in a superior arcuate scotoma (B)

Hence occurrence of these is considered an indication for the enhancement of glaucoma treatment.

Configuration of Vessels

The retinal vessels on the optic nerve head can provide clues about the tomography of the disc. Nasalization of the vessels and baring of circumlinear vessels can be seen in glaucoma as well as in other diseases of the optic nerve. Bayoneting of the vessels can be seen if the rim is absent or very thin. This causes the vessels to pass under the overhanging edge of the cup and then make a sharp bend as they cross the disc surface. This convoluted appearance of the vessels is called "bayoneting".

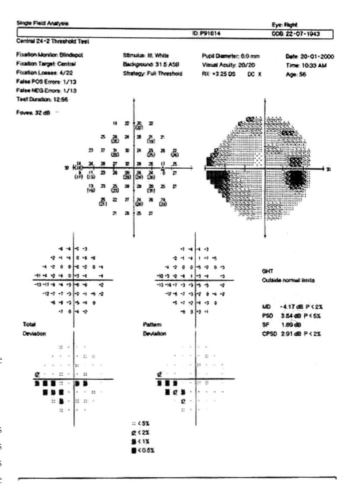

Fig. 7.4: Inferior neuroretinal rim hemorrhage (↑) and an adjoining nerve fiber layer defect (⇑) with the resultant nasal step on perimetry

Peripapillary Atrophy

The zone closer to the optic nerve head with retinal pigment epithelium (RPE) and choroidal atrophy and baring of sclera is called zone β. The more peripheral zone with only RPE atrophy is called zone α (Figs 7.5A and B). A highly significant correlation has been reported between the location of peripapillary atrophy and visual field defects. Since these changes may represent a congenital anomaly, especially in myopic eyes, appearance of these changes de novo or their presence in small, non-myopic discs should be viewed with suspicion. Peripapillary atrophy may be focal or circumferential (Fig. 7.6).

Retinal Nerve Fiber Layer Abnormalities

Examination of the nerve fiber layer is often useful in detecting early glaucomatous damage among patients of ocular hypertension with normal disc appearance and normal visual fields. The neuroretinal rim is formed by axons converging from the retina to the scleral canal. Since the axons are spread out in a thin layer in the retina, even minor losses of the axons can be observed in the retinal nerve fiber layer. In healthy eyes, the nerve fiber layer appears opaque with radially oriented striations. The small retinal blood vessels have a blurred and crosshatched appearance, as they lie buried in the nerve fiber layer. The best way to see the nerve fiber layer defect is through a dilated pupil with a stereoscopic lens, at the slit lamp, using white or green light and a wide slit beam. In the presence of nerve fiber layer atrophy, the small retinal blood vessels become more clearly visible and appear unusually sharp, clear and well focused. The fundus in the affected area appears darker and deeper red in contrast to the silvery or opaque hue of the intact nerve fiber layer (Fig. 7.7). Defects may be in the form of focal defects, slit areas of nerve fiber layer drop out or more diffuse areas of atrophy.

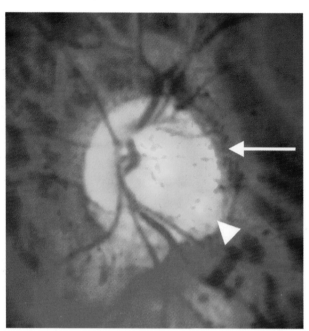

Fig. 7.6: Disc photograph showing loss of the inferior neuroretinal rim and inferior peripapillary chorioretinal atrophic changes (◄)

Myopic Changes versus Glaucoma

Myopic discs can present difficulty in evaluation for glaucoma due to the tilted discs, peripapillary atrophy and shallow

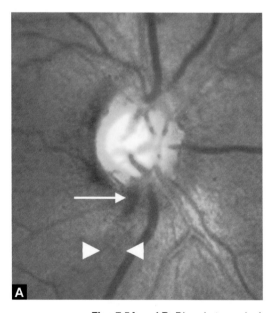

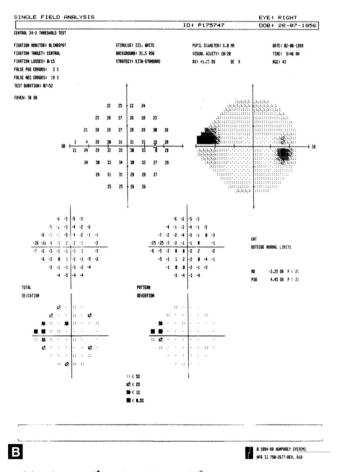

Figs 7.5A and B: Disc photograph showing the peripheral zone α (↑) and central zone β (⇑)

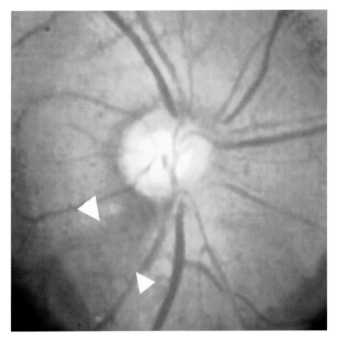

Fig. 7.7: Disc photograph showing inferior nerve fiber layer defect (◀)

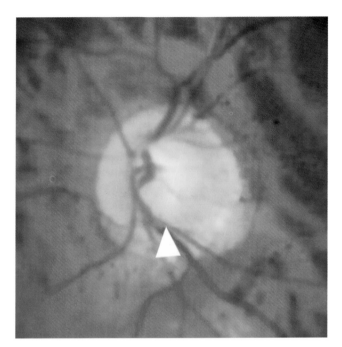

Fig. 7.8: Myopic disc with an inferior notch (◀) masked by the peripapillary changes

cupping. One needs to carefully examine the disc to look for changes in the contour of the blood vessels, as well as carefully delineate the disc margin from the peripapillary changes (Fig. 7.8).

Differential Diagnosis

In addition to glaucoma, other abnormalities can cause excavation and pallor of the optic disc and it is very important to rule these possibilities before making the diagnosis of glaucoma.

Physiological Cupping

Assessment of the size of the optic disc, careful examination of the neuroretinal rim and the retinal nerve fiber layer can help distinguish physiological cupping from glaucomatous damage in most cases.

Optic Nerve Coloboma

Optic nerve colobomas typically demonstrate enlargement of the papillary region, partial or complete excavation, blood vessels entering and exiting from the border of the defect and a glistening white surface. The visual field defects can be in the form of generalized constriction, centrocecal scotomas, altitudinal defects, arcuate scotomas, and enlargement of the blind spot and ring scotomas that can mimic those found in glaucomatous eyes.

Morning glory syndrome is a variant of optic disc coloboma and is characterized by large excavated disc, central core of white or gray glial tissue surrounded by an elevated annulus of variably pigmented sub-retinal tissue. The retinal vessels appear to enter and exit from the margins of the disc, are straightened and often sheathed.

Congenital Optic Disc Pit

Congenital optic disc pits appear gray or yellowish white, round or oval, and with localized depression within the optic nerve. They are located within the temporal aspect of the disc in over half of the cases and centrally in about one third. Involvement is usually unilateral in about 80% cases and the optic disc is larger on the involved side. Approximately 55% to 60% of the eyes have a field defect in the form of arcuate scotomas, paracentral scotoma, altitudinal defect, generalized constriction, and nasal or temporal steps.

Anterior Ischemic Optic Neuropathy

A history of acute visual loss, initial swelling of the optic disc, absence of marked cupping, rise in erythrocyte sedimentation rate, and presence of centrocecal scotoma or altitudinal defects can help differentiate it from glaucoma.

Neurological Causes

Pallor disproportionate to cupping, normal intraocular pressure or unusual history of onset, progression and age should arouse suspicion of a neurological cause for disc changes.

Optic Nerve Imaging in Glaucoma

The conventional method of diagnosis and follow-up of glaucoma has been a thorough stereoscopic examination of the optic nerve head and the retinal nerve fiber layer, serial fundus photography coupled with conventional white-on-white perimetry. However, detectable retinal nerve fiber layer and optic disc abnormalities have been shown to precede typical glaucomatous loss on conventional white-on-white perimetry. In the last decade or so, new imaging techniques have been introduced, which allow objective, quantitative evaluation of the optic nerve head and retinal nerve fiber layer and thus may have an important role to play in diagnosing preperimetric glaucoma as well as progression of the glaucomatous disease process.

The imaging techniques used to measure various optic nerve head and retinal nerve fiber layer parameters are:

- Confocal Scanning Laser Tomography (HRT-Heidelberg instruments, Heidelberg Germany; TopSS, Laser Diagnostic Technologies Inc., San Diego, CA, USA).
- Scanning Laser Polarimetry (GDx, Laser Diagnostic Technologies Inc., San Diego, CA, USA).
- Optical Coherence Tomography (OCT, Humphrey Systems Inc., Dublin, CA, USA).

Primary Congenital Glaucoma

Sushmita Kaushik, Surinder S Pandav

INTRODUCTION

Primary congenital glaucoma (PCG) is a potentially blinding disease of children, which if untreated, would result in a lifetime of blindness. It occurs due to obstruction of the drainage of the aqueous humor caused by a primary developmental anomaly at the angle of the anterior chamber. The onset of the disease is in the neonatal or infantile period, and is manifested by symptoms of raised intraocular pressure (IOP) and corneal edema, such as excessive tearing, photophobia, and an enlargement of the globe (buphthalmos). The consequences of persistently raised intraocular pressure on the optic nerve are far more serious, manifesting as axonal damage and eventual irreversible blindness.

Although primary congenital glaucoma is the most common glaucoma seen in infancy, it is still an uncommon disease. The variable incidence in various ethnic groups points towards a genetic basis for the disease.

Most cases of primary congenital glaucoma occur sporadically, but in approximately 10% of cases, an autosomal recessive hereditary pattern is evident. The PCG gene has been mapped to three different genetic loci: GLC3A (2p21), GLC3B (1p36); and GLC3C (14Q24.3). The first gene to be implicated in the pathogenesis of PCG was the human cytochrome P450 gene (CYP1B1). The involvement of CYP1B1 varies from 20% in Indonesians and Japanese, to 50% among Brazilians, and nearly 100% among Saudi Arabians and Slovakian Gypsies. In a study involving South Indian patients, 30.8% of 138 PCG cases were found to be positive for one of six mutations of the CYP1B1 gene. Ethnic differences and geographical variations may be associated with different mutation patterns.

Most studies on the molecular biology of PCG have investigated only the coding region of the gene, though it is known that mutations in the noncoding regions could lead to changes in gene expression or splicing, which in turn have the potential to alter gene function.

Epidemiology

This condition is now recognized worldwide, but the incidence of the disease varies substantially in different ethnic groups from 1:1,250 births in Slovakian Roms to 1:20,000 in Scandinavian regions. In the West, the average incidence is about 1:10,000 births, but appears to be higher in Asians. In Saudi Arabia, it is reported to be 1:2,500, while Indian data have indicated an incidence of 1:3,300, and the disease was responsible for 4.2% of blindness in the pediatric population.

Inheritance

Most cases of PCG are sporadic in occurrence. Recessive inheritance of some cases of PCG is proved by (1) a high frequency of parental consanguinity; (2) the presence of the disease in about 25% of sibs of probands; (3) the presence of the disease in all children of a marriage between 2 affected persons; and (4) the occurrence of glaucoma in collaterals of both parents in some families.

In approximately 10% of cases in which a hereditary pattern is evident, inheritance is usually believed to be autosomal recessive with variable penetrance.

The universal validity of the autosomal-recessive model has been challenged by reports of disease transmission in successive generations, unequal sex distribution among the affected individuals, and a lower-than-expected number of affected siblings in the familial cases. These observations have raised the possibility that PCG is a genetically heterogeneous disorder. The first molecular evidence for this possibility came from the genetic linkage studies by identifying two separate genetic loci associated with the disease, thus confirming that PCG is indeed genetically heterogeneous. Most of the PCG families were linked to the GLC3A locus on 2p21. However, few other families were linked to the GLC3B locus on 1p36. The existence of linkage between the GLC3A locus and PCG phenotype was subsequently confirmed in PCG families from Saudi Arabia and Romany Slovakians.

Genetic Defects

According to the Human Genome Organisation (HUGO) Nomenclature Committee, loci for congenital glaucoma are designated by GLC3, and letters are added to distinguish specific loci in order of their discovery. Till date, 3 genetic loci have been linked to PCG:GLC3A at chromosome locus 2p21; GLC3B at chromosome locus 1p36; and GLC3C at chromosome locus 14q24.3. Of these, only the GLC3A locus has been linked to a specific gene. This gene is called CYP1B1, and is the largest known enzyme of the human cytochrome p450 pathway.

There are several known missense mutations within the CYP1B1 gene. Among these, the mutations identified are: G61E, Ter 223, P193L, E229K, R390C, R368H. A study on the genotype-phenotype correlation of these patients identified the frame shift mutation and R390C homozygous mutations as being associated with very severe disease and poor prognosis regardless of any treatment. It was postulated that there might exist a possible correlation between genotype and phenotype, knowledge of which may come in handy when evaluating the prognosis of the presenting patient.

Structural Defects and Clinical Features

The glaucomas are a heterogeneous group of insidious diseases associated with elevated IOP and optic nerve atrophy. Primary congenital (infantile) glaucoma (PCG; gene symbol, GLC3) is a specific, inherited developmental defect in the trabecular meshwork and anterior chamber angle, which manifests in the neonatal or infantile period and is more severe and difficult to manage than other types.

There has been some debate as to the exact nature of the structural changes in the angle that are associated with the disease. The early postulation of an imperforate mesodermal membrane covering the outflow channels has not been verified by electron microscopy. Several histopathological studies have observed that the iris insertion and anterior ciliary body overlaps the posterior portion of the trabecular meshwork. It was concluded that during anterior chamber development, the iris and ciliary body failed to recede posteriorly. The juxtacanalicular area was found to be markedly thickened and consisted

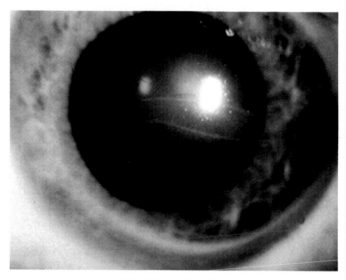

Fig. 8.1: Haab's striae

of many layers of spindle-shaped cells with surrounding extracellular matrix. In general, structural studies agree that the developmental defect affects all areas of the trabecular meshwork.

These developmental anomalies of the anterior chamber angle prevent drainage of aqueous humor, thereby elevating IOP.

During the first three years of life, the collagen fibers of the eye are softer and more elastic than in older individuals. Thus, elevation of IOP in children younger than 3 years of age (infantile glaucoma) causes rapid enlargement of the globe. The globe enlargement occurs primarily at the corneoscleral junction. As the cornea and limbus enlarge, the endothelium of the cornea and Descemet's membrane are stretched. This stretching can result in a linear rupture of the Descemet's membrane (Haab's striae) (Fig. 8.1). The Descemet's membrane rupture may occur acutely, causing an influx of aqueous into the stroma and epithelium, resulting in sudden corneal edema. Clinical features of PCG typically include tearing, photophobia, buphthalmos (enlargement of the globe), and clouding of the cornea (Figs 8.2 to 8.4). The more serious consequence of elevated pressure is that it can rapidly lead to axonal loss and permanent visual impairment in untreated children.

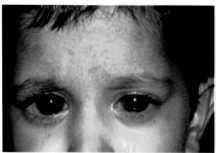

Fig. 8.2: Primary congenital glaucoma present with watering and photophobia

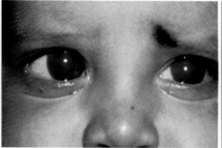

Fig. 8.3: Primary congenital glaucoma present with large eyes and hazy corneas

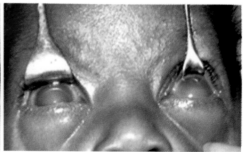

Fig. 8.4: Primary congenital glaucoma present with scarred corneas

Table 8.1: Severity index for grading primary congenital glaucoma phenotypes

Clinical parameters used for grading	Normal	Mild	Moderate	Severe/V Severe
Corneal diameter	Up to 10.5	>10.5–12	>12–13	>13
Intraocular pressure	Up to 16	>16–20	>20–30	>30
C/D ratio	0.3–0.4	>.4–.6	>.6–.8	>.8
Last recorded visual acuity	20/20			<20/200:<20/400–no light perception
Corneal clarity	No edema	Mild edema	Severe edema	Severe edema + Haab's striae

Management

The management of congenital glaucoma starts with parental counseling, which should include a discussion of what is glaucoma; the need for surgery and possibilites of multiple surgeries; the need for life-long follow-up; and the combination of problems to be tackled (IOP, amblyopia management, refractive correction, possible keratoplasty).

Examination under anesthesia is the first step to gauge the severity of the disease and extent of glaucomatous damage that has occurred. The parameters to be evaluated include corneal edema, IOP and cup-disc ratio. Panicker and associates have graded the severity of glaucoma depending upon the clinical features as given below in Table 8.1.

Tonometry

General anesthetics usually lower the IOP except for ketamine, which may increase IOP. Intraocular pressure should be checked in the early stage of anesthesia to reduce errors. The Schiötz tonometer should be avoided because it is not as accurate as the Perkins hand-held applanation tonometer. The Tono-Pen is convenient and easy to use.

The normal IOP in infants under anesthesia is usually in the low teens. A pressure of 20 mm Hg or more should be considered abnormal. Elevated IOP alone is not sufficient to confirm a diagnosis of congenital glaucoma. Other signs of this disease (e.g. corneal haze, increased corneal diameter, and increased optic disc cupping) are as important as elevated IOP.

Corneal Diameter

Accurate measurement of corneal size is important in the diagnosis and follow-up examination of children with glaucoma. Using calipers for this purpose, the corneal diameter measurement should be taken from limbus to a similar point 180° away at the opposite limbus. The 95% ranges of normal corneal diameters are: 9.4 mm to 11.0 mm at age 1 month, 10.5 mm to 11.7 mm at age 6 months, and 10.8 mm to 12.0 mm at age 12 months. In congenital glaucoma, the diameter of cornea may enlarge to as much as 17 mm. Changes in corneal diameter less than 0.5 mm in the follow-up examination should be interpreted cautiously.

Gonioscopy

A 14 mm Koeppe lens provides a clear view of the angle of the eye, and a hand-held microscope with a Barkan light or any type of illuminator is necessary for gonioscopy during anesthesia. If the cornea is cloudy, removing the corneal epithelium clears the view. During gonioscopy, the site of iris insertion should be evaluated carefully. In congenital glaucoma, the iris usually is inserted anterior to scleral spur, and the angle recess is poorly formed.

Fundoscopy

Dilated fundus examination and disc evaluation are essential in diagnosing congenital glaucoma. Cupping of the optic disc occurs much faster in infants than in adults. Optic disc cupping larger than 30% of disc diameter, especially if asymmetric between two eyes, is strong evidence that the disc is under pressure and may be glaucomatous. Changes in the optic disc occur readily with changes in IOP in infants. Early response of the infant disc to elevated IOP was recorded several decades ago. These findings demonstrate the greater vulnerability of the infant optic disc to increased IOP compared to the adult disc.

When congenital glaucoma is diagnosed at birth, there is often a significant degree of optic disc cupping. If IOP is not controlled, increased cupping can be demonstrated in 4 to 6 weeks. This early rapid change in disc contour may be related to mechanical distortion in the disc supporting elements, and in its initial stages may not represent neuronal loss. Thus, posterior bowing of the lamina cribrosa is a late occurrence in adult glaucoma, but it occurs early in infants.

Glaucomatous cupping in infants, unlike in adults, is usually reversible after normalization of IOP. Marked decreases in cupping commonly are seen at 4 to 6 weeks after normalization of pressure. The younger the child, the faster is this reversibility. Such a rapid change in optic disc cupping is probably related to mechanical changes cited earlier. Improvement in the amount of cupping may be limited by many factors, including the extent of nerve fiber loss.

Surgical treatment: The treatment of PCG is surgical. Medical management has a role as a temporizing measure until the

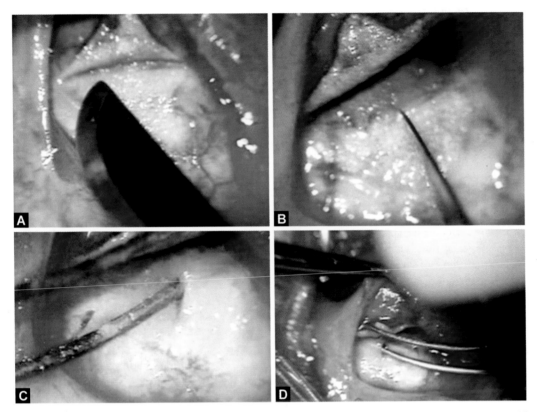

Figs 8.5A to D: Trabeculotomy with trabeculectomy being performed under general anesthesia. Partial thickness scleral flap raised (A) Schlemm's canal dissected (B), Schlemm's canal cannulated with Harms' trabeculotome (C and D)

child can be posted for general anesthesia. The surgical options include goniotomy, trabeculotomy and trabeculectomy with antifibrotic agents. A trabeculotomy-trabeculectomy combined surgery has been found to result in more favorable outcomes and many surgeons prefer that approach (Figs 8.5A to D).

The surgical success has been reported to be varied. In cases of refractory cases not responding to surgery, a repeat surgery is needed. Shunts in the form of valved and non-valved implants have been reported to be successful after failure of conventional surgery.

Chapter 9

Primary Angle-Closure Glaucoma

Harmohina Bagga, G Chandra Sekhar

INTRODUCTION

The angle-closure glaucomas are a diverse group of disorders characterized by iridotrabecular apposition and or adhesion, which can be caused by changes in the relative or absolute sizes or positions of anterior segment structures. Early detection of the angle-closure component is especially important because of the specific therapy (laser iridotomy, iridoplasty, etc.), which in most cases can halt, if not reverse, the chain of events leading to ultimate synechial angle-closure. Filtration surgery in this subgroup of patients requires certain special considerations and is associated with a higher rate of complications, such as uveal effusion and aqueous misdirection glaucoma.

Gonioscopy is one of the most important tools in the diagnosis, management and follow-up of these patients. A careful and accurate gonioscopy can clinch the diagnosis in most of the cases. Angle-closure glaucoma can sometimes be misdiagnosed as normal pressure glaucoma or as ocular hypertension. A careful gonioscopy in such cases can help identify subtle, but certain evidences of the episodes of angle-closure. Indentation gonioscopy is especially useful in evaluating the angle as it affords a dynamic view of the iris and the corneoscleral angle and help to differentiate appositional from synechial angle-closure. The grading systems introduced by Shaffer and Scheie have contributed to our understanding of the mechanism of glaucoma. The use of these systems can cause confusion as an angle graded, as "4" by the Shaffer's system is wide open while "IV" by Scheie's system is narrow. The system recommended by Philips, using descriptive words such as closed, narrow, wide is especially helpful if the exact anatomic structure seen in a particular quadrant of the angle is mentioned, e.g. Schwalbe's line, posterior trabecular meshwork, etc. along with certain specific features of the angle as pigmentation, iris processes, presence of pseudoexfoliative material, etc.

Epidemiology

Primary angle-closure glaucoma (PACG) is comparatively rare among whites with a prevalence rate of approximately 0.1% in individuals older than 40 years of age. The age adjusted prevalence for angle-closure glaucoma in the European population of over 40 years of age is 0.2% as opposed to 24.2% for open-angle glaucoma suggesting that the prevalence of angle-closure glaucoma is 11.4 times lower than open-angle glaucoma amongst the Europeans. Population-based surveys in the 40 years and older age group in different countries show that the prevalence of PACG is least in the Caucasians and highest in the Eskimos. Among the Eskimos, this prevalence rises to 2.6% in Alaska, 2.9% in Canada and 5% in Greenland. In Beijing, China, Hovsgol and Mongolia, population-based studies have reported prevalence of PACG of 1.4%, which is intermediate between the Caucasians and the Eskimos. In a population based study in the city of Vellore in southern India, the prevalence of PACG was reported to be 4.3%, i.e. five times more common than primary open-angle glaucoma. In the Andhra Pradesh Eye Disease Study (APEDS), which was a population-based study in the urban population of Hyderabad in southern India, among people 40 years of age or older, 1.08% had manifest PACG and another 2.21% had occludable angles without ACG. The difference in the prevalence of angle-closure glaucoma in the two studies could possibly be due to the use of different criteria for occludability and PACG. In the Vellore study, one half or more of the angle circumference had to be narrow for it to be considered occludable while the criterion for occludability in the APEDS was three quarters or more of the angle circumference to be narrow. Further, in the APEDS patients with occludable angles, but with intraocular pressure of < 22 mm Hg or without evidence of optic disc damage were not considered as having primary angle-closure glaucoma. Whereas, similar patients were included in the angle-closure group if there were synechiae in the angle in the Vellore study.

Risk Factors for Primary Angle-Closure Glaucoma

Family History

Studies have suggested that the oculometric parameters are controlled by polygenic variation. A 6-fold increase in risk for

PACG was found among subjects with any family history of PACG in a population-based survey in China.

Age

With the possible exception of India and China, PACG is rare in most populations below 40 years of age, reaching peak prevalence in the 50s and 60s. This is thought to be due to the thickening and slight forward movement of the crystalline lens throughout life, which is confirmed by the finding of progressively shallower anterior chambers and narrower angles with age.

Gender

Women are at an increased risk for angle-closure glaucoma over men by a ratio of 2-4:1 amongst almost all racial groups like the Caucasians, Blacks, Chinese and Eskimos. Among the Asians, reports suggest that the proportion of women in the population with narrow angles is significantly higher than men at all ages.

History of Symptoms

In contrast to a history of symptoms in only 9% of open-angle glaucoma patients; 80% of patients of angle-closure glaucoma reported some symptoms like headache, eye pain, haloes, etc. However, it is common for the East Asian eyes to progress to chronic angle-closure glaucoma without experiencing the symptoms of an acute attack.

Refractive Error

Angle-closure glaucoma and narrow angles have been reported to occur more frequently in emmetropic and hyperopic eyes.

Race

The prevalence of PACG is race dependent, being 20-40 times higher in the Eskimos as compared to the Caucasians. When the distribution of ocular parameters in the general population is compared, ethnic groups at greater risk for angle-closure glaucomas have smaller and more crowded anterior segment. Eskimos have shallower anterior chambers than the Caucasians of the same age. However, the correlation between population-based oculometry and angle-closure glaucoma prevalence is less clear among the East Asians. The higher prevalence of PACG among the Asians in the absence of clearly shallower anterior chamber depths could be because of a greater Asian tendency towards plateau iris.

Pathogenesis and Pathophysiology

Compared to normal eyes, eyes with PACG have certain specific structural characteristics such as:
- Smaller corneal diameter
- Smaller radius of anterior and posterior corneal curvature
- Smaller central and peripheral anterior chamber depth
- Thicker lens

- Steeper curvature of anterior lens surface
- More anterior lens position
- Smaller anterior chamber volume
- Shorter axial length
- Greater lens thickness/axial length factor.

In eyes with angle-closure glaucoma, the lens is 0.4–1.0 mm thicker and its relative position is more anterior as compared to normal eyes. Furthermore, there is an increase in these parameters with age. The increase in lens thickness by 0.7–1.1 mm along with its forward movement by 0.4–0.6 mm causes an increase in the lens thickness to axial length factor after 50 years of age. These factors cause "crowding" of the anterior segment making these eyes more prone to an acute attack. These biometric findings have been confirmed by ultrasound biomicroscopy (UBM).

The final common pathway in all cases of angle-closure glaucomas is iris apposition to the trabecular meshwork. In approximately 90% of the patients, the underlying mechanism is a relative pupillary block, which causes a functional block to the flow of aqueous from the posterior chamber into the anterior chamber through the pupil. The impedance in the flow of the aqueous causes its accumulation in the posterior chamber, which forces the peripheral iris anteriorly resulting in anterior iris bowing and iridotrabecular apposition leading to acute or chronic angle-closure glaucoma depending on the extent and suddenness of closure.

If the pupillary block is sufficient to cause appositional closure of a portion of the angle, peripheral anterior synechiae may gradually form leading to chronic angle-closure glaucoma. If the pupillary block is absolute, the peripheral iris is pushed forward to cover the entire trabecular meshwork causing a sudden rise in intraocular pressure and acute angle-closure glaucoma. Intermittent angle-closure glaucoma is caused by repeated brief episodes of iridotrabecular contact. It can result in the progressive formation of peripheral anterior synechiae leading to chronic angle-closure and elevation of intraocular pressure or it can suddenly convert into an acute angle-closure attack.

Pupillary block is the underlying mechanism for the majority of cases of primary angle-closure glaucoma and should always be suspected first. An iridectomy acts by equalizing the pressure between the anterior and posterior chambers and thus eliminating the pupillary block.

It is important to note that while performing indentation gonioscopy, one should take care to avoid pressure by the lens on the cornea, the room should be completely darkened and only a small square of light from a slit beam should be used to avoid stimulating the pupillary reflex, which may open an appositionally closed angle resulting in a false diagnosis.

Plateau Iris

Plateau iris is an uncommon form of angle-closure glaucoma. Though the occurrence of angle-closure in eyes with anterior chambers of relatively normal depth and flat iris plane has been noted as early as 1940, the term plateau iris was first used by Tornquist to describe the appearance of the iris of a 44-year-old man with angle-closure glaucoma who had normal anterior chamber depth, flat iris surface and a sharp backward curvature of the peripheral iris.

Plateau iris is characteristically used to define those eyes that continue to have appositional closure of the angles despite a patent peripheral iridotomy. Such patients tend to be younger, female and less hyperopic than those with pupillary block. The axial anterior chamber depth is usually normal while the peripheral anterior chamber depth is shallow. Gonioscopically, the body of the iris lies in a plane anterior to the iris root so that the approach to the angle is flat, but at the periphery the angle drops almost vertically to the site of insertion. This pre-iridotomy appearance of the anterior chamber with normal depth and flat iris plane, but an extremely narrow or closed angle gonioscopically is known as plateau iris configuration. Plateau iris syndrome is used to describe either spontaneous or mydriatic-induced angle-closure despite a patent peripheral iridotomy in eyes with plateau iris configuration.

However, it is important to exclude other conditions that can cause angle-closure in eyes with PACG following an iridotomy:

- Imperforate peripheral iridotomy
- Extensive synechial angle closure
- Malignant glaucoma
- Pseudo plateau iris (iris and ciliary body cysts, forward rotation of ciliary processes by choroidal effusion, scleral buckle, pan retinal photocoagulation)

True plateau iris syndrome is extremely rare. Many patients with plateau iris configuration have spontaneous or mydriatic induced angle-closure after laser peripheral iridotomy, but without a rise in intraocular pressure. Such patients can be divided into complete and incomplete plateau iris syndrome. Complete plateau iris syndrome is a rare condition in which there is a rise in intraocular pressure with angle-closure up to the Schwalbe's line spontaneously or following dilatation after an iridotomy. In the incomplete form, the intraocular pressure does not rise and closure of the angle occurs up to a point between Schwalbe's line and the scleral spur. The incomplete form is much more common and it is very important to identify such patients because they develop peripheral anterior synechiae years later either with the growth of the crystalline lens or its forward movement with age. Ultrasound biomicroscopy studies have shown that forward rotation of ciliary processes is responsible for forward displacement of the base of the iris.

It is important to remember that because an element of pupillary block can exist in eyes with plateau iris configuration, a diagnosis of plateau iris cannot be made until any component of pupillary block has been relieved by peripheral iridotomy.

In eyes with pupillary block, indentation gonioscopy opens the angle easily since the peripheral iris is displaced only by the aqueous in the posterior chamber. In eyes with plateau iris, the ciliary processes underlie the peripheral iris causing the iris to

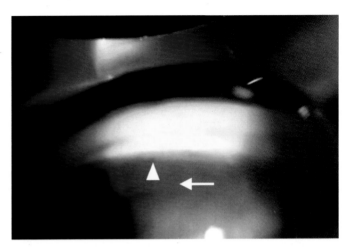

Fig. 9.1: Indentation gonioscopy in an eye with plateau iris shows the "sine wave sign"(←) and a goniosynechia in the angle (◀)

drape over the lens on indentation. Thus, the iris contour follows that of the lens, reaches its deepest point just peripheral to the lens and then rises upward again over the ciliary processes. This is known as the "sine wave sign" or the "double hump sign" (Fig. 9.1).

Controversies in Definition

Unfortunately, there is still considerable confusion regarding the terminology of PACG. The lack of an established nomenclature for classification and the mechanism of angle-closure glaucoma create confusion in diagnosing and treating these patients. The existing classification systems are full of misnomers.

Chronic Angle-Closure Glaucoma

The very entity "chronic angle-closure glaucoma" is associated with a lot of confusion. According to Shields, peripheral anterior synechiae and chronic elevation of intraocular pressure characterize chronic angle-closure glaucoma. According to Lowe and Ritch, chronic angle-closure is defined as an eye with any degree of peripheral anterior synechiae to the level of the trabecular meshwork resulting from a pupillary block mechanism irrespective of whether or not the intraocular pressure is elevated. Salmon and associates define chronic angle-closure glaucoma as intraocular pressure of more than 21 mm Hg or glaucomatous visual field loss in the presence of an occludable angle in an asymptomatic individual.

At the meeting Worldwide Glaucoma 2000, the following classification of angle-closure has been proposed:

1. Those with bilaterally narrow angles on gonioscopy, i.e. 270° or more of the angle with no view of the pigmented meshwork are called narrow angles.
2. Those with narrow angles, who in addition have intraocular pressure of more than 97.5 percentile for their population or who have peripheral anterior synechiae or who have signs of past attack by slit-lamp, but without any field loss are called primary angle closure.

3. Those with primary angle-closure with field defect and compatible disc changes are called primary angle-closure glaucoma.

Combined Mechanism versus Mixed Mechanism

Combined mechanism glaucoma refers to situations in which both open-angle and angle-closure components are present. The most common example is angle-closure glaucoma following laser iridotomy with persistently high intraocular pressures without the presence of peripheral anterior synechiae. Another common example is pseudoexfoliation syndrome with angle-closure glaucoma, which is successfully treated with laser iridotomy, but develops open-angle glaucoma later. However, in these cases, it is very difficult to assess the cause of reduction in outflow—whether it is primary or as result of past intermittent angle closure.

In mixed mechanism glaucoma, the rise in intraocular pressure is due to some element of pupillary block contributing to eyes with lens related glaucoma, malignant glaucoma or plateau iris. Mixed mechanism glaucoma or multi-mechanism glaucoma is especially common in China where approximately half of chronic angle-closure glaucoma cases may be caused by a variety of mechanisms.

Creeping Angle-Closure Glaucoma

Creeping angle-closure glaucoma is a variant of chronic angle-closure glaucoma. It is uncommon in whites, but much more prevalent in the Asians. The peripheral iris attaches first to the angle recess and then the peripheral anterior synechiae extend towards the Schwalbe's line. The closure gradually extends circumferentially so that over a period of time, the iris insertion becomes more and more anterior. The gradual shortening of the angle may either cause an acute attack to supervene or chronic elevation of intraocular pressure with glaucomatous disc and field changes.

The underlying mechanism for creeping angle-closure among the Asians and the Blacks is not clear. The thickness and rigidity of the iris have been postulated as possible mechanisms. The iris is reported to be inserted more anteriorly to the scleral wall in the Asians as compared to the Blacks and the Caucasians. These factors could predispose such eyes to develop peripheral anterior synechiae. According to West, a mechanism other than pupillary block may play a role as 9 of 30 eyes with creeping angle-closure glaucoma patients developed extension of peripheral anterior synechiae even after iridotomy. In plateau iris, the root as well as the mid-peripheral portion of the iris is redundant and thrown into folds, which can cause creeping of the redundant iris into the angle recess and towards the Schwalbe's line.

Clinical Presentation of Angle-Closure Glaucoma

Angle-closure glaucoma can present as an entire spectrum ranging from intermittent closure to the absolute stage. The onset and course of the disease is usually episodic and there is often an overlap in clinical presentation. For instance, repeated attacks of intermittent angle-closure may lead to progressive peripheral synechiae formation and eventually chronic angle-closure or may suddenly convert into an acute attack. Acute angle-closure may develop in the patients of chronic angle-closure glaucoma. Conversely, in patients with acute angle-closure, chronic PACG can develop soon after the resolution of the acute episode. The mode of presentation depends on the percentage of the filtering meshwork occluded, the suddenness of closure and the ease of reversal of the irido-trabecular block. Following are some examples of the mode of presentation of angle-closure glaucoma:

1. A 42-year-old lady was referred as a case of migraine because of complaints of frequent attacks of dull ache in and around the left eye and mild blurring of vision of 6 months duration. On further questioning, there was history of intermittent haloes around lights and relief of symptoms after sleeping for 2–3 hours. Her mother was a known patient of glaucoma and had undergone laser peripheral iridotomy in both eyes. Examination revealed best-corrected vision of 20/20, N6 in both eyes. The intraocular pressure by Goldmann applanation tonometry was 16 mm Hg in both eyes. Anterior chamber depth by Van Herick's test was grade 2 in both eyes. Rest of the anterior segment examination was unremarkable. On gonioscopy with a Sussman lens, pigmented trabecular meshwork could be visualized in only the temporal quadrant of the angle. On indentation, the angle opened up to the scleral spur. There were no peripheral anterior synechiae. However, an area of splotchy pigmentation was present in the inferior angle of the left eye along with an adjacent iris process (Fig. 9.2). Ultrasound biomicroscopy examination revealed narrow entry to the angle with posteriorly directed ciliary processes indicating pupillary block. A diagnosis of intermittent angle-closure was made. Laser iridotomy was done in both eyes. Following the iridotomy, the angle opened up to the scleral spur throughout its circumference. Dilated

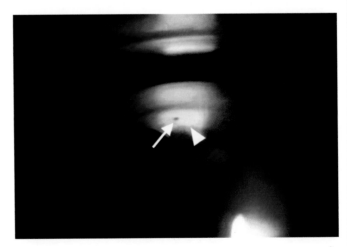

Fig. 9.2: Gonio-photograph shows peripheral blotch of pigment (↑), indicating past angle-closure. An iris process also is seen (◀) next to the pigment

fundus examination following the iridotomy revealed 0.3 cupping with healthy neuroretinal rim in both eyes. She has remained free of symptoms and the intraocular pressures have been normal.

The above case provides an example of how intermittent angle-closure can present with minimal or no signs and symptoms. A high index of clinical suspicion is necessary as symptoms of angle-closure can be mistaken for migraine. A careful gonioscopy without stimulating the pupillary reflex can clinch the diagnosis in such cases.

2. A 38-year-old lady came to the emergency service with complaint of nausea, severe headache and eye ache in her right eye for three days. She gave history of having had previous episodes of discomfort in her right eye off and on for one year. On examination, her vision was 20/100 in the right eye and 20/20 in the left eye. Intraocular pressure by Goldmann applanation tonometry was 42 mm Hg in the right eye and 18 mm Hg in the left eye. She had mild lid edema in the right eye, circumciliary congestion, moderate stromal corneal edema, shallow anterior chamber, dilated and fixed pupil, coagulum in the pupillary area and small white opacities in the anterior subcapsular region of the lens (Fig. 9.3). Examination of the left eye was within normal limits but for limbal anterior chamber depth by Van Herick's test of grade 1. On gonioscopy, details could not be visualized in the right eye owing to corneal edema. The left eye anterior chamber angle was open up to Schwalbe's line in the superior, nasal and temporal quadrants. The inferior quadrant was open up to the scleral spur. She was treated with intravenous injection of 20% mannitol tab., acetazolamide orally and timolol 0.5% eye drops in the right eye. Three days later, her intraocular pressure had reduced to 24 mm Hg in the right eye. The anterior chamber reaction had also reduced and she was subjectively more comfortable. Laser iridotomy was done in both eyes a week later. On gonioscopy, there were multiple goniosynechiae throughout

the angle in the right eye. The left eye angle had opened up to scleral spur in all the quadrants. Examination of the disc showed 0.3 cupping in both eyes. However, there was significant pallor of the disc in the right eye. She is being followed up at regular intervals and her intraocular pressure is under control in the right eye with timolol maleate 0.5% eye drops.

An acute attack of angle-closure glaucoma can sometimes be present with severe anterior chamber reaction and mimic acute iridocyclitis. However, the pupil will be usually constricted in acute iridocyclitis. If it is primary acute angle-closure glaucoma, the angle will be closed. In all cases of acute angle-closure glaucoma, a laser iridotomy should definitely be tried first as soon as the intraocular pressure is under control. Following the iridotomy, gonioscopy should be repeated to determine the status of the angle and the extent of peripheral anterior synechiae. Even if the intraocular pressure is elevated following the iridotomy, it may be due to the liberation of pigment in an already inflamed eye. It is advisable to treat these eyes medically till they become quiet before deciding on filtration surgery.

3. A 58-year-old lady came for a change of glasses. She had no other complaints. Her best-corrected visual acuity was 20/20, N6 in both eyes. Her intraocular pressure by Goldmann applanation tonometry was 26 mm Hg in the right eye and 28 mm Hg in the left eye. Anterior segment examination of both eyes was unremarkable except for grade 2 anterior chamber depths by Van Herick's method and 2 clock hours of sphincter atrophy in the right eye (Fig. 9.4). On gonioscopy, the angles were closed up to the Schwalbe's line and there were multiple goniosynechiae in the inferior and nasal angles on indentation (Fig. 9.5). A diagnosis of chronic angle-closure glaucoma was made and laser iridotomy was done in both eyes. She was started on timolol maleate 0.5% eye drops. A week later, her intraocular pressure was 18 mm Hg in both eyes. On gonioscopy,

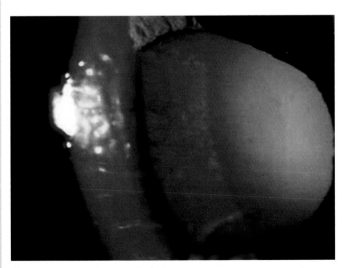

Fig. 9.3: Slit-lamp photograph showing glaucoma flecken in acute angle-closure glaucoma

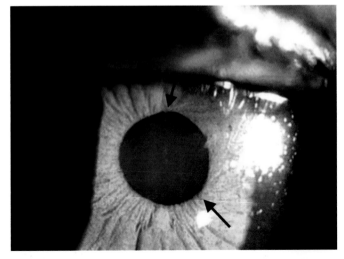

Fig. 9.4: Slit-lamp photograph showing sphincter atrophy form 12 to 5 o'clock position

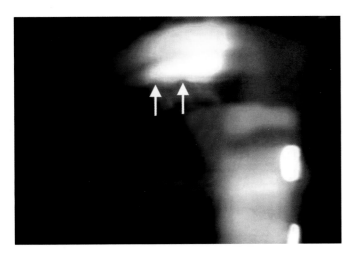

Fig. 9.5: Indentation gonioscopy showing a goniosynechia
in the inferior angle

the angle had opened till posterior trabecular meshwork in between areas of goniosynechiae. There was no appositional closure. Dilated fundus examination revealed 0.8 cupping with an inferior notch in the right eye and 0.7 cupping with thinning and pallor of the inferior rim in the left eye. Humphrey visual field examination showed a superior arcuate scotoma in the right eye and a superior nasal step in the left eye. She is being followed up at regular intervals. Her intraocular pressure is under control and fields are stable on timolol maleate 0.5% eye drops.

Silent chronic angle-closure glaucoma can present with relatively deep anterior chamber and disc cupping and be very easily mistaken for open-angle glaucoma unless a careful gonioscopy is done. Indentation gonioscopy is very important to determine the presence and extent of peripheral anterior synechiae. A laser iridotomy is indicated in all cases followed by a post-laser gonioscopy to determine the extent of opening of the angle by the iridotomy. A large number of these cases remain stable on medical treatment. If filtration surgery is required, certain special considerations are required.

4. A 55-year-old lady came in 1992 with the complaint of gradual diminution of vision in the right eye for six years. She was diagnosed as a case of glaucoma elsewhere and was on pilocarpine therapy at the time of presentation. On examination, she had a vision of inaccurate projection of light in the right eye and 20/20 (6/6), N6 in the left eye. Her intraocular pressures were 54 mm Hg and 16 mm Hg in the right and left eye respectively. Anterior segment examination of the left eye was unremarkable. In the right eye, she had moderate epithelial and stromal edema of the cornea, semi-dilated and fixed pupil with early rubeosis of the iris. Gonioscopy revealed 360° synechial closure of the angle in the right eye and an open angle with a narrow entry that revealed few scattered goniosynechiae in the left eye on indentation gonioscopy. Based on the above findings, a diagnosis of chronic angle-closure glaucoma in both

eyes with absolute stage in the right eye was made. Laser iridotomy was done in both eyes. Dilated fundus examination revealed total cupping in the right eye and 0.2 cupping with healthy neuroretinal rim in the left eye. She was called for follow-up after 3 months. However, she was lost to follow-up. She presented seven years later with the complaint of gradual blurring of vision in the left eye of two years duration. On examination, her vision was no perception of light in the right eye and 20/80, N8 in the left eye. The intraocular pressure was 10 and 43 mm Hg in the right and left eye respectively. The peripheral iridotomy was patent in both eyes. Gonioscopy revealed 360° synechial closure on indentation. She was advised to use tab. acetazolamide 250 mg tid, timolol maleate 0.5% eye drops bid and pilocarpine nitrate 2% eye drops tid in the left eye. When seen 2 days later, her intraocular pressure had reduced to 9 and 14 mm Hg in the right and left eye respectively. Dilated fundus examination revealed total cupping in the right eye and a bipolar notch in the left eye. Humphrey visual field examination of the left eye showed biarcuate scotoma. On ultrasound biomicroscopy, the angle was closed and the ciliary processes were directed anteriorly. A diagnosis of plateau iris syndrome was made. She is under regular follow-up now and is stable with pilocarpine and timolol eye drops.

5. A 33-year-old lady was referred for management of flat anterior chamber in the left eye following trabeculectomy done elsewhere 11 days ago. On examination, she had wound leak with total cataract, hypotony and choroidal detachment in the left eye. She was managed conservatively with bandage contact lens. We shall be discussing only the right eye since it is more relevant to the discussion here. Her best corrected vision in the right eye was 20/20, N6. Intraocular pressure by Goldmann applanation tonometry was 14 mm Hg. Anterior segment examination was within normal limits except for grade 2 anterior chamber depth by Van Herick's method. On gonioscopy, the angle was open, but with a narrow entry. In view of the occludable angle, laser iridotomy was done in the right eye. Post-laser gonioscopy showed appositional closure (Fig. 9.6A) with opening of the angle to the level of posterior trabecular meshwork on indentation (Fig. 9.6B). Dilated fundus examination showed 0.4 cupping with healthy neuroretinal rim. Her post dilatation intraocular pressure remained under 18 mm Hg on all visits. Humphrey visual field examination was within normal limits. Based on the above findings, a diagnosis of incomplete plateau iris syndrome was made. She has been on follow-up on a regular basis for six years. Her intraocular pressure and fields are stable without any treatment. Periodic gonioscopy at 6-month intervals did not reveal any goniosynechiae.

6. A 54-year-old gentleman came for a regular check up. His best-corrected visual acuity was 20/20, N6 in both eyes. Intraocular pressure was 26 and 28 mm Hg in the right and left eye respectively. Anterior segment examination was

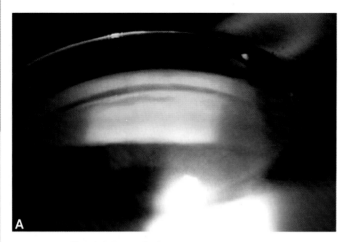 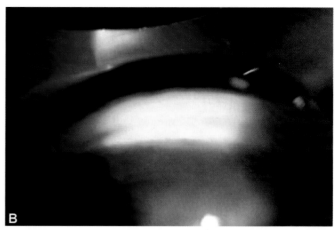

Figs 9.6 A and B: Gonioscopy without (A) and with indentation (B) showing narrow angle that opens following indentation

unremarkable except for Van Herick's grade 2 peripheral anterior chamber depth. On gonioscopy, the angles were open in both eyes, but with narrow entry. He was diagnosed as a case of subacute angle-closure glaucoma. Laser peripheral iridotomy was done in both eyes. Post-laser gonioscopy showed appositional closure in both eyes. Disc examination revealed 0.1 cupping in both eyes. There was a rise in post-dilatation intraocular pressure by 2 mm Hg in the right eye and 5 mm Hg in the left eye. Ultrasound biomicroscopy examination showed narrow angles throughout the circumference of the angle in both eyes with anteriorly directed ciliary processes. The diagnosis was revised as incomplete plateau iris syndrome. He was followed up at regular intervals. His intraocular pressure remained under control in both eyes with pilocarpine nitrate 2% eye drops at bedtime. Gonioscopy was repeated a year later. At this time, the angles were open to the level of anterior trabecular meshwork, opening up to the posterior trabecular meshwork on indentation. There were multiple goniosynechiae in the superior angles in both eyes. Hence a decision to perform iridoplasty was taken. Following the iridoplasty, the angles have opened to the level of the posterior trabecular meshwork and the intraocular pressure is under control.

The above cases demonstrate the varied spectrum in which plateau iris can present. Post-laser gonioscopy with indentation is absolutely essential in all cases of angle-closure glaucoma. It is important to rule out appositional closure following the iridotomy because in cases of primary pupillary block treated by iridotomy, there is no possible reason for appositional closure. If appositional closure persists after an iridotomy, plateau iris has to be ruled out. Undiagnosed cases of plateau iris can cause creeping angle-closure as was seen in the first example. Since these cases can develop peripheral anterior synechiae even after iridotomy, periodic gonioscopy to look for new peripheral anterior synechiae is a must. Iridoplasty can help in preventing progressive angle closure, especially if weak miotic therapy is not helpful.

MANAGEMENT OF ANGLE-CLOSURE GLAUCOMAS

The management of angle-closure glaucoma depends on the cause, type and duration of angle closure, the intraocular pressure control and the associated disc damage.

Medical Treatment

Medical treatment in angle-closure glaucomas is limited to the control of intraocular pressure before definitive laser or surgical treatment and to control of residual uncontrolled intraocular pressure following laser or surgery. Increasing the outflow or decreasing the inflow may decrease the pressure. Drugs, which can be used to decrease the inflow are beta-blockers, alpha-2 agonists and carbonic anhydrase inhibitors. The drugs, which act by increasing the aqueous outflow either through the conventional route or through the uveoscleral outflow, comprise of miotics, adrenergics and prostaglandin analogs. Hyperosmotic agents act by dehydrating the vitreous and may also have a central mechanism of action. These medications are very useful in the management of high intraocular pressure in acute or chronic glaucoma.

Beta-blockers are commonly used in the long-term therapy of chronic angle-closure glaucoma. Since they can be associated with serious and even life-threatening complications, it is very important to rule out asthma, cardiac arrhythmia and congestive heart failure in these patients.

Brimonidine is an alpha 2 agonist, which can be used for the treatment of residual glaucoma following laser or surgery. However, it is important to keep in mind that it can cross the blood-brain-barrier and cause sedation, headache and disorientation in some patients.

Pilocarpine has been routinely used for the management of acute angle-closure glaucoma attacks. It acts by causing mechanical traction on the scleral spur by the ciliary muscle contraction and opens the trabecular meshwork. It also relieves the pupillary block by causing miosis. However, in certain situations, it may actually increase the pupillary block by causing release of zonular tension and forward movement of the crystalline lens. It is important to perform gonioscopy on all patients off pilocarpine as it can cause artifactual narrowing of the angle.

Adrenergic agents should be avoided as they cause pupillary dilatation and can cause precipitation of an attack of angle-closure glaucoma even after peripheral iridotomy in cases of plateau iris syndrome.

Dorzolamide, a topical carbonic anhydrase inhibitor and Latanoprost, a prostaglandin analog can also be used to control the intraocular pressure following laser treatment or filtration surgery.

Laser Treatment

Laser iridotomy

Laser peripheral iridotomy is the definitive treatment for all forms of angle-closure in which pupillary block is the underlying mechanism either totally or in part. It is safe and effective. All the complications of intraocular surgery are avoided with the added advantage that the conjunctiva is left untouched in case filtration surgery is required in the future. The indications of laser iridotomy are:

- Eyes with angle-closure glaucoma
- Fellow eyes
- Chronic angle closure
- Occludable angles especially if frequent pupillary dilatation is required.
- Aphakic/pseudophakic pupillary block
- Nanophthalmos
- Suspected malignant glaucoma

Complications are few and minor consisting of bleeding from the iridotomy site, an acute transient rise of intraocular pressure and mild iritis.

Laser iridotomy is contraindicated in:

- Flat anterior chamber
- Corneal edema
- Closed angle caused by primary synechial closure as in iridocorneal endothelial syndrome, neovascular glaucoma and uveitis in which pupillary block is not the underlying mechanism.

Though iridotomy can be performed with argon laser, Nd:YAG in the pulsed mode is preferable as it is easier to achieve a full thickness iridotomy, which is less likely to close as compared to the iridotomy by argon laser. Nd:YAG laser in the pulsed mode is a photo-disruptive laser, which acts by creating plasma of free ions and electrons at the site of optical breakdown, which results in the release of shock waves that mechanically cause tissue rupture. Use of 2% pilocarpine nitrate eye drops at 10-minute intervals for half an hour before the procedure, stretches and thins the iris making penetration easier. The Nd:YAG laser is generally used at 1–4 pulses/ burst and 1–10 mj per burst. It is best to place the iridotomy anywhere between 11 and 1 o'clock, about three-fourths of the distance between the pupil and the root of the iris, at the base

of an iris crypt. Placing the iridotomy at the periphery allows it to clear the equator and thereby relieve the pupillary block. It is best to begin with a single pulse of 3–4 mj. He-Ne laser is used to impart red color to the aiming beams, as Nd:YAG laser is invisible. The aiming beams are joined to form a single spot when the laser beam is focussed on the surface of the iris. It is important to see that the laser is delivered perpendicular to the surface of the lens. If the spots cannot be brought together, it is due to malposition of the lens, which should be moved slightly to join the beams. Improper focus can also occur due to flexing of the neck by the patient in an attempt to look down. Moving it towards the patient so that the beams separate minimally then defocuses the laser slightly posteriorly. This technique focuses the laser below the surface of the iris allowing maximal use of the shock wave. The patient should be evaluated an hour after the iridotomy to determine the patency and measure the intraocular pressure. Depending on the intraocular pressure, the severity of disc damage, treatment with topical steroids and antiglaucoma medication is given. A week later pre- and post-dilatation intraocular pressure measurement and gonioscopy should be done to rule out plateau iris.

Argon Laser Peripheral Iridoplasty

Argon laser peripheral iridoplasty serves to open appositionally closed angles in situations in which peripheral iridotomy is ineffective in eliminating appositional closure due to underlying mechanisms being other than pupillary block. It consists of placing a ring of contraction burns of long duration, low power and large spot size in the extreme periphery of the iris so as to contract the iris stroma between the angle and the site of the burn thereby opening the angle. The basis of the modern technique of argon laser peripheral iridoplasty was given by Kimbrough and associates. Continued appositional closure in the presence of a patent peripheral iridotomy suggests plateau iris. In all such patients with a patent iridotomy and angle-closure with raised intraocular pressure, it is very important to determine if the angle is narrow, appositionally closed or closed by peripheral anterior synechiae. It's only in cases with a patent iridotomy and appositionally closed angles that iridoplasty is indicated. If the angle is closed due to peripheral anterior synechiae, then there is not sufficient functional angle to keep the intraocular pressure under control. If the intraocular pressure is elevated, but if there is no true functional closure and the access simply looks narrow, then the angle is basically functionally open. Iridoplasty in these cases provides more insult to the angle due to release of pigment and inflammation. So a thorough knowledge of indentation gonioscopy is essential to differentiate the indications from the contraindications of iridoplasty.

Pretreatment with pilocarpine stretches and thins the iris. The laser parameters that are used are: 500 μm spot size, 0.5 sec duration and 200–400 mW power. It is better to start with 200 mW for dark irides and 300 mW for lighter ones and then adjusts the power as necessary to obtain visible stromal contraction. The power should be reduced in case of bubble formation or release of pigment into the anterior chamber. Usually 24–36 spots are given all over the circumference of the angle leaving approximately 2 spot diameter between each spot. Contraction burns are placed perpendicular to the most peripheral portion of the iris through Abraham lens or angled mirrors of Goldmann or Ritch lens. The most common complications that are encountered with the procedure are mild iritis and a transient increase in intraocular pressure. Retreatment may be required in some cases although there have been no long-term prospective studies to determine the success and retreatment rate of iridoplasty.

Filtration Surgery

Filtration surgery in angle-closure glaucoma is usually required for uncontrolled intraocular pressure or progressive glaucomatous optic nerve cupping and visual field loss. A few important points to consider in the filtration surgery are:

- Malignant glaucoma is a definitive possibility and should be kept in mind.
- Preoperative intraocular pressure should be reduced if necessary with IV mannitol to minimize the risk of expulsive hemorrhage.
- Preferably, pilocarpine should be substituted with other topical or systemic agents in order to reduce the postoperative inflammation.
- It is desirable to discontinue aspirin, aspirin containing compounds and nonsteroidal anti-inflammatory drugs 3–6 weeks before surgery to reduce excessive intraoperative bleeding.
- In eyes with previous intraocular surgery, it is important to plan the site of surgery and evaluate conjunctival mobility.
- Paracentesis is especially important in spherophakia and in pseudophakic eyes where flat/shallow anterior chamber postoperatively would be hazardous. It allows reformation of the anterior chamber, to confirm patency of the sclerectomy, adequate closure of the scleral flap and absence of conjunctival wound leaks.
- The scleral flap should be dissected relatively anteriorly to ensure that the entry site of the sclerostomy is anterior to the scleral spur and the ciliary body.
- The scleral flap should completely cover the sclerostomy. An overlap of 1 mm on either side of the sclerostomy opening is recommended.
- The peripheral iridectomy should be wide enough at the base to prevent obstruction of the sclerostomy. One is usually able to see the ciliary processes after the iridectomy.
- Use of cycloplegics intraoperatively after completion of scleral flap closure helps to reduce the chances of flat/shallow anterior chamber postoperatively.
- It is very important to continue the treatment and monitor the fellow eye following surgery. It is not uncommon to see the fellow eye develop acute angle-closure glaucoma attack while all concentration is on the operated eye. It is also important to monitor the intraocular pressure in order to detect steroid-induced response due to drug crossover in the fellow eye.

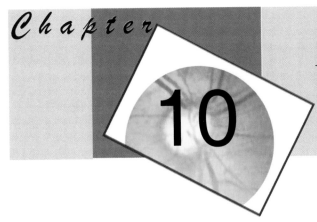

Chapter 10

Primary Open-Angle Glaucoma

M Baskaran, Arun Narayanaswamy, Lingam Vijaya

INTRODUCTION

Primary open-angle glaucoma (POAG) has been reported to be a predominant of glaucoma according to various epidemiological studies conducted so far. The burden of glaucoma is being estimated to be approximately 60.5 million by 2010 and 44.7 million are likely to have POAG. Table 10.1 summarizes important studies depicting the prevalence of POAG world wide. The estimated prevalence of glaucoma in India is 11.9 million. Recent studies in India have reported the age standardized prevalence of POAG to be 3.46% in the urban population and 1.58% in the rural population. Increasing age was reported to be a consistent risk factor. The reasons for differences between urban and rural populations is not clear, but could be possibly related to environmental and lifestyle patterns.

In this context, an ophthalmologist should be well versed with the varied risk factors, examination techniques and management options in such a blinding disease. The aim of this chapter is to give an overview on the clinical methods and management aspects in dealing with POAG and also the pitfalls in these methods.

DIAGNOSIS

Primary Open-Angle Glaucoma

Primary open-angle glaucoma, as defined by the American Academy of Ophthalmology (2005), is a chronic, generally bilateral and often asymmetrical disease, which is characterized (in at least one eye) by all of the following:
- Evidence of glaucomatous optic nerve damage from either or both the appearance of the disc or retinal nerve fiber layer or the presence of characteristic abnormalities in the visual field.
- Adult onset.
- Open, normal appearing anterior chamber angles.
- Absence of known other (secondary) causes of open-angle glaucoma (in which intraocular pressure (IOP) is usually raised and identified as a major risk factor).

The South East Asia Glaucoma Interest Group (SEAGIG) guidelines (2008) use the following criteria to define POAG:
- Chronic progressive optic neuropathy.
- Typical glaucomatous changes in optic nerve.

Table 10.1: Comparison of prevalence of primary open-angle glaucoma in various populations

Source (Period)	Ethnic group	Age range	Prevalence (per 100)
Framingham (1980)	White Americans	52–86	2.20
Beaver Dam (1991)	White Americans	43–84	2.10
Baltimore (1991)	White Americans	40 and older	1.29
Baltimore (1991)	Black Americans	40 and older	4.74
Blue Mountains (1992-1994)	White Australians	49–97	2.4
Barbados (1994)	Black Barbadians	40–84	7.00
Rotterdam (1994)	White Dutch	55 and older	1.10
Mongolia (1995)	Asians	40 and older	0.50
ACES (1997)	Indians	40 and older	1.7
APEDS (1997)	Indians	All ages	2.56
CGS (2003)	Indians (Rural)	40 and older	1.62
CGS (2003)	Indians (Urban)	40 and older	3.51

- Typical visual field defect may or may not be present.
- Open angle.
- Absence of secondary cause.

It is important to note that the focus of defining glaucoma is predominantly related to the pathological changes in the optic nerve head and IOP is only a risk factor and may not always be elevated in initial examination. This emphasizes the need for a careful comprehensive examination of every patient to rule out the presence of glaucoma.

Ocular Hypertension

Ocular hypertension vs. primary open-angle glaucoma: As many as 10% patients over age 40 are found to have IOP more than 21 mm Hg. Ocular hypertension (OHT) is a condition in which the following criteria is present:

- An intraocular pressure greater than 21 mm Hg in one or both eyes as measured by applanation tonometry on 2 or more occasions.
- No glaucomatous defects on visual field testing.
- Normal appearance of the optic disc and nerve fiber layer.
- Open angles on gonioscopy.
- Absence of any ocular disease contributing to the elevation of pressure.

All patients with elevated IOP alone need not be treated since long term studies have proved that only 1% among those group of patients between 21 and 30 mm Hg develop visual field damage each year. The ocular hypertension treatment study (OHTS) was designed to evaluate efficacy of lowering IOP in individuals with who met the criteria listed above. It was a multicenter, prospective and randomized clinical trial where in patients were randomly assigned to close observation versus treatment with topical medication to lower IOP by 20% from baseline. The major findings of the study were as follows:

- Lowering IOP by 20% reduced the incidence of glaucoma end points (confirmed by visual field defects or optic nerve changes).
- Baseline characteristics predictive of increased risk of glaucoma included higher IOP, older subjects, increased cup-to-disc ratio and lower central corneal thickness.
- Individuals with thinner corneas were at greater risk of converting to POAG. The study recommended that central corneal thickness (CCT) be measured in patients with ocular hypertension to assess risk better.
- A patient with OHT is assessed for risk characteristics mentioned above before instituting therapy. The amount of IOP lowering is generally less aggressive than in treating an established glaucoma patient with masterly follow-up.

ETIOPATHOGENESIS

In essence, scientists have till now not understood the definite etiology of glaucoma. Current research and clinical data only lead to a gray path possibly towards the various mechanisms of the elevated intraocular pressure and the changes that occur in

the trabecular meshwork and optic nerve due to glaucoma. The molecular (neuroprotection concepts), racial and genetic level understanding has given new dimensions to the etiopathogenesis, but cannot account for all the clinical situations. From the above discussion, it may be clear that primary open-angle glaucoma is possibly a multifactorial disorder with factors having variable involvement. The factors may influence the patient's condition at different time intervals in his/her life (e.g. genetic mutation and aging are factors with varying chronological involvement), which makes it even more difficult to unravel the mystery of this disease.

Causes of Elevated Intraocular Pressure

Most of the findings are related to accelerated and exaggerated aging changes, which occur in the Schlemm's canal, uveoscleral pathways, trabecular meshwork and juxtacanalicular tissue. The changes are summarized as:

- Loss of trabecular endothelial cells–there is increase of abnormal lattice collagen in the trabeculae with swelling and lamination of the basement membrane.
- Pigment accumulation within the trabecular endothelial cells–source of it is from the pigmented epithelial cells of the ciliary body and iris.
- Thickening and fusion of trabecular lamellae.
- Thickening of the scleral spur–occurs as a result of hyalinization and/or atrophy of the ciliary muscle along with collapse and condensation of the uveal trabecular meshwork.
- Increase in extracellular (plaque) material in the juxtacanalicular zone.
- Loss of ability to form giant vacuoles along the inner wall of Schlemm's canal.
- Proliferation of endothelial cells into the lumen of the Schlemm's canal.
- Aqueous humor from glaucomatous eyes may have an increasing level of transforming growth factor β_2 (TGF β_2), which promotes deposition of components of the extracellular matrix.
- Glaucoma subjects have decreased collagenase activity compared to controls.
- Alpha-crystalline from the lens cells can obstruct the trabecular meshwork.

Changes in the Optic Nerve Head

Abnormal levels of IOP can eventually cause compression of the scleral laminar sheets and distortion of laminar pores. There is evidence that during remodeling of the optic nerve, extracellular matrix degenerative changes occur with the activation of astrocytes. Backward displacement of the laminar sheets leads to excavation of the optic nerve. All these changes can mechanically compress the ganglion cell axons and the capillaries. This leads to blockage of axonal transport, which over time leads to apoptotic ganglion cell death. This cell death leads to the further loss of tissue and enhanced cup. The scleral lamellae are believed to be weaker in the superior pole of the optic nerve, which makes it vulnerable for early damage. There is also evidence to suggest the loss of elastin and presence of abnormal connective tissue, which leads to easier susceptibility in certain individuals. Some or most of the above factors could be genetically predetermined, the presence of which may determine the preponderance of nerve fiber IOP.

Mechanical and Vascular Theories

Mechanical theory suggests that IOP can have direct effect on the optic nerve to cause the damage. The fact that normal tension glaucoma and IOP at lower ranges cause optic nerve damage cannot be explained by this theory alone. The vascular theory is based on the concept that the autoregulation to the retinal and optic nerve head is hampered so that there is ischemia to the axons, which are rendered nonfunctional. The evidence for this comes from the presence of normal tension glaucoma; risk factors such as diabetes, anemia and migraine; ischemic patterns seen in fluorescein angiograms; peripapillary atrophy suggesting circumpapillary choroidal ischemia and reduced ocular blood flow compared to normal subjects as demonstrated with ocular blood flow measurements. However appealing the vascular theory is, there is no direct evidence to prove this beyond doubt. Flow chart 10.1 gives a diagrammatic

Flow chart 10.1: Possible mechanisms and interventions in primary open-angle glaucoma

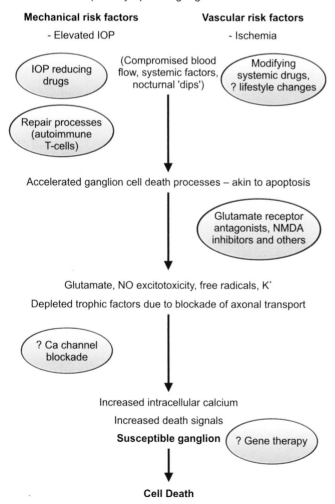

representation of theories involved in glaucoma and possible therapeutic interventions.

Genetics and Glaucoma

Roughly 25 to 50% of POAG patients have a positive family history of glaucoma. The pedigree structure of majority of families used in genetic linkage analysis suggests autosomal dominance with reduced penetrance. A family history of POAG is a high-risk factor for developing the disease. The incidence of open-angle glaucoma in first-degree relatives with the disease has been reported to be five times greater than that in the general population. The mapped genes are located so far as–2cen-q13, 3q21-q24, 8q23, 10p15-p14 and 7q35-q36. The locations have been named GLC1B, GLC1C, GLC1D, GLC1E and GLC1F respectively. The trabecular meshwork inducible glucocorticoid response (TIGR) protein gene mutations are linked to the corticosteroid response gene and the link to POAG is uncertain. However the first set of mutations were found in a family of juvenile open-angle glaucoma among Afro-American patients to a 3-cM region associated with 1q23-25 named GLC1A. There is another mutation found in the myocilin (MYOC) gene located identically with the TIGR gene. While TIGR protein is located in the TM and the ciliary body, the myocilin protein is located in the photoreceptors of the retina. It is found that 8% of the juvenile glaucoma pedigrees have mutations in the TIGR/MYOC gene.

Autoimmunity–Does it have a role?

Various studies with rhodopsin antibodies and molecular mimicry, heat shock protein 60, glycosaminoglycans (GAG) autoantibodies and HLA associations have shown evidence for a possible autoimmune neuropathy as one of the etiological factors in the pathogenesis of glaucoma. However this is more common in patients with normal tension glaucoma than primary open-angle glaucoma.

APPROACH TO DIAGNOSIS AND TREATMENT OF PRIMARY OPEN-ANGLE GLAUCOMA

Even though there are simple guidelines to diagnosis, such as elevated IOP, open angles and visual field defects, very often we come across patients for whom reaching a conclusion becomes difficult. The reason being, the variability of presentations and the relative ambiguity in the diagnostic procedures available. Besides all, elevated IOP subjects are not to be considered glaucoma patients and all normal visual field patients are not normal subjects. Early diagnosis in glaucoma being the most important factor in the treatment of this blinding disorder, the clinician must know the finer elements of proper and accurate diagnostic approach. Unfortunately, we do not have a single authentic clinical tool to diagnose glaucoma. However much is the pathogenesis complex, so is the investigative approach. We need to put in a lot of clinical information with adequate history to come to a conclusion. The risk factors in the history and clinical examination serve a major purpose in this regard.

Risk Factors

Before discussing the signs of the disease, the risk factors in favor of glaucoma development are as follows: Advanced age, black race and positive family history. Previously considered risk factors, such as high or low blood pressure and diabetes mellitus have been questioned in recent studies.

Other ocular risk factors could be steroid response, elevated IOP, large physiological cups, high myopia, glaucoma in one eye and retinal vein occlusions. As we have seen in the pathogenesis, the development of glaucoma is closely related to advanced age. While patients above 35–40 years of age are advised routine screening for glaucoma, the risk of POAG is increased in patients above 60 years of age.

Elevated IOP as a Risk Factor

IOP elevation more than 21 mm Hg along with short- and long-term fluctuation and asymmetric IOP recordings more than 4 mm Hg between two eyes is the most important risk factor for glaucoma. Diurnal variations more than 6 mm Hg should raise suspicion of glaucoma. Glaucoma subjects show a diurnal fluctuation of 10 to 15 mm Hg. Steroid responders have a tendency to develop glaucoma and this response is mostly genetically determined. Myopes and diabetic patients were found to have steroid response more than normal. Seven percent of the large cups have a risk of developing glaucoma over long-term follow-up. Retinal vein occlusions need careful follow-up and baseline visual fields will go a long way in fine-tuning the early diagnosis.

History

A positive family history should be sought for and it has to be re-evaluated in subsequent visits when the patient has more information in this regard. The type of glaucoma, response to drugs and surgical outcome in relatives should be documented. Previous steroid response, trauma, history of intermittent or subacute attacks of angle-closure, systemic illnesses especially cardiac and respiratory illnesses and medications should be enquired in detail.

History on previous IOP readings both baseline and maximum IOP, visual field reports, and response to medications and allergic reactions have to be sought for in possible situations. Previous medications with concentration of drugs, last application, compliance and tolerance of the patient to drugs have to be asked for and documented. The extent to which the patient is affected by the disease, whether he/she is able to work in his present job with existing vision, reading and writing capabilities– all form part of evaluation of the patient's quality of life which need to be thoroughly evaluated.

Symptoms

Primary open-angle glaucoma is an asymptomatic disease till the late stages. Very rarely, patients complain of loss of peripheral vision and subsequently loss of central vision also.

Signs

The hallmark signs of POAG are glaucomatous disc changes with associated visual field loss. For diagnostic purposes, POAG patients should have IOP above 21 mm Hg on diurnal phasing and open angles with a normal appearing trabecular meshwork on gonioscopy. POAG can present asymmetrically, but almost always bilateral.

While the above three parameters can be individually not confirmative of glaucoma, a correlation of all the factors will yield a good positive prediction. The most debated yet most useful of them is the IOP measurement, which is as of now the only treatable parameter in glaucoma. In this part we will discuss the methods used with their advantages in brief and the controversies related to IOP as a tool in diagnosis.

Clinical Examinations

Intraocular Pressure Assessment

When the initial population-based studies concluded that IOP more than 21 mm Hg by applanation tonometry is seen in less than 5% of the normal population, it was interpreted as all patients above that level of IOP may have glaucoma, which confused the interpretation of causal relationship. However all studies have proven that people with IOP more than 21 mm Hg have higher risk for developing glaucoma than general population. The glaucoma population has an IOP more than 21 mm Hg at the time of presentation in almost 50% and the rest have the so-called normal IOP.

The various instruments used for measuring IOP are based on indentation or applanation methods. The instruments are: Schiotz tonometer, Goldmann tonometer (which is the gold standard and recommended), Perkins hand-held tonometer, Noncontact air-puff tonometer, Tono-Pen, MacKay-Marg tonometer and pneumotonometer. Water drinking test and tonography have become out of practice because of very little true contribution to diagnosis by them. Indentation tonometer is no longer recommended for glaucoma diagnosis and follow-up, because lot more factors than in applanation method influence it.

The IOP measurements have a lot of physiological, clinical and artifactual variables, which can influence the outcome and one has to ensure that these erroneous influences are either overcome or have been accounted for. IOP can vary during the day and between days. Usually the peak IOP levels are found in the early mornings, but peak in the evenings or twice during the day are also observed. The peak IOP can be varied by medications. This makes unilateral therapeutic trial inconvenient and necessitates multiple readings. A baseline diurnal variation (conveniently can be done on different days at different time of the day-office diurnal variation) during most of the day is recommended before commencing treatment. The diagnosis of normal tension glaucoma demands a diurnal variation invariably. IOP can rise during systole and went even up to 4 mm Hg.

Lying posture can increase IOP by 2 to 3 mm Hg (can be the reason for Schiotz readings in lying posture to be higher than applanation readings in sitting posture). A decrease in the blood flow to carotid arteries can decrease IOP while Valsalva maneuver can increase IOP (akin to breath holding by the patient). Exercise can decrease IOP in POAG and stopping the exercise can bring IOP back to original levels in 3 weeks period. If the patient is not asked to fix for infinity, accommodation can cause IOP rise more so in the young patients.

The ocular hypertension treatment study showed CCT to be a powerful predictor of development of glaucoma. Eyes with corneal thickness of 555 μm or less (i.e. eyes with relatively thin corneas) had a three-fold greater risk of developing glaucoma than those who had corneal thickness of more than 588 μm. It has been found that with thicker corneas IOP may be overestimated with the Goldmann tonometer and in thinner corneas IOP may be underestimated. The applanation tonometer by Goldmann is calibrated for 520 μm of central corneal thickness and there is a widespread variation of the same in races, this can influence the estimated IOP. Correction factors, which can approximately calculate the error, were estimated to be between 0.19 mm Hg for 10 μm and 0.71 mm Hg for every 5 μm. Though there have been no recommendations to use correction factors, a comprehensive workup of a glaucoma suspect must include measurement of CCT by an ultrasound pachymeter so as to guide the clinician if there is a strong possibility of either IOP being overestimated or underestimated.

A patient with systemic beta-blockers can have low IOP at the presentation and diagnosis of glaucoma can be missed or can be misdiagnosed as normal tension glaucoma. In children due to the lower scleral rigidity, IOP can be falsely low, but in children more than age 10, Goldmann applanation is reliable. Following formula is used to note the amount of underestimation of IOP by applanation in children below 10 years of age: $T_a = 0.71$ age (years)$+10$ (T_a=True Applanation). Pneumotonometer has better accuracy in children. Contact lenses worn during applanation can overestimate IOP.

However inaccurate IOP correlation is at present with glaucoma, it is exclusively the tool used by clinicians to monitor the disease. It can be used to develop a baseline, monitor short- and long-term fluctuations. An asymmetric IOP can give more clues than symmetric elevated IOP readings.

Some of the controversies, viz. safest IOP levels in ocular hypertensives and intervention time are being studied in ongoing trials, such as the OHGC and early manifest glaucoma trial (EMGT).

Pupillary Evaluation

It is important to assess the direct and indirect papillary response along with Marcus Gunn phenomenon in all patients. Relative afferent pupillary defect (RAPD) in one eye can influence surgical decisions in the presence of significant media opacity.

Biomicroscopy

A careful slit-lamp examination to exclude the other causes of open-angle and angle-closure glaucomas should be a routine process. Pre- and post-dilatation examination is important in the context of pseudoexfoliation glaucoma and lens assessment in cases of coexisting cataract. Apart from this, corneal edema, pigment on the posterior surface of the cornea and AC, AC reaction, keratic precipitates, iris color, contour, defects, pupillary ruff defects, exfoliation flakes, transillumination defects, iris atrophy, neovascularization, shape and thickness of crystalline lens, and marks of previous trauma are signs for secondary glaucoma.

Optic nerve head evaluation is described in another chapter. The essential changes that can happen with primary open-angle glaucoma are dealt in Table 10.2. The optic disc area is not constant among individuals, but shows inter individual variability of about 0.80 to 5.50 mm². Depending on the methodology used, mean optic disc area in a normal Caucasian population measures 2.69 mm² with a standard deviation of ± 0.70 mm². Abnormally large optic discs, larger than the mean plus two-fold standard deviations (>4.10 mm²), have been termed macrodiscs and abnormally small optic discs, smaller than the mean minus twofold standard deviations (<1.29 mm²), have been called microdiscs. Two percent of normals have 0.7 CD ratio while symmetrical CD ratio is found in 99.5% of the normal population. Contour cup rather than color cup should be used to assess CD ratio for which the point of deviation of small blood vessels have to be taken into consideration. Average CD ratio is 0.4 and vertical CD ratio is 0.2 more than horizontal. Vertical elongation is seen in 4% of normals and 33% of glaucoma patients. Pallor of the rim is 94% specific for

Table 10.2: Optic nerve head (ONH) evaluation and changes

Optic nerve evaluation	ONH changes in POAG
Instruments: Hruby, 90D, 78D, 60 D, 20 D	Concentric enlargement of the cup
Goldmann fundus contact lens	Focal narrowing of the rim
Photos- 35 mm (stereo preferred)	Asymmetric cupping
Red free photography	Disc hemorrhages
Planimetry	Acquired parapapillary atrophy
	Baring of the circumlinear vessel
Method of assessment: (documentation)	
Disc size: Small, medium, large	Anomalous discs (dilemmas)
Rim color: Pink or pale	Drusen
CD ratio: Vertical and horizontal	Tilted disc
Type of cup: Shallow, deep, sloping	Oblique insertion of disc
	Congenitally full disc
Disc hemorrhages: Location and extent	Megalopapillae
	Physiological cups
Notch: Location and extent	Optic disc coloboma
Peripapillary area: Zone α and β-clock hrs	Optic disc pit
	Myopic disc
NFL defects: Slit, wedge, diffuse	Hypoplastic discs
Vessels: Abnormal loops, collaterals	

non-glaucomatous defects while obliteration of the rim is 87% specific for glaucoma. Nerve fiber layer hemorrhages can be frequently seen in primary open-angle glaucomas also. It occurs in 2% to 23% of glaucoma patients and disappears in 6 weeks, more commonly in the inferior pole. It is supposed to indicate progression and needs aggressive management. It may form nerve fiber layer defects on follow-up which can usually be seen in a maximum period of 2 months. Peripapillary atrophy with prominent beta zone is significant for diagnosis of glaucoma. It is also being correlated with visual field changes and systemic risk factors. If done properly, optic nerve head evaluation has sensitivity of 85% and specificity of 85% and forms one of the vital diagnostic tools.

The examination is preferably done with slit-lamp biomicroscopic technique with a high convex noncontact lens (60, 78, 90D) preferably under dilatation both with routine and red free illumination. During initial examination, if optic nerve changes are observed, drawings or disc photography (preferably stereo photography) is done for follow-up. Photographs can be manually measured under magnification for various parameters and there are several systems being evaluated. This is mainly used nowadays in epidemiological studies rather than in clinical practice–this method is termed optic nerve head planimetry. Computerized planimetry is also available, but has inaccuracies, which need to be corrected before using clinically. Table 10.3 summarizes the approach to a patient with glaucoma.

Gonioscopy

Evaluation of the angle by gonioscopy has a pivotal role in the diagnosis of any glaucoma. There is an alarming trend of assuming the angle to be open based on anterior chamber depth. This practice is often misleading and can lead to diagnostic errors. The diagnosis of primary open-angle glaucoma has to be a diagnosis of exclusion after a detailed gonioscopy to rule out all secondary causes of glaucoma. Gonioscopy can be done using a Goldmann two-mirror lens or a Sussman four-mirror lens or similar prototypes. A protocolled approach of evaluating the angle systematically in dim illumination followed by bright illumination and high magnification of each quadrant will ensure that subtle characteristics like inflammatory precipitates in angle, occult early neovascularization, blood in the Schlemm's canal and abnormal pigmentation all of which are mostly associated with various entities of secondary glaucoma are not missed. It is very important to reason the presence any of these features in the angle before arriving at a final

Table 10.3: Approach to diagnosis and treatment of primary open-angle glaucoma

- Identify the risk factors
- Demonstrate a definite elevation of IOP (Diurnal) with applanation methods
- Careful optic nerve evaluation and documentation
- Confirm visual field loss with automated perimetry
- Educate the patient regarding glaucoma and the role and side effects of therapy
- Institute therapy: Single medication with least side effects and most convenient dosage–consider unilateral trial
- Emphasize on compliance
- Switch over to alternative therapy rather than adding in nonresponders
- Surgery considered: If maximum tolerable medical therapy (MTMT) fails or in an extremely noncompliant patient

conclusion of open-angle glaucoma. Documentation of the morphological characteristics of the angle should include angle width, iris contour, and trabecular pigmentation. Gonioscopic grading systems (Table 10.4) have been used as a guideline to systematically document findings and a practice of adopting any one of the systems consistently will minimize errors. Typically the open-angle glaucoma is associated with a featureless normal angle, however the normal has innumerous variations of width, trabecular pigmentation and prominence of iris processes (Figs 10.1 A to D). Gonioscopy has a learning curve and repeated gonioscopy on every patient presenting to the practice will help add to the expertise of differentiating a normal versus an abnormal angle. Gonioscopy characteristics may change with time and periodic evaluation of patients diagnosed with glaucoma is an important aspect of comprehensive management of a glaucoma patient.

Spaeth gonioscopic grading system is shown in Table 10.5.

Table 10.5: Spaeth gonioscopic grading system

Parameter	Criteria
Iris insertion	**A**nterior to Schwalbe's line **B**ehind Schwalbe's line **C**entered at scleral spur **D**eep to scleral spur **E**xtremely deep/on ciliary band
Angle width:Slit	10° 20° 30° 40°
Peripheral iris configuration	queerly concave regular steep
Trabecular meshwork pigment	**0** (none) to **4** (maximal)

Table 10.4: Gonioscopy grading systems

Grade	0	I	II	III	IV
Shaffer	Closed	10°	20°	30°	40°
Modified Shaffer	Schwalbe's line not visible	Schwalbe's line visible	Anterior trabecular meshwork is visible	Scleral spur is visible	Ciliary band is visible
Scheie	Ciliary band is visible	Last roll of iris obscures Ciliary body	Nothing posterior to the trabecular meshwork is visible	Posterior portion of trabecular meshwork is hidden	No structures posterior to Schwalbe's line visible

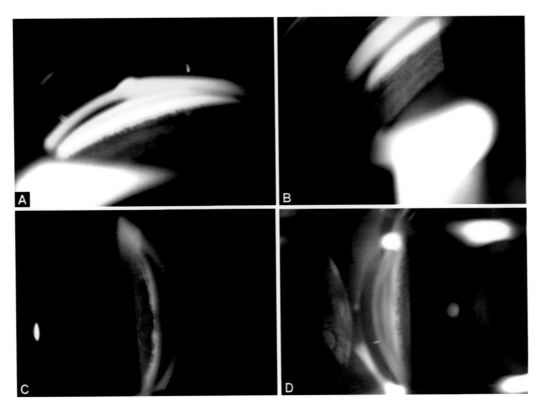

Figs 10.1A to D: Open Angle—Variations in width and pigmentation

Optic Nerve and Nerve Fiber Layer Imaging

During the last decade or so computerized imaging technologies have evolved and been extensively refined for clinical assessment of the optic nerve and retinal nerve fiber layer (RNFL). These technologies have the ability to provide objective and quantitative measurements of the optic nerve and retinal nerve fiber layer. The quantitative measurements have been shown to have good correlation with the status of optic nerve structure and function thereby facilitating glaucoma diagnosis and monitoring. All these technologies can only serve as adjuncts and data generated by these are best used with comprehensive information derived from clinical evaluation of the patient.

The following technologies are currently the mainstay of optic nerve and nerve fiber layer imaging:
- Confocal scanning laser ophthalmoscopy (Heidelberg retinal tomograph (HRT); Heidelberg Engineering, Heidelberg, Germany)
- Scanning laser polarimetry (GDx VCC; Carl Zeiss Meditec, Dublin, CA, USA)
- Optical coherence tomography (OCT; Carl Zeiss Meditec, Dublin, CA, USA)

Visual Field Changes

The demonstration of visual field defects serves as a major factor in the diagnosis of glaucoma. However, present clinical tools have the capacity to detect field loss only after at least 20% of the ganglion cell loss has occurred. The field defects include: Generalized constriction or depression; focal defects in the form of nasal step or Seidel's scotoma; enlargement of

blind spot in the mild form of the disease; superior or inferior arcuate defects in the moderate stage of the POAG; and biarcuate defects with or without central 10° involvement in the advanced stage. White-on-white perimetry is the gold standard. The advantages of blue on yellow perimetry and frequency doubling perimetry are described elsewhere in this book. The other perimetry processes are described here. Most of the perimetric tests involve a specific set of ganglion cells and does not give overall information regarding the patient's visual function (Table 10.6). Other psychophysical tests are not used in clinically practice in routine practice.

Table 10.6: The visual function testing in glaucoma

Type of cells	Visual function test
P-cells	Visual acuity, high pass resolution perimetry
K-cells	SWAP
M-cells	Flicker perimetry, motion perimetry, frequency doubling

High-pass resolution perimetry (developed by Lars Frisen): A total of 14 target sizes (in equal 0.1 log unit or 1 dB steps), which are rings with high-pass spatial frequency are filtering on a video monitor incorporating a light circular center and a dark annular surround. The stimulus design corresponds to the center-surround arrangement of retinal ganglion cell receptive fields. The progression of glaucomatous damage is seen 1.5 years before the routine automated perimetry.

Flicker Perimetry

Rapid flicker in glaucoma patients are affected which is mediated by the M-cells. There are several methods of doing this testing under evaluation. This seems to have more resistance to the optical degradation (blur, cataract) than conventional perimetry.

Motion Perimetry

Again a function mediated by M-cells, this is not affected by optical degradation, background illuminance and pupil size. However the machine is as yet not commercially available.

Detection and Resolution Perimetry

Detection means detection of the smallest grating stripe on a uniform background. Resolution is detecting the orientation. It works on detecting the damage to visual function affected by the P-system.

Pattern ERG is another form of subjective way of detecting the retinal sensitivity, however it has a long way before being clinically acceptable. At present none of the newer perimeters have replaced the white-on-white perimeter, however an ideal technique is being on the hunt.

MANAGEMENT OF GLAUCOMA – PRINCIPLES

Generally, POAG is treated medically first. Argon laser trabeculoplasty and selective laser trabeculoplasty can be considered in appropriate situations either as first line or second line management options. Surgery is reserved for patients who cannot tolerate maximum tolerable medical therapy (MTMT). The concept of Target IOP is introduced in this context since all measures as of now are for controlling IOP.

Principles of Medical Therapy for Glaucoma

At present, therapy for glaucoma consists of lowering IOP. There is good correlation between the level of IOP and progression of visual field loss in the majority of people. Advanced glaucoma intervention trial showed that IOP lowered below 18 mm Hg can decrease the chances of visual field progression over a period of 5 years. It is very important to remember that the best treatment does not always work and some people lose vision despite best efforts. Tables 10.7A and B contains drugs

Table 10.7 A: Medication classes approved for the chronic treatment of glaucoma before 1993 and used widely at present

Class	Generic name (Trade name)	IOP reduction	Concentrations and dosing	Major adverse reactions	Mechanisms of IOP reduction
1. Nonselective beta₁./beta₂. adrenergic antagonists	Timolol Hemihydrate (Betimol)	20–30%	0.5%, 0.5% qid, bid	Bradycardia Bronchospasm Fatigue Impotence Hypotension	Decreases Aqueous humor Production
	Levobunolol Hydrochloride (Betagan)		0.25%, 0.5% qid, bid		
	Timolol maleate (Timoptic**)		0.25%,0.5% qid, bid		
	Timolol maleate Gel-forming Solution (Timoptic XE)		0.25%,0.5% qid, bid		
2. Selective beta₁-adrenergic antagonist	Betaxolol Hydrochloride (Betoptic)		0.5% bid	Bradycardia Bronchospasm Fatigue	Decreases aqueous humor production
	Betaxolol Hydrochloride Suspension (Betoptic–S)		0.25% bid		
3. Parasympathomimetics	Pilocarpine Hydrochloride (Isopto Carpine)		0.25%,0.5%,1% 2%,3%,4%,6% 8%,10% qid	Brow ache Diminution of vision Fluctuating vision Gastrointestinal disturbance Headache Induced myopia Miosis Retinal detachment	Increases traditional outflow facility
	Pilocarpine Gel (Pilo-Hs gel)		4%		
4. Oral carbonic anhydrase inhibitors	Acetazolamide (Diamox)		125 mg, 250 mg qid	Anemias Electrolyte Imbalance Fatigue	Decreases Aqueous humor
	Acetazolamide Sustained Releasables		50 mg, 100 mg bid		

Nonselective alpha-and beta adrenergic agonists, Cholinesterase inhibitors – Not used anymore widely

Table 10.7B: Medications in glaucoma (newer class of drugs)

Class	Generic name (Trade name)	IOP reduction	Concentrations and dosing regimen	Major side effects	Mechanisms of IOP reduction
1. Topical carbonic anhydrase inhibitors	Dorzolamide (Trusopt) Brinzolamide (Azopt)	15–26%	2% bid, tid 1% bid, tid	Bitter taste Blurred Vision	Decreases aqueous humor production Decreases aqueous humor production
2. Combination product	Dorzolamide timolol (Cosopt)		Dorzolamide 2% Timolol 0.5% bid	Bitter taste Fatigue	Decreases Aqueous humor production
3. Selective alpha$_2$-adrenergic agonists	Apraclonidine (Lopidine)	18–27%	0.5%, 1%* bid, tid	Allergic blepharo-conjunctivitis Dry mouth Fatigue	Decreases Aqueous humor Production
	Brimonidine (Alphagan, Alphagan P)	24–27%	0.2% bid, tid 0.15% bid, tid	Dry mouth Fatigue	Decreases Aqueous humor Production and increases uveoscleral outflow
4. Prostaglandin analog	Latanoprost* (Xalatan)	27–34%	0.005% qhs	Cystoid macular edema Increased iris pigmentation(8–15%) Eyelash lengthening and darkening Uveitis	Increases uveoscleral outflow
	Unoprostone (Rescula)		0.002% tid	-do-	-do-
7. Others	Travoprost (Travatan) Bimatoprost** (Lumigan)	33% 33%	0.004% od 0.03% od	Similar to Prostaglandins	Increases uveoscleral outflow

Combinations of PG analogs are also available: e.g. Xalacom*, Ganfort**, etc.

approved in the recent past and before 1993 for glaucoma treatment. It gives the mechanism of action and a comprehensive list of adverse events associated with the drugs.

There are five basic steps one should follow while treating:

A. Establish a good baseline.

B. Set a reasonable goal for intraocular pressure.

C. Lower the pressure.

D. Follow-up the patient to see if the pressure goal is maintained with stable optic nerve head and visual fields.

E. Modify the pressure goal and treatment depending on patient's course.

In the initial examination there will be multiple visits, during those visits patient should be educated about the chronic nature of the disease, irreversible nature of glaucomatous visual loss and value of pressure reduction to avoid progressive damage. Patient education is most important aspect of chronic care of glaucoma because effective management depends not in the prescription of therapy, but in the use of therapy consistently for long time.

A. *Establish a baseline:* A good baseline consists of the following:

Intraocular pressure: Intraocular pressure varies from day-to-day over the course of the day. For a good baseline, ideally recommendation is a diurnal record of IOP, alternatively multiple readings at different times of clinic visits can be compiled to obtain a baseline.

Angle appearance: By definition, primary open-angle glaucoma should have open angles.

Optic disc examination: Evaluation of optic disc after dilatation with 90 D or 78 D lens, using slit-lamp biomicroscopy is very important. After examination it should be documented either with drawings or photography.

Visual fields: A good reliable field should be used as a baseline field. More than two sets of fields may be necessary to establish baseline free of learning curve artifacts.

B. *Setting a pressure goal:* There are two important concepts that help to assess given patients risk of damage from elevated pressure (i.e.) estimated threshold for damage and the presence of non-pressure risk factors.

Threshold for damage: We cannot determine a person's threshold for damage, but the visual fields at the time of presentation provides clues. Based upon extent of damage one should set target pressure. The concept of a target pressure presumes that by attaining an adequately low IOP the optic nerve will be protected from further damage and the patient from further visual field loss. How to get the target pressure? The answer is part science and part empiric. Generally the target pressure should be at least 20% lower than the mean pretreatment pressure. In addition the target is dictated by the cause of the disease and the degree of optic nerve damage. Target pressure should be reassessed from time to time. A general guideline for the target IOP is given in Table 10.8.

Table 10.8: Guidelines for target IOP

Visual field loss	Initial average IOP (mm Hg)			
	50	40	30	20
Mild	30	25	23	16
Moderate	25	25	20	14
Severe	20	20	15	10

Non-pressure risk factors: There are factors other than pressure that contribute to optic nerve damage and determine an individual's susceptibility to harm from pressure, but they are unknown. Greater the degree of damage, higher the chances of these risk factors to be present. Better the unknown factors; more IOP should be lowered because it is the only treatable risk factor.

So setting the pressure goal mainly depends on the extent of damage – the greater the damage, the greater should be the attempt to lower IOP.

C. *Lowering intraocular pressure:* Several general principles contribute to the goal of maximizing the therapeutic effect of each topical medication while minimizing side effects.

1. Start with least offensive drug first, considerations here are ocular and systemic side effects, cost and dosage frequency. Currently the prostaglandin derivatives qualify these requirements and is mostly accepted as first line therapy.
2. Treat unilaterally first to assess effect.
3. Encourage lid closure after drop use. Gentle lid closure with nasolacrimal duct occlusion for few minutes after instilling drops helps in more medication entry into the eye and less entry into systemic circulation.
4. Use fixed combination of drugs when multiple drug therapy is required. Combine drugs that have complimentary modes of action (e.g. Xalacom: Combination of timolol and latanoprost. Timolol reduces aqueous production where as latanoprost enhances aqueous outflow).
5. Give written instructions and inform clearly possible side effects. Glaucoma is usually an asymptomatic disease, so it may be difficult to continue the patient to take the medication regularly; there is very high chance for poor compliance. To improve compliance it is very important to explain the disease process, demonstrate visual field loss and how following the prescribed treatment plan may reduce the risk of visual loss.

D. *Follow-up:* When patient comes for follow-up, following determinations should be made:

1. Determine if the patient is taking and tolerating the medication, check for any side effects and record when patient took last medication.

2. Determine if the medication is lowering IOP or not. If IOP is not lowering, better to discontinue it and switch to another one.
3. If the medicine is lowering IOP determine whether lowering is effective or not. If the lowering is not sufficient enough–consider alternatives. The aim is to do a detailed examination to determine whether the disease process is stable or not. If not stable check for compliance and the target pressure should be reset. A table for disease progression and intervention strategy is given as a general guideline (Table 10.9).

E. *Modified pressure goal and treatment:* The follow-up guidelines for a glaucoma suspect and glaucoma patients are given below:

Untreated glaucoma suspect with stable optic nerve evaluation and intraocular pressure status: Once stability of IOP and optic nerve has been established, follow-up evaluation can be annual.

Untreated high-risk glaucoma suspect with stable optic nerve evaluation and intraocular pressure status: Follow-up evaluation should be performed every 3 to 12 months depending on severity of risk.

Treated high-risk glaucoma suspect with newly established control of IOP: Depending on the level of the intraocular pressure and presence of other risk factors visits may be required as often as every 3 months and may decrease to as few as once a year when stability is demonstrated on repeated examinations. Follow-up protocol for glaucoma patients is given in Table 10.9.

Table 10.9: Disease progression and follow-up

1. Mild disease – Both C/D ratio ≤ 0.4 and no more than mild field loss
2. Moderate – C/D ratio < 0.8 – no more than moderate field loss
3. Severe – C/D ratio → 0.8 – severe field loss

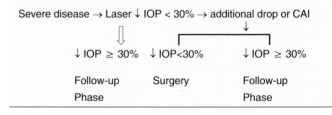

Laser Therapy

Argon Laser Trabeculoplasty (ALT)

This procedure is indicated in patients with MTMT and need further lowering of IOP without surgical intervention. More than 67% initial success is recorded in patients with POAG, PXF glaucoma and pigmentary glaucoma. It is contraindicated in patients with corneal pathology and angle-closure glaucoma.

Ritch four-mirror lens is widely used to perform the laser procedure. The laser settings are given in the Table 10.10.

ALT enhances aqueous outflow by changing the mitotic and metabolic activity of the trabecular endothelial cells. The response is apparent only after 6 to 8 weeks. It is estimated that 50% of the patients have failure of the procedure by the end of 5 years and so it is reserved for patients who need a temporary solution before surgery. The major side effect is a transient rise in IOP postoperatively.

Table 10.10: Argon laser trabeculoplasty–parameters

Argon Laser Trabeculoplasty: (Wise and Witter 1979)
Argon Green 515 nm using Goldman or 3-mirror Ritch trabeculoplasty lens
- Approximately 500 to 800 mW
- 360° – 70 to 100 burns
  or
  180° – 40 to 50 burns
- 50 µm spot size
- 0.1 sec

Junction of the anterior non-pigmented and posterior pigmented trabecular meshwork

Selective Laser Trabeculoplasty (SLT)

Selective laser trabeculoplasty offers benefits of ALT, without the irreversible damage that ALT causes. SLT uses a q-switched, 532-nm Nd:YAG laser (Coherent's Selecta 7000) to irradiate the trabecular meshwork. This triggers a biological response that causes increased outflow. SLT has several noteworthy characteristics: It is selective, nonthermal, repeatable and is effective for patients who have had prior treatment with ALT. The mechanism that allows SLT and ALT to lower IOP appear to be different. The thermal damage resulting from ALT causes tissue contraction, which results in widening of passages for aqueous flow. SLT does not have this effect. However, both treatments appear to attract macrophages to the treated tissue by triggering the release of cytokines. The selective targeting of melanocytes also acts to increase outflow.

Other Laser Procedures

Diode cyclophotocoagulation: It has been used in end stage and refractory glaucomas with low-visual potential. As of now, none of the studies have proven its safety as a primary procedure.

Surgery

The gold standard in surgery is as of now partial thickness trabeculectomy. There are several modifications that have evolved over years, since it was described by Cairns (1957). The basic technique has not changed however the use of filtering surgery as a primary procedure in POAG remains the same though the use of limbal vs fornix-based flap, use of antimetabolites in primary procedures differ with variations in the clinical practice. The use of single site vs two-site procedure for combined cataract and filtering procedures differs with practice setting.

A filtering surgery alone should be restricted to cases where cataract is not significant. Trabeculectomy is effective and safe, but is associated with progression of preexisting cataract. In planned two-stage surgeries, in cases with cataract, phacoemulsification with a temporal section is the preferred method irrespective of whether performed before or after the filtering surgery. Combined surgery (glaucoma-triple-procedure) refers to one-stage surgical procedure, which tackles both cataract and glaucoma.

The newer developments, which have evolved in the recent past with respect to trabeculectomy per se, are quite exciting:
- Wound modulation concepts and the use of 5-FU and mitomycin-C
- Newer antifibrotic agents–TGFβ
- Releasable suture techniques
- Argon laser suture lysis
- Modification of trabeculectomy: T-cut and scleral tunnel, reverse trabeculectomy

Phacotrabeculectomy

Phacoemulsification combined with trabeculectomy using mitomycin-C appears to be an effective approach to the management of cataract in patients with glaucoma. It offers potential for good improvement in visual acuity as well as long-term control of IOP. Potential vision-threatening complications, specifically hypotony maculopathy and late-onset bleb leaks should be considered in the decision to use mitomycin-C.

Discontinue pilocarpine before surgery and substitute with acetazolamide if required. There is no need to discontinue any other glaucoma medication. A tunnel incision from the 12 o'clock position can be used or a separate access with temporal clear-corneal incision can be gained. A limbal or fornix-based conjunctival flap is made. A 4 mm x 4 mm rectangular or 4 mm triangular partial thickness scleral flap (1/2 to 2/3rd thickness of the sclera) is raised and advanced to the limbus. A temporal clear-corneal tunnel is dissected, phacoemulsification is performed and an IOL is implanted in the capsular bag. The trabeculectomy and basal iridectomy are performed and the scleral flap is closed by 10-0 monofilament nylon sutures. The conjunctival flap is closed. Postoperative management should be custom-tailored, based on the response to surgical intervention, IOP levels and the occurrence of complications. Antiglaucoma medications should not be given unless high IOP is documented.

With well-designed glaucoma trials giving us further insight into the pathogenesis of glaucoma and stronger evidence into the newly developing interventional strategies, time will come when a glaucomalogist is armed with the right answer in terms of early diagnosis, genetic assessment and manipulation, newer therapeutic agents, including neuroprotective drugs and safer surgical procedures which last longer ultimately enhancing the quality of life of a glaucoma patient.

Newer Surgical Techniques: Non-penetrating Filtering Procedures

Non-penetrating filtering procedures are designed to avoid full thickness penetration of the anterior chamber. In theory this would minimize complications related to overfiltration, hypotony, antimetabolites and large avascular blebs. Viscocanalostomy and deep sclerectomy are two procedures currently being practiced. Both procedures involve removal of a deep scleral flap to de-roof the Schlemm's canal and expose a trabeculo-Descemet's window for aqueous to percolate into a scleral lake. The viscocanalostomy further involves the injection of high molecular weight viscoelastic substance into the Schlemm's canal. This ensures that aqueous from scleral lake exits into the widened Schlemm's canal and exits through the episcleral collector channels. The resultant effect is a low bleb in deep sclerectomy and an absent bleb in viscocanalostomy. Non-penetrating procedures have been reported to be less effective in reducing IOP to lower teens. Recent prospective randomized controlled trials have reported an IOP of less than 16 mm Hg at 2 years in less than 15% of subjects after deep sclerectomy in comparison to 30% observed in the viscocanalostomy group. This is far lesser than that of a standard trabeculectomy with antimetabolites.

Aqueous drainage implants have been used by a very few clinicians as primary procedure and is used as a tertiary glaucoma procedure. Molteno implant, Ahmed glaucoma implant and Baerveldt implant are the currently used implants of interest.

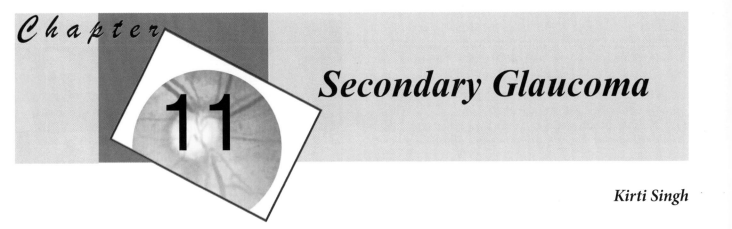

Chapter 11

Secondary Glaucoma

Kirti Singh

Glaucoma comprises a diverse group of conditions with characteristic optic nerve head damage and corresponding visual field defects with some relation to intraocular pressure. Secondary glaucomas are those conditions for which another ocular pathology accounts for the glaucoma. The mechanism in secondary glaucoma may be open angle, angle closure or both. In addition to the lowering of intraocular pressure by using the entire antiglaucoma armamentarium the underlying ocular pathology also needs to be treated.

PSEUDOEXFOLIATION SYNDROME

Introduction

Pseudoexfoliation is characterized by the deposition of homogenous grey white material, which is produced by the abnormal basement membrane of epithelial cells of trabecular meshwork, lens capsule, iris and deposited in various ocular structures. The material is composed of protein core surrounded by glycosaminoglycans. Initially identified by Lindberg, in 1917, this disorder of the elderly has a prevalence of 2.3% to 6%. Cataract is the commonest presentation in this condition. Glaucoma prevalence in pseudoexfoliation ranges from 7.5% to 14%. The condition is often under diagnosis and the patient is treated as primary open-angle glaucoma.

Both prevalence and bilaterality of pseudoexfoliation increase with age, almost doubling by 15 years. The prevalence has been reported to increase from 0.6% in 52–64 years, to 5% by 75–85 years of age. Genetic studies suggest that inheritance is by maternal transmission (mitochondrial X-linked inheritance).

A bilateral disorder, it frequently manifests asymmetrically. Long term follow-up reveals that 25 to 40% of those presenting with unilateral manifestation develop bilateral disease within 5–10 years. Almost 20% present with glaucomatous changes, of the remainder 10 to 15% develop glaucoma over a period

of 10 years. The risk of pseudoexfoliation patients developing glaucoma is 10 times that of normal population.

Etiopathogenesis

Pseudoexfoliative material (related to amyloid P protein and elastin), pigment and fragmented zonular fibrils block the intertrabecular spaces, long-term exposure of which overwhelms the outflow pathway. A vascular hypothesis has been postulated where a vascular event leads to endothelial dysfunction with the subsequent impairment of blood aqueous barrier. Homocysteine, a recognized marker of vascular insult and endothelial dysfunction is elevated in aqueous humor and plasma of pseudoexfoliation patients. Increased level of this chemical marker gives credence to the hypothesis of vascular injury with subsequent alterations and accumulation of extracellular matrix. Amyloid angiopathy is the histological manifestation of the ischemic etiology. Orbital blood flow studies corroborate the ischemic component. Transient ischemic attacks and aortic aneurysm are often the systemic manifestations of the vascular endothelial dysfunction in pseudoexfoliation patients.

Glaucoma is classically of the open-angle variant, however angle-closure element can occur due to pupil block. Pupil block in pseudoexfoliation patients occurs either due to zonular instability and subsequent anterior displacement of lens iris diaphragm or due to posterior synechiae associated with a rigid non-dilating pupil.

Clinical Features

Usually asymptomatic, pseudoexfoliation is often noted as an incidental finding. The condition presents in seventh decade or later and the severity of glaucomatous damage is proportional to the extent of pseudoexfoliation material in trabecular meshwork. Pseudoexfoliation material a grayish white fibrillogranular dandruff-like particles that are seen on the lens, pupil border, ciliary body, zonules, anterior hyaloid face, extraocular muscles, vortex veins and optic nerve sheath (Fig. 11.1). On the crystalline lens the material is characteristically seen in three zones:

a. *Central disc:* A translucent disc with scrolled edges, this zone may not always be present.

b. *Clear intermediate zone around central disc:* Due to the physiological contractions of iris the pseudoexfoliation material is wiped off the intermediate zone (windshield wiper effect).

c. *Outer peripheral zone of pseudoexfoliation material:* Granular material deposition with radial striations comprises this zone, which is always present. A dilated examination of eye is mandatory to check this zone if a patient is suspected to have pseudoexfoliation (Figs 11.2 and 11.3).

Iris features include atrophy with transillumination defects, pseudoexfoliation material at pupil border and a miosed pupil. Loss of pupil ruff is characteristic and is known as moth eaten pupil margin. The trabecular meshwork is often hyperpigmented and in addition may show presence of pseudoexfoliation material. Another characteristic gonioscopic picture is of pigmented Schwalbe's line called as Sampaolesi's line.

Patient often has concomitant cataract, which has fragile zonules. The zonular weakness manifests as phakodonesis, lens subluxation or dislocation. Corneal endothelial loss disproportionate to age is associated thus before undertaking a cataract surgery zonular stability and specular microscopy should be assessed. The blood aqueous barrier is disrupted so inflammation after surgery or laser treatment is more intense and prolonged necessitating corticosteroids to be prescribed more frequently and for a longer time. Optic nerve damage in pseudoexfoliation is disproportionate to the intraocular pressure (IOP) thus it has been proposed that the structural integrity of optic nerve head is decreased in this disorder.

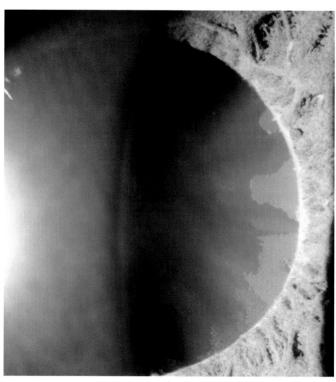

Fig. 11.2: Peripheral band of pseudoexfoliation material on the lens surface

Differential diagnosis includes pigment dispersion syndrome, capsular delamination, healed iridocyclitis and sphincteric atrophy due to angle-closure glaucoma.

Treatment

The condition is more resistant to medical management compared to open-angle glaucoma. The first line drugs remain aqueous suppressants. Theoretically, miotics use would decrease

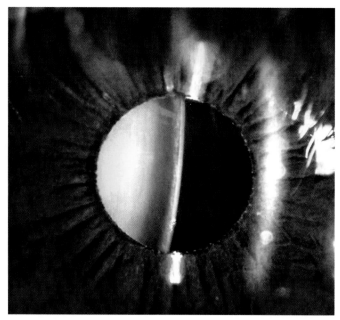

Fig. 11.1: Pseudoexfoliation material at the pupillary border

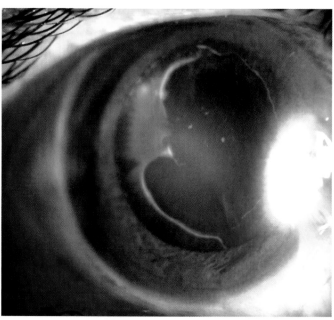

Fig. 11.3: Pseudoexfoliation material in the outer peripheral zone

iris movement and subsequent pigment/pseudoexfoliation liberation, but the concomitant risk of developing posterior synechiae/anterior rotation of subluxated lens and angle closure would necessitate close monitoring with their usage. Laser trabeculoplasty is more effective than in open-angle glaucoma, but the effects are transient.

Cataract is commonly associated so combined surgery is often indicated. Cataract surgery in these cases has some inherent problems. Foremost among them is inadequate pupil dilatation. In addition, the zonules weakened by the accumulation of pseudoexfoliation material often give way, thereby causing high incidence of zonular dehiscence and lens subluxation/dislocation. Vitreous loss is 5–10 times more in pseudoexfoliation patients. Iris hooks, capsule tension rings must always be at hand while doing surgery in these cases. Altered blood aqueous barrier leads to increased postoperative inflammation and posterior synechiae formation is common. Frequent topical steroid and cycloplegics need to be deployed in the postoperative period. Due to zonular instability the risk of late decentration of the intraocular lens (IOL) is a possibility. Trabecular aspiration, a technique of modified intraocular aspiration by a specialized probe in the inferior 180 degree of the angle after IOL implantation has been combined with cataract extraction to control the IOP.

Pseudoexfoliation glaucoma is more resistant to treatment and results of trabeculectomy alone or combined surgery is poorer with higher incidence of failure.

PIGMENTARY GLAUCOMA

Introduction

This type of bilateral secondary open-angle glaucoma results from disruption of iris pigment epithelium. Deposition of pigment occurs throughout the anterior segment. First described by Sugar and Barbour in 1949, it was Campbell in 1979 who postulated the accommodation theory wherein friction generated by the zonules during accommodation rubs pigment off from iris neuroepithelium.

Inherited as an autosomal dominant disorder, it has greater phenotypic expression in myopes and males (male:female ratio–3:1). Genetic mapping has identified chromosome 7q35-q36 as the locus. The disease intensity diminishes with aging and the onset of presbyopia. Decreased posterior iris bowing often results in resolution.

The disease is relatively uncommon in darker races namely the Asians and the Africans.

Etiopathogenesis

Anatomic factors associated with the etiopathogenesis of pigmentary glaucoma are larger iris in male patients or those with myopia, combined with a characteristic mid peripheral back bowing, which increases during accommodation. This increase in posterior iris bowing in the accommodated state induces a reverse pupillary block. Normally each blink forces aqueous from the posterior chamber into the anterior chamber. In predisposed individuals when the peripupillary iris presses against the lens, a ball valve mechanism prevents back flow, susceptible iris then bows back, rubs against lens zonules and pigment dispersal occurs. Exercises like jumping or running increase the iris activity with subsequent pigment showers, associated with IOP spikes, manifesting as intermittent colored haloes with or without pain.

Flattening of the iris following laser iridotomy for pigment dispersion syndrome decreases both the posterior concavity and iris-lens contact and helps in controlling the glaucoma.

Clinical Features

A bilateral asymmetric disorder is present in third to fourth decade. The classic triads of ocular manifestations are:

a. *Krukenberg's spindle:* This is seen as a vertical line of pigment deposition on the back surface of corneal endothelium (Figs 11.4A and B).

b. *Mascara line:* Heavy homogeneous pigmentation of trabecular meshwork, it needs to be differentiated from the patchy pigmentation seen post-uveitic or angle-closure attack resolution. A pigmented Schwalbe's line (Sampaolesi line) is often associated. (Figs 11.5A and B). Pigmentation is more pronounced in young age, later due to phagocytosis and decrease in pigment showers, the extent of pigmentation decreases.

c. *Midperipheral iris pigment epithelium loss:* It leads to radial spoke like transillumination defects (church-window defects). These may not be visible in the thick iris of the Indian subcontinent. To rule out transillumination defects a sclerotic scatter examination in addition to retro illumination must be done on the slit lamp. Partial loss of pupil ruff is also seen, this needs to be differentiated from markers of angle closure attacks. Sometimes, Zentmayer's line (pigmentation at zonular insertion site near equator of crystalline lens) is seen after pupil dilatation.

The IOP in pigment dispersion syndrome is very labile and undergoes large fluctuation, thus multiple IOP readings need to be taken to diagnose the underlying glaucoma.

Differential Diagnosis

Pigmentary glaucoma has to be differentiated from pseudoexfoliation syndrome which is seen in older individuals and has typical fibrillogranular pseudoexfoliation material deposits. Other differentials include healed iridocyclitis, melanosis, melanoma, post-cataract or intraocular surgery, and post angle closure glaucoma attacks. The latter would have narrow angle recess and patchy pigmentation along with some areas of peripheral anterior synechiae.

Treatment

Medications: Miotics flatten and tighten iris, straighten its back concavity and reduce pigment showers. However, they are poorly tolerated in the young patients of pigment dispersion

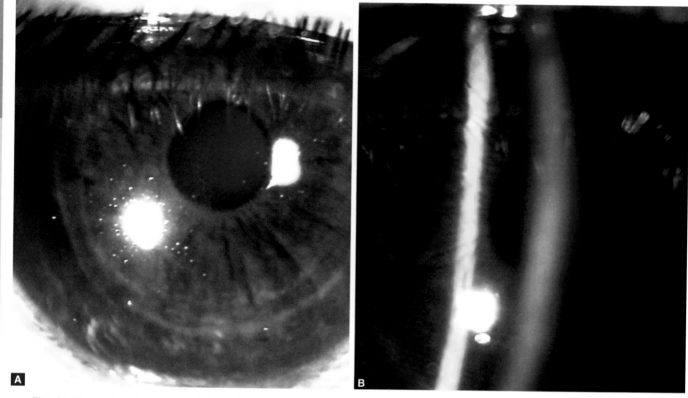

Figs 11.4A and B: Krukenberg's spindle. A. Krukenberg's spindle at back surface of cornea in a case of pigment dispersion syndrome B. Krukenberg's spindle is seen on high magnification

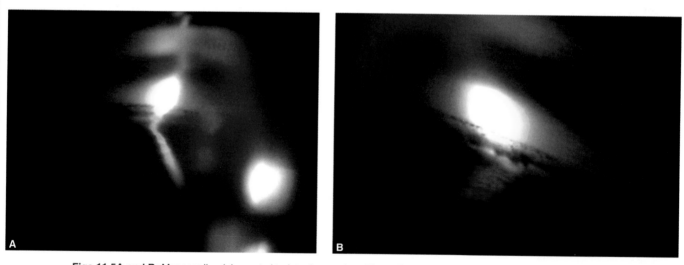

Figs 11.5A and B: Mascara line (pigmented trabecular meshwork) and Sampaolesi's line (pigmented Schwalbe's line)

glaucoma since they induce myopia. Myopes, in addition, run the risk of retinal detachment with pilocarpine usage.

Argon laser trabeculoplasty: This procedure has a good therapeutic response, as pigment facilitates laser absorption thereby increasing efficacy. However, the effect is short-lived.

Selective laser trabeculoplasty: Selective laser trabeculoplasty is associated with significant post-laser IOP elevations in deeply pigmented trabecular meshwork, thus must be performed preparing for this eventuality.

Surgery: The response to glaucoma filtration surgery or trabecular aspiration is good.

Peripheral iridectomy theoretically should eliminate posterior bowing of iris and does cause a planar configuration of the iris, however, it has not proven itself in aborting the transition of pigment dispersion syndrome into pigment dispersion glaucoma thus pure peripheral iridectomy may not accomplish a complete cure.

Prognosis

Pigment dispersion syndrome manifests at 25 years, gradually peters out after 45–50 years, as with onset of presbyopia the loss of accommodation leads to decrease in relative pupil block.

Although pigment dispersion syndrome burns out with age, patients need to be followed meticulously with yearly checkup of IOP and optic nerve head.

LENS-RELATED GLAUCOMA

Phacomorphic Glaucoma

The condition is due to an intumescent cataract, which combines an increase in equatorial girth (which relaxes zonules leading to forward movement of lens iris diaphragm) with an increased anteroposterior dimension (increasing iridolenticular contact) leading to secondary angle closure and pupil block respectively. Thus phacomorphic glaucoma is a variant of secondary angle-closure glaucoma.

Clinical Features

The patient presents with an acute rise in IOP, along with painful red eye and often nausea and vomiting (features of angle-closure attack). There is history of painless progressive diminution of vision over a period of months suggesting worsening cataract. Corneal edema, high IOP (30–40 mm Hg), circumcorneal congestion, swollen white mature cataract, and shallow anterior chamber more in center, all conclusively point to the diagnosis. Lens induced glaucoma can also occur due to rupture of cataractous lens, but the mechanism for glaucoma here is inflammatory trabeculitis, blockage of trabecular meshwork by lens matter (Figs 11.6A and B).

Treatment

In the emergency IOP has to be lowered by intravenous mannitol, systemic acetazolamide and topical beta-blockers. Topical corticosteroid at 4–6 hourly intervals are added to reduce inflammation prior to performing cataract surgery.

Most of these patients are elderly so mannitol must only be given after assessing the blood pressure and cardiac status. A circulatory overload induced by mannitol can prove lethal in cardiac compromised patients.

Lens removal by any surgical means either manual small incision or phacoemulsification is recommended once IOP has been controlled medically. A surgical iridectomy must also be done with the cataract surgery. If the attack has persisted for over a fortnight, then a combined glaucoma cataract surgery is advisable as peripheral anterior synechiae would have damaged the angle structures irreparably and filtration would be impaired. Sometimes if medical management fails to lower IOP sufficiently, a laser iridotomy may be required to break the pupil block prior to performing a definitive combined surgery.

Phacolytic Glaucoma

Described in 1900 by Gifford, it was Flocks in 1955 and Epstein in 1978 who actually demonstrated that phagocytosed lens particles/protein overwhelmed the filtration pathways and caused phacolytic glaucoma.

Clinical Features

Patient presents with an acutely painful red eye, preceded by gradual decrease of vision due to increasing cataract. The signs and symptoms are similar to lens induced glaucoma except the pupil block element. Flocculent lens material is sometimes seen as a pseudohypopyon. The anterior chamber is classically deep with a mild to moderate flare. The cataract is often mature or hypermature, but not intumescent (Fig. 11.7).

Etiopathogenesis

Macrophages laden with phagocytosed lens material and heavy molecular weight soluble lens protein block the trabecular meshwork and cause a secondary open-angle glaucoma.

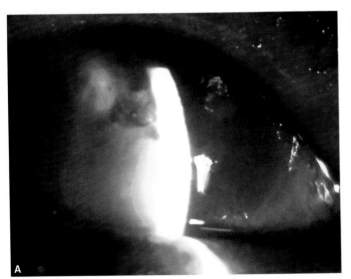 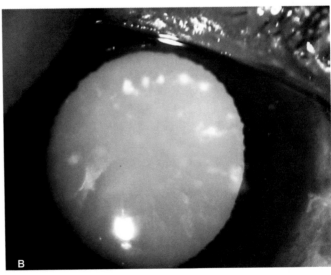

Figs 11.6A and B: Lens induced glaucoma (A) Glaucoma secondary to ruptured dislocated mature cataract. (B) Glaucoma secondary to hypermature intumescent cataract

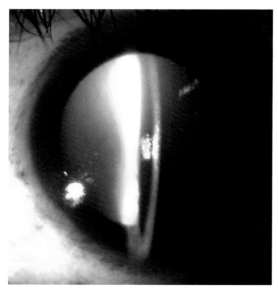

Fig. 11.7: Hypermature morgagnian cataract

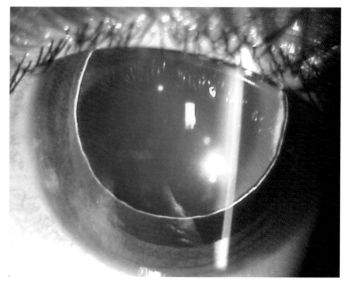

Fig. 11.8: Microspherophakia

Treatment

The IOP is controlled by intravenous mannitol, systemic acetazolamide and topical β blockers. In addition topical corticosteroids are prescribed to control inflammation prior to performing cataract surgery. Lens removal by any surgical means followed by meticulous anterior chamber wash is curative. Postoperatively systemic steroids are useful to reduce the inflammation induced by lens protein challenge.

Phacoantigenic/Phacoanaphylactic Uveitis

Release of lens protein through ruptured lens capsule after cataract surgery/trauma initiates a granulomatous uveitis occurring a few days after surgery/trauma. Patient presents with a painful red eye with flare, cells and keratic precipitates on the IOL and/or on corneal endothelium. Treatment is by intensive topical steroids and antiglaucoma drugs. Meticulous lens cortex aspiration during the primary surgery goes a long way in preventing this entity.

Ectopia Lentis Glaucoma

The anterior/posterior dislocation or subluxation of lens can cause glaucoma by inducing pupil block as seen after trauma and microspherophakia (Weill-Marchesani syndrome) (Fig. 11.8). Trauma, a very common denominator in lens dislocation, causes concomitant trabecular meshwork damage by angle recession, hyphema, inflammation or concussion. Ruptured lens material in addition adds the phacolytic element to the glaucoma load.

The causes of spontaneous ectopia lentis are Marfan's syndrome, homocystinuria, Weill-Marchesani and ectopia lentis et pupillae.

Ocular Features

The patient presents with signs and symptoms of pupil block glaucoma. Corneal edema is often disproportionate to the IOP due to corneolenticular touch. If lens is allowed to remain in the anterior chamber, persistent lenticulocorneal contact causes irreversible endothelial damage.

Treatment

Miotics worsen pupil block in microspherophakia by further relaxing the loose zonules. Cycloplegics are the drugs of choice as they tauten the zonules and push the lens posteriorly thereby relieving pupil block.

Surgical extraction of the truant lens must be performed once IOP is medically controlled. In young patients with residual zonular attachments remaining, limbal lensectomy with the pupil miosed (pilocarpine being used both preoperatively and intracamerally) is the solution. In older individuals intracapsular cataract extraction with wire vectis usually suffices. A thorough anterior vitrectomy along with surgical iridectomy must be done and anterior chamber IOL placed/or patient left aphakic depending on the fellow eye, age and associated pathology.

PSEUDOPHAKIC/APHAKIC GLAUCOMA

Post Congenital Cataract Surgery

Children who develop aphakic glaucoma are often those who have had surgery performed before 2 years of age. The causes of glaucoma are the stretch of capsular bag by disproportionate sized rigid polymethylmethacrylate lens causing a forward vaulting of optic contributing to pupil block and haptics pushing the iris root forward leading to trabeculitis. Glaucoma incidence increases with time elapsed since surgery and ranges from 6 to 25%. A very recent study from London reports a 12% incidence of glaucoma over a two-year follow-up in children whose cataract surgery was performed within 1 year of life along with in the bag IOL placement and posterior capsule capsulorhexis. The risk factors identified for glaucoma development are sulcus fixated IOL, protracted surgical trauma, chronic inflammation and the development of peripheral anterior synechiae. Lifelong follow-up is needed to screen for glaucoma in children operated for cataract.

Treatment

Medical management is with beta-blockers and carbonic anhydrase inhibitors. Miotics are not very useful and alpha agonists are contraindicated in young children. Glaucoma filtering surgery is ultimately needed and should be combined with adjunctive antifibrotics.

Epithelial and Fibrous Ingrowth

Inadequate wound closure after an intraocular surgery or penetrating trauma leading to wound leak is the inciting factor for both these conditions. In epithelial ingrowth; epithelium of bulbar conjunctiva origin, grows as a grey translucent/transparent membrane with thickened scalloped leading edge, over the posterior cornea, angle and iris structures causing corneal edema and refractory angle-closure glaucoma. The incidence was 0.09 to 0.12% after extracapsular cataract surgery; however after the advent of self-sealing valved incisions the incidence is much less.

Fibrous ingrowth is due to fibroblasts from subepithelial connective tissue entering through a breach in the Descemet's membrane and proliferating in the anterior chamber. A fibrous often vascularized membrane grows over corneal endothelium, iris and angle structures. It is less destructive and less aggressive than epithelial ingrowth.

The clinical picture is characteristic and specular microscopy is diagnostic of the conditions. Argon laser application is used to differentiate the two conditions, in case of epithelial ingrowth the laser marks will turn white.

Treatment requires radical excision of the ingrowth, vitrectomy and penetrating keratoplasty. Glaucoma is best treated by tube shunts although the membrane has a tendency to recur and block the tube if few viable cells have been left behind. Direct cryoapplication to affected sites to destroy the residual epithelial cells has been advocated in the past by Maumenee.

Complicated Cataract Surgery

With the popularity of phacoemulsification pseudophakic glaucoma related to large and poor incision construction is relatively less common. Both open- and closed-angle mechanism glaucoma can occur after cataract surgery. Incidence varies from 2 to 11% with the higher end of spectrum being reserved for anterior chamber or iris fixated IOL. In the bag placement of IOL has least chance of inducing iridocyclitis, erosion into ciliary body and subsequent glaucoma.

Etiopathogenesis

a. *Early intraocular pressure rise:* In the era of extracapsular cataract surgery (ECCE), limbal incisions caused distortion of the angle. An internal white ridge at the inner margin of the corneoscleral incision was documented. It was postulated to be due to corneal stromal edema and caused peripheral anterior synechiae formation, which led to transitory increase in IOP. The cause of glaucoma was both angle closure (due to peripheral anterior synechiae) combined with open-angle element (inflammatory debris clogging up the trabecular meshwork).

In the current era of valved, suture less incisions the cause of early IOP rise is due to residual viscoelastics, inflammatory debris, lens matter and pigment dispersion which overwhelm the trabecular outflow pathway. Thus it is now primarily an open-angle mechanism.

Pupil block element occurs after intracapsular cataract extraction, in eyes left aphakic wherein an intact anterior vitreous face blocks the pupil and after anterior chamber/iris supported IOL with an inadequate peripheral iridectomy. A large peripheral iridectomy (PI) is thus an essential component of intracapsular cataract surgery (ICCE), with anterior chamber / iris supported IOL to prevent this complication. Pupil block is also seen post congenital cataract surgery where the inflammatory fibrinous exudate is severe enough to cause occlusio and seclusio pupillae. In performing congenital cataract surgery a large PI (peripheral iridotomy) must always be performed to prevent pupil block glaucoma.

b. *Late intraocular pressure rise:* Wound leak due to inadequate wound closure may cause shallow anterior chamber, the latter if allowed to persist leads to peripheral anterior synechiae and angle-closure glaucoma (Fig. 11.9). Epithelial ingrowth, fibrous proliferations are the extreme manifestations of persistent wound leak and lead to intractable glaucoma. A complicated surgery incites intraocular inflammation with subsequent peripheral anterior synechiae induced glaucoma, IOL capture and after cataract (Figs 11.10 and 11.11). These complications are more frequent after congenital and traumatic cataract surgery.

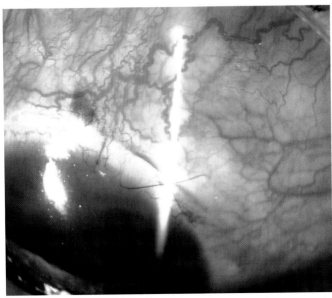

Fig. 11.9: Wound leak due to inadequate wound closure in a case of extracapsular cataract extraction

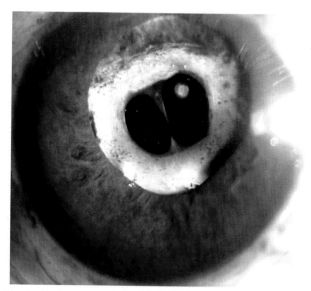

Fig. 11.10: Dense after cataract with extensive posterior synechiae

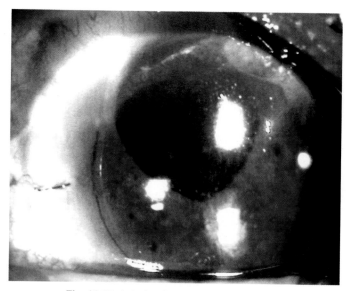

Fig. 11.12: Anterior chamber IOL with updrawn pupil and secondary glaucoma

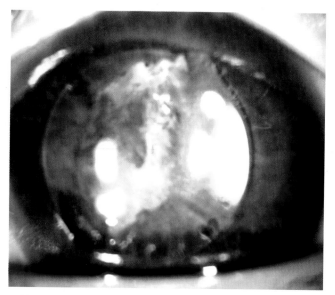

Fig. 11.11: Lens capture with dense after cataract and extensive synechiae. IOL capture with extensive peripheral anterior synechiae

Intracameral bleed from new vessels growing at limbal incision site, or a sulcus-fixated IOL eroding into adjacent tissues, or edges of a rough anterior chamber IOL (once notorious for causing uveitis glaucoma hyphema syndrome) also contribute to the formation of goniosynechiae and gradual zipping of the angle (Fig. 11.12).

Treatment

Meticulous aspiration of viscoelastic substances and intracameral injection of pilocarpine at the end of cataract surgery blunts the early postoperative IOP spike.

To prevent pupil block glaucoma a large surgical peripheral iridectomy must be performed in all cases with anterior chamber IOL implantation. Treatment of pupil block necessitates the use of cycloplegics, antiglaucoma medications and laser iridotomy (more than 1 site is preferred).

Glaucoma due to residual lens matter needs to be individualized; significant lens matter especially nuclear fragments need to be re-aspirated, however, minimal amount of cortical matter resorbs over time.

Medical therapy is same as for primary glaucoma except that usage of prostaglandin derivatives is avoided in early postoperative period in pseudophakic/aphakic eyes for fear of inducing cystoid macular edema and inflammation. Glaucoma filtering surgery when required is usually performed with antifibrotics.

NEOVASCULAR GLAUCOMA

Neovascular glaucoma results from the growth of a fibrovascular membrane over the trabecular meshwork in the anterior chamber angle. Also known as rubeotic glaucoma, it was documented as early as 1871 by Pagenstecher, however, it was only in 1906 and 1937 that Coats and Salus described new vessel formation on the iris in eyes with central retinal venous occlusion and diabetic retinopathy respectively.

Diabetic retinopathy is the most common cause of rubeosis iridis, accounting for one-third cases. The incidence of rubeosis in diabetic patients ranges from 0.25 to 20%, rising to 50% in cases with proliferative diabetic retinopathy (Figs 11.13A and B). Risk factors for developing neovascular glaucoma in diabetic retinopathy are pars plana vitrectomy, after cataract surgery especially if complicated with posterior capsule rupture, post-laser capsulotomy and poor glycemic control. Protective factors are completely attached retina, adequate anterior or peripheral photocoagulation after vitrectomy and use of intraocular silicone oil.

Vascular occlusions are the next common cause of rubeosis iridis. Central retinal vein occlusion (CRVO) accounts for almost 30% of cases, followed by central retinal artery occlusion in 18 % cases (Fig. 11.14). Branch retinal artery/vein occlusion rarely leads to rubeotic glaucoma (Fig. 11.15).

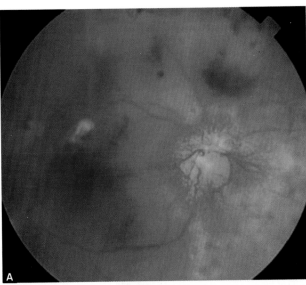

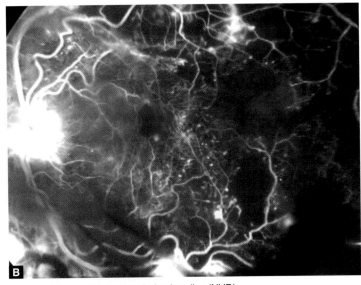

Figs 11.13A and B: (A) Proliferative diabetic retinopathy with neovascularization disc (NVD) and elsewhere (NVE) (B) Fluorescein angiogram

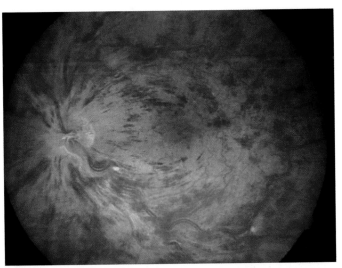

Fig. 11.14: Central retinal vein occlusion

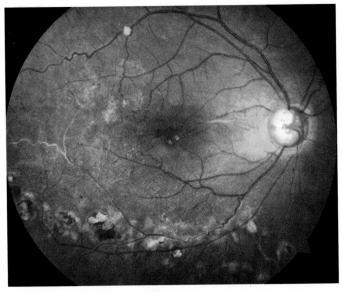

Fig. 11.15: Secondary glaucomatous cupping in lasered branch retinal venous occlusion

Neovascular glaucoma occurs in 40% to 50% of ischemic variant of CRVO within 2-weeks to 2 year period, usual time of onset is within 3 months giving rise to the popular terminology of 90/100 day glaucoma. Non-ischemic type usually does not develop into neovascular glaucoma. Fluorescein angiography is the most important modality to differentiate the two types; however, the differentiation is not sacrosanct as almost 15% of non-ischemic CRVO's convert to ischemic type over a period of 6 months. Therefore, a single angiogram does not rule out any risk of developing neovascular glaucoma in future. A reliable clinical test indicating an ischemic component predicting rubeosis is a relative afferent pupil defect.

The other causes of neovascular glaucoma are chronic retinal detachment associated with proliferative vitreoretinopathy, Eales' disease, chronic recalcitrant uveitis, retinopathy of prematurity, Coat's disease, sickle cell retinopathy, radiation-induced retinopathy, Leber's congenital amaurosis, persistent hyperplastic primary vitreous, carotid artery occlusive disease, temporal (giant cell) arteritis, intraocular tumors, sympathetic ophthalmitis and endophthalmitis (Fig. 11.16).

Etiopathogenesis

Tissue hypoxia caused by diabetes or vascular occlusions is the initiating event, which causes chronic dilatation of iris vessels and subsequent new vessels formation. Vasoproliferative factors namely vascular endothelial growth factor (VEGF), interleukin-6 liberated primarily by Müller cells of the pathological retina diffuse to the anterior segment and induce neovascularization of iris (NVI). The vasoinhibitory balancing factors are formed in the vitreous, lens and retinal pigment epithelial cells. When these vasoinhibitory elements are damaged by vitrectomy or lensectomy, the risk of developing rubeosis increases. Neovascular tissue grows into intertrabecular spaces leading to peripheral anterior synechiae formation, which cover trabecular meshwork. Microfibrils in the new vessels exert a

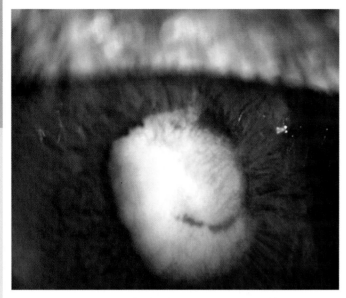

Fig. 11.16: Rubeosis iridis in a post endophthalmitis case

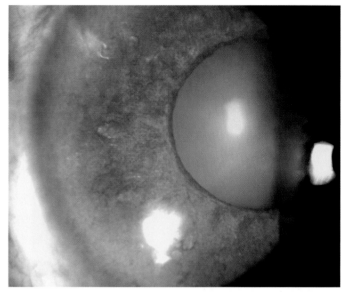

Fig. 11.17: Neovascular glaucoma–rubeotic stage

contractile force, distorting iris tissue causing more peripheral synechiae and ectropion uvea. Eversion of the pigmented posterior epithelium of the iris at the pupillary margin is called as ectropion uvea.

Ocular Features

a. *Rubeosis stage* is characterized by tiny, neovascular tufts present at pupillary margin. The IOP at this stage is essentially normal. It is important at this stage to differentiate abnormal vessels from normal vessels, which may sometimes be visible through stromal atrophy. Normal vessels always lie within the iris stroma, follow a radial pattern and are not associated with ectropion uvea whereas abnormal vessels lie on the surface of iris, have an irregular network and are associated with ectropion uvea due to contractile myofibrils present in the vessels (Fig. 11.17).

b. *Secondary open-angle glaucoma stage* is characterized by NVI, new vessels at angle (NVA) and fibrovascular membrane blocking the trabecular meshwork. The IOP is elevated in this stage. (Fig. 11.18).

c. *Secondary angle-closure glaucoma stage* occurs when the fibrovascular membrane starts to contract and zips up the angle. This stage is characterized by acute severe pain, headache, nausea, vomiting and photophobia; reduced vision and elevated IOP. Its other associated signs are circumcorneal congestion, corneal edema and hyphema.

d. *Advanced/late stage* is characterized by severe rubeosis, synechial angle closure, aqueous flare, hyphema, retinal neovascularization or hemorrhage with optic nerve head cupping, and fixed, mid-dilated pupil with ectropion uvea (Figs 11.19 and 11.20).

In this type of aggressive glaucoma prevention is the watchword. In those patients at risk factors like diabetic retinopathy, vascular occlusions, and Eales' disease periodic slit-lamp

examination and gonioscopy to pick up early signs of rubeosis and synechiae is mandatory. Regular fluorescein angiography to rule out capillary non-perfusion areas, conversion of non-ischemic occlusions into ischemic must be clubbed with the assessment of leakage of fluorescein dye at pupillary margin (which may need an undilated pupil). Dye leakage at pupillary margin is the first sign of incipient NVI.

Differential diagnosis includes angle-closure glaucoma, glaucoma with anterior uveitis, Fuchs heterochromic iridocyclitis, pseudoexfoliation syndrome, iridocorneal endothelial syndrome and the cases of old trauma.

Treatment

Identification of underlying etiology is of paramount importance as treating the cause of hypoxia will ultimately treat the glaucoma. A systemic work up to evaluate status of diabetes,

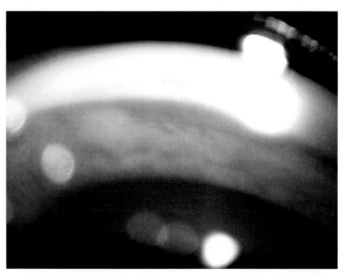

Fig. 11.18: Neovascular glaucoma–neovascularization at the angle

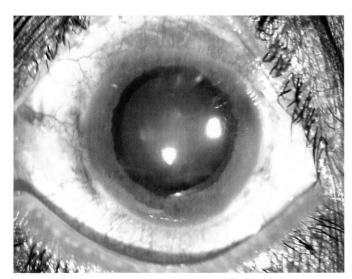

Fig. 11.19: Late-stage neovascular glaucoma–the pupil is fixed and dilated, ectropion uvea and circumcorneal congestion is seen

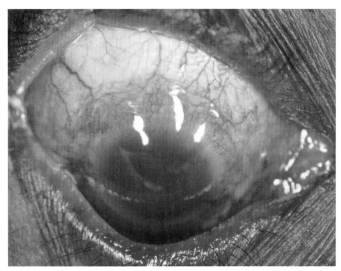

Fig. 11.20: Late-stage neovascular glaucoma–circumcorneal congestion and hyphema due to bleeding of new vessels

tight glycemic control and exclusion of other causes of vascular occlusions is done for every case.

Prevention, the mainstay of treatment is done by retinal ablation–pan retinal photocoagulation or cryotherapy in the case of media opacities, once rubeosis is detected. Goniophotocoagulation may work in the initial stages of NVA combined with a retinal ablation. Panretinal photocoagulation must also be planned prior to vitreous surgery in proliferative diabetic retinopathy cases. Anterior retinal cryopexy is done if media opacities prevent panretinal photocoagulation. Using a 2.5 mm retinal cryoprobe, cryoapplication burns are placed in 3 rows, with 8–12 spots in each quadrant between two rectus muscles. The first row has 3 spots, placed just anterior to the equator, 2 additional rows are placed posterior till the major vascular arcades. Around 32–54 cryoapplications at -70 degrees C , for 8–10 seconds, are given preferably under direct visualization after a 360 degree conjunctival peritomy and isolation of the rectus muscles is done. However, the procedure can be performed without a peritomy over intact conjunctiva. The rule of 8 applies here–minimum 8 spots per quadrant, starting 8 mm from limbus (location of equator) and freeze duration of 8–10 seconds. Regression of neovascularization and control of IOP in almost 80% to 99% cases has been documented. In addition anterior retinal cryopexy also hastens in the clearing of vitreous hemorrhage.

Medications

Atropine ointment decreases ocular congestion and provides relief in pain. Topical corticosteroids decrease inflammation and antiglaucoma medications like topical beta-blockers, bromonidine and carbonic anhydrase inhibitors are used. Pilocarpine is contraindicated as are prostaglandin derivatives since they increase intraocular inflammation.

Surgical Intervention

Surgical intervention is limited to those eyes with potential for useful vision and must only be done after adequate panretinal

photocoagulation/anterior retinal cryopexy. Photocoagulation is followed by a 3–4 weeks interval to allow the new vessels to regress. Atropine, steroids, antiglaucoma medications are used in this interval to keep the patient comfortable. Subsequently, trabeculectomy with antifibrotic regimen like mitomycin-C or 5 fluorouracil is performed. Extensive conjunctival scarring cases may benefit from glaucoma tube shunts like Ahmed, Molteno, Krupin valve (Fig. 11.21). Complications like postoperative hypotony and blockage of internal/external fistula by the new vessels have to be guarded.

Photodynamic therapy (PDT) with verteporfin reduces NVI and NVG, and controls glaucoma (Photodynamic Therapy Study Group). Ongoing trials evaluating efficacy of anti-VEGF therapy include use of bevacizumab (Avastin), pegaptanib (Macugen) and ranibizumab (Lucentis). Anecdotal reports of 1.0 mg of intracameral/intravitreal injections of humanized anti-VEGF monoclonal antibody, bevacizumab, ranibizumab

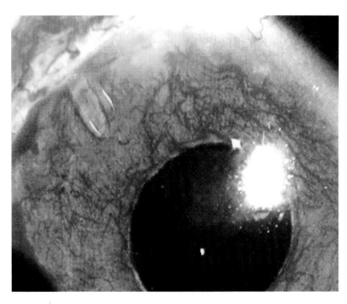

Fig. 11.21: Ahmed glaucoma tube shunt in a neovascular glaucoma case

0..5 mg causing regression of angle neovascularization have been published and VISION trial (VEGF inhibition studies in ocular neovascularization) evaluating 0.3 mg pegaptanib has indicated efficacy of the drug in arresting age-related macular degeneration. However, the jury is still out and final verdict on efficacy, sustainability and safety is awaited.

Cyclodestructive procedures namely cyclocryotherapy, Nd:YAG laser transscleral photocoagulation and diode laser transscleral cyclophotocoagulation are reserved for those with no potential of useful vision. Diode laser transscleral cyclophotocoagulation is being tried by author in eyes with useful vision with good short-term results. In late stages of the disease primary goal of treatment is pain control for which retrobulbar alcohol is a viable option when other modalities fail. Complications documented with its use are external ophthalmoplegia and blepharoptosis. Enucleation remains the last resort for intractable pain associated with neovascular glaucoma.

UVEITIC/INFLAMMATORY GLAUCOMA

Ocular inflammation can cause glaucoma both during active uveitis and after its resolution.

Etiopathogenesis

Depending on the aqueous production, which varies at the different stages of evolution of uveitis, the IOP in uveitic glaucoma fluctuates. The types and causes of glaucoma in uveitis are:

- Secondary open-angle mechanism: Blockage of trabecular meshwork by inflammatory debris and prostaglandin-induced trabeculitis impairs the conventional outflow pathway. Additional causes are the blockage of unconventional uveoscleral pathway by scarring and corticosteroid usage in the treatment of uveitis.
- Secondary closed angle: Peripheral anterior synechiae occur as a consequence of organized inflammatory debris or after peripheral iridotrabecular contact seen during shallow anterior chamber arising after an ocular surgery. Posterior synechiae arising due to inflammatory exudation may cause seclusio pupillae. Both types of synechial closure contribute to angle-closure glaucoma and occur during the later phase of inflammation or during the resolving phase (Figs 11.22 and 11.23).
- Preexisting predisposition to glaucoma in a previously shallow anterior chamber uveitis-induced ciliary body edema causes a forward shift of lens iris diaphragm. This coupled with hyperviscous aqueous overwhelms the inflamed trabecular meshwork. This type of glaucoma usually occurs during the acute phase of uveitis.
- An inflamed ciliary body with decreased aqueous production can lead to hypotony and may mask the glaucoma in the initial phase.

Ocular Features

Typical signs of iridocyclitis ranging from aqueous flare, cells, keratic precipitates, muddy iris, and posterior and peripheral anterior synechiae are visible depending on the severity and duration of the uveitis. All types of anterior uveitis and some types of posterior uveitis can cause secondary glaucoma. Seclusio pupillae is a condition where annular posterior synechiae create a pupil block mechanism for glaucoma (Fig. 11.24). Iris atrophy of varying grades is a clue to prior episodes of iridocyclitis and gonioscopy must be performed in such patients to rule out peripheral anterior synechiae (Figs 11.25 and 11.26).

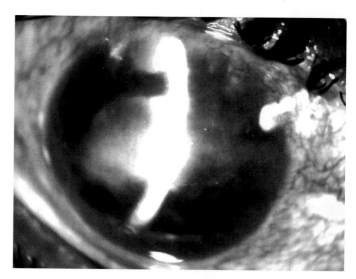

Fig. 11.22: Closed-angle glaucoma mechanism in uveitic glaucoma. Note the iris bombe'formation, the superior peripheral iridectomy blocked by organized inflammatory exudate

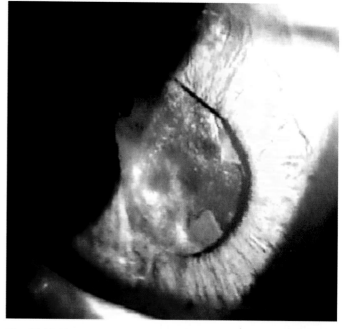

Fig. 11.23: Few posterior synechiae seen, extensive peripheral anterior synechiae cause impaired aqueous outflow

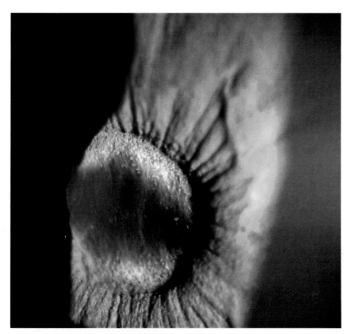

Fig. 11.24: Closed-angle glaucoma mechanism in uveitic glaucoma—seclusio pupillae

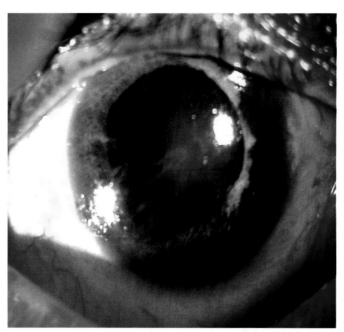

Fig. 11.26: Post-uveitic sphincteric and iris atrophy signifying recurrent angle-closure glaucoma attacks

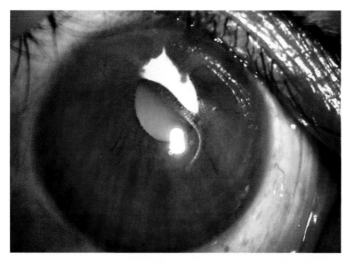

Fig. 11.25: Dense posterior synechiae with iris atrophy with evolving angle-closure glaucoma. Updrawing of pupil due to pull of superior peripheral anterior synechiae is seen

Some Specific Entities

Acute Anterior Uveitis

The commonest cause of recurrent anterior uveitis, glaucoma in these cases is linked to the intensity of inflammation. The HLA-B27 positive variant has more severe disease form. However, glaucoma in this disease usually responds well to antiglaucoma drugs.

Juvenile Rheumatoid Arthritis/Juvenile Idiopathic Arthritis

Glaucoma incidence in these young children ranges from 14 to 27% and has a poor prognostication. In addition, the chronic requirement of topical steroids exacerbates the glaucoma.

Treatment in this disease should never aim at total resolution of aqueous flare, since abnormal iris hyperpermeability does not permit the flare to resolve completely. Steroid usage must thus be limited to topical pulse steroid therapy. The therapy should be used to control acute exacerbations and never for the elimination of aqueous flare.

Pars Planitis

Glaucoma incidence is almost 8% in these cases, thus a dilated retinal exam with indentation to rule out this entity must be undertaken if an explained IOP rise occurs in a uveitis suspect case.

Glaucomatocyclitic Crisis (Posner Schlossman Syndrome)

The disease is characterized by mild recurrent episodes of uniocular iridocyclitis associated with markedly elevated IOP not commensurate with the extent of inflammation. This idiopathic condition occurs in young to middle aged adults, the attack duration varies from few hours to weeks and patient is totally asymptomatic in between the attacks. Dilated pupil, anisocoria, quiet eye, open angles, very high pressures, and mild discomfort relieved by topical corticosteroids or by itself are hallmarks of this condition. This condition needs to be differentiated from angle-closure glaucoma. Probable etiology is herpes simplex infection; some believe it is to be a precursor of open-angle glaucoma.

Fuchs Heterochromic Cyclitis

A uniocular mild, asymptomatic iridocyclitis seen in third to fourth decade, this condition is so asymptomatic that the presenting complaint is most often cataract. Heterochromia of iris (lighter color from fellow eye) noted during cataract assessment gives a clue to this entity. Fine stellate keratic precipitates may be observed along with iris transillumination defects. It is important to diagnose this condition and prescribe intensive preoperative steroids to prevent postoperative inflammation and hyphema. Open-angle glaucoma occurs in 13 to 59% later on in the disease course and persists after the uveitis has subsided. The glaucoma is often unresponsive to medications and requires surgical intervention.

Treatment

Treatment aims to control inflammation completely and as rapidly as possible to curtail the harmful effects of uveitis sequel. Topical corticosteroids usually contain the inflammation, but they are incapable of altering the underlying cause of uveitis, which must be treated at its own merit. Often the inflammation recurs on the withdrawal of steroids thus low-dose steroid may need to be given for long time. The route of administration is topical, but if despite frequent administration the inflammation is not controlled subconjunctival, subtenon and even systemic corticosteroids need to be given. The propensity for steroids to cause IOP rise in steroid responsive patients must always be kept in mind and drugs with less propensity to cause steroid response namely fluorometholone, medrysone, clobetasone and loteprednol etabonate need to be prescribed more often. Nonsteroidal anti-inflammatory drugs like rimexolone, flurbiprofen, indomethacin and diclofenac sodium must be substituted as early as possible. However, these drugs are not as potent as corticosteroids in controlling inflammation. Thus the ophthalmologist needs to strike a balance and fine tune the treatment.

Filtration surgery in these patients has a very poor prognosis and must never be undertaken during the acute uveitis. Filtration fails due to inflammatory sequel blocking the sclerostomy and/or iridectomy (Fig. 11.27). Tube shunts may be tried once trabeculectomy with antifibrotics fails.

STEROID-INDUCED GLAUCOMA

Steroid responsiveness concept was introduced by the landmark studies of Armaly and Becker in mid 1960's. Based on IOP response to topical betamethasone/dexamethasone (0.1%) used qid for 3–6 weeks in normal subjects, they classified three categories of steroid response–high responders where IOP rose to > 15 mm Hg (4%), intermediate responders with IOP increase of 6–5 mm Hg (1/3 rd) and low responders with IOP increase of < 5 mm Hg (2/3 rd). They postulated that steroid response is an inherited condition and that high responder prevalence was more in primary open-angle glaucoma patients.

Etiopathogenesis

Steroids by stabilizing lysosomal membranes reduce their catabolic effect on glycosaminoglycans, and inhibit phagocytosis of trabecular endothelial cells. This increases resistance in the outflow pathway. Effect on cyclic adenosine monophosphate (AMP) and abnormal response of hypothalamic pituitary adrenal axis are some of the other theories, which attempt to explain the increased sensitivity to plasma cortisol levels in these patients. A genetic propensity definitely exists.

Ocular Features

A history of persistent corticosteroid use and abuse is the common denominator. Ocular pathologies like vernal catarrh and post-refractive and ocular surgeries are the reasons for which the patient uses over-the-counter steroids for a long time (Fig. 11.28). Uveitis is a pathology for which steroids are both the rescuer and the enemy if not used judiciously. Concomitant cataract due to steroid abuse is often associated.

In post keratorefractive surgery cases reduced corneal thickness masks the IOP rise, with the tonometer giving a falsely low-pressure reading. Correction algorithms must be used to accurately assess the IOP.

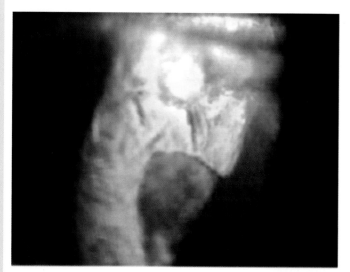

Fig. 11.27: Failed trabeculectomy in uveitic glaucoma. Sclerostomy and iridectomy are blocked by the inflammatory membrane

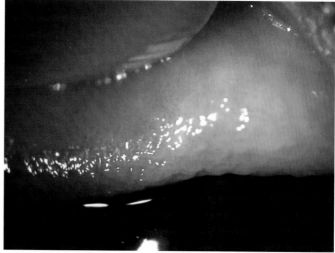

Fig. 11.28: Long-standing use of topical corticosteroids. Vernal catarrh

Topical steroids have a greater propensity for IOP rise than systemic usage. The periocular injections of depot preparations are the most dangerous and often the repository steroid (triamcinolone acetonide) has to be manually excised to control the IOP. The IOP enhancing effects are proportional to the anti-inflammatory potency and the dosage of steroid preparations.

Treatment

The discontinuation of steroids is often the solution and if not possible substitution with a nonsteroidal and noninflammatory drug is the answer. The acute form of glaucoma resolves within days and the chronic form requires 2–4 weeks. If the glaucoma persists despite steroid withdrawal antiglaucoma medications are tried and sometimes excision of depot steroid is necessary. Rarely surgery is warranted. The pathological conjunctiva of eyes suffering from chronic allergy of chronic allergy eyes along with poor tear film complicates the trabeculectomy postoperative course and bleb failure is quite common in these patients.

RETINAL CONDITIONS CAUSING GLAUCOMA

Retinopathy of Prematurity

The glaucoma presents at 3–6 months of age once the cicatricial phase starts. Contracture of retrolental mass causes anterior chamber (AC) shallowing and angle-closure glaucoma. The child presents with nausea, vomiting and is often misdiagnosed as a gastric episode. In addition, longstanding retinal detachment causes rubeotic glaucoma. Trabecular dysgenesis is another cause for glaucoma in some cases. The cornea in these children is small, steep, with a convex iris and shallow AC. Continued contraction of retrolental membrane may cause a spontaneous deepening of AC and resolution of glaucoma. Continued vigilance is needed as glaucoma can intervene at any stage later on in life.

Treatment

A large peripheral iridectomy is warranted as smaller peripheral iridectomy often closes. A prophylactic peripheral iridectomy in severe retinopathy of prematurity with shallow anterior chamber is now recommended.

Medical therapy is often ineffective, cycloplegics and steroids may be tried to reduce the cicatricial element. Lensectomy with vitreoretinal surgery may save the vision however, the surgery itself can be complicated by the development of glaucoma.

Nanophthalmos

Described as the phakic patient wearing aphakic glasses, this condition is characterized by high hyperopia due to abnormally small ocular dimensions, microcornea, shallow anterior chamber, high lens-eye volume, narrow angle, along with

retinal pigmentary dystrophy and cystic macular degeneration. Angle-closure glaucoma usually manifests in the fourth to fifth decade. An altered glycosaminoglycans and fibronectin metabolism causes the sclera to become abnormally thick, which causes compression of vortex veins. During intraocular surgery the lowering of IOP causes abrupt pressure changes across the vortex veins leading to leakage, uveal effusion and exudative retinal detachment. Prophylactic lamellar sclerotomy over the vortex veins for decompression is done before entering the chamber, to reduce this sight-threatening complication. Laser iridectomy/gonioplasty should be tried to treat the glaucoma as they often prove effective. Subsequent lens extraction alone may control the glaucoma.

Retinal Detachment /Surgery

Retinal detachments are usually associated with low IOP however, in certain conditions glaucoma may supervene. An idiopathic open-angle glaucoma can occur in 4 to 6% of retinal detachment, which is unrelated to myopia or use of miotics. Schwartz syndrome is a condition wherein unilateral retinal detachment, aqueous cells and flare are associated with open-angle glaucoma. Obstruction of trabecular meshwork with the damaged outer segment of photoreceptors and inflammatory cells is the postulated mechanism for this glaucoma. Angle-closure glaucoma can occur due to ciliochoroidal effusion in a case of retinal detachment.

Pars Plana Vitrectomy

a. *Acute rise of IOP:* In the early postoperative period after a fluid gas exchange IOP rises in 20 to 26% cases, due to gas expansion. Scleral buckling may cause the transient shallowing of AC, occlusion of vortex veins, and congestion and forward rotation of ciliary body leading to high IOP.

A high index of suspicion is warranted as glaucoma is often overlooked due to falsely low IOP due to reduced scleral rigidity and inadequacy of tonometric measurement in gas filled eyes. Tono-Pen or Goldman applanation tonometers are the more reliable instruments.

b. *Late rise of IOP:* Vitreous hemorrhage-induced ghost cell glaucoma, emulsified silicone oil, uveitis, rubeosis due to failed retinal detachment surgery are some of the late causes of glaucoma (Figs 11.29 and 11.30). With the use of silicone oil glaucoma incidence varies from 5 to 50%. Both angle-closure pupil blocks due to silicone oil in AC and open-angle glaucoma due to silicone bubbles/macrophages with phagocytosed silicone blocking the trabecular meshwork can occur.

Treatment and Prophylaxis

Since the specific gravity of silicone oil is less than water, it rises up and blocks a conventional superior peripheral iridectomy. Thus Ando recommended an inferior intraoperatively peripheral iridectomy concomitant with silicone oil that used to prevent

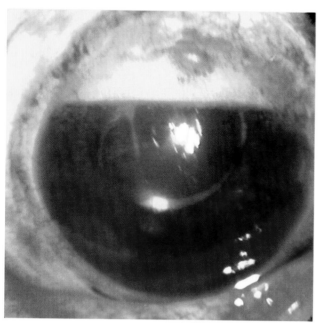

Fig. 11.29: Silicone oil in the anterior chamber. Inverse pseudohypopyon due to emulsified silicone oil, blocking a superior peripheral iridectomy

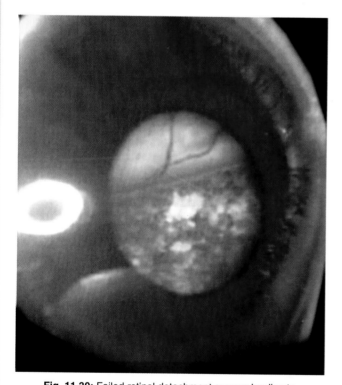

Fig. 11.30: Failed retinal detachment surgery leading to neovascular glaucoma

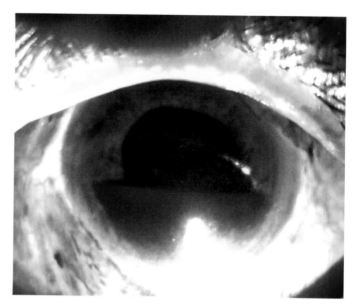

Fig. 11.31: Post-traumatic hyphema resulting in glaucoma

POST-TRAUMATIC GLAUCOMA

Blunt injuries constitute almost 40% of ocular trauma cases and primarily affect young productive individuals in whom the consequences of vision loss are more pronounced and debilitating. The underlying eye is often totally healthy therefore timely and appropriate management of these injuries may restore vision to a greater extent than in those with underlying primary pathology. Glaucoma complicates the situation in many such injury events, timely management of which restores the productive vision of the individual.

a. *Acute onset:* After concussional trauma, glaucoma may occur due to acute inflammation, hyphema with or without angle recession, traumatic iridocyclitis, and lens dislocation/rupture/ intumescence (Figs 11.31 and 11.32). Hyphemas are caused by the distortion of anterior chamber angle with subsequent rupture of iris or ciliary body vessels. Clot retraction starts after 3–5 days and may be associated with re-bleeding. Hypotony associated with cyclodialysis cleft or retinal detachment may mask the glaucoma in the early phase of trauma.

A large hyphema (total or eight-ball hyphema) causes increased IOP by blocking the aqueous outflow and causing pupil block with subsequent symptoms of acute angle-closure glaucoma.

b. *Late onset*
    i. *Angle recession:* Described in 1962 by Wolff and Zimmerman, this condition occurs due to tear in ciliary body between longitudinal and connecting circular and oblique fibers resulting in fibrosis and the scarring of trabecular meshwork. Hydrodynamic forces generated during trauma forcefully push aqueous against ciliary body causing the tear. The tear is peripheral to arterial arcade of ciliary body and disrupts branches of anterior

pupil from blocking glaucoma. For glaucoma due to emulsified silicone oil, vitrectomy with oil removal needs to be done.

Post Photocoagulation

Self-limiting ciliary body swelling with outpouring of fluid leading to exudative retinochoroidal detach can cause a transient rise in IOP.

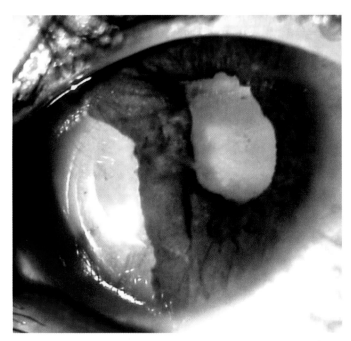

Fig. 11.32: Post-traumatic glaucoma. Iridodialysis with traumatic intumescent cataract

sphincter tears, lens and posterior segment injury are often associated and determine the final visual prognosis.

ii. *Ghost cell/khaki cell/hemolytic glaucoma:* A condition where distorted, non-pliable, khaki-colored RBCs migrate from a resolving vitreous hemorrhage (2–3 week old) and block the trabecular meshwork. Red blood cells trapped in vitreous transform as they age within 1–3 weeks from pliable, biconcave cells to rigid, spherical, khaki-colored cells due to partial loss of hemoglobin. Residual intracellular hemoglobin denatures into Heinz bodies, which characterizes these cells. These rigid khaki-colored RBCs lower outflow facility three times more than fresh RBCs. The patient presents with history of trauma, more than two weeks ago, with a mildly inflamed eye, vitreous hemorrhage, disruption of anterior hyaloid phase and elevated IOP (Fig. 11.34). The RBCs layer down in the anterior chamber in tan-colored stripes and can be confused with a hypopyon. If there is concomitant fresh blood then the ghost cells occupy the tan stripe in background of fresh red RBCs, which presents as "Candy stripe" sign.

iii. *Siderosis:* Retained iron foreign body can also be a cause for post-traumatic glaucoma.

Management

Gonioscopy is the clinching investigation and would delineate angle recession, peripheral anterior synechiae (PAS), or as the cause of glaucoma. It must, however, not be performed in acute phase (within 4 weeks) for risk of causing further bleeding due to manipulation with the goniolens. Angle recession is visible as wide ciliary body band, sometimes as a distinct scleral spur or posteriorly displaced iris root. Associated features are torn iris

and posterior ciliary arteries leading to hyphema. On gonioscopy angle recession presents as irregular widening of ciliary body band, which has a slate grey appearance (Fig. 11.33). Trauma history may often be vague and the angle recession is not commensurate with the intensity of injury. However, glaucoma is commensurate with extent of clock hours of angle recession. Incidence of angle recession in traumatic hyphema is high (55–70%), but incidence of glaucoma varies from 4%, if less than 6 clock hours are affected, to 20%, if more than 6 clock hours are involved. The IOP rise occurs as early as few months and as late as 40 years after injury. In those presenting late, angle recession merely unmasks a predisposition to open-angle glaucoma. The life-time risk of developing glaucoma in the fellow non-traumatized eye is 50% thus trauma probably initiates the glaucoma damage cascade in the genetically predisposed eyes. Iris

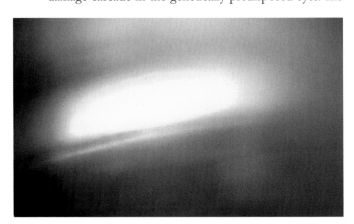

Fig. 11.33: Wide slate grey ciliary body band is visible

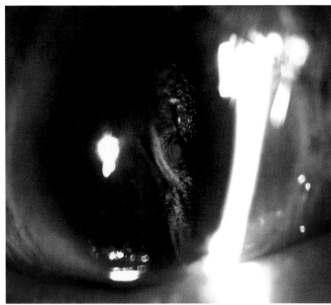

Fig. 11.34: Post-traumatic glaucoma. Resolving vitreous hemorrhage with glaucoma

processes and pigment clumps on trabecular meshwork (Fig. 11.35). In ghost cell glaucoma the angle is open and discolored due to the khaki cells in the meshwork.

A dilated anterior segment exam must be performed after gonioscopy to rule out the subtle evidence of zonular dialysis and indirect ophthalmoscopy with indentation must be done to rule out peripheral retinal dialysis or breaks.

Hyphema: The patient of hyphema is advised restricted activity and sleeping in head elevated position. Use of aspirin or nonsteroidal anti-inflammatory drugs, which hinder platelet activity are restricted. Topical corticosteroids are used judiciously; their anti-inflammatory activity has to be weighed against their propensity to increase IOP in steroid responders. They are prescribed at 4–6 hourly intervals and tapered once inflammation resolves. Use of aminocaproic acid to prevent re-bleeding is controversial. The risk of re-bleeding is variable and the evidence that aminocaproic reduces its incidence anecdotal. This antifibrinolytic agent prevents clot from dissolving early by the inhibiting conversion of plasminogen to plasmin, if given the dose is 50 mg/kg every four hours with maximum dose of 30 g/day for 5 days.

Topical β blockers, adrenergic agents and carbonic anhydrase inhibitors are the drugs commonly used to control the IOP. Pilocarpine, sympathomimetic or prostamide group of antiglaucoma drugs are avoided due to their propensity to increase inflammation. Use of systemic acetazolamide is contraindicated in sickle cell disease patients as this drug is known to cause metabolic acidosis thereby increasing sickling of the RBC in anterior chamber.

Indications for surgical drainage are specific namely – IOP of more than 50 mm Hg for 5 days, more than 35 mm Hg for 7 days, total "eight ball" hyphema not resolving for 9 days, or early signs of corneal blood staining. Surgical drainage is accomplished by simple paracentesis, washout of anterior chamber, viscoexpression of clot or automated extraction. Usually a two port entry is performed and a total removal must not be aimed at.

Angle recession: For angle recession glaucoma treatment protocol is similar to that of primary open-angle glaucoma. Miotics are contraindicated as they reduce uveoscleral outflow, which is the main pathway of aqueous outflow in these patients. Both eyes of an angle recession patient need to be examined annually, life long to detect early glaucoma change. Glaucoma surgery is more likely to fail, thus adjunctive antifibrotic are used when filtering surgery is needed.

For ghost cell glaucoma medical treatment usually suffices as the condition is usually transient, rarely vitrectomy along with anterior chamber wash out is required to control recalcitrant glaucoma.

Penetrating Injury

Initial IOP is always low due to open wound, but after repair it may rise due to lens intumescence, inflammation or hyphema. In the late phase inflammatory sequel like extensive PAS, angle recession, epithelial ingrowth, sympathetic ophthalmia, retained foreign body with subsequent siderosis or chalcosis also cause glaucoma (Fig. 11.36).

Meticulous wound closure with removal of incarcerated uveal tissue, removal of foreign body, lens aspiration if integrity of anterior capsule is doubtful, the adequate reformation of anterior chamber minimizes glaucoma propensity in these patients. Adequate systemic antibiotics with judicious steroids both topical and systemic (if ciliary zone involvement) prevent visually disabling consequences of the injury.

Before attempting heroic surgeries to control the glaucoma it is always wise to evaluate the posterior segment thoroughly, wherever possible. A large central choroidal rupture, maculopathy, optic nerve avulsion would preclude any visual recovery thus necessitating a rethink in glaucoma management strategy (Fig. 11.37).

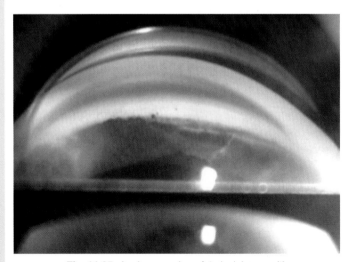
Fig. 11.35: Angle recession of 4 clock hours with increased trabecular pigmentation

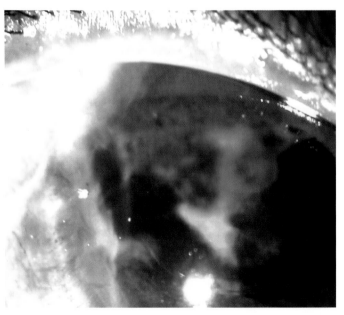
Fig. 11.36: Perforating injury repair with angle recession glaucoma

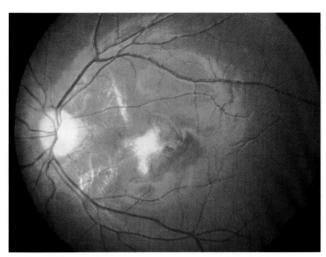

Fig. 11.37: Choroidal rupture with macular edema in a case of concussion injury and angle recession glaucoma

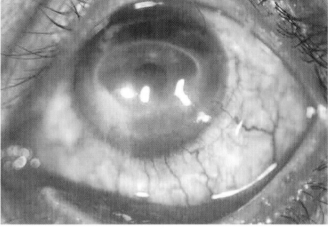

Fig. 11.38: Case with 360 degree vascularization, dry eye and glaucoma in the case of chemical burn

Chemical Burn

Glaucoma can occur both in the acute and late setting. Alkali burn patients have a greater propensity to develop secondary glaucoma.

Ocular Manifestations

Acute stage: The sequence of events of keratocyte coagulation, mucopolysaccharide lysis, collagen shortening, anterior chamber inflammation and shrinkage cause a variable IOP response. Intraocular pressure elevation occurs in a bimodal pattern. An initial rise due to collagen fibril hydration, longitudinal shortening of collagen fibers and the distortion of angle is followed with a second rise within a few hours. The second spike is due to obstruction of outflow channels by increased episcleral pressure, prostaglandin mediated inflammatory trabeculitis and uveitis.

Late stage: In the healing phase, the IOP varies depending on the extent of burn. It is balanced by decreased aqueous secretion due to ciliary body damage versus continued conjunctival scarring/shrinkage contributed to obstructed outflow pathway. Development of peripheral anterior synechiae, fibrous in growth and increase in episcleral pressure contributes to glaucoma (Fig. 11.38).

The inevitable sequel of dry eye, conjunctival scarring, symblepharon and fornix shortening make treatment of glaucoma with medical or surgical means a Herculean task (Fig. 11.39).

Treatment

The focus is on reducing the chemical insult by copious wash and decreasing inflammation by the judicious use of corticosteroids. Glaucoma is managed by aqueous suppressants. Miotics and prostamides may increase intraocular inflammation thus are best avoided. The prognosis for such patients is often poor, but timely trabeculectomy can save the eye if performed once the active phase has resolved. Symblepharon with subsequent fornix shortening may prevent trabeculectomy or tube shunt

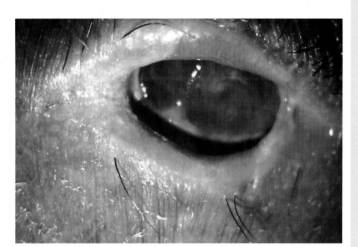

Fig. 11.39: Post-chemical burn symblepharon. Shortened fornix with secondary glaucoma is present

from being performed, in such situations laser cyclophotocoagulation remains the only option.

Raised Episcleral Venous Pressure

Goldman's equation defines as IOP to be the sum of secretion of aqueous ÷ facility of outflow + episcleral venous pressure, thus any increase in episcleral venous pressure from normal 8–10 mm Hg would raise the IOP. Episcleral venous pressure is affected by body posture, drainage in ophthalmic veins, external jugular vein, and cavernous and petrosal sinus. Impedance in the venous drainage at any of these sites leads to the stagnation of venous blood and retrograde transmission of the increased venous pressure to eye, which translates into increased IOP. The cause may be venous obstruction or arteriovenous abnormality. Thyroid ophthalmopathy, Sturge-Weber syndrome, cavernous sinus thrombosis, jugular vein obstruction and superior vena cava syndrome are causes of venous obstruction whereas carotid cavernous fistula, dural cavernous fistula, or orbital varixes are the etiologies of arteriovenous abnormality.

Etiopathogenesis

Raised episcleral venous pressure automatically translates into IOP rise as per Goldman equation. The other mechanisms for glaucoma includes trabecular damage after chronically elevated episcleral pressure, angle-closure component due to venous stasis in vortex veins causing choroidal detachment and neovascular element after prolonged ocular ischemia due to reduced arterial flow.

Clinical Features

Raised episcleral venous pressure commonly manifests as engorged dilated episcleral veins. The other presentations range from proptosis, chemosis, hemorrhagic choroidal detachment, and the signs of ischemia like rubeosis iridis. The port wine stain of Sturge-Weber syndrome is unmistakable (Figs 11.40 and 11.41). Gonioscopy reveals an open angle with occasional evidence blood in Schlemm's canal (an inconsistent finding) (Fig. 11.42).

The differential diagnoses are dilated blood vessels seen in conjunctival inflammations/infections, episcleritis, scleritis, and intraocular tumors. In raised episcleral venous pressure the blood vessels are larger in caliber, more diffuse and criss cross in pattern.

Systemic Associations

Comorbidity due to associated systemic associations is high and the eye sign is a clue to a graver underlying disorder.

- *Thyroid ophthalmopathy*: A very common cause of exophthalmos in the middle age, the disease is characterized by the deposition of mucopolysaccharides and lymphocytes in the

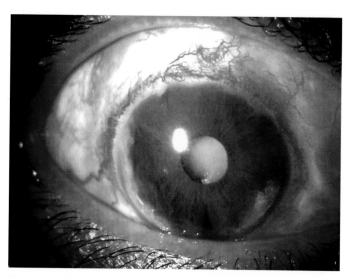

Fig. 11.41: Presence of secondary glaucoma in Sturge-Weber syndrome

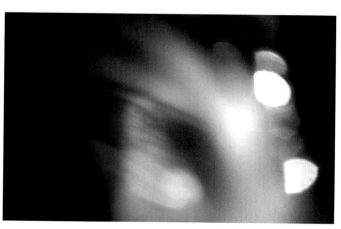

Fig. 11.42: Blood in Schlemm's canal

extraocular muscles causing restrictive myopathy. The inferior rectus muscle is affected most frequently, leading to a restriction in upgaze with classical increase in IOP during the upward deviation of the eyeball. Orbital congestion causes elevated episcleral venous pressure and the deposition of mucoplysaccharide deposits in trabecular meshwork reduces outflow facility. Visual loss occurs more often due to optic nerve compression and exposure keratopathy than glaucoma (Fig. 11.43).

- *Carotid cavernous fistula*: It is an idiopathic or post-traumatic condition caused due to fistula created between internal carotid artery and cavernous sinus, it presents as spontaneous pulsating proptosis. An accompanying bruit is often heard. The ocular features are dilated tortuous blood vessels with congested swollen extraocular muscles presenting as a quiet red eye. Glaucoma can occur as a result of increased episcleral pressure, angle closure secondary to increased intraorbital pressure and secondary to iris neovascularization (Fig. 11.44).
- Bronchogenic carcinoma casing superior vena caval obstruction and subsequent increased episcleral pressure. It can be complicated by otitis media, cavernous thrombosis in addition to glaucoma.

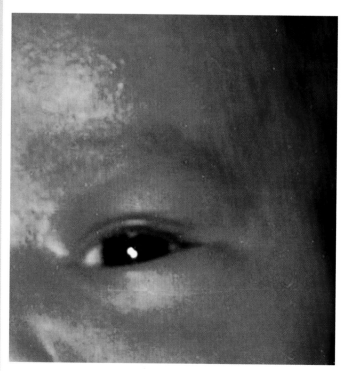

Fig. 11.40: Port wine stain in Sturge-Weber syndrome

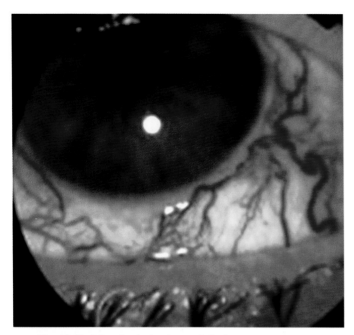

Fig. 11.43: Dilated episcleral vessels in thyroid exophthalmos

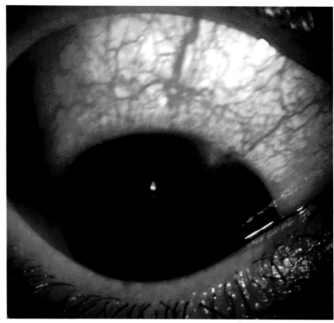

Fig. 11.44: Dilated episcleral vessels in carotid cavernous fistula

Treatment

As for all secondary glaucomas, the treatment of underlying condition is necessary to treat the IOP. The underlying etiologies often cause mortality and take precedence over glaucoma management. Thyroid ophthalmopathy often requires systemic corticosteroids or orbital decompression in addition to controlling the hormonal levels. Steroids are prescribed if patient develops primary gaze glaucoma; gaze dependent IOP rise due to infiltrative myopathy does not justify systemic steroid therapy. In recalcitrant glaucoma orbital decompression should be attempted before resorting to filtration surgery. Carotid cavernous fistula needs embolization for treatment whereas low-flow dural cavernous fistulas may undergo spontaneous closure.

Topical beta-blockers, carbonic anhydrase inhibitors or alpha agonists are the first choice antiglaucoma drugs. Prostaglandins act on uveoscleral outflow pathway, which is deranged thus in these types of glaucomas their role is limited. Glaucoma filtering surgery is often associated with choroidal effusion or hemorrhage. Preoperatively lowering of IOP, prophylactic sclerostomy or placing an anterior chamber maintainer are some of the safeguards used to prevent choroidal effusion. Trabeculectomy with releasable sutures should be done as a controlled IOP release is very important postoperatively.

MALIGNANT GLAUCOMA

Identified by the indefatigable von Graefe in 1869 this recalcitrant glaucoma gets its name due to its poor response to any therapy. Re-christened as aqueous misdirection syndrome/ciliary block, it often complicates the postoperative course of trabeculectomy in angle-closure glaucoma almost to the tune of 2 to 4%. It is also known to occur after cataract surgery, after miotic therapy and laser procedures. Eyes with short axial length, e.g. hyperopia, nanophthalmos are more susceptible to this condition.

Etiopathogenesis

Relative pupil block leads to the trapped aqueous getting misdirected into vitreous cavity wherein it forms pockets, subsequently leading to the inflammatory swelling and anterior rotation of ciliary body, cilolenticular/cilovitreal block followed by anterior movement of lens iris diaphragm, and shallow anterior chamber. Abnormal slackness of lens zonules contributes to the forward movement of iris lens diaphragm.

Clinical Features

The glaucoma is accompanied by extremely high IOP, pain and an extremely shallow anterior chamber (Fig. 11.45). The patient has often undergone a glaucoma/cataract surgery few days or weeks ago. The event is usually precipitated by the cessation of cycloplegics. The anterior chamber is uniformly flat and the IOP is in the range of 30's to 40's. A patent peripheral iridectomy, flat bleb, no choroidal detachment, and no evidence of wound leak are the hallmarks of this entity. Ultrasound may pick up the aqueous pockets in the vitreous cavity along with an anterior rotation of ciliary body. A high index of suspicion is necessary and pupil block glaucoma must always be ruled out before diagnosing malignant glaucoma. Pupil block glaucoma has irregular anterior chamber (AC), which is deeper in the center, shallow in the periphery, iris bombe, and a blocked or inadequate PI. Whereas in malignant glaucoma the anterior chamber is diffusely shallow. Sometimes if a PI is not seen, it is worthwhile to perform one and malignant glaucoma diagnosis is confirmed only once the AC does not deepen after patent PI.

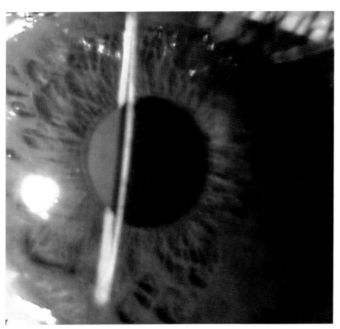

Fig. 11.45: Diffusely shallow anterior chamber in a case of malignant glaucoma

The other differential diagnosis is suprachoroidal hemorrhage where the choroidal elevation can be seen on direct ophthalmoscopy and confirmed on ultrasound.

Treatment

Strong cycloplegics like atropine sulfate need to be initiated along with topical steroids. Atropine relaxes the cilary muscle and enables the lens iris diaphragm to move backwards. Antiglaucoma drugs like beta-blockers, alpha agonists and carbonic anhydrase inhibitors are employed to reduce aqueous secretion. Intravenous mannitol 1–1.5 g/kg is used to shrink the vitreous and allow the lens iris diaphragm to fall back. Systemic acetazolamide is also given. The patient needs to be maintained on cycloplegic therapy for months/years and even indefinitely since the condition often recurs on withdrawal of therapy. Miotics are contraindicated.

In pseudophakic or aphakic patients, a Nd:YAG laser is used to break the anterior hyaloid face/posterior capsule to release the sequestered aqueous in the vitreous. More than one opening needs to be made without compromising the stability of the IOL. The PI must also be enlarged with the laser. In addition the anterior chamber needs to be reformed with viscoelastic through a paracentesis. The side port made at the time of glaucoma or cataract surgery comes in handy for this purpose. If these procedures fail pars plana vitrectomy is performed to remove the sequestered aqueous and allow the lens iris diaphragm to fall back.

Medical and laser therapy is successful only in 50% of cases and in case of no response within 3–5 days surgical intervention is done. In phakic eyes very often a lensectomy vitrectomy is required, however, all efforts must be made to give lens sparing vitrectomy a trial.

In the fellow eye the risk of malignant glaucoma occurring after an intraocular surgery is very high, thus it is recommended to perform a prophylactic laser PI prior to doing an intraocular surgery in the fellow eye. Cycloplegics must be started immediately after surgery in an attempt to abort malignant glaucoma.

GLAUCOMA ASSOCIATED WITH CORNEAL AND UVEAL CONDITIONS

Iridocorneal Endothelial Syndrome

Iridocorneal endothelial syndrome (ICE) is a group of disorders wherein abnormal corneal endothelium grows over the iris and angle structures. Over time, this membrane contracts causing corneal edema, iris atrophy and secondary angle-closure glaucoma. Three different entities comprising ICE syndrome are: Chandler's syndrome, essential iris atrophy and iris nevus (Cogan-Reese) syndrome. This unilateral condition manifests in third to sixth decade and commonly afflicts females. Intraocular pressure is not always commensurate with the amount of angle closure.

Clinical Features

Corneal edema, glaucoma and iris hypoplasia are the hallmarks of this unilateral disease. Slit-lamp biomicroscopy reveals abnormal endothelium posterior to a normal Descemet's membrane giving rise to a fine hammered silver appearance of the posterior cornea. Specular microscopy demonstrates typical ICE cells, which demonstrate loss of hexagonality along with pleomorphism. The typical ICE endothelial cells have a central clear zone, an intervening dark area, surrounded by a light peripheral perimeter just within the cell boundary. The condition needs to be differentiated from Fuchs' dystrophy, which is bilateral, seen in older individuals and is characterized by a thickened Descemet's membrane and endothelial guttata. High PAS are rampant in the anterior chamber angle, they occur due to the contraction of the abnormal corneal endothelial layer (Fig. 11.46). These subsequently zip up the angle and secondary angle-closure glaucoma occurs almost in 50% of the ICE cases. The contraction of the abnormal corneal endothelial layer also causes iris hole formation in the area opposite to the PAS formation. The iris nodules in Cogan-Reese syndrome are composed of iris stroma, which has been pinched out by the contracting, proliferating abnormal corneal endothelial layer.

Initially painful blurred vision episodes occur early in the morning after the pathological cornea has been subjected to the hypoxia occurring during sleep, however, later on the edema persists throughout the day. Iris atrophy may assume different patterns ranging from polycoria, heterochromia, ectropion uvea, and corectopia or stromal atrophy. The three variants differ in the proportion of iris or corneal changes. In Chandler syndrome, corneal element is more prominent whereas the iris atrophy element is more evident in essential (progressive) iris atrophy. A less aggressive pattern of iris atrophy coupled with

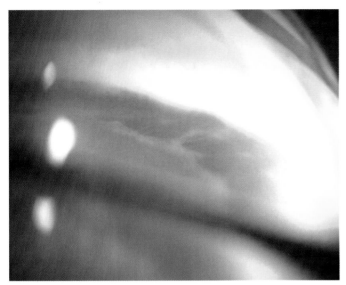

Fig. 11.46: Gonioscopic view of a case of essential iris atrophy demonstrating high peripheral synechiae with iris atrophy

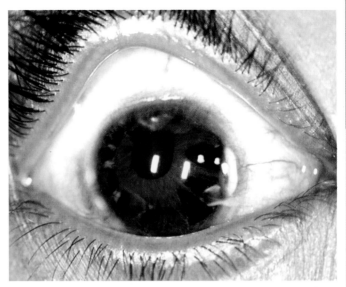

Fig. 11.47: Axenfeld-Rieger syndrome with iris stromal thinning and corectopia

tan colored nodules on anterior iris surface suggests Cogan-Reese (iris nevus) syndrome.

Treatment

Hypertonic saline preparations are used to control corneal edema and once secondary glaucoma intervenes antiglaucoma drugs are added. Miotics are usually ineffective. Trabeculectomy when required often fails due to blockage of sclerostomy due to ICE membrane regrowth. Glaucoma tube shunts can also be tried.

Fuchs Endothelial Dystrophy

It is an aging bilateral disorder that is present with visual loss, in sixth to seventh decade with a predilection for women. An autosomal dominant pattern has been described. The etiology is abnormal corneal endothelium, which causes the thickening of Descemet's membrane. The identifying features are endothelial guttata, which are dark areas overlapping cell borders, reduced cell count and polymegathism. Current view states that glaucoma is not so common an association and is more often angle closure subtype, rather than the previously thought open angle. Differential diagnosis includes ICE and pseudoexfoliation syndromes.

Treatment

Medical management usually suffices, an angle-closure component warrants an iridotomy to arrest the progress.

Axenfeld-Rieger Anomaly

It is an autosomal dominant bilateral developmental disorder that occurs due to abnormality in the neural crest development. A part of neurocristopathies, the disorder occurs due to disorder in neural crest cell migration, differentiation or regression.

Neural crest cells differentiate into corneal stroma and endothelium, sclera, trabecular meshwork, iris stroma in addition to giving rise to bones and cartilage of upper face, dental papillae, and mesenchyme of forebrain and pituitary gland. In Axenfeld-Rieger's anomaly residual primordial endothelium is retained over angle and iris. This endothelium contracts causing the high insertion of iris, stromal thinning and hole formation of iris. Secondary glaucoma occurs in almost 50% cases and is due to both angle closure and trabecular dysgenesis elements. If glaucoma and/or systemic malformations are associated, the entity is known as Axenfeld-Rieger's syndrome. It usually presents within the first two decades of life.

Ocular Features

Posterior embryotoxon (prominent anteriorly displaced Schwalbe's line) is the almost ubiquitous finding on gonioscopy. Sometimes, it is so anteriorly placed that it is visible as opaque white ring on the posterior surface of the cornea internal to the limbus. Irido-corneal adhesions arising from the Schwalbe's line may obscure the angle details. Iris hypoplasia of variable extent is almost always present with iris holes, corectopia, and polycoria and ectropion uvea. The component of iris hypoplasia is the Rieger's part of the anomaly (Fig. 11.47).

Associated features are high refractive errors, deprivation amblyopia and cataract, in addition to glaucoma. Glaucoma filtering surgery is often required to control the glaucoma, but the visual prognosis for these children is often poor.

Systemic Associations

Since neural crest development is defective, the other structures derived from neural crest like facial bones, teeth and mesenchyme of pituitary gland are also involved. Dental defects like microdontia (peg like teeth), hypodontia (decreased number of teeth), anodontia, maxillary hypoplasia, telecanthus, micrognathia and mandibular prognathism are associated (Fig. 11.48). It, sometimes, even leads to middle-ear deafness, heart defects, mental deficiencies and empty sella syndrome. A mutation of PITX2 gene is associated with this condition.

Peter's Anomaly

Peter's anomaly represents the extreme spectrum of anterior chamber developmental disorder wherein a central corneal endothelium, Descemet's and post-stromal deficient defect is associated with corneal opacity, iris adhesions to the defect and often keratolenticular contact. It maybe bilateral or unilateral and presents at birth. Sporadic in occurrence, an autosomal recessive and dominant mode have also been documented. Almost 50% patients ultimately develop glaucoma. Systemic associations include hearing defects, craniofacial dysostosis, spinal defects, and cardiac and genitourinary abnormalities.

Treatment requires a penetrating keratoplasty along with glaucoma filtering surgery, but the visual prognosis in these infants is very poor.

Aniridia

A rare bilateral congenital condition characterized by the underdevelopment of the iris, the term is a misnomer as a rudimentary iris stump is visible on gonioscopy (Fig. 11.49). It is associated with the poor development of the retina and poor vision. The commonest mode of transmission is autosomal dominant followed by sporadic (associated with Wilms' tumor). A mutation in PAX6 gene located in the short arm of chromosome 11 is associated with WAGR syndrome, acronym for Wilms' (nephroblastoma), aniridia, genitourinary abnormalities and mental retardation. Rarely autosomal recessive type of

inheritance occurs, which is associated with cerebellar ataxia in addition to mental retardation.

Ocular Manifestations

Aniridia is associated with foveal/disc hypoplasia, nystagmus, strabismus all of which contribute to the decreased vision. A progressive corneal pannus, microcornea, localized lenticular opacity, poor zonular integrity are the associated features. Photophobia is a predominant complaint and is linked to the extent of aniridia. Progressive contracture of peripheral iris strands causes posterior synechiae, which compound the initial trabeculodysgenesis. Glaucoma occurs in almost 50 to 75% of aniridia patients due to progressive synechial closure (angle closure), which manifests in late childhood or adolescence.

Treatment

Glaucoma filtering/tube shunt surgery is often required as medical therapy proves to be inadequate in controlling the glaucoma. The concomitant use of antifibrotics is beneficial as most of the glaucomas is present at a young age.

Postkeratoplasty Glaucoma

Secondary glaucoma occurring in a penetrating keratoplasty patient has a double impact on vision. Not only does it damage the optic nerve, but it also impairs the clarity of the grafted cornea and causes graft failure. The incidence of IOP raises postkeratoplasty ranges from 30% in the early postoperative period to 18% in the late postoperative period. Suturing induced distortion of angle structures, inadequate wound closure, wrong sized graft, long-term use of corticosteroids, preexisting glaucoma propensity, keratoplasty combined with

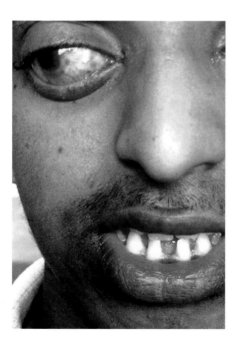

Figs 11.48: Dental anomalies of microdontia and hypodontia in Axenfeld-Rieger syndrome

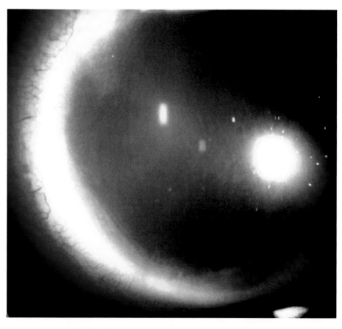

Fig. 11.49: Aniridia with secondary glaucoma

cataract surgery/vitrectomy, graft rejection and repeat graft are the common causes of secondary glaucoma in these patients.

Ocular Manifestations

In the early postoperative period uveitis, retained viscoelastics, hemorrhage and shallow anterior chamber leading to peripheral anterior synechiae all contribute to glaucoma. A unique mechanism of glaucoma is due to collapse of trabecular meshwork due to incision of the Descemet's membrane leading to the loss of anterior support and compression of angle. Corneal edema due to endothelial damage is associated with variable extent of PAS. Graft rejection, PAS, epithelial in growth and long-term usage of topical steroids are some of the causes for rise of IOP in the late postoperative period.

The measurement of IOP is further complicated with most of the tonometers giving erroneous readings on the edematous, thickened grafted cornea. Tono-Pens or pneumotonometers are more useful measuring tools in this condition.

The surgical modifications to prevent glaucoma are donor graft disparity using a 0.5 mm larger donor size than the host in an attempt to decrease angle compression, loose, deep and short suture bites, meticulous wound closure in addition to adequate formation of anterior chamber after surgery.

Treatment

The choices of medical drugs to lower IOP are limited. Carbonic anhydrase inhibitors with their propensity to impair corneal endothelial function, prostamides with their doubtful effect on graft clarity, miotics with their limited action once angle is zipped up leaves only beta agonists and alpha adrenergic agonist to fight the glaucoma. Laser trabeculoplasty and iridoplasty may be tried and has benefited few cases. Filtration surgery enjoys lower success in aphakic eyes and graft failure can compound the surgery. Tube shunts often save the day, but their placement must be meticulous and the tube trimmed such that it does not lead to corneal touch (Fig. 11.50). Laser

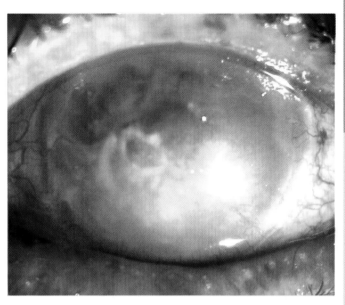

Fig. 11.51: Herpetic keratouveitis with secondary glaucoma

cyclodestruction is an option which is reserved once filtering surgery fails. Diode laser cyclophotocoagulation works with more than one sitting required and may save vision and the graft.

Corneal Infections

Keratitis of all types may be associated with trabeculitis and iridocyclitis both of which contribute to rise in IOP. In herpetic keratouveitis especially disciform or interstitial types IOP elevation has been documented in almost 28% cases. Herpes zoster ophthalmicus is associated with almost 40% incidences of acute uveitic glaucoma (Fig. 11.51). Sectorial iris atrophy is a common coexisting finding (Fig. 11.52).

Glaucoma medications are usually sufficient to control the IOP in addition to the judicious use of anti-inflammatory drugs like steroids to reduce trabeculitis and cycloplegics. Steroids must be used under antiviral cover in these cases to prevent

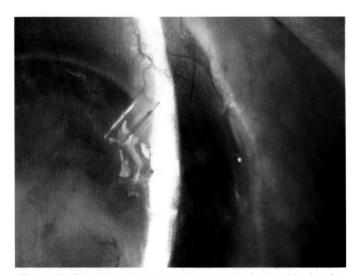

Fig. 11.50: Postkeratoplasty case with operated tube shunt implant for secondary glaucoma. Note failed graft secondary to the glaucoma

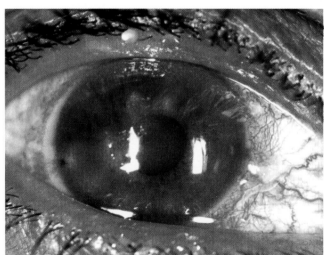

Fig. 11.52: Sectorial atrophy in healed herpetic keratouveitis

a flare up of herpetic infection. Almost 10 to 12% cases will require filtration surgery to control the glaucoma, the use of steroids post-trabeculectomy again needs to be used judiciously under antiviral cover for the fear of viral reactivation.

Corneal Ulcer with Glaucoma

Cases with acute corneal ulcer may often develop IOP rise especially in non-resolving infection (Fig. 11.53). Control of infection invariably controls the glaucoma of acute onset however if glaucoma is a sequel to healing/healed corneal ulcer, then more aggressive antiglaucoma management needs to be pursued. Antiglauoma drugs are often sufficient, but sometimes a trabeculectomy is required to control the glaucoma (Fig. 11.54). Rarely a perforated corneal ulcer heals and forms a vascularized retrocorneal membrane, which leads to neovascular glaucoma (Fig. 11.55).

Pseudophakic Bullous Keratopathy

Patients of bullous keratopathy often have secondary glaucoma compounding the corneal edema. A preparatory trabeculectomy followed by keratoplasty is the usual protocol in treating these cases (Fig. 11.56) Patients with poor visual prognosis would benefit from cyclodestructive procedures.

Ocular Tumors

The location of tumor determines the mechanism of glaucoma. Choroidal melanoma, retinoblastoma, neurofibroma associated with optic nerve glioma/meningioma, cavernous hemangioma, lymphangioma, metastasis, cause secondary angle-closure glaucoma due to the anterior shift of lens iris diaphragm. Inflammation secondary to tumor necrosis, infiltration of angle with tumor cells or liberated pigment,

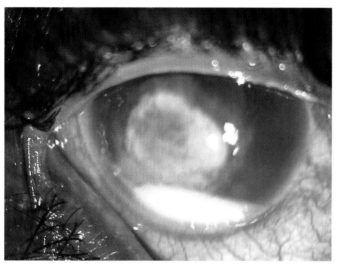

Fig. 11.53: Acute fungal corneal ulcer with secondary glaucoma

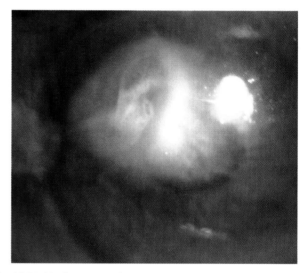

Fig. 11.55: Healing stage of corneal ulcer with retrocorneal membrane, rubeosis of lens and glaucoma

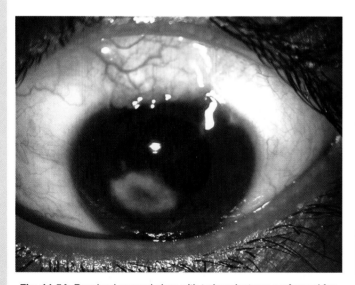

Fig. 11.54: Resolved corneal ulcer with trabeculectomy performed for uncontrolled secondary glaucoma

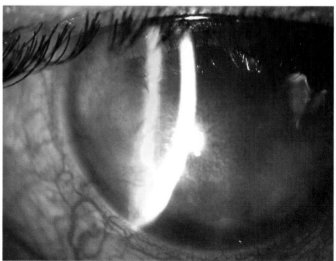

Fig. 11.56: Pseudophakic bullous keratopathy with secondary glaucoma

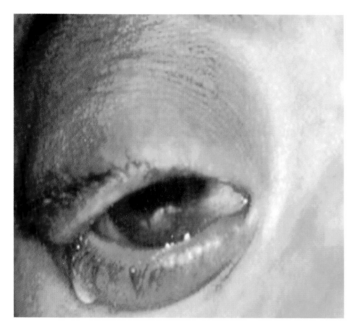

Fig. 11.57: Neurofibromatosis with secondary glaucoma and exposure keratitis in a 5-year-old child

Ocular Features

Yellow brown iris hamartomas (Lisch nodules) are the hallmark of the disease (Fig. 11.58). Chororetinal hamartomas may also be present. Glaucoma is associated in the peripheral variant and occurs when neurofibroma of the ipsilateral eyelid is present. Primary trabeculodysgenesis, angle infiltration by neurofibroma and growth of a fibrovascular membrane are the causes of glaucoma.

Treatment

Since it affects children or young adults, medical therapy may not always be curative. Trabeculectomy/trabeculectomy with trabeculotomy with the adjunctive use of antifibrotics like mitomycin-C are often required, but the prognosis is grim. Excision of neurofibroma should not be attempted.

Ocular Manifestations

The tumor manifestations are usually fully manifested by the time glaucoma intervenes. The cause of glaucoma is open-angle mechanism (tumor cells infiltrating the angle) or closed-angle mechanism (anterior push mechanism by posterior tumor/rubeosis leading to zipping of angle) (Figs 11.59 to 11.61). In pigmented tumors melanoma lytic glaucoma is a condition when macrophages, which ingest pigment liberated from tumor cells, block the trabecular meshwork. The dense pigmentation seen in the angle needs to be differentiated from pigment dispersion syndrome. The latter is bilateral, has fine pigment and iris atrophy. In advanced stage where the tumor has spread to surrounding structures both outflow pathways are obstructed in addition to anterior push of the lens iris diaphragm (Fig. 11.62).

Treatment

Treatment is dependent on the type of ocular tumor. Glaucoma is a poor prognosticator and often predicts a fatal outcome. Glaucoma management takes second seat to control the tumor.

direct compression and rubeosis iridis are the other factors responsible for glaucoma.

Neurofibromatosis (von Recklinghausen's Disease)

An autosomal dominant condition this systemic disorder is characterized by neurofibromas of skin, central and peripheral nervous system, iris, viscera, bony defects, specific pigmented skin lesions, the café-au-lait spots in the peripheral variant and bilateral acoustic schwannomas in the central variant (Fig. 11.57). Associated orbital bony defects transmit intracranial pulsations causing a pulsatile proptosis, with intermittent increases in IOP.

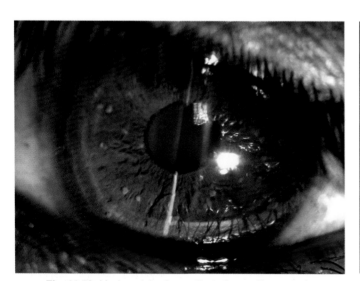

Fig. 11.58: Lisch nodules in a patient of neurofibromatosis

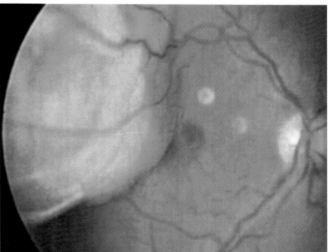

Fig. 11.59: Large choroidal melanoma causing an anterior lens iris shift

215

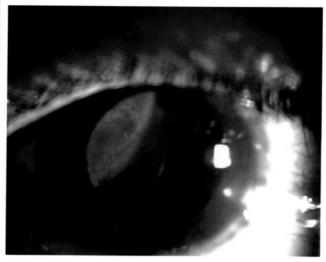

Fig. 11.60: Ciliary body melanoma

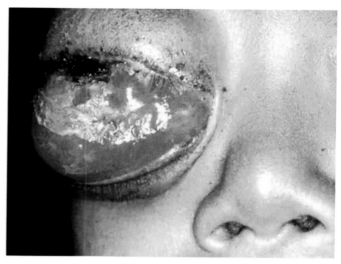

Fig. 11.62: Retinoblastoma with extraocular spread

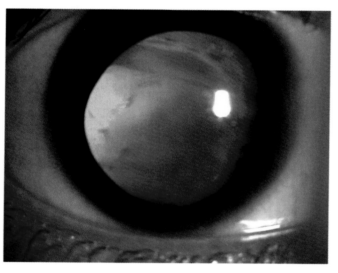

Fig. 11.61: Retinoblastoma with retinal detachment

Medical palliative therapy is usually the mainstay of treatment as by the time glaucoma has developed tumor is relatively advanced. Very often enucleation needs to be done to save patients' life.

In salvageable eyes conventional filtration surgery after treating the tumor is performed, however, this scenario is quite uncommon and is reserved for iris tumors where both tumor and glaucoma are diagnosed early on. Cyclodestructive procedures are the usual modality for treating the glaucoma in ocular neoplasms as the visual prognosis is poor. Ultrasonography and imaging modalities need to be done to differentiate the tumor and systemic evaluation to detect extent of spread if any.

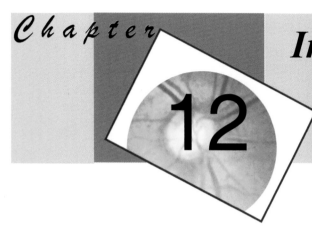

Chapter 12

Investigative Techniques Helpful in Glaucoma Surgeries

Tanuj Dada, Parul Sony

INTRODUCTION

Advanced newer investigative techniques like ultrasound biomicroscopy (UBM), optical coherence tomography (OCT), scanning laser polarimetry (SLP) with fixed and individualized custom compensation (GDx-VCC), and confocal scanning laser ophthalmoscopy (CSLO; Heidelberg retinal tomography; HRT) have been shown to have useful application in the diagnosis of glaucoma. Some of these modalities also have useful implication in preoperative evaluation and postoperative follow-up of patients undergoing glaucoma surgery.

ULTRASOUND BIOMICROSCOPY

Ultrasound biomicroscopy is a high-resolution ultrasound technology that allows imaging of structural details of the anterior ocular segment at near microscopic resolution in vivo. This diagnostic modality provides exceptionally detailed two-dimensional gray-scale images of the various anterior segment structures.

Principle

Ultrasound biomicroscopy uses a scan transducer with a frequency of 50 MHz. This is a much higher frequency than the transducer frequency of conventional diagnostic ultrasound instruments (7.5 to 10 MHz). This provides much higher image resolution of ultrasound biomicroscopy (approximately 25–50 μm of lateral and axial resolution) compared to the conventional B-scan ocular ultrasonography. However, improved image resolution is associated with a limited depth of penetration, of up to 5 mm, and a smaller angular field.

Uses of Ultrasound Biomicroscopy in Glaucoma Surgery

Preoperative Applications

Quantification of the anterior chamber angle in primary glaucoma: With the ultrasound biomicroscopy direct, precise and objective measurement of the angle recess is possible. It helps to determine the exact degree of angle closure and assess whether a patient is predisposed to angle closure. Hence it helps in planning further management. In addition, imaging of the anterior segment structures is possible even in eyes with corneal edema or corneal opacification that precludes gonioscopic assessment (Fig. 12.1).

Application in secondary glaucomas: Ultrasound biomicroscopy has been able to differentiate between primary angle-closure and secondary angle-closure due to processes, such as lens swelling and dislocation, massive hemorrhagic retinal detachment pushing the lens and iris anteriorly, and multiple neuroepithelial cysts of the iridociliary sulcus (Figs 12.2A to G).

Post-traumatic glaucoma: In eyes with blunt ocular trauma, ultrasound biomicroscopy can be used to evaluate iris-angle abnormalities associated with and possibly obscured by hyphema, including angle recession, iridodialysis and cyclodialysis, and to illustrate the presence and extent of blood clots. On ultrasound biomicroscopy, angle recession is characterized by posterior displacement of the point of attachment of the iris to the sclera. In the acute stage, the post-traumatic recess is usually filled with blood (Figs 12.3A and B).

Malignant glaucoma: Ciliary block or aqueous misdirection presents the greatest diagnostic challenge. Ultrasound biomicroscopy is an important tool in this condition. Imaging shows an extremely shallow anterior chamber, occluded angle, and forward rotation of the ciliary body with or without fluid in the suprachoroidal space.

Angle-closure glaucoma—evaluation of cysts and tumors: Ultrasound biomicroscopy can be used to determine the internal character of the anterior segment lesion (solid or cystic), to ascertain whether the lesion involves the anterior ciliary body or is restricted to the iris, and also to measure the full extent of the lesion. Ultrasound biomicroscopy can reveal whether the lesion involves only partial thickness or full thickness of the stroma and can thereby aid in surgical planning (Figs 12.4A and B). It

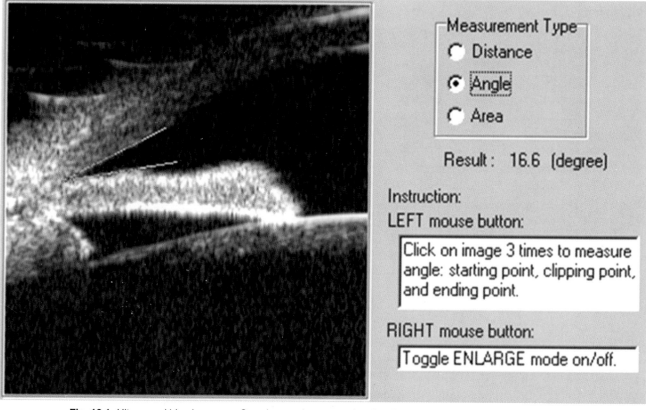

Fig. 12.1: Ultrasound biomicroscopy. Scan image shows anterior chamber angle quantification prior to surgery

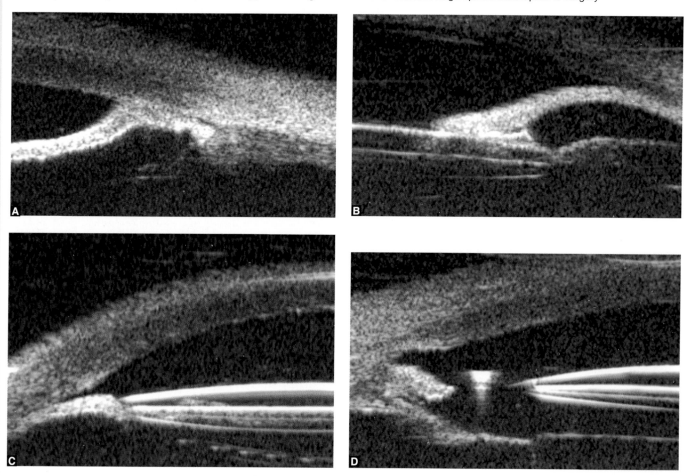

Figs 12.2:A to D

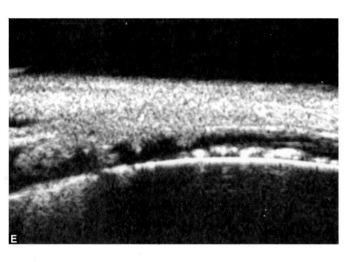

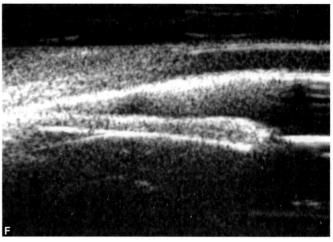

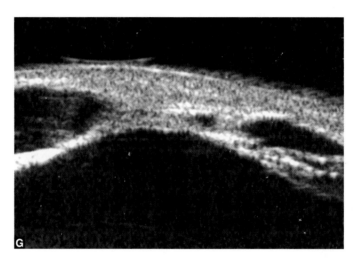

Figs 12.2A to G: Scan shows relation of anterior segment structure and there role in pathogenesis of secondary glaucoma (A) peripheral anterior synechiae with dense iridocorneal adhesion; (B) pupillary block with iris bombe; (C) secondary angle closure with anterior chamber intraocular lens; (D) pupillary capture of intraocular lens; (E) and (F) postvitrectomy silicone oil induced glaucoma; (G) secondary glaucoma associated with adherent leucoma, ultrasound biomicroscopy shows the extent of adhesion, status of anterior chamber, angle and lens

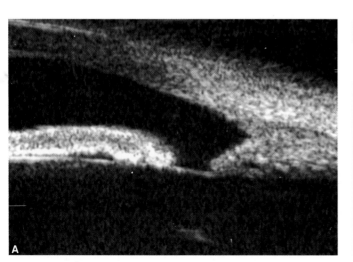

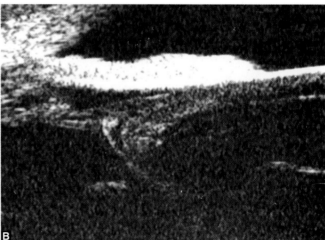

Figs 12.3A and B: Eyes with post-traumatic glaucoma shows (A) iridodialysis; (B) preoperative assessment of zonule status

allows measurement of the lesion's thickness and determination of the presence or absence or intraocular invasion.

Postoperative Applications

a. Filtration surgery
b. Trabeculectomy

After trabeculectomy ultrasound biomicroscopy scan can be used to know:

Whether the sclerostomy aperture is patent or blocked internally.

Whether the peripheral iridectomy is open or blocked.

Grading of the bleb according to intrableb reflectivity, visibility of route under the scleral flap, formation of cavernous fluid filled space, and the bleb height. Following four grades have been described:

- *Low reflective* L
- *High reflective* H
- *Encapsulated* E
- *Flat* F

Eyes with good intraocular pressure control mainly have "**L**" type blebs. These have low to moderate intrableb reflectivity, visible intrascleral route and higher intrableb height. Flat and encapsulated blebs generally denote a surgical failure

(Figs 12.5A and B). The position of the tip of the tube, after shunt surgery, can be determined. It can also be known whether its orifice is open or plugged (Fig. 12.6).

Non-Penetrating Deep Sclerectomy

Ultrasound biomicroscopy may be used in eyes with non-penetrating-deep sclerectomy:

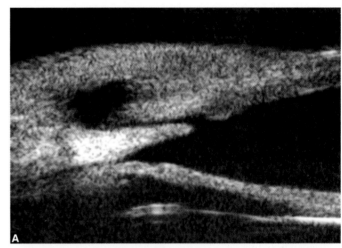

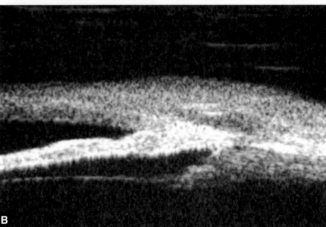

Figs 12.5A and B: Postoperative ultrasound biomicroscopy. Scan shows bleb status. (A) type E bleb; (B) type F bleb

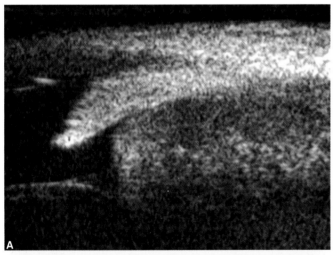

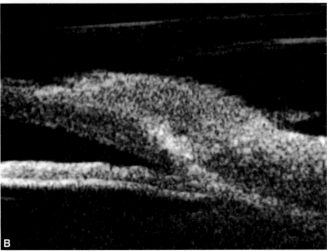

Figs 12.4A and B: Eyes with intraocular tumor and secondary glaucoma shows (A) tumor induced angle-closure; (B) depth and extent of involvement

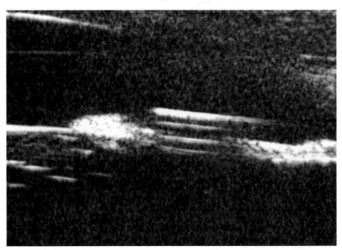

Fig. 12.6: Tip of the drainage device is visualized

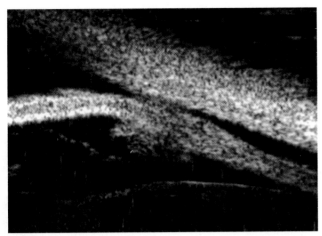

Fig. 12.7: Scan in an eye with hypotony reveals choroidal effusion

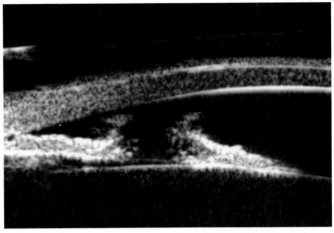

Fig. 12.8: Scan shows patent peripheral iridotomy

i.   To evaluate the thickness and to demonstrate a non-perforated continuous trabeculo-Descemet's membrane.

ii. To evaluate the height and length of collagen implant. It has been shown on ultrasound biomicroscopy that these collagen implants dissolve slowly leaving a tunnel in the sclera. The usual dissolution time is between 6 and 9 months.

iii. A grading of bleb similar to the trabeculectomy bleb has also been used for non-penetrating deep sclerectomy blebs.

Evaluation of Postoperative Complications after Trabeculectomy

After any type of glaucoma filtering surgery, ultrasound biomicroscopy can be used to detect and evaluate the extent of postoperative complications, such as ciliochoroidal effusion and cyclodialysis (Fig. 12.7).

In ciliochoroidal effusion, ultrasound biomicroscopy shows the ciliary body to be edematous and separated from the sclera by a sonolucent collection of supraciliary fluid. Many ciliochoroidal effusions that are too limited in extent to be detectable by indirect ophthalmoscopy and slit-lamp biomicroscopy can be imaged by ultrasound biomicroscopy. In cyclodialysis, ultrasound biomicroscopy shows a well-defined separation between the uveal tissue and the sclera in the region of the scleral spur.

Laser Iridotomy

After Nd:YAG laser iridotomy for angle closure, ultrasound biomicroscopy can demonstrate whether the iridotomy is partial thickness or full thickness and whether the plane of curvature of the peripheral iris has changed compared to the pretreatment status (Fig. 12.8). It can also identify any lenticular damage induced by the laser.

OPTICAL COHERENCE TOMOGRAPHY

Optical coherence tomography is a noncontact, noninvasive diagnostic technique and has a useful application in the evaluation of eyes with glaucoma. Role of optical coherence tomography in evaluating the glaucomatous retinal nerve fiber damage is now well established. The latest version of the optical coherence tomography, OCT-3 (STRATUS, Zeiss Humphrey, Dublin, CA, USA) allows a detailed quantitative evaluation of the optic nerve head.

Principle

Optical coherence tomography is based on the principle of Michelson interferometry. Low-coherence super luminescent infrared diode (830 nm) light coupled to a fiber-optic travels to a beam splitter and is directed through the ocular media to the retina and to a reference mirror, respectively. Light passing through the eye is reflected by structures in different retinal tissue layers. The distance between the beam-splitter and reference mirror is continuously varied to produce an interference pattern. The interference pattern is detected and then processed into a signal. The optical coherence tomography image can be displayed on a false color scale where different colors correspond to different degrees of reflectivity. Optical coherence tomography being noncontact and noninvasive can be easily used in the evaluation of postoperative eyes.

Uses of Optical Coherence Tomography in Glaucoma Surgery

Hypotonous Maculopathy

Hypotony and hypotonous maculopathy are the well-documented complication of glaucoma filtering surgery. Optical coherence tomography in eyes with hypotonous maculopathy shows an increased macular thickness when compared to the fellow eye or preoperative macular thickness measurements (Figs 12.9A and B). Optical coherence tomography is able to detect minor changes and increase in thickness in eyes with vision loss associated with low postoperative intraocular pressure even when the macula looks normal on clinical examination or even fluorescein angiography. Macular thickness as measured with

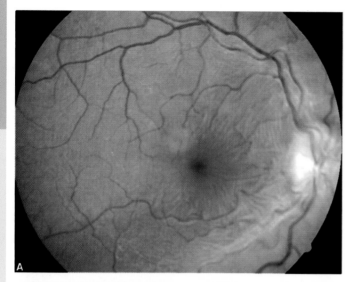

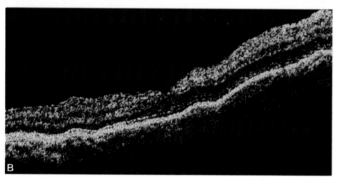

Figs 12.9A and B: Line scan through macular area shows increased macular thickness with increase reflectivity of the inner macular layers in an eye with hypotonous maculopathy

optical coherence tomography has been shown to correlate well with visual acuity in these eyes. Increase in macular thickness in eyes with hypotonous maculopathy has been shown to be associated with poor visual acuity, which shows recovery with decrease in macular thickness. Optical coherence tomography helps to confirm the structural changes both qualitatively and quantitatively in hypotonous maculopathy and also helps to demonstrate its reversal following treatment.

Cystoid Macular Edema

Optical coherence tomography serves as a useful diagnostic tool in eyes that develop postoperative cystoid macular edema and helps to differentiate it from hypotonous maculopathy if it is coexisting (Figs 12.10A and B). It can be used to study

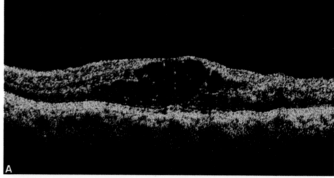

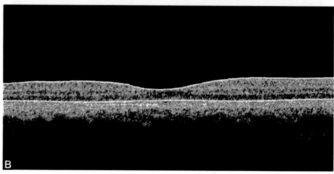

Figs 12.10A and B: Optical coherence tomography (A) Macular line scan showing occurrence of cystoid macular edema with use of latanoprost; (B) disappearance of macular edema with discontinuation of latanoprost drops

the evolution and follow-up of eyes that develop cystoid macular edema as a side effect of prostaglandin analogs like latanoprost.

Retinal Nerve Fiber Layer Thickness Measurements

Optical coherence tomography allows direct measurement of peripapillary retinal nerve fiber layer thickness by in vivo visualization of retina and retinal nerve fiber layer (Figs 12.11A to E). A high reflectance layer located just under the inner surface of the retina that corresponds to the retinal nerve fiber layer is measured using a computer-fed algorithm to generate the retinal nerve fiber layer measurement. Optical coherence tomography generated morphologic findings in experimental animals have been shown to correspond very well with histological findings. Many studies available in literature have shown that optical coherence tomography generated parameters possess high sensitivity and specificity in distinguishing eyes early glaucomatous visual field defects from normal.

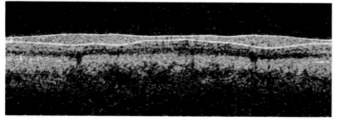

Fig. 12.11A: Peripapillary retinal nerve fiber layer scan showing normal retinal nerve fiber layer thickness (average retinal nerve fiber layer thickness of 99 μm)

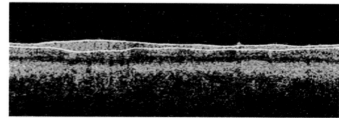

Fig 12.11B: Peripapillary retinal nerve fiber layer scan showing decreased retinal nerve fiber layer thickness in an eye with moderate glaucomatous visual field defect (Anderson's criteria, average retinal nerve fiber layer thickness of 64 μm)

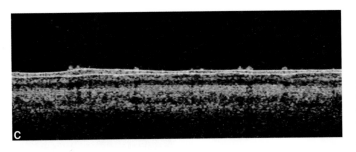

Fig. 12.11C: Peripapillary retinal nerve fiber layer scan showing marked thinning of retinal nerve fiber layer in an eye with advanced glaucomatous visual field defect (Anderson's criteria, average retinal nerve fiber layer thickness of 42 µm)

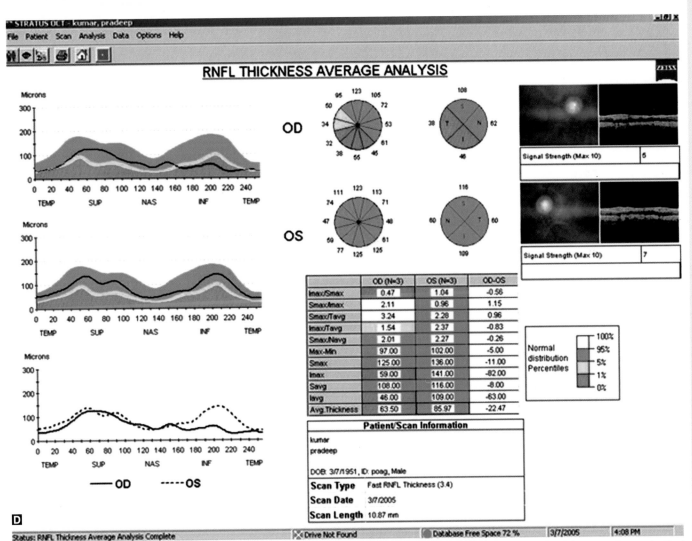

	OD (N=3)	OS (N=3)	OD-OS
Imax/Smax	0.47	1.04	-0.56
Smax/Imax	2.11	0.96	1.15
Smax/Tavg	3.24	2.28	0.96
Imax/Tavg	1.54	2.37	-0.83
Smax/Navg	2.01	2.27	-0.26
Max-Min	97.00	102.00	-5.00
Smax	125.00	136.00	-11.00
Imax	59.00	141.00	-82.00
Savg	108.00	116.00	-8.00
Iavg	46.00	109.00	-63.00
Avg.Thickness	63.50	85.97	-22.47

Patient/Scan Information

kumar
pradeep

DOB: 3/7/1951, ID: poag, Male

Scan Type Fast RNFL Thickness (3.4)
Scan Date 3/7/2005
Scan Length 10.87 mm

Fig. 12.11D: Retinal nerve fiber layer thickness analysis printout showing mild decrease in retinal nerve fiber layer in the right eye and normal retinal nerve fiber layer thickness in the left eye

Assessment of the retinal nerve fiber layer after filtration surgery shows significant increase in the overall mean nerve fiber layer thickness following surgery. Segmental analysis shows a significant increase in nerve fiber layer thickness in the nasal, superior, and temporal quadrants. Intraocular pressure reduction results in the less posterior bowing of the lamina cribrosa resulting in changes in the optic nerve head and increase of retinal nerve fiber layer thickness. This may reflect the recovery of the compressed retinal nerve fiber layer which regains its original shape. However, its function in the terms of visual field defect as documented by perimetry remains unchanged.

Optic Nerve Head Analysis

A detailed analysis of the optic nerve head is also possible with the optical coherence tomography and one can document progression of the cupping and any reversal after trabeculectomy (Fig. 12.12).

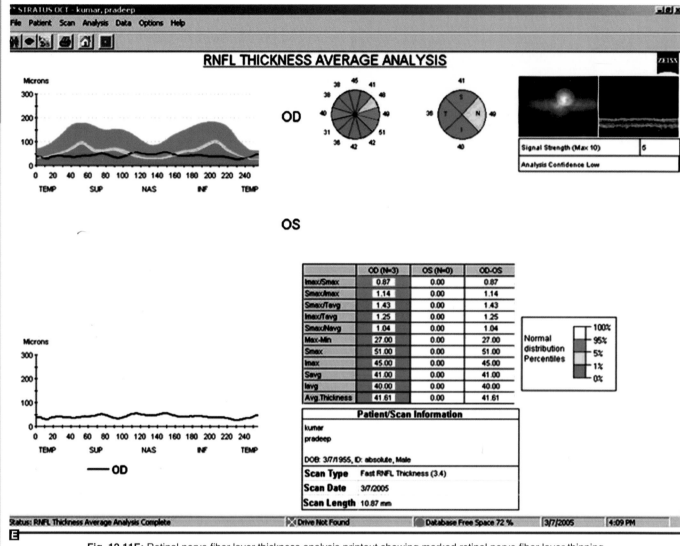

Fig. 12.11E: Retinal nerve fiber layer thickness analysis printout showing marked retinal nerve fiber layer thinning

High-Speed Corneal and Anterior Segment Optical Coherence Tomography

High-speed corneal and anterior segment optical coherence tomography uses a wavelength of 1310 nm and provides high resolution, detailed and cross sectional visualization of anterior segment structures. Images generated by high-speed corneal and anterior segment optical coherence tomography are easy to interpret. It gives similar details as that of ultrasound biomicroscopy, with an additional advantage of being noncontact. It provides a detailed view of cornea; angle and angle recess; sclera and scleral spur; iris and its root; ciliary body band and the limbus. Sclera and the scleral spur are seen as highly reflective structures and ciliary body is seen as a hypo-reflective structure. It allows a direct measure the anterior chamber angle, and with real-time imaging the canal of Schlemm is also visible.

The imaging information provided by high-speed corneal and anterior segment optical coherence tomography equates well with the ultrasound biomicroscopy findings. The biggest advantage of high-speed corneal and anterior segment optical

coherence tomography over ultrasound biomicroscopy is that the former being noninvasive and noncontact and it can be used in the imaging of the angle in immediate postoperative period and also in eyes with anterior segment trauma. Anterior segment optical coherence tomography, after non-penetrating deep sclerectomy, provides information regarding the status of bleb, trabeculo-Descemet's membrane and bleb height.

SCANNING LASER POLARIMETER

A scanning laser polarimeter (GDx Laser diagnostic technologies, Inc, San Diego, CA, USA) is a confocal scanning laser ophthalmoscope with an integrated ellipsometer to measure retardation. Retinal scanning laser polarimetry determines the retinal nerve fiber layer thickness, point-by-point in the peripapillary region, by measuring the total retardation in the light reflected from the retina. The GDx VCC (GDx-VCC; Laser Diagnostic Technologies, Inc, San Diego, CA, USA) measures and individually compensates for anterior segment birefringence for

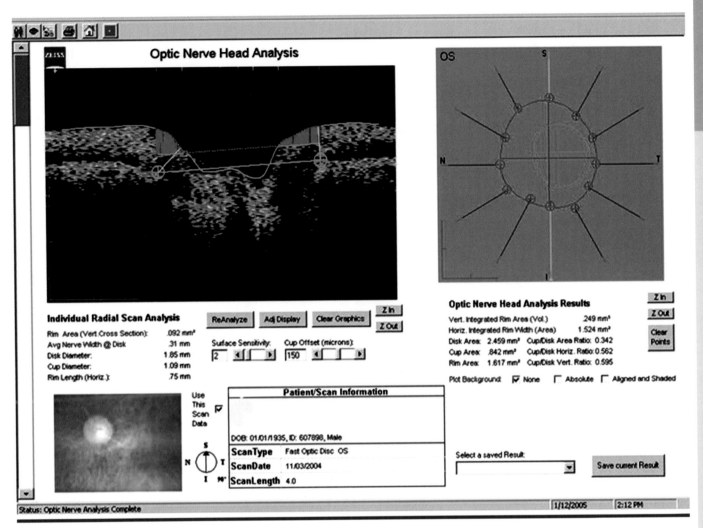

Fig. 12.12: Disc analysis in optical coherence tomography

each eye and gives retinal nerve fiber layer values that are not affected by the anterior segment birefringence.

Serial retinal nerve fiber layer thickness analysis helps in assessing retinal nerve fiber layer change over time. The first exam is the baseline or reference exam, and all follow-up exams are compared to this baseline exam. The deviation from reference map displays the retinal nerve fiber layer difference, pixel by pixel, of the follow-up exam compared to the baseline exam. If the difference exceeds 20 μm at any pixel, the pixel is color coded according to the legend retinal nerve fiber layer change is color coded in 20 micron increments, where the first 20 micron change is coded dark green, a 40 micron change is coded light blue and 60 is dark blue. The areas of retinal nerve fiber layer change shown on the deviation from reference map will frequently correspond to the areas of loss detected by the deviation map (Fig. 12.13).

This analysis may serve as a useful guideline in decision making especially when it demonstrates progressive retinal nerve fiber layer loss with medical management and apparently controlled intraocular pressure, thus indicating a need to further lower the intraocular pressure with surgical intervention.

CONFOCAL SCANNING LASER OPHTHALMOSCOPY

Optic nerve head changes have been documented on confocal scanning laser ophthalmoscopy (HRT) after trabeculectomy. Most of the available reports document that 40% or more intraocular pressure lowering following surgery is associated with a significant increase in the rim area and rim volume; and a significant decrease in the mean cup area, cup volume and cup-to-disc ratio. These changes may be documented up to 3 months to 2 years after surgery. A lesser tight intraocular pressure control, i.e. less than 25% of intraocular pressure reduction may not be associated with any reversal of the optic nerve head morphology, thus postoperative intraocular pressure should be kept low to permit reversal of optic disc changes. A significant correlation has been found between the changes in the optic disc parameters and the reduction of intraocular pressure. The improvement is confined to the nasal hemi disc and the adjacent retinal nerve fiber layer as this area is least affected by the disease, so the retinal nerve fiber layer compression is not longstanding as is on the temporal side. Intraocular pressure reduction following surgery releases the compression

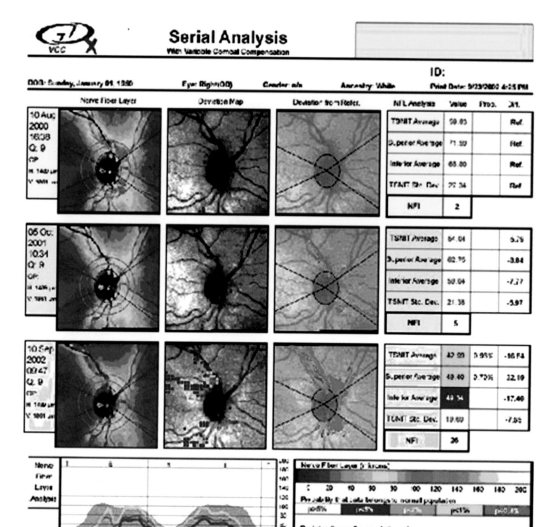

Fig. 12.13: GDx-VCC serial analysis. Progressive loss of retinal nerve fiber layer despite good medical control of intraocular pressure is seen. This may be an indication for surgical interval to further lower the intraocular pressure

and retinal nerve fiber layer on nasal side may regain its original shape and thickness.

The confocal scanning laser ophthalmoscopy provides a detailed analysis of the optic nerve head (Fig.12.14). The HRT employs a standard reference plane. The cup shape, cup volume below the surface, the mean cup depth, maximum cup depth and disc area are independent of the reference plane. The disc cup is the structure beneath the reference plane, but within the contour line. The neuroretinal rim is the structure above the reference plane, but within the contour line. Any abnormality in the disc is inferred by the Moorfields regression analysis, which divides optic nerve head into six sectors. Each sector result is represented by the following symbols with crossed sectors representing areas with abnormally thin neuroretinal rim:

- √ within normal limits
- ! borderline
- x outside normal limits

Progression of glaucoma can also be documented on the confocal scanning laser ophthalmoscopy. A change probability map uses red and green color coding on a reflectance image to signify height changes with red representing significant depression and green representing significant elevation. Red areas within the optic disc margin carry maximum significance while green areas carry less significance.

VISUAL FIELDS

Successful surgery with adequate and good postoperative intraocular pressure control is able to prevent further progression of glaucomatous visual field defect. Lowering of

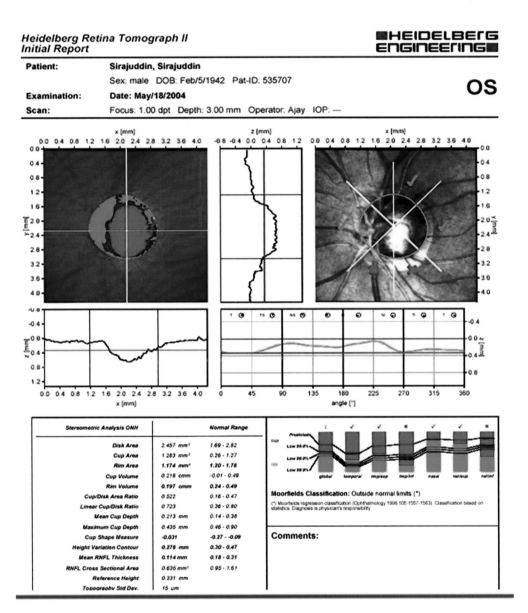

Fig. 12.14: Disc evaluation in confocal scanning laser ophthalmoscopy

intraocular pressure, improvement of optic nerve head topography and retinal nerve fiber layer thickness may be associated with improvement of visual field indices and visual function. However, occurrence or worsening of cataract, which is one of the known complications of glaucoma surgery may result in visual disturbance or the worsening of visual field defect earlier more so with blue on yellow perimetry (Short-Wavelength Automated Perimetry, SWAP).

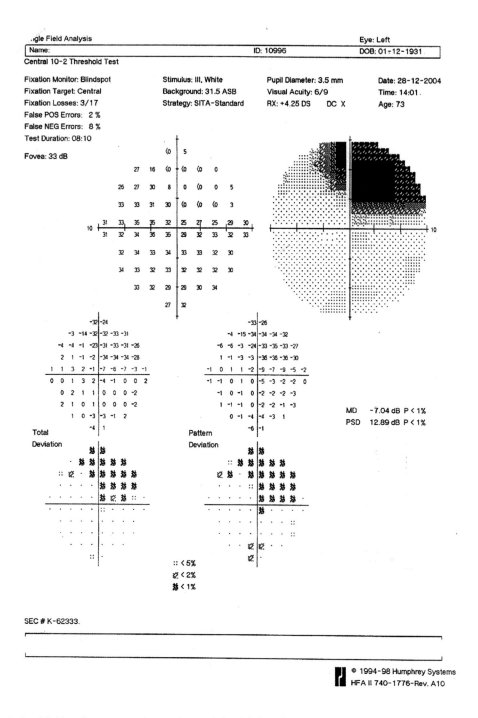

© 1994-98 Humphrey Systems
HFA II 740-1776-Rev. A10

Fig. 12.15: 10–2 visual field testing strategy shows advanced visual field defect with macular split as seen on the pattern deviation plot

Macular split (Fig. 12.15) and advanced visual field defects on white on white standard automated perimetry have higher association of immediate and permanent loss of central vision following an uncomplicated and otherwise successful glaucoma surgery. In patients with advanced visual field defects, sudden loss of visual field is not experienced if the central vision is spared at the time of surgery.

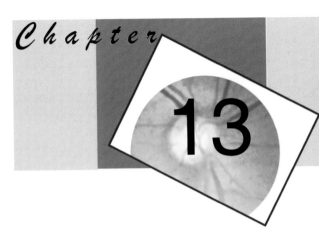
Glaucoma Surgeries

Lingam Vijaya, M Baskaran, Ronnie George,
Arun Narayanasamy, Sachi Devi, Aditya Neog

APPLIED ANATOMY FOR GLAUCOMA SURGERY

Thorough knowledge of the corneoscleral or limbal anatomy is essential for performing glaucoma surgeries. The surgical limbus is a blue-gray transition zone between the parallel collagen fibers of the peripheral cornea and those of the anterior sclera. The color of the blue zone results from facilitation of light transmission by the oblique insertion of the clear cornea into the sclera. The junction between the cornea and sclera, the external scleral sulcus, appears as a slight depression due to the union of two different radii of curvature and is bounded anteriorly by the slightly protruding peripheral edge of the Bowman's membrane. The conjunctiva tethers here anteriorly and hence in a limbus-based flap anterior dissection of the conjunctiva should stop here to avoid disinsertion of the conjunctiva. As there is an abrupt change in the curvature at this junction, the plane of the dissection should be adjusted to this curvature while making a scleral flap to avoid a premature entry into the anterior chamber. The Tenon's capsule, a loose fibrovascular layer is usually easily separable from the overlying conjunctiva and inserts into the connective tissue at the limbus 0.5 to 1.0 mm posterior to the conjunctival insertion.

Corneolimbal Junction

The corneolimbal junction, the anterior boundary of the limbus, is the termination of the Bowman's membrane and is approximately 0.5 mm anterior to the insertion of the conjunctiva. The conjunctiva inserts more anteriorly in the superior and inferior quadrants and hence the limbus is wider in these quadrants. The conjunctiva and Tenon's capsule cover the limbus, and these have to be reflected to visualize the posterior boundary of the limbus. During trabeculectomy, a circumferential incision at the corneolimbal junction enters the anterior chamber just anterior to the trabecular meshwork.

Sclerolimbal Junction

The sclerolimbal junction, also called the posterior limbus, is the junction between the opaque white sclera posteriorly and the translucent bluish-gray zone anteriorly. This is an important landmark as the scleral spur is situated just posterior to it and Schlemm's canal just anterior to it. The ciliary body attaches to the posterior portion of the scleral spur. A radial incision in the posterior portion of the blue-gray zone just anterior to the sclerolimbal junction will reveal the Schlemm's canal during a trabeculotomy.

Blue Zone Transition

The blue zone transition from a white sclera to the clear cornea is displaced more posteriorly in the deeper layers of the sclera than on the scleral surface because the corneoscleral interface is oblique with corneal fibers inserting obliquely into the sclera. This configuration creates an impression that the scleral dissection is sufficiently anterior and can lead to premature entry into anterior chamber. Hence, scleral flap dissection should extend into the clear cornea.

In addition to the arteries and veins running in the recti muscles, perforating scleral blood vessels (Axenfeld loops) are encountered during dissection. The scleral flap is placed in such a manner that would avoid these vessels.

- Defining the edges of the adjacent recti muscles before conjunctival dissection in cases of limbus-based flaps helps to maintain orientation and accurate placement of the scleral flap.
- In eyes with narrow angles the lamellar dissection of the scleral flap is extended farther into the clear cornea than is usually required to avoid injury to the ciliary body, which is often anteriorly situated in these eyes.
- Preservation of Tenon's insertion anteriorly prevents anterior dissection of the filtering bleb and a thin cystic bleb. This can be done by dissecting a partial-thickness scleral flap without disrupting the Tenon's insertion.
- Variations in the anatomy in infants and children and in the anomalous formation of angle structures should be kept in mind.

SURGICAL INSTRUMENTS FOR GLAUCOMA SURGERY

Apart from the routine instruments used in the cataract surgery, the following instruments are needed for a routine trabeculectomy and external trabeculotomy. The implant surgery requires special instruments, such as the tube holder, extender, etc. which are available commercially. However, many surgeons do not routinely use them.

Kelly-Descemet Membrane Punch

It is used to excise the block of tissue to make a sclerostomy during trabeculectomy. It is designed to produce a clean hole without any tissue tags; each bite makes an opening 0.75 mm in diameter. The instrument has to be held vertically to avoid shelving the tissue. Alternatively, Vannas scissors can be used to make the stoma. It is very convenient to use the punch in phacotrabeculectomy since use of Vannas scissors will require an additional step of opening the flap before making the stoma (Fig. 13.1).

Harms Trabeculotome

It comes as a pair, one for the right and left side respectively. It has two curved arms, 9 mm long. The tip is blunt. One arm is inserted into the Schlemm's canal, while the second arm guides the surgeon regarding the direction of movement. It is used in external trabeculotomy for congenital glaucoma (Fig. 13.2).

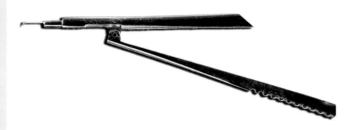

Fig. 13.1: Kelly-Descemet membrane punch

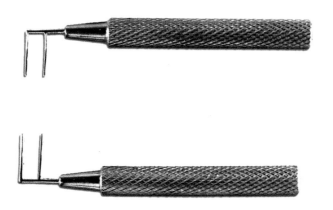

Fig. 13.2: Harms trabeculotome

TRABECULECTOMY

Trabeculectomy, the most commonly performed glaucoma surgery involves creation of a fistula, which drains the aqueous into the subconjunctival space thereby reducing intraocular pressure (IOP).

Usually, the superior nasal quadrant is chosen. Ease of surgical approach, more space for elevated blebs, better protection and surface lubrication by the eyelids and less likelihood of shadow images form a basal iridectomy make superior blebs preferable to the blebs at other sites. Superior nasal quadrant or superior 12 o'clock site is preferable so as to spare one quadrant for future use.

Exposure of the Surgical Site

A superior rectus bridle suture or a traction suture with 8-0 polygactin or a 8-0 silk in the peripheral superior cornea just anterior to the site of proposed scleral flap is used to turn the globe inferiorly and achieve maximum visualization of the surgical field (Fig. 13.3).

Conjunctival Flap Dissection

Limbus-based Flap

Dissection can either be initiated in the subconjunctival plane or in the sub-Tenon's space. Conjunctiva alone or along with the underlying Tenon's is gently lifted with a non-toothed forceps and a circumferential cut is made through the conjunctiva with a sharp Westcott scissors at least 8 mm posterior to the limbus. The incision is extended at least for two clock hours in the selected quadrant maintaining the distance from the limbus. The anterior lip of the wound is held with a toothless forceps and a dull Stevens scissors or a blunt-tipped Westcott's scissors is introduced into the plane of dissection and the flap is dissected anteriorly to the limbal conjunctival insertion (Figs 13.4 to 13.6).

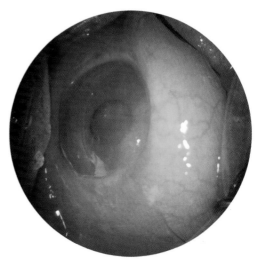

Fig. 13.3: Superior quadrant chosen for trabeculectomy

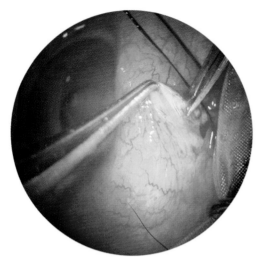

Fig. 13.4: Conjunctival flap (limbal based)

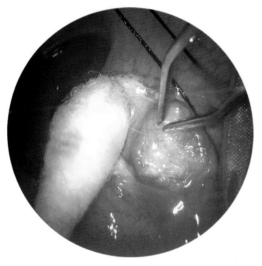

Fig. 13.5: Hemostasis at the scleral bed

Fornix-based Flap

Limbal peritomy is done for about three clock hours in the selected quadrant using Pierce-Hoskins forceps and Westcott's scissors. With a dull Stevens' scissors, tunneling is done posteriorly and on either side of the peritomy to create a potential space for filtration of aqueous.

After conjunctival dissection, meticulous hemostasis is achieved with an underwater coaxial diathermy. Care is taken to avoid contact of the thermal cautery with the conjunctiva (Fig. 13.7).

Use of Antimetabolites

A micro sponge made of methylcellulose or polyvinyl acetal soaked in either 5-fluorouracil (5-FU) or mitomycin-C are applied underneath the conjunctival flap while the conjunctival flap is gently lifted up with a nontoothed forceps. The concentrations and the duration of application of antimetabolites are titrated for each case. Thorough irrigation with isotonic solutions is done after the application of antimetabolites.

Fashioning Scleral Flap

Partial-thickness incisions with a sharp blade are made to outline the extent of the scleral flap. Since the shape of the flap has no bearing with the IOP control, the flap can be of any geometrical shape. The size of the flap should not be less than 2.5 × 2.5 mm size and should be of at least 1/3 thickness of the sclera to produce enough resistance to aqueous humor outflow. A straight Pierce-Hoskins forceps is used to grasp the edge of the flap which is lifted upwards and forwards towards the pupil and the flap is dissected anteriorly with a no. 67 Beaver blade or no. 15 B-P blade into the clear cornea. High magnification and flap bed hemostasis with dry cellulose sponges facilitates visualization (Figs 13.8 to 13.12).

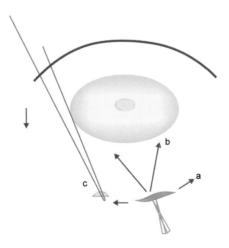

Fig. 13.6: Steps of trabeculectomy (limbal flap): (a) Direction of conjunctival opening; (b) Direction of Tenon's dissection; (c) Superior rectus bridle suture

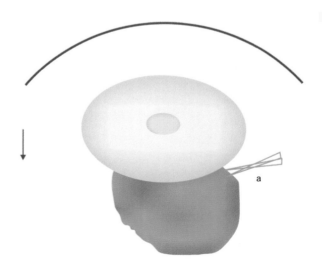

Fig. 13.7: Steps of trabeculectomy: (a) Fornix-based flap

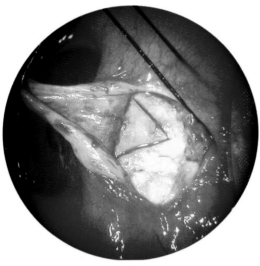

Fig. 13.8: Triangular flap area marked

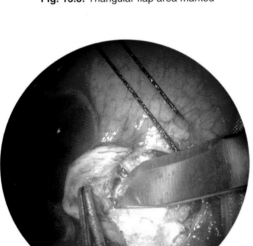

Fig. 13.9: Triangular flap dissected till limbus (half thickness of sclera)

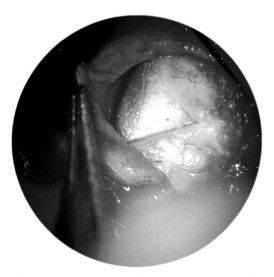

Fig. 13.10: Exposure of the blue limbus and completion of triangular flap

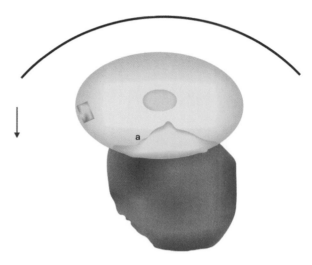

Fig. 13.11: Steps of trabeculectomy: (a) Triangular shaped scleral flap

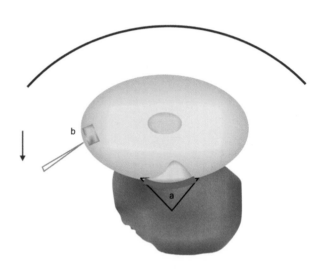

Fig. 13.12: Steps of trabeculectomy: (a) Dissection till limbus (b) Paracentesis

Removal of the Inner Block: Sclerectomy

It can be accomplished either with Vannas scissors or with Kelly-Descemet punch.

Inner Block Removal with Scissors

While the scleral flap is gently retracted towards the pupil, two radial incisions of 1.5 mm in length and 1.5 mm apart are made extending from the anterior base of the scleral flap to the sclerolimbal junction extending not beyond the scleral spur. A third incision is made parallel to the limbus connecting the anterior ends of the two radial incisions. This free block of tissue is held and excision is completed by cutting the posterior attachment with fine scissors, such as Vannas scissors.

Inner Block Removal with Descemet's Punch

An ab externo through-and-through incision parallel to the limbus of at least 2 mm is made in the most peripheral portion of the cornea at the anterior base of the scleral flap with a mini sharp blade. While retracting the scleral flap the Kelly's punch is introduced vertically through the incision with the cutting edge facing posteriorly. Closing the punch completes the sclerectomy. One or more bites not extending beyond the scleral spur may be required. A tissue block of approximately 0.75 mm is removed with each Kelly's punch bite (Figs 13.13 to 13.15).

Peripheral Iridectomy

The iris is grasped through the scleral window with a straight Pierce-Hoskins forceps and the iridectomy is performed either with an iris scissors, angled Vannas or with Westcott's scissors keeping the blades parallel to the limbus. The size of the iridectomy should be comparable to the size of the inner sclerectomy to avoid blockage of the stoma by the iris tissue. Patency of the iridectomy is confirmed either by inspecting the excised tissue for the presence of posterior pigment epithelium or by visualizing the anterior capsule of the lens through the iridectomy. After the iridectomy the iris can be repositioned either by

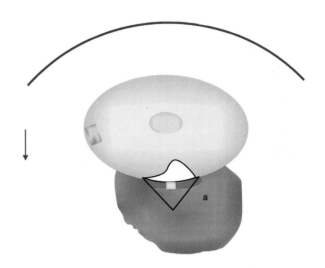

Fig. 13.15: Steps of trabeculectomy: (a) Trabecular stoma within the flap using Kelly's punch or van Hoss' scissors

irrigating the sclerostomy site or by gently stroking the cornea towards the pupil with a blunt instrument (Fig. 13.16).

Closure of the Scleral Flap

The scleral flap is reposited onto its bed and sutured with 10-0 nylon sutures; the number of sutures are titrated according to the size of the flap and the amount of aqueous run-off is noted intraoperatively. Releasable sutures either apical or basal can be taken, the number and position of which are at the discretion of the operating surgeon (Figs 13.17 to 13.20).

Conjunctival Closure

Limbus-based Flap

Conjunctiva and the underlying Tenon's capsule are sutured with 8-0 vicryl in a running horizontal mattress fashion either in two layers or in a single layer to achieve a watertight closure (Figs 13.21 A, B and C and 13.22).

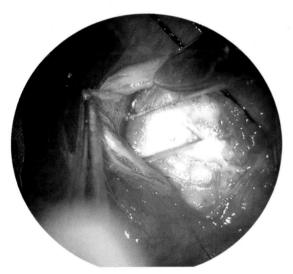

Fig. 13.13: Anterior chamber entry with blade knife

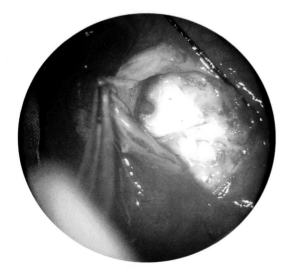

Fig. 13.14: Completion of trabeculectomy stoma (Kelly's punch used)

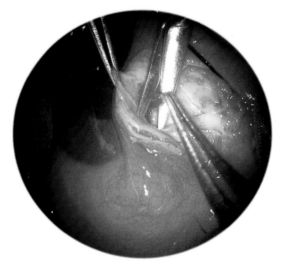

Fig. 13.16: Basal iridotomy using de Wecker's scissors

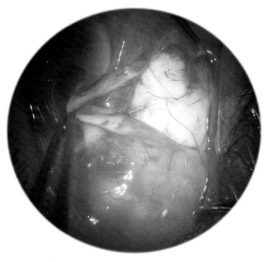

Fig. 13.17: Apical releasable suture application

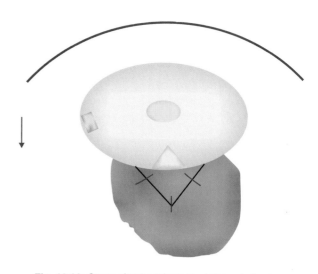

Fig. 13.20: Steps of trabeculectomy: interrupted sutures

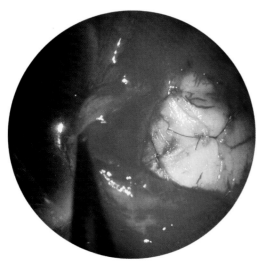

Fig. 13.18: Completion of suturing of the flap

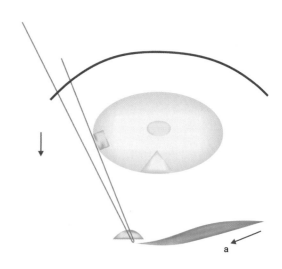

Fig. 13.21A: Steps of trabeculectomy: limbal-based flap direction of suturing (a)

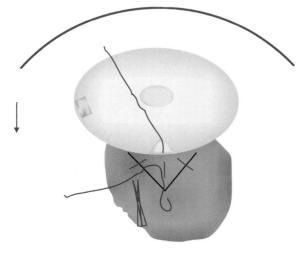

Fig. 13.19: Steps of trabeculectomy: apical releasable suture application

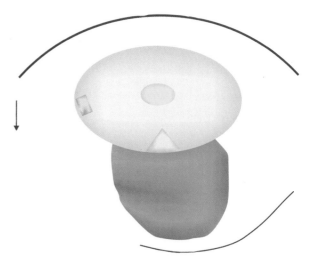

Fig. 13.21B: Steps of trabeculectomy: limbal-based flap—final appearance

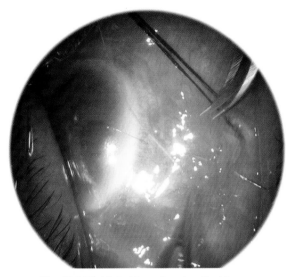

Fig. 13.21C: Limbal-based conjunctival flap

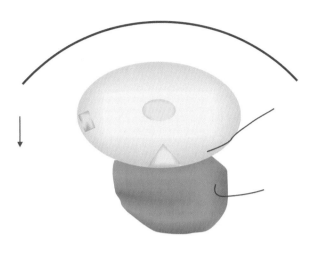

Fig. 13.23: Steps of trabeculectomy (fornix-based): wing suture application for conjunctival flap

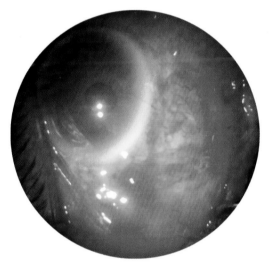

Fig. 13.22: Final appearance at completion of surgery

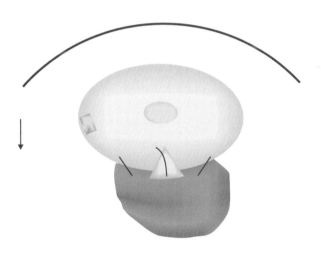

Fig. 13.24: Steps of trabeculectomy: final appearance in fornix-based flap

Fornix-based Flap

This is closed by two wing sutures of 10-0 nylon taken at the two edges of the incision. Firm bites are taken in the sclera and the peripheral cornea so that the anterior edge of the conjunctiva is tightly stretched over the peripheral cornea (Figs 13.23 and 13.24). Comparison of fornix-based versus conjunctival-based flap is shown in Table 13.1.

Technique

- The superior quadrant is usually chosen as it is a convenient site to operate on and superior limbus is the widest.
- Superonasal quadrant is chosen so as to preserve the other quadrant for future use.
- Avoid areas of conjunctival scarring and areas of scleral thinning.
- Conjunctival mobility can be assessed preoperatively or intraoperatively with a moist cotton-tip applicator.

Table 13.1: Fornix-based versus conjunctival-based flap

Fornix-based conjunctival flap	Limbus-based conjunctival flap
Advantages	*Advantages*
• Exposure better	• Tenonectomy easier
• Technically easier	• Postoperative procedures convenient and more safe
• More diffuse bleb since there is no posterior limit	• Better long-term control of IOP
• Less conjunctival manipulation	
• Wound closure is easier	
• Same technique for a combined cataract and glaucoma surgery	
Disadvantages	*Disadvantages*
• Wound leaks	• Technically difficult
	• Conjunctival buttonholes

- Cauterization of the vessels should be optimum as inadequate cautery results in bleeding and promotes subconjunctival fibrosis, whereas excessive cautery results in tissue necrosis and results in inappropriate apposition.
- In cases where antimetabolites are used, the conjunctival edge is pulled over the sponge so as to avoid contact with the antimetabolites.
- Scleral flap dissection is by a combination of tearing and dissection.
- A triangular-shaped flap is easy to dissect and close.
- Pre-placed sutures can be taken to avoid prolonged shallow anterior chamber intraoperatively.
- Corneal paracentesis made before making the inner sclerostomy will help to form the anterior chamber at the end of the surgery, to decide the degree of filtration and to irrigate the anterior chamber of pigments or blood.

Complications of trabeculectomy are shown in Table 13.2.

Table 13.2: Complications of trabeculectomy

Intraoperative	Postoperative
• Retrobulbar hemorrhage	• Shallow or flat anterior chamber
• Choroidal effusion and hemorrhage	• Wound leak
• Hyphema	• Hypotony
• Conjunctival buttonholes	• Aqueous misdirection
• Amputation of the scleral flap	• Inflammation and infection
• Damage to the lens	• Failure of the surgery
• Vitreous loss	• Cataract
• Choroidal detachment cleft	• Choroidal effusion and hemorrhage
	• Loss of central island of vision

COMBINED CATARACT AND GLAUCOMA SURGERY: TECHNIQUES

In cases with visually significant cataract and glaucoma, combined cataract and glaucoma techniques are possible. Depending on the density of the cataract and the available facilities, the surgeon could combine glaucoma filtering techniques with a conventional extracapsular cataract extraction (ECCE), phacoemulsification (PE) or a manual small incision cataract surgery (SICS). The SICS technique is referred to here as the Blumenthal technique.

Extracapsular Cataract Extraction Combined with Trabeculectomy

Preoperative Precautions

It is vital to ensure a soft globe prior to starting surgery. Preoperative hyperosmotic agents, digital massage/Honan's balloon can be used to achieve this. Adequate pupillary dilatation is equally important.

Intraoperative Procedure

A superior rectus bridle suture is taken after retracting the lids. A superior fornix-based flap is created. The conjunctiva is incised using a sharp-tipped Westcott's scissors. The peritomy is extended superiorly for 160°. The posterior conjunctiva is then dissected using a blunt-tipped Westcott's scissors, to ensure adequate mobility of the conjunctiva. Bleeding points are cauterized using the minimal cautery power that is effective. If antimetabolite use is planned, a Weck-Cel sponge or filter paper soaked in antimetabolite is placed on the bare scleral bed. It is important to ensure that the conjunctival edges do not touch the sponge. The exposed area is flushed thoroughly with saline prior to the next step. A partial-thickness limbus-based triangular scleral flap approximately 2.5 mm wide and 2 mm in height is raised at the 12 o'clock position. The flap is dissected anteriorly into the clear cornea. A curvilinear groove is then made on both sides of the flap parallel to the limbus.

The anterior chamber is entered with a 15 degree knife through the groove. Alternatively, a separate stab incision can be made for capsulotomy. The capsulotomy is then performed under viscoelastic cover. The cataract section is then extended and the nucleus delivered. It is safer to place stay sutures immediately after nucleus delivery following which cortex is extracted conventionally. The intraocular lens is then implanted. The cataract section is closed excluding the trabeculectomy flap region. The flap is reflected onto the corneal surface. The trabeculectomy block is then removed from the inner edge internal wound lip using Vannas scissors or Kelly-Descemet punch. A peripheral iridectomy is performed through the trabeculectomy stoma using de Wecker's scissors. The flap is sutured with 10-0 monofilament using one apical and 2 or more basal sutures. Any of these could be a releasable suture. The anterior chamber is reformed using saline. Ensure that the anterior chamber is formed and that the trabeculectomy is filtering adequately. The conjunctiva is then mobilized and anchored to the limbus nasally and temporally using two-wing sutures ensuring that it is stretched across the cornea. A central horizontal mattress suture may be required to anchor the conjunctiva firmly. Additional sutures may be required for watertight closure. The bridle suture is then removed. A subconjunctival steroid injection is given.

Precaution

Placement of a lens in sulcus is avoided such that its haptic is in the area of the peripheral iridectomy due to the possibility of fracturing the haptic while doing the iridectomy.

Extracapsular Cataract Extraction: Variations

Trabeculectomy can be done at one edge of the cataract section if the surgeon so desires. Another variation to the technique is the combination of a corneal section for the cataract extraction with a conventional fornix or limbus-based trabeculectomy. In this technique, a limbus-or fornix-based conjunctival peritomy is performed initially with the application of antimetabolites if required. Care should be taken to thoroughly flush out the area after antimetabolite application prior to starting the cataract surgery. The trabeculectomy flap is then created as for a conventional trabeculectomy. The trabeculectomy stoma is not created at this time. Extracapsular cataract surgery is then performed through a corneal section. After the cataract procedure has been completed the trabeculectomy block is excised from the bed of the trabeculectomy flap, and the flap and the conjunctiva are closed conventionally.

Phacoemulsification Combined with Trabeculectomy

A superior rectus bridle suture is taken. A superior fornix-based flap is created. The conjunctiva is incised using a sharp-tipped Westcott's scissors. The peritomy is extended 4 to 7 mm (depending on the size of the cataract section) using a blunt-tipped Westcott's scissors; the posterior conjunctiva is dissected to ensure adequate mobilization of the conjunctiva. Bleeding points are cauterized using the minimal cautery power that is effective (Fig. 13.25).

A Weck-Cel sponge or filter paper soaked in antimetabolite is placed on the bare scleral bed. It is important to ensure that the conjunctival edges do not touch the sponge (Fig. 13.26).

The exposed area is flushed thoroughly with saline prior to the next step. A scleral groove is marked approximately 1.5 to 2 mm posterior to the limbus. The scleral tunnel is created with careful dissection into the clear cornea (Fig. 13.27). Care should be taken not to make a very anterior entry. Cataract surgery is performed as planned. Once surgery is completed and the intraocular lens (IOL) is implanted, the trabeculectomy block is removed from the internal edge of the inferior wound lip using a Descemet's punch (Figs 13.28 and 13.29). An iridotomy is done through the same opening (Fig. 13.30). The section is closed using 10-0 monofilament interrupted sutures (Fig. 13.31). Depending on the extent of overlap and the width of the section, 2 to 3 sutures may be required. Any of these sutures can be a releasable suture. After checking for adequate filtration from the wound, the conjunctiva is mobilized, stretched across the superior cornea and anchored to the limbus using 2-wing sutures. A central horizontal suture may be required. The bridle suture is then removed. A subconjunctival steroid injection is given (Fig. 13.32).

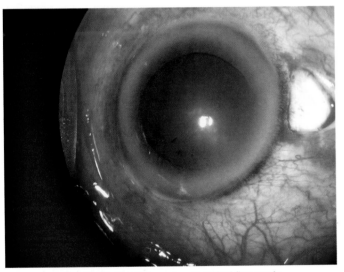

Fig. 13.25: Fornix-based conjunctival flap made

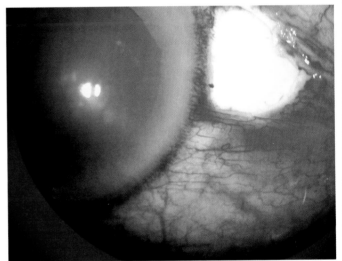

Fig. 13.27: Scleral tunnel made

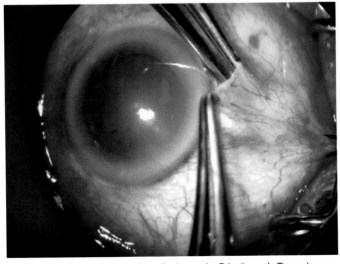

Fig. 13.26: Sponge application of mitomycin-C in the sub-Tenon's spa

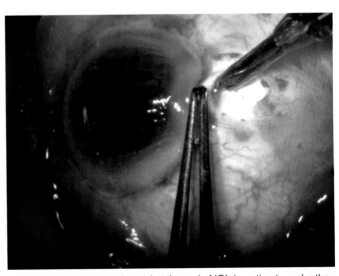

Fig. 13.28: Kelly's punch used at the end of IOL insertion to make the stoma

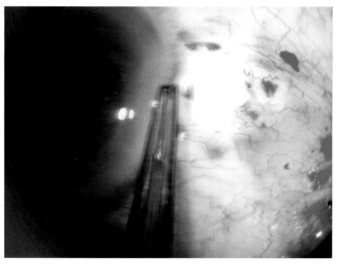

Fig. 13.29: Completion of trabeculectomy stoma

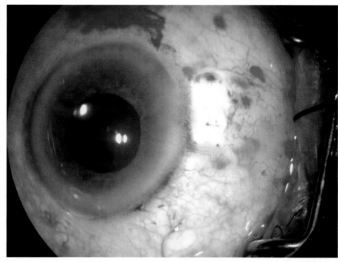

Fig. 13.31: Interrupted sutures applied to the tunnel

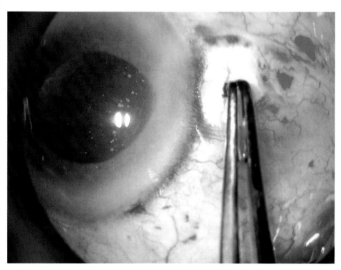

Fig. 13.30: Basal iridectomy made

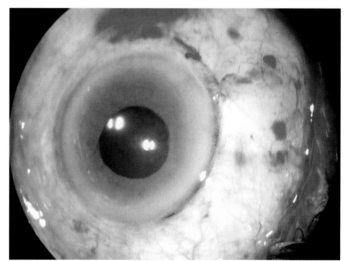

Fig. 13.32: Fornix-based flap sutured with wing sutures

Phacoemulsification Combined with Trabeculectomy: Variations

A separate site trabeculectomy can be performed along with a corneal or scleral section phacoemulsification. A limbus- or fornix-based conjunctival peritomy is performed initially, away from the planned site of the cataract extraction, with the application of antimetabolites if required. Care should be taken to thoroughly flush out the area after antimetabolite application prior to starting the cataract surgery. The trabeculectomy flap is then created as for a conventional trabeculectomy. The trabeculectomy stoma is not created at this time. Phacoemulsification with IOL implantation is then performed through a corneal or scleral section. The trabeculectomy stoma is then excised and the trabeculectomy and conjunctiva are closed conventionally. The effect of single site versus twin site phaco-trabeculectomy is debatable, however, few meta-analysis show evidence for a minimal difference in favor of twin site phacotrabeculectomy. One should weigh the ease of a single site versus the advantage of twin site before adopting either technique, and we need further studies to conclusively prove this difference (Fig. 13.33).

Blumenthal Surgery Combined with Trabeculectomy

A superior rectus bridle suture is taken after retracting the lids. A superior fornix-based flap is created. The conjunctiva is incised using a sharp-tipped Westcott's scissors. The peritomy is extended for 7 to 8 mm (depending on the size of the cataract section). Dissect the posterior conjunctiva using a blunt-tipped Westcott's, to ensure adequate mobility of the conjunctiva. Bleeding points are cauterized using the minimal cautery power that is effective.

A Weck-Cel sponge or filter paper soaked in antimetabolite is placed on the bare scleral bed. It is important to ensure that the conjunctival edges do not touch the sponge. The exposed area is flushed thoroughly with saline prior to the next step. The scleral groove is marked approximately 1.5 to 2 mm posterior

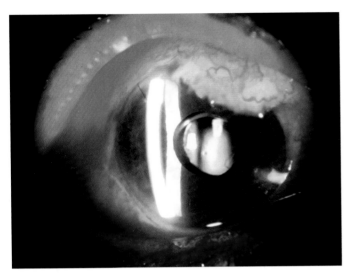

Fig. 13.33: Superotemporal clear-corneal phacoemulsification done in a patient with a pre-existing bleb

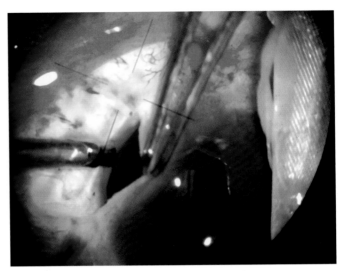

Fig. 13.35: Trabeculectomy stoma made at the internal lip of the tunnel after completion of intraocular lens insertion

to the limbus with the back cuts extending 1.5 to 2 mm posteriorly. Dissect into the clear cornea to create the scleral tunnel (Fig. 13.34). Care should be taken not to make a very anterior entry. Cataract surgery is performed as planned. Once surgery is completed and the intraocular lens is implanted, the anterior chamber maintainer fluid infusion height is reduced and the trabeculectomy block is from the internal lip of the posterior wound bed removed using a Descemet's punch (Figs. 13.35 and 13.36). An alternative technique is to make a stab incision in the wound bed approximately 1 mm from the posterior wound lip, extend it 1 mm on both sides and using a straight Vannas scissors make a radial incision in the wound bed through this stab incision till the anterior wound entry. Using the Vannas scissors the scleral flap is excised from the bed of the wound. If this technique is used, it is simpler to make the stab incision after the tunnel is dissected; and prior to entering the anterior chamber with the keratome, the stab incision can

be extended sideways and the trabeculectomy block excised after completing cataract surgery. An iridotomy is done through the same opening.

The section is closed using 10-0 interrupted sutures, depending on the extent of overlap and the width of the section 2 to 3 sutures may be required (Fig. 13.37). Any of these sutures can be a releasable suture. After checking for adequate filtration from the wound, the conjunctiva is mobilized and anchored to the limbus using 2-wing sutures after stretching the conjunctiva across the superior cornea. A central horizontal suture may be required.

The bridle suture is then removed. A subconjunctival steroid injection is given (Fig. 13.38).

Complications related to phacotrabeculectomy are similar to routine trabeculectomy except the IOL related problems and the excessive postoperative inflammation associated with cataract surgery.

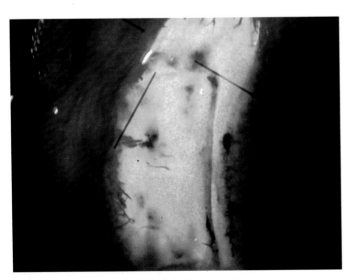

Fig. 13.34: Small incision tunnel made

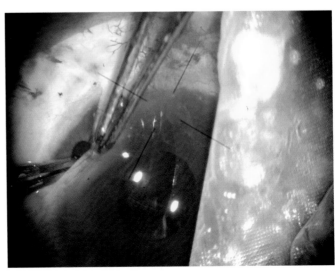

Fig. 13.36: Basal iridectomy made

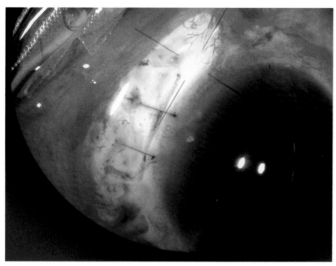

Fig. 13.37: Interrupted sutures to the tunnel applied after anterior chamber wash

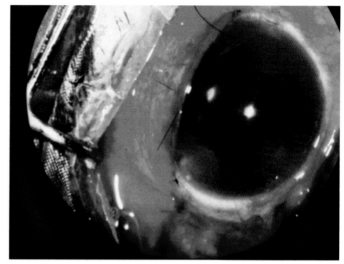

Fig. 13.38: Final appearance after conjunctival flap dissection

WOUND MODULATION

Antimetabolites

Filtering surgery adequately lowers IOP in most glaucoma patients. However, the prognosis is less favorable for aphakic patients with glaucoma or glaucoma in phakic eyes following unsuccessful filtering operations. Failure of filtering surgery is usually attributed to the proliferation of fibroblasts at the filtering site. Mitomycin-C and 5 fluorouracil (5-FU) are the two antimetabolites used as wound modulators. Other antimetabolites, such as anti-TGF beta 2, CAT-152 are under investigation. Beta irradiation is also used by some centers postoperatively for wound modulation.

Mitomycin-C

Mitomycin-C was first developed in 1955 by Hata and associates, from *Streptomyces caespitosus*. Mitomycin-C inhibits cell mitosis by interrupting DNA synthesis, and probably also acts on the vascular endothelium. Kunitomo first introduced this agent to ophthalmology as a topical drop for prevention of recurrent pterygium. In 1981, Chen was the first to use mitomycin-C intraoperatively for refractory glaucoma.

Adjunctive mitomycin-C application during filtering surgery has since been popularized for refractory glaucoma, and has been reported to maintain the filtering effect in patients with childhood glaucoma and secondary glaucoma, as well as when used in initial surgical approaches for primary open-angle glaucoma. However, such procedures are not without complications.

The first reported adverse effects of mitomycin-C were scleral changes, such as scleral melting in cases of pterygium excision. Complications may appear early, or as late as 15 to 20 years after mitomycin-C application. Mitomycin-C can also cause ocular complications and toxicity in glaucoma surgery. Eye surgeons must, therefore, exercise caution to avoid serious complications when performing mitomycin-C procedures.

In 1990, Chen and associates demonstrated that intraoperative mitomycin-C application is indicated for the treatment of patients for whom filtering surgery carries a high risk of failure. Their study of mitomycin-C and fibroblast inhibition indicated that activated fibroblasts are one of the major factors leading to failed filtering surgery.

The indications for mitomycin-C set forth in their series included failure of previous filtering operations, previous intraocular surgery, high-scar tendency related to race, and a strong inflammatory reaction in patients with secondary glaucoma. However, a recent study indicated that intraoperative application of mitomycin-C can increase the success rate of initial trabeculectomy for patients with primary glaucoma, even for younger age groups. The indications for adjunctive mitomycin-C application in filtering surgery may, therefore, expand to include treatment of childhood glaucoma.

Complications

Past studies of postoperative application of mitomycin-C eye-drops in pterygium excision provide a valuable insight into the potential complications of intraocular mitomycin-C use. In subtropical areas, such as Taiwan, recurrent pterygium is so common that 0.04% mitomycin-C solution is usually applied 4 times daily after pterygium excision. Poor wound healing, scleral ulcer, and even perforations may occur as early complications of mitomycin-C therapy. Serious long-term complications, usually appearing more than 10 years later, in the original pterygium excision site include scleral melting and necrotizing scleritis. Such scleral complications prompted Rubinfeld and associates to suggest that mitomycin-C should not be used to prevent pterygium recurrence in patients with poor ocular healing, as in those with Sjögren's syndrome, herpetic keratitis or keratoconjunctivitis sicca.

With increasing experience of the application of intraoperative mitomycin-C during the past decade, the minor complications of punctuate corneal erosion, poor conjunctival wound healing or leakage, and elongation of postoperative wound reaction have become almost negligible.

The most serious complications of mitomycin-C application include ciliary body toxicity and long-term hypotony of less than 5 mm Hg, which may induce macular change. Our stereoscopic fluorescein angiography study in 1992 showed only 2 cases of maculopathy in 30 eyes 18 months after mitomycin-C surgery. Moreover, mitomycin-C-related maculopathy might be reversible. The reported frequency of hypotony after mitomycin-C treatment ranges from 1.5 to 35%, while approximately 4 to 10% of patients develop hypotonous maculopathy following various forms of mitomycin-C application. Such hypotonous maculopathy is seen frequently in young and myopic patients. The treatments for hypotonous maculopathy include auto-blood bleb injection, scleral patching, and cryotherapy. However, the best approach is to prevent hypotony by regulation of the concentration and duration of mitomycin-C application, which can be accomplished with the use of releasable sutures or other methods.

Dose and Duration of Mitomycin-C Application

Chen and associates originally reported that application of mitomycin-C at a concentration of 0.2 to 0.4 mg/ml for 5 minutes is adequate, and poses little risk of severe complications, such as hypotony. However, Chen and associates also suggested that 0.2 mg/ml for 5 minutes may be the safest effective dose. In North America, an initial report indicated that application of 0.5 mg/ml mitomycin-C for 5 minutes could result in severe hypotony associated with maculopathy. The dose of mitomycin-C for intraoperative application ranges from 0.2 to 0.3 mg/ml with durations ranging from 2 to 5 minutes according to the risk factors for bleb closure; these risk factors include patient age, previous operation, duration of antiglaucoma drug medication, and a tendency for wound scarring.

It is encouraging that a lower concentration of 0.02% twice daily has been recommended for prevention of recurrent pterygium. In addition, some institutes have shortened the duration of mitomycin-C application to 2 minutes when used for adjunctive trabeculectomy.

Because of the high prevalence of primary angle-closure glaucoma in Asia, trabeculectomy with releasable sutures is probably safe for treatment of shallow anterior chamber glaucoma, with the goal of early restoration of the anterior chamber. Therefore, the concentration and duration of mitomycin-C application are also important in trabeculectomy for primary angle-closure glaucoma. Mitomycin-C application can also yield effective bleb formation after restoration of the chamber followed by releasing suture and digital pressure.

Subconjunctival Injection

With intraoperative application and washing techniques, the amount of mitomycin-C left in the eye is quite variable; it may also vary considerably among surgeons. Because of the potential adverse effects of mitomycin-C in pterygium surgery, as well as the possible cytotoxicity of mitomycin-C in the ciliary body, a variety of approaches have been tried to precisely control the mitomycin-C dose. Although drug carriers and controlled delivery implants have been used in an attempt to control the mitomycin-C dose more precisely, simple subconjunctival injection appears to be the most practical and least invasive method.

In 1992, Wang and associates first reported the use of simultaneous sclerostomy and subconjunctival mitomycin-C injection. The sclerostomy was performed with a THC: YAG laser probe subconjunctivally in rabbits, and IOP and bleb survival were monitored. This procedure proved to be effective in enhancing bleb filtration. A similar rabbit experiment was reported in 1994 by Karp and associates.

The most important consideration in preoperative subconjunctival mitomycin-C injection for filtering surgery is optimization of the mitomycin-C dose. Ando and associates showed that when 0.2 mg/ml mitomycin-C is injected subconjunctivally, followed by thorough washing 5 minutes later, approximately 3 µg of mitomycin-C remains in the eye. Subconjunctival administration of mitomycin-C prior to filtering surgery appears to be a safe and easy procedure. Its advantages include exact control of the amount of mitomycin-C delivered, prevention of back-flow of mitomycin-C intracamerally via a fistula during intraoperative use, and the fact that it improves the ease of the fornix-based conjunctival flap procedure. However, the procedure can be difficult in patients with a very thin conjunctiva or thick conjunctival scarring, and mitomycin-C can be difficult to place in the intrascleral lamella.

Mitomycin-C at a concentration of 0.1, 0.2, 0.4 mg/ml is used for 0.5, 1, 2, 3, and 5 minutes by various surgeons intraoperatively by a sub-Tenon's sponge application. Even though the success rates improved with trabeculectomy, the hypotony rates, bleb-related complications increased as compared to conventional procedure. We use 0.2 mg/ml for 1 minute and in resurgeries, 0.4 mg/ml is used. However, use of antimetabolites in primary surgeries is controversial and is sparingly advocated by many surgeons.

5-Fluorouracil

The use of 5-fluorouracil (5-FU), an antimetabolite, has been shown to inhibit the proliferation of fibroblasts in tissue culture, and in preliminary studies it increased the success of filtering surgery in a nonhuman primate model. Fluorouracil filtering surgery study was undertaken to determine whether postoperative subconjunctival injections of 5-FU increases the success rate of filtering surgery in patients at high risk for failure after standard glaucoma filtering surgery.

Fluorouracil Filtering Surgery Study

The Fluorouracil Filtering Surgery Study was a randomized, controlled clinical trial comparing the success rate of standard glaucoma filtering surgery to the success rate of standard surgery with adjunctive 5-FU treatment.

Another element of this study was to evaluate the frequency and severity of possible adverse effects related to 5-FU injections. Detailed preoperative and postoperative examinations of the cornea, lens, and retina were performed. Systemic toxicity was assessed by preoperative and postoperative hematologic studies.

After the investigators performed the filtering surgery and determined that the new outlet channel was working, patients were randomized to receive either 5-FU injections or standard postsurgical care without 5-FU. The patients treated with 5-FU received subconjunctival injections of 5 mg of 5-FU twice daily on postoperative days 1 through 7 and once daily on postoperative days 8 through 14. There were 213 patients recruited into the study, 162 with previous cataract extraction and 51 with previous filtering surgery.

All patients were examined at 1 month, 3 months, 6 months, 1 year, 18 months and 2 years postoperatively and at yearly intervals thereafter until 5 years postoperatively. Possible concomitant risks of 5-FU treatment, such as toxic effects to the cornea, lens or retina, were monitored.

The data demonstrate improved surgical control of glaucoma using 5-FU in patients at high risk for trabeculectomy failure. At 1 year, the cumulative success rates as calculated by survival analysis were 80% for the 5-FU group and 60% for the standard surgery group; at 3 years, the success rates were 56% for the 5-FU group and 28% for the standard group; at 5 years, the success rates were 48% in the 5-FU group and 21% in the standard. Success was defined as no reoperation for the IOP control and no IOP over 21 mm Hg at or after the 1-year visit.

Visual acuity results (logMAR scale) in the 5-FU group were worse than results in the standard therapy group at 1 month; however, the visual acuity change from the qualifying visit was better in the 5-FU group at 1, 2 and 3 years. The difference was not statistically significant at 4 or 5 years. This study showed that, regardless of the treatment group, patients with controlled IOP had less visual acuity loss than patients whose IOPs were not controlled. No difference between treatment groups was found in change in visual field sensitivity. Patients who underwent re-operation showed more visual field loss than those who did not undergo re-operation; the results also suggest that visual field loss is associated with high IOPs. Both treatment groups lost visual acuity and visual field throughout the 5 years of the study.

Risk factors other than treatment that clearly affect success are the preoperative IOP, the number of previous ocular procedures with a conjunctival incision, and the time interval between the last ocular surgery and the study filtering surgery.

The development of a late-onset leak in the filtering bleb was more likely to occur in the 5-FU group (9%) than in the standard therapy group (2%). No other long-term adverse effects were significantly different between the two groups. Two cases of endophthalmitis developed in the 5-FU group versus one case in the standard group.

The risk of a suprachoroidal hemorrhage was not related to 5-FU. However, an important finding concerning suprachoroidal hemorrhage after filtering surgery is that the risk of hemorrhage was strongly associated with the preoperative IOP.

The association between high preoperative IOP and acute postoperative hypotony was not suspected as a risk factor for the development of suprachoroidal hemorrhage prior to this study. This observation has contributed to a change in ophthalmic surgical practice. Patients with very high preoperative IOPs now undergo trabeculectomies either with multiple tightly tied sutures or with releasable sutures in the scleral flap placed to minimize postoperative hypotony. Postoperative argon laser suture lysis or removal of releasable sutures may reduce the likelihood of large postoperative IOP fall and subsequent hypotony.

The fluorouracil filtering surgery study group recommends the use of subconjunctival 5-FU after trabeculectomy in eyes that have undergone previous cataract surgery or unsuccessful filtering surgery. However, because of a higher risk of late-onset wound leaks, which may increase the risk of endophthalmitis, the study group cautions against the routine use of 5-FU in patients with good prognoses.

Preservation of visual function was associated with IOP control in both treatment groups, providing additional evidence to support IOP lowering in patients with glaucoma.

The technique of 5-FU injection is given in Table 13.3. Intraoperative sponge application for 1 to 5 minutes is described, and whether it replaces the injection method or not is a debatable issue.

Table 13.3: Technique of 5-FU injection

- Topical anesthesia is followed.
- The injection is administered at the slit lamp.
- 5 mg 5-FU (0.1 ml of 50 mg/ml 5-FU) is loaded in a tuberculin syringe with 25-gauge needle.
- 30-gauge needle is subsequently used.
- At least 5 mm of subconjunctival track is ensured.
- Ideally a site is chosen 180° away from the bleb.
- Alternatively adjacent to the bleb.
- 1–2 injections/day for 5 to 7 days.
- Watch for complications is kept (superficial punctate keratopathy, epithelial defects).
- Injections are stopped if complications occur.

Releasable Sutures

Releasable or adjustable sutures are the preferred intraoperative method for postoperative wound modulation due to the ease of the procedure and the amount of IOP reduction that can be achieved in the immediate postoperative period.

Technique

Apical or basal releasable sutures are applied as per the surgeon's comfort. However, basal sutures can be avoided when tight wound closure need to be achieved as in angle closures and retrabeculectomy.

The 10-0 nylon sutures are used and the first bite is placed in the corneal side and the second bite at the base of the flap with care taken not to go to full thickness to avoid wound leak, third bite is taken at the apex of the flap (in case of apical suture in a triangular flap) and finally at the scleral side. The loop formed is used to apply a loop knot tightly to oppose the flap to the scleral bed (Figs 13.39 to 13.44).

The free end can be trimmed at the end of the procedure, which can be removed approximately 1 to 4 weeks when the IOP spikes are noted with healing. The aim is to lift the scleral flap with minimal force and facilitate the aqueous to form a barrier for healing of the flap to the bed enabling the formation of bleb. The procedure can be supplemented with 5-FU injections if further healing is noted.

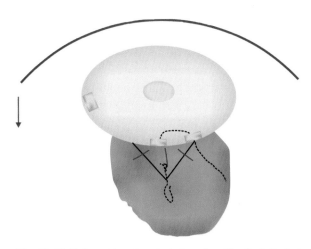

Fig. 13.41: Releasable suture technique (modification): Buried releasable suture–free end of the suture in conjunctival side

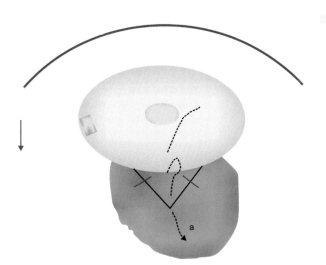

Fig. 13.39: Releasable suture technique: (a) Direction of apical releasable suture

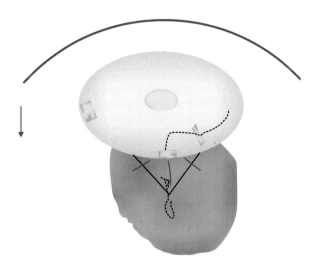

Fig. 13.42: Releasable suture technique (modification): Buried releasable suture–free end of the suture under cornea

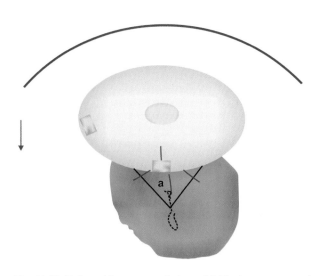

Fig. 13.40: Releasable suture technique: (a) Final appearance of releasable suture

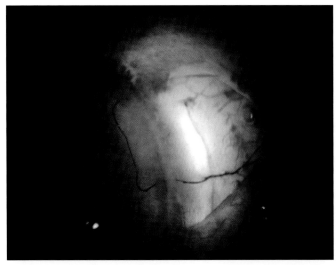

Fig. 13.43: Buried releasable suture in-situ at the end of surgery

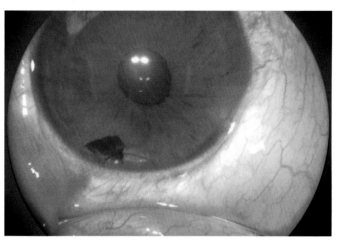

Fig. 13.44: Buried releasable suture appearance after conjunctival closure

Modifications

The free end can be taken through the sclera, then cornea and the routine procedure followed or buried through cornea only to avoid the windshield wiper effect due to the free end of an open-ended suture (Fig. 13.45).

Argon Laser Suture Lysis

Instead of a releasable suture, interrupted sutures also can be cut using short pulse argon laser (Table 13.4). However, this procedure requires partial tenonectomy to visualize the suture. Any subconjunctival hemorrhage can preclude the procedure due to visibility and laser delivery (Figs 13.46A and B).

GLAUCOMA IMPLANTS

To ensure that aqueous drainage through the artificial implanted devices forms a bleb away from the limbus, the implants are placed in between the extraocular muscles. The encapsulation around the equatorially located plate made of silicone or

Table 13.4: Argon laser suture lysis

- Topical anesthesia is followed.
- Hoskin's or Mandelkov's lens is used to blanch the congestion at the site of laser delivery.
- 50 micron spot size; 50-100 ms pulse; 0.1–0.4 W are usually required for the suture lysis.
- The IOP is monitored at the end of 1 hour to decide on further intervention.
- Possible complications include overfiltration, subconjunctival hemorrhage, shallow anterior chamber, rarely buttonholing of conjunctiva if excess energy is used.

polypropylene will ensure the formation of a bleb. The anterior chamber is connected to the plate through a silicone or silastic capillary tube to the device.

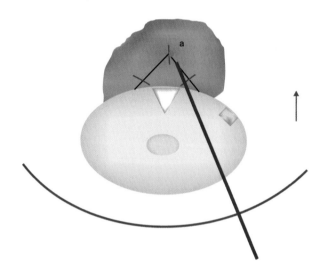

Fig. 13.46A: Argon laser suture lysis—Hoskin's lens or Mandelkov's lens can be used to blanch vessels before the procedure (not depicted in the figure)

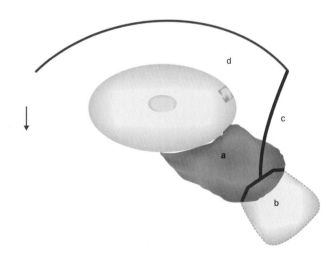

Fig. 13.46B: Steps of glaucoma implant surgery: (a) limbal or fornix-based flap. (b) implant inserted in superotemporal quadrant after adequate dissection. (c) tube in place after tuning. (d) paracentesis example given is Ahmed glaucoma valve implant

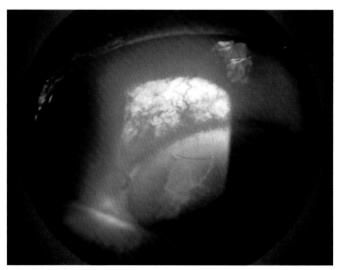

Fig. 13.45: Routine-free end releasable suture causing windshield wiper effect

Indications

1. Refractory glaucoma (neovascular glaucoma, inflammatory glaucoma, glaucoma associated with aphakia and pseudophakia, postvitreoretinal surgery or penetrating keratoplasty glaucoma).
2. Failed trabeculectomy (single or multiple).
3. Pediatric glaucomas (to avoid an exposed bleb).
   Some centers use the implants as primary procedure itself.

Choice of Implant

The choice of implant is according to the comfort of the surgeon while Ahmed glaucoma valve implant (New World Medical Inc, Rancho Cucamonga, CA, USA) and Baerveldt implant (Pharmacia Iovision Inc, Irvine, CA, USA) have gained popularity in recent times. Molteno implant (STAAR Surgical Co, Monrovia, CA, USA) is still being practiced in many centers. Ahmed and Krupin implants are closed valve implants while Molteno and Baerveldt are non-valved open tube implants which need a suture within or around the tube to limit the aqueous flow until the encapsulation surrounds the plate. Krupin has a slit valve, while the Ahmed has a venturi-type valve.

The surface area of the bleb can be enhanced by actual increase of the plate size (Krupin, Baerveldt) or by single or double plates (Molteno and Ahmed).

Surgical Technique

(Mainly for the Ahmed Glaucoma Valve Implant)

1. Local or general anesthesia is used.
2. Clear-corneal traction or a superior rectus bridle suture is used.
3. Fornix- or limbal-based incision in single or double quadrants (for double plate implants) is given. Superotemporal quadrant is preferred.
4. Priming of implant is done in valve implants to check device patency with 30-gauge cannula through the tube.

5. Placement of plate (single plate) is relatively easy with blunt dissection carried out posteriorly. With double plate and Baerveldt implants, the quadrant needs to be prepared and the muscles retracted using silk sutures to create adequate space to position the plate. The plate's anterior edge is placed at approximately 8 to 9 mm behind the limbus and anchored with 5-0 nylon sutures.
6. One-stage versus two-stage procedure: With valved implants, one-stage procedure with direct placement of the tube in the anterior chamber is used. With non-valved implants, the tube is placed in the sub-Tenon's space and after encapsulation occurs over the equatorial plate; usually, after 4 to 6 weeks, the tube is placed in the anterior chamber. This procedure will avoid immediate postoperative hypotony.
7. The tube is then trimmed so that the bevel faces upwards and the proposed internal length of the tube should be approximately up to the mid-iris level (2 to 3 mm) (Figs 13.47A and B).
8. The tube insertion is done at the limbus so that the internal entry is at the level or just anterior to the trabecular meshwork. If the direction of entry is parallel to the iris, this can be achieved. A paracentesis can be made before, and some surgeons prefer to use an anterior chamber maintainer or high-molecular-weight viscoelastic solutions to maintain the anterior chamber to prevent sudden hypotony.
9. If a non-valved implant is used, internal or external tube ligation is achieved using 5-0 or 7-0 polyglactin absorbable sutures or alternatively 10-0 vicryl sutures for external ligation. Some surgeons use both to avoid hypotony. The free end of the internal ligating suture can be withdrawn from the equatorial plate and left in the temporal or inferior subconjunctival space to be removed later when the IOP spikes at the end of 4 to 9 weeks.
10. A 22- or 23-gauge needle is used to make the entry into the anterior chamber. The tube is then held with a nontoothed forceps, such as Pierce-Hoskins forceps, and directed into the anterior chamber. The direction of entry is critical for

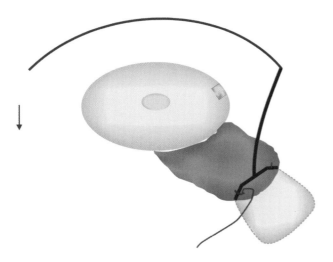

Fig. 13.47A: Steps of glaucoma implant surgery: Suturing of the equatorial plate

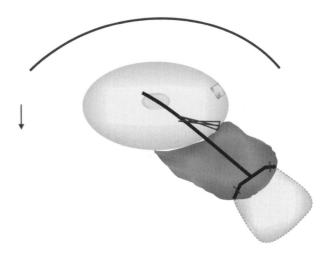

Fig. 13.47B: Steps of glaucoma implant surgery: Trimming the tube for proper sizing before insertion into the anterior chamber

the proper placement of the tube in anterior chamber (Figs 13.48 and 13.49).

11. Once the tube is secured, donor sclera (or preserved pericardium) can be sized to cover the length of the tube from the equatorial plate and anchored to the sclera with 5-0 nylon sutures. Few surgeons prefer to insert the tube under a half-thickness scleral flap, which may not be ideal since the chances of erosion, and exposure of the tube is common with this method (Figs 13.50 and 13.51).

12. The limbal end of the tube can be secured or fixed with the sclera so that future migration can be avoided. A 10-0 nylon horizontal mattress suture is used to fix the tube in this manner.

13. The anterior chamber is formed at the end of the procedure to ensure adequate firmness and the conjunctiva is sutured with 8-0 vicryl double or single layered, continuous, horizontal mattress sutures (Figs 13.52 to 13.55).

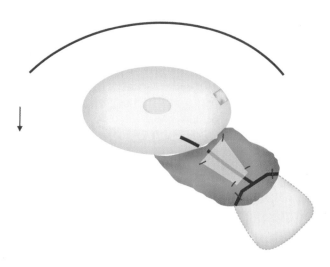

Fig. 13.50: Steps of glaucoma implant surgery: Suturing of scleral patch graft over the tube length

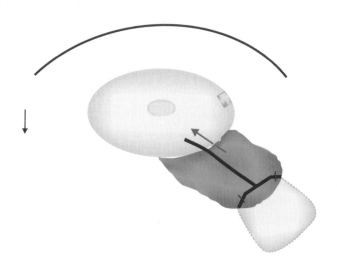

Fig. 13.48: Steps of glaucoma implant surgery: Direction of AC entry with 23-gauge needle

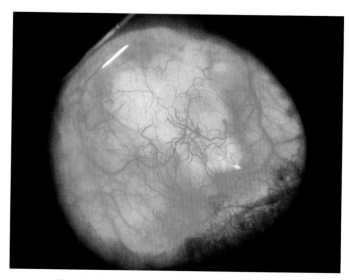

Fig. 13.51: Scleral patch graft over the tube in place

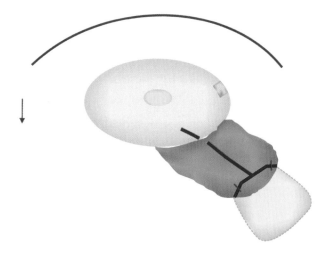

Fig. 13.49: Steps of glaucoma implant surgery: Tube in anterior chamber—note that the tube tip goes until the mid iris

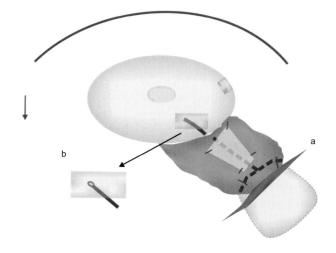

Fig. 13.52: Steps of glaucoma implant surgery: (a) Conjunctival closure, (b) Tube tip in magnification for the shape of bevel

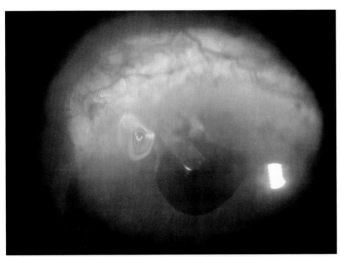

Fig. 13.53: Tube in anterior chamber after completion surgery

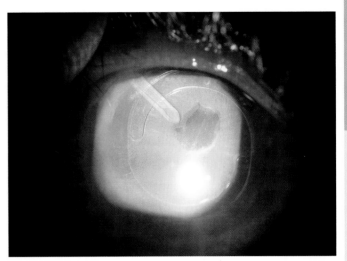

Fig. 13.55: Tube in the anterior chamber in the presence of an anterior chamber intraocular lens

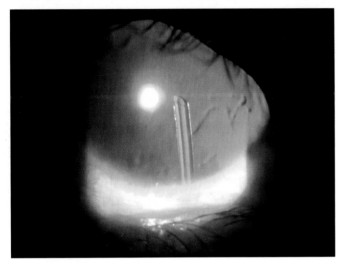

Fig. 13.54: Inferior implantation of drainage device showing tube inferiorly (rarely performed)

Other Modifications in Implant Surgery for Glaucoma

1. The tube can be extended with an angioplasty catheter or customized extension tubes available (Tube extender).
2. The donor sclera can be replaced by preserved pericardium, dura or alternatives available.
3. Nonocclusive ligatures and/or fenestrations are made in the proximal end of the tube to avoid postoperative spike in open tube shunts with tube ligatures.
4. Many investigators have proposed use of mitomycin-C before implant insertion; however, the chances of hypotony are variable with this technique unlike the trabeculectomy.
5. Use of 5-FU injections have been proposed by some of the investigators with mixed success.
6. The Ahmed and Baerveldt implants come with a pars plana modification (pars plana clip), which allows the implant to bend without kinking. This will require the eye to be aphakic or pseudophakic and pars plana vitrectomy is mandatory for this procedure. However, long-term results of this procedure are not available to recommend this procedure widely.

Implant Specific Instructions

Molteno Implant

Single or double plate implants are used. Single plate can be inserted as given for any implant, but the tube needs to be ligated to avoid hypotony.

Double plate Molteno implants need to be inserted negotiating the extraocular muscles usually the superior rectus.

Baerveldt Implant

The implant is of a larger surface area, and it needs to be inserted with tagging of the superior and lateral rectus. Tube ligation is a must in this type of implant.

Postoperative Care for Modification of Intraocular Pressure in Implant Surgery

1. Postoperative hypotony can be taken care with anterior chamber reformation with viscoelastics (usually high molecular weight) and steroids.
2. Hypertensive phase (56%) occurs between 4 and 9 weeks during which time antiglaucoma medications are needed. Some surgeons have reported that the phase continues in majority of subjects (70%) and they continue with antiglaucoma medications. If medications do not control the IOP, partial capsule removal over the equatorial plate is attempted at a later stage.
3. Blood clots, vitreous, posterior capsule or iris plugging the tube (in case of aphakia where inadequate vitrectomy is performed), can be managed with irrigation of the tube, intracameral tissue plasminogen activator injection or argon laser vitreolysis near the tube end without damaging the tube (Fig. 13.56).
4. Few surgeons prefer using 5-FU injections in the lower fornix as in the case of trabeculectomy.

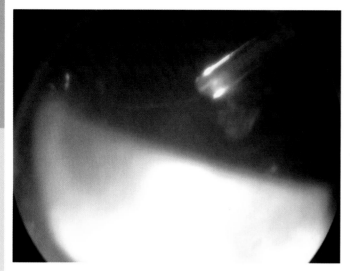

Fig. 13.56: Vitreous blocking the tube elevating intraocular pressure

5. Pseudocapsule excison, tube repositioning, choroidal drainage, re-implant are aggressive methods required in difficult and complicated situations mentioned elsewhere (Table 13.5).

Success rate of implants varies from 57 to 80% with various studies over a 5-year period.

Other implants such as Optimed, ACTEB, Joseph, White are used rarely now, and therefore, have not been mentioned.

Complications

See Table 13.6.

Table 13.5: Implant materials and relevant details

S. No	Implant	Tube material	Plate material	Surface area (mm²)
1.	Ahmed	Silastic	Polypropylene/ Silicone	184, double plate 364
2.	Baerveldt	Silicone	Silicone	250, 350, 425, 500
3.	Molteno	Silicone	Polypropylene	135, double plate 270, 180
4.	Krupin	Silastic	Silicone	180, 300 (360 band)

Table 13.6: Short- and long-term complications related to implant surgery (Fig. 13.57)

- Immediate postoperative hypotony—choroidal detachment (7–33%)
- Prolonged hypertensive phase (10–70%)
- Tube-related complications (10%)
  - —Tube blockage
  - —Tube migration
  - —Tube erosion
  - —Tube endothelial touch
- Encystment of equatorial bleb
- Corneal decompensation (6–50%)
- Melting of patch graft

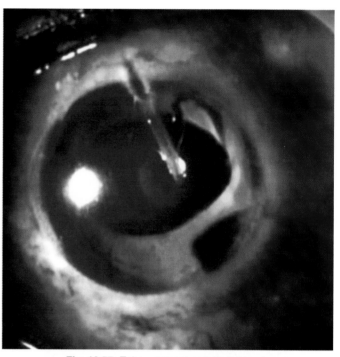

Fig. 13.57: Tube—corneal endothelial touch

External Trabeculotomy

External trabeculotomy is usually performed in the management of congenital glaucomas. It can also be performed in the developmental glaucoma, wherein the success rate is much lower than in congenital glaucomas. It involves rupturing of the inner wall of Schlemm's canal and trabecular meshwork by a blunt-tipped probe. It is a good alternative in cases of cloudy cornea wherein goniotomy cannot be performed successfully (Fig. 13.58).

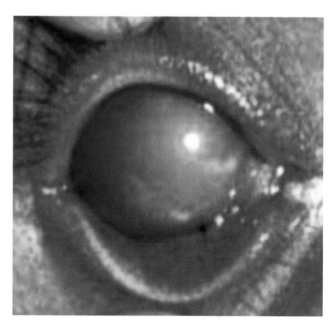

Fig. 13.58: Buphthalmic eye (severe corneal edema)

After the induction of anesthesia, a thorough examination is done to confirm the findings. The surgical site is exposed as described for trabeculectomy. Usually, the superior quadrant is selected because of ease of identification of the anatomical structures, especially in buphthalmic eyes.

Conjunctival Flap

Conjunctival flap is similar to the one described for trabeculectomy. A fornix-based flap is usually preferred (Figs 13.59A and B).

Partial-thickness Scleral Flap

The partial-thickness scleral flap is fashioned as described for trabeculectomy (Fig. 13.60). Usually, a triangular-shaped flap is made as it provides adequate exposure without excessive dissection. A thick flap of approximately 80% thickness is made to facilitate identification of Schlemm's canal (Figs 13.61 and 13.62).

Exposing Schlemm's Canal

The key anatomic landmark is the scleral spur, a circumferential band of white fibers in the scleral bed, wherein randomly arranged scleral fibers become circumferential. A radial scratch incision is made in the exposed scleral bed with a blade knife across the sclerolimbal junction anterior to the scleral spur initiated approximately 1 mm anterior to the corneolimbal junction. The incision is carefully extended through the deeper layers to cut the external wall of the Schlemm's canal until blood or aqueous reflux is seen in its lateral wall (Fig. 13.63).

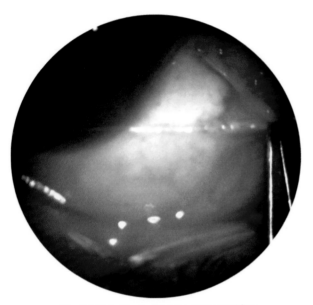

Fig. 13.59A: Fornix-based conjunctival flap

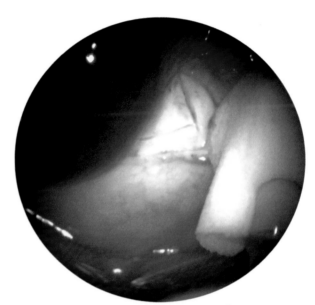

Fig. 13.60: Triangular scleral flap

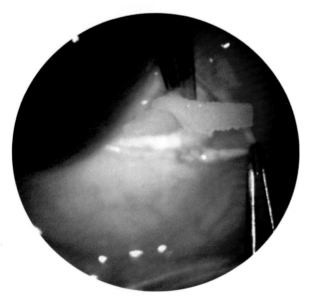

Fig. 13.59B: Use of intraoperative mitomycin-C (in the event of conversion to combined trabeculectomy)

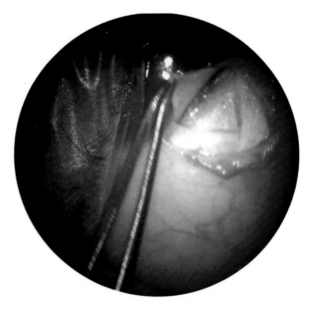

Fig. 13.61: Completion of scleral flap and exposure of limbus

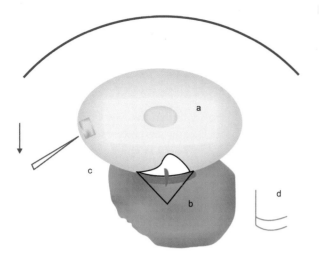

Fig. 13.62: External trabeculotomy: (a) Corneal edema (b) Radial section at the blue limbus (c) Paracentesis (d) Harms trabeculotome

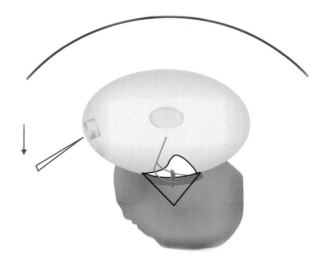

Fig. 13.64: External trabeculotomy: Trabeculotomy performed through the Schlemm's canal

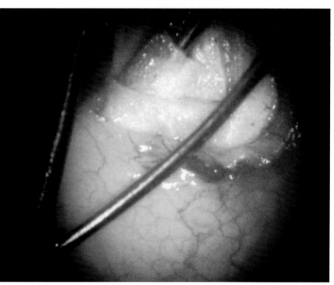

Fig. 13.65: Use of Harms trabeculotome to open the Schlemm's canal to AC

Trabeculotomy

The internal arm of the trabeculotome is introduced at one end of the incision and is fully engaged into the Schlemm's canal (Figs 13.63 and 13.64). If the probe is properly positioned, it cannot be moved posteriorly and the anterior rotation should be without any resistance. It is then swept gently towards the center of the anterior chamber by rotating the probe about the axis of the handle with the external parallel arm as a guide maintaining the position of the blade parallel to the iris plane. A similar procedure is repeated at the other end of the incision. Scleral flap is closed with three to five 10-0 nylon sutures in a fluid tight fashion. Conjunctiva is closed as described for trabeculectomy (Figs 13.65 and 13.66A and B).

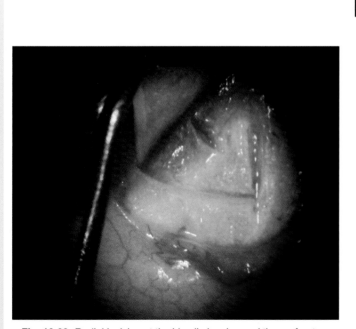

Fig. 13.63: Radial incision at the blue limbus beyond the perforators

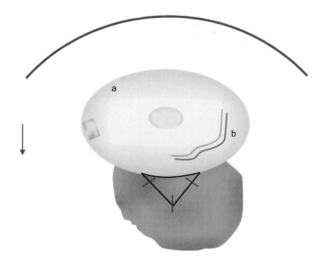

Fig. 13.66A: External trabeculotomy (final appearance): (a) Resolved corneal edema (b) Haabs' striae

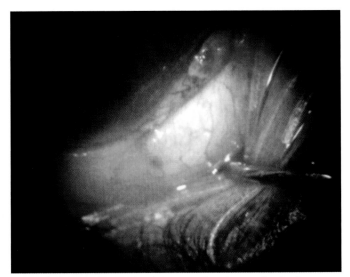

Fig. 13.66B: Final appearance after closure of scleral and conjunctival flap

Complications

- Hyphema
- Peripheral anterior synechiae
- Descemet's membrane stripping
- Injury to the iris
- Increase in lenticular opacity
- False passages into anterior chamber
- Iridodialysis
- Cyclodialysis
- Choroidal detachment
- Postoperative infection
- Anatomy is often altered in buphthalmic eyes; hence, identifying the scleral spur is essential.
- A 5-0 or 6-0 nylon can be passed through the cut end of the Schlemm's canal and confirm if resistance is encountered, the suture is not probably in Schlemm's canal.
- A paracentesis can be made before passing the probe as sometimes anterior chamber may collapse after entering on one side and the other end entry would be difficult.

PROCEDURES RELATED TO COMPLICATIONS FOLLOWING TRABECULECTOMY

Glaucoma surgery has been associated with a significant morbidity right from its evolution. There is a fine balance that one needs to achieve for a successful outcome with the least possible complications. Surgeries have a learning curve but experience and keen judgment are essential to manage the postoperative course.

Most patients will assume visual improvement as the goal of the surgery, adequate patient counseling is a necessary measure with regards to the aim of the surgery, possible complications and visual outcome.

Prevention of Complications

Attention to detail will go a long way to minimize complications and ensure both short- and long-term success of filtration surgery. A meticulous approach with strict adherence to protocol listed in Table 13.7 will help achieve desirable results.

Table 13.7: Approach protocol

- Adnexal problems should be treated prior to surgery
- Anticoagulants should be stopped 3 to 5 days before surgery
- Topical treatment is stopped and oral carbonic anhydrase inhibitors are substituted if required
- High risk eyes (high myopes, children, raised episcleral venous pressure, nanophthalmos) should be identified
- Strict protocol for antimetabolites should be followed
- Gentle tissue handling

Intraoperative Complications

Anesthesia Related

Since most often surgery is done under peribulbar or retrobulbar anesthesia, acute retrobulbar hemorrhage is a rare, but possible complication that is of most concern to the glaucoma surgeon. Eyes with advanced glaucomatous damage are at the risk of ischemic complications resulting in macular wipe out. Immediate measures to reduce the IOP will include administration of intravenous 20% mannitol (1 g/kg body wt) in addition to a lateral canthotomy. Surgery is postponed to a later date.

Topical anesthesia in combination with intracameral lidocaine or sub-Tenon's injection is recommended to avoid these complications.

Traction Sutures

We use superior rectus traction suture routinely. Bleeding at this site is a possible complication. Postoperative ptosis can result, especially in elderly patients. Both conditions are self-limiting and one can consider corneal traction suture as an alternative.

Corneal traction sutures may cut through if too superficial and will result in the shallowing of anterior chamber if the track is deeply placed. The first situation will need either a careful re-pass just below the earlier pass or to switch to a superior rectus traction suture.

Conjunctival Complications

Bleeding is rarely excessive in routine surgeries. It is of concern in extremely vascular beds as in patients with raised episcleral venous pressure. Controlled cautery and avoiding incision at sites where perforating vessel exit would minimize the risk. Excessive bleeding as well as excessive usage of cautery cause increased inflammation at the surgical site.

Conjunctiva needs delicate handling and meticulous care. Avoidance of conjunctival tears and holes is integral to every glaucoma surgery. Non-toothed forceps and blunt dissection tools are the instruments of choice for glaucoma surgery.

The risk of accidental perforation and buttonholing is greater in limbus-based flaps and in eyes undergoing repeat surgeries. In case of repeat surgeries, the preoperative assessment of conjunctival mobility with cotton-tipped applicator under slit lamp guidance is a must. Good mobility lowers the risk of buttonholing. Small holes are best managed with horizontal mattress or purse string suture using a tapered point needle (to avoid slicing along the suture track). Large buttonholes will necessitate either relocation of surgery site or conjunctival free grafts. It is essential to ensure watertight closure on table. Sterile fluorescein can be used over the surgical site to confirm the same.

Scleral Flap Complications

Flap complications are rare and more likely while managing thin sclera as seen in pediatric population and eyes with prior surgery. If flap amputation occurs prior to the creation of stoma, it is ideal to change the site of surgery. If the amputation occurs after the creation of stoma or there is no alternative site possible, a scleral patch graft from an adjacent area will have to be created. It is anchored with horizontal mattress sutures.

Suprachoroidal Hemorrhage

Suprachoroidal hemorrhage is a rare, but serious complication occurring in eyes at risk (high myopes, aphakia, elderly people, nanophthalmos and raised episcleral venous pressure). Intravenous mannitol preoperatively is likely to reduce the sudden effects of decompression and thereby possibilities of suprachoroidal hemorrhage. It commonly occurs on table in an acute fashion, but can occur in the first postoperative week. Inability to form the anterior chamber, loss of fundal glow and progressive pain are indications. The problem must be immediately recognized, and the surgeon's priority would be to ensure a quick wound closure in order to prevent prolapse of intraocular contents. Intravenous mannitol on table and posterior sclerotomy should be considered if wound closure is difficult. Eventually, drainage of the hemorrhage with the assistance of a vitreoretinal surgeon would be the best way to manage this sight-threatening complication.

Hyphema

When the entry into the anterior chamber inadvertently occurs posterior to the scleral spur, bleeding into the anterior chamber occurs. This is due to damage to the major arterial circle. It may occur when the ciliary processes are inadvertently cut during basal iridectomy. Both the problems can be avoided if adequate care is taken to ensure an anterior entry. If the bleeders are visible, unipolar wet diathermy can be used. Hyphema less than 30% to 40% are self-resolving while the remaining patients may require anterior chamber wash.

Early Postoperative Complications (Day 2–6th Week)

The second phase of complications is essentially related to the amount of aqueous run-off from the filtration procedure. It could be excessive, inadequate or misdirected resulting in various scenarios.

Low Intraocular Pressure with Shallow Anterior Chamber

This situation is likely in the first few days of filtration surgery. It is generally associated with:
- Overfiltration
- Wound leak
- Cyclodialysis cleft

Overfiltration: It is an obvious diagnosis when the bleb is large and the IOP is below 6 mm Hg with a shallow anterior chamber. The management depends on the status of chamber depth (Table 13.8). The clinical picture can change within the next few days when choroidal detachment sets in as a sequelae and bleb size decreases due to a gross decrease in the IOP and outflow. A close meticulous follow-up in the postoperative period is a must to guide the surgeon to decide on a timely and effective intervention. Seidel's test to detect the presence of a leak should be done before intervention for a shallow anterior chamber with or without choroidal detachment (Figs 13.67 to 13.69).

Table 13.8: Decision to intervene in the presence of shallow anterior chamber and choroidal detachment

Anterior chamber shallow (no iridocorneal touch)
- Hourly steroids (waking hours) and strong cycloplegics for two weeks and then tapered
- Usually response in 2 weeks with complete stabilization in 6 weeks

Anterior chamber shallow (peripheral iridocorneal touch)
- Patching for 24 to 48 hours
- Followed by frequent steroids and strong cycloplegics
- The patient is observed for 2 weeks for stabilization of chamber depth and intraocular pressure
- Anterior chamber reformation +/– choroidal tap is done if no response is observed

Anterior chamber flat (lenticulocorneal touch)
- Gentle patch for 24 hours is done
- Anterior chamber reformation is done if no improvement in 24 hours
- Choroidal drainage is performed in presence of large choroidal detachment

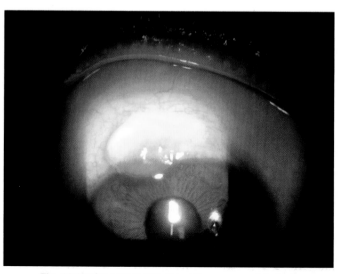

Fig. 13.67: Siedel's test to detect the presence of a leak

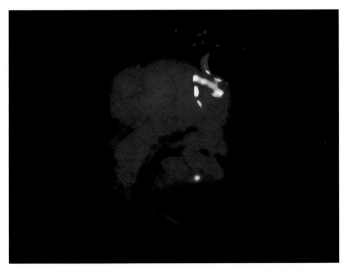

Fig. 13.68: Siedel's test to detect the presence of a leak

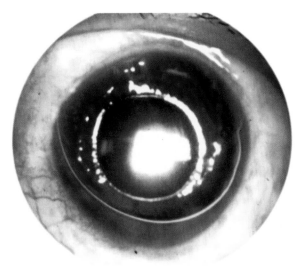

Fig. 13.70: Anterior chamber reformation

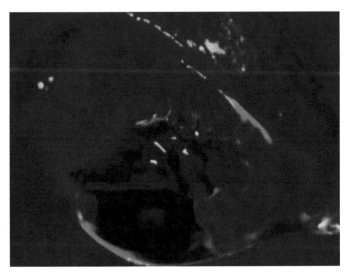

Fig. 13.69: Siedel's test to detect the presence of a leak

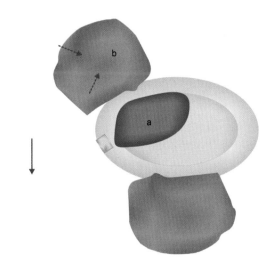

Fig. 13.71: Steps of choroidal drainage: (a) Choroidal detachment, (b) Drainage site (inferotemporal)

Anterior Chamber Reformation (Fig. 13.70)

- Topical anesthesia is followed by povidone-iodine 5%.
- Operating room is ideal
- Lid speculum is placed and anterior chamber entered with a beveled track at the limbus. Sodium hyaluronate is injected. (Air/BSS/20% SF6/C3F8 are alternatives for sodium hyaluronate)
- Moderate deepening of anterior chamber is desired
- Patch 24 hours followed by topical steroids and antibiotics

Choroidal Drainage (Figs 13.71 and 13.72)

- General anesthesia is preferred, alternatively a parabulbar block is safe and effective.
- Sterile draping procedures and topical 5% povidone iodine is applied.
- Anterior chamber is deepened with balanced salt solution (BSS) and an inferior corneal traction suture is taken.
- Drainage sites can be inferotemporal or inferonasal or both

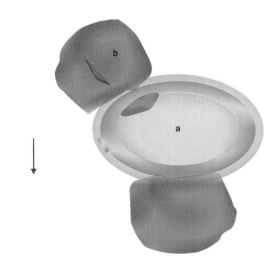

Fig. 13.72: Steps of choroidal drainage: (a) Air in anterior chamber, (b) Drainage site (inferotemporal)

- Conjunctival periotomy is performed 3 mm from limbus followed by a 3 mm radial scleral incision (50 to 70% thickness).
- Gentle cuts are made to reach suprachoroidal space, indicated by ooze of straw-colored fluid.
- Lips of scleral wound is cauterized.
- The IOP is raised by forming anterior chamber with BSS allowing fluid to egress through sclerotomy.
- Scleral wound is left open and conjunctiva is sutured with 10-0 nylon or vicryl sutures.

Wound leak: It must be suspected if the bleb is shallow and IOP is low (< 6 mm Hg) with or without shallow anterior chamber. Seidel's test must be done with sterile fluorescein painted over the bleb surface and suture areas. If the leak is small, patching with antibiotic ointment is recommended for two days. Persistent leaks are best sutured under topical anesthesia. Horizontal mattress sutures with a tapered point needle will suffice for a small hole, while purse string sutures are ideal for larger holes. However, necrotic or avascular blebs may not heal with routine methods. Various techniques, including the use of autologous blood injection, conjunctival patch graft with or without scleral grafts are used in noncompliant situations (Figs 13.73 to 13.77).

Cyclodialysis cleft: It can occur if the anterior chamber entry is posterior to the scleral spur. It is more common with the use of a scleral punch to create the stoma. It is difficult to diagnose it in the early postoperative period and is usually a cause for persistent late hypotony. An ultrasound biomicroscopic examination is helpful in demonstrating the communication between the anterior chamber and suprachoroidal space. Conservative treatment over a prolonged period with cycloplegic agents or else argon laser to the cleft would be ways to manage a nonresponsive cleft.

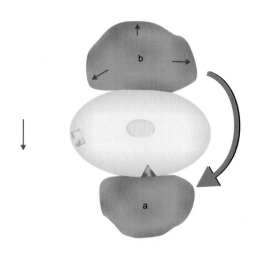

Fig. 13.74: Steps of conjunctival patch graft: (a) Dissection of the diseased conjunctiva, (b) Graft harvesting from inferior fornix

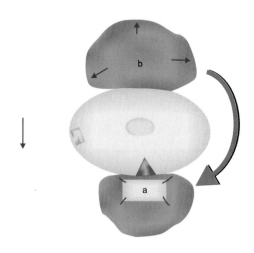

Fig. 13.75A: Steps of conjunctival patch graft: (a) Scleral graft (used when flap is necrosed), (b) Bare area

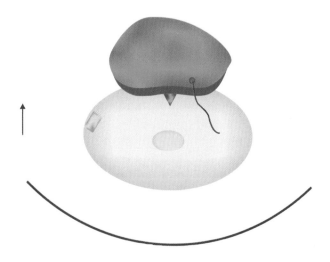

Fig. 13.73: Steps of conjunctival patch graft: Bleb leak with gross hypotony requiring patch graft

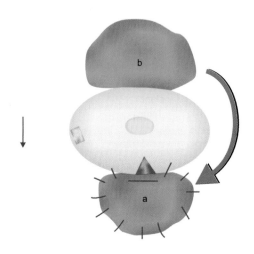

Fig. 13.75B: Steps of conjunctival patch graft: (a) Graft in place, (b) Bare area

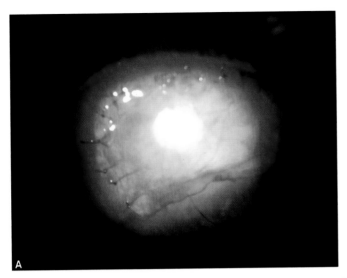

Figs 13.76A and B: Conjunctival patch graft

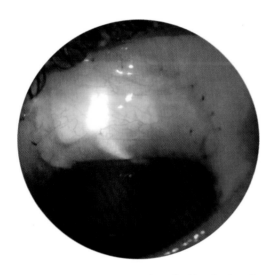

Fig. 13.77: Conjunctival patch graft with scleral graft

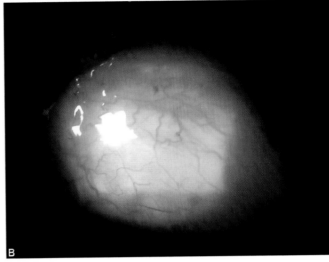

Fig. 13.78: Malignant glaucoma

Elevated Intraocular Pressure with Shallow Anterior Chamber

This complication can occur in the early postoperative situation or as a delayed long-term complication. It could be due to:

- Pupillary block
- Malignant glaucoma
- Suprachoroidal hemorrhage

Pupillary block: It can occur if the iridectomy is not patent. It is generally associated with moderate central AC depth and shallow to flat peripheral anterior chamber due to peripheral ballooning of the iris. Re-establishing patency with Nd:YAG laser is usually curative. Rare situations require surgical iridectomy.

Malignant glaucoma: Malignant glaucoma due to aqueous misdirection can be precipitated following surgery usually in hyperopic eyes and in eyes with chronic angle-closure glaucoma. The IOP is usually elevated, but could be normal, the anterior chamber is flat with a clearly visible and patent iridectomy and bleb is shallow or absent (Fig. 13.78). Few cases respond to aggressive medical treatment with a combination of strong cycloplegics like atropine thrice daily, frequent steroids, beta-blockers and carbonic anhydrase inhibitors. Most often, breaking the anterior hyaloid face with Nd:YAG laser in pseudophakic eyes through the iridectomy or visual axis will help establish communication between anterior and posterior chambers. Vitrectomy ensuring disruption of anterior hyaloid with anterior chamber reformation is the definitive answer, but reserved for failed medical treatment. Ultrasound biomicroscopy helps decide between surgical intervention and conservative management. Eyes with shallow choroidal detachment in the periphery respond better to medical therapy and could be observed for a while; whereas cases without it could be subjected to early surgery.

Elevated Intraocular Pressure with Normal Anterior Chamber

Glaucoma surgery is unpredictable with the outcome being variable through the initial and late postoperative periods. Surgery may appear successful during the initial few days and may start to fail later even as early as two weeks. A vigilant watch is necessary for progressive rise in the IOP and vascularization of the bleb, which is indicative of:

- Bleb failure
- Encapsulated bleb

Bleb failure: It is a likely complication in spite of wound modulation, especially in high-risk eyes (chronic inflammation/medical therapy, repeat trabeculectomy). In the initial phases of failure, gonioscopy has to be done to ensure stomal patency. If there is any obstruction due to fibrin, hemorrhage or membrane, digital massage over the inferior or superotemporal aspect of the globe should be tried. This maneuver may help clear the stoma. The Nd:YAG laser to clear the stoma is also recommended.

In the presence of a patent stoma and progressive evidence of failure, it is recommended that the frequency of topical steroid be increased and 5-FU injections be given subconjunctivally. The technique of injection has been described subsequently. Digital massage can be continued at a frequency of 5 times a day for up to two weeks.

Late bleb revision (> 6 weeks–3 months) is an option if all measures fail. The procedure involves re-establishing stomal patency and relieving the fibrosis along the scleral walls using an internal approach under viscoelastic cover. The fibrosis in the subconjunctival space is also relieved by an external approach similar to a needling procedure. Supplemental 5-FU injections are given over 5 to 7 days.

Encapsulated bleb: It may be sequelae of a failing bleb, wherein a fibrosed Tenon's cavity overlies the filter site encapsulating the aqueous. The cyst is an extension of the anterior chamber, but is nearly impervious to aqueous. Clinically, a vascular, tense, white elevation at the filter site with an increased IOP is the presenting situation. Conservative approach usually involves aqueous suppressants to reduce the IOP and await for spontaneous resolution, which may occur in 2 to 3 months. Needling is an option where the IOP is uncontrolled with medication. It is done under peribulbar or topical anesthesia. The cyst is approached sub-conjunctivally with a 25-gauge needle ensuring a track of at least 5 mm to avoid leaks and also to avoid double perforation. The tip of the needle is advanced into the wall of the cyst and multiple slicing perforations are made. It is usually supplemented with 5-FU injections. Topical steroid and antibiotics are tapered over a few weeks (Fig. 13.79).

Technique of Needling of Bleb:

- Surgery is performed under topical anesthesia
- Slit lamp or operating microscope is used
- 5 mg 5-FU (0.1 ml of 50 mg 5-FU) is loaded in tuberculin syringe with 25-gauge needle or 0.001 mg/ml of mitomycin-C used.

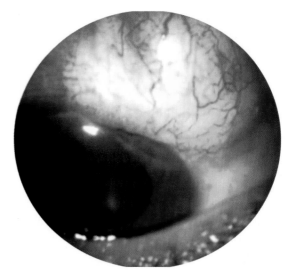

Fig. 13.79: Encysted bleb

- 30-gauge needle is subsequently utilized
- Alternatively, some surgeons do not use antimetabolites
- At least 5 mm of subconjunctival track is ensured
- With the bevel up, the capsule is cut with sharp edges and the sub-Tenon's fibrosis is dissected under visualization through the conjunctiva.
- Similar procedure is used in failed blebs to ensure the patency of subconjunctival filtration. This is followed by 5-FU injections.
- Watch for complications (superficial punctate keratopathy, epithelial defects) is kept.

Late Complications

Bleb Leak

Wound modulation with 5-FU and mitomycin–C has increased the risk of late bleb leakage. Strict protocol, which has been discussed earlier, plays an important role in reducing the risk. Thin-walled blebs are at higher risk for trivial injuries followed by leak and may present in the early months or even years later. In the presence of small leaks, patients are typically asymptomatic or may have drop in visual acuity with the low IOPs (< 6 mm Hg). It is necessary to check for bleb leakage by a Seidel's test if there is an unusual drop in the IOP during follow-up. Large leaks may present with the shallowing of anterior chamber and choroidal detachment. Small leaks can be treated by patching for 1 to 2 days followed by topical antibiotics. Leaks that do not respond to this method will need alternative measures like autologous blood injections or a bleb excision with conjunctival free graft. Alternatively, large diameter soft contact lenses, fibrin tissue glue and cyanoacrylate glue have been tried.

Conjunctival free graft is considered when measures as described above fail. The procedure is done under peribulbar anesthesia. The aim is to excise the ischemic thin-walled bleb and to mobilize adequately sized free conjunctival tissue from temporal or an inferior site. This then is anchored with interrupted 10-0 nylon sutures with limbal orientation maintained. Alternatively, sliding or mobilizing superior conjunctiva can be considered if there is adequate mobility of superior tissue.

Autologous Blood Injection (Figs 13.80A to F)

- Surgery under topical anesthesia, under operating microscope
- Topical 5% povidone-iodine is used
- Lid speculum is applied
- Venous blood is drawn from the patient with a butterfly needle by an assistant.
- Prompt switch over to a 26-gauge needle is done and bleb is entered with it ensuring a 5 mm subconjunctival track.
- Blood may enter anterior chamber which may be washed via paracentesis if required.
- Patching is done for 24 hours
- Postoperative antibiotics

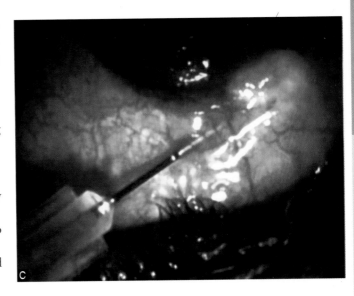

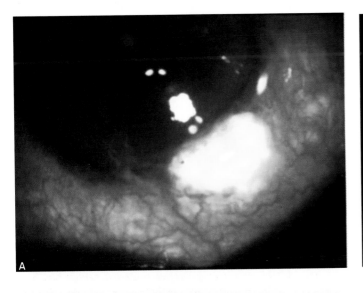

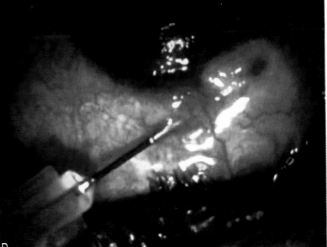

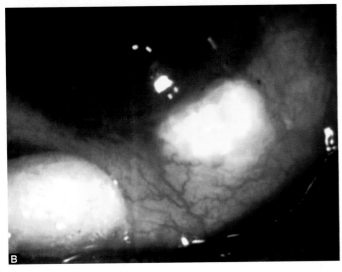

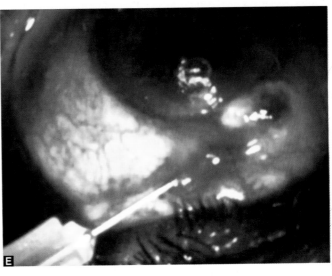

Figs 13.80A to E

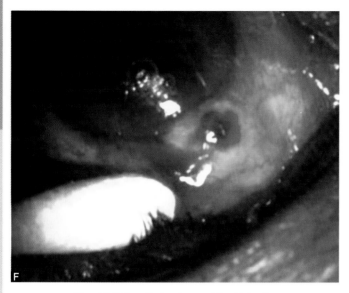

Figs 13.80A to F: Autologous blood injection

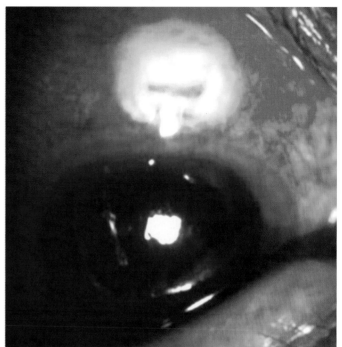

Fig. 13.81: Blebitis with leak

Bleb-related Ocular Infection

As with bleb leaks, wound modulation has increased the risk of bleb-related ocular infection. Blebitis is referred to an infection limited to the bleb wall and anterior chamber. All patients should be made aware of symptoms and signs of a possible infection (pain, redness, decreased vision) to ensure prompt intervention, a delay would result in a rapid downhill course and eventual visual loss. At this stage, ultrasound to rule out vitreous inflammation is done followed by a conjunctival swab for culture and sensitivity. Treatment regimen includes hourly fortified antibiotics (Cephazolin/Cephaloridine 50 mg/ml) and fluoroquinolones (Ciprofloxacin/Ofloxacin). A close watch for improvement on a daily basis is followed by gradual tapering. Long-term daily basis antibiotic ointment may be considered in high-risk cases (thin-walled blebs, repeated leaks). The antibiotics are altered every month.

Blebitis untreated can rapidly progress to endophthalmitis. Any evidence of vitreous involvement is best managed with the help of a vitreoretinal surgeon like any other case of endophthalmitis.

There is a possibility of bleb failure and increased IOP as the acute episode subsides, which is best managed medically (Figs 13.81 and 13.82).

Blebesthesia

Overfiltration or exuberant bleb can form an air pocket in some subjects and be very painful, which is termed as blebesthesia. Usually, it is treated with topical tear supplements. The condition can be cosmetically disfiguring and may require procedures such as compression sutures (parallel and crossed) or in certain extreme cases conjunctival patch graft (Figs 13.83 to 13.87C).

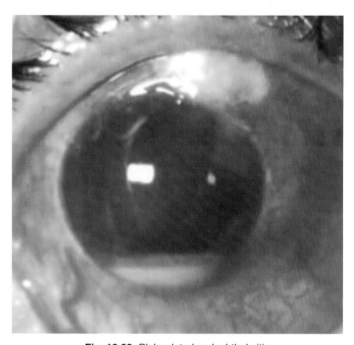

Fig. 13.82: Bleb related endophthalmitis

VISCOCANALOSTOMY

Viscocanalostomy is a relatively new surgical technique developed for glaucoma surgery and it was first proposed in 1991. Whereas a trabeculectomy creates a "flap" in the eye, allowing the aqueous humor to drain directly from the anterior chamber of the eye to form a bleb under the conjunctiva, viscocanalostomy does not involve making a

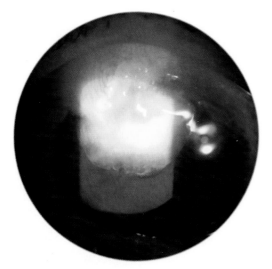

Fig. 13.83: Exuberant bleb

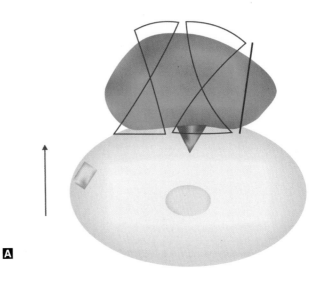

A

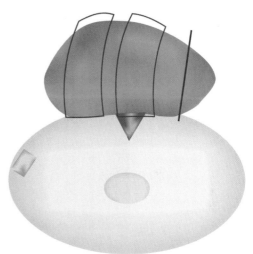

B

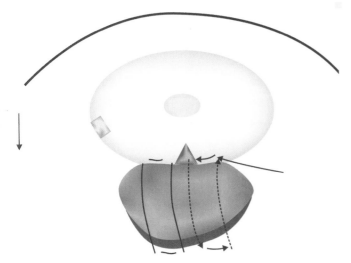

Fig. 13.84: Compression suture technique (for overfiltering bleb) vertical compression sutures

Figs 13.86A and B: Compression suture technique (for overfiltering bleb) (A) Crossed compression sutures (B) Vertical compression sutures

full-thickness hole into the anterior chamber. Instead, the surgeon removes a block of sclera to leave a thin membrane (Descemet's membrane) through which the aqueous humor percolates. The aqueous humor then drains away either through Schlemm's canal (in the natural way) or under the conjunctiva. During the surgery, a thick fluid (viscoelastic) is injected into Schlemm's canal, hence the name of the operation—viscocanalostomy.

There is a theoretical advantage over trabeculectomy with less complications likely, however, the amount by which the IOP is lowered is not usually as great with viscocanalostomy as with trabeculectomy.

SUCCESS RATES FOR GLAUCOMA SURGERY

Trabeculotomy has been widely used in the management of congenital glaucoma. Success rates for the procedure have

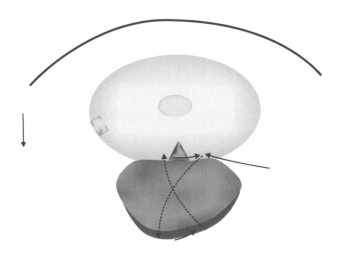

Fig. 13.85: Compression suture technique (for overfiltering bleb) crossed compression sutures

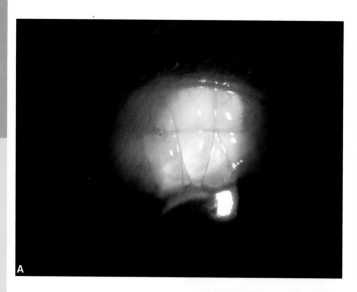
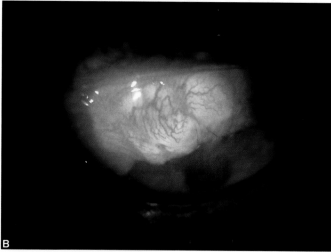
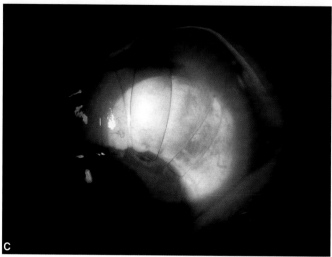

Figs 13.87A to C: Compression sutures

ranged from 92.3% at six months 1 to 72.0 to 83.3% at 2 years. Long-term success has been 92.5% at 5 years and 76.5% at 10 years when multiple surgeries were included.

There are a variety of aqueous drainage devices available today. The reported success rates for primary glaucoma surgery with the Ahmed glaucoma valve (69.8%) was comparable to trabeculectomy (68.1%) at a mean follow-up of 41 months. Success rates for the conventional indications for aqueous drainage devices ranged from 33 to 73.8%.

Trabeculectomy is probably the most widely practiced glaucoma surgical procedure. Its success rates depend on a number of factors including age at surgery, duration from surgery, type of glaucoma and use of antimetabolites. Trabeculectomy for primary glaucoma has been reported to have success rates ranging from 85 to 89% depending upon the type of glaucoma. With success defined as an IOP level of 15 mm Hg or less, Beckers and associates report a success rate of 83.3% in the first year, dropping to 60% in the sixth year following

trabeculectomy with mitomycin. Early results have been similar for other studies using mitomycin ranging from 82 to 85.4% at one year to 70 to 78% at two years. Trabeculectomy is not as successful in the longer term with 5- and 10-year success rates to be, 70%, and 67% respectively, with mean duration of the IOP control (IOP < 21 mm Hg) being 88 months. A 12-year follow-up reported success rates of 50.4% in for trabeculectomy with antimetabolites.

Trabeculectomy combined with cataract surgery has shown varied results. Trabeculectomy combined with the ECCE succeeded in reducing the IOP to less than 20 mm Hg in 82% of patients. Ninety five percent of patients undergoing phacoemulsification combined with trabeculectomy had postoperative IOP reduced to less than 20 mm Hg with similar mean follow-up of 23 months. Blumenthal SICS combined with trabeculectomy has been shown to have similar success rates as a phacotrabeculectomy (Mitomycin being used in both groups).

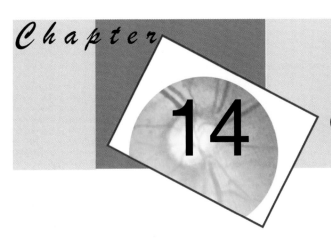

Non-Penetrating Glaucoma Surgeries

Kirti Singh

INTRODUCTION

Non-penetrating glaucoma surgeries, namely deep sclerectomy and viscocanalostomy, work by enhancing the natural aqueous outflow channels by reducing outflow resistance. Outflow resistance to aqueous is constituted by trabecular meshwork, which contributes 75% of resistance and by outer wall of Schlemm's canal, which constitutes rest of 25%.

Non-Penetrating Deep Sclerectomy (NPDS)

Fydorov and Koslov are credited with creating resurgence in non-penetrating deep sclerectomy during 1980s. In non-penetrating deep sclerectomy deep scleral flap, outer and inner wall of the Schlemm's canal and juxtacanalicular meshwork are removed thereby removing the main sources of outflow resistance. Corneal stroma, anterior trabeculum and Descemet's membrane are left behind, which constitute the trabeculo-Descemet's membrane, the creation of which is a critical step in this surgery. Aqueous humor leaves the anterior chamber through the intact trabeculo-Descemet's membrane and reaches the scleral lake (which is a consequence of the volume loss due to excision of deep scleral layer). The major advantage of non-penetrating deep sclerectomy is that precludes the sudden hypotony that occurs following trabeculectomy by creating progressive filtration of aqueous humor from the anterior chamber to the subconjunctival space, without perforation of the eye. Consequently chances of shallow anterior chamber, cataract, macular edema and other sequel of hypotony are minimized. The long-term control of intraocular pressure (IOP) is, however, more efficient in trabeculectomy. Deep sclerectomy surgery is still in its evolving phase and many reports are being published advocating good IOP control over long-term follow-up.

How Does it Work?

In open-angle glaucoma the main site of aqueous outflow resistance is the juxtacanalicular meshwork, therefore removing this tissue after deroofing Schlemm's canal along with floor (inner wall) of Schlemm's canal strikes at the core of the problem. Aqueous subsequently flows through the thin trabeculo-Descemet's membrane, which offers a little resistance to aqueous outflow, allowing a slow fall in IOP. The resistance offered by trabeculo-Descemet's membrane is low enough to ensure a significantly low IOP and simultaneously high enough to maintain anterior chamber depth. After percolating through trabeculo-Descemet's, aqueous momentarily collects in the reservoir created by loss of scleral volume (excision of deep scleral flap) and then gets absorbed gradually. This slow run-off of aqueous prevents a large subconjunctival bleb from forming, unlike that in trabeculectomy.

From scleral lake aqueous gets absorbed through four proposed pathways:

a. *Subconjunctival filtering bleb*: A low diffuse, shallow subconjunctival bleb.

b. *Intrascleral bleb*: The empty scleral space beneath the superficial scleral flap is left behind which transforms into an intrascleral bleb over time with a volume of almost 1.8 mm^3. To maintain this intrascleral bleb various implants namely collagen, hyaluronate, etc. have been used. Aqueous humor from this space is absorbed by new/existing aqueous drainage vessels.

c. *Subchoroidal passage:* The residual thinned scleral bed (10% of original thickness) allows aqueous to permeate into suprachoroidal space. Persistent localized choroidal detachment beneath the deep sclerectomy detected by ultrasound biomicroscopy in almost 45% cases many years after surgery lens credence to this outflow mechanism.

d. *Episcleral drainage via Schlemm's canal*: On either side of deep sclerectomy the two surgically created ostia of Schlemm's canal drain the aqueous into the episcleral veins.

Status of this Surgery

Indications

• Currently due to *safety concerns* post-trabeculectomy, surgical option is offered as last resort to glaucoma patients who do not show an adequate response to medical management. Deep sclerectomy having a much lower complication rate than trabeculectomy can be offered as an earlier option.

- Conjunctiva and trabecular meshwork subjected to cumulative effect of antiglaucoma drugs are altered histologically and react poorly to any filtering surgery and form unhealthy blebs. Virgin conjunctiva forms the best functional bleb, thus an early surgery option like deep sclerectomy is the need of the hour.
- In developmental glaucoma where concern of the cumulative side effects of long-term glaucoma drugs, evidence base validating filtering surgery as the better treatment option, earlier safer surgery is the holy grail. Deep sclerectomy is useful in such patients.
- In high myopia/Sturge-Weber syndrome where abnormal scleral thickness, ocular dimensions entail a higher risk of developing choroidal detachment and shallow chamber after trabeculectomy deep sclerectomy is the better option.
- In both pigmentary and pseudoexfoliation glaucomas, the blocked trabecular meshwork is targeted and pseudoexfoliation material/pigment is peeled away after exposing the trabecular meshwork, which re-establishes filtration.
- In aphakic/pseudophakic glaucoma vitreous herniates through the peripheral iridectomy and blocks the sclerostomy. Adjunctive vitrectomy needs to be performed, which increases risk of tractional retinal detachment. Deep sclerectomy is the surgery of choice in such conditions. However, sometimes Schlemm's canal and trabecular meshwork in aphakia is collapsed, scarred and dysfunctional. Thus, the decision to perform deep sclerectomy is made intraoperatively after viewing extent of aqueous percolation through trabeculo-Descemet's membrane. If the outflow is felt to be insignificant then deep sclerectomy is converted into trabeculectomy. A large wide peripheral iridectomy encompassing the entire length of sclerostomy should be made.

Contraindications

The surgery should not be attempted in cases where the trabecular meshwork is too dysfunctional to allow it to function after deep sclerectomy or where the pathology is proximal to the trabecular meshwork like in narrow-angle glaucoma, rubeotic glaucoma, extensive peripheral anterior synechiae or post-laser trabeculoplasty.

Need for an Implant

The main nemesis of filtering surgery is subconjunctival and subscleral fibrosis, which ultimately leads to the failure of the drainage surgery. Antimitotics, such as mitomycin-C, 5-fluorouracil, daunorubicin have come to play a major role in high-risk cases to minimize the risk fibrosis, however, these drugs are a double edged sword in that they come armed with inherent dangers. In deep sclerectomy too the sclerocorneal space is prone to collapse and fibrosis. To keep this surgically created intrascleral space open Kozlov and associates, in 1990,

proposed the use of an intrascleral collagen implant. Since then various materials have been used for this purpose. After complete resorption of implant over few months, aqueous lake is entrenched enough to maintain patency of the scleral space. Implants have been found to enhance success rates, provide significantly lower IOP levels and lower the need for postoperative medications/goniopunctures.

A multitude of absorbable and nonabsorbable implants have been designed.

Absorbable

- Collagen implant (Aquaflow, Starr Surgical AG, Switzerland): This is a purified biologically inert, porcine scleral collagen, 2.5 by 1 mm in dimension. The device swells 2-3 times to its dry size, after placement in the subscleral space and exposure to ocular fluids. The water content of the hydrated device is 99%, and its complete resorption occurs within 6–9 months.
- Reticulated cross-linked sodium hyaluronate implants (SK-Gel, Corneal Laboratories Paris, France): This is a biosynthetic triangular implant. It is available in two sizes 3.5 and 4.5 mm.
- Autologous sclera
- Amniotic membrane: It creates anatomic barrier by keeping the potentially adhesive surfaces apart, amniotic membrane also prevents fibrosis of the decompression space. It has anti-fibrotic properties owing to the down regulation of TGF-β (responsible for fibroblastic activation in wound healing), and the avascular stroma of amniotic membrane inhibits in the growth of new vessels.

Nonabsorbable

- T-Flux: This 0.2 mm thick T-shaped hydrophilic acrylic implant with 38% water content is placed with two arms inside the cut ostia of the Schlemm's canal. It is anchored to the sclera with 10 zero monofilament nylon suture through a preplaced hole in the implant.
- T – bar: This is made of stainless steel.
- Mermoud X/polymethylmethacrylate implants

Adjunctive Use of Antifibrotics

Mitomycin-C has been successfully used as an adjunctive to prolong survival of deep sclerectomy, and several researchers have vouched for its efficacy in producing lower IOP consistently and reducing the need to perform goniopunctures. The dose used is 0.2 to 0.4% and it is placed both under the superficial scleral flap and in the sub-conjunctival space for 2–3 minutes. The application needs to follow the safe surgery protocol as its use is associated with a high incidence of avascular blebs and transconjunctival ooze/leak.

Technique

A limbal-based/fornix-based conjunctival flap is created. Hemostasis is ensured with minimal wet-field bipolar cautery, taking care to avoid any of the aqueous draining channels. The key is to use the cautery to a minimum to avoid damage to collector channels and aqueous veins (Fig. 14.1). Excess tenon tissue is excised. A 5 × 5 mm rectangular/parabolic, one-third scleral thickness flap is made (330 μm) and dissected 1–1.5 mm anteriorly into clear cornea with a disposable crescent knife.

A wide dissection is needed as large trabeculo-Descemet's membrane needs to be created for adequate percolation (Figs 14.2 and 14.3). Mitomycin-C may be applied at this stage. Dose of 0.2–0.4 mg/ml, for a duration of 2–3 minutes is used. The author prefers the use of amniotic membrane over mitomycin-C. The former acts both as an implant and antifibrotic. Magnification increased to 16-20X and a second 3 × 3 mm, deep scleral flap of approximately 90% of scleral thickness is dissected. The larger superficial flap covers the smaller deeper flap by a small margin on each side. If dissection plane is right, bluish-brown choroid would shine through the thin residual layer of sclera of 10% depth. The dissection is carried anteriorly into the clear cornea for about 2 mm, with a disposable crescent knife. In the posterior part of the scleral dissection, scleral fibers are laid in a random fashion; anteriorly they become more organized, eventually forming a gleaming ligament parallel to the limbus, namely the scleral spur. Usually

Schlemm's canal lies just anterior to this. Thus, the circular ligament serves as a landmark for the identification of Schlemm's canal (Fig. 14.4).

At this stage it is advisable to lower IOP by a paracentesis to reduce the risk of perforation. Alternatively an anterior chamber maintainer can be deployed, which gives adequate control of anterior chamber depth and IOP. It is switched off during the opening of the Schlemm's canal. Schlemm's canal is then deroofed. Subsequently sclerocorneal dissection is carried forward for 1–1.5 mm to remove the sclerocorneal tissue in front of the anterior trabeculum, and inner wall of the Schlemm's canal. A special trabecular meshwork scraper (carbide impregnated metal tip) scrapes off the juxtacanalicular meshwork, which is then peeled with a Mermoud's trabecular peeler forceps. Alternatively blunt diamond knife and capsulorrhexis forceps can be used. Before peeling the inner wall of SC, the area must be thoroughly dried. The end point is when the aqueous starts percolating through the remaining thin trabeculo-Descemet's membrane. The anterior chamber maintainer can be switched on to objectively assess aqueous percolation. The deep scleral flap is then excised at the base, including the corneoscleral tissue overlying anterior trabeculum using a Vannas scissors or diamond knife (Fig. 14.5). A simple

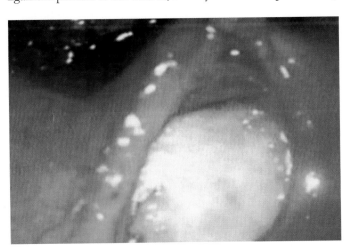

Fig. 14.1: Limbus-based conjunctival flap is created

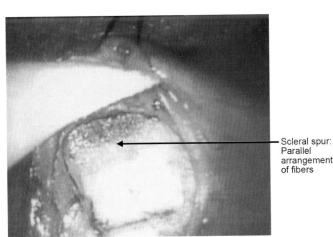

Fig. 14.3: End point of superficial scleral flap

Scleral spur: Parallel arrangement of fibers

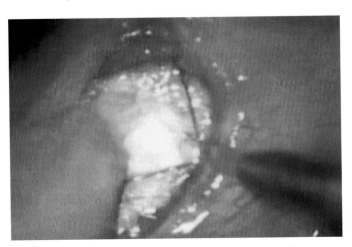

Fig. 14.2: Superficial scleral flap is being dissected

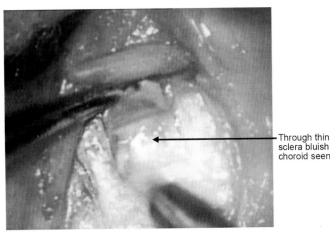

Through thin sclera bluish choroid seen

Fig. 14.4: Deep scleral flap is dissected

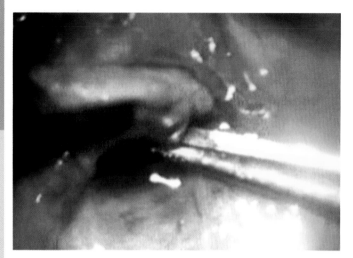

Fig. 14.5: Cutting of deep scleral flap is being performed.
Note aqueous percolation

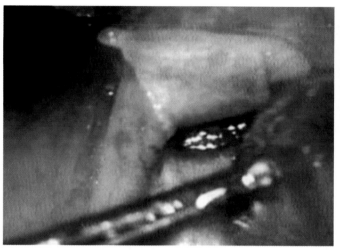

Fig. 14.6: Amniotic membrane is being placed from
a spatula onto scleral bed

yet novel modification is to insert the trabeculotome through a vertical cut at one end of the deeper scleral flap, just anterior to the scleral spur (anterior to the circumferential band of scleral fibers and just at the posterior end of the translucent blue gray zone). This is made after complete superficial flap dissection and once the deep flap has been marked out.

The trabeculotome is then introduced horizontally into the Schlemm's canal. At the other edge of the 3 × 3 mm deeper scleral flap, a direct vertical incision is made over the trabeculotome, and the instrument tip is allowed to exit. The handle of the trabeculotome is then rested on the surface. With the trabeculotome in place, deeper flap is dissected and the Schlemm's canal is opened along its posterior wall thereby exposing the steel arm of the trabeculotome. This technique enables easy identification of Schlemm's canal. An implant or 10 × 6 mm amniotic membrane with the epithelial side up is then placed over the deep scleral bed. The amniotic membrane does not need to be sutured (Fig. 14.6). Alternatively an implant-collagen, T–Flux, etc. is placed on the scleral bed and anchored with one to two 10 nylon sutures. The superficial scleral flap is secured to the scleral bed with two loose interrupted 10-0 nylon sutures and the knots are buried (Fig. 14.7). Conjunctiva and tenon capsule are closed in two/single layers in limbal based technique whereas limbal anchorage with 2–3 sutures is sufficient in the fornix-based technique.

At the start of the deeper flap dissection, Mermoud recommends that the beginning of the posterior cut is made till 100% depth; this induced microperforation gives an estimate of the scleral thickness. The sclera is then held with a non-toothed forceps from one corner, dissection plane is created a hair breadth above the induced microperforation with a crescent blade. The correct plane is where the bluish-brown choroid is hazily visible at the base of the bed.

Postoperatively, antibiotic steroid drops are prescribed for 2 weeks till IOP stabilizes at ≤10 mm Hg, after which nonsteroidal anti-inflammatory drugs may be substituted and prescribed for 4–8 weeks.

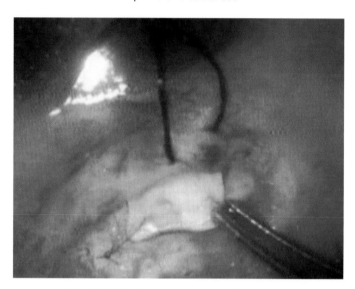

Fig. 14.7: Suturing superficial scleral flap is done
with two loose 10-0 nylon sutures

Postoperative Course and Need for Goniopuncture

Visual acuity returns to baseline within 7–10 days and there is virtually no anterior chamber inflammation. Hypotony on first day is usual and a recent study predicts the success of the surgery, based on first postoperative day IOP. First day pressure of ≤5 mm Hg, favorably predicts the longevity and success of deep sclerectomy with fewer requirement for post-surgery laser goniopuncture.

Goniopuncture needs to be performed in more than half (51 to 63%) of deep sclerectomy patients. It is performed when the aqueous percolation is insufficient as demonstrated by the poor control of IOP. The mean time of goniopuncture has been documented to occur between 3–21 months after surgery. Almost 50% patients require it at the end of 12 months. The procedure is performed with a Nd:YAG laser, using a gonioscopic mirror lens—CGI from LASAG/Haag-Streit lens. The aiming beam is focused on the thinned out less pigmented trabeculo-Descemet's membrane with a power of 2–4 mJ.

Around 5–15 shots may be required at the level of Schwalbe's line both above and below. Air bubbles may be generated during the procedure and a dramatic fall in IOP within hours is usual. Spontaneous iris prolapse with subsequent IOP rise is a common complication which needs treatment with pilocarpine, laser goniosynechiolysis, or rarely surgical revision. The final IOP achieved after deep sclerectomy is usually in mid teens.

Longevity of Non-Penetrating Deep Sclerectomy

As in trabeculectomy, non-penetrating deep sclerectomy also shows a waning effect with time and supplemental medications and/or repeat surgery are required in more than 50% after 4–5 years. In a six year follow-up, qualified success rate was 80% and 67% without supplemental medications.

Combined with Cataract Surgery

Primary combined phacoemulsification with NPDS, with or without implant or antimitotics is an effective modality with almost 85% cases achieving target IOP. The most frequent observed complications are conjunctival wound leakage, severe inflammatory reaction and hyphema. Compared to phacotrabeculectomy, deep sclerectomy combined scores in visual rehabilitation, but lags in IOP control.

Modifications

Laser-assisted deep sclerectomy: Lasers like CO_2/Er:YAG/excimer have been employed to aid in regular and smoother microsurgical dissection of deep lamellae. The surgery is virtually bloodless; tissue coagulation at wound has the possible advantage of the inhibition of healing at the wound edge and keeping the scleral lake patent. Carbon dioxide laser has the additional unique characteristic is that it does not function when it comes in contact with liquid, thus the dissection stops automatically when aqueous percolation occurs, thereby avoiding trabeculo-Descemet's membrane penetration.

Viscocanalostomy

It was first proposed in 1991 by Robert Stegman of South Africa, as a safer surgical option for people living in poor hygienic conditions, with poor adherence and accessibility to medical care. The surgery entails same steps as for deep sclerectomy till Schlemm's canal is deroofed. Then by a paracentesis the IOP is lowered, the two cut ends of Schlemm's canal are canulated with a special 165 μm blunt needle and high–molecular-weight sodium hyaluronate is slowly injected into the canal. Almost 1–2 clock hours of the canal are dilated atraumatically, with slow injection of Healon GV, which is repeated six to seven times on each side. The rest of the procedure is same as deep sclerectomy except that the outer scleral flap is tightly secured with 6–7 10–0 nylon sutures to ensure that the intrascleral chamber is created. Healon GV is left beneath the superficial scleral flap.

Complications

I. *Intraoperative*
   a. Perforation of the trabeculo-Descemet's membrane
   b. Hemorrhage
   c. Transient corneal edema due to Descemet's detachment after forceful viscoelastic injection in viscocanalostomy.
   d. Early rise of IOP indicating inadequate dissection.

II. *Early postoperative*
   a. Wound leak
   b. Hyphema
   c. Inflammation
   d. Hypotony
   e. Shallow or flat anterior chamber
   f. Decreased visual acuity
   g. Cataract formation

III. *Late postoperative complications*
   a. Fibrosis of subconjunctival bleb
   b. Increased intraocular pressure
   c. Late rupture of trabeculo-Descemet's membrane

Non-penetrating deep sclerectomy scores over trabeculectomy in safety issues as it does not cause shallow anterior chamber, inflammation, cataract and bleb-related issues. However, it only works in variants of open-angle glaucoma and should not be attempted in angle-closure glaucoma.

Nd: YAG Laser Iridotomy, Selective Laser Trabeculoplasty and Cyclophotocoagulation

Sushmita Kaushik, Surinder S Pandav

ND:YAG LASER IRIDOTOMY

Introduction

Von Graefe introduced surgical iridotomy for glaucoma in 1857. Meyer-Schwickerath, in 1956, demonstrated that iridotomy could be created, without the need of an incision, using xenon arc photocoagulation. Neodymium:yttrium-aluminium-garnet (Nd:YAG) iridotomy has essentially replaced surgical iridectomy in the vast majority of cases. Laser iridotomy is the established procedure of choice for angle-closure glaucoma associated with papillary block, whether primary or secondary or acute, intermittent or chronic (Fig. 15.1).

Indications

Laser iridotomy is indicated for the following types of glaucomas:

- Acute angle-closure

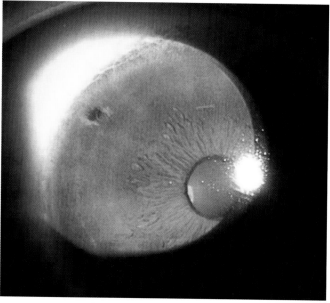

Fig. 15.1: Nd:YAG laser iridotomy

- Chronic (creeping) angle closure
- Phacomorphic with element of papillary block
- Iris bombe
- Pigmentary dispersion syndrome
- Prophylaxis of occludable angle.

Laser iridotomy also aids in the diagnosis of aqueous misdirection and plateau iris syndrome (in a non-pupillary block narrow angle).

Procedure

A drop of pilocarpine (1%) is instilled twice, 5 minutes apart; miosis helps to stretch and thin the iris. Apraclonidine (0.5%) or brimonidine (0.2%) is used 30 minutes preoperatively to prevent postoperative IOP elevation. Proparacaine (0.5%) drops are instilled immediately before the procedure.

Abraham lens and Wise lens are used that help to limit eye movements and blinking. They also help to concentrate the energy delivered, magnify the target site and act as a heat sink to minimize the risk of superficial corneal epithelial burns. The Abraham lens has a 66 D plano-convex button. The Wise lens has a 103 D plano-convex button. The iridotomy is placed in the peripheral iris under the upper eyelid to avoid ghost images that may arise through the iris hole. The superotemporal position at 11 o'clock and 1 o'clock is the best position to use. The Q-switched mode is used, which allows treatment independent of pigmentation. Iris blood vessels are avoided. The red laser aiming beam is brought to focus when multiple beams are brought into a single spot, aimed through the center of the contact lens. The energy used is 3–8 mJ, there are 1–3 pulses per shot, and one or more shots are used as required for penetration. One patent iridotomy is sufficient to relieve papillary block. Theoretically, functional failure can be avoided with a peripheral iridotomy diameter of at least 50 μm; an iridotomy with a diameter of 100–200 μm is ideal. In rare instances in which the long-term patency of the opening is uncertain or in the presence of inflammatory papillary block, a second iridectomy may be made at the same sitting.

The patient is ambulatory immediately. Prednisolone eye drops are administered four times daily for 4–7 days. If the peripheral iridotomy remains patent after 4–6 weeks, the opening usually remains open unless an active inflammatory response is present.

Complications

Elevated intraocular pressure (IOP) occurs in approximately one-third of eyes after treatment, but the use of apraclonidine (0.5%) or brimonidine (0.2%) significantly decreases the risk. Transient iritis may occur due to the breakdown of aqueous-blood barrier. Occasionally, inflammation may be quite severe. An iridotomy may fail because the opening created is too small or because perforation is not achieved, with a residual iris pigmented layer present. Diplopia or "ghost images" is an occasional complaint, especially when the peripheral iridotomy is placed in the horizontal meridians. Post-laser hyphema is usually minimal and self-limited. Brisk bleeding may be stopped by applying direct pressure to the cornea using the contact lens to tamponade the bleeding site temporarily. The lens may be rarely damaged directly due to laser irradiation or indirectly because of deficient nourishment of the lens. Focal laser damage to the epithelium, Descemet's membrane or endothelium may occur and is usually transient. Post-laser rare complications include malignant glaucoma, lens-induced uveitis and retinal burns.

SELECTIVE LASER TRABECULOPLASTY

Introduction

The trabecular meshwork has been targeted by laser application since the early 1970's. The conventional argon laser trabeculoplasty (ALT) was first described by Worthen and Wickham in 1973, and modified by Wise and Winter in 1979. Krypton lasers, continuous wave neodymium lasers and diode lasers can be effectively used to perform trabeculoplasty.

Selective laser trabeculoplasty is a new alternative to ALT for the treatment of open-angle glaucoma, and achieves about the same level of pressure lowering compared with ALT.

Indications

Selective laser trabeculoplasty (SLT) indications are similar to that of ALT. Patients with failed ALT (in whom scarring of trabecular meshwork precludes further ALT) may also benefit from SLT. Selective laser trabeculoplasty can be considered for primary treatment for newly diagnosed glaucoma, as an adjunct to medication, as an alternative for poorly compliant patients or for patients who are intolerant to antiglaucoma medications, or as an end-stage treatment to avoid surgery in patients who are on multiple medications. Selective laser trabeculoplasty has also been effectively used in pseudoexfoliation glaucoma, pigmentary glaucoma, juvenile open-angle glaucoma, aphakic glaucoma, normal tension glaucoma and inflammatory glaucoma (which are considered a relative contraindication for ALT).

Principle

Selective laser trabeculoplasty is based on the principle of selective photothermolysis. It selectively targets the pigmented trabecular cells with short laser pulses of low energy, to generate a photochemical rather than coagulative reaction. The thermal relaxation time of a chromophore is the time required by it to convert absorbed electromagnetic energy to heat energy. During an SLT procedure, the 3-nanosecond pulse of the Q-switched laser and 1-microsecond thermal relaxation time of melanin cause minimal thermal dissipation to the surrounding tissues. Selective laser trabeculoplasty is therefore called "cold laser trabeculoplasty".

Mechanism of Action

Histologic studies of the trabecular meshwork after SLT have revealed no evidence of scarring or coagulative damage to the trabecular meshwork, unlike ALT. This indicates that mechanical effects are likely of limited therapeutic value in SLT. Biologic effects may be more important. These include the induction of an immune reaction with cytokine release and macrophage recruitment, affecting the aqueous outflow directly or indirectly. Hence, SLT stimulates the intrinsic system to remodel the trabecular meshwork, rather than mechanically or thermally damaging it.

Instrumentation

Selective laser trabeculoplasty uses a Q-switched, frequency-doubled, neodymium:yttrium-aluminium-garnet pulsed laser emitting at a wavelength of 532 nm with 3-nanosecond pulse duration and a spot size of 400 μm, coupled to a slit-lamp delivery system. The commercially available laser can deliver pulse energies ranging from 0.2 to 1.7 mJ.

Procedure

A drop of apraclonidine (0.5%) is instilled 1 hour before the procedure, to prevent transient post-SLT IOP spike. The procedure is done under topical anesthesia. With the patient seated at the SLT laser slit-lamp system, a Goldmann 3-mirror goniolens or Latina SLT lens is coupled to the eye with methylcellulose (1%). The aiming beam is focused on the pigmented trabecular meshwork. The power is initially set at 0.8 mJ. Lower power is used for more heavily pigmented trabecular meshwork. Unlike in ALT, blanching or large bubble formation within the trabecular meshwork is not seen as an end-point in SLT. However, tiny "champagne" bubble formation is used as an end-point for setting the power in SLT. If no champagne bubbles are seen, the power may be increased by increments of 0.1 mJ (can reach up to 1.2 mJ/pulse). Bubble formation is monitored with each pulse. Small champagne bubbles should be seen in at least 50% of the spots.

The standard regimen is to treat 180° of the trabecular meshwork with approximately 50 adjacent, but nonoverlapping laser spots at 0.6–1.0 mJ.

The pretreatment antiglaucoma medications may be resumed post-SLT. Topical anti-inflammatory drugs are used for post-treatment prophylaxis. The IOP-lowering effect of SLT may be seen as early as 1 day post-laser, or frequently, within 4–6 weeks.

Selective Laser Trabeculoplasty versus Argon Laser Trabeculoplasty

A number of prospective randomized clinical trials comparing SLT to ALT have shown SLT to have equal or more favorable outcomes. Selective laser trabeculoplasty has been shown to be effective in both pseudophakic and phakic patients, unlike ALT which has been less effective in pseudophakic eyes. Compared to ALT, better tolerance and less discomfort have been seen with SLT. Selective laser trabeculoplasty avoids the coagulative damage of argon, theoretically conferring repeatability.

Complications

Low energy levels account for low complication rates with SLT. The most commonly reported complications of SLT are a transient elevation of IOP and anterior chamber inflammation. The incidence of blurred vision, corneal edema, and appearance of a corneal lesion is less than 1%. No scarring or peripheral anterior synechiae have been seen after SLT. Although transient and uneventful, hyphema and bleeding can occur during the procedure.

Selective laser trabeculoplasty is equivalent to ALT in terms of IOP lowering, and is a safe and effective in several forms of open-angle glaucoma. With the potential for repeatability, initial therapy with SLT may prove beneficial. A large spot size enables an easy focus on the trabecular meshwork and makes the technique simple. Selective laser trabeculoplasty can be considered as a treatment option in patients who are intolerant or noncompliant with their antiglaucoma medications.

CYCLOPHOTOCOAGULATION

Introduction

Cyclodestructive procedures for intractable glaucoma that are unlikely to benefit from surgery, have evolved in the last 70 years from penetrating cyclodiathermy, cyclocryotherapy, ultrasound for ciliary body ablation and laser cyclophotocoagulation. Cyclocryotherapy was initially shown to reduce IOP in 1950, and was shown to be a reasonably safe and effective treatment that was less destructive and more predictable than cyclodiathermy. But problems did exist with cyclocryotherapy, e.g. severe postoperative pain, IOP rise, hemorrhage, marked inflammatory reaction, hypotony and severe visual loss. Ultrasound for ciliary ablation was briefly utilized, but it was abandoned because of marked scleral thinning and ectasia at the treatment site. Subsequently, transscleral cyclophotocoagulation (TSCPC) was reported using a ruby laser (693 nm) and since then a wide range of wavelengths have been used.

Indications

Cyclodestructive procedures, in their various forms, have been traditionally restricted to eyes with end-stage glaucoma, which are some of the most difficult to control with conventional glaucoma filtration surgery (Fig. 15.2). These are neovascular glaucoma, advanced developmental glaucoma, inflammatory glaucoma, glaucoma associated with corneal transplantation, silicone oil-induced glaucoma, and glaucoma in eyes with intractable chronic angle closure glaucoma. Cyclophotocoagulation is also used in eyes with limited visual potential, in urgent situations with dangerously elevated IOP, or for pain relief in eyes with no visual potential.

Mechanism of Action

Cycloablation lowers IOP by destruction of the ciliary body epithelium and stroma, thus reducing aqueous production. Experimental reports have described ciliary body atrophy with abnormal ciliary epithelium four weeks after cyclophotocoagulation.

Current Cyclophotocoagulation Techniques

Currently available cyclophotocoagulation (CPC) techniques include:
1. Transscleral cyclophotocoagulation
   a. Noncontact Neodymium: yttrium-aluminum-garnet (Nd:YAG) laser.
   b. Contact Neodymium yttrium-aluminum-garnet (Nd:YAG) laser
   c. Semiconductor diode laser (DLCP)
2. Transpupillary cyclophotocoagulation
3. Endoscopic cyclophotocoagulation.

Transscleral Cyclophotocoagulation (TSCPC)

The most frequently used lasers for this modality of treatment are the 1064 nm Nd:YAG laser and 810 nm semiconductor diode. Both wavelengths can produce thermal tissue damage, and there is evidence that the semiconductor diode laser with 810 nm wavelength exhibits considerably greater absorption by melanin compared to the 1064 nm Nd:YAG laser. The clinically significant effect is that the energy needed to produce comparable lesions is less with the diode laser than that required with Nd:YAG laser. Due to the same reason, less laser energy has

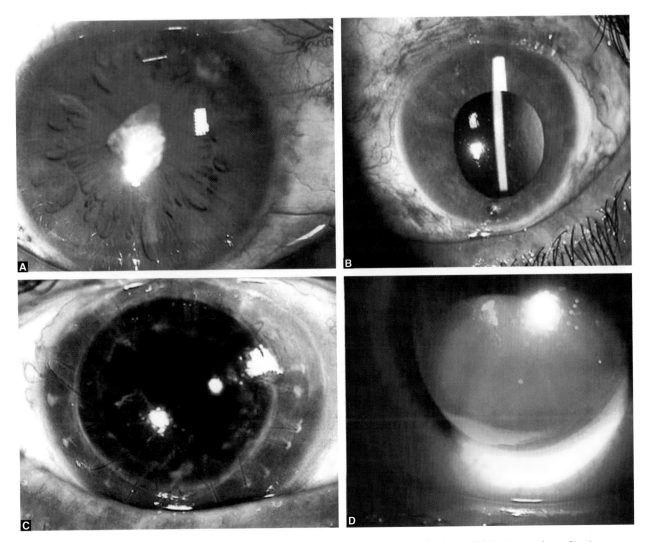

Figs 15.2A to D: (A) Post-uveitic glaucoma with bound-down pupil and complicated cataract; (B) Post-pars-plana-vitrectomy glaucoma; (C) Post-penetrating keratoplasty glaucoma; and (D) Neovascular glaucoma with hyphema

also been reported to be needed in pigmented eyes compared to produce the same effect.

Though there are numerous reports describing the effectiveness of TSCPC, an accurate comparison of different techniques based on published studies is difficult because of the wide variation in treatment parameters and the lack of uniform definition of success.

Semiconductor Diode Laser

A semiconductor solid state diode laser system (IRIS Oculight SLx, IRIS Medical Inc., Mountain View, CA, USA) with an 810 nm wavelength exhibits less scleral transmission (~35), but considerably greater absorption by melanin than the 1064 nm Nd:YAG wavelength. The 810 nm semiconductor diode laser appears to offer a better method of cycloablation with potentially fewer complications as there is better absorption of this wavelength by the pigmented tissues of the ciliary body causing coagulation necrosis of the ciliary body stroma. Initial

reports suggest a lower incidence of the complications seen with other cyclodestructive techniques, such as phthisis, hypotony, uveitis, pain, and loss of visual acuity. These advantages, combined with the compact and portable nature of the diode, make it an attractive treatment modality and currently the most favorite one in use. An overall success rate between 35 and 85% observed with TSCPC. However, risks and prognostic factors other than the type of glaucoma (e.g. age of patients) are yet to be determined.

The laser energy is delivered through a 600 μm diameter quartz fiber with a flat, polished tip oriented by a hand piece (G-probe) designed to center treatment 1.2 mm behind the surgical limbus with the fiberoptic approximately parallel to the visual axis. Maximum power from the system is 3.0 watts for 9.9 seconds duration.

The probe hand piece footplate that comes in contact with the sclera is curved spherically to match the scleral contour. The anterior, curved edge of the footplate is designed to overlie and match the surgical limbus during laser application (Fig. 15.3).

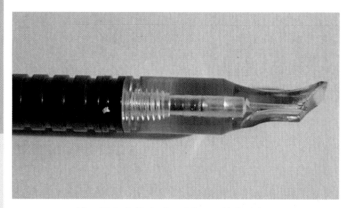

Fig. 15.3: G-Probe handpiece with footplate

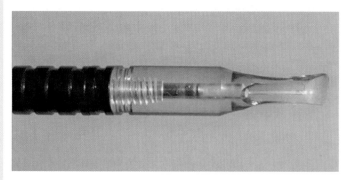

Fig. 15.4: G-Probe handpiece with laser energy "on". Note the fiber-optic tip, which protrudes 0.7 mm beyond the contact surface of the footplate

The probe hand piece has a fiberoptic tip, which protrudes 0.7 mm beyond the contact surface (Fig 15.4). The protruding fiberoptic indents the conjunctiva and the sclera to enhance laser light transmission.

Principle and Technique

A wavelength of 810 nm is particularly effective for energy transmission across the sclera and into the structures containing melanin pigment in the ciliary body epithelium and stroma. Diode laser transscleral cyclophotocoagulation is known to achieve its IOP-lowering effect via two independent mechanisms: By direct thermal destruction of the ciliary epithelial cells that produce aqueous, and by inducing inflammation that may in turn lead to decreased aqueous production and/or increased uveoscleral outflow. The former mechanism should produce relatively permanent IOP reduction, while the latter may result in transient IOP reduction that disappears as the inflammation clears.

Local anesthesia is given by peribulbar injection of lidocaine hydrochloride in combination with bupivacaine hydrochloride. The laser is set at an initial power of 1750 mW, and duration of 2 seconds. If there is no sound denoting tissue disruption (a "pop" or "snap" sound from within the eye), the power is titrated upwards till a "pop" is heard when the power is reduced by increments of 250 mW till no pop is heard. Each laser application is spaced approximately 2 mm apart, using

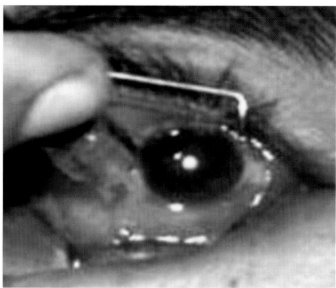

Fig. 15.5: Diode laser cyclophotocoagulation procedure in progress

the half width of the G-probe footplate as the guide, to produce burns in the ciliary processes. About 20 applications are required in the inferior 270°. Superior quadrant is usually spared from laser (Fig. 15.5).

Post-laser treatment: The patients should be given topical steroids and cycloplegics, along with oral analgesics, as required. One can wait for a minimum of 4 weeks for the full IOP effect of the first TSCPC to stabilize. After 4 weeks, if the IOP under medical treatment is persistently high on 2 consecutive visits separated by an interval of at least 1 week, a second session of diode laser TSCPC can be given in the same inferior 270°.

Currently, the G-probe is sold as a single-use, disposable instrument. Despite its marketing as a single-use, disposable instrument, the IRIS diode laser G-probe has demonstrated reusability. To reuse the G-probe, care should be taken to minimize debris accumulation and tip damage by cleaning with alcohol wipes. However, anecdotal evidence points to some decrease in the clinical effectiveness of the G-probe with reuse.

Histopathologic studies comparing Nd:YAG laser to diode found that treatment with diode CPC required less energy, and tended to cause less blanching, and deeper ciliary body contraction and coagulation.

Limitation of Transscleral Cyclophotocoagulation

With noncontact or contact Nd:YAG and semiconductor diode lasers predictability is limited by the inability to visualize target tissue. In lieu of direct visualization, transillumination may be used to identify the location of the ciliary body, especially in eyes with abnormal anatomy or enlarged eyes (congenital glaucoma). An ocular transilluminator is placed against the posterior globe and directed towards the ciliary sulcus. In a darkened room, the diffuse illumination will demarcate the ciliary body, which can be marked externally.

Complications

Complications seen with all modes of cyclodestruction include pain, intraocular hemorrhage, prolonged ocular inflammation, hypotony, phthisis bulbi, visual loss, postoperative pain, and the need for retreatment. Potential complications of transscleral diode CPC include conjunctival surface burns that heal quickly. Another potential complication is intraocular disruption ("pop"), which is characterized as an intraocular uveal microexplosion and represents boiling of tissue water. Postoperative iridocyclitis is more severe with an increased number of pops observed. Malignant glaucoma and atonic pupil may occur following the laser treatment. There is high risk of graft failure in patients undergoing diode laser CPC.

Cyclophotocoagulation is indicated for patients with refractory glaucoma who have failed trabeculectomy or tube shunt procedures, patients with minimal useful vision and elevated IOP, patients who have no visual potential and need pain relief, and patients with complicated glaucoma and conjunctival scarring from previous surgery. It is also useful in emergent situations, such as the acute onset of neovascular glaucoma.

Recent evidence shows that semiconductor diode systems appear to possess the best combination of effectiveness, portability, expense, ease of use at this time and predictability of the laser and tissue response along with the currently available cyclophotocoagulation techniques available. Unlike endoscopic CPC, transscleral treatment can usually be performed in an office setting. However, visualizing the treatment target tissue directly is impossible with transscleral treatment and can potentially cause more collateral tissue damage.

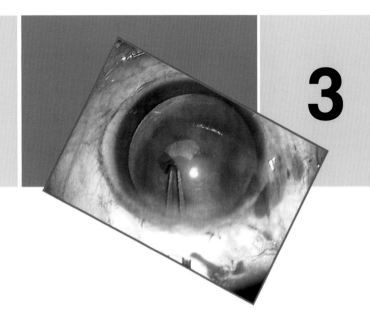

S e c t i o n

3

Cataract

Technological Advances in Intraocular Lenses and Instrumentation

Jagat Ram, Gagandeep S Brar

The small incision cataract surgery has fascinated ophthalmologists just as keyhole surgery for appendix removal. Credit for invention and first intraocular lens (IOL) implantation is given solely to Harold Ridley who performed the first IOL implantation on November 29, 1949, at the St. Thomas Hospital in London.

Phacoemulsification has become the standard of care for cataract surgery in the industrialized world and is rapidly gaining popularity in developing countries. In a survey carried out by David Leaming, among the American Society of Cataract and Refractive Surgery Surgeons, the number of cataract surgeons performing phacoemulsification has increased from 12% in 1985 to 97% in 1998. The turning point was 1990 and the main reasons were introduction of continuous curvilinear capsulorrhexis, hydrodissection and use of newer nucleus dividing techniques for safer phacoemulsification. At present, majority of the eye specialists in developing world perform large incision intracapsular and extracapsular surgery and phacoemulsification accounts for approximately 10% of cataract surgery.

INTRAOCULAR LENS MATERIALS AND DESIGNS

The acrylic polymer, polymethylmethacrylate (PMMA), used in Ridley's first implantation is still the most popular material for IOL optic and haptics, but the preference for foldable IOLs is steadily increasing. The anterior chamber lens was developed by Choyce and subsequently refined by Kelman, while the first practical posterior chamber implant was proffered by Shearing and Pearce and further modifications were made by Sinskey, Simcoe and others. The progress has led to the configuration that we now recognize as the modern posterior chamber IOL. The introduction of phacoemulsification by Charles Kelman in 1967 stimulated the research for newer IOL materials and designs to provide advantages of small incision phacoemulsification. The idea of using soft foldable IOLs began in the 1950s. By the mid-1970s, Mazzocco, Epstein and others had begun implanting soft IOLs in humans and now, at the beginning of new century, use of foldable IOLs has eclipsed the rigid IOLs.

Beside refinement of surgical techniques, recently, attention has been focussed on the optimal configuration of an intraocular lens optic design and material to improve the optical performance of the IOL and to eliminate important complications of phacoemulsification or extracapsular cataract surgery, i.e. posterior capsule opacification and decentration of IOLs.

The biconvex IOL optic is most suitable in providing superior optical performance and in reducing the image degradation with tilt or decentration and in reducing posterior capsule opacification (PCO) by providing maximum posterior capsule contact and barrier effect when the IOL is in the capsular bag.

Square Edge Effect

Intraocular lenses with square edge optic profile for enhancing the barrier effect reduce migration of lens epithelial cell onto the posterior capsule. The available IOL designs are acrylic (Alcon AcrySof, AMO Sensar) and silicone IOLs. Several studies have emphasized the efficacy of barrier effect of square edge optic in reducing PCO.

Intraocular Lens Haptics

Polymethylmethacrylate haptics are preferred over polypropylene haptics as the former has better memory and fixation quality. The latter is associated with biodegradation, bacterial adherence and inflammation. Anterior angulation of the IOL haptics (between 5–10°) is considered to provide tight contact of IOL optic with the posterior capsule, thus providing the barrier effect in reducing PCO.

Intraocular Lens Materials

Polymethylmethacrylate, acrylic, silicone, hydrogel, memory lenses, toric lenses and many more IOL designs and materials are available for implantation. Obvious advantages of small incision phacoemulsification, such as low-induced astigmatism, rapid visual rehabilitation, and less intraoperative and postoperative complications have led to increase in the use of foldable IOLs. Intraocular materials can be divided into two groups:

- Acrylate/methacrylate polymer, and
- Silicone elastomers.

Acrylate/Methacrylate Polymer

The first group contains rigid PMMA IOLs and foldable acrylic and hydrogel IOLs. Altering the side groups of the standard methacrylate polymer backbone has developed the foldable acrylate/methacrylate polymers. These IOLs differ in refractive indices, water content, folding and unfolding behavior and surface properties.

Rigid Polymethylmethacrylate Intraocular Lenses

The examples of methacrylate polymers are PMMA and heparin surface-modified PMMA IOLs. The heparin surface modification (HSM) may render the surface of PMMA implants more hydrophilic and improve the biocompatibility. PMMA lenses continue to hold a significant percentage of the worldwide market and this material is standard and time-tested with which other biomaterials are compared. Newer designs allow lens insertion through a 5 mm incision. Ovoid lens design of 5 × 6 mm has become less popular due to unwanted edge glare. One-piece, all PMMA designs provide maximum fixation stability and memory and are therefore ideal for patients with weakened zonules and/or compromised capsule. PMMA IOLs are suitable for highly myopic eyes and unusually large eyes.

Foldable Intraocular Lenses

Soft acrylic intraocular lenses: Popular acrylic IOLs in clinical use namely hydrophobic Alcon AcrySof and Allergan AMO Sensar AR40 are examples of acrylic IOLs. Acrylic lenses have been manufactured in both one-piece and three-piece designs. AcrySof IOL has 5.5 mm or 6 mm optic sizes and PMMA haptics. Currently, one-piece acrylic IOLs are also available for clinical use. Because of its elasticity, soft acrylic IOLs unfold more slowly than silicone. Its refractive index is highest (1.55) of any available IOL. Since this material is not compressible, therefore, insertion of an acrylic IOL requires slightly larger incision compared to silicone IOLs. The tacky surface of acrylic IOL tends to adhere to surgical instruments and wetting the lens or coating it with viscoelastic may manage this. Acrylic IOLs have lower rate of posterior capsule opacification, which is likely to be a function of lens design, especially the truncated square edge optic (Fig. 16.1).

Hydrogel intraocular lenses: Hydrogel IOLs are unusual in that they tend to swell in contact with water. The monomer 2-hydroxyethylmethacrylate (HEMA) has been used successfully in copolymerization as a foldable IOL. By varying the polymerization and the side chains, this material may be rendered quite hydrophilic, with a high refractive index (1.47). Currently, FDA-approved soft hydrogel lenses are based on a thermoelastic combination of PMMA and HEMA. The IOL is available in 6 mm optic with either propylene or PMMA haptics of 13.0 mm or 12.5 mm overall size. Once this IOL is implanted, it slowly unfolds in the warm intraocular environment. Its hydrophilicity

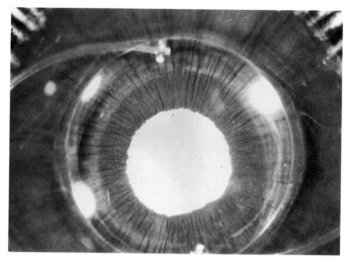

Fig. 16.1: Miyake-Apple view in an eye obtained postmortem with Alcon AcrySof IOL with acrylic optic and blue PMMA haptics in the capsular bag

makes this lens highly compatible. Clinically, minimal anterior and posterior capsule opacification is observed with this material.

Silicone Elastomers

The second group of IOLs is made up of foldable polysiloxanes. The silicone-oxygen molecule backbone confers mechanical flexibility and the apparent organic groups, e.g, methyl and pheny ; determine properties, such as refractive index, mechanical strength and clarity. Silicone elastomers have been refined, overcoming the earlier problems, such as discoloration or browning. Currently available generation of silicone lenses have higher refractive indices thus allowing thinner profile and smaller incisions. Silicone IOL will adhere to all biomaterials to some degree, though its highest proclivity is to silicone elastomers. Impaired visualization secondary to condensation from intraocular gases and air seems to be more pronounced with silicone implants. These factors should be taken into consideration while selecting IOL biomaterial for use in-patients predisposed to posterior segment diseases.

Several manufacturers offer an option of 5.5 mm or 6 mm optic. Prolene haptics have been replaced with PMMA haptics in most of the newer silicone IOLs (Fig. 16.2) Single piece plate haptic designs have enjoyed popularity because of both ease of insertion and minimum incision size. This lens is designed strictly for capsular bag implantation. Absolute contraindication for use of silicone plate haptic IOLs are anterior or posterior capsule tear and significant zonular dehiscence. Relative contraindications include weak zonules, pseudoexfoliation syndrome and large eyes

Toric intraocular lenses: FDA has approved silicone plate haptic design as the first toric implant. Two cylinder powers are available: a 2.0 diopter model that corrects 1.25 diopters of astigmatism at the spectacle plane and a 3.5 diopter model that corrects 2.25 diopters of astigmatism.

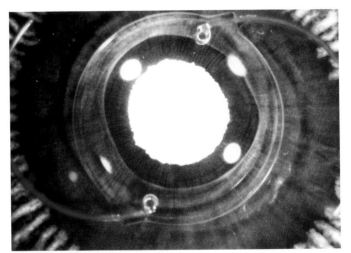

Fig. 16.2: Miyake-Apple view in an eye obtained postmortem with Allergan SI 30NB IOL with silicone optic in the capsular bag. Note blue prolene haptics. In the newer IOLs, such as SI40NB and SA40NB, the prolene haptics are replaced with PMMA material

Multifocal lenses: Multifocal IOLs have advantages of providing ability to focus at distant, near or intermediate distance without any significant decrease in contrast sensitivity and quality of vision. A number of multifocal IOLs designs are available, such as diffractive, refractive and aspheric blends.

IOL IMPLANTATION TECHNIQUES

Implantation of Rigid IOLs

A PMMA lens is inserted though an incision of 5–6.5 mm, using implantation forceps. The leading haptic is placed in the capsular bag and the trailing haptic is then rotated into position. In patients with zonular dehiscence, placing the haptic into the capsular bag in the area of stress helps to expand and strengthen the capsular bag. In eyes with posterior capsular tear, haptics should be placed away from the defect. In eyes where posterior capsule support is lacking or deficient but the anterior capsulorhexis is intact, IOL haptics (preferably PMMA) should be placed in the ciliary sulcus.

Foldable Lens Delivery Systems

Advancement in the refinement of IOL delivery system is allowing insertion of foldable IOLs into the capsular bag through progressively smaller incisions.

Cartridge Injector System

The cartridge injector system is now available for all foldable IOL designs. There are several advantages of cartridge injector system, which includes controlled IOL implantation, sterility and ease of folding and implantation through a smaller incision.

BASICS OF PHACOEMULSIFICATION

The pace of innovation seems to be accelerating in cataract surgery where, the ophthalmologists are refining their surgical

techniques to optimize benefits to the patients. The evolution of technology from surgical technique to intraocular lens design has been amazing. The innovations in phaco surgery are in the field of surgical techniques, phacodynamics and in intraocular lens designs. Innovations in phacodynamics are discussed in the section on innovations in phacomachines.

The goal of phacoemulsification is to remove cataract through a small incision to achieve rapid visual rehabilitation. Three important factors, which help in achieving this goal are: accurate biometry, perfect craftsmanship and application of principles of phacodynamics. Understanding fundamental principles of phaco machine and their utilization is most important to achieve perfect surgical results. The basic functions of the phacomachine are irrigation, irrigation and aspiration and ultrasonic emulsification.

Ultrasonic Handpiece

Piezoelectric crystals that convert electric energy into mechanical vibration in the phaco handpiece produce phaco or ultrasonic power. This phaco power is transmitted along the ultrasonic handpiece into the phaco tip. The phaco needle is hollow with a distal opening functioning as the aspirating port and the irrigation fluid flows through two ports located 180° apart on the silicone sleeve. Ultrasonic frequency used in phacoemulsification is usually between 40,00–60,000 Hz.

Mechanism of Phacoemulsification

The conventional view of phacoemulsification is that the process of mechanical cutting emulsifies the lens. Mechanical cutting is determined by stroke length. The phaco tip's high acceleration breaks frictional bonds within the lens material. This effect of solid on solid produces mechanical cutting and this is the major part of ultrasound energy produced by phacoemulsification.

A second form of energy generated by the ultrasound is termed as cavitation, the formation of a cavity. Cavitation can be considered as the sonological effect of ultrasound. The physical process that creates, enlarges and ultimately implodes gas and air cavities in a liquid produces the effect. The sonological effect occurs because all sound waves, including ultrasound emit cycles of compression and decompression. Each cycle of sound causes the cavity to grow greater than it shrinks, thus the cavity continues to grow. When the cavity no longer maintains itself, it implodes. Heat is generated, but the region is so small that the heat dissipates quickly. The implosion also creates tremendous negative pressure (up to 70,000 negative PSI), which results in ultrafine emulsification of lens particles. The ultrasound plays an important role in cavitation. Cavitations also produce air bubble formation in the tubings and in the anterior chamber.

Irrigation Aspiration Handpiece

The irrigation-aspiration tip is a smooth and rounded tip with single aspirating port on one side of the tip. The irrigation ports are placed most commonly 90° away from the aspirating port. The silicone sleeve fits around the irrigation-aspiration tip. Most commonly used irrigation-aspiration tip is 0.3 mm. In addition to the straight irrigation-aspiration tip, 45° and 90° tips are available. The 45° and 90° irrigation-aspiration tips allow access to cortex around 12 o'clock position.

Aspiration Pump

Aspirating pumps are used to control aspiration and vacuum. The most commonly used are peristaltic pump and venturi pump.

It is essential to understand the terms flow rate, vacuum and rise time.

Flow rate is the amount of fluid pulled out of the eye per minute from the irrigation tubing or instrument tip. The flow rate is measured in cc/minute. The vacuum is a negative suction force created by the pump, which helps in holding or attracting material toward the phaco or irrigation-aspiration port. The rise time is a measure of how rapidly the vacuum builds on occlusion of the aspirating port. The flow rate is an important factor in the rise time.

Peristaltic Pump

This is a simple design popularized by the heart-lung machine used in open-heart surgery. The incoming aspirating tubing pinches against the pump roller as the pump head rotates (Fig. 16.3). The continued rotation creates a pressure differential and as the aspirating port is occluded by the nucleus, vacuum is produced in the aspirating tubing. At higher flow rate, vacuum is produced in the tubing even without an occlusion of the aspirating port.

The vacuum build up is slow in peristaltic as compared to rapid vacuum rise in venturi pump. In peristaltic system, one has to approach the nuclear fragments to produce occlusion

and then vacuum will rise in contrast to venturi pump where rapid rise in spontaneously created vacuum pulls nuclear materials toward phaco tip on pressing the foot pedal. The peristaltic pump allows zero and high vacuum phaco.

Venturi Pump

The venturi pump is driven by compressed gas, which generates vacuum. The production of vacuum is related to flow of gas, which is regulated by a valve (Fig. 16.4). The vacuum build up is almost instantaneous from zero to preset level on pressing the foot pedal and does not depend on the occlusion of the aspirating port. This provides good followability of tissue. As a result of rapid rise in vacuum with this pump, there is increased risk of posterior capsular rupture and iris trauma, particularly by the beginner.

Diaphragmatic Pump

In this pump, a flexible membrane within a cassette is used to generate vacuum. This is similar to venturi pump sharing both relatively fast flow rates and rapid rise in vacuum.

Concentrix Pump

Millenium microsurgical system is available with concentric fluidics control technology. This helps to provide chamber stability, surge control and fluidic precision. The rigid scroll elements, noncompliant tubing and in-line transducer of concentrix reduce flow loss and fluid pulsing to protect against chamber fluctuation.

Foot Pedal

The foot pedal has four positions. The position 0 is the resting and this is fully upright point of the foot pedal. In this position

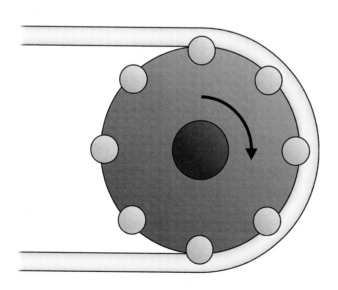

Fig. 16.3: Peristaltic pump. The incoming aspirating tubing pinches against the pump roller as the pump head rotates

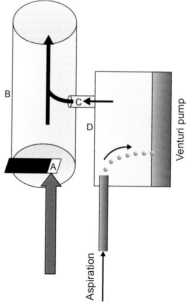

Fig. 16.4: Venturi pump. This pump is driven by compressed gas, which generates vacuum. A valve regulates the flow of gas

no fluid flows. All the other positions refer to the travel of foot pedal to a particular range. In position 1, the plunger slides away from the tubing and only irrigation fluid flows. As the position 2 is entered, pump head begins to rotate and irrigation and aspiration occur simultaneously. The position 3 of the foot pedal represents a point in which ultrasonic power is active. In this position, irrigation, aspiration and ultrasonic power are present. Most of the modern phaco machines have a foot pedal reflux control in which fluid is pushed from the aspiration line to the eye to push back the engaged iris or capsule. Some phaco machines have similar pedal setup for both phaco and irrigation-aspiration mode while others combine the travel of the position two and three into a single longer excursion for position two in irrigation-aspiration mode.

SPECIFICATION OF A BASIC MODEL PHACO MACHINE

An ideal phaco machine should have the following specifications:
1. Phaco machine should have preset linear and pulse modes in phaco mode.
2. It should have facility for preset vacuum and flow rate.
3. It should have a multifunction foot switch.
4. A minimum vacuum range between 0–201 mm Hg (desirable 0–400 mm Hg) in the ultrasonic (US) mode provides sufficient vacuum for phaco chop techniques.
5. Reflux facility should be present in the foot pedal to disengage capsule or iris from the aspiration tubing.
6. The monitor should be provided with a panel display of parameters, such as phaco power, irrigation, aspiration, IA minimum, IA maximum, vacuum, flow rate, bottle height, etc.
7. Phaco machine should ideally have facility for wet field diathermy and anterior vitrectomy.
8. The monitor should display total phaco power and effective phaco power used to emulsify cataract.
9. The surgeon should be able to feed the memory with the parameters of at least phaco power, vacuum and flow rate to emulsify different density of cataracts.
10. The machine should have the scope for reusable tubings and cassettes.
11. It is desirable to have auditory feedback in phaco machine. It may indicate the different functions by auditory electronic sound.
12. It is desirable to have a remote control, which can be kept in a sterile area to change parameters during phacoemulsification.
13. Monitor panel should display the error or any fault arising in the phaco machine.

It is the primary responsibility of the surgeon to have full knowledge of the functioning of the machine. Knowledge of proper machine setup is essential for its functioning and to take the full advantages of the machine's capabilities.

Burst and Pulse Mode Phaco

Burst mode is useful for performing phaco on the hard cataract. At foot position 3, each burst will occur at the preset value. Each burst may be 40, 60 or 80 millisecond. In burst mode, while pressing the foot switch in position 3, each burst is 2 ½ seconds apart and as the foot pedal is pressed further, bursts get closure and on pressing the foot switch fully, power becomes continuous. Continuous phaco is mostly required while making a groove in the nucleus. After fracturing the nucleus into various quadrants, emulsification of nucleus quadrants is done using pulse phaco, which separates the phaco power delivery on to the nucleus.

Power Modulations in Phacoemulsification

In the late 1980s, as phacoemulsification was increasing in popularity, most phacoemulsification surgeons desired systems with increased power to address increasingly hard cataracts. In the 1990s, this became available, as did other important technical innovations, such as high-vacuum tubing and cassettes, microprocessor controls integrated with central onboard computers and downsized tips with better holding power and increased followability. Presently, techniques use the pulse mode to remove nuclear material, which decreased chattering and increased holding power of the nuclear material. Many modulations in the delivery of power are now available. Power modulation in phacoemulsification takes advantage of technologies to significantly reduce the amount of ultrasound energy placed into the eye and enhance the rapidity and level of visual rehabilitation in patients.

Cold Phacoemulsification

Cold phacoemulsification, a term was coined by David Chang, MD, refers to a novel technology that decreases the chances of thermal tissue injury during phacoemulsification relative to traditional ultrasonic equipment. Cold phacoemulsification technology utilizes an emulsifying tip that does not exceed a 45° operational temperature. Traditional ultrasonic needles vibrate axially between 25,000 and 60,000 times a second, leading to deleterious heat buildup from friction with the surrounding intraocular fluid. This can especially occur when the incision compresses the surrounding silicone irrigating sleeve against the vibrating needle. This frictional heat needs to be dissipated by the surrounding cool irrigating fluid, which acts as a heat sink. The heat is also dissipated when the ultrasound is inactive and the needle is not vibrating.

Ultrasonic power modulations of pulse mode and burst mode have the advantage over continuous power modes of "off" cycles that allow for thermal relaxation of incisional protein as well as improve followability and decrease overall phacoemulsification time. In order to combine the advantages of both pulse and burst modes while limiting their disadvantages, Alcon (Fort Worth, TX, USA), Bausch & Lomb (Rochester, NY, USA), and Advanced Medical Optics (AMO, Santa Ana, CA, USA) have developed a modified pulse mode known as "Hyper Pulse". This term was also coined by Dr Chang. The Alcon Infiniti terms it "Hyper Pulse", while the AMO Sovereign calls it WhiteStar. This new mode is a variation of pulse mode that retains the linear control of ultrasound power, but also allows the choice of shorter duty cycles to enable longer "off" periods, which facilitates improved followability and thermal protection. In comparison to the 15–20 maximum pulses per second of traditional pulse mode, "Hyper Pulse" allows up to 120 pulses per second with adjustable pulse durations as short as 4 msec. These rapid short pulses produce relatively more transient cavitation that increases ultrasonic efficiency of emulsification.

AquaLase (Alcon Laboratories, Fort Worth, TX, USA) effectively offers some advantages of laser systems, including a thermally safe probe. It achieves emulsification via a deflected stream of warmed balanced salt solution that is ejected at the tip, with emulsified particles aspirated within the tip's lumen just as with traditional ultrasound. These four microliter fluid pulses are rapidly dampened by the surrounding aqueous fluid, providing a good safety margin for surrounding tissues, such as iris and capsule. AquaLase is not suited to dense nuclei, may play an increasingly important role with the softer nuclei.

Torsional Phacoemulsification

Torsional phacoemulsification utilizes side-to-side oscillations of an angulated bent phaco tip to change the energy profile of the tip and its surgical efficiency. The Kelman tip provides the greatest displacement and shearing action wherein the energy created at the incision is sufficiently less than at the distal end of the tip. The cutting is by shearing action. There is a continuous contact between the phaco tip and the nucleus. The continuous contact reduces the chatter, flow and turbulence that decrease the number of loose nuclear pieces at the side port incision. Torsional phaco requires footswitch handling dexterity to attain optimum energy delivery and fluidics. It is an efficient and faster method with no half cycle wastage. One stroke of the tip, one side to another and back, is like two strokes making it effectively 64 kHz. There is decreased ultrasound time, decreased energy production at the incision site and reduced ultrasonic play in position 3 to embed the nucleus. Stable anterior chamber is an advantage because the cold incision site permits working in a tight incision. Significantly lesser amount of fluid is required because continuous contact allows lesser fluid transfer through the eye. Lower fluidic parameters and lesser procedure time decrease fluid consumption. Torsional phacomulsification has clearer corneas because of minimal repulsion, decreased turbulence with the better retention of viscoelastic, remarkable chamber stability, improved followability, thermal injury free profile, reduced fluid consumption and deeper plane of emulsification.

Instruments used for Incisions

Metal blades, disposable keratomes, and sapphire and diamond knives are used for preparing phaco incisions. Metal blades may be disposable or reusable and are most commonly used. Reuse of these blades may lead to inconsistent sharpness. Diamond blades are very sharp and are affected less by tissue resistance and are reusable. The incisions made with diamond blades are more precise. Disadvantage is the higher cost of diamond blades. The sapphire blades provide almost same advantages as diamond blades, but offer more tissue resistance during incision construction. These blades are available in 15°, 2.8 mm, 3 mm and 3.2 mm sizes.

Phaco Choppers

Nagahara introduced the phaco-chop technique in May 1993. At the 3rd American-International Congress on Cataract, IOL and Refractive Surgery meeting at Seattle in his grand prize award-winning film "Phaco-Chop" introduced a new concept of nucleus disassembly named "Phaco Chop". In Nagahara's original technique, the nucleus is fractured using a bent chopper. In this technique, the phaco tip is embedded in the center of the nucleus after the superficial cortex is aspirated. A second instrument, the chopper is then passed to the equator of the nucleus beneath the capsulorhexis margin and embedded in the nucleus and then drawn toward the phaco tip to fracture the nucleus. The procedure is repeated to dissemble the nucleus into the small pieces before each can be emulsified. Koch and Katzen modified this technique by creating a central groove and then the nucleus is cracked into two halves. The chopper is used to divide each half into many small pieces. Each small piece of nucleus is then emulsified. Vasavada and Desai modified the phaco-chop technique, which they named as "Stop, Chop, Chop and Stuff", which is utilized for hard cataract using vacuum of 150–200 mm Hg, aspiration flow rate 18 cc/minute and phaco power of 60% or more. Phaco choppers used vary from a simple Sinskey hook to its various modifications. The choppers are available in stainless steel and titanium. The chopper has a shaft and tip. The tip is about 1.5–2.5 mm, bent usually at 90 degree. The tip is usually blunt with a sharp inner surface. Some of the phaco choppers have a sharp tip. Phaco choppers named after their modifiers are—Nagahara phaco chopper, Nichamin chopper, Fine-Nagahara phaco chopper, Shepherd Tomahawk chopper, Seibel nucleus chopper and Davidoff ambidextrous nucleus chopper.

Phaco Tips

The phaco needle is made of titanium and has a hollow distal opening, which acts as an aspirating port. Phaco tip is attached to the phaco handpiece and is the cutting part of the machine. The efficiency of the phaco tips is related to the type of the phaco handpiece and type of phaco tip. A silicone sleeve surrounds the phaco tip to reduce the effect of heat on corneal tissue.

Standard phaco tip: The standard phaco tip has a straight shaft of 19-gauge and usually requires a 3 to 3.25 mm incision. Phaco tips have variable beveled angle between 0°, 15°, 30°, 45° and 60°. The 0° flat tip has minimum sculpting power, but has strong holding power. This tip is occluded most easily and is used for phaco-chop techniques. The 45° tip has sharp cutting power, but poor holding power and is used for sculpting. The beginner most commonly uses the 30° tip as it has balanced sculpting and holding power.

Kelman tip: Kelman tip is a 19-gauge needle, which has the advantage of increased cutting ability. It has 180° cutting edge, which can be dangerous because it can cut toward the periphery of the lens. The other features of this tip are circular cutting, higher stroke length and increased frequency leading to more energy delivery and high-incision burn rate. This tip is efficient if used with a thermal protective sleeve.

Microflow tip: This tip is also a 19-gauge needle with a groove in the outer shaft. It has the advantage that the grooves in the outer shaft help to cool down the phaco tip. Smaller incision size is required for this tip varying between 2.8–3.2 mm.

Microseal tip: It is a 19-gauge needle with an insulated sleeve. It has advantage of having thicker sleeve providing less thermal effect and closes down the fluid outflow, which helps in maintaining anterior chamber better.

Masket ergo tip: It is a 19-gauge needle with an insulated sleeve. It is bent at the hub for more control. It is safer than Kelman tip and has less chances of thermal damage to cornea.

Cobra tip: It is a 19-gauge needle and has increased size at the end of the needle shaft. It is used for magnetorestrictive handpiece, which has tendency to heat up faster than piezoelectric handpiece. It is not commonly used.

Mackool tip: The Mackool tip is a 21-gauge needle. It has an insulated sleeve with thermal protection. It requires smaller incision: a 2.75 mm or 2.8 mm clear corneal incision. There is less chance of corneal burn with this needle.

Mackool-Kelman tip: Mackool-Kelman tip is a 21-gauge needle. This needle has an advantage of having smaller gauge with efficient cutting ability. It has a bent tip with greater cutting space and an oscillating stroke length. The insulated sleeve reduces thermal damage to the cornea.

Endocapsular Ring

Recent advancement in handling cases of complicated cataract surgery with subluxated cataracts or zonnular dehiscence in trauma cases, pseudoexfoliation syndrome and others such as Marfan's syndrome, homocystinuria, is use of a capsular tension ring. The capsular tension ring is made up of PMMA and is available in sizes of 10, 11, 12 and 13 mm (Fig. 16.5). The endocapsular ring is introduced after continuous curvilinear capsulorhexis into the capsular bag before emulsification of nucleus. Endocapsular ring helps to stretch the capsular bag and reduces stress on the equatorial zonule-ciliary body complex.

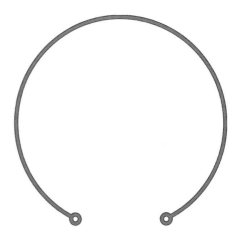

Fig. 16.5: PMMA endocapsular ring. This ring is used during phacoemulsification for subluxated cataracts, zonular dehiscence or pseudoexfoliation syndrome

VISCOELASTIC SUBSTANCES

Viscoelastic substances (ophthalmic viscoelastic device; OVD) play an important role in successful outcome of cataract surgery. Viscoelastic substances have proved to be useful adjuncts for extracapsular cataract surgery and phacoemulsification with intraocular lens implantation. Viscoelastic agents offer the following advantages in extracapsular cataract surgery or phacoemulsification:

- It helps to maintain deep anterior chamber during surgical manipulation.
- It flattens the convex anterior surface of lens during capsulorhexis and helps in its completion and prevention of radial capsule tear.
- It protects corneal endothelium from surgical or mechanical trauma.
- Injection of viscoelastic substance into anterior chamber facilitates anterior capsulotomy formation, cortical aspiration, managing posterior capsule tear and intraocular lens implantation into capsular bag. Viscoelastic agents are irrigated out of the anterior chamber at the completion of surgery.
- Viscoelastic agents also help in combating the vitreous pressure.

Properties of viscoelastic substances: Viscoelastic substance should have the following properties:

- It should be optically clear, sterile, inert and iso-osmotic.
- It should possess high viscosity and pseudoplasticity (ability to pass through small canula 26-- to 30-gauge).
- Hydrophilic: It should be possible to irrigate it out completely from the anterior chamber at the end of surgery.
- It should have ability to protect corneal endothelium.

Toxicity of Viscoelastics

Although viscoelastic substances help in the safe completion of various steps of phacoemulsification or cataract surgery, but residual viscoelastic in the anterior chamber at the end of surgery can produce increase in intraocular pressure. This rise in intraocular pressure occurs between 2– to 24 hours after cataract surgery with a peak about 6 hours after surgery. Obstruction of trabecular meshwork by the viscoelastic agent is the main cause of this pressure rise. Inflammatory reaction and endothelial toxicity has been reported with certain preparations of methylcellulose and sodium hyaluronate.

Types of Viscoelastics

- Viscoadaptive viscoelastic
  Healon 5 (sodium hyaluronate 2.3%)
- Viscocohesive viscoelastics
  Healon GV (sodium hyaluronate 1.4%)
  Healon (sodium hyaluronate 1%)
  ProVisc (sodium hyaluronate 1%)
  Amvisc
- Viscodispersive viscoelastics
  OcuCoat (hydroxypropyl methylcellulose 2%)
  VISCOAT (sodium chondroitin sulphate 4%, sodium hyaluronate 3%)

Even though all viscoelastic substances protect the corneal endothelium, some viscoelastics may provide better protection than others. Viscoat is a dispersive viscoelastic with low viscocity at zero shear rate. The dispersive nature causes the better adherence of the viscoelastic to the corneal endothelium resulting in better protection of corneal endothelium. Viscoelastics with cohesive property are helpful for performing capsulorhexis. If there is increased convexity of the anterior surface that is associated with positive vitreous pressure or a shallow anterior chamber, high viscosity viscoelastic like Healon GV or Healon 5 are preferred. During phacoemulsification, a viscoelastic that persists in the anterior chamber and provides protection to the corneal endothelial cells is required. Viscodispersive agents tend to persist in the anterior chamber. For intraocular lens implantation, cohesive viscoelastic agents are suitable as they maintain the space better and are easy to remove.

Viscoanesthesia

Mixing lidocaine with viscoelastics prolongs the action of anesthetic agent.

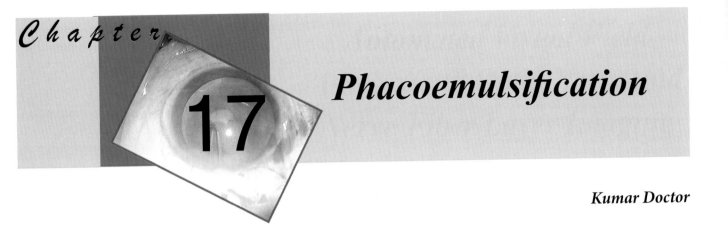

Chapter 17

Phacoemulsification

Kumar Doctor

INTRODUCTION

Cataract surgery is uniquely demanding and ever-changing. Over the last few decades, ophthalmology has witnessed profound technological advancements, adding new qualitative dimensions to cataract surgery. Charles Kelman, with his invention of ultrasound phacoemulsification, virtually transformed cataract surgery. With revolution in technology, there has to be evolution in technique to make the procedure safe, easy and reproducible—"a quantum leap towards perfection".

LENS HARDNESS GRADING SYSTEM IN CATARACT

Grading the density of the nucleus in a cataractous lens is important for setting the parameters of the machine for effective phacoemulsification. In an attempt to develop a uniform, comprehensive classification and photographic standards to set up various grades of each type of cataract have been published. The grades are based either on density and color (in the case of nucleus) or according to the anatomic area of the cataract.

Lens Opacities Classification Systems

The Lens Opacities Classification Systems (LOCS) I–III are in vivo systems, with which in clinical grading, the observer may directly compare the patient's lens as seen on the slit lamp (Fig. 17.1) with the photographic standard grades. LOCS grading may also be applied to standardized photographs of the lens.

LOCS I: It uses a reference set of standard photographs that define the extent of opacification in cortex (C) and posterior subcapsular (P) zones and the intensity of opalescence (NO) in the nuclear zone, grading nuclear color (NC) separately from opalescence. Grade 0 implies no lens opacities, grade 1 implies presence of early opacification and grade 2 implies definite cataract. Subcategory 1a includes minor clinically insignificant and 1b early cortical cataract. A set of standard photographs consisting of one color slit-lamp photograph used to grade nuclear opalescence and nuclear color, and 3 black-and-white

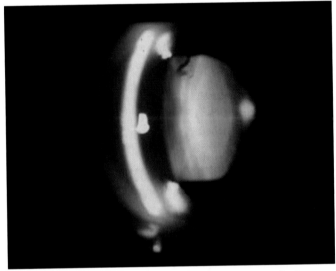

Fig. 17.1: Lens opacity observed in the slit-lamp examination

retroillumination photographs used for posterior subcapsular and cortical classifications are placed on a light box located at eye level behind the patient's right shoulder while examining on slit lamp with maximally dilated pupil.

LOCS II (Modified) and LOCS III: The lens opacities observed in the slit-lamp examination are evaluated using colored photographic standards modified from the Lens Opacities Classification System II. Quantification is helpful and should correlate with the degree of visual acuity reduction. LOCS standards exist for the years 1988, 1989 and 1993. A summary of the 1989 Standard (LOCS II) is listed below (Table 17.1). LOCS II is an expanded version of LOCS I to further differentiate degrees of cortical, subcapsular and nuclear opacification. LOCS II uses 4 nuclear standards for grading nuclear opalescence, 5 cortical and 4 subcapsular standards. Using low magnification view of the slit lamp with the slit beam oriented 45° to the patient's visual axis, with height and brightness set to equal those in the standard photograph: If the color is less yellow than the standard, it is graded 0; if similar, then grade 1;

and if darker yellow, then grade 2. While grading nuclear opalescence (NO), average opalescence of nucleus is estimated and compared with standard, for example, if more than NO, but less than or equal to N-I standard, the grade is N-I. When grading a cortical (C) or posterior subcapsular (P) opacity, the grade estimates whether the area of opacity is less than or equal to the area of opacity in a particular standard. The classification envisions an aggregate opacity by clumping contiguous and noncontiguous opacities into one zone and compares with standard. In the LOCS classification, the cortical and posterior subcapsular zones are graded individually as C and P respectively. The C zone includes the subcapsular anterior, cortical anterior, equatorial and posterior and supracapsular zones of American CCRG in vitro classification. The P zone includes subcapsular posterior zone. It is recorded on a form that contains guidelines for classifying each type.

Table 17.1: LOCS grading intervals (1989)

Nuclear color (NC)	0, 1, 2
Nuclear opalescence (NO)	0, I, II, III, IV
Cortical cataract (C)	0, I, II, III, IV
Posterior subcapsular (P)	0, I, II, III, IV

The improved lens opacities classification system, LOCS III, with its expanded sets of reference photographs (six slit-lamp images for grading nuclear color and nuclear opalescence, five retroillumination images for grading cortical cataract and five retroillumination images for grading posterior subcapsular cataract) and decimalized grading, LOCS III provides a more sensitive grading than LOCS II, when applied to photographic images of cataracts. With 0.1-unit intervals, NC and NO scores summarize the nuclear color or opacity of the lens in one numeric dimension between 0.1 (colorless or clear) and 6.9 (brunescent or very opaque). In cases of cortical and posterior subcapsular cataract, the scale ranges from 0.1 to 5.9.

ANESTHESIA

Ophthalmic anesthesia, over the last two decades, has evolved from the days of retrobulbar and facial anesthesia to topical anesthesia with intracameral anesthesia.

Topical Anesthesia

Topical anesthesia offers considerable potential advantages by eliminating life-threatening complications, traumatic and painful orbital injections and the debilitating effects of systemic sedation required before giving injections (Table 17.2). The keys to successful use of topical anesthesia are preoperative patient assessment and intraoperative surgeon-patient communication. Topical anesthesia is a continuum that begins with the patient's first contact with the surgeon's office and ends the morning after the surgery. The successful implementation of topical anesthesia helps make cataract surgery minimally discomforting

and maximally rehabilitating experience. It allows patients to immediately begin enjoying the restoration of their vision.

Table 17.2: Risks of injection anesthesia

- Damage to optic nerve.
- Retrobulbar hemorrhage
- Ocular penetration/perforation
- Central nervous system anesthesia
- Apnea
- Unintended bilateral ocular anesthesia
- Damage to extraocular muscles/diplopia
- Aesthetic blemish

Fichman first used topical tetracaine hydrochloride in phacoemulsification in 1992. Commonly used topical anesthetic agents are 4% xylocaine (lignocaine), 0.5% tetracaine, 0.5% proparacaine, 0.75% and 0.5% bupivacaine, and 2% lignocaine jelly.

Intracameral Anesthesia

A 0.5 ml 1% preservative free lignocaine or 0.4 ml 2% mepivacaine, or 0.5 ml 0.5% preservative-free bupivacaine can be used intraoperatively safely if the patient gets pain or is uncomfortable, with topical anesthesia alone. Some surgeons prefer to routinely use it with safety. The iris is not particularly sensitive to touch or minor manipulation, but there is pain in the event of prolapse. The ciliary muscle appears to be sensitive to minute changes in tension on the zonular fibers, e.g. sudden deepening of anterior chamber. The manipulations stretch zonules in anterior-posterior direction; and also, alteration of depth of anterior chamber, sculpting or rotating nucleus may tangentially pull them. Ciliary muscles have painful proprioception and can cause an immediately painful spastic reflex, particularly in younger patients. Analysis of aqueous humor with gas chromatography techniques showed higher concentration with use of 1% tetracaine topical and 0.5 ml. A 1% preservative free lignocaine compared to 1.0 ml. 2% lignocaine peribulbar block, serum lignocaine concentration was below detectable level of 100 ngm/ml as seen after 0.5 ml 1% preservative-free intracameral lignocaine. Topical 4% lignocaine instilled 3 times in 30 minutes and 6 times in 60 minutes showed mean aqueous humor concentration of 8.68 microgram/ml $\pm$ 2.3 and 23.21 microgram/ml $\pm$ 8.87 respectively with negligible blood levels. Advantages and contraindications of topical/intracameral anesthesia are shown in Tables 17.3 and 17.4.

Table 17.3: Advantages of topical/intracameral anesthesia

- Avoids pain, blemish and risk of injection anesthesia
- Allows immediate useful vision after surgery
- Eliminates need for patch after surgery
- Reduces anxiety and/or heavy sedation associated with injection anesthesia
- Compatible for patients on anticoagulants
- Patients can aid the surgeon by moving eye for favorable exposure

Table 17.4: Contraindications to topical/intracameral anesthesia

- Patients with hearing or language problems
- Anticipated difficult surgery
- Poorly cooperative patient (apprehensive and uncooperative)
- Dementia
- Mental retardation, cough, tremors
- Ocular problems—coarse nystagmus
- Inability to see microscope light

CATARACT INCISION

Side Port Entry

This incision is required to introduce a spatula or a hook into the anterior chamber. While using the two-handed phaco technique, the site of incision is at 90° away from the basic incision for phaco probe entry at approximately 2 o'clock. This clear-corneal incision is always self-sealing and is made with a narrow keratome or a needle 1.5 mm, inside the clear cornea, parallel to the iris surface (Fig. 17.2).

Scleral Flap Incisions

The scleral flap incision has three dimensions (Figs 17.3 to 17.5). Depth is the thickness of the flap. Width is the perpendicular distance from the scleral groove to the line of entry into the anterior chamber. Length is the distance between the length of the incision measured along the contour of the incision.

Depth: Sclera is on an average 0.6 mm thick at 2.0 mm posterior to limbus. Flap depth can be determined accurately using a guarded calibrated diamond knife held perpendicular to the scleral surface for the initial groove. Optimal depth is 0.2 mm, i.e. 1/3rd thickness.

Width: To avoid astigmatism, external incision should be as posterior as possible, to reduce the effect of sutures. Astigmatism is indirectly proportional to the surface area of the flap since the internal pillars of the wound help support the existing shape. Maximum practical limit for going back is 4.0 mm. To avoid bleeding, width of 1.5 to 2.0 mm is preferable.

Length: An incision of 3 mm or less minimally disturbs circumferential corneal ring and as there is no wound sag and no against-the-rule astigmatism is produced.

Different Types of Scleral Incisions

Curved parallel to the limbus: The limbus parallel curvilinear incision (Figs 17.6 to 17.9) is unstable because it does not fit within the incisional funnel. The anterior edge has no support and can be displaced toward limbus creating wound slide and against-the-rule astigmatism.

Technique

1. Few drops of the anesthetic agent are applied 2 to 3 times at 3 to 4 minutes' intervals, nearly 5 to 10 minutes before surgery.
2. During the draping process, one should communicate with the patient about the operative process. The patient should be told that he will feel slight pressure from the lid speculum and that he will need to fixate on the light of the microscope. He is informed that requests to look up, down, etc. should be achieved by moving the eye and not the head. He should be reassured that no pain will be felt.
3. Surgery is begun with the microscope light at low level of illumination, sufficient only to perform a paracentesis. A volume of 0.2 cc of nonpreserved lidocaine HCl is placed in the anterior chamber, which replaces the aqueous. The anesthetic is washed out as the viscoagent fills the chamber. Slowly, the microscope illumination is increased and routine surgical procedure is continued.

Bloomberg Supernumb Anesthetic Ring

The ring is used to avoid toxic effect on corneal epithelium in prolonged procedure and to maintain the level of topical anesthesia. The ring has a diameter more than that of cornea and is soaked in anesthetic agent and placed on the eye around the cornea against conjunctiva for two minutes before surgery and kept intraoperatively (except in patients with small or deep-set eye).

Deep Topical Nerve Block Anesthesia

An absorbent pledget soaked with a high concentration of anesthetic is placed deep in the fornices and pressurized (Honan's balloon) to encourage absorption in adjacent tissues and posteriorly thus inducing a nerve block. External pressure enhances the absorption of medication across conjunctiva, since the tissue pressures have additive effect with both passive and active transport mechanisms.

Lignocaine Jelly

Two percent jelly applied once, has an effect similar to topical and applied twice has effect similar to intracameral anesthesia.

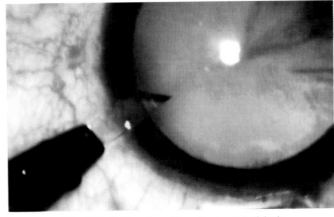

Fig. 17.2: Self-sealing sideport entry at 2 o'clock

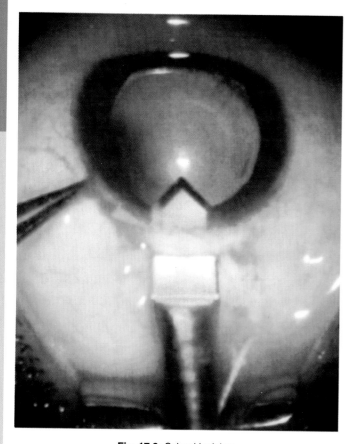

Fig. 17.3: Scleral incision

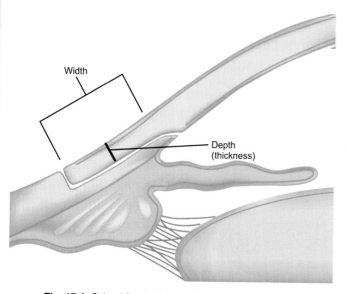

Fig. 17.4: Scleral flap incision—depth, width and length

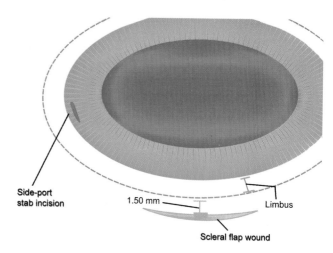

Fig. 17.5: Scleral flap and sideport incision

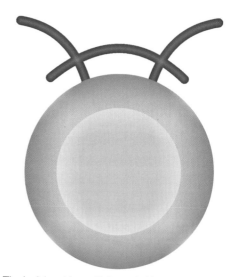

Fig. 17.6: The incisional funnel is bounded by a pair of lines whose shape is based upon the relationship between astigmatism and two characteristics of incision: Length and the distance from the limbus. Incision made within this funnel will be astigmatism equivalent. A curvilinear incision made parallel to the limbus crosses out of the incision funnel and is unstable

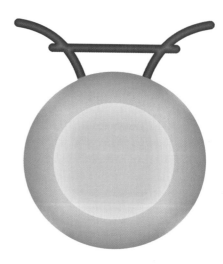

Fig. 17.7: The straight incision placed at the same distance still folds outside the funnel, but not as stable as the frown or chevron incisions

Straight and tangential to the limbus: This incision is more stable than the previous incision and can lie within the incisional funnel, if made far enough from cornea. This increases the length of scleral tunnel and interferes with instrument movements in eye (oarlock mechanism).

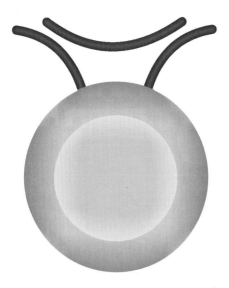

Fig. 17.8: Incision, which lies entirely within the funnel

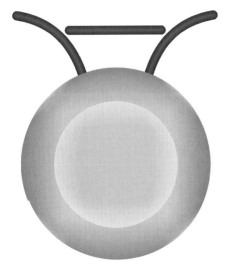

Fig. 17.9: Moving the linear incision further away from the limbus will make it more stable, but also hampers surgery by increasing the length of the tunnel and restricting movements of the instruments

Frown incision (Singer's): The chord length is made 1 to 1.5 mm less than the optic diameter of the intraocular lens (IOL), while the scleral tunnel and internal opening are made 0.5 mm greater than the optic diameter. It is 2 mm from the edge of peripheral corneal vascular arcade at the anterior most point. If a line is drawn tangential to the vascular arcade that is closest to the incision, then the ends should be 4 mm from it, regardless of the chord length. It confines incision in imaginary funnel up to 7 mm (Fig. 17.10). It straightens and deforms during IOL insertion and so lens slides into the eye freely. One mm straight extension at ends increases the length by 2 mm (Dr Sugita's modification).

Corneal Valve Incision

In this procedure, a 3.2 mm vertical groove 400 μm in depth (600 μm in hinge incision) is made in the clear cornea, close to the limbus, with a diamond knife. Before entering into the anterior chamber, dissection is carried out in the corneal stroma in a second plane, approximately parallel to the iris plane. The process involves exactly the same mechanism as the scleral tunnel, except that the beginning of the incision is made in the clear cornea rather than in the sclera. This two-plane incision produces a corneal valve at the internal site of entry. The valve thus made in the cornea allows the incision to self-seal. As the intraocular pressure (IOP) builds up, the sealing effect of the corneal valve increases. The vertical part of the corneal incision should be deeper than the horizontal part. This allows free movement of the internal lip of the wound to seal very well when pressure is put on the cornea, but leaks with pressure, distal to the incision (Fig. 17.11).

Technique

To construct a corneal valve incision, an angled blade with bevel up curved edge is used to dissect the tunnel into clear cornea. Then a triangular bevel up keratome blade or slit-knife is entered through the tunnel until its tip is 1.0 to 1.5 mm into

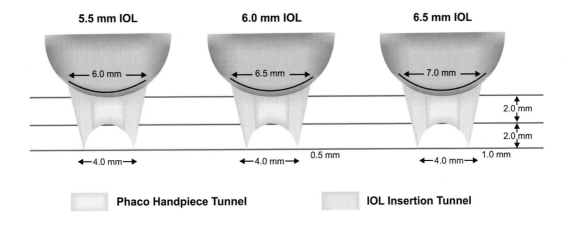

5.5 mm IOL   **6.0 mm IOL**   **6.5 mm IOL**

6.0 mm   6.5 mm   7.0 mm

2.0 mm

2.0 mm

4.0 mm   4.0 mm   0.5 mm   4.0 mm   1.0 mm

☐ **Phaco Handpiece Tunnel**   ☐ **IOL Insertion Tunnel**

Fig. 17.10: Frown incision (Singer's) modified by Dr Sugita: A semicircular frown incision is made with a radius of 2 mm in the sclera, 4 mm away from the position of the corneal incision. A scleral tunnel is made for the phaco handpiece. Internal flap is cut following the shape of the corneal limbus (smile incision). Depending on the IOL's optic diameter, the frown radial incision and the smile incision are modified

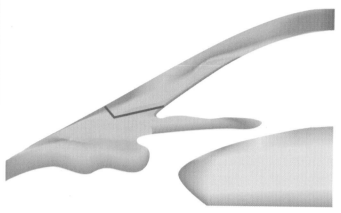

Fig. 17.11: Corneal valve incision

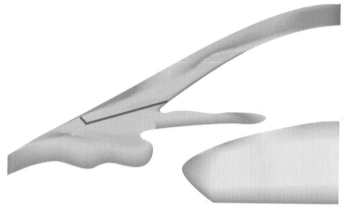

Fig. 17.12: Limbal incision

the clear cornea. A corneal dimple is created, by dipping the blade posteriorly, so that it is pointed towards the center of the pupil. The slit-knife is slowly advanced until its tip enters the anterior chamber and then oriented parallel to the plane of the iris before inserting the remaining cutting edge. Under view, a horizontal linear cut through Descemet's membrane about 1.5 mm into the clear cornea is produced. Having made the incision, while removing the diamond blade, the same plane is maintained. The width of the incision depends on the tip to be used (a lamellar flow tip needs a smaller incision). Width also depends on whether it is created with a diamond/stainless steel knife. Advantages of the corneal incision are shown in Table 17.5.

Table 17.5: Corneal valve incision

Advantages

- Rapid visual rehabilitation and high patient satisfaction.
- Very little postoperative inflammation, with good cosmetic effect.
- Minimal invasiveness and accompanying trauma.
- Reduced operating time and cost, not only because the time in the operating room is shorter, but also because the procedure can be performed under topical anesthesia.
- No bleeding, as the groove is made anterior to the limbal vascular arcade.

Disadvantages

Higher rate of complications than with the scleral tunnel incision. The main ones are endophthalmitis, iris prolapse, flap chamber and hypopyon.

Limbal Incision

Limbal incision has four advantages over true corneal incisions: Wound stability, wound healing, patient comfort and refractive stability (Fig. 17.12).

1. *Wound stability:* Wounds located in the limbus are 30% to 100% stronger than those just 0.5 mm anterior to this location. The reason may be the construction of the lamella in the limbus. In the cornea, lamellae are arranged in a radial fashion for visual clarity. In the limbus the arrangement is more irregular and resembles a meshwork. This arrangement appears to give the limbus more strength and may also explain why the limbal tissue is "stretchable" unlike the corneal tissue.

2. *Speedy healing:* Because limbal incision is so much closer to the vascular supply (often involving terminal arterioles of the vascular arcade of the conjunctiva), it heals much more quickly.

3. *Patient comfort:* Corneal incision, with vertical component, often leads to postoperative discomfort. The cornea absorbs the fluid like a sponge, resulting in swelling on either side of the groove, with a trough in the middle. This trough is covered by epithelial cells, it results in a ridge that can persist up to 8 months, which can result in foreign body sensation. This does not occur with limbal incision.

4. *Refractive stability:* The square incision has been found to be the most stable from a refractive standpoint based on corneal topography. Stable topographies were seen in limbal incisions up to a maximum width of 4 mm, while a true corneal paracentesis incision is stable only up to a width of 3 mm. Beyond 3 mm, a true corneal incision requires a stepped or hinged component. It is then stable refractively up to a maximum width of 3.5 mm.

Wound Architecture

Wound geometry: The more closely incision width matches the tunnel length, the stronger the incision. Studies show that square corneal or corneoscleral wounds will withstand external pressure up to and over 525 mm Hg. If the IOP is low (10 to 15 mm Hg), a 3.2 mm by 2 mm corneal wound will leak, with just 1.3 lbs of pressure. Such wounds also gape by as much as 0.5 mm, a significant amount, considering that the maximum length of a corneal tunnel is only 1.5 to 2 mm.

Wound design: Beveled or paracentesis wounds are the weakest. Stepped incisions are stronger and hinged incisions like Langerman's hinge are the strongest. Hinged, step limbal incisions provide all the speed and aesthetics of the so-called "clear" corneal incisions and the strength of traditional scleral tunnel incision.

Temporal Limbal Incision

Physiological advantages of locating the wound at the temporal limbus—temporal limbal incisions and oblique limbal incisions are more astigmatically neutral than superior limbal incisions. The reason is the arrangement of the collagen fibers across the limbus. The fibers of the inferior and superior limbus are arranged radially, they connect the cornea and the sclera in an almost straight line. Since superior limbal incisions are perpendicular to the fibers, the incision crosscuts a large number of these fibers. Also, temporal limbus is farthest from the visual axis. This cross-cutting of corneal scleral fibers explains why superior incisions begin inducing against-the-rule drift once their length exceeds 3 mm.

Admittedly, oblique limbal incisions offer near astigmatic neutrality, because the fibers in the oblique area, course circumferentially. So, a 6 mm oblique incision induces very little induced astigmatism because very few fibers are crosscut. But access can be a problem with an oblique incision, particularly in a patient with a prominent brow or a right-handed surgeon attempting to do an oblique incision on a left eye. Temporal limbal incisions have none of these access drawbacks. Because the fibers of the temporal and nasal limbus are arranged less radially than they are at the superior limbus, one can use any incision length and any IOL, without causing much wound instability. In addition, no against-the-rule astigmatism is induced and with-the-rule astigmatism is actually encouraged. This is because a with-the-rule shift will enhance the patient's uncorrected depth perception (Tables 17.6 and 17.7).

Table 17.6: Tips for transition to temporal incision

- Visit a surgeon who is successfully, consistently performing temporal incisions.
- Start slow with easy cases
- Have a chalkboard session with the staff; prepare them by explaining the advantages of the surgery.
- Communicate the value of providing a more consistent operation, lessening the likelihood of capsular rupture.
- Tell them what they'll be going through is worth the effort.
- Perform dry runs to acclimate yourself and the staff to a different operating room setup.
- Use the anesthesia you are most comfortable with

Table 17.7: Advantages of temporal incision

- Superior rectus stitch is not necessary as no need to turn eye down.
- Red reflex is enhanced with better visualization, as iris plane is parallel to light of microscope.
- Irrigation fluid drains naturally due to proximity to lateral canthus and no pooling of fluid.
- Better access as compared to 12 o' clock incision
- Affection of corneal curvature along visual axis is lesser than 12 o' clock incision.
- More stable as gravity and eyelid blinks, which tend to create drag on superior incision are neutralized because temporal incision is parallel to the vector sources.
- With-the-rule astigmatism is induced

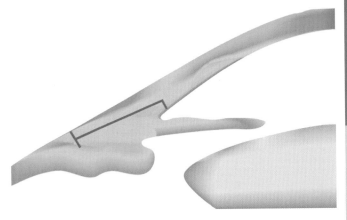

Fig. 17.13: Hinge incision

Hinge Incisions

In cases of corneal/limbal incision, the external wound remains exposed, hence an additional safety mechanism is required.

Langerman's hinge: This wound employs not just one, but two independent components, one that is self-sealing and another that prevents leak when pressure is applied to the posterior lip. This keeps aqueous from flowing out and prevents contaminants from flowing in. Even if one of the seals fails, there is always an independent back-up seal that remains intact (Fig. 17.13).

Creating the hinge: First the groove is made with a diamond knife set at 600 μm. It is important to make the groove perpendicular to the corneal curvature. The groove can be 2.6 mm and 3 mm, 3.2 mm or 3.5 mm, depending on the type of phaco tip and IOL; the width of the groove should ideally match the width of the tunnel. Groove is made at the anterior limbus and the tunnel is made perpendicular to the groove at one-third stromal depth. The tunnel follows the corneal curvature for 2 mm and then enters into the anterior chamber.

Careful examination of all the incisions at the completion of surgery is mandatory in any sutureless case.

CAPSULORHEXIS

Continuous circular (curvilinear) capsulorhexis (CCC) was developed by Gimbel and Neuhann, for in-the-bag phacoemulsification. Diameter of an adult lens is 9.5 to 10 mm, with 6 mm zonule-free area on the anterior capsule, hence the ideal size is 4 to 5.5 mm (it can stretch up to 60% and hence size can be 2/3rd size of the IOL). The single most important step in phacoemulsification is making a continuous tear capsulorhexis. Capsulorhexis can be round, ovoid or elliptical. Ovoid or elliptical capsulorhexis can be positioned to allow access to the superior cortex at 12 o' clock, making the removal of this most difficult area simpler to perform during aspiration.

Mechanics

Tearing by Stretching

The plane of force is in the plane of material. One must exert a force sufficient to overcome maximum strength of capsule. The direction of force is kept perpendicular to the desired direction of the tear. One must pull free flap of capsulorhexis towards the center of the lens capsule. It can tear in the undesired direction with less force than is needed to tear in the desired direction (Fig. 17.14).

Tearing by Shearing

As with paper cutter, the applied force is in the direction of the least resistance of the planer material (perpendicular to its plane), so only minimal force is needed to tear it. The direction of application of force is in the direction in which one wants it to tear, so one can easily lead tear in the desired direction. Because force for desired "force" needed is minimal, the tear will only proceed slowly and in the intended direction, as with forceps (Fig. 17.15).

Forceps capsulorhexis: Capsulorhexis is undertaken with an Utrata forceps or a Kershner forceps. An initial flap is formed with a blunt cystitome. The incision is pushed sideways with the broad side profile of the cystitome. However, if it cuts into the capsule, a linear incision will be made, which will move towards the equator. During capsulorhexis, the capsule is re-grasped every three clock hours. Attempts to pull the capsule more than three hours with a single grasp leads to the capsule going-off course and heading for the equator of the lens.

Needle capsulorhexis: Capsulorhexis in a closed chamber can also be done with a bent needle. Initial cut is made centrally. Tear is spiraled to enlarge the capsulotomy in circular manner by gentle traction with the needle tip. If it starts extending peripherally, it can indicate positive vitreous pressure. Introducing viscoelastic

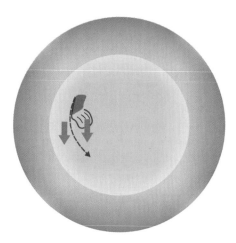

Fig. 17.15: Mechanics of continuous circular (curvilinear) capsulorhexis: Tearing by shearing. The force is in the plane of least resistance. Force must be directed parallel to the desired direction of tearing. Once started, this type of tear will proceed slowly and can easily be controlled

in the anterior chamber counteracts it. Best control is achieved by grasping the developing capsular flap where the capsule is tearing at that time. Placing tip of instrument peripheral to advancing tear will direct it outwards, while placing the tip of instrument central to the tear will direct it towards the center.

Two-staged CCC is used in patients with small pupil and for corneal endothelial protection in intercapsular and endocapsular phacoemulsification. Firstly, continuous curvilinear capsulorhexis is just big enough to introduce the phaco tip. Secondly, continuous curvilinear capsulorhexis is started with a tangential snip on one side, first with scissors and then with forceps. Advantages of capsulorhexis and comparison between anterior capsulotomy and capsulorhexis are shown in Tables 17.8 and 17.9.

To point out the difference between the needle and the forceps technique, the following example might be appropriate. To turn over a page of a book, one can take the sheet between two fingers and turn it from one side to the other (i.e. what one does with the forceps), or one can take a moistened finger and turn it over (i.e. what one does with the needle, the counterhold is the cortex).

Special Circumstances

Intumescent Cataract

The initial steps of fashioning the anterior capsular flap and lens decompression are done under the microscope's high magnification and non-coaxial oblique illumination. Filling the anterior chamber with a viscoelastic agent controls intralenticular pressure. Once the lens is decompressed, the capsulorhexis is completed with forceps that allows controlled capsulorhexis in eyes with intumescent cataract.

Milky White Cataract

Trypan blue 0.1% or indocyanine green 0.5% can be used to stain the capsule for better visualization of tear, as the capsule

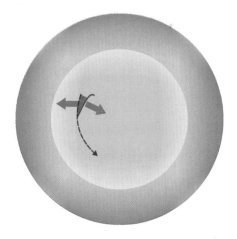

Fig. 17.14: Mechanics of continuous circular (curvilinear) capsulorhexis: Tearing by stretching. The force is in the plane of the maximum resistance. Force must be directed perpendicular to the desired direction of tearing. Once started, this type of tear will proceed very rapidly and can easily get out of control

Table 17.8: Advantages of capsulorhexis

- In-situ phacoemulsification is facilitated and the ultrasonic turbulence is contained within the lens capsule.
- IOL implantation and verification of the "in-the-bag" implantation is greatly facilitated because of the visible rim.
- IOL rotation is possible with no chance of decentration caused by loops coming out of bag.
- No capsular tags or V-shaped tears are left that can extend up to the posterior capsule, under even minimal mechanical stress.
- In the event of a ruptured posterior capsule, a capsulorhexis permits implantation of the IOL in the sulcus. Chances of posterior synechiae formation are reduced.
- In-the-bag IOL implantation is facilitated in the very elastic capsular bag of children.

Table 17.9: Anterior capsulotomy: Can-opener versus capsulorhexis

Can-opener	Capsulorhexis
Advantages	
• Consistent	• Resistant to tearing
• Easily learned; desired diameter easily achieved	• Good containment of nucleus during phacoemulsification
• Facilitates superior nuclear prolapse	• Excellent PC IOL centration
• Easier to use in small pupil cases	• Zonular stress may be less than during can-opener capsulotomy
• Appropriate for mature and hypermature and cataracts with compromised red reflect	• No capsular tags, which may interfere with cortical clean-up during I/A.
• Viscoelastic not necessary	
• Removal of 12 o' clock cortex easier	
• Easier to dial PC IOL into the capsular bag through a large capsulotomy	
Disadvantages	
• Prone to anterior capsular radial tears	• Limits nuclear prolapse
• High zonular stress during procedure	• ECCE more difficult
• Skip areas with incomplete anterior capsulotomy more ikely	• Limits access to superior nucleus during phacoemulsification
• IOL dislocation more likely with anterior (pea-podding) and posterior (sunset syndrome) capsular tears	• More difficult to learn
• Poor support for IOL implantation if posterior capsules breaks	• Not safe for small pupil cases
• Capsular tags may occlude I/A port during cortex removal	• Removal of 12 o' clock cortex difficult.
	• Difficult in the presence of compromised red reflex
	• Viscoelastic usually necessary
	• Tendency for diameter to shrink
	• Capsular bag distention syndrome

stains blue and green respectively. Radiofrequency endodiathermy has been tried in such cases.

HYDROPROCEDURES

Terminology and Classification

Hydrodissection: Hydroseparation of the subcapsular region from the capsule by injection of fluid into the subcapsular plane is known as hydrodissection. However, some surgeons extend it to include the hydroseparation of the superficial cortex from the epinucleus as well. The former is more specifically termed cortical cleaving hydrodissection, while the latter is termed conventional hydrodissection (Figs 17.16 and 17.17).

Hydrodelineation: Separation of the inner hard-core endonucleus from the overlying epinucleus by fluid injection is known as hydrodelineation (Fig. 17.18). The term hydrodemarcation is also used for this separation.

Hydro-free dissection: In this cortical cleaning hydrodissection is done, but preceded by lifting and tenting of the anterior capsule at the margin of the anterior 2/3rd and posterior 1/3rd and fluid wave is injected while sweeping the tip of the hydrodissection cannula along the potential subcapsular space. Gimbel propagated this technique. Hydro-free dissection is thought to produce a cleaner dissection in the corresponding quadrant (Fig. 17.19).

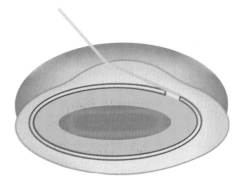

Fig. 17.16: Hydroprocedure: Conventional hydrodissection

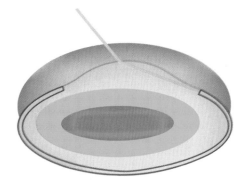

Fig. 17.17: Hydroprocedure: Cortical cleaving hydrodissection

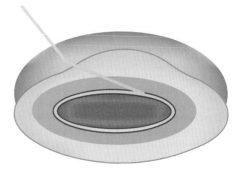

Fig. 17.18: Hydroprocedure: Hydrodelineation

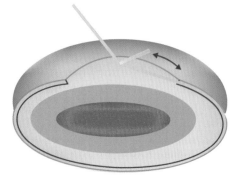

Fig. 17.19: Hydroprocedure: Hydro-free dissection

Hydrosonic hydrodelineation: In this method developed by Aziz Anis, simultaneous jets of ultrasound and water are used from a special handpiece to decompact and hydrate the posterior nucleus. The aim is to decrease phaco time by achieving a softening of the hard-core nucleus.

Role of hydromaneuvers is shown in Table 17.10.

Table 17.10: Role of hydromaneuvers

- Facilitates nucleus manipulation and rotation. This decreases the risk of zonular dialysis and posterior dislocation of the nucleus during phacosurgery.

- Hydrodelineation increases the safety during phacoemulsification. It allows the hard-core nucleus to be emulsified over the protective cushion of the epinucleus. This decreases the risk of posterior capsular tear.

- The epinuclear shell also has a shielding effect. By its presence, it keeps the capsular bag stretched and prevents its collapse, thus decreasing the risk of capsular zonular rupture.

- Decreases the use of irrigation-aspiration handpiece by leaving lesser amount of cortical matter after epinucleus removal.

- Enables linear phacoemulsification to be undertaken

- Hydrodissection also has a polishing effect on the capsule. This decreases the incidence of posterior capsular opacification and the risk of lens-associated uveitis.

Technique of Hydrodissection and Hydrodelineation

Hydrodissection

A hydrodissection cannula (26-gauge cannula) mounted on a 2-cc syringe with frictionless movement of its piston is used. If one prefers hydrodissection first at the 12 o'clock, a "J" shaped cannula is mounted onto the syringe. The cannula is introduced through the scleral or corneal tunnel into the viscoelastic filled anterior chamber. With the microscope sharply focused on the anterior capsule and the capsulorhexis margin, the tip of the hydrodissection cannula is guided along the subcapsular plane in the desired quadrant. Having steadied the cannula with a gentle grip over its hub, with the other hand, a jet of irrigating fluid is injected. This normally amounts to 0.1 to 0.3 cc only. The fluid wave dissects the subcapsular plane and spreads in a fan-shaped manner. The wave next passes between the forniceal capsule and superficial cortex and finally reaches the potential space between the posterior capsule and posterior cortex (Figs 17.20 and 17.21). Fluid dissection by a gentle pressure wave is undertaken in all quadrants. For hydro-free dissection as advocated by Gimbel, the surgeon sweeps beneath the capsule mechanically before injecting the fluid. When hydrodissection is complete, the surgeon notices a symmetric, uniform

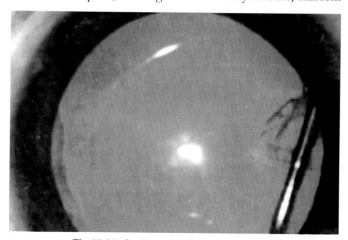

Fig. 17.20: Cortical cleaving hydrodissection

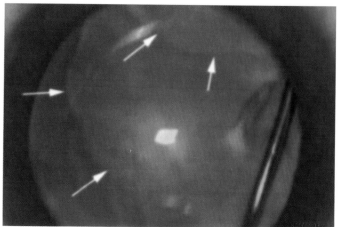

Fig. 17.21: Cortical cleaving hydrodissection: Spreading fluid wave in subcapsular space

shallowing of the anterior chambers. If this goes unnoticed and the surgeon continues to inject fluid, the lens may prolapse into the anterior chamber or the posterior capsule may give way. A safer approach is to stop hydrodissection when it is still incomplete (asymmetric shallowing of the anterior chamber) and then decompress the nucleus in the center, which results in the fluid wave to come anterior and breakage of the equatorial capsulocortical adhesions. This in turn completes the hydrodissection, which is very essential during phacosurgery.

Hydrodelineation

For effective hydrodelineation, it is necessary first to find the cleavage between the endonucleus and the epinucleus. This can be achieved by one of the two techniques. Aspiration of the superficial cortex and overlying epinucleus is done so as to reach that part of the lens, which cannot be aspirated any further. This, as we know, is the hard-core endonucleus. Hydrodelineation can now be performed by guiding the cannula between the epinucleus and the endonucleus and then by injecting 0.1 ml of irrigating fluid. This method can be followed during conventional extracapsular cataract extraction or manual small incision surgery. The other approach, more commonly used in phacosurgery, is to identify the epinuclear-endonuclear junction by the method of differential resistance to penetration. Here the hydrodelineation cannula penetrates first through the superficial cortex with no resistance, the anterior epinuclear shell with a small degree of resistance and gradually, the resistance becomes appreciably significant at a certain depth. This, we know by the nature of the lens architecture, cannot be anything other than the endonucleus. The cannula is now fractionally withdrawn and then fluid is injected along this plane. This fluid pressure wave dissects the epinuclear-endonuclear junction, spreading out in a fan-like manner. The fluid entrapped between the two, appears to the surgeon as the golden ring when hydrodelineation reaches completion. Golden ring formation marks the end of hydrodelineation. However, the dissecting wave may also appear as a dark ring instead of a golden color (Tables 17.11 to 17.13).

Table 17.11: Endpoints during hydroprocedures

- Shallowing of the anterior chamber
- Free rotation of the nucleus
- Golden ring reflex

Table 17.12: Complications during hydromaneuvers

- Extension of a noncapsulorhexis capsulotomy or of an irregular capsulorhexis (threat to integrity of the capsular bag).
- Rupture of posterior capsule by fluid wave under pressure.
- Prolapse of the nucleus and at times the entire lens out of the capsular bag.

Table 17.13: Contraindications to hydrodissection

- Intumescent cataract
- Post-traumatic cataract
- Noncapsulorhexis capsulotomy (e.g. endocapsular)
- Irregularity in capsulorhexis

NUCLEOFRACTIS TECHNIQUES

Principles of Phacoemulsification

The essential principles of the processes involved in the phacoemulsification are outlined as follows.

Isolation of Phacoemulsification Tip into Manipulation, Cutting and Suction

The phaco tip may be utilized for all the above-mentioned functions by alteration in the surgical technique. In manipulation mode, phaco is utilized to move the nuclear fragments or to crack the posterior plate. In this mode, the foot-pedal is placed in position.

Only irrigation is on and no vacuum or phaco power is used.

In cutting mode, nuclear material is shaved away. A 45° tip is best for the procedure as the chances of tip occlusion are minimal. Here a high phaco power and a low vacuum and moderate flow rate are required.

In the suction mode, the tip of either 30° or 15° is best for suction. A high vacuum and low phaco settings are required for the purpose (Table 17.14 and Fig. 17.22).

Table 17.14: Various properties of tips depending upon the angle of the cutting edge

60° tip	Very sharp cutting edge with minimum holding power.
45° tip	Sharp cutting with good cutting ability and less holding power.
30° tip	Balanced cutting and holding power, suitable in most of the phaco procedures.
15° tip	Less cutting and more holding power, suitable for improving followability.
0° tip	Flat tip with minimum cutting power but very strong holding power, most suitable for phaco chop techniques.

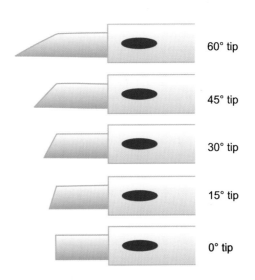

Fig. 17.22: Phaco tips with different bevel angles

Nuclear Rotation

The segments of the nucleus to be acted upon have to be manipulated inferiorly as all maneuvers are easier to perform in the inferior half. The nucleus is rotated clockwise when rotating while trenching and counterclockwise when rotating the broken nucleus fragments for emulsification.

Nuclear Segmentation

The nucleus requires to be broken into smaller fragments (the size of the pieces of cataract depends on the size of the continuous curvilinear capsulorhexis) for being engaged into phaco tip and emulsified. Cracking of the quadrants is performed with a two-handed technique utilizing the phaco probe and the nucleus rotator. The instruments are placed deep in the trench and cracking initiated by a cross movement. The direction of force being lateral and posterior.

Nuclear Fragment Removal

The removal of broken nuclear fragment involves low phaco power with high vacuum. It is preferable to engage the tip of the nuclear fragment by lifting it away from the posterior capsule by pressing on the peripheral broader part of the fragment. This eases the process of emulsification decreasing nucleus rotation and chattering, which has the potential for damaging the posterior capsule.

Broad guidelines for settings of various parameters are given in Table 17.15. These settings, of course need to be varied for individual cases and according to the surgeon's preferences.

Table 17.15: Principle and suggested settings for different stages of phacoemulsification process

Stage	General principle	Flow (cc/min)	Vacuum (mm Hg)	Mode
Preparing Quadrants	Low flow/low vacuum	10–20	0–15	Linear
Removing Quadrants	High flow/high vacuum	25–30	75–100	Pulse/Linear
Removing Epinucleus	Low flow/high vacuum	8–12	75–100	Pulse/Linear
Cortex I/A	Medium flow/high vacuum	12–15	400+	Linear

ENDOCAPSULAR PHACOEMULSIFICATION

Techniques that are currently favored can be divided into the following categories:

Endocapsular Phacoemulsification without Nuclear Cleavage

These techniques involve emulsification of the nucleus while working entirely within the capsular bag; however, there is no attempt to separate the inner nucleus from outer nucleus. Examples of this type of phacoemulsification technique without nucleus cleavage include in-situ emulsification, capsular bag emulsification with minimal lift technique and cutting and suction for soft nuclei.

Endocapsular Phacoemulsification with Nucleus Cleavage

Endocapsular phacoemulsification with nucleus cleavage is currently one of the most favored techniques of phacoemulsification as this has greatly increased the safety of the phaco procedure. Techniques of endocapsular phacoemulsification with nucleus cleavage include "the chip and flip technique" and its variant the "spring surgery".

Chip and Flip Phacoemulsification

This is a technique for in-the-bag phacoemulsification, which allows the phacoemulsification tip to be consistently far away from the posterior capsule thus increasing safety and control for phacoemulsification (Figs 17.23 to 17.25). This technique avoids any need for sculpting near the posterior capsule, in the capsular fornix or under the iris.

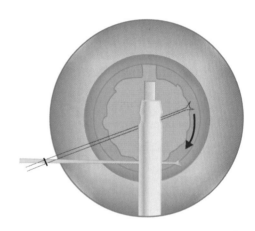

Fig. 17.23: Chip and flip technique: Pulsed phaco is used to remove entire rim of the inner nuclear bowl, while nucleus rotator pushes the nucleus towards 11 o'clock (arrow) under the phaco tip

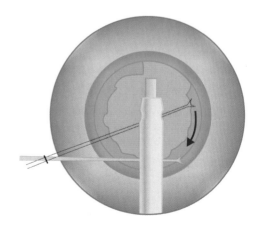

Fig. 17.24: Chip and flip technique: The rim of the inner nuclear bowl is removed at 6 o'clock

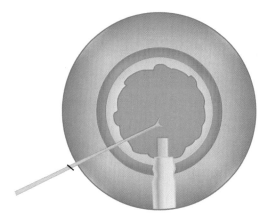

Fig. 17.25: Chip and flip technique: Inner nuclear chip is elevated into the center of the capsular bag and removed by phacoemulsifier

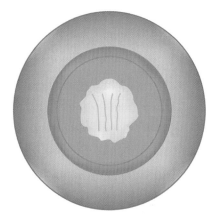

Fig. 17.26: Spring surgery: Nuclear core is sculpted out leaving fairly wide "handles" on either side of the sculpted area

Technique: Phacoemulsification is initiated by moderate central sculpting. The nucleus rotator is then introduced into the anterior chamber and the nucleus is pushed towards 12 o'clock. The inner rim of the nuclear bowl is removed from the 5 to 6 o'clock position. The nucleus is then rotated and similarly the nuclear rim is removed all around leaving a chip of nuclear plate posteriorly.

After the removal of the inner rim of the nuclear bowl, the nucleus rotator is brought into the cleavage plane between the nuclear chip and the epinucleus chip and swept under the chip, elevating it into the center of the capsular bag. The chip is engaged into the phaco tip and emulsified. Pulsed phacoemulsification adds a measure of control, which avoids breaking through to the outer nuclear bowl, and also, dramatically reduces "chattering" of the chip. The 5 to 6 o'clock rim is then mobilized towards 12 o'clock by using the phaco tip aspiration, simultaneously pushing the bottom of the nuclear bowl towards 5 to 6 o'clock with the second handpiece to tumble or flip the outer nucleus bowl. Flipping the bowl away from the capsule ensures safer removal either with aspiration alone or with low phaco power. This is followed by cortical aspiration. The recommended settings of parameter for various phases of procedure as recommended by the author is shown in Table 17.16.

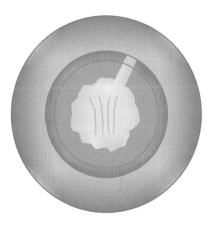

Fig. 17.27: Spring surgery: The first nucleotomy is made by placing the phaco tip of the nuclear girdle at 7.30 o'clock and going into gentle aspiration/ emulsification. An entire tunnel of the nucleus comes to the tip

Table 17.16: Parameters for sculpting and chip removal

Function	Phaco power (%)	Vacuum (mm Hg)	Flow rate (cc/mm)
Sculpting	70	20	18
Chip removal	50	100	18

Spring Surgery

Spring surgery is a form of endocapsular phacoemulsification that has evolved from Fine's chip and flip method (Figs 17.26 to 17.35). This is a very useful technique for removal of soft and medium density cataracts. The name SPRING is an acronym for "Sequential Pulsed Removal of the Inner Nuclear Girdle"

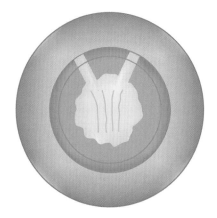

Fig. 17.28: Spring surgery: The island of tissue between the two nucleotomies is not attached to anything on the left or the right; the bottom surface is separated because of the hydrodissection planes. It is only attached at the posterior plate. The capsular bag cannot be aspirated because it is held fully stretched by the rest of the nucleus

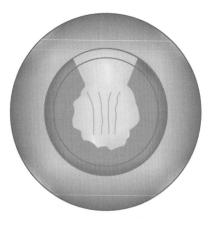

Fig. 17.29: Spring surgery: The phaco tip is placed at the base of the island. Gentle aspiration and retraction causes the island to snap-off at its base and is easily emulsified

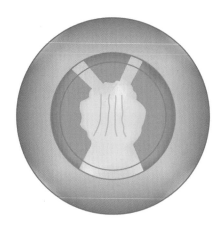

Fig. 17.32: Spring surgery: Another nucleotomy is made at 4.30 o'clock

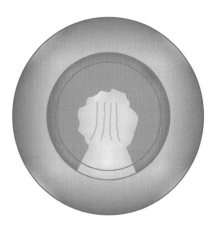

Fig. 17.30: Spring surgery: The nucleus is then rotated 180° to bring previously untouched tissue to the working area at 6 o'clock

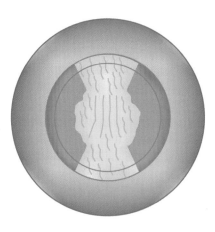

Fig. 17.33: Spring surgery: The island of tissue between the two nucleotomies is aspirated, retracted, snipped-off and emulsified

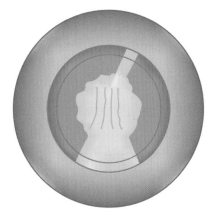

Fig. 17.31: Spring surgery: A new relaxing nucleotomy is made at 7.30 o'clock

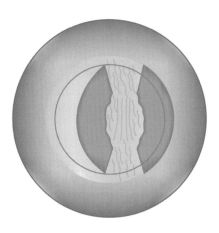

Fig. 17.34: Spring surgery

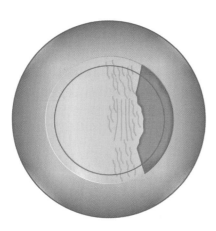

Fig. 17.35: Spring surgery: The peripheral aspiration and removal maneuver is repeated in the mirror image; the other nuclear handle is aspirated and then drawn away from the capsular bag for emulsification

and also denotes the natural spring action of the physiological trampoline constituted by the capsular bag and zonular ring.

Technique: Spring surgery is based on the premise that sculpting remains the easiest and most effective way to remove the nuclear tissue. Phacoemulsification is initiated by performing deep and relatively broad sculpting removing a good amount of inner nucleus leaving a firm structurally intact nuclear girdle. The phaco tip is next placed on the inferior nucleus at the 6 o'clock position and a relaxing nucleotomy is made around inferior two clock hours about 2 mm deep. The phaco tip is kept near the edge of the capsulotomy allowing the nuclear material to come into the tip during the maneuver.

When the tip is held at the inferior part of the nucleus and aspiration is initiated, the contents of the capsular bag move up stretching the inferior zonules. When the rigid inner nucleus moves towards the tip, the upward pull compresses the cleavage between the hydrodissected nuclear layers and the inferior zonules pull back on the nucleus (physiological trampoline). When the tension in the zone overcomes the force of aspiration, there is a natural rebound of the nucleus away from the tip. The result is that the nucleus will normally "chug" back and forth towards the stationary phaco tip (spring effect). Once enough of nucleus is removed, the compressive forces are not adequate and the trampoline will not have the same pressure on it, the lens will cease to rebound away from the tip. If the nucleus keeps coming towards the phaco tip and does not move back even when the aspiration is switched-off during relaxing nucleotomy, the zonules have broken. Zonular rupture is not likely to occur during relaxing nucleotomy with pulse mode and low-aspiration settings, as long as the phaco tip is held steady. The next step is peripheral aspiration and removal of the two-to-three clock hours of the inner nuclear girdle adjacent to relaxing nucleotomy. It involves aspirating the nucleus with phaco tip, drawing it centrally and emulsifying it safely in the middle of the bag. The aim is to widen the area of the relaxing nucleotomy creating two distinct handles of nucleus with

enough room between them for handles to be folded inwards. The nucleus is then rotated through 180°. Another relaxing nucleotomy is made and several clock hours of inner nucleus are removed using the same maneuvers. After wide relaxing nucleotomies are completed, what is left are the two nuclear handles separated by a thin plate of posterior nucleus. This central plate of nucleus is shaved some more, until it is very thin. The two nuclear handles are then pulled into the middle of the capsular bag and emulsified. After removal of the nucleus, the epinucleus is removed as described earlier and cortical removal is completed.

ENDOCAPSULAR EMULSIFICATION TECHNIQUES WITH NUCLEUS CRACKING

Nucleus emulsification involving the various cracking techniques is a great leap in safe phacoemulsification (Table 17.17). The various cracking techniques include the following:

Phacoemulsification by Divide and Conquer

Howard Gimbel is considered the father of all nuclear cracking operations. His divide and conquer technique is the prototype for all operations that break the nucleus into several small pieces for removal through a small capsulorhexis opening. Divide and conquer is the most commonly practiced technique for emulsification. This reduces the phaco power and time thus making the procedure safer.

Four-Quadrant Cracking

This method of four-quadrant cracking is a modification of the technique originally described by John Shepherd.

Table 17.17: Parameters for trenching and quadrant emulsification

Function	Phaco power (%)	Vacuum (mm of Hg)	Flow rate (cc/mm)
Trenching	70–80	18	10–20
Quadrant emulsification	50–60	100	25–30

Technique

Surgery is initiated with a moderate amount of sculpting with some trench digging. The aim is to make the nucleus bare to create a narrow gully right down the middle of the cataract (Fig. 17.36). The trench should be as deep as possible and about two phaco tips wide. This width is necessary for attainment of the adequate depth (2 to 3 mm deep) of the groove and for placement of the two instruments required during the cracking operation. At the initial stage, it is not possible to attain the required depth of the trench as the uncut tissue in the subincisional area prevents the phaco tip from getting down to clean out the bottom of the trench. After the first trench is made, the nucleus is rotated through 90° clockwise with a nucleus rotator/spatula (Figs 17.37 to 17.48). Another trench is then made, in the inferior nucleus similar to the first trench, as deep as possible, beginning the process of quartering the nucleus. After the second trench is dug, the nucleus is rotated clockwise another 90°, and the third trench is made. It is now possible to remove the tissue, which was originally in

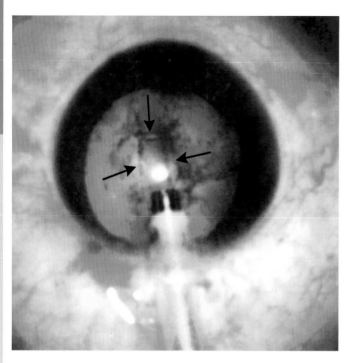

Fig. 17.36: Initial groove width

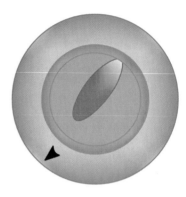

Fig. 17.39: Trench divide and conquer: 90° rotation

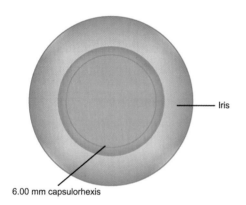

Fig. 17.37: Trench divide and conquer: 6 mm capsulorhexis

Iris

6.00 mm capsulorhexis

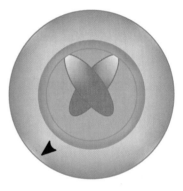

Fig. 17.40: Trench divide and conquer: Second linear sculpting

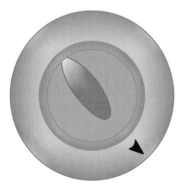

Fig. 17.38: Trench divide and conquer: First linear sculpting

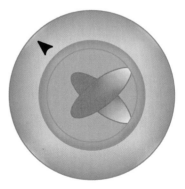

Fig. 17.41: Trench divide and conquer: 90° rotation

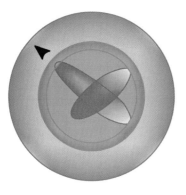

Fig. 17.42: Trench divide and conquer: Third linear sculpting

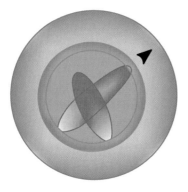

Fig. 17.43: Trench divide and conquer: 90° rotation

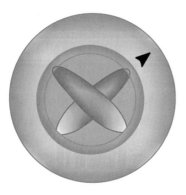

Fig. 17.44: Trench divide and conquer: Fourth linear sculpting

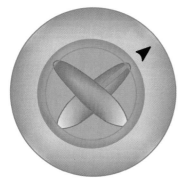

Fig. 17.45: Trench divide and conquer: First cracking

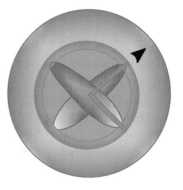

Fig. 17.46: Trench divide and conquer: Second cracking

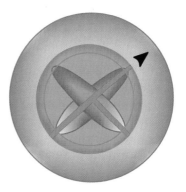

Fig. 17.47: Trench divide and conquer: Third cracking

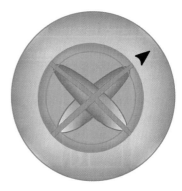

Fig. 17.48: Trench divide and conquer: Fourth cracking

the subincisional area. This will allow completion of the first trench. The trench should be made from 12 o'clock all the way to 6 o'clock and should be of adequate depth. The nucleus is rotated through 90° once more, and the fourth trench is made. The second trench is also completed at this setting, cleaning out the bottom of the gully as deep as possible. Clockwise rotation of the nucleus keeps the trench on the opposite side from the spatula entry point thus making further rotation easy. Brightening of the glow acts as a guide for the assessment of the depth. Phaco tip width can also be used as a guide. Formation of a cross, as described, isolates the four quadrants of inner nucleus separated by a thin bridge of posterior nuclear plate. This trenching removes the hardest part of any cataract, which is the endonucleus. The length of the trench should be equal to the continuous curvilinear capsulorhexis or little beyond. The maximum use of phaco energy is in trenching. It is important that the trenches are of adequate depth and width as this ensures an easy cracking of the nucleus.

Cracking the nucleus: Phaco tip is placed in the inferior trench and pressed against the left-hand wall. Spatula is inserted through the sideport incision and pressed against the right-hand wall of the trench. Using a cross-section, the two walls are separated. This will crack the posterior plate. If it does not crack, another attempt is made. If it still does not crack, the posterior plate needs to be shaved thinner. A special effort is necessary to thin out the posterior plate centrally, because it is the thickest part of the cataract. While making the first crack, the separations should extend right down to the crossroads past the middle of the cataract. Deep placement of the instruments ensures the proper direction of force application for easy cracking. It is helpful to momentarily bring the foot-pedal to position 1 when the actual event of cracking is being carried out as this helps in the nucleus moving anteriorly resulting in the phaco tip and the nucleus rotator being buried deeper into the trench. The nucleus is rotated one-quarter turn counterclockwise, and another separation is carried out. Counterclockwise rotation of the nucleus at this stage keeps the intact pieces of the nucleus on the opposite side of the eye from the spatula easing manipulation.

With the completion of the second cracking, quarter of nucleus (between 3 and 6 o'clock) is completely isolated from the rest of the cataracts and pushed towards 4:30 o'clock position. This lifts the posterior apex of the quadrant up, away from the posterior capsule. The tip is placed right up against this corner and the fragment is engaged and emulsified. This maneuver avoids the tendency for the fragment to spin or tumble. After the first quarter of the nucleus has been emulsified, the nucleus is rotated another 90° counterclockwise and the posterior plate is cracked in the trench that is now at the 6 o'clock. The nuclear quadrants are emulsified in a similar fashion.

Fractional 2:4 Phaco

This is another variant of the divide and conquer technique where the nucleus is initially divided into two halves followed by division into quadrants and emulsification. Maloney popularized this technique of nucleus cracking. This is the technique that the author favors the most. The procedure is initiated by removal of the superficial nuclear plate to make the nucleus bare. A trench is then made in the inferior half of the nucleus extending up to 6 o'clock. The trench should be as deep as possible and two phaco tips wide. The nucleus is then rotated through 180° and the trench completed and deepened leaving just a thin plate posteriorly.

Cracking the Nucleus

After deep trenching it is fairly easy to crack the nucleus. The cracking is performed and the nucleus is rotated through 180°

and the cracking movement is repeated to ensure complete division of the nucleus. The nucleus is now rotated through 90°. The quadrants are then engaged into the phaco tip and emulsified one by one. After emulsification of the inferior half, the superior half is rotated down broken into 2 quadrants and emulsified similarly. Alternatively, the emulsification may be delayed till cracking into 4 quadrants is completed. The phaco-emulsification settings for the various procedures in this technique are same as those in four-quadrant cracking.

Crater Divide and Conquer

Nucleofractis technique changes with the densing of lenses. In moderately hard to very hard nuclei, including brunescent cataracts, the crater divide and conquer nucleofractis techniques can be employed as described by Gimbel. In this technique, a deep central crater is made in the nucleus (Figs 17.49 to 17.54). A trough is not used in these cases because it does not sufficiently weaken the lens nucleus enough to fracture easily and also the resulting segments are too large to manage safely. Therefore, a crater is cored deep enough to penetrate the posterior part of the nucleus. Once central sculpting and coring of the lens is accomplished, the nuclear rim is systematically

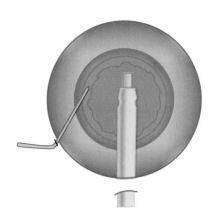

Fig. 17.49: Crater divide and conquer: A deep crater is cored, leaving a thin posterior shell of nucleus

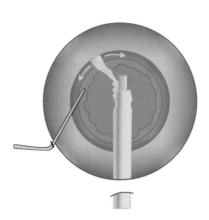

Fig. 17.50: Crater divide and conquer: The nuclear rim is fractured using a bimanual technique

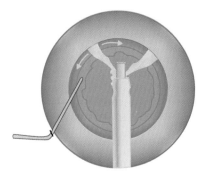

Fig. 17.51: Crater divide and conquer: The lens is rotated and a second crack is made isolating a pie-shaped section

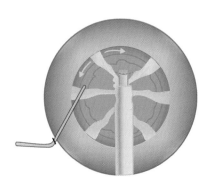

Fig. 17.52: Crater divide and conquer: Sequential multiple fractures of the nuclear rim are made without removing the sections until all fractures are completed

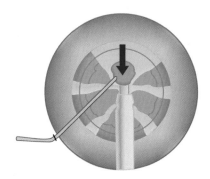

Fig. 17.53: Crater divide and conquer: Each pie-shaped piece is then emulsified

divided. However, rather than emulsification of each section immediately, the sections are left in place. This is the variation, so that the fractured lens material continues to fill up the capsular bag and hold the nuclear pieces in place, in order to facilitate complete fracturing of the nuclear rim. Once this has completed, each pie-shaped piece of the nuclear rim is brought to the center of the capsule where phacoemulsification is safer. The ultrasonic turbulence is still continued within the lens and absorbed by the lens and capsule for all except the last one or two fragments.

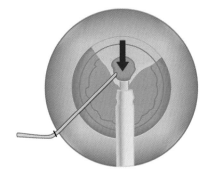

Fig. 17.54: Crater divide and conquer: Alternatively, the first sections can be removed before the rest of the fracturing to allow more space for the separation of tissue during fracturing

V-Style

Kelman suggested the division of nucleus into 3 fragments, by 2 diverging grooves like "V". As grooves are in the softer part of lens, this requires less phaco time. Since only one nuclear rotation is required, there is reduction in zonular stress and trauma to the endothelium, as firm central nucleus is emulsified from bottom to top.

Down Slope Sculpting

Using a 30° phacoemulsification tip, the down slope technique begins with a shallow trench sculpted slightly to the right of and just past the center of the lens surface (Figs 17.55 and 17.56). The lens is stabilized and the nucleus is nudged inferiorly with the second instrument to accomplish down slope sculpting, going very deeply to the posterior pole of the lens. Hydrodissection is essential to obtain down slope sculpting because the nucleus is not attached to the peripheral cortex and capsule and can be displaced in the capsular bag. Once the instrument tips are deep in the center of the lens, fracturing is accomplished with irrigation and aspiration only, without ultrasound power, by pushing toward the right with the phaco tip as the cyclodialysis spatula is pushed to the left. The lens will

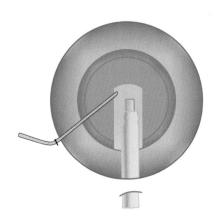

Fig. 17.55: Down slope sculpting: Down slope sculpting start with deep central trough as the lens is nudged inferiorly with the second instrument

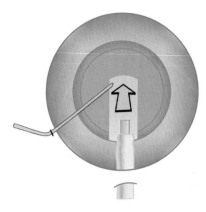

Fig. 17.56: Down slope sculpting: With the second instrument stabilizing the lens, down slope sculpting proceeds parallel and close to posterior capsule

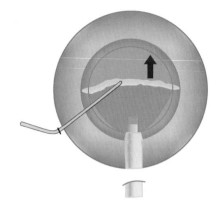

Fig. 17.58: Using downslope sculpting and phaco-sweep, a horizontal fracture is created

usually split from the center to the superior and inferior rim of the nucleus, if the instruments are held deep in the center. After the first crack has been obtained, the depth of position in the lens can be determined and how much deeper the surgeon must sculpt for further fracturing is easily gauged. In all, but brunescent nuclei, usually three to five sculpting passes will allow one to get deep enough into the lens to start fracturing.

Phaco-sweep

Another variation, on the theme of sculpting, is a technique the author calls "phaco-sweep". In traditional sculpting techniques, the phaco tip is moved from the superior to the inferior portion of the nucleus to create a groove. By using the phaco tip in a lateral motion (nasal to temporal and back again), the central nucleus can be sculpted quickly and deeply while maintaining constant visualization of the tip of the instrument (Figs 17.57 and 17.58).

As sculpting proceeds to deeper layers, the phaco tip is moved in a lateral sweeping motion. It is important to avoid occlusion of the tip during this procedure. The lens is stabilized inferior to the groove with a second instrument through the paracentesis. After lateral sculpting is sufficiently deep, a horizontal fracture is created. Phaco-sweep is a variation of down slope sculpting, which enhances visualization of the phaco tip and results in increased safety for the removal of central nuclear material. In addition, the motion of the probe remains parallel to the posterior capsule, diminishing the risk of its inadvertent rupture.

Multidirectional Divide and Conquer Technique

Down slope multidirectional nucleofractis is begun by debulking the superior part of the lens (Figs 17.59 to 17.61). The phaco-sweep technique is initiated with small lateral movement of phaco tip at the bottom of the previously formed groove. The Kelman tip works very well for this side-to-side movement to create a deep groove horizontally. The phaco tip is then used to stabilize the upper portion, while the spatula pushes inferiorly against the wall, creating a horizontal fracture. This horizontal fracture is a combination of separation and shearing. The second instrument pushes towards 6 o'clock and the phaco tip pushes down and away so that these opposing forces result in the splitting of the nucleus as the horizontal fracture.

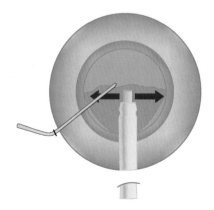

Fig. 17.57: Phaco-sweep: The phaco-sweep technique is accomplished with small lateral movements of the phaco tip at the bottom of the previously formed groove. Nuclear depth can easily be judged with phaco-sweep

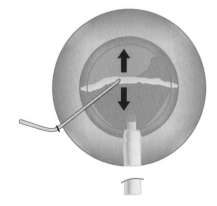

Fig. 17.59: Multidirectional divide and conquer: After phaco-sweep is done, the phaco tip is used to stabilize the upper portion, while the spatula pushes inferiorly against the wall creating a horizontal fracture

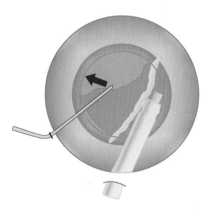

Fig. 17.60: Multidirectional divide and conquer: The phaco tip is used to engage the inferior hemisection and multiple pie-shaped sections are fractured using second instruments to stabilize the nucleus

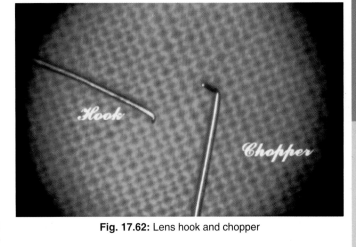

Fig. 17.62: Lens hook and chopper

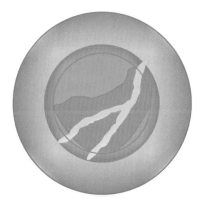

Fig. 17.61: Multidirectional divide and conquer: Multidirectional fracturing is accomplished without rotating the nucleus

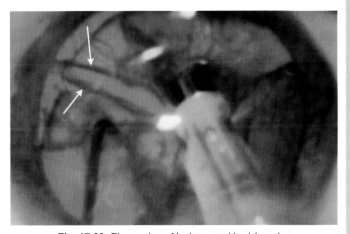

Fig. 17.63: Phaco-chop: Nuclear cracking/chopping

Multidirectional nucleofractis occurs when the phaco tip is used to engage the inferior hemisection and multiple pie-shaped sections are fractured using the second instrument to stabilize the nucleus. The sections are brought into the central pupillary zone for safe emulsification. The multidirectional fracturing is accomplished without rotating the lens. With the natural fault lines in the lens, this can be accomplished very easily without the chopping technique through the use of two-instrument separation.

The superior hemisection is rotated inferiorly and emulsified in a similar fashion. Alternatively, the superior section is nudged inferiorly with the spatula and the phaco tip is burrowed into the bulk of the nucleus, which is fractured without rotation.

Phaco-chop

Nagahara, who introduced the phaco-chop, brought a real breakthrough in the splitting techniques. This is one technique, which has changed the direction of the phaco surgery for a long time to come. It is a very effective method of reducing the phaco energy used and shortening the total energy time as compared to the divide and conquer of Gimbel and 2:4 quadrantic cracking of Shepherd. The phaco-chop uses a zero degree phaco tip and a chopping instrument, principle being similar to chopping wood; the nucleus is fractured along longitudinal fibers using appositional forces rather than parallel. Every motion pulls the nucleus in toward the middle of capsular bag moving it out of capsular for nix. The phaco tip is placed as far superiorly as possible and firmly holds the nucleus to prevent movement. A modified lens hook (chopper; 1.5 mm bent tip) (Figs 17.62 and 17.63) is introduced from sideport as down as capsulotomy permits in the nucleus and pulled towards phaco tip ripping a narrow groove. When both approach each other, they are moved apart gently, chopper to left and phaco tip to right, chopping nucleus into 2 pieces. The nucleus is rotated by 90° and chopping is repeated. Danger of radial capsular tear is avoided by directing chopper in cortex. Effective phaco time needed is reduced. This leads to lesser endothelial cell loss.

Stop and Chop

Disadvantage of phaco-chop was lack of space in the bag to remove the broken fragments, which stuck into one another and made it very difficult to remove a single piece. Stop and chop modification by Paul Koch in 1993 made chopping much easier by creating an initial central space by sculpting.

Modification of Stop and Chop

Various newer modifications of the stop and chop technique have been described in the literature. In stop, chop, chop and stuff technique described by Vasavada and associates, the heminucleus is chopped into smaller fragments, which are then stuffed into the phaco tip and emulsified bit by bit using minimal phaco power. This technique is particularly useful in eyes with hard nuclei. In another modification for leathery hard cataracts, Vasavada and associates have described a "Step-by-step chop in-situ" technique. Complete division of the bottom plate is accomplished in step-by-step fashion by repeated lateral movements of the chopper at different sites along the length of the trench/crater. This stepwise division eliminates stress on the capsular bag.

Quick Chop

In this technique, deep central space is created pulling silicone sleeve back exposing more needle. Using low-aspiration flow rate with appropriate vacuum pulse mode, the surgeon impales into the central nucleus and then chops down on top of the lens in front of or besides impaled phaco needle, instead of making the potentially dangerous step of peripheral excursion with the chop instrument during traditional phaco-chop.

Prerequisite

Pulling the silicon sleeve back exposes the phaco needle more, allowing one to impale the nucleus more deeply. Low power, high vacuum and flow rate is used to help evacuate the chopped segments. Pulse mode is used to avoid corneoscleral burns. Chopper with a more pointed or faceted distal tip is preferable.

Adequate hydrodissection is ensured before starting nuclear disassembly. Hydrodelineation is optional. When the chop instrument is pressed down, it is important to use the sideport incision as a fulcrum. In other words, just the tip moves downwards. The heel of the instrument, outside of the eye, actually moves upwards. If this fulcrum method is used at the sideport with the phaco tip as countertraction, the procedure becomes very efficient. In cases of very dense lenses, some sculpting or central debulk is done because it simply takes too much mechanical energy to start the initial cleavage plane with two passive instruments. An initial bowl is sculpted and then the chopper is impaled further out peripherally to create the first quick-chop. Hence, there is the less bulk of lens material to be divided.

Other modifications like horizontal and vertical chop techniques are depicted in Figs 17.64 to 17.69.

Autocrack Chop

The autocrack technique uses the Autocrack Cobra phaco tip with 15° bevel and 15° curve upward, modified hexagon external shape with circular lumen and high vacuum to induce stress and strain near the "Y-sutures", resulting in a lensquake that propagates radially along the natural fault lines in the nucleus.

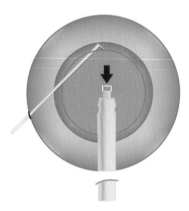

Fig. 17.64: Horizontal chop: A horizontal chop is performed by hooking the nucleus with a chopper and impaling phaco tip with burst mode

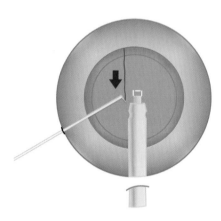

Fig. 17.65: Horizontal chop: The chopper chops the nucleus against the phaco tip

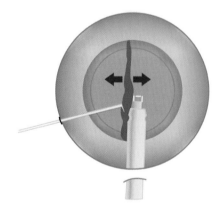

Fig. 17.66: Horizontal chop: The chop continues as the lateral motion completes the nucleus split

Phaco parameters include a low-flow rate (3 to 5 cc/min) and a vacuum of 200 mm Hg. Using the ultrasound, the tip is driven into the nucleus at a steady pace. When the top of the hexagon is completely buried, leveling off of the entry angle is begun as the port is advanced at the level of the central nucleus and its bottom point at ½ nuclear depth. Ultrasound is kept

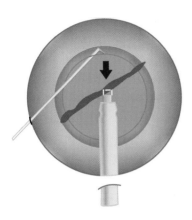

Fig. 17.67: Horizontal chop: The chop is repeated after rotation of the nucleus

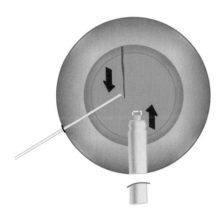

Fig. 17.68: Vertical chop: A vertical chop is performed as quick chopper depresses and phaco tip elevates the nucleus

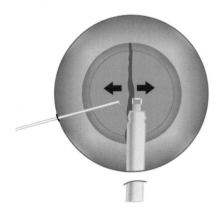

Fig. 17.69: Vertical chop: The nucleus splits into hemisections

on mute, the surgeon stays in foot switch position 2 holding the phaco tip, while the vacuum builds. During the vacuum rise or shortly thereafter, a lensquake occurs, which propagates from the Y-sutures to the equator along nuclear fault lines. This technique works well for 1+ to 2+ nuclei, but with nuclei 3+ or more, it may be necessary to induce the lensquake with the nucleus manipulator. After the vacuum is allowed to

build, the manipulator is placed directly above the phaco tip. Then it is moved down the side of the phaco tip to produce an earthquake-like fault. The two instruments are separated while moving the phaco tip slightly forward and the nucleus manipulator slightly backward. This ensures the complete propagation of the autocrack to the posterior pole and the proximal equator. This technique is useful particularly in situations where we want to decrease the stress on zonules.

Choo-Choo Chop and Flip Phacoemulsification

The choo-choo chop and flip phacoemulsification is a chopping technique that uses power modulations and high vacuum along with specific maneuvers to minimize the amount of ultrasound energy in the eye and maximize safety and control (Table 17.18).

After clear-corneal incision, cortical cleaving hydrodissection is performed in the two distal quadrants followed by hydrodelineation. After the two hydro steps, the nucleus should rotate easily within the capsular bag. The Mackool/Kelman microtip on the Legacy is introduced bevel down to aspirate the epinucleus uncovered by the capsulorhexis and is then turned bevel-down tip is used throughout endonuclear removal. The Fine-Nagahara chopper is placed in the golden ring and is used to stabilize the nucleus by lifting and pulling towards the incision slightly after which the phaco tip lollipops the nucleus. With the energy set as in the Table 17.18, we minimize ultrasound and energy into the eye and maximize our hold on the nucleus as the vacuum builds between pulses of bursts. Because of the decrease in cavitational energy around the tip at this low pulse rate or in burst mode, the tunnel in the nucleus in which the tip is embedded fits the needle very tightly and gives us an excellent hold on the nucleus, thus, maximizing control of the nucleus as we score and chop it in foot position.

The Fine-Nagahara chopper is grooved on the horizontal arm close vertical "chop" element with the groove parallel to the direction of the sharp edge of the vertical element. In scoring the nucleus, the instrument is always moved in the direction of the sharp edge of the wedge-shaped vertical elements is facing (as indicated by the groove on the instrument), thus facilitating scoring. The nucleus is scored, by bringing the chopper to the side of the phaco needle. It is chopped in half by pulling the chopper to the left and slightly down while moving the phaco needle, still in foot position 2, to the right and slightly up. Then the nuclear complex is rotated. The chop instrument is again brought into the golden ring and the nucleus is again lollipopped, scored and chopped, with the resulting pie-shaped segment now lollipopped on the phaco tip. The segment is then evacuated, using high vacuum and short bursts or pulse mode phaco at 2 pulses/second. The nucleus can be scored, chopped and removed essentially by the high vacuum assisted by short bursts or pulses of phaco. The short bursts or pulses of ultrasound energy continuously reshape the pie-shaped segments that are kept at the tip, allowing for occlusion and extraction by the vacuum. The

Table 17.18: AMO sovereign surgical parameters

Mode	Parameter	Settings Phaco 1 (Central Groove)	Phaco 2 (Heminuclear Removal)	Phaco 3 (Epinuclear Removal)
Phaco unoccluded	Max power	30%	30%	5%
	Power delivery	Cont.	Burst cont.	Cont.
	Max vacuum	30 mm	300 mm	250 mm
	Aspiration rate	22 cc/min	26 cc/min	30 cc/min
Phaco occluded	Max power	30%	30%	5%
	Power delivery	Short pulse 6 pps	Short pulse 6 pps	Long pulse 6 pps
	Vac threshold		80 mm	80 mm
	Aspiration rate	22 cc/min	26 cc/min	22 cc/min
I and A	Aspiration rate	28 cc/min		
	Max vacuum	500 mm		

size of the pie-shaped segments is customized to the density of the nucleus, with smaller segments for denser nuclei. Phaco in burst mode or at this low pulse rate sounds like "Choo-Choo-Choo", ergo the name of this technique. With the burst mode or the low pulse rate, the nuclear material tends to stay at the tip rather than chatter as vacuum holds between pulses. The chopper is used to stuff the segment into the tip or keep it down in the nuclear shell. After evacuation of the first heminucleus, the second heminucleus is rotated to the distal portion of the bag and the chop instrument stabilizes it while it is lollipopped. It is then scored and chopped. The pie-shaped segments can be chopped a second time to reduce their size if they appear too large to easily evacuate.

Petalloid Phacoemulsification

In this technique of Dada and associates sequential chopping like petals follows partial central debulking.

Akahoshi Pre-Chopping Technique

By employing Akahoshi's method of pre-chopping the nucleus, prior to phacoemulsification, surgeons can reduce phaco time and minimize the risk of posterior capsule rupture. Unlike the traditional phacoemulsification technique of grooving the nucleus, this technique effectively "cuts" the nucleus into two, then four pieces before the phaco tip is even introduced. Reduced phaco time results in a better self-sealing wound, by minimizing thermal damage and manual movement of the entry port. Available with an angled tip for scleral tunnels, a straight tip for clear corneal, temporal wounds and curved shafts for 12 o'clock approach, the Akahoshi's pre-chop is effective on both hard and soft nuclei.

EPINUCLEUS MANAGEMENT

Epinucleus management is depicted in Table 17.19 and Figures 17.70 and 17.71.

Table 17.19: Epinuclear management

1. Legacy
   standard tubing
Trim	Flip
Pulse Mem 2	Pulse Mem 3
50–70	50–70
16	16
100	50
Pulse 8/sec	Pulse 8/sec
70	70

2. Max vaccum (Hi-vac)
Trim	Flip
Pulse Mem 2	Pulse Mem 3
40–50	40–50
16/18	12
120/140	100/180
Pulse 4/8 sec	Pulse 4/8 sec
72	72

3. 0.9 SIS with Standard Tubing
Trim	Flip
Pulse Mem 2	Pulse Mem 3
50	50
20/18 (4 + nucleus)	16
180/200 (4 + nucleus)	120
Pulse 2/sec	Pulse 2/sec
72	72

4. Mackool System Hi-Vac
   "Choo-choo chop and flip"
Trim	Flip
Mem 2 Pulse	Mem 3 Pulse
35	35
20/18	22
180	180
Pulse 7/sec	Pulse 7/sec
72	72

5. Max-Vac SIS
Trim	Flip
Pulse 2	Pulse 3
50	50
25	25
200	250
Pulse 8/sec	Pulse 8/sec
78	78

Flow chart 17.1: Approach to safe cortical clean-up

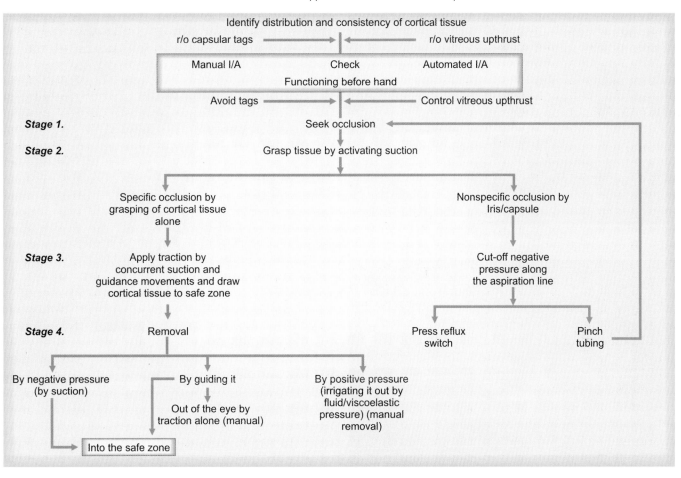

Flow chart 17.2: Management of subincisional cortical matter

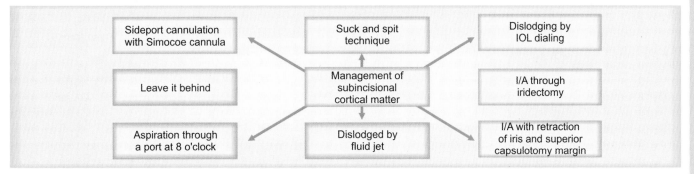

CORTICAL CLEAN UP

Strategies for cortical clean-up are depicted in Flow charts 17.1 and 17.2.

FOLDABLE LENS INSERTION

Technique

Foldable lens insertion technique needs specially designed instruments as mentioned above. Any of these can be chosen ensuring that they provide fumble-free IOL loading insertion through an unenlarged 3 mm phaco incision, which is the bottom line in any delivery system and finally should ensure symmetrical unfolding of the IOL is in the capsular bag. Lens insertion using a folding forceps can be done. The lens can be folded by using either of the two principles. Horizontal or longitudinal principle, which allows for a two-step implantation technique, ensures control and safety. This is folding along the 6 to 12 o'clock meridian. Vertical or transverse principles, which allow the lens to be placed in one maneuver by an experienced surgeon. However, plenty of space in the anterior chamber and capsular bag is required. This is folding along the 3 to 9 o'clock

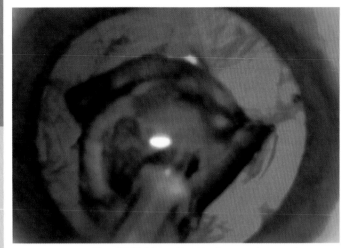

Fig. 17.70: Epinuclear shell removal

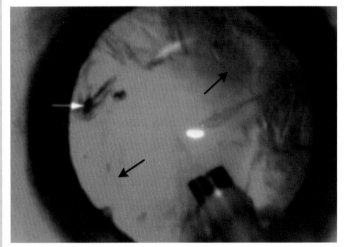

Fig. 17.71: Epinuclear shell removal completed. Intact capsulorhexis margins (black arrows) and residual cortical matter (white arrow) are seen

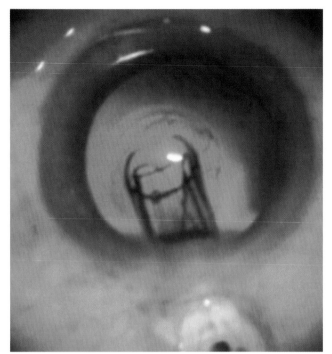

Fig. 17.72: Intraocular lens insertion with injector

meridian. The IOL insertion with injector cartridge is the most commonly practiced technique (Fig. 17.72).

COMPLICATIONS AND MANAGEMENT

Various complications can occur during phacoemulsification. Their management is discussed as follows:

Wound Construction

A well-constructed wound is the key to a strong sutureless wound. A poorly constructed wound can be a source of astigmatism, filtration, irritation, hemorrhage and corneal trauma despite a satisfactory wound disclosure.

A scleral incision is usually made at a distance of 2.0 to 3.0 mm from the limbus. It is essential to measure the distance each time because there is a tendency for "corneal creep" to occur with scleral incisions. Posterior incisions create more bleeding and take a little extra time. Because of the longer tunnel created, a further posterior incision binds the phacoemulsification tip so that it is more difficult to move towards the right or left portions of the pupil. Anterior or nonbeveled

incisions have a thin area of contact and do not approximate well. The depth of the scleral flap is important in incision making. A very thin flap causes buttonholing of the scleral tissues. On the other hand, the dissection of the scleral flap, which has been too steep relative to the curvature of the scleral and cornea, may cause a premature entry into the anterior chamber, with troublesome iris prolapse or Descemet's tears. The tendency to be too shallow or too deep can be prevented in part by remembering that the radius of curvature of the cornea is shorter than that of the sclera with transition occurring at the limbus. Incisions should enter the anterior chamber well above the iris plane to prevent iris prolapse.

Hyphema

Incision construction and closure also affect the postoperative hyphema formation. A uniformly smooth lamellar scleral incision requires the use of a precisely beveled knife for dissection. If an incision is closed, by placing the suture at its edge, blood is trapped in the tunnel. Blood oozing from the scleral bed can flow only in one direction into the anterior chamber. In a corneal valve incision, blood cannot flow in the anterior chamber because the closure is between the bleeding point and the anterior chamber. As a result, all blood must flow through the external incision. Thus, hyphema is a more common complication with scleral incision without a corneal valve than with corneal incision. Blood oozing towards the sclera is a sure sign that the incision is watertight.

Anterior Capsulotomy

The single most important step in phacoemulsification is making a continuous tear capsulotomy. Too small a capsulotomy will increase the risk to anterior capsular remnant and posterior capsule opacification. It will also cause optical problems later. Anterior capsulotomy shrinkage occurs further as the anterior capsular remnant undergoes the contraction of epithelial cells and fibrosis. Ultrasonic removal or cryopexy of the anterior capsular epithelial cells have been advocated for such purposes.

If the bent portion of the capsulotomy needle is fairly small, a single incision usually develops. However, if a pupil parallel pattern is not observed at every moment, a straight line will start to develop. This may result in a capsulotomy that is too small or one that gets lost among the zonular fibers in the equatorial zone. Moreover, frequent repositioning of the needle tip is required so that it is never more than 2 mm from the active peripheral tear edge, in order to prevent the peripheral extension of the capsulotomy.

Corneal Complications

Postoperative superior corneal edema is generally present in cases of phacoemulsification. However, it is transient. Moreover, adequate incision construction, proper instrumentation and avoidance of false passages prevent its occurrence and subsequent early resolution. Incisional burns can be avoided by avoiding too tight an incision, using cold balanced salt solution (at 4°C) as irrigating solutions and obtaining a minimum phaco time. Diffuse corneal haze or loss of corneal clarity is a common problem encountered during phacosurgery. This can be prevented, by avoiding corneal exposure, especially after peribulbar anesthesia or facial block. The topical drugs should be used optimally, as prolonged and frequent instillation may simulate superficial punctuate keratitis. Moreover, corneal hydration should be maintained at all times during surgery and any mechanical trauma or excess irrigation be prevented.

Descemet's detachment and Descemet's tears may also occur infrequently. The anterior tip of the incision should be lifted up when the instruments are inserted. Descemet's tears can be also prevented, by using sharp instruments. The phaco tip should be inserted with the bevel down. The side port entry should also be made by the beveled instrument similarly and any mechanical damage to the Descemet's membrane should be avoided. Corneal endothelium can further be prevented from damage by decreasing the effective phacoemulsification time and confining the procedure to the posterior chamber and with the nucleus so that the attenuation of the acoustic trauma occurs in the nucleus. The infusion sleeve sideport should remain parallel to the iris plane. Moreover, the flow should not be directed anteroposteriorly, but laterally. Better viscoelastics like sodium hyaluronate and irrigating fluids like balanced salt solution should be used, and endotheliotoxic drugs like adrenaline and pilocarpine should be avoided.

In the event of a postoperative corneal decompensation, IOP should remain low on antiglaucoma medication. Anti-inflammatory agents should be used to decrease inflammation

and ciliary body rest should be given by the use of cycloplegics. Hyperosmotics should be used when indicated. In the effect of irreversible endothelial damage, however, keratoplasty may be undertaken.

Iris Injury

The iris can be injured inferiorly or superiorly. Inferior iris injuries can occur and can be prevented by avoiding phaco in a small pupil or shallow anterior chamber. Iris flutter should always be prevented. While doing the phacoemulsification, the bevel of the phaco probe should be upwards and should remain parallel to the iris plane. Superior iris injuries are not disfiguring and no active intervention is required. Iris injuries can be prevented by ensuring that phaco is performed in central 5 to 6 mm zone. The capsulorhexis should never be crossed and the phaco tip should be inserted with the tip bevel downwards.

Vitreous Loss

Zonular dehiscence may occur if an attempt is made to rotate the nucleus after an inadequate hydrodissection, capsulorhexis does not stretch with the rotation of the nucleus and, therefore, the zonules give way. In the event of a posterior capsular rent with no vitreous loss, vitrectomy may not be required. Nevertheless, the flow rate and infusion should be decreased. However, in cases of vitreous loss, a proper vitrectomy is mandatory. A single vitrectomy tip with a coaxial cannula should generally be avoided in favor of a bimanual vitrectomy with separate infusion and cutting tip. Coaxial infusion rips open the posterior capsule, permitting more vitreous into the anterior chamber. With the bimanual technique, the main body of the vitreous should not be disturbed and vitreous should be aspirated downwards below the plane of the posterior capsule. Irrigation should be gentle and limited to the anterior chamber. Following vitrectomy, an IOL may be placed on the anterior capsule if an adequate rim is present. Vitreous loss can be prevented by not attempting to phacoemulsify posterior to the nucleus. The phaco area decreased to the central 5 mm peristaltic pump is better in these settings. However, one must not hesitate to convert to the routine procedure of cataract extraction in case of vitreous loss. Monitoring of the anterior chamber depth is depicted in Flow charts 17.3 and 17.4. Management of rupture of the posterior capsule, during phacoemulsification is shown in Flow chart 17.5.

Conversion to Extracapsular Cataract Extraction

Conversion to extracapsular cataract extraction is merely an alternative to attain the primary goal, i.e. functional visual acuity. Conversion should be undertaken preferably before excessive, endothelial damage occurs and before the posterior capsule ruptures. "Planned conversion to extracapsular cataract extraction is a better alternative to forced conversion".

Flow chart 17.3: Management of shallow anterior chamber during phacoemulsification

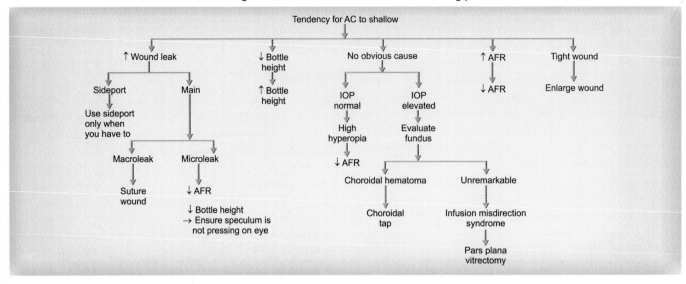

Flow chart 17.4: Management of deep anterior chamber during phacoemulsification

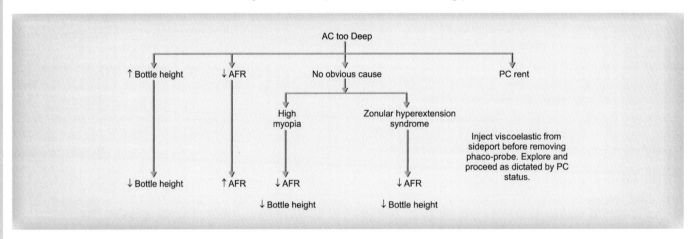

CHALLENGING SITUATIONS

Intraocular Lens Power Calculation after Refractive Surgery

Previous corneal refractive surgery changes the architecture of the cornea such that the standard methods of measuring the corneal power cause it to be underestimated. Radial keratotomy causes a relatively proportional equal flattening of both the front and back surface of the cornea, which leaves the index of refraction relationship the same. On the other hand, photorefractive keratectomy and laser-assisted intrastromal keratomileusis (LASIK) flatten only the front surface. This changes the refractive index calculation creating an underestimation of the corneal power by about 1 D for every 7 D of refractive surgery correction obtained.

The major cause of error is the fact that manual keratometers measure at the 3.2 mm zone of the central cornea, which often misses the central flatter zone of effective corneal power. There are two methods to better estimate the corneal power in these refractive surgery eyes.

Clinical History Method

This method is based on the fact that the final change in refractive error, which the eye obtains from surgery is due only to a change in the effective corneal power. If this change (at the corneal plane) is added to the presurgical corneal power, we will obtain the present effective corneal power.

Warning: All patients having corneal refractive surgery should be given the following data to maintain in their personal health records. They should be told to give it to anyone planning to perform cataract/IOL surgery on them—preoperative corneal power, preoperative refractive error (spectacles with vertex distance or contact lens power) and postoperative healed refractive error (before lens changes affected it).

All attempts should be made to obtain the above information from the refractive surgeon records. Each spherical equivalent refractive error (R) should be vertex (v) corrected to the corneal plane (0 mm) using:

$$Ro = Rv/1 - V \times Rv \text{ or}$$
$$\text{using vertex of 12 mm: } Ro = R_{12}/1 - 0.012 \times R_{12}$$

Flow chart 17.5: Approach to management of posterior capsular rupture during phacoemulsification

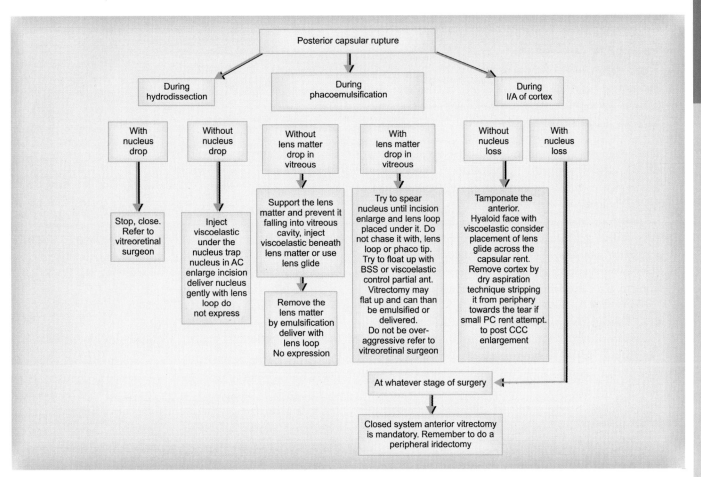

The estimated effective corneal power (K) can be calculated using the following formula:

$$K = K_{PREOP} + R_{PREOPo} - R_{POo}$$

Contact Lens Method

This method is based on the principle that if a hard contact lens (CL) of plano power (P) and a base curve (B) equal to the effective power of the cornea, is placed on the eye, it will not change the refractive error of the eye, and the difference between the manifest refraction with the contact lens (R_{CL}) and without it (R_{NoCL}) is zero. The formula to calculate the estimated corneal power is:

$$K = B + P + R_{CL} - R_{NoCL}$$

The refractive errors should also be vertex corrected. Several computer IOL power calculation programs calculate these two methods automatically when needed.

If the results of both methods are different, use the lowest estimated corneal power. Rarely are such eyes myopic after the IOL surgery. Obviously, the former method cannot be used if the historical data is not available and the latter is impossible if the cataract precludes performing refraction. In such cases, it might be wise to delay the IOL implantation and calculate the secondary implant power using the aphakic refractive error in the refraction formula or a piggyback lens or phakic refractive lens to correct any deficiency.

It is recommended that the third generation IOL power calculation formula (but not a regression formula) be used. SRK/T formula is more accurate for corneal plane calculations, while SRK-II formula is for spectacle plane calculations.

Intraocular Lens Power Calculation in Corneal Transplant Eyes

A problem also arises when attempting to predict what the corneal power will be after a corneal transplant. Some have suggested using the corneal power of the other eye (if it is available) or using an average of one's post-transplant corneal powers, but published reports show a very large range of prediction and refractive errors using these attempts. Performing the IOL implantation after the corneal transplant has settled down was suggested by the author in 1986 and in 1990. Geegel reported excellent refractive results using this two-stepped approach (66%, 6/12 or better acuity without correction). A secondary piggyback IOL or phakic refractive lens is another alternative to correct residual ametropia.

Hard Nucleus

Hard cataracts are the nightmares for all phaco surgeons. For hypermature white cataracts with hard nuclei, hydrodissection is not necessary because nuclei are mobile and rotation is easily directly achieved. Importance of performing delamination is mentioned in Table 17.20.

Table 17.20: Importance of delamination

If delamination is not performed:

- The epinucleus follows the nucleus in phaco.
- Exposes the bag in that quadrant.
- Once the nuclear material is removed the bag becomes floppy.
- No protection to posterior capsule.

Until now, there are two main techniques for dealing with hard cataracts:

1. Creating a deep central bowl and proceeding with the phaco-chop technique.
2. Creating four cross-grooves and proceeding with the chop. In both these techniques, most of the phaco energy is utilized in creating a bowl or the grooves in the endonucleus, which is the hardest part of any cataract. To overcome this problem, the author introduced two techniques:
   i. Mechanical delineation in-situ, and
   ii. To manage the central nuclear core a new technique—the central flip.

The authors prefer to increase the power to 80% for all grade IV nuclei. The sleeve has to be moved slightly backwards for slightly more exposure of the tip. The authors do find a need to increase the vacuum to 250 mm Hg. We use a new generation phaco machine, where we use burst mode with high vacuum tubing.

The Central Flip

Small linear groove is performed using a 30-degree phaco tip. The groove is only in the epinucleus and smaller than the continuous curvilinear capsulorhexis. Using a sharp tip chopper, the phaco-chop technique is performed and the nucleus is rotated. The chopping is repeated. This chopping is performed 360° round the nucleus without removing any nuclear piece. It was soon realized that the initial chops met underneath the hard central core. This central core could easily be flipped out and it is fed into the handpiece (Fig. 17.73) without using phaco energy. This new technique, the central flip, i.e. separating the endonucleus and flipping the central core, results in reducing the effective phaco time to less than 30 seconds. Advantages of this technique are that it creates a cushion on the posterior capsule and no stress is transmitted to the posterior capsule. It has also kept the effective phaco time low. The next step is to perform "mechanical delineation in-situ". As there are firm adhesions between the epinuclear shell and the central endonucleus, hydrodelineation in such cases is impossible. Once the central core is removed, the small individual pieces of nuclei are held and the epinuclear shell is mechanically separated with the help of the sharp tip chopper in the nondormant hand. The epinuclear shell is repositioned into the bag. The nuclear piece is held and a burst of phaco energy is applied. This continues till all the nuclear pieces are engulfed. Advantages of mechanical delineation in-situ are shown in Table 17.21.

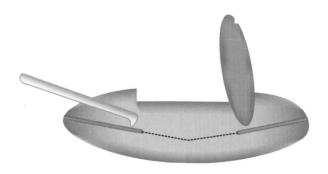

Fig. 17.73: Central flip

Table 17.21: Advantages of mechanical delineation in-situ

- Protective cushion of epinucleus created
- Keeps the bag on stretch
- Can be used in any grade of nucleus—II, III, IV
- Epinuclear shell is free
- Chopper assisted

Other Technique

Dr Kammann developed a technique called four-before-phaco for red-brown nuclei that employs mechanical division of the nucleus without ultrasound energy combined with reversed tip-and-snip phacoemulsification (Figs 17.74 to 17.77).

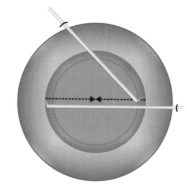

Fig. 17.74: Four-before-phaco for hard cataract: A vertical ditch is created by moving the hooks from the periphery to the center, which separates the nucleus into halves

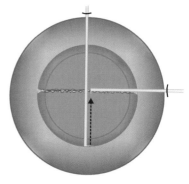

Fig. 17.75: Four-before-phaco for hard cataract: The nasal half is separated into two quarters

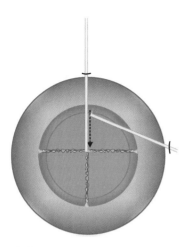

Fig. 17.76: Four-before-phaco for hard cataract: The temporal half is separated into two quarters

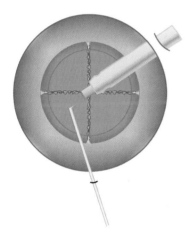

Fig. 17.77: Four-before-phaco for hard cataract: Phacoemulsification of each nuclear quarter is achieved with the reversed tip-and-snip technique

Method: Three paracenteses, at the 12 o'clock, 9 o'clock and 3 o'clock positions, are necessary to perform four-before-phaco and the subsequent phacoemulsification. Preparation of the conjunctiva and frown-incision of the sclera are performed in the upper temporal quadrant. After the instillation of viscoelastic, a 5 to 6 mm capsulorhexis is performed with Utrata forceps. The subsequent steps are facilitated by a large capsulorhexis.

Loose cortex fragments and the epinucleus above the nuclear center are aspirated to acquire a better view for the four-before-phaco procedure. Viscoelastic is injected once more and two 2.5 mm long Sinskey hooks are inserted through the 12 o'clock and temporal paracenteses. The temporal hook is moved forward under the anterior capsule to the lens equator at the 12 o'clock position. The 12 o'clock hook is extended likewise to reach the 6 o'clock position. Then both hooks are pulled from the periphery to the center, dividing the nucleus, by creating a vertical ditch. The 12 o'clock hook then steadies the nasal half of the nucleus while the temporal hook produces a horizontal ditch that divides the nasal half into two quarters. The horizontal ditch is completed when the 12 o'clock hook is

pulled from the equator to the center, while the temporal hook fixates the temporal half. The nucleus is thus divided into four parts and both hooks are removed. Advantage of this technique is the nucleus separation which is achieved with a few manipulations without using ultrasound energy.

Phaco in White and Black Cataracts

White and black cataracts pose special problems in phacoemulsification.

White Cataract

During capsulorhexis, the white color of the cortex and the presence of dispersed liquefied cortex can obstruct your vision during surgery. Additionally, fragile and fibrotic capsules can increase the chance of radial tears.

Capsulotomy techniques: (i) Grasp technique: After viscoelastic is injected into the anterior chamber, use Utrata forceps to grasp the anterior capsule and hold onto the anterior capsule flap with the forceps and continuous curvilinear capsulorhexis is completed. If the liquefied cortex is so dispersed to hamper visualization, it is aspirated. Viscoelastic is reinjected into the anterior chamber both above and within the capsular bag and continuous curvilinear capsulorhexis is completed; (ii) Oblique illumination; (iii) A fiber-optic light pipe, introduced into the anterior chamber, can enhance the view of the tearing capsule considerably; (iv) Capsular staining as described in capulorhexis section previously can be used, and (v) A radiofrequency endodiathermy can be used.

When a radial tear occurs, there are multiple methods to manage it:

- Microscissors can be used to cut the capsule and start the tear in a new direction.
- A bent needle can be used to make a new tear in another site on the capsule.
- Anterior vitrector with a separate infusion port can be used to cut the remaining capsule in a circular pattern. This technique can also be used in the cases of fibrotic or calcified capsules.

Hydrodissection step can be skipped, because most of these nuclei will already rotate freely. Instead, irrigate and aspirate out the remaining cortex to improve visualization.

For nucleus removal, use an elevate-and-chop technique. After removal of the liquefied cortex, the phaco tip is embedded into the central nucleus. One side of the nucleus is elevated until its equator is up over the pupillary plane, then a chop is performed from the equator to the central nucleus (Table 17.22). Advantages of the elevate-and-chop technique include good visualization during the chop; ease of chopping and cracking from the equator towards the central nucleus; decrease chance of capsular rupture by the chopper; and no streching of the capsule and zonules. The technique can be performed in the cases of radial tear and in eyes with small pupil. After the chopping and cracking are done, the pieces of nucleus can be emulsified in the posterior chamber.

Other technique: Stop, chop, chop and stuff technique with two-stage continuous curvilinear capsulorhexis can also be done, as described by Vasavada and associates.

Table 17.22: Parameters for phacoemulsification

White cataract	Parameters
Phaco power	50 to 60%
Flow rate	30 cc/min
Vacuum	150 to 250 mm Hg
Phaco time	2 to 4 minutes
Operating time	15 to 30 minutes
Black cataract	*Parameters*
Transverse cracking	
Phaco power	50 to 60%
Flow rate	20 cc/min
Vacuum	60 to 80 mm Hg
Serial-chop	
Phaco power	50 to 60%
Flow rate	30 cc/min
Vacuum	150 to 250 mm Hg

Black Cataract

Problems with brunescent and black cataracts include hard and sticky nucleus fibers; thin capsules and weak zonules and a large mass of nucleus and epinuclues. The large mass of the nucleus means we encounter an increase in the anterior-to-posterior diameter of the nucleus, some degree of capsular stretching and limited space for manipulation. A technique to address these problems called the transverse cracking and serial chop can be employed. To begin, central sculpting of the nucleus is performed. Then a transverse crack is made. The phaco tip is embedded in the upper part of the nucleus with pull on the lower part with a Sinskey hook or chopper. This makes the nucleus separate into two pieces. Then a serial chop is performed. In this method, embed the phaco tip and perform a chop, then embed the tip again and perform a second chop and then a third chop, resulting in three small pieces of the nucleus. It is easy to manipulate the third piece of the nucleus; first, because it is moved into the center more easily than the other pieces. The author refers to it as the connecting effect emulsifying the third, second and first pieces sequentially. After having emulsified the first three pieces, a chop or elevate- and-chop technique is used to manage the remaining nucleus. Advantages of transverse cracking are that it decreases the mass of the core nucleus, which increases space for manipulation and destroys the hard and sticky nucleus fibers in the core nucleus; and it divides the nucleus without rotation. Advantages of the serial chop are that it destroys the core nucleus with multiple embeddings of the phaco tip; rotation of the nucleus occurs automatically. Using these techniques, phaco time, operative time and the number and severity of complications can be significantly reduced.

Subluxated Lens

Preoperative Evaluation

Assessment of the extent of subluxation and determine the cause (pseudoexfoliation, myopia, trauma, etc).

Anesthesia

Both general and local anesthesia enable the creation of scleral windows and trans-scleral suturing of the capsular ring or of the IOL to be performed if necessary.

When using 1% intracameral lidocaine, there is a risk of its passage through the zones lacking zonular fibers and transitory loss of sight resulting from retinal toxicity, as described in the cases of capsular rupture, is theoretically possible. Topical anesthetic may also provide insufficient analgesia if either trans-scleral suturing of the capsular ring or the IOL becomes necessary.

Incision

The incision should be made in the zone opposite to the subluxation to minimize the traction on the zone of zonular disinsertion. If this is not possible, incision may be performed at 90° of the subluxation, according to its location. As a rule, incision in the zone of subluxation should be avoided because of the inherent risks of enlargement of the subluxation or vitreous loss, among others. The surgical approach may be scleral or corneal. In either case, it is advisable to precut a scleral window preoperatively when it may be necessary to suture the IOL or capsular ring to the sulcus. The scleral window must be created in the zone of zonular disinsertion, where a trans-scleral suture is likely to be needed and before intraocular entry, considering the well-known difficulty of dissecting the scleral window when the eyeball is open and hypotonic.

Capsulorhexis

If vitreous is present in the anterior chamber, the gel must first be isolated. Coaxial vitrectomy systems hydrate the vitreous at the level of zonular dehiscence and can extend vitreous loss. The two-port systems enable isolation of the vitreous. Capsulorhexis, which is especially difficult in these situations, must be performed in such a way that traction is minimized not on the zone of zonular dehiscence itself, where zonular fibers have already been lost, but on the ends of the zone, with the goal of not extending the dehiscence.

It is helpful to begin in a zone where the zonule is whole and where the capsule offers sufficient resistance. Folds frequently form in the anterior capsule when an attempt is made to open it. Repositioning the anterior chamber with sufficient viscoelastic facilitates the first step of the capsulorhexis. The use of needle and forceps and the exercising of controlled movements, preferably begun away from the zone of disinsertion, enable this crucial step to be completed. When necessary, traction on the capsule in the zone must be toward the zone of zonular dehiscence and never in the opposite direction.

Performing capsulorhexis is a prerequisite for implantation of a capsular ring and if centration of the lens in the pupil with a disposable nylon hook with adjustable silicone retaining sleeve is desired. The capsulorhexis size should be as large as possible.

Hydrodissection

Hydrodissection must be meticulously performed to ensure the correct freeing of the lens nucleus. A 27-gauge cannula is inserted well through the incision or sideport paracentesis in the direction of the zone of disinsertion rather than in the opposite direction, which would enlarge the disinsertion. When this has been completed, the nucleus should rotate freely within the capsular bag. As a consequence, the rotational movements, which are required during nuclear phacoemulsification, are minimized, thus, limiting the risk of increasing the zonular dehiscence.

Implantation of the Capsular Ring

The use of capsular rings provides different advantages, among which is the maintenance of circular contour of the bag despite zonular dehiscence, preventing asymmetric retraction, increased phacoemulsification safety and efficiency (even prevention of vitreous where zonular dehiscence co-exists), inhibition of cell proliferation of the posterior capsule with the resultant better quality of vision and possible prevention of capsulorhexis contraction syndrome in which the opening is small. If the lens is manifestly unstable and nuclear phacoemulsification cannot be safely performed, capsular ring implantation can be considered and may prove sufficient. However, if the instability is greater, then transcapsular suturing of the ring may be appropriate.

Phacoemulsification Technique

With soft nuclei, the "chip and flip" technique enables limited traction to be exerted on the capsular bag. With moderate or hard nuclei, when it is necessary to use cracking techniques, the Kelman's V technique limits the need for rotating the nucleus and may prove especially useful. In general, phacoemulsification in these situations may be considered a safe alternative if performed by low vacuum, low aspiration and low infusion.

Cortical Aspiration

In these cases, manual cortical aspiration is preferred because it may be more controllable. When performing cortical aspiration, tangential traction movements are advised, and not radial.

Implantation of Intraocular Lenses

Endocapsular implantation of the IOL is done with the haptics in the zone of disinsertion. It is desirable to implant a large diameter lens—greater than 6 mm to minimize symptoms if lens decentration were to occur. The lens may be implanted in the bag or in the sulcus. In either case, rotational maneuvers must be avoided. Some authors advocate supporting the haptics in the sulcus, where zonular support may still exist, capturing the lens optics by the means of capsulorhexis in the same way that a button is passed through a buttonhole.

Small Pupil

The most important goal in small pupil cataract surgery is to limit serious surgical complications. A small pupil is generally between 2 and 5 mm in diameter (pseudoexfoliation syndrome, chronic miotic therapy, uveitis, etc). Various factors, which contribute to the surgeon's decisions to change the size of the pupil and various pupil-enlarging techniques, have been depicted in Tables 17.23 and 17.24.

Anterior capsulotomy: A smooth capsulorhexis border can be made slightly larger than the small pupil by guiding the tear under the iris; at the same time, observing a fold at the edge of the capsule flap. A two-stage capsulorhexis can also be done.

Hydrodissection: The cannula is taken under the pupil and just posterior to the edge of the capsulotomy; and with gradual pressure, the balanced salt solution is gradually, but firmly injected.

Hydrodissection would be noted to be complete once there is anterior movement of the lens/iris diaphragm with egress of viscoelastic. There is enlargement of the pupil with this

Table 17.23: When to enlarge a small pupil

Factors which contribute to a surgeon's decision to change the size of the pupil:

1. The hardness of lens material relative to the size of the pupil.
2. Status of zonular support meshwork—patients older than 90 years and pseudoexfoliation have weak zonules.
3. Status of anterior chamber—shallow anterior chamber increases the difficulty in maneuvering the phacoemulsification tip.
4. Status of cornea—patients after penetrating keratoplasty and Fuchs' dystrophy benefit from larger pupils.

Table 17.24: Management of small pupil

Nonsurgical treatment of small pupil

1. Viscoelastic injection, which enlarges the pupil during capsulotomy.
2. Pupil can also be stretched using iris hooks through the surgical wound.

Surgical treatment of small pupil

1. Sphincterotomy or pupilloplasty
2. Midperipheral (partial sector) iridectomy: This begins with mid-stromal, full-thickness iridectomy; viscoelastic is placed above and below the iris and incisions are used to enlarge the iridectomy to the pupillary aperture.
3. Radial iridectomy
4. Keyhole iridectomy
5. Multiple sphincterotomies can be done in patients on chronic miotic therapy to dilate the pupil.
6. Iris hook and pupil dilators

maneuver. If necessary, it is important that the rotation of the lens is checked using two hooks prior to insertion of the phacoemulsification tip.

Nucleus removal: A phacoemulsification chop technique can be used as a secondary maneuver to decrease the size of each quadrant. Once the quadrant is caught in the phacoemulsification tip, this is then brought more centrally and the second instrument used to chop the individual quadrant into two smaller pieces. This enables easier phacoemulsification of each smaller individual piece with even less movement of the phacoemulsification tip.

Cortical clean up: It is important that the port of the cannula be always visible to the surgeon. The cannula must be placed deep in the capsular bag, to prevent any incarceration of the iris. To deepen the capsular bag it may be necessary to raise the height of the irrigating solution bottle.

The individual quadrants of the pupil can be retracted using a second instrument. Cortex is then grasped with the cannula and aspirated once the cannula is brought into view within the pupillary area. The most difficult area to remove cortex, especially in small pupils, is subincisional cortex. The problems include overhanging pupillary margin and the anterior capsulotomy edge. A two-instrument technique is used here whereby a 90° curved irrigation aspiration cannula is used with the retraction of the iris superiorly using a second instrument. The second method is to use an aspiration cannula through the sideport incision and irrigating cannula placed in the cataract incision. Vasavada has described phaco with step-by-step chop in-situ and lateral aspiration of the nucleus with minimal or no pupil widening maneuvers, restoring the preoperative pupil configuration.

Postvitreoretinal Surgery

Patients who have had prior vitreoretinal surgery may be particularly challenging to the cataract surgeon. Careful attention to details, however, often enables the surgeon to perform phacoemulsification in these cases with good results.

The spectrum includes patients who have had incidental rupture or resection of the posterior capsule by the vitreoretinal surgeon. If the anterior segment surgeon is not aware of this unintended rent, the lens drop can occur during hydrodissection or phaco. Therefore, the anterior segment surgeon should be aware of the potential for damage to the posterior capsule and to the zonules. The absence of the vitreous, particularly in cases with damage to the posterior capsule or zonules, may allow the infused fluid used during cataract surgery to more readily percolate to the back of the eye. This increases the risk for cystoid macular edema or other forms of maculopathy if epinephrine or certain antibiotics are used in the infusing bottle.

Precaution: Avoid epinephrine and aminoglycoside antibiotics in the infusate for patients who have had prior vitrectomy. Also, avoid intracameral lidocaine in such cases.

Operative fluidics: It is very challenging in eyes with total vitrectomy. The lens/iris diaphragm tends to move extensively so that the chamber may shallow and the iris may come forward and prolapse into the incision. Alternatively, the chamber may become excessively deep, making visualization very difficult. In these cases, the surgeon must always be aware of chamber depth and titrate the level of the infusing bottle.

Implant choice is very significant in patients with silicone oil. Studies have shown that silicone oil may irreversibly damage silicone lens implants after the posterior capsular disruption.

Also, lens implant power calculations in eyes with silicone oil require a different ultrasound speed. When the standard speed (1,550 meters per second) is used, the eyes read disproportionately long. A speed of 1,000 meters/second is used. Silicone oil also changes refraction with PMMA intraocular lenses. A standard IOL calculation would result in an even higher degree of postoperative hyperopia in the presence of silicone oil.

Silicone oil refractive effect: The second problem that arises when the vitreous is replaced with silicone oil is that the refractive index of the oil is much less than that of vitreous and it acts as a negative lens in the eye, which must be offset with more power in the IOL. This effect is dependent upon the shape factor of the back surface of the IOL such that a biconvex IOL creates the worst problem and a concave posterior lens causes practically none. In between the two is the planoposterior lens, which is recommended in these cases. With a plano-convex lens, 2 to 3D must be added to the IOL power to compensate for this issue. The modification of an existing scleral buckle makes the final postoperative refractive error even more problematic.

SECONDARY INTRAOCULAR LENS IMPLANTATION

Indications for secondary IOL implantation are shown in Table 17.25.

Table 17.25: Indications for secondary intraocular lens implantation

- Dissatisfaction with the visual rehabilitation of aphakic spectacles
- Contact lens intolerance
- Dry eye syndrome
- Herpetic keratitis
- Eyes with large filtering blebs
- Occupational or environmental problems
- Difficulty with contact lens manipulation
- Arthritis
- Tremors
- Senility
- Visual deficits as seen in age-related macular degeneration

18

Microincision Cataract Surgery

Kumar Doctor, Chanda Hingorani

INTRODUCTION

The term microincision cataract surgery (MICS) was created by Jorge Alio in 2001, aiming to identify a specific trend of cataract surgery towards incisions of less than 2 mm. The technique is known as microincision or bimanual microincision or phakonit or microphako.

Microincision cataract surgery can be performed with different types of instruments with different types of energy, using different instruments, but ultimately involves three main issues:

- To decrease the incision size to the minimum level now, in real practice, in the range of 19–21 gauge.
- To make a global transformation of the surgical procedure towards minimal aggressiveness.
- To separate the functions of irrigation and aspiration through two independent incisions handled bimanually.

Today, the average MICS incision is 1.7 mm and the lower limit is 0.7 mm (21- gauge). We now have lenses that can be implanted through sub 2.0 mm incisions, although lenses that will fit through a sub 1 mm incision are not yet available.

BIMANUAL MICROPHACOEMULSIFICATION

With the development of new phacoemulsification technology and power modulations, we are now able to remove the cataract without the generation of significant thermal energy. Thus, the removal of the cataract through two separate incisions is now a viable alternative to traditional coaxial phacoemulsification. Machines, such as the AMO WhiteStar, Alcon Infiniti with NeoSonix, Stellaris Vision Enhancement System by Bausch & Lomb, and STAAR Sonic has the potential for offering cold lens removal capabilities and the capacity for bimanual cataract surgery.

Advantages of Bimanual Phacoemulsification

1. *Astigmatic-neutral incisions:* Bimanual phaco offers the potential for truly astigmatic-neutral incisions and the eye has normal integrity immediately at the end of the surgery. Incision size has direct effect on patient satisfaction, postoperative comfort, wound integrity and safety, endothelial cell loss, postoperative corneal clarity, and reflux of ocular surface debris into the eye that causes endophthalmitis.

2. *Decreasing surgical trauma:* There is consistent evidence to state that MICS decreases effective phaco time by decreasing total phaco power used for cataract extraction up to grade 4, thereby increasing the surgical control and decreasing the surgical trauma.

3. *Better control of surgical steps:* Bimanual phaco may increase a surgeon's access to nuclear material. The angle of attack can be steepened with a shorter tunnel, and also, a shorter tunnel undergoes less distortion, reducing the dimple-down effect of the cornea and providing better visibility.

4. *Ideal fluidics and better cortical clean-up:* The separation of irrigation from aspiration allows for improved flow ability by avoiding competing currents at the tip of the phaco needle. Perhaps the greatest advantage of the bimanual technique lies in its ability to remove subincisional cortex without difficulty. By switching infusion and aspiration handpieces between the two microincisions, 360° of the capsular fornices are easily reached and cortical clean-up can be performed quickly and safely (Figs 18.1A and B).

5. *Decreased hydration of cornea:* Using a sleeveless phaco probe also offers the advantage of decreased hydration of the corneal stroma surrounding the tunnel incision. A sleeved probe has two irrigating holes in its side that allow balanced salt solution (BSS) to flow tangentially from the probe and directly hydrate the corneal tunnel incision stroma. The secondary whitening of the stroma can obstruct the view of the surgeon intraoperatively, and postoperatively the patient may complain of peripheral blurring. A sleeveless probe obviously reduces corneal stromal hydration.

6. *Increased efficiency of phacoemulsification:* The small incisions increase the efficiency of phacoemulsification by changing the movement of the currents within the anterior chamber so that the separated irrigation pushes material toward the

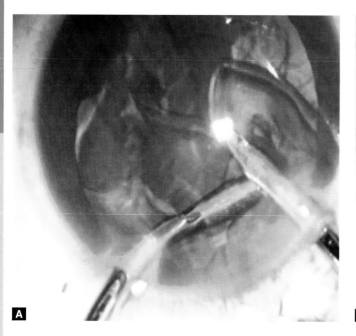
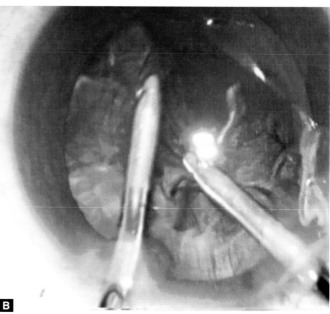

Figs 18.1A and B: Bimanual phacoemulsification

sleeveless phaco tip. The lack of a sleeve also draws material toward the phaco tip. Increasing the effectiveness of phaco reduces the power delivered to the anterior segment, which translates to faster recoveries, less corneal edema, and less endothelial cell loss.

7. *Short and safe learning curve:* We have found the learning curve in making the transition to this technique to be relatively short and safe. The same coaxial technique (either chopping or divide-and-conquer) can be performed bimanually, differing only in the need for an irrigating chopper for chopping methods (Fig. 18.2). If difficulty arises during the procedure, conversion to a coaxial technique is simple and straightforward, accomplished by the placement of a standard clear corneal incision between the two bimanual incisions.

Advantages of Bimanual MICS in Difficult Situations

1. *Zonular weakness or dialysis:* Bimanual MICS offers improved fluidics along with enhanced chamber stability, and it greatly minimizes incisional outflow so that it approaches the ideal scenario of operating in a completely closed system with low inflow/outflow volumes, a situation ideal for subluxated cataract.

2. *More controlled irrigation aspiration system:* Bimanual MICS is fabulous to remove residual cortex from the capsular bag in the presence of an open posterior capsule.

3. *Post-radial keratotomy:* Another approach of bimanual phacoemulsification is the ability to perform easier post-radial keratotomy (RK) incisions by going between radial incisions. By avoiding proximity to RK incisions with the 1.2 mm bimanual incisions, the risk of an RK dehiscence is theoretically lessened.

4. *Floppy iris syndrome:* These cases can also be better controlled because the incision are smaller, so the iris comes to the incision but does not prolapse and because the irrigation is held above the plane of the iris and iris is kept back.

5. *Microcornea or microophthalmus:* Bimanual MICS is a great help in the presence of microcornea or microophthalmus, as smaller instruments in the eye result in less distortion of the cornea and better visualization of intraocular structures.

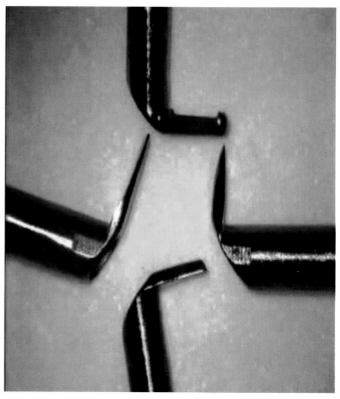

Fig. 18.2: Irrigating choppers

6. *Refractive lens exchange:* This is the procedure of choice for refractive lens exchange. It is considered to be the safest and least invasive technique available.

7. *Recurrent microhyphema:* In the case of recurrent microhyphaema due to iris neovascularization, cauterization is achieved under direct visualization with a microcautery through one of the microincisions and pinching the tubing of the irrigating handpiece through the other.

8. *Reduced risk of retinal detachment:* Bimanual MICS may reduce the risk of retinal detachment. It is especially beneficial in high myopic eyes because the irrigating instrument can be kept in the eye throughout the procedure and never trampoline the vitreous face.

Disadvantages of Bimanual MICS

A standardized technique has not been developed yet for cataract surgeons to use with bimanual phacoemulsification, so the technology requires a certain sense of adventure and creativity. The main disadvantage is that, compared to conventional phacoemulsification, the procedure is less forgiving with respect to incision size (must be exact), fluidics (easier to experience surge), and chopper maneuverability (more cumbersome and one can lose inflow when retracted).

1. *Incision size is critical:* An incision that is too large compromises chamber stability and one that is too tight restricts the movement of the instruments. Wounds must be tight in order to prevent intraoperative leakage.

2. *Capsulorhexis:* The problem involved is performing a capsulorhexis through a 1.0 mm incision. As lot of surgeons stopped doing a full-needle capsulorhexis sometime back and been using forceps since so it is either a question of re-learning how to use the needle or finding some forceps to do the capsulorhexis through a microincision (Fig. 18.3).

3. *Maneuvering through incision:* Maneuvering through 1.2 mm incisions can be awkward early in the learning curve.

Because the instruments move so tightly through the incisions, there are the issues of "oarlock", in which any lateral movement of the instrument tends to move the entire eye and distorts the cornea.

4. *Chopper:* The nondominant hand holds the chopper and carries out most of the work. The increased diameter and weight of the irrigating chopper somewhat limits the mobility and the user must avoid retracting the chopper so far that the irrigation port slides out of the anterior chamber.

5. *Surgeon's natural reflex:* When finishing a case or encountering trouble, the surgeon's natural reflex is to remove the second instrument (hook or chopper), first before removing the sleeved extraction probe. This technique prevents the eye from collapsing, but it must be reversed when using an irrigating chopper.

6. *Fluid flow:* By nature of the size of these incisions, less fluid flows into the eye than occurs with coaxial techniques. It is a low inflow/outflow technique. Most current irrigating choppers integrate a 20-gauge lumen that limits fluid inflow. This can result in significant chamber instability when high vacuum levels are utilized and occlusion from nuclear material at the phaco tip is cleared. Using high vacuum is more difficult and requires a machine that allows changing vacuum memory settings on the fly with the foot pedal.

7. *Needle spray:* There is a considerable amount of spray from the phacoemulsification needle, particularly the hub. Not as in conventional phacoemulsification, where the sleeve covering the needle prevents the spray. Additionally, there are times when the material being emulsified will actually spindle on the sleeveless phaco tip. The tip will puncture right through the fragments, which will then slide down the tip, forcing the surgeon to pull the tip back and immobilize the fragment in order to access it.

8. *Intraocular lens limitations:* The current limitations in IOL technology, perhaps the greatest disappointment are the need to place a relatively large 2.5 mm incision between the two microincisions in order to implant a foldable IOL.

Intraocular Lenses for MICS

Bimanual MICS requires extremely thin, flexible IOLs that can be rolled up small enough to be inserted through a sub 2 mm opening.

Advantages of Ultrathin Lenses

1. They can be inserted through smaller incisions.
2. They are potentially more optically perfect, since optical aberrations increase with lens thickness.

Technical Challenges for Bimanual MICS Lenses

1. These lenses must be soft enough to roll into a small tube, yet sturdy enough to resist decentration or other movement in the eye.
2. They must be thin enough to roll up small while retaining enough refractive power to be useful for a wide range of patients.

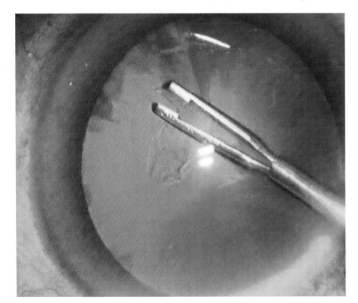

Fig. 18.3: Capsulorhexis in bimanual microphacoemulsification

3. They should offer optical performance and resistance to posterior capsular opacification (PCO) comparable to existing standard lenses.

Acri.Tec Intraocular Lenses

These lenses were founded in 1997 by Dr Christine Kreiner. The rollable Acri.Smart lens was first implanted through a 2.0 mm incision in 2000. Wide range of these lenses are available, including spheric, aspheric, optimized aspheric, bitoric and bifocal versions in powers from 0 to +32 diopters.

The lens is typically implanted through incisions of 1.5 to 1.7 mm depending on the technique. The lens is made of hydrophilic acrylic material with a high refractive index. However, the surface of the lens is a hydrophobic compound to discourage the growth of endothelial cells and calcification.

ThinOptx Rollable Intraocular Lenses

ThinOptx, the company that manufactures these lenses, has patented technology that allows the manufacture of lenses with plus or minus 30 diopters of correction on the thickness of 100 μm (Fig. 18.4). The thickest part of the lens is 350 μm and the Haptic part of the lens is as thin as 50 μm. The lens is made from off-the-shelf hydrophilic material, which is similar to several IOL materials already on the market. The key to the ThinOptx lens is the unique optic design and nano-precision manufacturing. The basic advantage of this lens is that they are ultra-thin lenses. These lenses are called the Ultrachoice 1.0 lenses.

ThinLens Optics

The drawing illustrates the optical characteristics of the ThinOptx lens (Fig. 18.5). The front surface is a curve that approximates a radius. The back curve is a series of steps with concentric rings. The back surface can be concave, convex or plano. The combination of steps with the front radius corrects for spherical aberrations. The convex and plano back designs can be used for positive power lenses. The concave or meniscus back surface is used for negative powered lenses.

The lines intersecting the lens represent parallel light (Fig. 18.6). The light is bent at the intersection of the lens surface in accordance with Snell's law. When light strikes the lens surface, the light is bent toward the central axis. The light travels to the

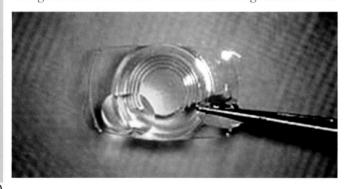

Fig. 18.4: ThinOptx lens

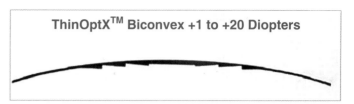

Fig. 18.5: ThinOptx optics

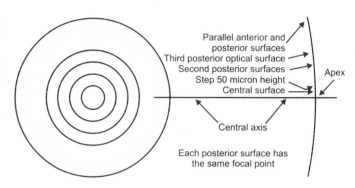

Fig. 18.6: Lines intersecting the ThinOptx lens represent parallel light

back edge of the lens and again is bent toward the central axis. All the parallel light rays entering the back of the lens come to focus at approximately the same point; therefore the lens is a refractive lens.

Tips to Transition to Bimanual MICS

1. Every surgeon with expertise in standard ultrasonic phacoemulsification can easily make the transition to bimanual MICS.

2. For their initial cases, surgeons should choose a posterior subcapsular cataract with a 1+ or 2+ nuclear hardness to build confidence. They can easily convert to their usual technique to prevent any complications.

3. Performing bimanual microincision phaco requires one to rethink the cataract surgery process.

4. An important step in the process of converting to a bimanual procedure is learning to use the irrigation and aspiration instruments for bimanual irrigation and aspiration. Use two 1 mm paracenteses on either side and develop bimanual dexterity.

5. Holding onto a heavier instrument with one's nondominant hand is something that every surgeon should practice before trying bimanual phaco.

6. The viscoelastics used during the procedure need to be managed differently from during a standard procedure, in that there must be fluid egress during hydrodissection to avoid rupturing the posterior capsule, which can easily be done when using high-density cohesive viscoelastics.

7. With the new technology, the surgeon will learn the fluidics, because the bottle height, vacuum and flow must be adjusted with the new bimanual technology.

8. The procedure can be performed with virtually any newer generation phaco machine, and with adequate instruments, by any phaco surgeon over a fast and smooth learning curve.

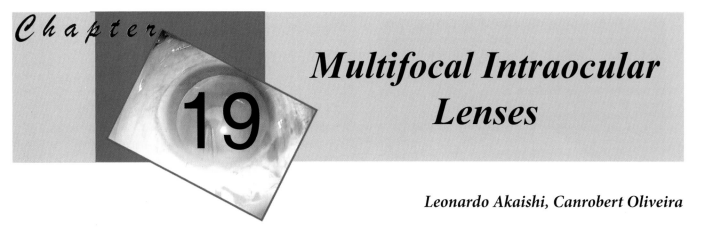

Multifocal Intraocular Lenses

Leonardo Akaishi, Canrobert Oliveira

INTRODUCTION

Multifocal intraocular lenses are developing as the appropriate answer to freedom from spectacles after cataract surgery. One should custom match multifocal intraocular lenses so as to provide the best intraocular lenses for each kind of patient. Sometimes two kinds of different intraocular lenses have to be mixed to find solution to patient's need. In these years, with the multifocal intraocular lens, one has to understand the patients' expectations, because the goal is patient's satisfaction. There is not a perfect intraocular lens yet.

Types of Multifocal Intraocular Lenses

Multifocal intraocular lenses are of two types:
* Refractive type
* Diffractive type.

Refractive Multifocal Intraocular Lens

* ReZOOM lens by AMO, USA (Figs 19.1A to 19.2)
Refractive multifocal intraocular lenses are of various types:
* Two zone
* Three zone
* Five spherical curve.

Diffractive Multifocal Intraocular Lens

* ReSTOR multifocal intraocular lens, Alcon, USA. (Fig. 19.2), and

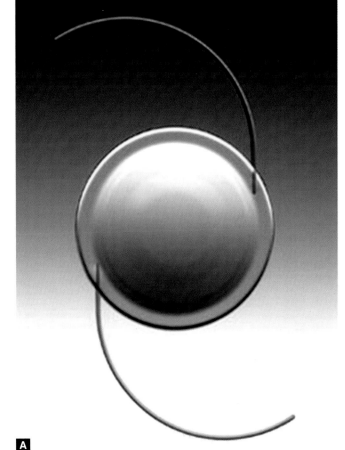

A

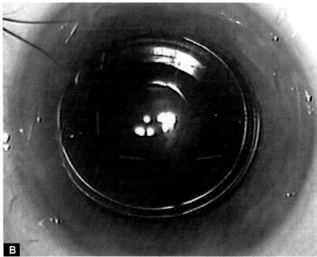

B

Figs 19.1A and B: ReZOOM multifocal intraocular lens

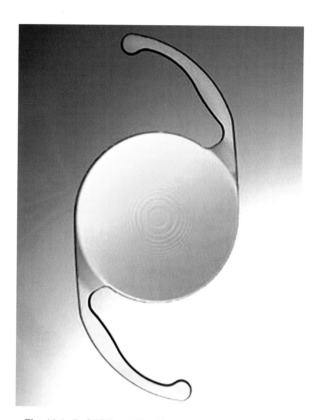

Fig. 19.2: ReSTOR multifocal intraocular lens, Alcon, USA

- Tecnis multifocal intraocular lens, AMO, USA (includes diffractive mutifocal design and modified prolate anterior surface optic).

The diffractive multifocal intraocular lenses consist of refractive and diffractive part. The two parts separate near and distant vision. The central portion of the lens has series of steps that are carved in a very precise arrangement with varying step heights and distances between steps. Each of the steps of this diffractive optic bends the incoming light differently, creating a near focus that is quite separated from the distance focus formed by the remaining refractive portion of the lens. This large separation between the two images allows for less artifacts or distortion in either of the images (Fig. 19.3). The ReSTOR diffractive apodized multifocal intraocular lens has really been a great advancement for multifocal intraocular lenses. Visual acuity with ReSTOR multifocal intraocular lens for distance probably is better than other multifocal intraocular lenses due to the apodization (4.0 mm pupil size, 70% of energy goes for distance vision) and the periphery of the part optic is refractive (work as monofocal intraocular lens). ReSTOR multifocal intraocular lenses, in the last few years have provided very good near and distance vision (Fig. 19.4). However, some patients complain about the lack of intermediate vision, especially among computer users. Some of them complain about the requirement of clearer lighting conditions to read, and some others complain about halos and starbursts at night. The ReSTOR multifocal intraocular lens has addition of +4.00 D for near vision. Some patients with ReSTOR/Silicone piggyback intraocular lenses have an improved intermediate vision,

without increasing photic phenomena. ReSTOR multifocal intraocular lens in capsular bag and a silicone intraocular lens in the sulcus are shown in Figure 19.5.

ReZOOM or Tecnis have better intermediate visual acuity than ReSTOR. ReZOOM has good vision for distance (best MTF-modulation transfer function) and intermediate vision is noticed, but with a deficient reading vision concerning speed and clearness. In Tecnis diffractive aspheric multifocal intraocular lenses, the distance and near vision are very similar to ReSTOR intraocular lenses, with intermediate vision being 85% better than J5. However, still very few patients complain about intermediate vision, especially while using computers.

Numerous patients with a monofocal lens in one eye, and a multifocal ReSTOR or Tecnis multifocal implant in the fellow eye, are all happy and less dependent on spectacles. These patients tolerate that mix (multifocal/monofocal), because

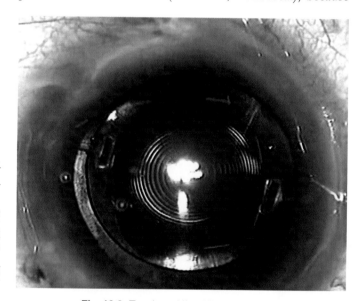

Fig. 19.3: Tecnis multifocal intraocular lens

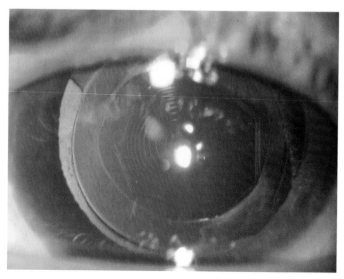

Fig. 19.4: ReSTOR intraocular lens after Nd:YAG capsulotomy, the reflex of cornea should be in the center of central ring. This is how to verify the intraocular lens centralization

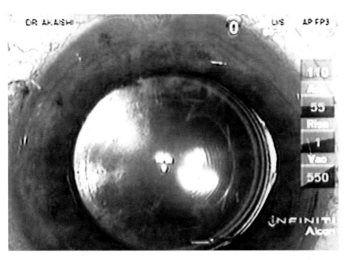

Fig. 19.5: ReSTOR (Alcon) in the bag and Clariflex (AMO) in the sulcus

diffractive apodized lens have a distance visual quality very similar to monofocal, also providing near vision, as well.

Comparison between diffractive and refractive multifocal intraocular lenses is shown in Table 19.1.

Table 19.1: Comparison between diffractive and refractive multifocal IOLs

Diffractive Multifocal IOL	Refractive Multifocal IOL
Excellent reading vision and very good distance vision	Excellent intermediate and distance vision
Fair intermediate vision	Near vision: Fair, but may not be sufficient to see very small print
Less dependant on pupil size	More dependant on pupil size
Patients who do lots of computer work may not accept it well	Patients who read for prolonged periods of time or in poor lighting may experience eye fatigue

Comparison of Multifocal Intraocular Lenses

By the experience with three multifocal lenses, it can be concluded that diffractive lenses are better for near vision. Refractive lenses are better for intermediate vision, and cause more night halos. Both refractive and diffractive intraocular lenses present a good acuity at distance (Table 19.2).

With the introduction of refractive and diffractive and/or apodized multifocal intraocular lenses, pupil diameter role becomes important for presurgical evaluation. This importance is justified not only by the effect determined by corneal aberrations on the optical behavior after refractive and diffractive intraocular lenses implantation (especially asymmetrical aberrations towards axis, such as coma), but also because some

intraocular lenses are pupil-dependent, in addition to the focus depth concerning miosis. Multifocal lenses, notably the diffractive lenses, have shown high sensitiveness to small ametropias and also a restraint on focus depth, compromising vision in medium distances.

Refractive multifocal lenses (ReZOOM) depend on larger pupil diameters for a better near vision (in eyes with smaller pupillary diameters, near vision is significantly compromised).

Diffractive lenses (ReSTOR) provide a better near vision with smaller pupillary diameters and their reading efficiency can be compromised in larger pupil diameters). The diffractive Tecnis intraocular lens is really nondependent of pupil size. If the final refraction is +0.50 D, there is a increasing of vision for intermediate.

Additionally to these observations, we must take into account that the pupil diameter reduced with age and the pupil behavior seen by the time of surgery can change with time.

One of the stimuli for accommodative miosis is the blurring of a retinal image in an attempt to focus those remote points to near vision. Thus, with the ciliary muscle contraction, a pupil sphincter contraction will also occur. It is not known exactly if the absence of the accommodation reflex caused by retinal image sharpness provided by a refractive intraocular lens would significantly change the accommodation reflex, and, therefore, the magnitude of accommodative miosis.

Another point of considerable importance is the sensorial adjustment with diffractive intraocular lens implantation. It is not uncommon that people with a significantly difficult intermediate vision at immediate postoperative period manifest a higher level of satisfaction or a lower degree of restraint as months pass by, which follows neurosensorial plasticity that is seen with the reduction of complaints about night halos.

By realizing the fact that we are not always able to get the same outcomes using the same multifocal intraocular lenses, we have started to implant multifocal intraocular lenses having different diffractive/refractive optics or vice versa. There are some characteristics, which may be taken into consideration, such as occupation, night driving, hobby, computer use, reading and sports.

Multifocal Intraocular Lens Selection and Mixing and Matching of Intraocular Lenses for Spectacle Independence

Mixing and matching different intraocular lenses allows surgeons to combine the advantages of both refractive and diffractive lens technologies. It also offers selected patients a

Table 19.2: Characteristics of multifocal intraocular lenses

	Far vision	Intermediate vision	Near vision	Halos	Pupil size dependent	Light level
ReSTOR	+++++	+	++++	+	++	+++
*ReZOOM	+++++	+++	++	++	+++	−
Tecnis	++++	++	+++++	++	−	−

unique way to gain spectacle independence and fulfill more of their lifestyle expectations.

After 15 days of surgery, the patient is reassessed regarding the presence of desired emmetropia, centered intraocular lens. With no complaints of insufficient near vision one may choose to implant a diffractive lens with the purpose of improving vision to 30 cm. If another patient presents with characteristics for near vision, a diffractive multifocal intraocular lens is implanted, and if, after 15 days, the patient is not happy with his/her vision for using a computer, a refractive multifocal intraocular lens is then implanted in the fellow eye.

Refractive lenses are ideal for light to moderate readers who drive mostly during the day. Patients who play sports, use a computer frequently or enjoy activities, such as playing cards—activities that all rely heavily on intermediate vision—will benefit from refractive lenses.

Diffractive intraocular lenses, such as Alcon's ReSTOR lens and AMO's Tecnis multifocal intraocular lens, offer excellent near and distance vision with good reading speed. They are pupil-independent so patients experience fewer night vision problems. However, a gap in intermediate vision and a loss of transmitted light exists and therefore there is a loss in contrast sensitivity with these lenses. These diffractive lenses are ideal for patients who spend a lot of time reading or doing detailed craft work. Those who like to go to the movies or those who drive often at night are also good candidates for these lenses because they function independently of pupil size.

The combination of the refractive and diffractive multifocal lenses offers a complete refractive solution because it offers a full range of vision in all light conditions. Using intraocular lenses that complement each other, patients achieve a higher rate of spectacle independence. Mixing and matching refractive

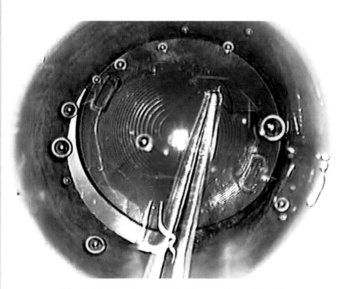

Fig. 19.6: Small capsulorhexis must be enlarged

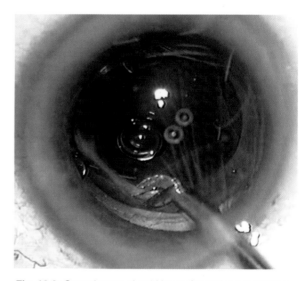

Fig. 19.8: Capsulotomy should be performed to centralize a decentered multifocal intraocular lens

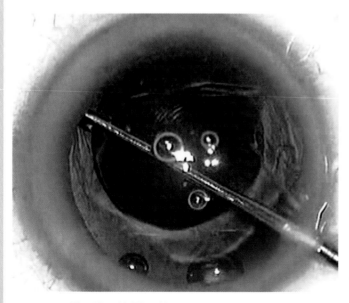

Fig. 19.7: Multifocal intraocular lens should be centered after capsular contraction

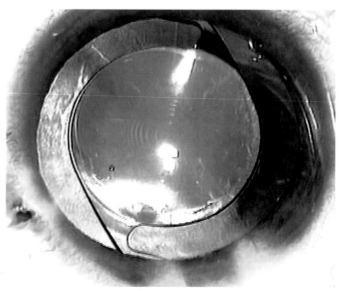

Fig. 19.9: Decentralized light reflex out of the concentric rings of multifocal intraocular lens

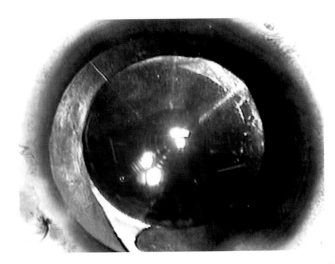

Fig. 19.10: Good centralization of light reflex in the concentric rings of the multifocal intraocular lens

and diffractive intraocular lens styles can offer patients binocular vision that is excellent at all distances, including near, intermediate and far.

Special Considerations

Multifocal intraocular lens should always remain well centered. Small capsulorhexis must be enlarged (Fig. 19.6). Multifocal intraocular lens should be centered after capsular contraction (Fig. 19.7). Capsulotomy should be performed to centralize a decentered multifocal intraocular lens (Fig. 19.8). Figures 19.9 and 19.10 show decentralization and a well centered light reflex in a multifocal intraocular lens.

Patient should be guided to not compare the vision separately, the faster the patients get used with both the eyes, the quicker the patient will adapt. A multifocal intraocular lens should never be explanted before 6 months.

Chapter 20

Small Incision Cataract Surgery

Albrecht Hennig, Vinita Singh

INTRODUCTION

The degree of revolution seen by cataract surgery in the last decade is unparalleled, with the result the cataract surgeon is persistently facing the pressure to keep pace with fast developing technology often driven by commercial forces and community pressure to provide quality care at affordable prices. The high prevalence of cataract blindness is an important factor to be considered in choosing the technique best suited for providing cost-effective quality care to the masses. The estimated global magnitude of visual impairment due to cataract is approximately 50 million, which is increasing annually by addition of new cases. The annual surgical rate is approximately 7 million. This situation calls for surgery of about 20 million by the year 2010, and 30 million by the year 2020 in addition to the surgery for the annual incidence, to clear the cataract backlog. There has to be at least a two-fold increase in the annual surgical rate to effectively deal with the magnitude of cataract blindness by the year 2020. The estimated cataract backlog in India (WHO-NPCB survey report 1990) is approximately 20 million blind eyes (10 million people) with an annual incidence of approximately 3.8 million and annual surgical rate of approximately 1.6 to 1.9 million. The cataract backlog is increasing per year by 1.9 to 2.2 million. The need is to increase, almost double, the annual surgical rate to 3 to 4 million.

The technique of cataract surgery has advanced rapidly in the past 20 years from simple intracapsular extraction, which required hospitalization of about 10 days and use of thick aphakic glasses to extracapsular lens extraction or emulsification and aspiration with implantation of artificial lens, which requires almost no hospitalization.

ADVANCES IN CATARACT SURGERY

The advancements have been possible mainly due to better visualization with the help of modern operating microscopes. These have been three-fold, lens removal technique, incision and intraocular lens (IOL) design, each being interdependent.

Lens Removal Techniques

- Intracapsular cataract extraction (ICCE)
- Extracapsular cataract extraction (ECCE)
- Phacoemulsification and small incision cataract surgery (SICS): The development of operating microscopes has made it possible to dissect within the layers of the lens thereby separating the central nucleus from the surrounding epinucleus and the cortex thus isolating just the small central hard piece that can then be either emulsified and aspirated (phacoemulsification) or removed in one piece through a small incision.

Intraocular Lens Designs

- Anterior chamber intraocular lens (AC IOL)
- Posterior chamber intraocular lens (PC IOL) (6.5 mm, 6.0 mm and 5.5 mm optic)
- Foldable posterior chamber intraocular lens. Folded width approximately 3.5 mm (unfolded optic 6.5 mm, 6.0 mm).
- Rollable intraocular lens requiring an incision size of approximately 2 mm or less.
- Multifocal intraocular lens

Incision Site, Design and Size

Site

- Superior or temporal
- Scleral, limbal or corneal

Design

- Straight or curved: Frown or smile.
- Uniplanar, biplanar or triplanar.

Size

The incision size is largely governed by the technique of nucleus removal and the IOL optic size. The incision size can be smaller in foldable or rollable lenses. Scleral tunnel with self-sealing corneal valve is usually 3.5 mm to 6.5 mm and 7 to 7.5 mm in selected cases. Clear-corneal incision is usually 3 to

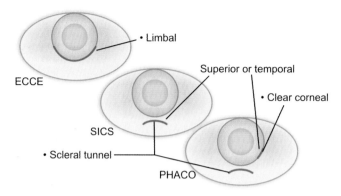

Fig. 20.1: Incisions in modern cataract surgery

3.5 mm. With recent development of Phakonit and rollable IOLs, the surgery can be performed through a sub-2 mm incision (Fig. 20.1).

Thus, we see that the choice for site, size and design of the incision has a lot of variation and depends, apart from the surgeon's choice, on the technique of lens removal and type of IOL to be implanted.

Most of the surgeons perform conventional extracapsular cataract surgery through a limbal incision that needs about 5 sutures. The incision is limbal from 10 to 2 o'clock. This incision is less stable than a frown incision and hence calls for hospitalization and is associated with incision and stitch-related complications.

In developing countries, many centers still perform cataract surgery by the intracapsular technique. This is a comparatively simple method of cataract surgery with no risk of posterior capsular opacification. This remained the method of choice for cataract surgery for several decades prior to the advent of modern cataract surgery. The incision is limbal from 9 to 3 o'clock. This incision is the least stable and hence calls for longer hospitalization and is associated with larger astigmatism and maximum incision and stitch-related complications. This technique leaves the anterior vitreous phase unprotected and is associated with vitreous-related complications.

Some surgeons placed in tertiary care hospitals or high-profile private practices do machine-dependent phacoemulsification. It has its limitations due to cost, dependence on machine and technician and related complications long learning curve and unsuitability for community settings.

Community need and pressure for a large number of cataract surgeries plus pressure for sutureless surgery with early rehabilitation calls for the development of safe, simple and cheap sutureless techniques with short learning curve. This led to the development of sutureless nonphaco-dependent small incision cataract surgery. This is being developed and accepted the world over with the aim of providing quality cataract surgery at affordable costs at a large scale to the community. The lower cost and shorter learning curve is an encouraging factor for the surgeons to adopt this technique. In order of chronology, small incision cataract surgery was developed after phacoemulsification and became popular for reasons discussed above.

THE TECHNIQUE OF SMALL INCISION CATARACT SURGERY

The Incision

Fashioning a good triplanar stable incision, which can be secure without sutures, is the first basic step for performing a sutureless cataract surgery. Starting from a curved frown shaped, 6.5 mm long, partial-thickness incision in the sclera 1.5 to 2 mm away from the limbus at the center, lamellar dissection is done within the layers of the sclera to fashion an inverted funnel-shaped, tunnel ending anteriorly in the cornea 1 mm inside the limbus. The depth of the lamellar dissection is such that the crescent knife is just visible throughout the tissues. The inner corneal lip acts like a self-sealing valve. The ideal dimensions length, width and depth of the sclerocorneal tunnel is 6 to 7 mm (the length of the incision may be 7 to 7.5 mm in large brown nuclei), 3 to 4 mm and 0.2 to 0.3 mm respectively (Figs 20.2 and 20.3).

Problems During Wound Construction

- Too deep groove may require dissection too close to the ciliary body and may be associated with risks like premature entry and cycloasthenia (Fig. 20.3).

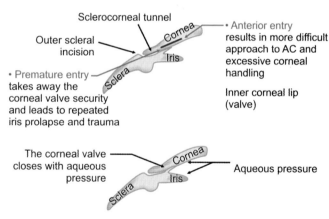

Fig. 20.2: The incision—the lateral view

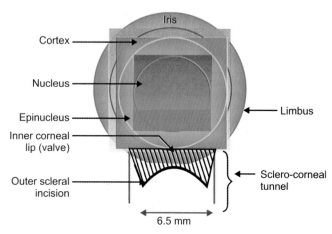

Fig. 20.3: The incision—anteroposterior view

- Too shallow groove may lead to thin scleral flap, buttonholing and insecure wound. The thin flap should be handled carefully and sutured later if necessary.
- Sometimes there may be excessive bleeding. This usually can be taken care of by cautery. Bleeding from the edges of the tunnel may be difficult to touch with the cautery point. This can be dealt with by cold irrigation, gentle pressure and allowing time.
- Premature entry into the anterior chamber before completion of the triplanar tunnel is a complication that makes the rest of the surgery very difficult. It leads to repeated prolapse and trauma to the iris during rest of the procedures and results in an unstable wound. If detected early, change the plane and enter the anterior chamber at another site in the tunnel and complete the rest of the surgery through this entry. If unable to change the plane and site of entry, then complete the surgery through the initial entry while handling the prolapsed iris carefully, suture later or convert to conventional ECCE.
- Anterior entry can be prevented by dipping the keratome while entering the anterior chamber. If detected early, change the plane, otherwise complete the surgery carefully and be prepared for postoperative keratitis.
- It is possible and safe to convert to conventional extracapsular cataract surgery at any stage of incision.

Capsulotomy

- The direction of approach and working inside the anterior chamber is different through a sclerocorneal tunnel as compared to a conventional limbal incision. This feel has to be experienced and learnt.
- Depending upon its size, the nucleus can be delivered through an appropriate anterior capsulotomy.
- Capsulorhexis is performed with a cystitome, fashioned out of a 26-gauge needle. A capsulorhexis forceps is usually helpful in completing the capsulorhexis. A 5 to 6 mm capsulorhexis may allow sufficient space to deliver a small nucleus. Two relaxing incisions at 10 and 2 o'clock are usually enough for delivery of larger nuclei.
- While developing confidence with small incision cataract surgery and in large brown nuclei, it is safer to do a can-opener or an envelop capsulotomy as they permit easier nucleus prolapse and cortical clean-up. The envelope technique ensures better protection to the corneal endothelium.
- Can-opener capsulotomy allows easier clean-up of the 12 o'clock cortex.

The Hydroprocedures

The hydroprocedures are done to separate the cortex from the capsule and the epinucleus from the nucleus so as to facilitate rotation and prolapse of the nucleus and delineate the central hard nucleus for removal through the capsulotomy and small incision. It also helps in cleaning the cortex subsequently. In

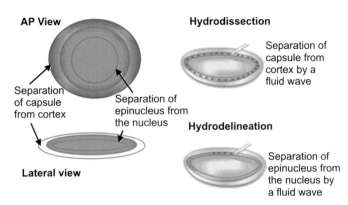

Fig. 20.4: Hydrodissection and hydrodelineation

small incision cataract surgery, the hydroprocedures may be done before or after extending the incision (Fig. 20.4).

Hydrodissection

Using a hydrodissection cannula, 0.2 to 0.3 ml of saline/Ringer's solution is injected slowly under the edge of the anterior capsulotomy and the fluid wave is allowed to sweep all around. It may be done at one or multiple points to separate the capsule from the cortex all around.

Hydrodelineation

Using a sharper cannula, fluid is injected in the deeper planes to dissect between the epinucleus and central hard nucleus. In immature cataracts, this line of cleavage can be observed as a golden ring.

Viscoelastic is injected into the anterior chamber, the nucleus is now free for rotation and delivery.

Nucleus Prolapse

- Using a Sinskey hook, the nucleus is rotated gently while slightly tilting forwards to bring the upper part out of the capsule and in front of the upper iris.
- Viscoelastic is injected both in front and behind the nucleus to protect the cornea and push the iris and capsule back.

Nucleus Delivery

- An irrigating vectis is gently inserted below the nucleus taking care not to engage the iris or the capsule, this is facilitated by prolapsing only the upper edge of the nucleus out of the capsule.
- The nucleus is pulled out, taking care of the corneal endothelium and avoiding excessive pull. The posterior lip of the tunnel is gently pressed backwards while delivering the nucleus. A second instrument may be used if needed to facilitate the nucleus delivery.
- Viscoelastic is injected into the anterior chamber and capsular bag. The bed is now ready for the IOL (Fig. 20.5).

Other Options for Nucleus Delivery

- Hydroexpression or viscoexpression in patients with small nuclei.

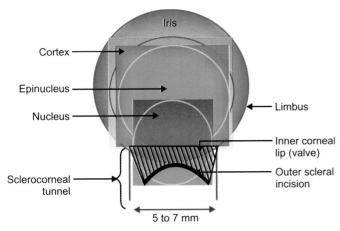

Cortex

Epinucleus

Nucleus

Iris

Limbus

Inner corneal lip (valve)

Outer scleral incision

Sclerocorneal tunnel

5 to 7 mm

Fig. 20.5: Removal of the nucleus

- Fishhook and bimanual sandwich technique can be used.
- Nucleus fracture at tunnel, nucleus bisection or trisection can be used for harder/bigger nuclei or to deliver through smaller incisions.
- All these maneuvers require greater manipulation in the anterior chamber, hence are unsuitable while at the beginning of the learning curve.

Problems in Nucleus Delivery

- In very soft nuclei, it may be difficult to manually rotate it, instead there may be peeling or fragmentation of epinucleus as shreds. This is also called cheese wiring of the nucleus. It is easier to remove the nucleus, in such situations, by gently tumbling it into the anterior chamber and removing it by hydroexpression.
- In large brown or black nuclei, where the cortical support is less, the nucleus may keep rotating half in and half out of the bag. Injection of viscoelastic underneath the superiorly prolapsed nucleus allows space to pass the irrigating vectis below the nucleus so as to bring it out.
- In large nuclei, shaving off the peripheral soft part of the nucleus is easier and often safer than bisection through the more hard central part. Nucleus trisection may thus be easier and cause fewer disturbances in the anterior chamber than bisection.

Delivery of the Epinucleus and Cortex Aspiration

After extraction of the endonucleus, there is a mixture of epinucleus and viscoelastic in the anterior chamber. A good hydrodissection allows the epinucleus to come out as a whole by hydroexpression. This may be facilitated by gently pressing the inferior scleral lip with the Simcoe cannula while irrigating. Pulling the superior rectus bridle suture when it has been applied helps in hydroexpression. In the case of difficulty, viscoelastic may help in the expression of the epinucleus.

The residual cortex is carefully aspirated with the help of Simcoe cannula. The 12 o'clock cortex is difficult to aspirate due to a posteriorly placed tunnel and capsulorhexis. This may

be facilitated by one of these techniques using a J-shaped cannula, dialing IOL in the bag, gently stroking the 12 o'clock iris or aspirating through the side port.

Intraocular Lens Implantation

The IOL optic size would depend upon the size of the tunnel through which the nucleus has been extracted. While implanting the IOL, it is important to fill the anterior chamber and bag with viscoelastic then place the inferior haptic in the bag. The IOL is then rotated clockwise to gently maneuver the remaining optic and the trailing haptic into the bag. The anterior capsulorhexis stretches to allow this and then comes back to its original shape.

The viscoelastic is then cleared from the anterior chamber and the bag. The anterior chamber is reformed with the irrigating solution.

Wound Closure

The primary purpose of a triplanar incision is to provide watertight self-sealing valve (Fig. 20.2) effect with the return of normal intraocular pressure (IOP) postoperatively. However, it is important to check the incision for water tightness by gentle pressure near the limbus on the nasal or temporal side. Usually, no sutures are required; but if one does feel insecure, central, vertical or horizontal sutures may be applied.

PRACTICAL TIPS FOR BEGINNERS

- While converting to small incision cataract surgery: Change gradually step by step.
- Case selection: The following should be preferred while selecting cases for small incision cataract surgery:
  - healthy cornea
  - moderately dense nuclei grade 1 or 2
  - intact zonules
  - avoid sunken eyes
- *Incision:* An anteriorly (0.5 to 1 mm from limbus) placed external incision makes manipulation in the anterior chamber easier. A straight or lesser frown and longer incision up to 7 to 8 mm facilitates delivery of the nucleus and conversion to ECCE, if needed. A single suture may be used to strengthen the incision.
- *Capsulotomy:* While beginning small incision cataract surgery, it is safer to do a can-opener or an envelope capsulotomy as they permit easier nucleus prolapse and cortex clean-up.
- *Hydroprocedures and nucleus handling:* Careful and gentle handling during hydroprocedures, and nucleus handling are essential in order to minimize the risk of injury to posterior capsule, iris and corneal endothelium and finally checking wound closure to minimize wound-related problems. While extracting the nucleus, care must be taken to protect the corneal endothelium. Gentle pressure on the posterior lip helps to minimize the risk of endothelial damage. Excessive pull

to bring out the nucleus may result in prolonged keratitis or corneal decompensation. It must be avoided, in such a situation, it is safer to enlarge the incision. Viscoexpression may be useful when difficulty is encountered in hydroexpression.

THE FUTURE

Success in the struggle for more sophistication in manual fragmentation techniques may allow smaller incisions, clear-corneal incisions and foldable IOLs in a larger number of patients.

Advantages of Small Incision Cataract Surgery

Though phacoemulsification is a more sophisticated method of cataract surgery, its application to meet the community need is limited by cost, longer learning curve and dependence on machine and trained personnel. In view of the community need, small incision cataract surgery was developed and promoted later in order of chronology. In certain respects, it has been found to be advantageous over extracapsular cataract surgery as well as phacoemulsification.

Advantages of Small Incision Cataract Surgery over Extracapsular Cataract Surgery

- Better wound stability
- Lesser astigmatism
- Greater patient comfort (no suture-related irritation)
- Early visual rehabilitation
- Better per operative anterior chamber stability
- Lesser complications
- Lesser postoperative visits
- Saving on suture time
- Saving on suture cost

Advantages of Small Incision Cataract Surgery over Phacoemulsification

- Shorter learning curve
- Lower initial and maintenance cost
- Lower dependence on machine, power and technician
- Applicable to all grades of nuclei
- Lesser time taking
- Lesser trauma to cornea
- Lesser chances of nucleus drop
- Equal visual reward
- Applicable in community settings

Besides, small incision cataract surgery offers a good experience for beginning and converting to phacoemulsification, as almost all the steps including plane of the incision are similar to phacoemulsification.

Advantages of Phacoemulsification

- Smaller clear-corneal incision with foldable IOL is possible with phacoemulsification. Though small incision cataract surgery is being performed through smaller scleral tunnels

with foldable IOLs, small incision cataract surgery surgeons are still struggling to offer the advantage of a postoperative white eye as seen with clear-corneal incision.
- In experienced hands causes minimal iris and sphincter trauma.
- Perhaps more feasible under topical anesthesia.

Disadvantages of Phacoemulsification

- The equipment is costly and incurs extra initial and recurring maintenance cost.

  It requires additional trained technician and hence additional expenditure on personnel.
- Longer learning curve.
- Higher incidence of complications like endothelial damage, burns and nucleus drop.
- Conversion to extracapsular cataract is difficult after the nucleus has been divided.
- Not suitable for all kinds of nuclei
- Not suitable for community settings where high volume surgery is a necessity.
- Incurs the entire above extra trouble and cost for no additional visual reward in the long term.

  The increasing cost of surgery due to the use of costly equipment supported by commercial forces is not easily affordable by most patients and many surgeons. This is contrary to the community need for quality care at low cost to deal with the magnitude of blindness due to cataract. Small incision cataract surgery provides quality care with the advantages of sutureless stable incision and shorter learning curve at affordable cost. It, therefore, appears to be the answer for community need and the cataract backlog.

SMALL INCISION CATARACT SURGERY: THE FISHHOOK TECHNIQUE

During the last decade, in industrialized countries phacoemulsification has largely replaced ab-externo ECCE with posterior chamber IOLs with sutures. The small self-sealing phaco incision provides rapid visual rehabilitation, and the surgery is increasingly done on an outpatient basis. However, in the developing countries, phacoemulsification is performed only on selected patients, usually those able to pay high treatment charges. This is mainly due to the cost of a phaco machine and consumables, such as foldable IOLs. Until now, phacoemulsification has played a very limited role in the reduction of cataract blindness in low-income countries. Therefore, eye surgeons in developing countries are searching for alternatives to phacoemulsification. Other small incision cataract surgical techniques are needed, which are easy to learn, provide an immediate good uncorrected visual outcome, and are affordable to most cataract patients. Such techniques would advance cataract surgery in low-income countries and contribute to reaching the goal of VISION 2020: The Right to Sight.

Small Incision Cataract Surgical Techniques

Already during the early 1980s, surgeons in the USA introduced a self-sealing tunnel incision and developed instruments and techniques to cut the nucleus into parts, for easy removal through a self-sealing sclerocorneal tunnel. These techniques are now partly revitalized in the developing countries.

There are different names given to techniques, where the whole nucleus, or the nucleus divided in parts, is removed through a self-sealing tunnel requiring no sutures, e.g. small incision cataract surgery, manual small incision cataract surgery, manual phaco and sutureless extracapsular cataract extraction with posterior chamber intraocular lens.

There are various ways how the nucleus can be removed through the tunnel. In most techniques, the nucleus first needs to be brought into the anterior chamber.

Cutting the nucleus into pieces before delivery requires additional instruments and careful manipulation within the anterior chamber. Instruments used are bisector, trisector, wire loop and others.

A more easy and straightforward approach is the removal of the whole nucleus either through hydroexpression with the help of an anterior chamber maintainer, or a Simcoe cannula, or an irrigation cannula or with a combination of irrigation/extraction using an irrigating vectis.

The Fishhook Technique

A different technique, the "Fishhook" extraction, was developed at Lahan Eye Hospital in Nepal in 1997; where, since then, it has become the routine cataract surgical procedure. Till February 2004, nearly 200,000 sutureless cataract surgeries have been performed in Lahan by this technique and many more in other eye centers around the world (Fig. 20.6).

Tunnel Construction

The tunnel can be done at 12 o'clock or temporal, ideally at the steepest corneal meridian to keep the postoperative astigmatism at a minimum.

The size of the tunnel depends on the age of the patient and the anticipated size of the nucleus. Very big brown nuclei in older patients (Fig. 20.7) may require an opening of 8 mm, whereas cataracts in younger patients need incisions only as large as the IOL.

The tunnel construction can be made with either conventional tunnel instruments (razor blade fragment, crescent knife, keratome) or with a diamond knife (Figs 20.8 to 20.14).

A good sclera holding forceps (Fig. 20.9) helps to perform the following three steps:

Frown incision: A "frown" shaped scleral incision goes halfway into the sclera. At its closest point, it should be 2 mm from the limbus (Figs 20.10 and 20.11).

Sclerocorneal tunnel: The sclerocorneal tunnel should be done in half scleral thickness and needs to end at least 1 mm into the clear cornea to ensure a self-sealing effect and no iris prolapse during surgery (Figs 20.12 and 20.13).

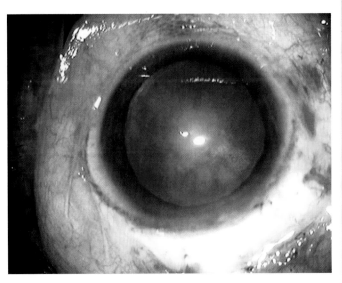

Fig. 20.7: Large brown cataract after fornix-based conjunctiva flap and scleral cauterization

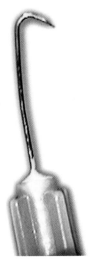

Fig. 20.6: "Fishhook" made from a 30-G ½ inch needle

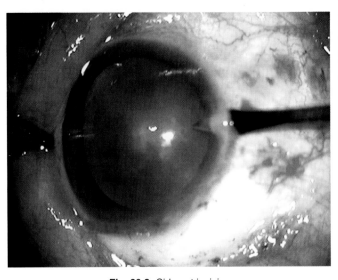

Fig. 20.8: Sideport incision

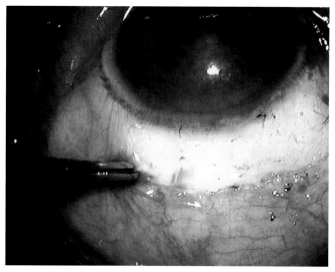

Fig. 20.9: Scleral fixation with forceps

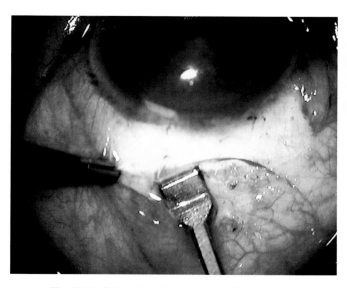

Fig. 20.12: Scleral tunnel preparation with penetration into the clear cornea—beginning

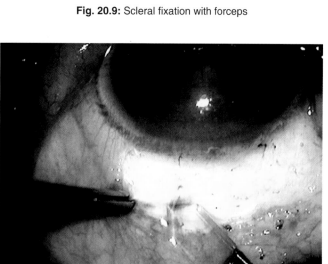

Fig. 20.10: Frown incision—beginning

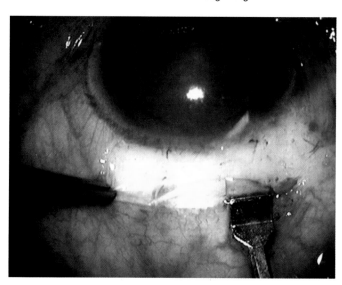

Fig. 20.13: Scleral tunnel preparation with penetration into the clear cornea—completed

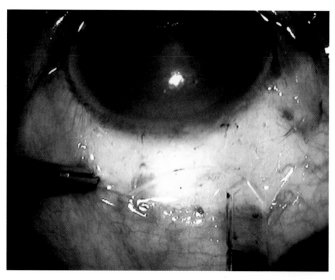

Fig. 20.11: Frown incision—completed

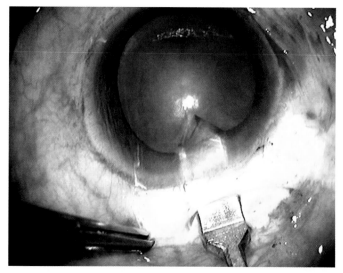

Fig. 20.14: Opening of the anterior chamber

Opening of the anterior chamber: The opening of the anterior chamber is performed with a sharp pointed instrument (keratome or diamond knife) with cutting movements from outside to inside (Fig. 20.14).

Capsulotomy

A linear capsulotomy can be performed with a cystitome, a keratome or a diamond knife.

Preferred, but more difficult is a continuous curvilinear capsulorhexis, which guarantees the best possible IOL centration. It needs to be large enough for the nucleus to get through.

In case of mature white cataracts, it is very helpful to stain the anterior capsule with "Trypan Blue". First, air is injected into the anterior chamber through a sideport incision (Figs 20.8 and 20.15) before the anterior capsule is stained with "Trypan Blue" (Figs 20.16 and 20.17). Then the air is replaced with viscoelastic solution, like methylcellulose (Fig. 20.18) and the continuous curvilinear capsulorhexis performed with Utrata forceps (Figs 20.19 to 20.25) or a cystotome.

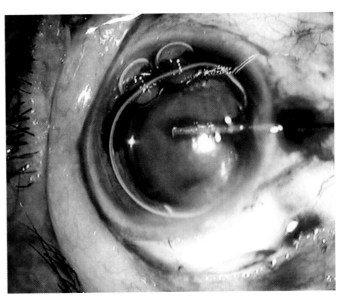

Fig. 20.17: Capsule staining with "Trypan Blue"—completed

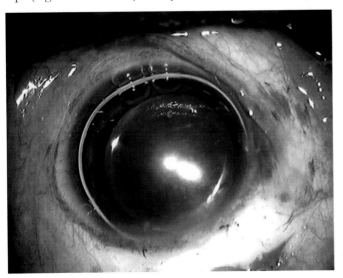

Fig. 20.15: Injected air in the anterior chamber

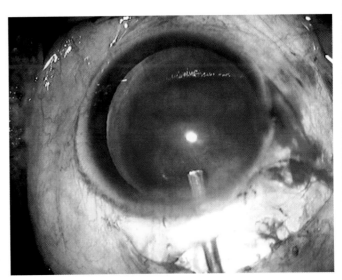

Fig. 20.18: Replacing the air with viscoelastics

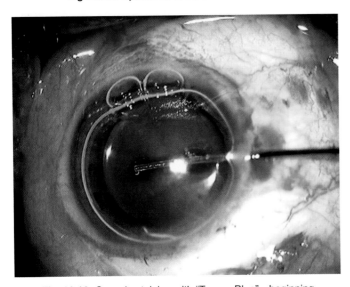

Fig. 20.16: Capsule staining with "Trypan Blue"—beginning

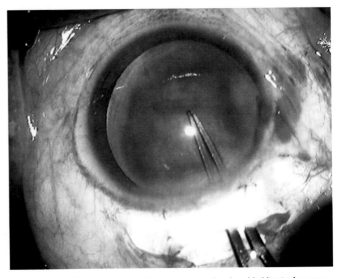

Fig. 20.19: Continuous curvilinear capsulorhexis with Utrata forceps

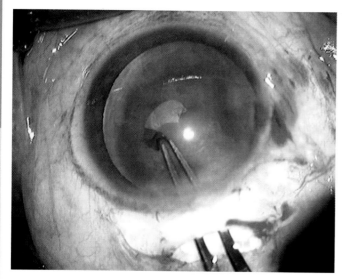

Fig. 20.20: Continuous curvilinear capsulorhexis—continued

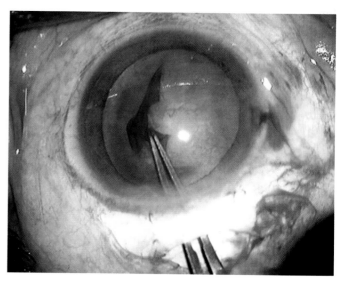

Fig. 20.23: Continuous curvilinear capsulorhexis—continued

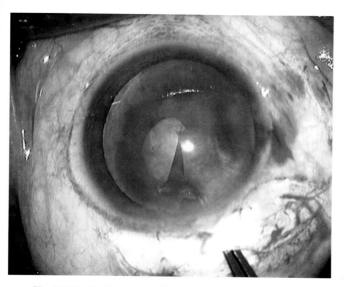

Fig. 20.21: Continuous curvilinear capsulorhexis—continued

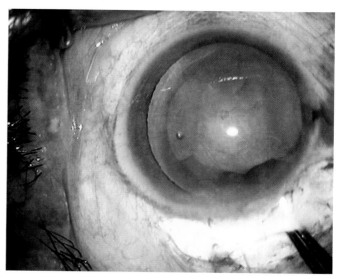

Fig. 20.24: Continuous curvilinear capsulorhexis—continued

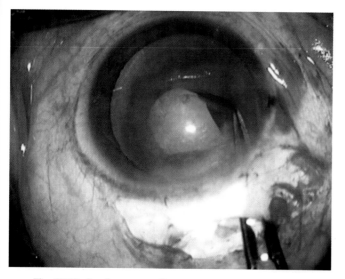

Fig. 20.22: Continuous curvilinear capsulorhexis—continued

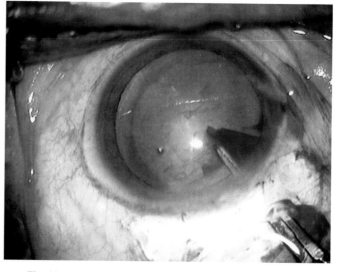

Fig. 20.25: Continuous curvilinear capsulorhexis—completed

Hydrodissection and Nucleus Extraction

In case of a linear capsulotomy, a forceful hydrodissection is done to mobilize the nucleus. Then the nucleus is slightly lifted at the side of the tunnel.

In case of continuous curvilinear capsulorhexis, a gentle hydrodissection is performed beneath the remaining anterior capsule (Fig. 20.26). The fluid pressure pushes a part of the nucleus out of the capsular bag (Fig. 20.27). Then the elevated nucleus is rotated towards the tunnel (Figs 20.28 and 20.29). After the injection of viscoelastics in front and behind the nucleus (Fig. 20.30), the fishhook is carefully inserted between nucleus and posterior capsule and the tip turned so that it inserts into the central lower nucleus. Without lifting the nucleus into the anterior chamber, it is just extracted out of the capsular bag and the tunnel (Figs 20.31 to 20.36).

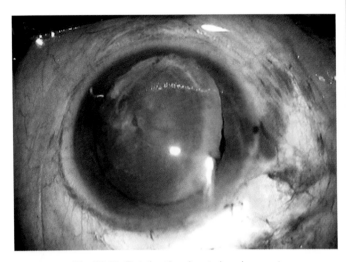

Fig. 20.28: Rotating the elevated nucleus part towards tunnel—beginning

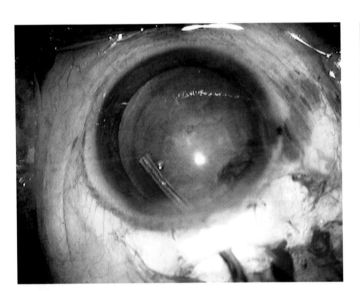

Fig. 20.26: Gentle hydrodissection beneath the remaining anterior capsule

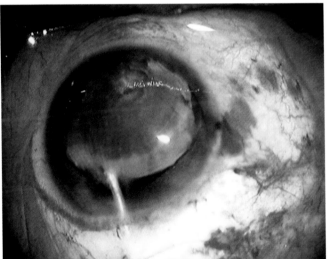

Fig. 20.29: Rotating the elevated nucleus part towards tunnel—completed

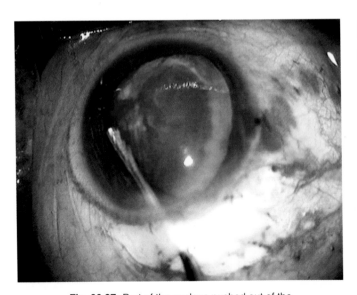

Fig. 20.27: Part of the nucleus pushed out of the capsular bag by fluid pressure

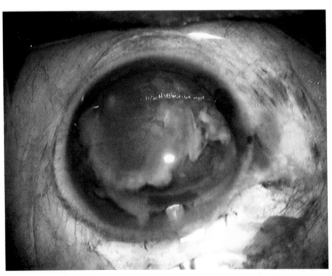

Fig. 20.30: Injection of viscoelastics between nucleus and posterior capsule and into the anterior chamber

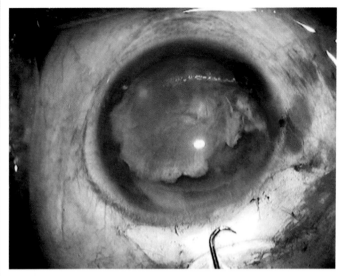

Fig. 20.31: The Fishhook before insertion

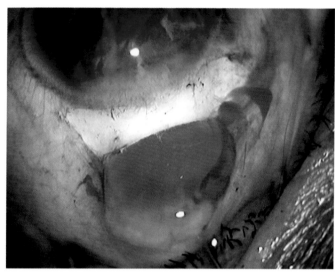

Fig. 20.34: The Fishhook extracting the nucleus—continued

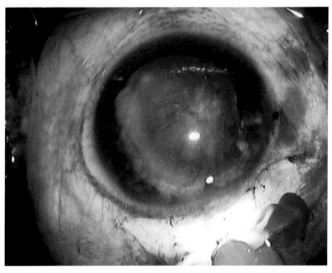

Fig. 20.32: The Fishhook inserted between nucleus and posterior capsule

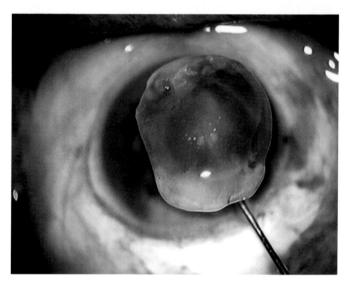

Fig. 20.35: Extracted nucleus

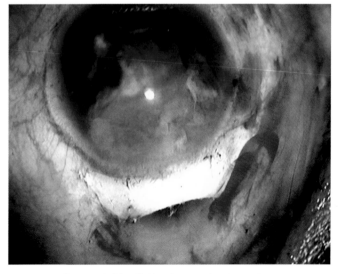

Fig. 20.33: The Fishhook extracting the nucleus

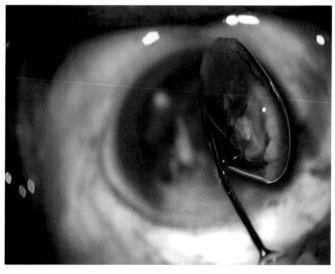

Fig. 20.36: Extracted nucleus, side view

Completing the Surgery

Remaining cortex is removed by hydroexpression and with the help of a Simcoe cannula (Figs 20.37 to 20.39). Figure 20.40 shows the clean capsular bag with a remaining posterior capsular plaque, which is commonly seen in advanced cataracts. A polymethylmethacrylate (PMMA) posterior chamber IOL is inserted into the capsular bag (Fig. 20.41).

Outcome

In the hands of experienced surgeons, sutureless cataract surgery with nucleus hook extraction has a very low complication rate and provides excellent immediate uncorrected postoperative visual acuity. This is underlined by another outcome study on

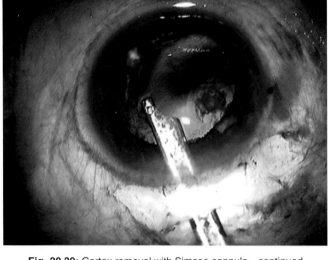

Fig. 20.39: Cortex removal with Simcoe cannula—continued

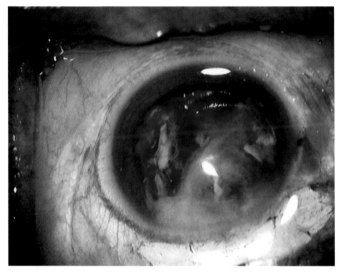

Fig. 20.37: Remaining cortex in anterior chamber before hydroexpression

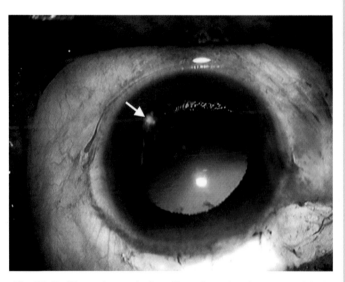

Fig. 20.40: Cleaned capsular bag. Note: Capsular plaque at 5 o'clock

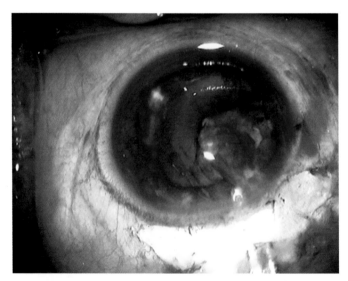

Fig. 20.38: Cortex removal with Simcoe cannula—beginning

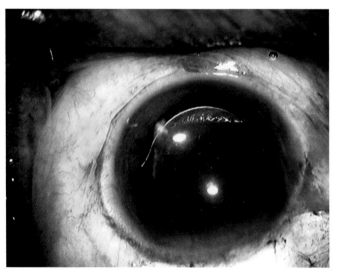

Fig. 20.41: Polymethylmethacrylate intraocular lens inserted in the capsular bag

high-volume surgery, where six surgeons performed 2,111 sutureless cataract surgeries within six days.

Transition from Sutured to Sutureless Cataract Surgery

There is no doubt that sutureless cataract surgery is more difficult to learn than ab-externo sutured extracapsular cataract surgery with posterior chamber IOL surgery. A self-sealing wound with minimum induced astigmatism requires a very accurate tunnel construction as well as good surgical skills and experience to work inside the eye through a narrow tunnel. Many surgeons are keen to convert from sutured to sutureless cataract surgery. It is best to wait until they feel entirely confident and have consistently good results with conventional cataract surgery with posterior chamber IOL surgery. Self-evaluation of the postoperative uncorrected visual acuity and surgical and postoperative complications is a reliable indicator.

Stepwise Approach

While converting from sutured to sutureless cataract surgery, a stepwise approach is an important key to success. The surgeon should:

- First practice hydrodissection, nucleus mobilization and nucleus hook extraction during conventional ab-externo extracapsular cataract surgery with posterior chamber IOL surgery.
- Select immature cataracts to start with so that the tip of the hook can be seen while inserting it into the nucleus.
- Start with a larger tunnel and smaller nuclei

Sutureless cataract surgery provides a rapid visual recovery. Other major advantages are a stable watertight wound without any suture-related problems. All types and sizes of nuclei can be removed through a self-sealing tunnel. The surgical time is short and the cost for consumables reduced. In addition, it has proved to be suitable for high-volume surgery. Thus, sutureless nonphaco cataract surgery will attract many patients and can play an important role in the reduction of worldwide cataract blindness.

Pediatric Cataract Surgery and Intraocular Lens Implantation

Jagat Ram, Gagandeep S Brar

INTRODUCTION

There are 1.5 million blind children (corrected visual acuity <20/400 in the better eye) in the world and one million of these live in Asia. Several studies report on blindness data in the pediatric population. The prevalence of blindness ranges from 1 to 4/10,000 children in industrialized countries to 5 to 15/10,000 children in the developing world. Whereas hereditary diseases, congenital cataract and retinopathy of prematurity (ROP) predominate in the industrialized world, causes of blindness and visual impairment are different in the developing countries. However, blindness due to ROP is now increasing in incidence even in developing countries due to survival of low birth weight babies as a result of intensive neonatal care. In countries with the very low incomes, malnutrition, particularly Vitamin A deficiency and infections, are responsible for half of all cases. In countries with intermediate incomes, cataract and glaucoma are important causes of blindness.

It is estimated that childhood blindness is responsible for 75 million blind years (number of blind x length of life).

Childhood Cataract

The prevalence of childhood cataract has been reported as 1 to 15 cases in 10,000 children. The prevalence of bilateral cataract in the industrialized world is estimated to be 1 to 3 cases in 10,000 births and this figure will undoubtedly be higher for developing countries because of various etiological factors, such as rubella infection. Assuming a birth rate of 2% (i.e. 20,000 per million population), approximately 4 children in a million of the total population of a country in a year will be born with bilateral cataract in the industrialized world. This estimate is much higher for the developing countries and most likely to be about 10 cases per million total population per year. It is estimated that globally, there are 200,000 children blind from bilateral cataract. The prevalence of cataract blindness amongst children in developing countries is probably 1 to 4 per 10,000 and approximately 0.1 to 0.4 per 10,000 children in the industrialized countries.

Etiology of Childhood Cataract

The main causes of infantile cataract are genetic, metabolic disorders, prematurity, intrauterine infections and others, i.e. cornea guttata. Other causes of childhood cataract in older children include trauma, drug-induced cataract, radiation therapy and laser therapy for ROP. Trauma is one of the commonest causes of unilateral cataract in the developing countries. Bilateral cataracts occur commonly due to the long-term use of topical or systemic steroid therapy. In industrialized countries, in approximately 50% of bilateral cases and virtually all of the unilateral cases, the underlying cause usually cannot be determined. Approximately 20% cases have a positive family history of isolated cataract with autosomal dominant disease being more commonly diagnosed than X-linked or autosomal recessive disease and the underlying cause of the remaining 30% is chromosomal abnormalities, systemic abnormalities, metabolic disorders, intrauterine infections, prematurity, or in association with other abnormalities. In a large series, 46% of congenital cataracts were found to be idiopathic.

Morphology

The morphologic types of childhood cataracts are broadly divided into following types:

a. *Zonular cataract* is the most common type of cataract. This is further divided into nuclear, lamellar, sutural or capsular.
b. *Polar cataracts* occur in the anterior or posterior polar region. The posterior lentiglobus is also a type of posterior polar cataract.
c. *Total or diffuse cataracts* are usually bilateral. The diffuse cataract may also start as partial cataract (Fig. 21.1).
d. *Membranous cataract* usually associated with congenital anomalies, such as microphthalmos, congenital rubella syndrome, Lowe syndrome and Hallermann-Streiff-Francois syndrome.
e. *Primary hyperplastic* persistent vitreous is usually a unilateral condition. It is associated with micro-ophthalmic eyes. Initially the lens may be clear, but opacifies slowly.

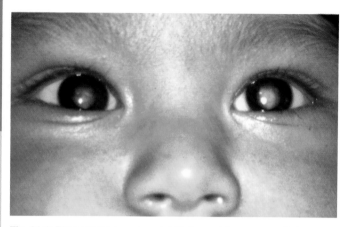

Fig. 21.1: Bilateral diffuse cataract: This type of dense congenital cataract is most often associated with deprivation amblyopia if surgical treatment is delayed

Ocular Examination

A thorough ocular and systemic examination is must in every child. Ocular examination should include visual acuity assessment, pupillary response and ocular motility. Biomicroscopic examination should be carried out in each case to evaluate the size, density and location of cataract to plan the surgical procedure. Fundus examination should be carried out after pupillary dilatation. A-scan helps to measure the axial length for calculating IOL power and monitoring the globe elongation postoperatively. A history from the parents is useful to understand whether the cataract is congenital, developmental or traumatic in origin. One must ascertain if there is any history of maternal drug use, infection or exposure during pregnancy. A pediatrician for thorough systemic work should examine each child up to rule out systemic associations, anomalies or congenital rubella. This is also essential as surgery in children is performed under general anesthesia.

Laboratory Work-up

The work-up includes fasting blood sugar, urine for reducing substance for galactosemia after milk feeding and urine amino acids for Lowe's syndrome. Plasma phosphorus, red blood cells transferase, galactokinase levels and calcium evaluation for hypothyroidism should be done. The titers for toxoplasma, rubella, cytomegalovirus and herpes simplex (TORCH titers) to rule out these disorders should be carried out. Genetic testing should be carried out for children with congenital cataract.

Cataract Surgery in Children

The timing of the surgery is most important. Visually significant cataracts not only produce a blurred image on the retina, but also affect the development of visual pathways. In the 1970s, it was customary to defer infantile cataract surgery until at least 6 months of age. In sharp contrast, presently more and more surgeons recommend that visually significant cataract should be removed at the earliest possible time as sensory deprivation due

to cataract in the first few months of life is critical. Unilateral cataract should be operated within first few months of life to prevent the development of deprivation amblyopia.

Most surgeons prefer to perform the surgery for visually significant cataract before 6 months of age. With modern cataract surgical techniques; we feel it is better to perform surgery for significant cataract as early as is safely possible to prevent amblyopia.

Options in the Management of Pediatric Aphakia

The rehabilitation of pediatric aphakia is must to prevent further amblyopia and changes in the visual pathways. The options in the management of pediatric aphakia include aphakic glasses, contact lenses, epikeratophakia and intraocular lens implantation.

Aphakic Glasses, Contact Lenses and Epikeratophakia

In the past optical correction of pediatric aphakia has been extremely challenging to the ophthalmologists. Aphakic glasses are unsatisfactory for rehabilitation because of several problems associated with their use, such as induced magnification, visual field restriction and prismatic effect beside poor compliance. Moreover use of aphakic spectacles for unilateral aphakia is impractical. Major goal of visual rehabilitation is to bypass the use of spectacles and strive for a much more practical regimen, the intraocular lens (IOL).

Several pediatric ophthalmologists have used contact lenses for rehabilitation. Although contact lenses offer several advantages over aphakic spectacles, such as full visual field and stereopsis, there are several problems associated with their use, such as the risk of infection, loss of the contact lens, higher cost and difficulty with compliance. Repeated insertion and removal of a contact lens may also be psychologically traumatic to the child.

Epikeratophakia for surgical rehabilitation of pediatric aphakia has been used by a few authors. The vagaries of the wound healing, including epithelial healing problems and interface scarring as well as nonavailability of lenticules and high cost for the procedure have led to the near abandonment of this procedure.

Intraocular Lens Implantation in Children

Presently, highly refined and perfected microsurgical techniques that have made lens implantation one of the most successful surgical techniques in history are now providing highly favorable results in the field of pediatric cataract surgery. There is a clear swing towards the implantation of IOLs over contact lenses for the management of cataracts among children. Early attempts at IOL implantation in the 50s and 60s failed, not because of the inherent problems with pediatric cataract, but largely because the techniques and lenses available at the time were still rudimentary and also not yet satisfactory for general adult IOL implantation.

Why is there an Increase in the Use of IOLs in Pediatric Cataract Surgery?

The main reason for the acceptance of IOL implantation for children is the refinement of microsurgical technique. The continuous, curvilinear capsulorhexis (CCC) provides an intact capsular bag for the safe fixation of capsular IOLs. Now, all polymethylmethacrylate (PMMA) capsular IOLs are available with the optic size of 5 to 6 mm, over all diameter of 11.5 to 12 mm, which is suitable for pediatric cataract surgery.

The number of surgeons using IOLs in children markedly increased between 1990–present. A survey conducted in 1994, among the ASCRS members, showed that 46% of the 234 pediatric ophthalmologists and 27% of the adult cataract surgeons were implanting the IOLs in children. At present, the number of surgeons using IOL in pediatric cataract surgery might have increased many folds. The relative contraindications for IOL implantation in children are microphthalmia, recurrent uveitis, aniridia, glaucoma and inadequate capsular support. However, a few reports have shown encouraging results of intraocular lens implantation in microphthalmic eyes.

Capsule management for anterior and posterior capsule have markedly improved the visual results. The anterior continuous curvilinear capsulorhexis ensures safe, bag-bag fixation of IOL and helps to provide centration.

Posterior capsulotomy with anterior vitrectomy or posterior CCC with optic capture has revolutionized pediatric cataract surgery by providing clear visual axis.

Despite major advances in the field of microsurgical techniques and available modern foldable IOLs designs, children less than two years have not fully benefited from these refinements.

How Does Pediatric Cataract Surgery Differ from Adult?

The specific characteristics of the pediatric eye especially in children less than two years of age are:
- *Intraoperative:* Scleral collapse, high intraoperative pressure, elasticity of capsule for CCC, miosis, fibrin release, etc.
- *Postoperative:* Uveitis, posterior capsular opacification (PCO), secondary membrane formation and amblyopia.
- *Long-term:* Growth of the eye and induced myopia.

A factor of important concern after the birth is the changing axial length of the globe. The eye of an adult is 40% to 50% larger than that of a child. The mean axial length of a newborn's eye is 17.0 mm compared to 23 to 24 mm in adult. The mean diameter of the crystalline lens is 6.0 mm at birth and 9.3 mm at 16 years. There is also change in the size of the capsular bag from 7 mm at birth to 9.0 mm at two years. Another major problem is IOL power calculation particularly for infantile cataract. Most of the authors suggest under correction to prevent myopic shift. In the growing eyes of monkeys and rabbits, lensectomy decreases the ocular growth as measured by axial length. In children less than 14 months of age with unilateral cataracts, the cataractous eye is shorter than the non-cataractous eye. In older children, (3 to 10 years) having lensectomy and IOL accelerate the growth of the eye.

Use of currently available adult size rigid IOLs, particularly in small eyes in the first two years of life is associated with the problems of oversizing. The need for downsizing of intraocular lens implants for infants to an overall diameter of 10 to 11 mm has been recognized. However, at present, all PMMA IOL designs with 5 to 6.0 mm with overall diameter of 11.5 to 12 mm are available for capsular placement in these young children. The incidence of postoperative complications, such as uveitis, secondary glaucoma and posterior capsular opacification are also much higher in the pediatric age groups.

SURGICAL PROCEDURE

The aim of the operation is to provide a long-term clear visual axis, to rehabilitate the aphakia with a compliant therapy and to prevent long-term complication, such as the development of induced myopia and amblyopia.

IOL Power Calculation

Intraocular lens power calculation for the growing pediatric eye poses several problems. Most reports have recommended the undercorrection of the IOL power for pediatric cataract, anticipating the myopic shift following IOL implantation. Several authors have reported myopic shift in the aphakic and pseudophakic pediatric eyes.

The axial length and keratometry readings should be measured for IOL power calculation in children. Four IOL formulas (1 regression formula SRK II) and 3 theoretical formulas (SRK-T, Holladay and Hoffer Q) have been suggested to predict mean refractive outcome within 1.4 D for pediatric IOL implantation. A very practical approach for younger children has been suggested. The IOL power calculations may be performed using axial length in children under one year of age and keratometry readings are not as crucial since these readings change rapidly from 52.00 ±4.00 D to 42.00±4.0 D in the first 6 months of life. The K-readings in the newborn are ignored and replaced by the average adult K-reading that is 44.00 D. Aiming for undercorrection in children between 2 to 8 years by performing biometry and undercorrecting by 10% has been suggested. For children younger than 2 years, perform biometry and undercorrect by 20% or use the axial length only. The IOL power suggested for 21 mm is (22.00 D), 20 mm (24.00 D), 19 mm (26.00 D), 18 mm (27.00 D) and for 17 mm axial length is 28.00 D. It has also been suggested to implant 21.0 D of adult IOLs in all pediatric cases. This may be acceptable for most of the children over 2 years, but will not be suitable for eyes with microphthalmos and infantile cataract.

IOL Selection

Currently available IOLs include the classic PMMA design, which is virtually the material used by Ridley in 1949 and modern foldable designs.

All-PMMA, single piece IOLs for capsular bag has an overall diameter of 11 to 12 mm with an optic size 5.5 to 6.0 mm and anterior haptic angulation 5° to 10°. Although these are "adult" sized IOLs, recent anatomic studies have shown that they are compatible for pediatric implantation.

Another IOL material now widely used for children is acrylic foldable, the design most readily approved in the USA being the Alcon AcrySof IOLs. The main advantage of the foldable designs is, of course, the ability to insert it through a small incision. This lens is also efficacious in lowering the incidence of posterior capsular opacification (PCO) (Fig. 21.2).

Most of the authors have used adult size lenses in children because of availability. Many complications are associated with the use of standard adult IOL having overall diameter of 12.5 to 13.5 mm. The small incision foldable designs acrylic-PMMA material may prove to be of choice in the near future.

Current Surgical Techniques

The aim of the surgical technique is to provide a long-term clear axis by preventing development of PCO or secondary membrane. The rehabilitation of aphakia should be performed with modalities having full-term compliance. Most of the pediatric cataract can be aspirated using two-way irrigation-aspiration (IA) cannula or automated IA; however membranous or calcified cataract may need phacoemulsification. The best current techniques for pediatric implantation are basically those perfected over the years for adult surgery, but modified to meet the specific characteristic of the infantile eye.

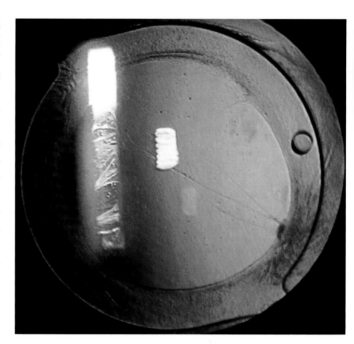

Fig. 21.3: Close up of right eye in a child aged 5 years. Capsular bag fixation of all PMMA IOL with a clear visual axis

Primary intraocular lens implantation should now be the target in every case. Intraocular lenses have the advantages of providing full term correction of an aphakic eye. A number of surgical techniques have been used to implant IOLs as a primary procedure in pediatric cataract. Capsular bag fixation of IOL is preferred to optimize centration and to reduce contact with the uveal tissue (Fig. 21.3). Continuous curvilinear capsulorhexis (CCC) technique introduced by Gimbel and Neuhann is used for pediatric cataract surgery. Now various techniques and models of CCC are available for pediatric cataract surgery. While the CCC works well in adults and older children, it is difficult to perform particularly in infants due to the elasticity of capsule and formation of radial capsular tear. The use of viscoelastic agents, such as sodium hyaluronate (Healon or Healon-GV) greatly facilitates the controlled capsulorhexis.

The Lensectomy and Anterior Vitrectomy Technique

Until recently, the basic surgical technique for pediatric cataract surgery has been lensectomy and anterior vitrectomy (LAV). This technique provides a clear visual axis, but needs rehabilitation of aphakia by use of the spectacle or contact lens. The approaches for LAV are either a limbal or pars plana approach. Most of the surgeons prefer limbal approach to minimize the risk of damaging the peripheral retina and to prevent vitreous from becoming incarcerated in the wound. This approach is particularly useful for the management of rubella cataract and infantile cataract associated with uveitis.

The lensectomy and anterior vitrectomy technique has been used by several authors for pediatric cataract surgery. The report of simultaneous bilateral surgery is rare due to the risk of postoperative endophthalmitis. Simultaneous removal of

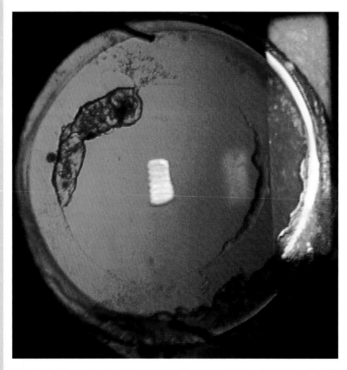

Fig. 21.2: Clear visual axis in an eye with a capsular bag fixated acrylic IOL AcrySof with primary posterior capsulotomy and anterior vitrectomy status 12 months postoperative. Note Soemmering ring formation peripheral to the IOL optic and lens epithelial cell accumulation on the capsulorhexis margins

bilateral infantile cataract may be performed in selected cases with high anesthetic risk.

Primary Posterior Capsulectomy, Anterior Vitrectomy with Intraocular Lens Implantation

Posterior capsular opacification is one of the major postoperative complications following primary IOL implantation, which necessitates secondary surgical procedures such as, surgical or Nd:YAG laser capsulotomy to achieve a clear visual axis. Until recently, primary opening of the posterior capsule was deemed mandatory in most of the cases by most surgeons. The major goal will be to improve the procedure so that this will not be mandatory in the future.

In 1983, primary posterior capsulotomy with anterior vitrectomy was advocated for pediatric cataract. Ideally, the posterior capsulotomy may be performed at the time of primary surgery. Several studies have reported an IOL dislocation rate of 3 to 20% with primary posterior capsulotomy.

Most of the authors at present prefer to perform primary posterior CCC with anterior vitrectomy to decrease the incidence of PCO. This technique is particularly useful for pediatric cataract in children younger than 8 years.

Posterior Circular Curvilinear Capsulorhexis with Optic Capture

Neuhann and Neuhann, in 1991, first suggested capturing of optic through a capsulorhexis opening in the posterior capsular tear in adult. The haptics of the IOL were placed in the ciliary sulcus and the IOL optic was placed through the anterior capsulorhexis to achieve optic capture. Subsequently, the same technique was also used for children, by Gimbel, using posterior CCC to capture the IOL optic to maintain clear visual axis. Many reports of primary posterior capsulorhexis with optic capture have shown encouraging results in terms of maintaining a clear visual axis with this technique in children.

Secondary Intraocular Lens Implantation

Since IOLs are now commonly implanted in infants during the first two years of life prior to the reaching of the adult size axial length of the eye, dioptric adjustment by the use of a secondary or exchange IOLs will become more common in the future.

Though low complication rates have been reported with Kelman-style, open-loop anterior chamber IOL implantation in adults, long-term effect of AC IOLs for pediatric cataract is not known. We do not recommend this technique for pediatric cataract. Other techniques for secondary IOL implantation are the placement of IOL in the sulcus-sulcus and bag-bag. There are several reports on the use of secondary IOL implantation for pediatric aphakia. A secondary posterior chamber IOL may be implanted in the sulcus or in the capsular bag if an intact bag can be salvaged and reopened at the time of secondary implants. The newly described piggy back technique, basically adding a new IOL with the appropriate power at the time of

secondary implantation into the grown eye represent a future possibility—another example of applying techniques from the adult procedure.

Operative Problems and Complications in Pediatric Cataract Surgery

There are several operative complications similar to cataract surgery in adults, but a few specific complications for pediatric cataract surgery are:

- Difficulty in capsulorhexis formation
- Positive intravitreal pressure
- Intraoperative miosis
- Wound leak

Most surgeons perform continuous curvilinear capsulorhexis (CCC) manually using needle cystotome or capsulorhexis forceps. Wilson and associates have reported good results with the use of vitrector for capsulotomy, which is called "vitrector rhexis". There are several newer techniques for CCC for pediatric age group. Can-opener capsulotomy should be avoided to prevent the occurrence of IOL decentration. For the beginner, it is relatively difficult to achieve CCC in younger children with age group less than 2 years due to elasticity of the anterior capsule. Use of viscoelastic agents with higher viscosity, such as sodium hyaluronate helps in achieving CCC. The high intravitreal pressure produced as a result of scleral collapse due to low scleral rigidity results in the forward movement of iris lens diaphragm. An appropriate hypotony can be achieved using hyperventilation anesthesia. Small incision and closed chamber techniques of surgery help to maintain intraoperative pressure. Constriction of pupil during surgery is a common problem in younger children. Pupillary dilatation is achieved using preoperatively topical phenyl-epinephrine hydrochloride 2.5% eye drops, cyclopentolate (0.5%), tropicamide (0.5%) and flurbiprofen (0.03%). Use of 0.3 ml of adrenaline (1:1000) in 500 ml of irrigating fluid also helps to maintain pupillary dilatation. Most surgeons prefer scleral incision to a clear corneal incision in children. Wound closure may be performed using 10-0 nylon. Wound leak with self-sealing incision have been found in the 25% of eyes (all younger than 11 years).

Postoperative Management

Postoperatively, a child's eye tends to show more tissue reaction. The inflammatory response can be managed with the use of intensive topical steroid (as frequently as six to eight times a day). The steroids are tapered over a period of six weeks. Topical antibiotics are instilled three times a day for 10 to 14 days. Cyclopentolate eye drops 0.5% or atropine eye ointment should be used for about 4 weeks to prevent posterior synechiae formation.

Postoperative amblyopia therapy should be instituted meticulously. Occlusion therapy for unilateral cataract after surgery should be instituted early as these children are at the higher risk of developing amblyopia.

Postoperative Complications in Pediatric Cataract Surgery

The risk of postoperative complications is higher due to greater inflammatory response after pediatric intraocular surgery. Close follow-up, early detection and the management of complication is a must.

Uveitis

Postoperative uveitis (fibrinous or exudative) is a common complication due to increased tissue reactivity in children. Uveitis results in fibrinous membrane formation pigment deposits on the IOL and posterior synechiae formation. As a result of microsurgical techniques, closed chamber surgery and capsular fixation of IOL, severe postoperative inflammation is becoming less significant. Frequent use of topical steroids and cycloplegics in the postoperative period helps to reduce uveitis-related complication.

Brady and associates recommend five units of intravenous heparin in 500 ml of irrigating solution. Many authors have used heparin surface modified PMMA IOLs in children to reduce postoperative uveitis. Mullaney and associates reported dissolution of pseudophakic fibrinous exudate with the use of intraocular streptokinase (500 to 1000 IU) without any adverse effect.

Posterior Capsular Opacification

Posterior capsular opacification is the most common complication after pediatric cataract surgery with or without IOL surgery. Posterior capsular opacification often occurs during the critical period of visual development and is amblyogenic (Fig. 21.4). In a thick PCO, surgical posterior capsulotomy combined with anterior vitrectomy is required to prevent amblyopia (Fig. 21.5). Nd:YAG laser has also been used to perform posterior capsulotomy in posterior capsule opacification. Use of newer surgical techniques like primary posterior CCC and anterior vitrectomy or posterior capsulotomy with endodiathermy of capsule or posterior capsulorhexis with optic capture have shown encouraging results in maintaining a clear visual axis.

Pupillary Capture

Pupillary capture occurs when a portion of the optic passes anterior to the iris. The incidence of pupillary capture among children is high, varying from 8.5% to 33%. Pupillary capture has been found in 28% of eyes in bag-sulcus or sulcus-sulcus fixated IOLs compared to none in the bag-bag-fixated IOLs. The pupillary capture can be left untreated if it is not associated with decreased visual acuity, IOL malposition or glaucoma. Pupillary capture is usually associated with PCO and may need posterior capsulotomy with anterior vitrectomy. Fixation of posterior chamber IOL in the capsular bag decreases the incidence of this complication.

Decentration of IOL

Capsular bag placement of IOL is mandatory to reduce this complication. Asymmetrical fixation bag-sulcus is to be avoided in order to minimize IOL decentration.

Glaucoma

The incidence of glaucoma following pediatric cataract surgery varies from 3% to 32 %. Glaucoma occurring soon after surgery is usually due to pupillary block or peripheral anterior synechiae formation while open-angle glaucoma may occur late,

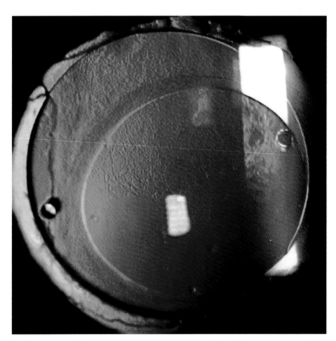

Fig. 21.4: Capsular bag fixated IOL in a 6-year-old child, status 12 months postoperatively. Note early posterior capsule opacification approaching in the visual axis

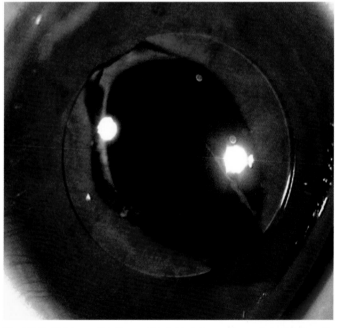

Fig. 21.5: Right eye of a 5-year-old child status post membranectomy with anterior vitrectomy for dense posterior capsule opacification following surgery for traumatic cataract. Note the clear visual axis and total optic capture

which emphasizes the need for the life-long follow-up of these children. A peripheral iridectomy may prevent pupillary block in pseudophakic glaucoma. Some surgeons believe that all children having posterior chamber IOLs should have a peripheral iridectomy when there is rupture of the posterior capsule or zonular dehiscence, which may predispose to vitreous plugging. Intraocular pressure should be periodically recorded to detect and treat this vision threatening complication.

Secondary Membrane Formation

Secondary membranes are commonly reported after pediatric cataract surgery, particularly after infantile cataract surgery. Nd:YAG laser capsulotomy is sufficient to open them in the early stage. Dense secondary membrane may need membranectomy and anterior vitrectomy.

Retinal Complications

Hemorrhagic retinopathy may occur following infantile cataract surgery. These hemorrhages are nonprogressive and resolve within a few weeks. Cystoid macular edema is a rare complication following pediatric cataract surgery probably due to healthy retinal vasculature. The incidence of retinal detachment following cataract surgery has been reported between 1% to 1.5%. Retinal detachments are usually a late complication of pediatric cataract surgery. The significant risk factors for an occurrence of retinal detachment are high myopia and repeated surgeries.

Amblyopia

Pediatric cataract may also be associated with strabismus and/or nystagmus. Amblyopia is one of the most important vision-threatening complications. The aphakic or pseudophakic child must be provided with suitable optical correction after surgery.

The postoperative occlusion therapy of the normal eye in the cases of unilateral congenital, developmental or traumatic cataract is done to achieve binocular vision and stereopsis (Fig. 21.6). In fact, it is noncompliance of occlusion therapy, which appears to be a major stumbling block in achieving satisfactory visual outcome.

Change in the Axial Length of the Globe and Refractive Errors

Many researchers have reported myopic shift following pediatric cataract surgery with or without intraocular lenses. However, animal models have shown that aphakic or pseudophakic eyes during infancy had less elongation than the fellow unmanipulated eyes. Animal models also have shown that severe visual deprivation secondary to lid suturing results in elongation of globe. The aphakic eye receives a blurred image and this reduction in pattern vision could explain an elongation of eye as shown in monkeys, kittens and humans. This effect could explain induced myopia following cataract surgery and IOL implantation.

Postoperative change of the axial length of the globe and expected myopic shift has convinced surgeons to use the undercorrection of the IOL power used for implantation. Dahan and associates prefer an IOL exchange and suggest the implantation of a second IOL, negative power in the sulcus over the top of primary IOL for high myopia.

Visual Outcome

Several studies have reported good visual outcome following intraocular lens implantation in children. Pandey and associates found 85.5% of eyes operated for traumatic cataract and having PC IOLs achieved 20/40 or better visual acuity. Birch compared the visual outcome of unilateral cataract cases operated during the first 6 weeks of life with those operated at the age of 2 to 8 years. The visual acuity of children operated during the first 6 weeks of life was 20/40 compared to 20/100 for children operated at the age between 2 to 8 years. Bradfort and associates found visual acuity of 20/80 or more in 61% of children with an average postoperative follow up of 6.3 years in dense bilateral congenital cataract after surgery. They found that preoperative nystagmus, age at the time of surgery and postoperative nystagmus were not prognostically significant in visual outcome. The visual outcome and academic performance is also influenced by the presence of systemic abnormalities and mental status. Jain and associates in a study reported that 33% of cases in children with congenital cataract who had mental retardation, frustrated attempts are to be managed. The high incidence of mental retardation, nystagmus, strabismus and systemic abnormalities should make us look congenital or developmental cataract as a part of generalized systemic disturbance. Gimbel and associates found very encouraging results of bilateral PC IOL implantation in children 4 years after surgery; 79.2% of the first eye and 66.7% of the second eye had 20/40 or better best corrected visual acuity.

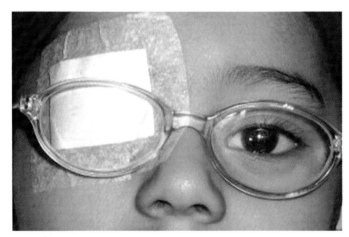

Fig. 21.6: Five-year-old child status post phacoaspiration with capsular bag fixation of posterior chamber intraocular lens in the left eye. This child had best corrected visual acuity of 20/80 in the left eye after surgery and underwent full time occlusion of the right eye (normal eye). After six months of follow-up, left eye achieved best-corrected visual acuity of 20/30

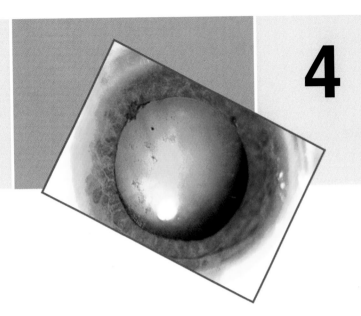
Uveitis

Chapter 22

Uveitis

Chinmaya Sahu, S Sudharshan, Jyotirmay Biswas

INTRODUCTION

The uveal tissue comprises of iris, ciliary body and choroid. The inflammation of uveal tissue is called as uveitis.

CLASSIFICATION

Anatomical Classification

A workshop held in Baltimore, Maryland, USA in 2004 under the aegis of International Uveitis Study Group (IUSG), devised a set of uniform criteria for the classification and grading of uveitis. This meeting was called Standardization of Uveitis Nomenclature (SUN). The classification and grading systems described here have been adopted accordingly (Table 22.1).

Anterior Uveitis: Subset of uveitis where the anterior chamber is the predominant site of inflammation.

Intermediate Uveitis: Subset of uveitis where the vitreous is the major site of the inflammation, and that the presence of peripheral vascular sheathing and macular edema should not change the classification.

Pars Planitis: Subset of intermediate uveitis where there is snowbank or snowball formation occurring in the absence of an associated infection or systemic disease (that is, "idiopathic"). If there is an associated infection (for example, Lyme disease) or systemic disease (for example, sarcoidosis), then the term intermediate uveitis should be used.

Panuveitis: Subset of uveitis where there is no predominant site of inflammation, but inflammation is observed in the anterior chamber, vitreous and retina and/or choroid (that is, retinitis, choroiditis or retinal vasculitis).

For the definition of panuveitis, structural complications, such as macular edema or neovascularization should not be considered in classifying the anatomic location of the uveitis.

Inflammation in the anterior chamber and vitreous (that is, more vitritis than in an iridocyclitis and more anterior chamber inflammation than in intermediate uveitis) should be referred to as anterior and intermediate uveitis and not as panuveitis.

Vasculitis: There was consensus that it is a descriptive term for those situations in which there is evidence of ocular inflammation and retinal vascular changes. The presence of occlusive retinal vasculopathy in the absence of visible inflammation, such as in the antiphospholipid antibody syndrome, should not be considered retinal vasculitis.

Clinical Classification

The onset of uveitis should be described either as sudden or insidious.

The duration of an attack can be:

Limited: If attack of uveitis is 3 months or less in duration.

Persistent: If attack of uveitis is greater than 3 months in duration.

The course of uveitis can be:

Acute: The term acute is used to describe the course of specific uveitic syndromes characterized by sudden onset and limited duration. For example, HLA-B27 associated acute anterior uveitis.

Chronic: The term chronic is used to describe persistent uveitis characterized by prompt relapse (within 3 months) of discontinuation of therapy.

Table 22.1: Standardization of uveitis nomenclature classification

Types	Primary site of inflammation	Includes
Anterior uveitis	Anterior chamber	Iritis, iridocyclitis, anterior cyclitis
Intermediate uveitis	Vitreous	Pars planitis, posterior cyclitis, hyalitis
Posterior uveitis	Retina/Choroid	Focal, multifocal, diffuse choroiditis Chorioretinitis, retinochoroiditis Retinitis, neuroretinitis
Panuveitis	Anterior chamber, vitreous and retina or choroids	

Table 22.2: Classification based on the types of immune reaction

	Nongranulomatous uveitis	Granulomatous uveitis
Onset	Well defined	Insidious
Course	Acute	Chronic
Pain	+++	+
Keratic precipitates	Fine	Mutton fat
Iris nodules	Absent	+

Recurrent: The term recurrent is used to describe repeated episodes of uveitis separated by the periods of inactivity without treatment, in which these periods of inactivity without treatment are at least three months in the duration.

Classification based on the types of immune reaction is shown in Table 22.2.

Etiological Classification

- Infectious: Bacterial, fungal, viral, protozoal
- Noninfectious
  - Known systemic association: Vogt-Koyanagi-Harada's disease
  - Not known systemic association: Serpiginous choroiditis
- Traumatic
  - Surgical: Intraocular lens-related uveitis
  - Nonsurgical
- Toxic
  - Chemical
  - Drug-induced: Rifabutin
- Masquerade syndrome

PATHOGENESIS

The understanding of pathogenesis of uveitis involves a basic understanding of immunology.

Immune Response

It is defined as a sequence of cellular and molecular events to get rid of an offending stimulus, usually a pathogenic organism, toxic substance, cellular debris or neoplastic cell.

Cells of the Immune System

The cells of the immune system include:
- *Leukocytes:* Neutrophils, basophils, eosinophils, B and T lymphocytes and mast cells
- *Tissue presenting cells:* Macrophages and histiocytes

Lymphocytes

The lymphocytes are divided into:
  T lymphocytes: Mature in the thymus.
  B lymphocytes: Mature in the bone marrow.

The T lymphocytes are further divided into:
- *CD 4 cells:* These T cells have the CD 4 marker on the cell surface and mainly respond to antigen antibody complexes assisted by various cytokines. They act by the release of

Table 22.3: Types of immunity

	Innate immunity	Adaptive immunity
Time of response	Immediate	Delayed
Specificity	Nonspecific	Specific
Memory	No memory	Memory present
Cells involved	Mediated by neutrophils and macrophages	Mediated by B and T lymphocytes
Response is elicited by	Occurs in response to stimulation from component of bacterial cell wall or toxin released by bacteria	Occurs in response to antigen–antibody complexes, viruses and tumors

various inflammatory mediators. They need the presence of HLA Class 2 molecules on the surface of the antigen presenting cell to react.
- *CD 8 cells:* These T cells have the CD 8 marker on the cell surface and respond to viruses and tumor cells by forming pores in their wall (by perforins) or by inducing apoptosis. They need the presence of HLA Class 1 molecules on the surface of the antigen presenting cell to react.
- *NK cells:* These are also the Non T and B cells because they do not have these cell markers on their surface. Thus, they can respond to viruses and tumors just like the CD 8 cells without the need for being presented with the HLA markers on the antigen presenting cells.

The B lymphocytes produce the various immunoglobulins by converting into plasma cells.

The immunoglobulins are further divided into IgA, G, M, D and E.

Types of immunity is shown in Table 22.3.

Major Histocompatibility Complex

It is present on short arm of chromosome 6. This region codes for proteins, which play a role in the presentation of antigens to the antigen processing cells.
- *Class I*   HLA-A, B, C
- *Class II*   HLA-DR, DP, DQ

Class I molecules on antigen presenting cells present antigens to CD8 T cells.

Class II molecules on antigen presenting cells present antigens to CD4 T cells.

HLA Association of Certain Uveitic Conditions

Certain diseases have HLA associations. The strength of the association between HLA type and disease is denoted by:

Relative Risk: Frequency of HLA haplotype in people with a particular disease.

Frequency of HLA haplotype in a disease free population is shown in Table 22.4.

Amplifiers of the Immune System

Cytokines

They are small proteins that communicate between cells

Table 22.4: Frequency of HLA haplotype in a disease free population

Disease	HLA marker	Relative risk
Birdshot Retinochoroidopathy	HLA–A 29	80–100 especially in a North American population
Reiter's syndrome	HLA–B 27	60
Ocular Histoplasmosis syndrome	HLA–B 7, DR 2	12
Acute anterior uveitis	HLA–B 27	8
Intermediate uveitis	HLA–B 8, –B 51, –DR 2, –DR 15	6
Behcet's disease	HLA–B 51	4–6
Vogt-Koyanagi-Harada	HLA–DR 4	
Sympathetic Ophthalmia	HLA–DR 4	
Sarcoidosis	HLA–B 8 –B 13	

They include:
- Interferons – IFN-α, IFN-β, IFN-γ
- Interleukins – IL-1 to IL-18
- Colony-stimulating factors
  – G-CSF, GM- CSF, M-CSF
- Chemokines
- Growth factors

Complements: They are endogenous amplifiers of immunity, as well as mediators of inflammatory response functions:
- C3b–phagocytosis
- Membrane attack complex (MAC) – cell lysis through pore formation
- Anaphylatoxins C3 a, C4 a, C5 a – recruitment of PMN's and induction of inflammation

Complements can be formed in response to antigen antibody complexes via the classical pathway or in response to microbial cell wall, plastic surfaces via the alternate pathway.

Sequence of Events in an Immune Response

Whenever a foreign antigen enters the body, it is attacked by the innate or adaptive or both immune systems. The cells of the immune system are assisted in this by the amplifiers like cytokines and complements.

Eye: A Site of Immune Privilege

Immune privilege refers to the better survival of tumor implants or allografts in the immunologically privileged regions.

    Sites in the eye: anterior uvea, subretinal space

    Other sites: brain, testes

Anterior uvea: Immune privileged to alloantigens (transplantation antigens), tumor cells, haptens, soluble proteins, bacteria, viruses and autoantigens.

Anterior Chamber Associated Immune Deviation (ACAID): It is an altered form of systemic immunity to a particular antigen following immunization of anterior chamber with the same.

This happens because of the following reasons:
- Functionally unique APC's – ACAID inducing
- Activation of suppressor T-cells in addition to helper T-cells and B-cells
- Immunosuppressive cytokines like TGF β2 in the aqueous and anterior uvea.

Mechanisms of Immune System Failure

- Hypersensitivity
- Autoimmunity
- Immunodeficiency

Hypersensitivity Reactions

They are of the following types:

Type 1: Whenever an antigen binds to the Ig E receptor on the surface of the mast cells leading to release of histamines and other inflammatory mediators.

Type 2: Whenever an antigen binds to a tissue and incites an antibody response, it can either attract complements or the Fc portion of the antibody can attract neutrophils (Antibody-dependent cellular cytotoxicity). For example, systemic lupus erythematosus.

Type 3: Whenever antigen antibody complexes get deposited in a tissue and attract damage through complements and other inflammatory mediators.

Type 4: Whenever there is a delayed response by the immune cells giving rise to granuloma formation.

There are two types of delayed hypersensitivity responses:

DH 1: Mediated by TNF β, IL 1 and 12, INF γ. They help the Ig G1 and 3. For example, sympathetic ophthalmia.

DH 2: Mediated by IL 4, 5 and 10. They help Ig A and E and lead to the formation of eosinophilic granulomas. For example, Toxocara granuloma.

Autoimmunity

To understand why the body's immune system wages an attack against its own cells, it is important to understand the concept of tolerance.

Tolerance

It is defined as sum total of mechanisms to prevent immune responses against self-antigen. Example of tolerance in uveitis: Extracapsular cataract extraction rarely causes autoimmune uveitis.

Mechanisms of Tolerance

Clonal deletion: Deletion of clones of lymphocytes that were autoreactive while they are maturing.

Clonal anergy: Reactive cells present but made incapable of responding to antigen.

Apoptosis: Programed cell death.

Suppression: Reactive T-cell is actively kept from carrying out its function by another cell.

The following are a list of uveitogenic antigens:
- Retinal S antigen (arrestin)
- Interphotoreceptor retinoid binding protein (IRBP)
- Recoverin
- Melanin protein
- Rhodopsin
- Phosducin

CLINICAL FEATURES

The patients can present with the following symptoms and signs:

Symptoms

Blurring of vision: It can be due to cells and fibrin in the anterior chamber (Fig. 22.1), cataract, vitreous haze and macular edema.
Floaters and scotoma
Redness

Pain:
It can be due to
- Inflammation of iris leading to release of mediators of pain
- Ciliary spasm, which radiates over a large area supplied by the trigeminal nerve
- Secondary glaucoma

Watering and photophobia: They occur when the cornea gets involved.

Signs

The signs include those which are of the underlying disease and those which occur because of uveitis.

Lid
- *Vitiligo:* It is seen in cases with Vogt-Koyanagi-Harada's disease and sympathetic ophthalmia (Fig. 22.2).
- Nodules

Conjunctiva
- Circumciliary congestion
- Nodules

Cornea
- *Keratic precipitates:* They are the deposits of inflammatory cells on the endothelium.
- *Distribution:* Generally, due to the convection currents in the anterior chamber the cells are seen in the lower part of the endothelium (von Arlt's triangle). They are very rarely seen dispersed throughout the endothelium (Fuchs heterochromic iridocyclitis).
- *Appearance:* Early on in the disease they are fine (Fig. 22.3). With time, they appear crenated, glassy or pigmented. Granulomatous inflammation is associated with large yellow keratic precipitates called as "mutton fat" keratic precipitates (Fig. 22.4).

Anterior Chamber Reaction

With increase in the permeability of the blood vessels in the uveal meshwork, there is an influx of cells in the anterior chamber. This gives rise to anterior chamber reaction, which can be described as:
- *Serous:* Protein influx
- *Purulent:* Polymorphonuclear leukocyte influx–Hypopyon (Fig. 22.5)
- *Fibrinous* (Fig. 22.6)
- *Sanguinous:* Inflammatory cells with red blood cells. (Fig. 22.7)
- *Cells:* The number of cells in the anterior chamber is seen in a 1 × 1 mm high-powered beam at 45–60 degrees angle on a slit lamp.

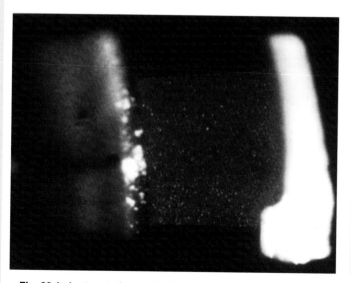

Fig. 22.1: Acute anterior uveitis: Slit-lamp photograph showing cells and flare in the anterior chamber

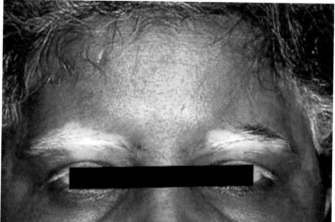

Fig. 22.2: Vitiligo: It is observed in cases with Vogt-Koyanagi Harada's disease and sympathetic ophthalmia

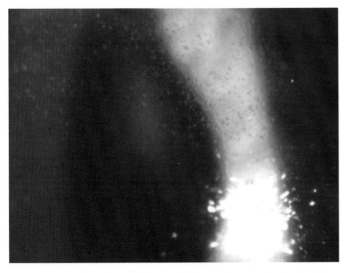

Fig. 22.3: Fine keratic precipitates: Slit-lamp photograph showing fine keratic precipitates in a case of nongranulomatous anterior uveitis

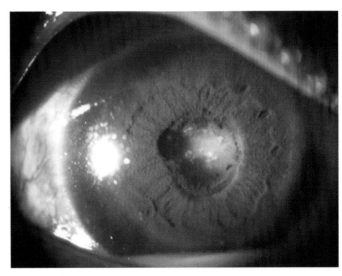

Fig. 22.5: Hypopyon. Slit-lamp photograph shows hypopyon uveitis

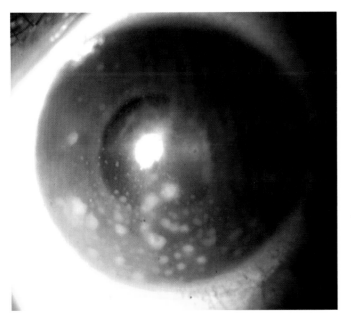

Fig. 22.4: Mutton fat keratic precipitates. Slit-lamp photograph showing mutton fat keratic precipitates in a case of granulomatous uveitis

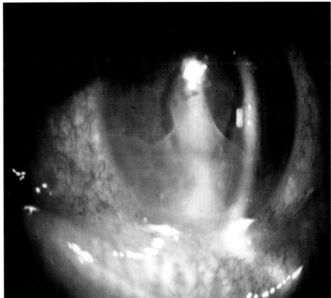

Fig. 22.6: Fibrinous anterior chamber reaction: Slit-lamp photograph shows fibrinous anterior uveitis

The SUN recommendation for grading of cells in the anterior chamber is shown in Table 22.5.

Table 22.5: Grading of cells in the anterior chamber

Grade	No. of cells
0	1
0.5	1–5
1	6–15
2	16–25
3	26–50
4	>50

• *Flare:* The SUN recommendation for grading of flare in anterior chamber is shown in Table 22.6.

Table 22.6: Grading of flare in the anterior chamber

Grade	Number of cells
0	None
1+	Faint
2+	Moderate (iris and lens details clear)
3+	Marked (iris and lens details hazy)
4+	Intense (fibrin or plastic aqueous)

Iris

• Nodules
• *Koeppe:* These are situated at the pupillary border (Fig. 22.8)
• *Busacca:* These are situated on the iris stroma away from the papillary border (Fig. 22.9)

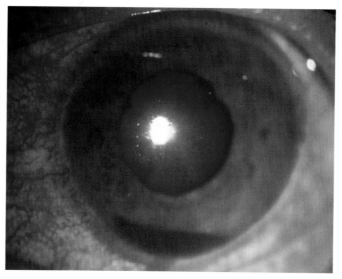

Fig. 22.7: Sanguinous anterior chamber reaction: Slit-lamp photograph showing hyphema in a case of acute anterior uveitis

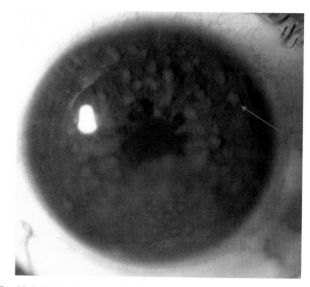

Fig. 22.9: Busacca's nodules: Slit-lamp photograph showing Busacca's nodules away from the pupillary margin (arrow)

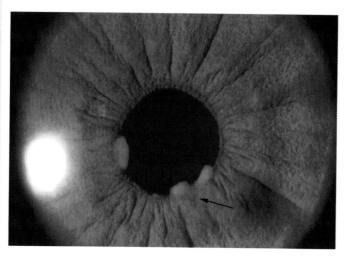

Fig. 22.8: Koeppe's nodules: Slit-lamp photograph shows Koeppe's nodules at the pupillary margin (arrow)

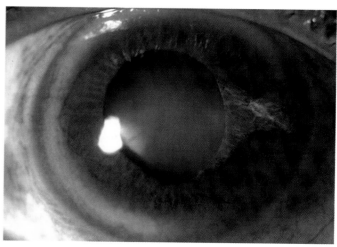

Fig. 22.10: Sectoral iris atrophy: Slit-lamp photograph shows sectoral iris atrophy in a case of viral uveitis

- Anterior and posterior synechiae
- Heterochromia
- Stromal atrophy (Fig. 22.10)
- Rubeosis iridis

The other signs will be dealt in the subsequent topics.

INVESTIGATIONS

A lot of options are available to the ophthalmologist while deciding on the investigations to be ordered.

Certain steps should be followed before ordering for tests.

- What is the most likely clinical diagnosis?
- What is the main purpose of ordering the test?
- What is the cost of the investigations and whether the patient can afford it?

Clinical Diagnosis

- Compare clinical characteristic with known uveitic entities
- Shortlist etiological possibilities

Reason for Ordering a Test

- *To identify presumed autoimmune disease*: Like HLA-B27 testing in the cases of acute nongranulomatous uveitis. If the test result is positive, it gives information that the person is likely to have further attacks of uveitis. Also, the patient is more likely to suffer from diseases like ankylosing spondylitis.
- *To identify specific uveitic entities*: If a patient has granulomatous anterior uveitis and typical periphlebitis (candle wax appearance), sarcoidosis is the most likely diagnosis. In such a case chest X-ray, serum ACE levels and serum calcium and phosphorus should be ordered. So, when the clinical

features are suggestive of a particular diagnosis, specific investigations should be done for the suspected disease.

- *To obtain therapeutic directions*: Many investigations are ordered to guide the therapy. If the patient is to be started on immunosuppressive therapy, then the routine hematological, hepatic and renal investigations have to be done to rule out any contraindication.

The investigations, which can be ordered can be divided on the basis of type of investigations:

Skin Tests

Mantoux test: It is practically the only skin test still being used. Kveim's test for sarcoidosis is no longer in vogue (Fig. 22.11). It involves the injection of purified protein derivative of mycobacterium tuberculosis intradermally. The response is checked after 48 hours. Mantoux test positive means that there has been erythema and induration around the injection site, which is at least 10 mm in the maximal diameter. Delayed hypersensitivity is supposed to be the basis for the reaction. It is found to be positive even in people who have been vaccinated and also in people who might harbor the bacilli but might not have active disease. It is found to be positive in 30–69% of the healthy Indians.

Serology

The blood investigations that can be ordered include:
- Routine
- Renal and liver function tests
- Tests for detection of specific substances
- Immunological tests

Routine: Blood hemoglobin (Hb), complete blood count (CBC), erythrocyte sedimentation rate (ESR) and random blood sugar (RBS) are the routine blood investigations. These tests give an idea of the condition of the patient and are important when the patient has to be started on immunosuppressive agents.

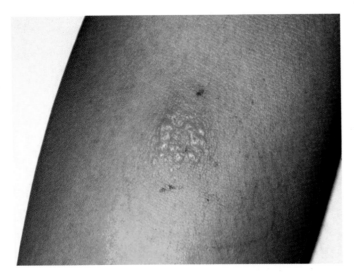

Fig. 22.11: Mantoux test: External photograph shows positive Mantoux test

Renal and liver function tests: Renal and liver function tests are ordered when immunosuppressive agents are to be started.

Tests for detection of specific substances: Tests for serum calcium, phosphoros, ACE or lysozyme are carried out when sarcoidosis is suspected. Tests for detection of serum homocysteine may also be done.

Immunological tests: These include enzyme-linked immunosorbent assay (ELISA). It is useful for the detection of both antigens and antibodies in the serum. If the particular antigen or antibody, which is being tested is present, then the antibody to it, which has been linked to an enzyme will go and bind to it. When the substrate is added, there will be a color change indicating the test is positive. There are different types of ELISA, such as indirect, sandwich, competitive and reverse method and device.

Other tests include:
- Complement fixation tests
- Hemagglutination tests
- Fluorescent antibody tests
- Interferon gamma assays

These tests can be ordered for diagnosing variety of diseases. The specific serological test to be ordered when a particular disease is suspected is discussed below.

Syphilis

VDRL (Venereal disease research laboratory test) and FTA (Fluorescent treponemal antibody) tests are done for detecting syphilis.

VDRL acts like a screening test while FTA is more specific.

Toxoplasmosis: Anti-toxoplasma IgM antibodies peak within two weeks and taper off by two months. While IgG antibodies start at two weeks, peak at two months and are present for life. Toxoplasmosis can be diagnosed by either detecting IgM antibodies or by detecting a 4-fold rise in IgG antibody titres repeated at 3 weeks interval. But, antibody titers might not correlate with ocular disease. Antitoxoplasma antibodies may be very low and should be tested in undiluted (1:1) samples, if possible.

Toxoplasma antibody titers can be determined by several techniques like:
- Enzyme-linked immunosorbent assay (ELISA)
- Indirect fluorescent antibody test
- Indirect hemagglutination test
- Complement fixation
- Sabin-Feldman dye test

The Sabin-Feldman test requires live *T. Gondii* organisms and hence is no longer used. ELISA is the most common test used because of the easy availability of the testing kit and the relative ease of performing the test.

Systemic lupus erythematosus: In most of the retinal vasculitis cases, antinuclear antibody testing should be done. The anti-double stranded DNA antibody is detected in a lot of collagen vascular disorders, including systemic lupus erythematosus. However, the antihistone antibody is positive only in systemic lupus erythematosus and is more specific for it.

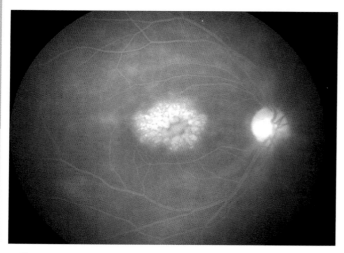

Fig. 22.12: Cystoid macular edema: Fundus fluorescein angiogram showing a typical flower petal pattern

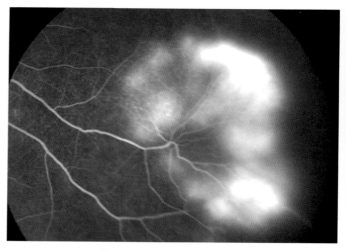

Fig. 22.13: Retinal vasculitis: Fundus fluorescein angiogram showing staining of the neovascular frond

Sarcoidosis: Serum ACE, lysozyme and calcium/phosphorus are ordered for in a case suspected of sarcoidosis.

Tuberculosis: QuantiFERON-TB Gold test is the latest test available in the market. It measures the release of interferon gamma from primed macrophages. The test report is available in a day and also it is more specific for mycobacterium tuberculosis compared to the Mantoux test. In this test, macrophages, which were primed by the BCG bacilli or most of the atypical mycobacteria will not be picked up. It just gives an idea that the person has the tubercle bacilli, but it does not mean that the patient has active tuberculosis.

Imaging

Fluorescein Angiography

- *Choroiditis:* In active choroiditis, the choroiditis patch appears hypofluorescent in the early phase and hyperfluorescent in the late phases.
- *Intermediate uveitis:* Cystoid macular edema is a common complication of intermediate uveitis. Cystoid macular edema has a typical petalloid appearance in the late phases of the angiogram (Fig. 22.12).
- *Vasculitis:* There is a staining of the vessel wall in the cases of active vasculitis. When ischemia occurs secondary to vasculitis, the first sign is the development of arterovenous shunts, then capillary nonperfusion areas and finally the formation of new vessels. Capillary non-perfusion areas appear as hypofluorescent patches and neovascularization is detected by the leakage of dye (Fig. 22.13).
- *Exudative retinal detachment:* There is staining of the disc and pooling of dye in the area of detachment.

Indocyanine Green Angiography

It is more useful for detecting choroidal pathologies as the indocyanine dye remains bound to the serum proteins and does not leak out of the choriocapillaris (Figs 22.14A and B). It is useful for picking up choroidal neovascular membrane, which can be a complication of uveitic conditions like histoplasmosis. It is very useful in detecting deeper choroidal pathologies especially conditions like multifocal white dot syndromes.

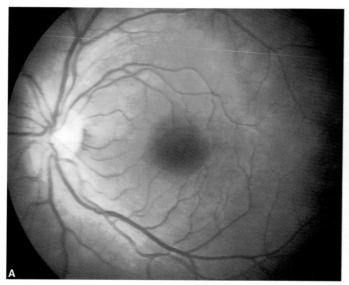

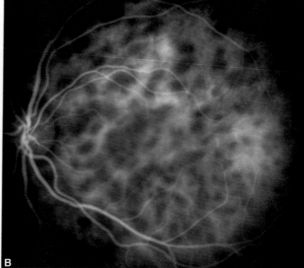

Figs 22.14A and B: Indocyanine green angiography: Deeper choroidal lesions more clearly visible

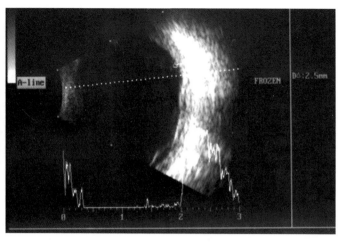

Fig. 22.15: Vogt-Koyanagi-Harada's disease: Ultrasonogram shows increased choroidal thickness

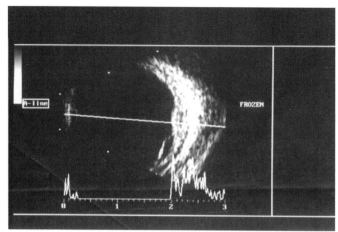

Fig. 22.17: T sign in posterior scleritis: Ultrasonogam shows localized choroidal thickening with widening of the sub-Tenon's space

Ultrasonography

Ultrasonography is a very useful tool in detecting lesions when the media is hazy, for example cataract, vitreous hemorrhage. It is useful in differentiating rhegmatogenous and exudative retinal detachment. It is useful in specific uveitic conditions like Vogt-Koyanagi-Harada's disease and choroidal abscess.

Vogt-Koyanagi-Harada disease: There is choroidal thickening in case of Vogt-Koyanagi-Harada's disease (Fig. 22.15). Normal choroidal thickness is around 1.1 mm.

Choroidal abscess: It appears as a chorioretinal mass with echolucent spaces within the mass along with localized widening of the sub-Tenon's space (Fig. 22.16).

There are various conditions, which can mimic a choroidal abscess.

- *Choroidal melanoma:* It appears as a chorioretinal mass with moderate surface reflectivity and variable low to moderate internal reflectivity. It also has other features like acoustic hallowing and choroidal excavation. It is associated generally with a shallow retinal detachment.
- *Choroidal metastases:* It appears as a chorioretinal mass with high surface reflectivity and uniform high to moderate internal reflectivity. Acoustic hallowing and choroidal

excavation are not present. It is generally associated with a large retinal detachment.

- *Posterior scleritis:* There is a localized choroidal thickening with widening of the sub-Tenon's space called the "*T*" sign (Fig. 22.17).

Optical Coherence Tomography

The conventional time domain optical coherence tomography (OCT) has a resolution of 10 μm and is useful for detecting macular edema (Fig. 22.18), epiretinal membrane and choroidal neovascular membrane. Spectral domain OCT has increased the resolution to 5 μm and gives a three-dimensional view enhancing its diagnostic potential.

Biopsy

Vitreous or samples of lesions sent for histopathology give confirmatory diagnosis in many conditions (Figs 22.19A and B).

Polymerase Chain Reaction

Whenever the etiology of retinitis or chorioretinitis is doubtful, polymerase chain reaction is a useful test. The aqueous or vitreous aspirate can be tested. Here, a particular segment of

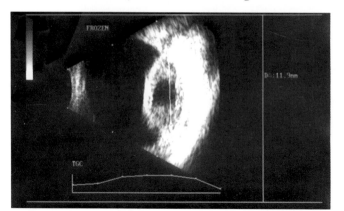

Fig. 22.16: Subretinal abscess: Chorioretinal mass with echolucent spaces within the mass is visible

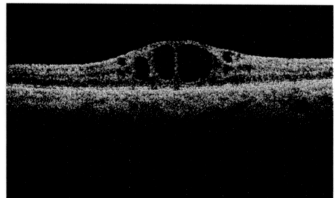

Fig. 22.18: Optical coherence tomography: Cystoid macular edema is observed in the case of intermediate uveitis

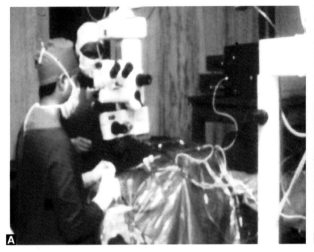
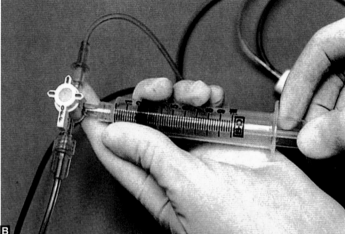

Figs 22.19A and B: Technique of vitreous biopsy

the genome is amplified using single stranded DNA as a template, DNA oligonucleotides as a primer and heat-resistant taq polymerase as an amplifier (Figs 22.20A and B). This gives an idea of the causative organism, helping in the management of the cases. In endophthalmitis, it might detect the exact organism and therapy can be oriented towards it.

TREATMENT

Medical Management

Mydriatic and Cycloplegic Agents

They are used to:
- Prevent the formation or break posterior synechiae
- Relieve the photophobia occurring due to ciliary spasm.

They include short acting cycloplegics like cyclopentolate or homatropine and long-acting drops like atropine. The choice of the cycloplegic agent depends on the severity of the anterior uveitis. The onset of cycloplegic action of cyclopentolate and homatropine is within 30–60 minutes and lasts for 6–8 hours. While, the onset of cycloplegic action of atropine is within 60–120 minutes and lasts for almost 10 days. The cycloplegic agents can thus cause blurring of vision. The choice of cycloplegic agent will depend on the severity of the inflammation and also on the effect, it is likely to have on the clarity of the patient's vision.

Corticosteroids

They are the mainstay of uveitis therapy.

Mechanism of action: Mechanism of action of corticosteroids is as follows:
- Inhibits arachidonic acid release from phospholipids
- Inhibit the transcription and action of cytokines
- Limits B- and T-cell activity.

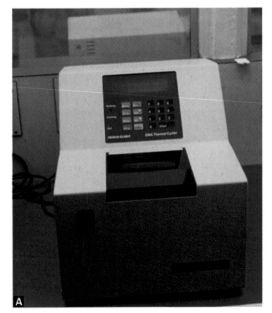

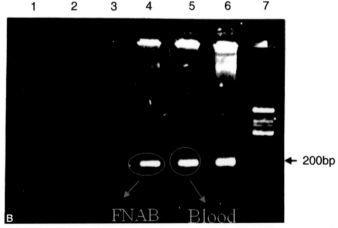

Ethidium bromide stained 2% agarose gel with amplification products from a case of subretinal abscess suspected to be tuberculous. Lane 1: Reagent control of the first round. Lane 2: Reagent controal of the second round. Lane 3: Aqueous humor-negative. Lane 4: FNAB specimen - positive. Lane 5: Blood - positive. Lane 6: Positive control M.tuberculosis (H37Rv), Lane 7: Phi X174 DNA/Hinf I digest

Figs 22.20A and B: Polymerase chain reaction: (A) DNA thermocycler used for polymerase chain reaction testing, (B) Gel photograph of polymerase chain reaction

Indications: They can be used for the following indications:
- They are used to control active inflammation in the eye. If the cause is infective, then they are used in combination with the anti-infective agent.
- They are used to prevent complications like cystoid macular edema in intermediate uveitis.

Routes of administration: Three routes of administration are available: topical, periocular and systemic. The best route and dose is determined for each patient, but the minimum amount needed to control inflammation should be used to reduce complications.
- Topical: For anterior uveitis, topical steroid drops are used. Depending on the severity of the inflammation being treated, the frequency can range from hourly to every other day. Prednisolone acetate 1% is preferred. Since this agent is a precipitate, the patient must vigorously shake the bottle before use. Sometimes, steroids can cause ocular hypertension; therefore, patients must be monitored at 4- to 6-week intervals. If the patient develops high intraocular pressure (IOP), then alternative steroid like fluorometholone can be used. Fluorometholone has less penetration into the anterior chamber and so is less likely to cause the increase of IOP. But anti-inflammatory action of fluorometholone is 10 times less compared to that of prednisolone. Hence, it should be reserved for very mild cases of uveitis or cases where the use of prednisolone has led to an increase in IOP.
- Periocular: When a more posterior effect is necessary or when compliance is an issue, periocular corticosteroids can be administered. Either a transseptal or a sub-Tenon approach (Fig. 22.21) works to deposit a long-lasting steroid (e.g. triamcinolone acetonide) around the eye. Initially, treating patients with a topical steroid for 3–4 weeks prior to the administration of a long-acting depot steroid may help to identify those patients who are steroid responders. Some evidence exists that deep transseptal injections cause less ocular hypertension than the sub-Tenon method. These injections should not be used in patients with infectious uveitis or scleritis because scleral thinning and possible perforation could result.
- Systemic: When systemic disease is present that also requires treatment or for vision-threatening uveitis that is poorly responsive to other methods of delivery, oral or intravenous therapy is necessary. Both the short- and long-term adverse effects of corticosteroid use should be discussed with the patient and may require the help of an internist. Prednisolone is the most commonly used oral corticosteroid.

Side Effects of Corticosteroids

Topical
- Increase in IOP
- Cataract formation, especially posterior subcapsular cataract.
- If infection is present, there can be worsening and in some cases there can be corneal thinning or perforation.

Periocular
- All the side effects as described above.
- Scleral perforation and hemorrhage can occur while giving the infection.
- While giving transseptal injection, ptosis can occur.
- Scarring of the conjunctiva and the Tenon's capsule can occur at the site of the injection.

Systemic
- Increase in IOP and cataract formation
- Hypertension and diabetes mellitus
- Peptic ulcers
- Increase in appetite and weight gain
- Mood changes
- Aseptic necrosis of the head of femur
- Menstrual irregularities
- Osteoporosis
- Impairment of wound healing
- Worsening of systemic infections

Immunosuppressive Agents

Include three main categories of therapy:
- *Antimetabolites:* Azathioprine, methotrexate, and mycophenolate mofetil
- *T-cell suppressors:* Cyclosporine and tacrolimus
- *Cytotoxic agents:* Cytotoxic agents are alkylating agents and include cyclophosphamide and chlorambucil.

Most agents take several weeks to achieve efficacy; therefore, they initially are used in conjunction with oral corticosteroids. Once the disease is under control, corticosteroids can be tapered.

Azathioprine

It is a nucleoside analog, which interferes with DNA replication and RNA transcription. It decreases peripheral T- and B-lymphocyte count and reduces lymphocyte activity. Its

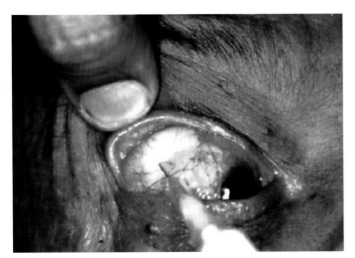

Fig. 22.21: Periocular corticosteroid: Photograph shows the technique of giving posterior sub-Tenon's injection of depot steroid

metabolism is dependent on xanthine oxidase. It may decrease proliferation of immune cells, which results in lower autoimmune activity.

Indications: Behçet's disease or chronic uveitis, especially with oral corticosteroids.

Dose: 1 mg/kg/d orally initially; not to exceed 2.5–4 mg/kg/day.

Side effects: Gastrointestinal upset, altered liver function and renal function, decreased bone marrow function, rarely pancreatitis and increased risk of neoplasia.

Complete blood count and liver function tests should be done once every two weeks.

Methotrexate

It is a folic acid analog and inhibitor of dihydrofolate reductase, which is the enzyme responsible for the conversion of dihydrofolate to tetrahydrofolate. It arrests DNA replication, inhibiting rapidly dividing cells, e.g. leukocytes.

Indications: It is used to treat various ocular inflammatory diseases, including vasculitis, panuveitis, intermediate uveitis, vitritis, and Behçet's disease or chronic uveitis, especially with oral corticosteroids.

Dose: 7.5–12.5 mg/wk orally initially; not to exceed 25 mg/wk; folate (1 mg/d) is given concurrently to minimize nausea.
Side effects: Increased fatigue, gastrointestinal upset, altered liver, hematological and renal function and rarely pneumonitis.

Complete blood counts and liver function tests should be done once every two weeks.

Mycophenolate Mofetil

It is a selective inhibitor of inosine monophosphate dehydrogenase, which interferes with guanosine nucleotide synthesis. It prevents lymphocyte proliferation, suppresses antibody synthesis, interferes with cellular adhesion to vascular endothelium and decreases the recruitment of leukocytes to sites of inflammation.

Indications: Various studies are ongoing to study effectivity in various inflammatory conditions.

Dose: 500 mg orally bid initially; not to exceed 1.5 g bid.
Side effects: Increased chance of infection, gastrointestinal upset like nausea, vomiting and diarrhea; altered liver, hematologic and renal functions; and reported incidence of leukopenia, lymphoma, and nonmelanoma skin cancers.

Complete blood counts, renal and liver function tests should be done once every two weeks.

Cyclosporine

It binds to the cytosolic protein cyclophilin (immunophilin) of immunocompetent lymphocytes, especially T-lymphocytes. This complex of cyclosporin and cyclophylin inhibits calcineurin, which under normal circumstances is responsible for activating the transcription of interleukin-2. It thus inhibits the

transcription of T lymphocytes that are in the G0 and G1 phase of their cell cycle, which blocks replication and ability to produce lymphokines.

Indications: Cyclosporine can be used in the cases of uveitis, which are not responding to treatment with steroids.

Dose: 2.5–5 mg/kg/day orally initially; not to exceed 10 mg/kg/day.

Side effects: Gingival hyperplasia, tremors, myalgias and hirsuitism; nephrotoxicity, hepatotoxicity and hypertension.

Complete blood count, renal and liver function tests should be done once every two weeks.

Cyclophosphamide

It is chemically related to nitrogen mustards. As an alkylating agent, mechanism of action of the active metabolites may involve cross-linking of DNA, which may interfere with growth of normal and neoplastic cells. It is cytotoxic to resting and dividing lymphocytes.

Indications: The main indication is Wegener's granulomatosis. It can also be used as second line in the management of cases not responding to steroids or other immunosuppresives.

Dose: 2 mg/kg/day orally initially; not to exceed 3 mg/kg/day.

Side effects: Hemorrhagic cystitis, severe nausea, vomiting, ovarian failure and testicular atrophy.

Complete blood counts, renal, liver function tests and routine urine examination should be done once every two weeks.

UVEITIS IN SPONDYLOARTHROPATHIES

HLA-B27 Association

It is a genome located on the short arm of chromosome 6. It is present in around 8% of the western population and 1% of the Asian population. But almost 50% to 60% of the patients with acute anterior uveitis are HLA-B27 positive. HLA-B27 positivity is generally associated with anterior non-granulomatous uveitis.

Pathogenesis

The actual role of HLA-B27 in triggering an inflammatory response causing disease is still not precisely known.

Molecular Mimicry

It is a process in which an autoimmune response initially is mounted against a peptide from an infectious agent and is subsequently directed against HLA-B27 itself due to epitopic similarities.

Arthritogenic Peptide

This theory states that HLA-B27 molecule acts as a peptide-binding molecule for infectious agents.

There are other theories also but the exact mechanism is still not understood. A group of seronegative spondyloarthropathies is associated with both acute anterior uveitis and HLA-B27 positivity.

These include:
- Ankylosing spondylitis
- Reiter's syndrome/postinfectious or reactive arthritis
- Inflammatory bowel disease
- Psoriatic arthritis
- Undifferentiated spondyloarthropathy.

Clinical Features

It is characterized by acute onset of unilateral alternating, non-granulomatous acute anterior uveitis, characterized by significant cellular and protein extravasation into the aqueous humor, including fibrin and hypopyon in the anterior chamber, with high tendency for recurrences, and significant association with other HLA-B27-related diseases.

There is a high frequency of recurrent episodes with a mean number of 0.6–3.3 attacks per year and a mean duration of each episode of 4–6 weeks. The interval between acute attacks is most commonly about 14–25 months. There may also be a decrease in the frequency of uveitis attacks with increasing duration of disease (Table 22.7).

ANKYLOSING SPONDYLITIS

Ankylosing spondylitis is a chronic, usually progressive, disease involving the articulations of the spine and adjacent soft tissues. The sacroiliac joints usually are affected. Involvement of the hip and shoulders commonly occurs, and peripheral joints are affected less frequently.

Age: The disease begins most often in the third decade.

Sex: Males are more commonly affected.

Incidence: HLA-B27 positivity is found in almost 90% of the patients with ankylosing spondylitis. Almost, 1 in 4 patients

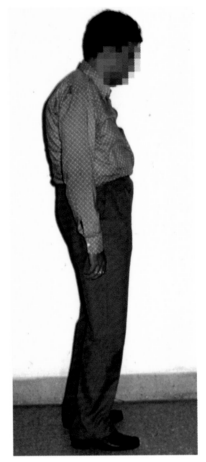

Fig. 22.22: Ankylosing spondylitis: Photograph shows a patient with ankylosing spondylitis

with HLA-B27 positivity will develop ankylosing spondylitis or anterior uveitis.

Clinical Features

Symptoms: Patient complains of lower back pain and stiffness (Fig. 22.22), which is worse after the periods of inactivity. But very often, patients might not complain of back pain.

Table 22.7: Clinical features of HLA-B27 positive and negative anterior uveitis

Clinical Features	HLA-B27 Positive Anterior Uveitis	HLA-B27 Negative Anterior Uveitis
Age at onset (years)	32–35	39–48
Sex	Male preponderance (1.5–2.5:1)	1:1
Eye involvement	Unilateral in 48–59%	Bilateral in 21–64%
	Unilateral alternating in 29-36%	
Pattern of uveitis	Acute in 80–87%	Chronic in 43–61%
Recurrence	Frequent	Uncommon
Keratic precipitates	Mutton fat keratic precipitates in 0–3%	Mutton fat keratic precipitates in 17–46%
Fibrin in anterior chamber	25–56%	0–10%
Hypopyon	12–15%	0–2%
Associated systemic disease	48–84%	1–13%
Familial aggregation	Yes	No

Investigations

Radiological: Radiographs of sacroiliac joints show sclerosis and narrowing of the joint space. This is followed by ligamentous ossification and osteoporosis. Both sacroiliac joints usually are involved, but findings may first appear on one side. Later on, there might be fusion of the lower vertebrae leading to the loss of curvature and giving rise to "bamboo spine" appearance (Fig. 22.23).

REACTIVE ARTHRITIS AND REITER'S SYNDROME

Reactive arthritis (ReA) refers to spondyloarthropathies, following enteric or urogenital infections and occurring in individuals who are HLA-B27 positive. Reiter's syndrome is included in this category.

Reiter syndrome is described as a triad of:
- Arthritis
- Nonspecific urethritis
- Conjunctivitis, often accompanied by iritis.

Age: It is generally seen in the young age group (20–40 years).

Sex: If the disease is acquired secondary to a gastrointestinal infection, it is seen equally in both males and females. If the disease is acquired secondary to a urogenital infection, it is more common in males.

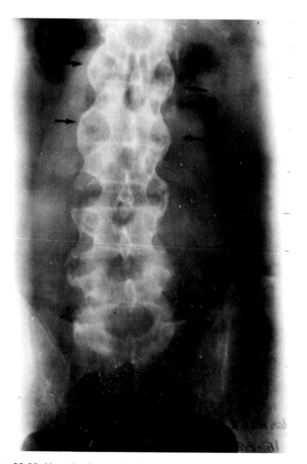

Fig. 22.23: X-ray lumbosacral spine: Bamboo spine appearance in ankylosing spondylitis

Incidence: Almost 75% of the patients with reactive arthritis are HLA-B27 positive.

Pathogenesis

As described earlier, molecular mimicry is thought to be the cause for the inflammatory response. The bacteria that have been implicated include *Salmonella* species, *Yersinia enterocolitica*, *Campylobacter jejuni*, *Chlamydia trachomatis*, *Chlamydia pneumoniae*, *Clostridium difficile* and *Ureaplasma urealyticum*.

Clinical Features

The syndrome usually begins with urethritis followed by conjunctivitis and rheumatological findings. The conjunctivitis is usually minimal and lasts for only a few days or weeks. It is mucopurulent and papillary.

Arthritis begins within the one month of infection in 80% of patients. It usually is acute, asymmetric, oligoarticular, involving predominantly the joints of the lower extremities (e.g. knees, ankles, feet and wrists). The arthritis usually is quite painful. Dactylitis or sausage digit is a diffuse swelling of a solitary finger or toe. This is a distinct feature of both reactive arthritis and psoriatic arthritis. Plantar fasciitis and Achilles tendonitis are also common. Sacroiliitis is present in as many as 70% of patients.

Punctate and subepithelial keratitis may occur rarely, leading to permanent corneal scars.

Acute nongranulomatous iritis recurs frequently in this condition. It may become bilateral and chronic and may result in blindness.

Mucocutaneous lesions like keratoderma blennorrhagicum, a scaly, erythematous, irritating disorder of the palms and soles of the feet, as well as circinate balanitis, a persistent, scaly, erythematous circumferential rash of the distal penis are known to occur.

Investigations

Reactive arthritis is a clinical diagnosis without definitive laboratory or radiographic findings. The diagnosis should be considered when an acute asymmetric inflammatory arthritis or tendonitis follows an episode of diarrhea or dysuria.

Inflammatory Bowel Disease

Ulcerative colitis and Crohn's disease are associated with acute anterior uveitis. Specifically, 2.4% of patients with Crohn's disease and 5% to 12% of patients with ulcerative colitis develop acute anterior uveitis. Patients with uveitis and inflammatory bowel disease alone tend to be HLA-B27 negative. Almost, 50% to 60% of the patients with spondyloarthropathies and inflammatory bowel disease with uveitis are HLA-B27 positive.

PSORIATIC ARTHRITIS

Psoriasis is a noncontagious disorder characterized by the presence of silvery white scales on the extensor surfaces of the body. Psoriasis precedes the onset of arthritis by months or years. Most patients have onychodystrophy, which includes onycholysis and ridging and pitting of nail beds. Twenty-five percent of patients develop a more severe symmetrical arthritis resembling rheumatoid arthritis. The proximal interphalangeal joints and distal interphalangeal joints commonly are involved with characteristic sausage-shaped digits. HLA-B27 positivity is present in cases where psoriatic arthritis is associated with spondylitis.

MISCELLANEOUS ANTERIOR UVEITIS

Fuchs Uveitis Syndrome

Fuchs heterochromic iridocyclitis (FHI) is a chronic, unilateral iridocyclitis characterized by iris heterochromia.

Age: It affects people between 20–60 years of age.

Sex: Males and females are equally affected.

Incidence: Nearly 2% to 3% of the patients with uveitis have Fuchs heterochromic iridocyclitis.

Pathogenesis

Sympathetic/neurogenic theory: This theory states that there is adrenergic dysfunction leading to iris hypopigmentation by reduced innervation to iris stromal melanocytes. Abnormal innervation to iris vasculature leads to breakdown in the blood-aqueous barrier with secondary leakage of proteins, cells and inflammatory mediators into the anterior chamber.

Infectious theory: A strong association between Fuchs heterochromic iridocyclitis and ocular toxoplasmosis has been documented. Rubella, HSV and Toxocara Canis are some of the other organisms associated with Fuch's heterochromic iridocyclitis.

Immunologic theory: T helper 1 (Th1)–subtype response has been implicated in Fuchs heterochromic iridocyclitis.

Clinical Features

Symptoms: The symptoms can vary from none to mild blurring of vision and discomfort.

Signs:
- The classic triad of Fuch's heterochromic uveitis is heterochromia, cataract and keratitic precipitates.
- Conjunctiva and sclera: In most patients, there is no ciliary congestion or conjunctival hyperemia.
- Cornea: Small, nonpigmented, translucent, stellate keratic precipitates with filamentous projections distributed over the entire endothelial surface is pathognomic of Fuch's heterochromic iridocyclitis (Fig. 22.24). Stellate keratic precipitates can also be seen in uveitis associated with toxoplasmosis, herpes simplex, herpes zoster and cytomegalovirus (CMV).
- Anterior chamber: There is minimal anterior chamber cells and flare. Paracentesis may result in the appearance of a filiform hemorrhage (Amsler's sign).

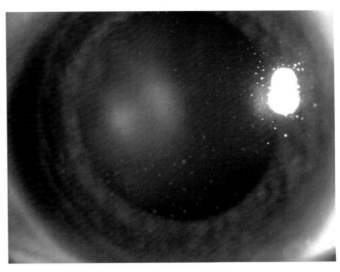

Fig. 22.24: Fuch's heterochromic uveitis: Slit-lamp photograph shows scattered stellate fine keratic precipitates in Fuchs uveitis syndrome

- Iris: Heterochromia is present in 75% to 90% of cases. In unilateral cases, the hypopigmented eye is usually the affected eye. It is difficult to comment in bilateral cases (5% to 10%). Normally, a lighter colored eye becomes darker when extensive loss of iris stroma occurs, exposing the darker pigment epithelial layer.

  Iris sphincter atrophy may cause an irregular-shaped pupil. White iris nodules may be seen along the pupillary border and in the iris stroma.

  Fine vessels may be seen on the iris surface, especially in the angle. Neovascularization of the iris and the anterior chamber angle (radial and circumferential) occurs in 6% to 22% of cases. Posterior synechiae are never present.
- Trabecular meshwork: Fine blood vessels may be seen on the trabecular meshwork. These may bleed unexpectedly when the intraocular pressure suddenly drops during surgery or paracentesis.
- Lens: Nearly, 80% to 90% of cases develop a posterior subcapsular cataract, which matures rapidly.
- Vitreous: Fine vitreous opacities are observed.
- Retina: The absence of cystoid macular edema distinguishes Fuch's heterochromic iridocyclitis from other uveitis syndromes with chronic vitritis. Chorioretinal scars have been reported in some patients.
- Intraocular pressure: Secondary glaucoma is a frequent complication and can be presented in 15% to 59% of cases.

Posner Schlossman Syndrome (Glaucomatocyclitic Crisis)

Posner Schlossman syndrome is characterized by recurrent episodes of unilateral uveitis associated with corneal edema and increase in intraocular pressure out of proportion to the uveitis.

Age: It typically affects people between the age of 20–50 years.

Sex: Males and females are equally affected.

Laterality: Generally, only one eye is affected at one time,

Pathogenesis

The exact etiology of glaucomatocyclitic crisis is not known.

Factors that have been postulated as contributors to the development of glaucomatocyclitic crisis and include the following: Abnormal vascular process, autonomic defect, allergic condition, cytomegalovirus (CMV), Herpes simplex virus and variation of developmental glaucoma.

Clinical Features

It is characterized by recurrent episodes of unilateral uveitis with elevation of IOP which is out of proportion and lasts from a period of hours to days.

Symptoms

Patient complains of blurring of vision with haloes and sometimes pain.

Signs:

- *Conjunctiva:* The eye is quiet with no or minimal ciliary flush.
- *Cornea:* If the IOP is above 40 mm Hg, the cornea can become edematous. Fine KPs can appear after 2–3 days of inflammation and resolve rapidly.
- *Anterior chamber:* Minimal flare might be present and cells are generally absent.
- *Iris:* Segmental ischemia may be present. Posterior synechiae may be present.
- *IOP:* It is generally elevated and in the range of 40–60 mm Hg. It is related to the number of days of uveitis and not to the severity of uveitis.

LENS-ASSOCIATED UVEITIS

Uveitis which results from immune reaction to lens material is called lens-associated uveitis. This can occur either through the leakage of lens material through intact capsule as occurs in hypermature cataract or following the rupture of lens capsule (traumatic or surgical).

Pathogenesis

It is thought to be an autoimmune reaction to lens protein because of altered tolerance. The first episode generally occurs insidiously but once the patient has got sensitized to the lens protein, e.g. following cataract surgery in one eye, the immune reaction occurs rapidly in the other eye following exposure to lens protein.

Clinical Features

Symptoms: Patient complains of redness, blurring of vision and pain.

Signs: Both, granulomatous (Fig. 22.25) and nongranulomatous uveitis may occur. The anterior chamber reaction may vary

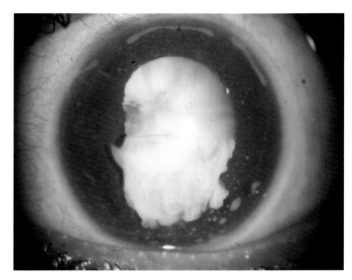

Fig. 22.25: Lens-induced uveitis: Slit-lamp photograph shows granulomatous reaction

from mild to severe depending on the amount of lens protein. Posterior synechiae formation occurs and IOP is quite often elevated.

INTERMEDIATE UVEITIS

Intermediate uveitis refers to inflammation localized to the vitreous and peripheral retina. According to the latest SUN criteria, the primary site of inflammation is the vitreous. The term intermediate uveitis includes pars planitis, posterior cyclitis and hyalites.

Pars planitis is considered a subset of intermediate uveitis and is characterized by the presence of white exudates (snow-banks) over the pars plana and ora serrata or by aggregates of inflammatory cells in the vitreous (snowballs) in the absence of an infectious etiology (e.g. Lyme disease) or a systemic disease (e.g. sarcoidosis). This primary form accounts for over 50% of patients with intermediate uveitis.

Age: Although intermediate uveitis can develop at any age, it primarily afflicts children and young adults. There is a bimodal distribution with one peak in the second decade and another peak in the third or fourth decade. Most of the patients are < 40 years.

In the pediatric age group, intermediate uveitis is associated with a worse presenting visual acuity. Poorer outcomes may be related to delayed presentation/diagnosis, the inherent difficulties of immunosuppression in children or a more aggressive disease.

Sex: Males and females are equally affected.

Laterality: It is bilateral in 80% of the cases.

Incidence: Intermediate uveitis accounts for almost 20% of pediatric uveitis cases. The incidence was found to be 2000/100,000 in one study.

Genetics: HLA-DR2 and B 8 have been associated with intermediate uveitis. Recently, there have been studies showing that cytokine gene polymorphisms may play a role in determining the prognosis of intermediate uveitis. The TT homozygote for Interferon-gamma may be at a higher risk for disease development and may also develop a more severe form of disease.

Pathogenesis

The inciting agent in intermediate uveitis is not known. It could be a variety of factor, which leads to an immune response against the self antigen. This leads to vasculitis or vitritis, which is responsible for intermediate uveitis.

Associations

Intermediate uveitis is idiopathic in a vast majority of the cases. It is also associated with MS, sarcoidosis and inflammatory bowel disease. Infectious etiologies include Epstein-Barr virus (EBV) infection, Lyme disease, human T-cell lymphotrophic virus type1 (HTLV-1) infection, cat scratch disease and Hepatitis C.

Clinical Features

Symptoms: Blurring of vision and floaters are the main complaints. The vision though reduced remains 6/12 in more than 80% of the cases. Pain and photophobia are characteristically absent.

Signs:

- Anterior uveitis is uncommon. Rarely, granulomatous anterior uveitis occurs in patients with sarcoidosis, especially in the pediatric age group.
- Aggregates of inflammatory cells may appear in the inferior vitreous as white or yellow tufts termed vitreous snowballs. (Fig. 22.26) Scleral depression is usually required to appreciate snowbanks, (Fig. 22.27), but sometimes they can be seen

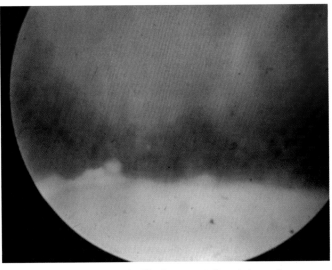

Fig. 22.27: Parsplanitis: Representative photograph shows snow banking

by asking the patient to look down and using an indirect ophthalmoscope without the 20 D lens.

- Often, a grayish white membrane might be seen extending inferiorly at the pars plana and is called snow banking. In certain cases, they may be more posterior and vascularized. For example, HTLV-1 infection. Vitritis is usually present. Periphlebitis may occur, but is often obscured by the vitritis. Periarteritis is less common. Peripheral retinal neovascularization can occur as a result of ischemia, causing vitreous hemorrhages; this occurs more commonly in children.

Complications

Cystoid macular edema occurs in 28% to 50% of cases. Epiretinal membrane formation may occur (Fig. 22.28). Optic nerve edema may occur especially in the pediatric age group. Anterior and posterior synechiae, band keratopathy (Fig. 22.29),

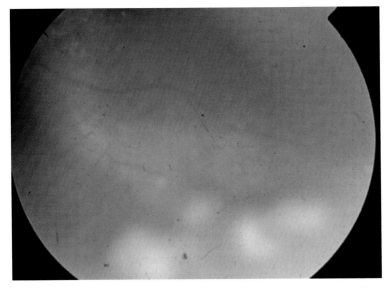

Fig. 22.26: Intermediate uveitis: Color fundus photograph shows snow ball vitreous opacities.

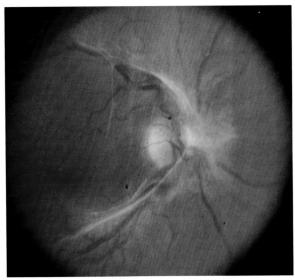

Fig. 22.28: Intermediate uveitis: Epiretinal membrane formation

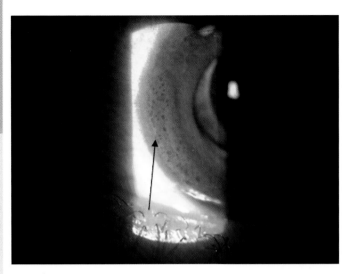

Fig. 22.29: Intermediate uveitis: Slit-lamp photograph shows band-shaped keratopathy (arrow) in a child

cataracts and glaucoma can occur. Glaucoma may be related to both the uveitis and/or corticosteroid use. Retinal detachment may occur in 3 to 22% cases. Some detachments may become complete, leading to a phthisical eye.

Investigations

Serological: This includes Serum ACE, serum lysozyme, serum calcium and phosphorous and QuantiFERON-TB Gold test.

Radiological: X-ray chest PA view, gallium scanning to rule out sarcoidosis. MRI brain is done to rule out multiple sclerosis.

Fluorescein angiography: If cystoid macular edema is present, then late stages will show typical petalloid edema.

Optical coherence tomography: To detect the presence of cystoid macular edema.

Histopathology

The snowbanks are predominantly a combination of collapsed vitreous, blood vessels, inflammatory cells (mainly lymphocytes), fibroblasts and glial elements.

Differential Diagnosis

Intermediate uveitis is a clinical entity that can occur in a variety of diseases or caused by a number of organisms. The following need to be kept in mind: multiple sclerosis, sarcoidosis, Lyme's disease, HTLV-1 infection and cat scratch disease.

Conditions that might not have snow ball opacities and snow banking, but might mimic intermediate uveitis because of the vitritis include intraocular lymphoma and Toxocara granuloma.

Management

Kaplan's modified four step approach is followed in the management of intermediate uveitis, which includes periocular steroids, oral steroids, immunosuppressives and finally cryotherapy or surgery.

Periocular Steroid

It remains the first line of management. Injection triamcinolone acetonide is given in the superotemporal sub-Tenon's space. The dose is 1 ml (40 mg) in adults and 0.5 ml (20 mg) in children.

A drop of paracaine and povidone iodine is instilled in the conjunctival cul-de-sac. The patient is asked to look down and towards the nose. An ear bud soaked in paracaine is held over the proposed site of injection. Then the 26-gauge needle is passed in the sub-Tenon's space with the bevel facing upwards and with side-to-side movements. If the eyeball starts moving with the movement of the needle, it is an indication that the needle is in the sclera.

The injection can be given 3–4 times at least four weeks apart. The intraocular pressure of the patient needs to be monitored as some patients might be steroid responders. Also, if the injection has been given anteriorly, there is the chance of cataract formation and in rare cases phthisis bulbi.

Oral Steroids

It can be given, if the patient has bilateral intermediate uveitis or the patient is not responding to periocular steroids. Steroids are given in the dose of 1mg/kg/day. It is generally tapered off by 10 mg every week and then maintained at a 10 mg dose for a period of at least 2–3 months. The tapering differs from case to case.

Immunosuppressive Agents

These are used only if the patient is not responding to the above lines of management. Azathioprine or cyclosporine is the drug mainly used. These drugs are given in the dose of 2–3 mg/kg/day and tapered slowly over a period of 4–6 months. The patient has to undergo complete blood counts, liver function tests and renal function tests every two weeks.

Topical Steroids

They have to be used, if the patient has anterior uveitis. Intravitreal triamcinolone acetonide, intravitreal bevacizumab and fluocinolone acetonide implant have been tried.

Newer drugs like daclizumab (monoclonal antibody against IL–2) are under study.

Management of the complications has to be done as and when they occur.

Prognosis

Most of the patients present with vision better than 20/40 and if treated on time most patients improve. The presentation and prognosis is worse in the pediatric age group.

WHITE DOT SYNDROMES

White dot syndrome comprises of a group of inflammatory conditions, affecting the retina and the choroids, which gives the appearance of multiple white dots.

Acute Posterior Multifocal Placoid Pigment Epitheliopathy

It is characterized by the appearance of multiple yellowish dot like lesions affecting the posterior pole. The disease is seen in younger age group (average age is 27 years), with no sex predilection. Generally, both the eyes are involved simultaneously. Almost, 1/3 of the patients have prodromal symptoms like myalgia, headache and sore throat.

Pathogenesis

It is believed to be due to obstructive vasculitis of the choroidal vessels.

Clinical Features

Symptoms: Generally, present with mild blurring of vision, especially if the posterior pole is involved. Anterior uveitis and vitreous cells are present in almost 50% of the cases.

Signs: There are presence of multiple yellowish-colored inflammatory lesions, affecting the retina, retinal pigment epithelium and choroid. Rarely, there can be serous retinal detachment. Disc hyperemia and papillitis with a neuroretinitis like picture can also be seen (Fig. 22.30A). The lesions resolve, leaving multiple chorioretinal scars.

Investigations

Fluorescein angiography: Multiple hypofluorescent spots in the early phase, which become hyperfluorescent in the late stage (Figs 22.30B and C).

Prognosis

Almost 50% of the patients have recurrences.

Treatment

These patients need a trial of corticosteroids.

Multiple Evanescent White Dot Syndrome.

Multiple evanescent white dot syndrome (MEWDS) is characterized by the appearance of multiple yellowish dot like lesions outside the macula at the posterior pole. The lesions are smaller compared to acute posterior multifocal placoid pigment epitheliopathy. It is seen in younger age group (average age is 27 years), more commonly in females. Generally, only one eye gets affected. Almost 1/3 of the patients have prodromal symptoms like myalgia, headache and sore throat.

Pathogenesis

It is believed to be due to viral etiology.

Clinical Features

Symptoms: Patients generally, present with mild blurring of vision especially if the posterior pole is involved.

Signs: There is the presence of multiple yellowish colored inflammatory lesions affecting the retina and retinal pigment epithelium. They range in size from 100–300 µm. Disc edema, vitritis and vasculitis can also occur. A characteristic feature of MEWDS is the presence of foveal granularity. The lesions resolve without leaving scars.

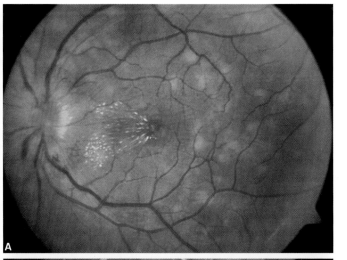

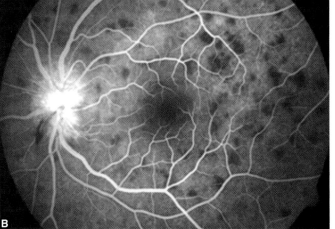

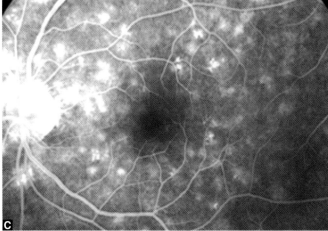

Figs 22.30A to C: Acute Posterior Multifocal Placoid Pigment Epitheliopathy. (A) Fundus photograph shows multiple placoid choroidal lesions with neuroretinitis like picture. (B and C) Fluorescein angiography shows early hypofluorescence with late hyperfluorescence

Investigations

Fluorescein angiography: Multiple areas of punctuate hyperfluorescence, which stain in the later phases.

Automated perimetry: Enlargement of the blind spot, which persists even after the resolution of the lesions.

Prognosis

The lesions resolve spontaneously in 4−8 weeks. Recurrences are uncommon.

Treatment

These patients do not need corticosteroids.

Birdshot Retinochoroidopathy

Introduction

It is also known as vitiliginous choroidopathy. It has strong HLA-A29 association. It is seen in middle age group (40−50 years), more commonly in females.

Clinical Features

Symptoms: Generally, present with mild blurring of vision, photopsiaes and loss of color vision.

Signs: Presence of multiple depigmented yellowish white-colored lesions radiating from the optic disc along the larger choroidal vessels (Fig. 22.31). Disc edema, vitritis and cystoid macular edema can also occur.

Investigations

Fluorescein angiography: Isofluorescent in the early phases and hyperfluorescent in the later phases is seen.

Prognosis

Multiple recurrences are known to occur.

Treatment

These patients need a trial of steroids.

Multifocal Choroiditis with Panuveitis

Multifocal choroiditis with panuveitis is characterized by the appearance of multiple yellowish dot like lesions and significant anterior uveitis and vitritis. It is seen in middle age group (average age is 33 years), more commonly in females and myopes. Bilateral involvement is common (up to 75%).

Pathogenesis

It is believed to be due to viral etiology (Epstein-Barr virus).

Clinical Features

Symptoms: Generally present with mild blurring of vision, photopsiae and floaters, especially if the posterior pole is involved.

Signs: There is the presence of multiple yellowish colored inflammatory lesions, affecting the retina, retinal pigment epithelium and choroid (Fig. 22.32). The lesions range in size from 100−1000 μm. They affect the mid periphery and the nasal quadrant. They can be arranged in clusters or in a linear pattern. Disc edema, vitritis, cystoid macular edema and vasculitis can also occur. The lesions resolve leaving variably pigmented chorioretinal scars.

Complications

Complications like choroidal neovascular membrane and peripapillary subretinal fibrosis can occur.

Investigations

Fluorescein angiography: Multiple areas of hypofluorescence, which hyperfluoresce in the later phases are present.

Prognosis

Recurrences are common.

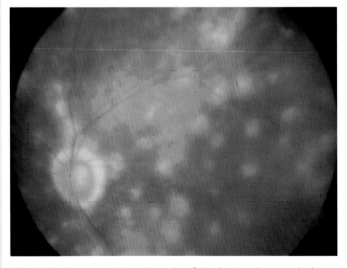

Fig. 22.31: Birdshot chorioretinopathy: Color fundus photograph shows multiple yellow choroidal lesions

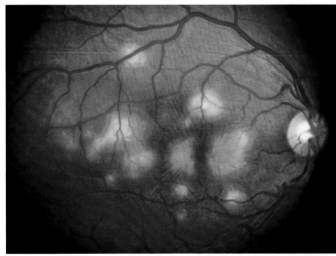

Fig. 22.32: Multifocal choroiditis: Fundus photograph shows multiple yellowish dot like lesions

Treatment

These patients need oral corticosteroids and topical steroids, if patient has cells in the anterior chamber. If patient develops choroidal neovascular membrane (Figs 22.33A to C) laser photocoagulation or anti-VEGF therapy may be required.

Punctate Inner Choroidopathy

It is characterized by the appearance of multiple yellowish dot like lesions characteristically at the posterior pole. It is seen in younger age group, more commonly in females and myopes. Bilateral involvement is common.

Pathogenesis

It is believed to be due to viral etiology (Epstein-Barr virus).

Clinical Features

Symptoms: Generally, present with mild blurring of vision, photopsiae, especially if the posterior pole is involved.

Signs: Presence of multiple yellowish-colored inflammatory lesions, affecting the retina, retinal pigment epithelium and choroid. They range in size from 100–300 μm. They affect the posterior pole. The lesions resolve leaving variably pigmented chorioretinal scars. Anterior segment inflammation, vitritis and cystoid macular edema are typically absent. Complications like choroidal neovascular membrane and peripapillary subretinal fibrosis can occur.

Investigations

Fluorescein angiography: Multiple areas of hypofluorescence, which stain in the later phases are seen.

Optical coherence tomography: Choroidal neovascular membranes are detected easily.

Prognosis

In 33% of cases, choroidal neovascular membrane may develop, hence the prognosis is variable.

Treatment

These patients need oral corticosteroids and topical steroids, if patient has cells in the anterior chamber. If patient develops

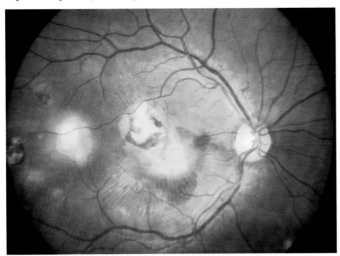

Fig. 22.33A: Multifocal choroiditis: Fundus photograph shows active choroidal neovascular membrane

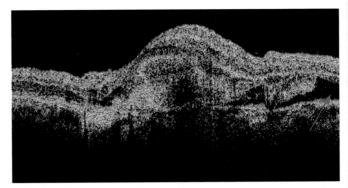

Fig. 22.33D: OCT scan passing through the CNVM shows disrupted retinal pigment epithelium with fibrovascular complex and scar. Note the PED (↑)

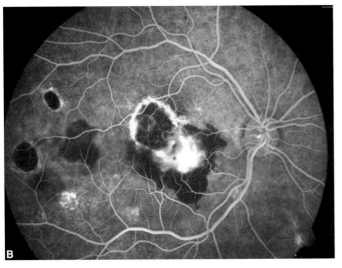

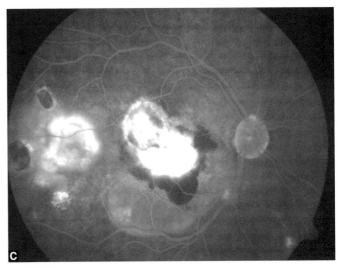

Figs 22.33B and C: Fluorescein angiography shows early hypofluorescence with late hyperfluorescence and leak in a case of active choroidal neovascular membrane

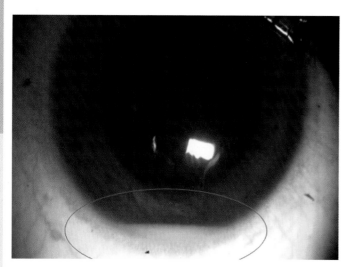

Fig. 22.34: Behçet's disease: Slit-lamp photograph showing hypopyon in the case of panuveitis

choroidal neovascular membrane, laser photocoagulation and anti-VEGF therapy may be us.

PANUVEITIS CONDITIONS

Behçet's Syndrome

It is a multisystemic autoimmune disorder, characterized by generalized occlusive vasculitis. The classic triad of Behcet's syndrome is acute iritis with mobile hypopyon, (Fig. 22.34) oral and genital ulcers.

Age: Generally affects people in the 2nd to 4th decade.

Sex: Males are more affected than females.

Distribution: It is more common in the people from Turkey and Japan and in the region of the "Old Silk route".

Incidence: The incidence is 80–370/100,000 in Turkey, 2–30/100,000 in East Asia and 0.12–0.33 in US.

Genetics: HLA-B51 positivity is seen in 55% of patients with Behcet's in Japan, but just the presence of HLA-B51 positivity does not increase the risk of having the disease. In addition, susceptible group is also required. For example, the relative risk of disease among HLA-B51 patients is 6.7 in Japan, but only 1.3 in US.

Pathogenesis

Microbial organisms like herpes simplex or Streptococcus sanguis triggers type 2 hypersensitivity and autoimmune reaction in a genetically susceptible patient.

Clinical Features

Oral and genital ulcers: (Figs 22.35 A and B) Oral ulcers are the commonest and the earliest sign of Behçet's disease. They are recurrent, round with surrounding erythema and pesudomembranous covering and painful. They heal in 10 days.

Skin manifestations: They are the second commonest after oral ulcers and were found to be present in 87% patients in one study. Erythema nodosum, a reddish painful nodule with subcutaneous induration commonly found on the legs, faces, arms and buttocks is the commonest skin presentation. They involute in 10–14 days without scarring and leave some hyperpigmentation. Other skin lesions include subcutaneous thrombophlebitis, acneiform lesions and follicular rash.

CNS involvement: It is seen in 10% patients and includes headache, meningismus, nystagmus, tremor, ataxia, speech disturbances, memory loss and dementia.

Sensorineural hearing loss, tinnitus and vertigo: These features may herald the onset of the disease. High frequency sounds are typically lost.

International Study Group Criteria

Presence of recurrent painful oral ulcers with at least any two of the following:
- Recurrent genital ulceration
- Eye lesions
- Skin lesions
- Positive pathergy test

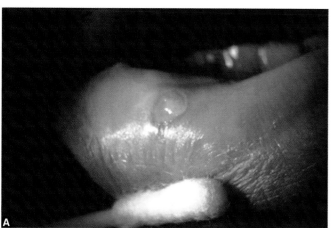

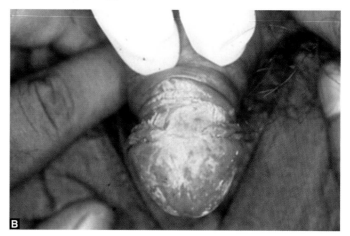

Figs 22.35A and B: Behçet's disease: Photograph shows aphthous and genital ulcers in a patient

Ocular Features

It can present with panuveitis. Hypopyon in Behcet's disease is typically transient and mobile. Both arteritis and phlebitis can be seen. It can have varied presentations, such as choroiditis, retinitis, occlusive vasculitis (Fig. 22.36), severe vitritis and disc edema.

Treatment

Cyclosporine is the drug of choice. Patients have to be treated on a long-term basis with systemic steroids and immunosuppressives.

SARCOIDOSIS

Sarcoidosis is an inflammatory multisystemic granulomatous disease of unknown etiology.

Although it predominantly affects the lungs, the illness often manifests within the eye.

The word "sarcoid" is derived from the Greek words, "sark" and "oid," which mean "flesh like" and were used to describe the skin lesions of sarcoidosis.

Age: Commonly affected age group is 20–40 years.

Sex: Females are said to be more affected than males.

Distribution: Sarcoidosis is a relatively common disease with worldwide distribution. Sarcoidosis tends to be more severe and chronic in the American blacks, with a higher risk of extrathoracic manifestations.

Incidence: The incidence ranges from 107 per 100,000 in African black women to 3–50 per 100,000 in Europe to 2 per 100,000 in Japan. Between 25% to 50% of the patients with sarcoidosis exhibit ocular inflammatory disease. Sarcoidosis accounts for 3% to 10% of all cases of uveitis.

Pathogenesis

It has been theorized to be due to immune dysregulation to a persistent antigen of low virulence that is poorly cleared by the immune system, leading to a chronic Th1 subtype response, which results in granuloma formation with increased B-cell activity with hypergammaglobulinemia.

Proposed Antigens

Infectious

Bacterial: M. tuberculosis, *Mycoplasma* spp, *P. acnes.*

Viral: Herpes simplex virus, hepatitis C virus, Epstein-Barr virus.

Fungal: Histoplasma species, *Cryptococcus* species

Environmental metals (e.g. zirconium, aluminum and beryllium)

Organic dusts (e.g. pine and pollen)

Inorganic dusts (e.g. clay, soil and talc).

Clinical Features

It is a noncaseating epithelioid granuloma that may affect any organ system, including

- *Skin, hair and mucosa:* Lupus Pernio, a plaque like lesion involving the face. Other skin lesions include nodules, plaques, psoriasiform lesions, papules, ulcerations and erythema nodosum (Figs 22.37A and B)
- *Central nervous system:* Sarcoid granulomas affect the basal leptomeninges in 5% to 10% patients. They can affect the cerebrum and lead to weakness, affect cranial nerves, affect hypothalamus and thalamus, affect spinal cord and lead to paralysis.
- *Pulmonary involvement:*
  Stage 1: Hilar lymphadenopathy
  Stage 2: Hilar lymphadenopathy and parenchymal involvement
  Stage 3: Only parenchymal involvement
  Stage 4: Pulmonary fibrosis
- Cardiac defects like conduction defects and arrhythmias occur in 5% patients.
- Hepatic, splenic and bone involvement may be there.
- Hypercalcemia, hypercalciuria in 17% patients and is associated with the increased risk of nephrocalcinosis.

Symptoms

Symptoms exacerbate during winter and early spring. Constitutional symptoms depend upon the system affected.

The commonest ocular manifestation of sarcoidosis is intermediate uveitis, which can present with blurring of vision and floaters.

Signs

- Conjunctival granulomatous nodules and keratoconjunctivitis sicca. Interstitial keratitis and band keratopathy and scleritis are rare although cataracts occur frequently.
- Anterior uveitis is seen in 6% of patients and patients have mutton fat keratic precipitates, Koeppe and Busacca nodules.

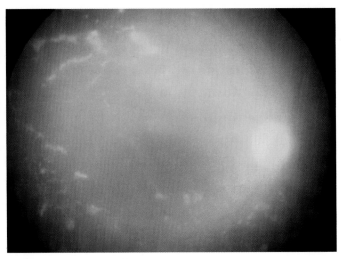

Fig. 22.36: Behçet's disease: Fundus photograph showing severe vitritis

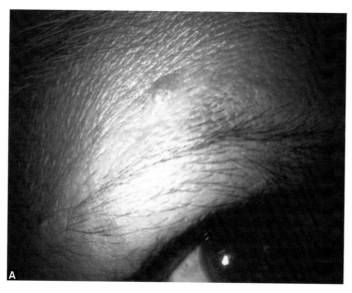 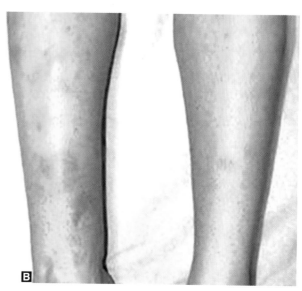

Figs 22.37A and B: Sarcoidosis: Skin lesions

- 360 degree posterior synechiae might be present leading to extensive iris bombe formation.
- Peripheral anterior synechiae may be present giving rise to narrow-angle glaucoma.
- Lacrimal gland involved in 15% to 28%.
- Snow ball opacities might be seen in the peripheral vitreous and snow banking might be present.
- Posterior segment involvement is rare compared to anterior segment involvement. Granulomas measuring 1/4 to 1 disc diameter are seen in both the retina and the choroid (Fig. 22.38).
- Multiple small or irregular large with ameboid pattern subretinal choroidal infiltrates might be present.
- Irregular nodular granuloma seen along the retinal veins gives rise to the "candle wax" or "tache de bougies" appearance (Fig. 22.39).

- Preretinal granuloma located inferiorly anterior to the equator is called "Lander's sign" (Fig. 22.39).

Some of the syndromes identified with ophthalmic sarcoidosis include:

Heerfordt Syndrome: Uveitis, which may precede parotid enlargement and occasionally papilledema.

Löfgren Syndrome: It includes erythema nodosum, bilateral hilar adenopathy and arthralgias.

Investigations

Serological: Serum ACE levels, serum calcium and phosphorous and serum lysozyme levels should be done. Though, they might be elevated in a lot of granulomatous conditions, a positive result along with clinical findings and positive chest X-ray is very helpful in clinching the diagnosis of sarcoidosis.

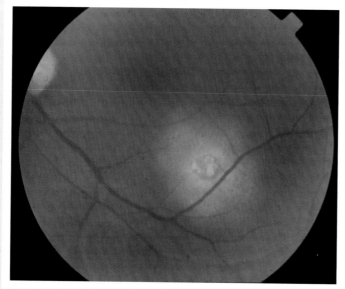

Fig. 22.38: Ocular sarcoidosis: Fundus photograph shows choroidal granuloma

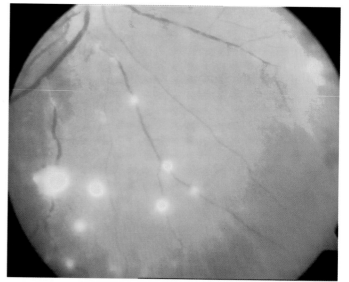

Fig. 22.39: Ocular sarcoidosis: Fundus photograph shows candle wax drippings and preretinal granulomata

Radiological: X-ray chest PA view should be done. Hilar lymphadenopathy of pulmonary granuloma can be detected. High-resolution computed tomography (HRCT) is more diagnostic. Gallium scan of the head and the neck might be useful.

Histopathology: A biopsy of the involved organ might show the presence of noncaseating epitheloid cell granuloma. The granuloma consists of epitheloid cells, multinucleated giant cells of the Langerhans type and a thin rim of lymphocytes. Inclusion bodies present in the cytoplasm of the giant cells include Schaumann bodies and Asteroid bodies.

Treatment

Mainstay of treatment is corticosteroid therapy. The controversy remains, however, concerning the efficacy of corticosteroids to alter the natural course of the disease. For refractory disease, methotrexate is reported to control the activity.

Current therapy is targeted at tumor necrosis factor, which has been shown to be highly expressed in patients with sarcoidosis. Evidence shows a high level of tumor necrosis factor in sarcoidosis (produced by alveolar macrophages). Successful therapy for sarcoidosis with either a corticosteroid or methotrexate has been associated with a decrease in the amount of tumor necrosis factor, released by alveolar macrophages. In a study of patients with refractory sarcoidosis who were not responding to corticosteroid therapy, tumor necrosis factor, released by alveolar macrophages was not suppressed by systemic therapy. This has lead to the use of anti-tumor necrosis factor biologicals, such as infliximab with good outcomes.

Vitrectomy is indicated in the following situations:
- Differentiation of sarcoidosis from intraocular malignancy
- Cases with persistent vitreous hemorrhage
- Resistant vitreous opacities.

The effect of the removal of the vitreous on intraocular inflammation and on cystoid macular edema has not yet been proved.

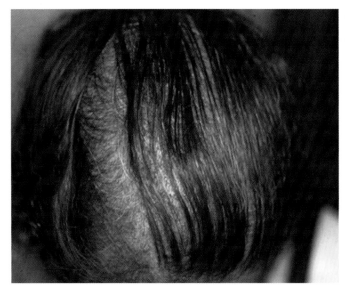

Fig. 22.40: Vogt-Koyanagi-Harada's disease: External photograph shows severe alopecia in a young female

VOGT-KOYANAGI-HARADA'S SYNDROME

Vogt-Koyanagi-Harada's syndrome (VKH) is so named after three different clinicians who described this clinical entity at different points of times.

It has been divided into complete VKH and incomplete VKH and diagnostic criteria have been set. It affects the following major organ systems: central nervous system (meningismus, cerebrospinal fluid: pleiocytosis), ear (dysacusis, tinnitus), skin-vitiligo (Fig. 22.2), alopecia (Fig. 22.40) and eye-panuveitis and poliosis (Figs 22.41A and B).

Pathogenesis

There is a strong HLA DR 4 association, especially in Japanese population. Development of autoimmunity against proteins like tyrosinase or S 100 protein present in the melanin has

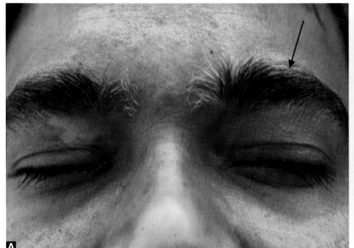
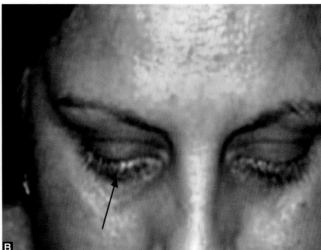

Figs 22.41A and B: Vogt-Koyanagi-Harada's disease: External photograph shows poliosis (arrow)

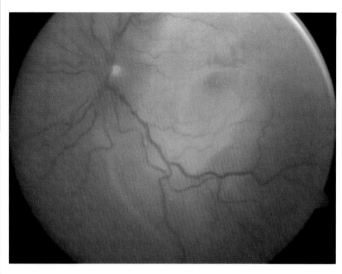

Fig. 22.42: Vogt-Koyanagi-Harada's disease: Fundus photograph shows disc edema with exudative retinal detachment

been implicated. This autoimmunity can be triggered by a viral infection or cutaneous injury.

Clinical Features

It has the following stages:

Prodromal stage: The patient experiences headache, nausea, dizziness and meningismus for a few days, followed by increased light sensitivity for 1 to 2 days.

Uveitic stage: Patient complains of blurring of vision and develops bilateral panuveitis. First, one is involved and very soon the other eye gets involved.

- There is thickening of the choroids and elevation of the retinochoroidal layer, especially in the peripapillary region (Fig. 22.42).
- There are multiple exudative retinal detachments.

- Fundus fluorescein angiogram shows pin point hyperflourescence in the early and mid phase and pooling in the subretinal space in the late phase (Figs 22.43A and B).
- There are also multiple areas of retinal pigment epithelium alteration, which are appreciated better on angiogram as areas of hyperfluorescence.
- Soon, the inflammation spills over to the anterior chamber and cells and flare can be detected.
- Rarely, mutton fat keratic precipitates and nodules are seen.

Chronic/convalescent stage: This occurs weeks to months after the uveitic stage. It is characterized by

- Depigmentation of the perilimbal area: Sugiura's sign.
- Depigmentation of the choroids, especially in the inferior mid periphery.
- Also, the disc becomes paler and the surrounding choroids appear yellowish orange giving rise to the "Sunset glow" fundus appearance (Fig. 22.44).

Chronic recurrent stage: This is characterized by recurrence of posterior uveitis without development of exudative detachments. Also, mutton fat keratic precipitates and iris nodules are seen. The patient may develop complications like cataract, glaucoma, subretinal fibrosis and choroidal neovascular membrane.

Pathology

Thickening of the peripapillary choroid is observed. This is associated with the presence of granulomatous infiltration of choroid. There is the presence of Dalen Fuchs nodules, which are focal aggregates of epithelioid histiocytes below the retinal pigment epithelium.

Differential Diagnosis

- *Sympathetic ophthalmia:* Shows the presence of the bilateral posterior uveitis, but can be distinguished by the history of trauma.

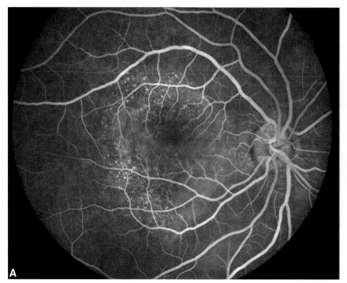

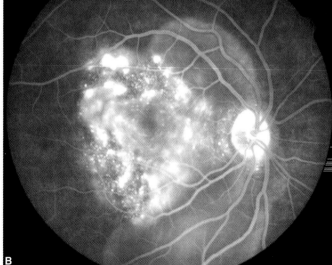

Figs 22.43A and B: Vogt-Koyanagi-Harada's disease: Fundus fluorescein angiogram showing early pinpoint hyperfluorescence and late pooling of dye

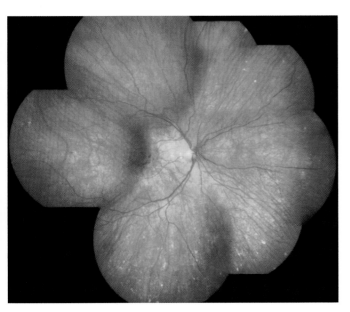

Fig. 22.44: Vogt-Koyanagi-Harada's disease: Montage fundus photograph shows sunset glow appearance in convalescent phase

- *Uveal effusion syndrome:* There can be the presence of exudative detachments, but there is characteristic absence of inflammatory cells.
- *Posterior scleritis:* Can be distinguished on ultrasonography by the thickening of the sclera and the widening of the sub-Tenon's space.
- Acute posterior multifocal placoid pigment epitheliopathy
- Intraocular lymphoma and
- Sarcoidosis.

Prognosis

Depends on the following factors:

- Initial visual acuity: Better the initial visual acuity, better the prognosis
- *Age:* More advanced the age, worse the prognosis
- *Duration of disease:* Longer the course of the disease, worse the prognosis
- Complications

Treatment

When the patient presents initially, IV methylprednisolone (1 gm/day) can be given to the patient. Patient is then put on a course of topical and oral steroids (1 mg/kg/day) with gradual tapering. The treatment has to be carried out for a period of at least 6 months with close monitoring. If the patient does not seem to be responding or develops complications to steroids then immunosuppressives like azathioprine (2.5 mg/kg/day) or cyclosporine (5 mg/kg/day) can be added to the regime. Complications need to be managed when they develop.

SYMPATHETIC OPHTHALMIA

Sympathetic ophthalmia is a bilateral inflammatory condition of the eyes that follows an inciting penetrating injury (Fig. 22.45) or surgery to one or both eyes. It almost invariably follows a penetrating wound involving uveal tissue produced by either ocular trauma or intraocular surgery. Sympathetic ophthalmia also may occur with laser ciliary ablation procedures, particularly direct contact lasers and after pars plana vitrectomy. It is called "sympathetic ophthalmia" as the normal eye is said to be sympathizing with the affected eye.

Age: Can occur at any age.

Sex: Males are more commonly affected as they are more likely to suffer from penetrating injury. Following surgery, males and females are equally affected.

Incidence: The incidence is variable and the reported incidence appears to be declining with time. This decline may be due to increased knowledge of the disease and enhanced ability to diagnose other ocular inflammatory diseases, which were wrongly attributed to sympathetic ophthalmia. The incidence appears to be 0.2% to 0.5% after penetrating ocular injuries and 0.01% after intraocular surgery.

Genetics: Expression of HLA-A11 antigen has been shown to be more frequently found in patients with sympathetic ophthalmia. HLA-DRB1*04, DQA1*03 and DRB1*04 have been shown to be associated with sympathetic ophthalmia among the Japanese, British and Irish patients. These data suggest that genetic predisposition may contribute to the development of the disease.

Pathogenesis

The etiology is not clearly understood. It is postulated that when an uveoretinal antigen, such as Retinal S-antigen is released either by penetrating injury or surgery, the immune system responds by delayed hypersensitivity reaction mediated by T-helper1 (Th1) cells. However, no antiretinal S-antigen antibody has been detected in patients with sympathetic ophthalmia. A curious finding in sympathetic ophthalmia is the lack of inflammation in the choriocapillaris. It is postulated that the

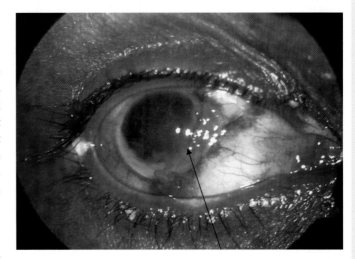

Fig. 22.45: Penetrating trauma: Clinical picture of the right eye with history of penetrating trauma shows corneoscleral tear, which has undergone primary repair

retinal pigment epithelium releases some factors that protect the choriocapillaris from the inflammatory mediators.

Clinical Features

After the inciting event, traumatic or surgical, bilateral intraocular inflammation has been reported to appear anytime between one week and 66 years. Eighty percent of cases manifest within three months and 90% occur within one year from the time of the initial insult.

Symptoms

They range from mild visual disturbance to significant visual loss. Near vision may be compromised, owing to change in accommodation.

Signs

Patients typically present with bilateral acute anterior uveitis associated with mutton-fat keratic precipitates. In the posterior segment, the extent of inflammation can vary. Patients may have vitritis, retinal vasculitis, choroiditis and papillitis. The extent of inflammation may sometimes be represented by serous retinal detachment and optic nerve swelling in affected patients (Figs 22.46A and B). White yellowish lesions can be seen at the level of the choroid in the peripheral fundus.

Complications

Cataract, glaucoma, choroidal neovascularization, subretinal fibrosis and atrophy of the optic nerve, retina or choroid.

Investigations

Fluorescein Angiography

If, Dalen-Fuchs nodules or vasculitis is present, lesions will fluoresce. Optic disc staining might be present in late stages even in the absence of clinical papillitis.

Indocyanine Green Angiography

It shows areas of hypofluorescence in intermediate phases, which disappear on treatment with steroids.

Histopathology

There is granulomatous inflammation throughout the uveal tissue, except for the choriocapillaris. The inflammatory cells involved are primarily lymphocytes, epithelioid cells and multinucleated giant cells. Dalen-Fuchs nodules, which are clumps of lymphocytes and epithelioid cells are found in approximately one-third of enucleated eyes just behind the retinal pigment epithelium. The retinal pigment epithelium generally remains normal.

Differential Diagnosis

The important differential diagnoses include Vogt-Koyanagi-Harada's syndrome, intraocular lymphoma and other conditions, which present as panuveitis. However, patient history recording will reveal previous penetrating ocular injury or intraocular surgery.

Vogt-Koyanagi-Harada's syndrome presents as bilateral granulomatous panuveitis with prominent choroidal involvement. Patients do not have a history of surgery or penetrating ocular injury. They have serous retinal detachment and optic nerve involvement more frequently than do patients with sympathetic ophthalmia. In addition, they may have skin and hair changes, such as vitiligo, alopecia or poliosis or such neurological symptoms as tinnitus, headache or mental status change.

Intraocular lymphoma, presents with vitreal cells and choroidal abnormality. If lymphoma is suspected, careful systemic workup, including neurological evaluation, should be performed. If necessary, a vitreous sample must be obtained for diagnostic purpose and IL-10/IL-6 ratio should be found.

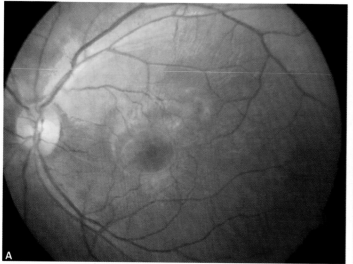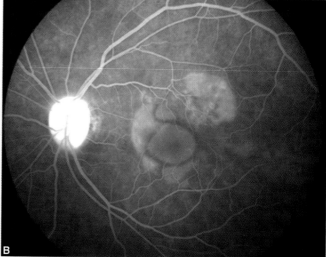

Figs 22.46A and B: Sympathetic ophthalmia: (A) Fundus photograph shows multiple pockets of fluid at the posterior pole, (B) Fluorescein angiography shows pooling of the dye in the late phase

Management

Prompt enucleation of the injured eye is known to be preventative of sympathetic ophthalmia. In general, the time frame required for this approach is believed to be within 2 weeks from the penetrating injury. The problem with this approach is that with current advanced surgical techniques, many eyes once considered nonviable may now have a fair prognosis. Furthermore, the incidence of sympathetic ophthalmitis from penetrating injury is decreasing.

The benefit of enucleation of the inciting eye, once the disease process is apparent in the sympathizing eye, is more controversial. Evaluation of the literature revealed reports of varying success rates.

The decision to enucleate a traumatized eye or an inciting eye should be made very cautiously. Not infrequently, the inciting eye may ultimately become the eye with the better vision.

Steroids are given intravenously, orally, topically and in the form of regional injection. Oral prednisone is most frequently employed. It is generally given at 1 to 2 mg/kg/day and tapered slowly over 3 to 4 months.

Successful use of cyclosporine-A in conjunction with prednisone has been reported. Favorable results with various combinations of cyclophosphamide, azathioprine and chlorambucil with or without steroids have also been observed. A combination of azathioprine and cyclosporine-A has been to be efficacious in the management of sympathetic ophthalmia.

UVEITIS ASSOCIATED WITH OTHER SYSTEMIC DISEASES

Juvenile Rheumatoid Arthritis

Juvenile rheumatoid arthritis is also known as juvenile idiopathic arthritis. Juvenile idiopathic arthritis, as defined by the American Rheumatism Association (ARA), is the presence of arthritis (chronic, seronegative and peripheral) before the age of 16 years, of at least 3 months duration, when other causes have been excluded (Fig. 22.47).

Classification

It is classified as follows:
1. *Oligoarticular (Pauciarticular) onset juvenile idiopathic arthritis* (40 to 60%): This is common in girls (5:1). Peak age of onset is at the age of 2 years. Four or fewer joints are involved during the first six months of the disease (often asymmetric). Oligoarticular onset commonly involves the knees and less frequently, the ankles and wrists. The arthritis may be evanescent, rarely destructive and radiologically insignificant. Approximately 75% of these patients test positive for antinuclear antibody. This mode of onset rarely is associated with systemic signs. A high risk for uveitis exists.
2. *Polyarticular onset juvenile idiopathic arthritis* (20 to 40%): This is common in girls (3:1). Peak age of onset is at the age of 3 years. It involves five or more joints during the first

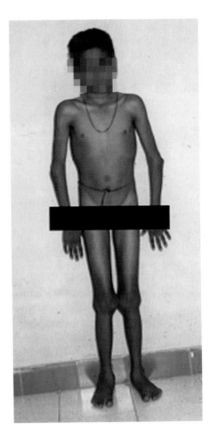

Fig. 22.47: Juvenile idiopathic arthritis: External photograph of a child with joint deformities

six months of the disease. Polyarticular onset juvenile idiopathic arthritis commonly involves the small joints of the hand and less frequently, the larger joints of the knee, ankle or wrist. Asymmetric arthritis may be acute or chronic and may be destructive in 15% of patients. Immunoglobulin M (IgM) rheumatoid factor is present in 10% of children with this juvenile idiopathic arthritis subgroup. It is associated with subcutaneous nodules, erosions and a poor prognosis.

Approximately 40% of these patients test positive for antinuclear antibodies. Systemic symptoms, including anorexia, anemia and growth retardation are moderate. An intermediate risk for uveitis exists.

3. *Systemic onset juvenile idiopathic arthritis* (10 to 20%): The disease occurs with equal frequency in boys and girls and can appear at any age. Symmetric polyarthritis is present and may be destructive in 25% of patients. Hands, wrists, feet, ankles, elbows, knees, hips, shoulders, cervical spine and jaw may be involved.

Antinuclear antibodies are positive in only 10% of the patients (Fig. 22.48). Systemic onset is associated with fever (high in evening and normal in morning), macular rash, leukocytosis, lymphadenopathy and hepatomegaly. Pericarditis, pleuritis, splenomegaly and abdominal pain less commonly are observed. A low risk for uveitis exists.

Risk factors for the development of uveitis in patients with juvenile idiopathic arthritis: Female gender, pauciarticular variety and antinuclear antibody positivity.

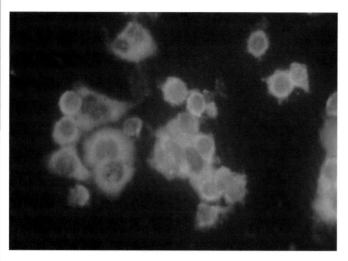

Fig. 22.48: Juvenile rheumatoid arthritis: Immunofluorescence study showing rim staining of antinuclear antibody

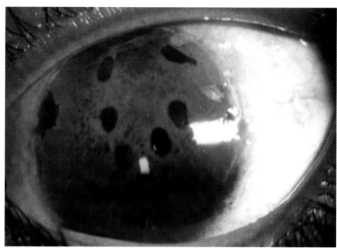

Fig. 22.49: Juvenile idiopathic arthritis with chronic uveitis: Slit-lamp photograph shows band-shaped keratopathy

Incidence: Around 10% of the cases with juvenile idiopathic arthritis develop uveitis.

Clinical Features

Symptoms

Patients complain of mild pain, photophobia and blurring of vision. Many a times, the patient is asymptomatic.

Signs

Anterior uveitis: The following signs can be observed in these cases:
- Cells and flare; chronic flare (very common)
- Nongranulomatous uveitis (> 90%)
- Bilateral (70% to 80%)
- Chronic smoldering or recurrent disease in greater than 90%

Conjunctiva and sclera: Most patients have no conjunctival injection even during acute exacerbations.

Cornea: The following signs can be seen in the cornea:
- Keratic precipitates—Small-medium, rarely mutton fat.
- Patient may develop band-shaped keratopathy with time (Fig. 22.49).

Iris: Signs such as posterior synechiae; pupillary membrane; and rarely Koeppe nodules may also develop.

Management

It includes the use of topical steroids and use of systemic steroids in cases, which are not responding to topical therapy. But, most patient have a chronic course and use of steroids can give rise to severe complications like growth retardation, hypertension and diabetes mellitus. So, steroid sparing agents like methotrexate are being tried in these patients.

Management of Cataract

Cataract surgery is contraindicated in young patients with juvenile idiopathic arthritis due to the high chances of severe postoperative inflammation and cystoid macular edema. Cataract surgery can be tried in older patients with juvenile idiopathic arthritis.

The following are few recommendations:
- Preoperatively the inflammation should have been absent for at least a period of three months.
- Heparin-coated intraocular lens should be used.
- Minimal intraoperative handling should be there.
- Combined lensectomy and vitrectomy can be tried in these patients.
- Postoperatively inflammation should be controlled aggressively and if required immunosuppressive therapy should be used.

PARASITIC UVEITIS

Toxoplasma Retinitis

Toxoplasmosis is caused by an obligate, intracellular protozoan *Toxoplasma gondi*. The cat is the definitive host that becomes infected by eating contaminated raw meat, wild birds or mice. The three forms of the protozoan, tachyzoites, bradyzoites and sporozoites are only present in the cat. Humans and other mammals are infected only by tachyzoites and bradyzoites.

Classification

Toxoplasmosis may be either congenital or acquired.

Congenital Toxoplasmosis

When a pregnant susceptible woman acquires primary toxoplasmosis, transplacental transmission of the parasite to the fetus may occur.

Acquired Toxoplasmosis

It can result from the following:

- Ingestion of tissue cysts from contaminated raw or under-cooked beef, lamb or pork.
- Ingestion of oocysts from soil, milk, water or vegetables.
- Inhalation of oocysts
- Contaminated blood transfusions, organ transplants and accidental inoculation acquired in the laboratory.

Age: Congenital toxoplasmosis generally presents after birth. Acquired toxoplasmosis can present at any time after birth though it has been reported to occur more commonly between the 2nd to the 4th decade.

Sex: Males and females are equally affected.

Laterality: No particular predilection for any eye has been noted.

Incidence: The incidence varies from place to place. Toxoplasmosis is said to be more common in hot and humid climates. Almost, 30% to 40% of the population has serum titres positive for toxoplasma antibodies.

Pathogenesis

When a cat becomes infected, the organism undergoes sexual reproduction in its intestine. As a consequence, a cat sheds millions of noninfectious unsporulated oocysts in its feces. Sporulation occurs in the next 3−4 days at room temperature. With sporulation, the oocyst becomes infective (sporozoite) for at least a year. Ingestion of the sporulated oocyst results in an acute infection.

The oocyst gives rise to tachyzoites, which reach the eye through the bloodstream. Here, depending on the host's immune status, a clinical or subclinical focus of infection begins in the retina. As the host's immune system responds and the tachyzoites convert themselves into bradyzoites, the cyst forms. The cyst is extremely resistant to the host's defenses and a chronic latent infection ensues.

If a subclinical infection is present, no funduscopic changes are observed. The cyst remains in the normal-appearing retina. Whenever the host's immune function declines for any reason, the cyst wall may rupture, releasing organisms into the retina and the inflammatory process restarts. If an active clinical lesion is present, healing occurs as a chorioretinal scar. The cyst often remains inactive within or adjacent to the scar.

Clinical Features

Symptoms: Blurring of vision and floaters are the main complaints. Rarely, the patient may complain of redness, pain and photophobia.

Signs: Congenital toxoplasmic lesion presents typically as a deep punched out scar sometimes mimicking a macular coloboma (Fig. 22.50).

Granulomatous and nongranulomatous anterior uveitis might be present with the distribution of the keratic precipitates

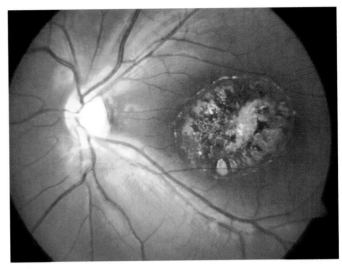

Fig. 22.50: Congenital toxoplasma retinochoroiditis: Fundus photograph shows a deep punched out scar

in the classic von Arlt's triangle. Some patients present with the stellate keratic precipitates pattern, characterized by a diffuse homogeneous distribution pattern and a stellate fibrillar keratic precipitates.

Dense vitritis may be present. The hallmark of the disease is a necrotizing retinochoroiditis, which is present at the posterior pole in more than 50% of the cases. This appearance is often referred to as the "headlight in the fog appearance" (Fig. 22.51). As the lesion heals, it appears as a punched-out scar, revealing white underlying sclera. This results from extensive retinal and choroidal necrosis surrounded by variable pigment proliferation.

Whenever, there is a recurrence, it usually occurs at the margin of the old chorioretinal scar (Figs 22.52A and B) (so-called satellite lesions) as live tissue cysts are located at the border of the scars.

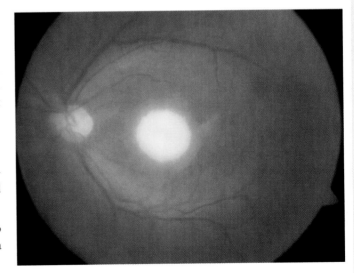

Fig. 22.51: Active toxoplasmic retinochoroiditis: Fundus photograph shows the classic "headlight in the fog" appearance.

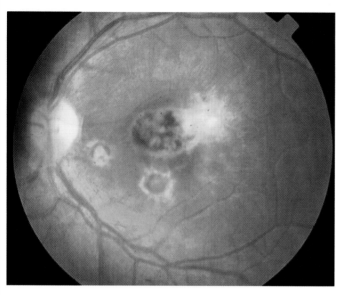

Fig. 22.52A: Recurrent toxoplasmic retinochoroiditis: Fundus photograph showing an active lesion adjacent to an old scar

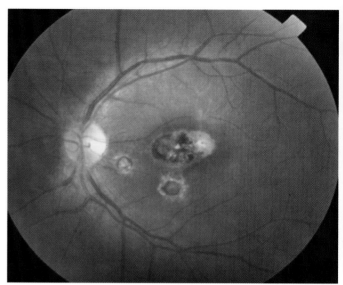

Fig. 22.52B: Resolving retinochoroiditis: Fundus photograph shows resolving retinochoroiditis at the edge of an old scar

When the optic nerve becomes involved by toxoplasmosis, the typical manifestation is optic neuritis or papillitis associated with edema, often called Jensen's disease.

Punctate outer toxoplasmosis has been described in the Japanese and American literature. This form of the disease is unique in that the classic large atrophic posterior lesions are not seen. Vasculitis may also be seen.

In immunocompromised patients, toxoplasmosis has an atypical presentation. There are multifocal areas of necrotizing retinochoroiditis.

Complications

Macular edema, neovascularization elsewhere, neovascularization of the disc and choroidal neovascularization may occur.

Investigations

Serological: Serum antitoxoplasma antibody titers can be determined by several techniques, which include the following:
- Enzyme-linked immunosorbent assay (ELISA)
- Indirect fluorescent antibody test
- Indirect hemagglutination test
- Complement fixation
- Sabin-Feldman dye test

Acute systemic toxoplasmosis has traditionally been diagnosed by seroconversion. Antitoxoplasma immunoglobulin G (IgG) titers present a 4-fold increase that peak 6–8 weeks, following infection, then decline over the next two years, but remain detectable for life.

Antitoxoplasma IgM appears in the first week of the infection and then declines in the next few months.

Antibody titers do not correlate with ocular disease. Antitoxoplasma antibodies may be very low and should be tested in undiluted (1:1) samples, if possible.

Polymerase chain reaction: The aqueous fluid can be sent for detection of toxoplasma organisms in suspected cases of toxoplasmosis.

Fluorescein angiography: The lesion shows hypofluorescence in the early stages and hyperfluorescence in the late stages.

Optical coherence tomography: Macular edema, choroidal neovasculariztion and epiretinal membrane formation can be ruled out.

Histopathology: It is rarely done but can show the tachyzoites.

Differential Diagnosis

Most panuveitic conditions, especially acute retinal necrosis and sarcoidosis may mimic the disease. Laser scars and cryotherapy scars can mimic the chorioretinal scar.

Management

- Triple drug therapy refers to pyrimethamine, sulfadiazine and prednisone.
- Quadruple therapy refers to pyrimethamine, sulfadiazine, clindamycin and prednisone.
- Pyrimethamine (75 mg oral qid or 50 mg oral bid loading dose, followed by 25 mg oral bid) should be combined with folinic acid to avoid hematological complications. The duration of treatment varies depending on the patient's response but usually lasts for 4–6 weeks.
- Clindamycin (300 mg qid) can be given for 3–4 weeks. It is the preferred drug.
- Azithromycin (500 mg orally day 1, followed by 250 mg/d for the next 4 days) is another drug that can be used.
- During pregnancy, spiramycin and sulfadiazine (2–4 gm orally single dose, loading dose, followed by 1 gm orally qid) can be used in the first trimester. Throughout the second trimester, spiramycin, sulfadiazine, pyrimethamine and

folinic acid are recommended. Spiramycin, pyrimethamine and folinic acid may be used during the third trimester.

Corticosteroids: Topical corticosteroids are used depending on the anterior chamber reaction. Systemic corticosteroids are used as an adjunct to minimize collateral damage from the inflammatory response.

Toxocariasis

Toxocariasis is an infection caused by the ingestion of larvae of the dog roundworm *Toxocara canis* or the cat roundworm *Toxocara cati*.

Age: Ocular toxocariasis is common in children and young adults.

Sex: There is no sex predilection.

Pathogenesis

Adult worms of the *Toxocara* species, which live in the small intestine of dogs and puppies release *Toxocara* eggs, which survive for years in the environment. Humans typically ingest the eggs via oral contact with contaminated hands. Once introduced into the human intestine, the eggs decorticate, releasing the larvae. The larvae penetrate the bowel wall and migrate through vessels to the muscles, liver and lung and sometimes to the eye and brain.

Once, it reaches the eye, it incites a delayed hypersensitivity response helped by IL 45, 10 and dominated by eosinophils. This gives rise to an eosinophilic granuloma.

Clinical Features

Signs: Toxocariasis gives rise to three ocular syndromes:
i. *Chronic endophthalmitis:* The age of onset is generally around 2–9 years. It is characterized by the presence of chronic unilateral uveitis and cyclitis.
ii. *Localized granuloma:* The age of onset is between 6–14 years. It is characterized by the presence of a solitary white elevated lesion around 1–2 disc diameter in size. It is generally found at the macula or the peripapillary region (Fig. 22.53).
iii. *Peripheral granuloma:* This can occur anytime between the ages of 6–40 years. It is characterized by the presence of a mass in the periphery with dense vitreous strands projecting into the vitreous and sometimes reaching the disc. They can give rise to heterotropia.

Treatment

Corticosteroids can be used in the active inflammatory phase. Antihelmintics like thiabendazole have not been found to be useful for the ocular disease and may in fact worsen the disease.

Onchocerciasis

Onchocerciasis is a chronic parasitic disease caused by the filarial nematode *Onchocerca volvulus*.

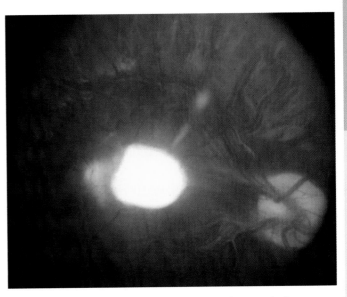

Fig. 22.53: Toxocara granuloma: Fundus photograph shows a granuloma at the posterior pole

Age and sex: Persons of all ages and of both sexes are equally predisposed to getting the infection.

Incidence: Onchocerciasis is believed to affect around 18 million people worldwide of which 2 million are blind. In hyperendemic areas, everyone above the age of 15 is affected and over half of them will turn blind before they die.

Pathogenesis

Humans are the only host of *Onchocerca volvulus*. The infective larvae of *O. volvulus* are transmitted through the bite of female black flies of the *Simulum* genus. As black flies breed in the fast flowing streams, the blindness caused by it is also known as "River blindness."

In the human host, the larvae molt twice to become male and female adult worms. This process occurs in subcutaneous nodules known as onchocercomata, and a mature female can produce microfilariae after 6–12 months.

Microfilariae are said to reach the eye through: direct invasion of the cornea from the conjunctiva, penetration of the sclera through the vascular channels and hematogenous spread.

Microfilariae live for 6–30 months; most die without completing their life cycle. Symptoms of onchocerciasis are caused by localized host inflammatory responses to the dead or dying microfilariae. In persons with heavy infection, as many as 100,000 microfilariae die each day. The predominant immune response is production of antibodies, but cellular responses, particularly those of eosinophils, are important.

Clinical Features

Symptoms: Patient complains of itching, redness and blurring of vision.

Signs:

Cornea
• Live microfilariae can be seen in the cornea

- Punctate keratitis and sclerosing keratitis.

Anterior chamber

- Live microfilariae can be seen in the anterior chamber
- Both granulomatous and nongranulomatous anterior uveitis can occur. This can lead to iris atrophy, inflammatory glaucoma and cataracts.

Posterior segment

- Lesions are also due to inflammatory responses to microfilarial death. This causes disturbances of the retinal pigment epithelium and can lead to chorioretinitis, chorioretinal atrophy and subretinal fibrosis. Only 5% of patients have active retinitis.
- Active optic neuritis may be due to infection or may develop after systemic treatment. Both optic neuritis and optic atrophy can cause blindness in up to 10% of some populations with onchocerciasis.

Investigations

The diagnosis of onchocerciasis is clinical. It can be confirmed by finding the microfilariae in the skin biopsy or in the eye.

Treatment

Ivermectin is the drug of choice. It binds to the glutamate gated chloride channels in the nerve and muscles and causes cell death. It kills the microfilariae but does not kill the worms.

Cysticercosis

Cysticercosis is a parasitic infection caused by the ingestion of *Cysticercus cellulosae,* the larva of *Taenia solium.*

Age and sex: No particular age or sex predilection.

Pathogenesis

The infection is acquired by eating food contaminated with eggs of the tapeworm.

Additionally, autoinfection may occur by means of fecal-oral contact and theoretically, by reverse peristalsis in the small intestines of individuals infected with adult worms.

In the stomach, oncospheres are liberated following digestion of the eggs' coats. Oncospheres invade and cross the intestinal wall, enter the bloodstream and then migrate to and lodge in tissues throughout the body, where they produce small (0.2−0.5 cm) fluid-filled bladders containing a single juvenile-stage parasite (protoscolex).

Although the cysticerci may infect any organ of the body (most often the eye, skeletal muscle and central nervous system are affected). Larvae may be seen in the subretinal space or vitreous in 15% to 46% of the infected patients.

Clinical Features

Symptoms: Patients might complain of decreased vision.

Signs: Death of the larvae leads to a severe inflammatory reaction, which is seen as anterior uveitis, vitritis and retinitis. Sometimes, retinal detachment can take place.

Treatment

Praziquantel (50 mg/kg/day) and laser can kill the larvae but these are associated with worsening of symptoms. The larvae can be removed surgically from the vitreous and the subretinal space by vitrectomy.

Diffuse Unilateral Subacute Neuroretinitis

Diffuse unilateral subacute neuroretinitis (DUSN) is a progressive parasitic disease affecting the outer retina and retinal pigment epithelium.

Age: It occurs most frequently in the second and third decades.

Sex: This condition occurs more frequently in males than in females.

Pathogenesis

The following organisms are implicated: *Ancylostoma caninum* and *Baylisascaris procyonis.*

Stationary or migrating nematodes have been identified deep in the retina or in the subretinal space. Later in the course of the disease, slowly progressive retinal pigment epithelial changes and optic atrophy may be observed, as well as narrowing of the retinal vessels.

Clinical Features

Symptoms: In the early stages, patient might present with mild-to-moderate visual loss, paracentral or central scotomas, floaters and redness, which might progress to severe visual loss.

Signs: The signs of DUSN are as follows:

- Visual acuity ranges from 20/30 to 20/200 or less.
- Conjunctival injection, ciliary flush, anterior chamber cells and flare, fine keratic precipitates and small hypopyon may be present.
- Posterior segment examination findings reveal mild-to-moderate vitritis, optic disc swelling, narrowing of the retinal arterioles, retinitis and nematodes.
- Retinitis is the most characteristic feature of this syndrome. Transient, multiple, focal, gray-white lesions of the deep retina or retinal pigment epithelium vary in size from 0.25−1 disc diameter and tend to develop in clusters over wide areas of the retina at various time periods. The active evanescent gray-white lesions fade within a period of 7−10 days as the nematode moves elsewhere in the eye, only to recur in an adjacent area or distant site over the ensuing weeks. Lesions typically resolve without any ophthalmoscopic or angiographic evidence of damage.
- Nematode: Identification of the subretinal worm is the pathognomonic finding in DUSN. The worm can be present in all layers of the retina, but it most frequently is found in the subretinal or outer retinal layers. The motile worm is more likely to be observed in the neighborhood of the active grayish-white retinal lesions. The worms appear smooth in outline, tapered on both ends and often assume an S-shaped, coiled or figure "8" configuration.

- Focal retinal and subretinal hemorrhages, perivenous exudates and vascular sheathing, localized serous detachments of the neurosensory retina, cystoid macular edema, retinal striae, and choroidal neovascularization may occur.

Investigations: Serologic studies for parasites, analysis of stool for ova and parasites and hematologic evaluation for eosinophilia are of limited value in establishing the diagnosis of DUSN.

Management

Laser photocoagulation of the nematode is the treatment of choice. No significant intraocular inflammation has been associated with this treatment.

Anthelmintic treatment is being used more frequently. Thiabendazole is the drug of choice for initial medical therapy. Successful treatment is characterized by the development of a localized area of intense retinitis and fading of the grayish-white retinal lesions within 10 days after completion of therapy.

Ivermectin may be considered if thiabendazole is not effective or cannot be tolerated.

VIRAL UVEITIS

HIV Microangiopathy

It is the most common ocular finding in patients with AIDS occurring in almost 50 to 70% of the patients.

Pathogenesis

The HIV antigen has been found in the retinal endothelial cells. It is believed that it causes a microvasculopathy and other hematologic abnormalities like increased leukocyte activation, which leads to thrombosis and consequent changes of ischemia.

Clinical Features

It is characterized by the presence of cotton wool spots, retinal hemorrhages and microaneurysms (Fig. 22.54). The cotton

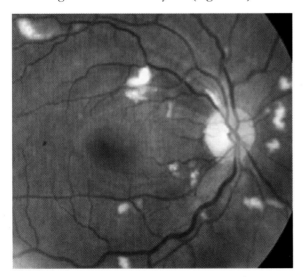

Fig. 22.54: HIV retinopathy: Fundus photograph shows multiple cotton wool spots

wool spots are generally oriented along the vascular arcades. The microaneurysms are also distributed along the nerve fiber layer and the inner retinal layers.

Cytomegalovirus Retinitis

Cytomegalovirus retinitis is caused by Cytomegalovirus, which is a double stranded DNA virus belonging to the Herpes group. It is seen mainly in immunocompromised patients like those with AIDS or those on immunosuppressive therapy. It is seen in patients with AIDS when the CD4 counts fall below 50 cells/cubic mm.

Mode of transmission: The infection is spread through infected body fluids, blood, transplanted organs and transplacentally.

The antibodies to the virus are present in 60% to 90% of the normal individuals.

Age: Most people are between 20–50 years of age

Sex: Males and females have equal chances of getting affected but it is more prevalent in males due to the higher incidence of HIV in males.

Laterality: Generally, affects one eye. If the patient does not receive treatment, in 50% of the patients, the other eye gets affected.

Clinical Features

In immunocompetent persons, it presents as a mild flu.

In immunocompromised patients, it presents as hepatitis, colitis, pneumonitis and encephalitis.

The ocular features generally occur once the CD4 count < 50 cells/mm cube and is seen in 15% to 40% patients, affected with AIDS.

The retina is divided into three zones to assess prognosis:
- *Zone 1:* A region 3000 μm from the center of the fovea and 1500 μm from the optic nerve head.
- *Zone 2:* Extends from the borders of Zone 1 to the ampullae of the vortex veins.
- *Zone 3:* Retina peripheral to Zone 2.

Cytomegalovirus causes a type of necrotizing retinitis and various morphological patterns are seen.

Brush-fire pattern: This is the commonest pattern where there is vasculitis leading to hemorrhages and exudates and later retinal whitening. This appearance is also called as the "pizza pie" appearance (Fig. 22.55).

The rate of progression is slow as compared to ARN and PORN and is 250–300 μm/week

Granular pattern: This is generally seen in the periphery. These lesions have a more granular appearance and hemorrhages are typically absent. When these lesions heal, satellite lesions occur in the nearby area.

Frosted branch angiitis: There is diffuse involvement of blood vessels with severe sheathing (Fig. 22.56).

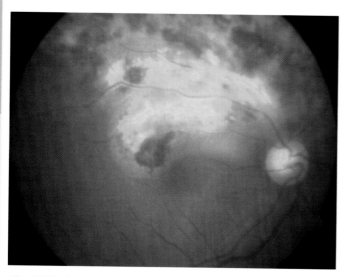

Fig. 22.55: Cytomegalovirus retinitis: Fundus photograph shows active pizza pie appearance

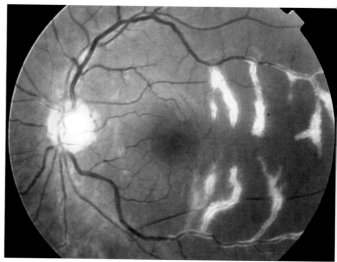

Fig. 22.56: Cytomegalovirus retinitis: Fundus photograph shows frosted branch angiitis

Cotton wool spots and vitritis: These are seen in immunocompetent patients.

The areas of hemorrhage can lead to fibrovascular proliferation and later lead to tractional retinal detachment.

Histopathology: It shows the presence of eosinophilic intranuclear inclusions and basophilic cytoplasmic inclusions.

Differential Diagnosis

- Acute retinal necrosis
- Toxoplasmosis

Investigations

- Complete blood count: Generally, the CD4 counts are below 50 cells/cubic mm.
- Testing for HIV: Most patients with CMV retinitis are HIV positive and it needs to be ruled out.
- Polymerase chain reaction for CMV from aqueous or vitreous aspirate.

Management

The treatment of CMV retinitis in patients of AIDS involves the use of antiviral agents and antiretroviral agents.

The treatment of CMV retinitis in immunocompetent patients includes just giving antiviral agents.

Antiviral Agents

Ganciclovir: It is a nucleoside (Guanine) analogue. It is active as a triphosphate. The deoxyguanosine kinase in the cell first forms Ganciclovir monophosphate, which is then activated by the cell kinases to G. triphosphate. This attaches to DNA polymerase inhibiting DNA synthesis. Route of administration, dosage and side effects of Gancoclovir are shown in Table 22.8.

Foscarnet: It is a trisodium salt of phosphonoformic acid. It is active in Ganciclovir resistant CMV and halts progression

of CMV retinitis in more than 80% patients. It inhibits DNA polymerase of CMV and reverse transcriptase of HIV. Foscarnet has anti-HIV activity but has more dose-limiting toxicity. Route of administration, dosage and side effects of Foscarnet are shown in Table 22.9. Both Cidofovir and Foscarnet should not be used in the same patient as both are nephrotoxic.

Table 22.8: Route of administration, dosage and side effects of ganciclovir

Route	Dosage		Side effects
	Induction	**Maintenance**	
Intra venous	5 mg/kg bid for 14–21 days	5 mg/kg daily indefinitely	Neutropenia, anemia, thrombocytopenia. Elevated liver enzymes
Intravitreal	0.2–2 mg in 0.05–0.1 ml once to twice weekly Vitrasert is an intravitreal ganciclovir implant. Releases drug at the rate of 1 µg/hr and it lasts for 6–9 months		
Oral	500 mg/kg for six days		

Table 22.9: Route of administration, dosage and side effects of foscarnet

Route	Dosage		Side effects
	Induction	**Maintenance**	
Intravenous	90 mg/kg BD or 60 mg/kg TDS for 14–21 days Hydrate with saline 1 l IV or 2 l orally twice daily	90–120 mg/kg/day	Nephrotoxicity
Intravitreal	1.2–2.4 mg in 0.05–0.1 ml once or twice a week		

Cidofovir: It is a nucleotide analogue that selectively inhibits viral DNA production in CMV and other herpes virus. Route of administration, dosage and side effects of Cidofovir are shown in Table 22.10.

Table 22.10: Route of administration, dosage and side effects of Cidofovir

Route	Dosage		Side effects
	Induction	Maintenance	
Intravenous	5 mg/kg IV a week for 2 weeks. Give 1 L of NS 1 hr before and after the infusion 2 gm Probenecid 3 hours prior to the infusion and 1 gm Probenecid 2 hours post cidofovir and another 1 gm 8 hours postinfusion	5 mg/kg IV every 2 weeks indefinitely	Nephrotoxicity Uveitis and hypotony in 40% patients

Valganciclovir: It is a valine ester of Ganciclovir. The bioavailability of Valganciclovir is 10 times that of Ganciclovir. Route of administration and dosage of Valganciclovir is shown in Table 22.11.

Table 22.11: Route of administration and dosage of Valganciclovir

Route	Dosage	
	Induction	Maintenance
Oral	900 mg BD for 21 days creates concentration Equivalent to that of 5 mg/kg Ganciclovir	900 mg OD

Fomivirsen: It is an antisense inhibitor of CMV. The role of this drug in the management of CMV retinitis is being studied.

Acute Retinal Necrosis

Acute retinal necrosis was earlier known as Kirasawa uveitis. The exact etiology is unknown but it is said to be caused by reactivation of Varicella Zoster, HSV 1 or 2.

Age: It generally affects people between the ages of 20 to 50. When HSV 2 is the causative agent, it is the younger age group people who are affected. When HSV 1 or Varicella zoster is the suspected cause, the older age group people are affected.

Sex: Males are more likely to get affected.

Genetics: HLA-DQ w7 positivity is found in > 50% patients

Pathogenesis: Acute retinal necrosis is said to occur by the reactivation of dormant viruses like HSV 1, 2 or Varicella-zoster virus in predisposed population. This includes people who are immunocompromised and people who are positive for HLA-DQ w7.

Clinical Features

Symptoms: Patient can complain of redness, blurring of vision and periorbital pain.

Signs: According to the diagnostic criteria by "The American Uveitis Society", clinical characteristics that must be present are as follows:
- Focal well demarcated areas of retinal necrosis that must be present in the retinal periphery outside the vascular arcade.
- Rapid circumferential progression of necrosis.
- Evidence of occlusive vasculopathy.
- Prominent inflammatory reaction in the anterior chamber and vitreous.

Characteristics that support, but are not required for the diagnosis of acute retinal necrosis are as follows:
- Optic neuropathy
- Scleritis
- Pain

Staging of acute retinal necrosis: The staging of acute retinal necrosis as follows:

Stage 1: Necrotizing retinitis
  Stage 1a: Discrete areas of peripheral retinitis
  Stage 1b: Confluent areas of peripheral retinitis (Fig. 22.57), papillitis, macular edema

Stage 2: Vitreous opacification or organization

Stage 3: Regression of retinal necrosis, secondary pigmentation of the lesion with condensation of the vitreous base.

Stage 4: Retinal detachment
  Stage 4a: Acute retinal tears or detachment with traction or proliferative vitreoretinopathy
  Stage 4b: Chronic retinal detachment

Treatment

Antiviral therapy: Acyclovir is the drug of choice. It acts against HSV 1 and 2. It does not act against CMV.

In the initial stage, the recommended adult dose is 1500 mg/sq meter every 8 hours for the first seven days. The regression is rapid and seen in four days. Following the initial dose, oral acyclovir is given at dose of 400–600 mg five times a day for six weeks. Usage of acyclovir reduces the incidence of recurrence.

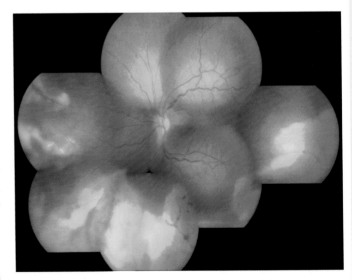

Fig. 22.57: Acute retinal necrosis: Montage fundus photograph

Anti-inflammatory therapy: Corticosteroids in dose of 60–80 mg/day for one week followed by tapering over 2–6 weeks is given to control the inflammation.

Prophylactic laser photocoagulation: Prophylactic laser photocoagulation is given posterior to the areas of active retinitis to prevent the future occurrence of retinal detachment.

Retinal detachment surgery: Scleral buckling is required with or without pars plana vitrectomy in the case of retinal detachment. Endolaser and intraocular gases may also be required.

Progressive Outer Retinal Necrosis

It is a rapidly spreading necrotizing retinitis caused by Varicella-zoster virus in a severely immunocompromised patient.

Age and Sex: No specific age or sex predilection

Clinical Features

Symptoms: Early blurring of central vision because of posterior pole involvement, metamorphopsia and floaters.

Signs: Patients present with outer retinal involvement without granular border with a typical cracked mud appearance (Fig. 22.58). Early macular involvement leads to decrease in vision early and also it progresses rapidly. Unlike acute retinal necrosis, patients do not have vasculitis, retinal hemorrhages and less chances of retinal detachment.

Management

It is similar to that of acute retinal necrosis but patients do not respond very well.

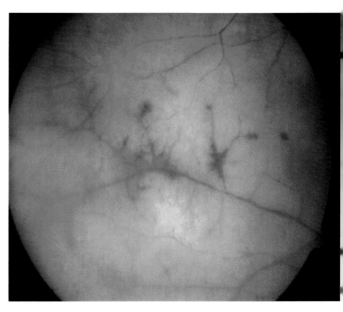

Fig. 22.58: Progressive outer retinal necrosis: Fundus photograph shows the typical cracked mud appearance in progressive outer retinal necrosis in a patient with AIDS

Prognosis

More than 50% of the patients with progressive outer retinal necrosis die within six months of being diagnosed.

Comparison between clinical features of acute retinal necrosis, progressive outer retinal necrosis and cytomegalovirus retinitis is shown in Table 22.12.

Table 22.12: Comparison between clinical features of acute retinal necrosis, progressive outer retinal necrosis and cytomegalovirus retinitis

	Acute retinal necrosis	Progressive outer retinal necrosis	Cytomegalovirus retinitis
Immune status	Healthy, rarely immunocompromised	Immunocompromised	Immunocompromised
Laterality	Bilateral in 30 to 80% cases	Bilateral in 70% cases	Bilateral 30 to 50% cases
Visual loss	Initially mild, later gross	Early loss of central vision	Variable, depending on involved site
Anterior chamber	Mild cells and flare	Mild cells and flare	Mild cells and flare
Intraocular pressure	Sometimes raised	Normal	Normal
Vitreous	Vitritis	Normal	Normal
Retinal involvement	Full thickness	Deep retinal involvement without granular border	Full thickness involvement with granular border
Pattern of involvement	Multifocal, mainly peripheral	Multifocal, early macular	Unifocal, fovea relatively spared
Classic appearance	Late Swiss cheese	Cracked mud	Cottage cheese
Vasculitis	Common	Uncommon	Seen but not common
Retinal hemorrhages	Common	Uncommon	Common in active lesion
Retinal detachment	Common	Common	Less common
Optic nerve involvement	Common	Uncommon	Seen but not common
Progression	Rapid	Rapid	Slow
Treatment	Responds to acyclovir	Does not respond to acyclovir well. 50% patients dead within 6 months of diagnosis	

FUGAL UVEITIS

Candida

Introduction

Candida albicans is a dimorphic fungus. Ocular candidiasis has increased recently due to widespread use of immunosuppressive therapy, hyperalimentation and intravenous drugs. It is the most common cause of ocular fungal infection.

Incidence: Endogenous *Candida* endophthalmitis is seen in 10% to 37% of the patients with Candidemia, if they are not receiving antifungal treatment. If antifungal treatment is given, the incidence drops to 3%.

Pathogenesis

The organism spreads hematogenously and reaches the choroid where fungal replication results in secondary vitreous and retinal involvement.

Clinical Features

Symptoms: The patient complains of blurring of vision and floaters mainly.

Signs: Multiple whitish circular lesions with fluffy borders ranging in size from 100–3000 μm in size are seen at the posterior pole. There is some extension into the vitreous cavity. Mainstay of the infection is chorioretinitis although endophthalmitis or panophthalmitis can also result. When the posterior pole is involved, they tend to mimic toxoplasmosis and when the periphery is involved, they tend to mimic pars planitis.

Investigations

- *Blood culture*
- *PCR:* The aqueous sample or the vitreous sample obtained can be sent for PCR evaluation.

Management

The treatment of choice is intravitreal amphotericin B 5–10 μg. Oral fluconazole has excellent ocular penetration on systemic administration. Systemic corticosteroids can be given 48 hours after starting antifungals. Vitrectomy may be useful in some patients with severe vitritis or endophthalmitis.

Presumed Ocular Histoplasmosis

Introduction

Presumed ocular histoplasmosis syndrome (POHS) is a syndrome characterized by peripheral atrophic chorioretinal scars, peripapillary scarring and maculopathy. It is believed to be caused by a dimorphic fungus *Histoplasma capsulatum*, which grows in soil, around chicken houses and places where bats abound like caves.

Incidence: This condition is endemic in the United States. Almost 2,00,000 to 5,00,000 infections occur every year.

Pathogenesis

Humans get infected by inhalation of spores of *Histoplasma capsulatum*. In a normal host, the initial infection is usually asymptomatic or feels like influenza. In a few patients, a chronic cavitary pulmonary disease may follow. In immunocompromised patients, a progressive, life-threatening, disseminated form can occur. Following initial infection, hematogenous spread to the rest of the body, including the eye, can occur. A focal granulomatous choroiditis is thought to occur. This phase seldom is observed in humans.

Clinical Features

Symptoms: The patient complains of sudden painless loss of visual acuity, micropsia and scotomas.

Signs:
- The anterior chamber and the vitreous are quiet.
- Punched-out chorioretinal scars (smaller in size than the optic nerve) also called "histo spots" are seen. These spots represent the focal, healed and punched out lesions from variable amount of scarring in the choroids and the adjacent layers of the retina. Black pigment may appear within or at the margins of these lesions. Linear streaks of atrophic scars in the mid periphery are observed in about 5% of patients with POHS.
- Peripapillary chorioretinal scarring is present.
- Macular CNV usually is observed as a gray-green subretinal lesion that is surrounded by subretinal blood and leads to a serous or hemorrhagic macular detachment. CNV is estimated to occur in 5% of eyes affected with POHS. The CNVM is Type 2 CNVM, which means it is subretinal.

Investigations

Fluorescein angiography: The active choroiditis lesion appears hypofluorescent in the early phase and hyperfluorescent in the late phases. While the choroidal neovascular membrane shows lacy hyperfluorescence early on in the study and goes on intensifying as the study progresses.

Management

- *Laser photocoagulation:* The macular photocoagulation study (MPS), a multicenter prospective randomized clinical trial, demonstrated that laser photocoagulation is indicated in the treatment of extrafoveal and juxtafoveal CNV secondary to POHS. It studied the role of Argon blue, Argon green and Krypton red laser in the treatment of CNVM. It found that treated patients (22%) are less likely to have a 6 line loss of vision compared to untreated patient (50%). It also found that argon green and krypton red are less likely to cause retinal injury. The goal of treatment is to obliterate the entire area of CNV. Despite its marginal benefits, the MPS recommended laser treatment of peripapillary CNV. Alternatively, pars plana vitrectomy and excision of the peripapillary CNV may be considered. Most surgeons recommend removal of recent subfoveal CNV but not peripapillary lesions. Pilot studies of laser photocoagulation of subfoveal CNV were inconclusive.

- *Photodynamic therapy (PDT):* Subfoveal CNV secondary to POHS is a labeled indication for PDT by the US Food and Drug Administration. An open-label, uncontrolled clinical study reported the median improvement of visual acuity of six letters after a mean of 3.9 PDT treatments in a 2-year follow-up with no serious ocular or systemic effects reported.
- *Submacular surgery:* Given that most CNV secondary to POHS grow in the subretinal space, uncontrolled studies have recommended surgical excision of subfoveal CNV via pars plana vitrectomy. The goal is to remove the CNV, but to leave the underlying RPE and choriocapillaris intact. The Submacular Surgery Trial (SST), a randomized multicenter prospective trial sponsored by the National Eye Institute (NEI), recently reported on the modest benefit in eyes with CNV secondary to POHS with a baseline visual acuity of 20/100 or worse.
- *Macular translocation:* Macular translocation surgery is another experimental surgical option to treat subfoveal CNV.

Cryptococcosis

Cryptococcus neoformans is yeast like fungus, which is ubiquitous in nature. It exists in the contaminated soil. The disease is acquired by the inhalation of the fungus, which results in pulmonary infection and secondary dissemination to central nervous system causing meningoencephalitis. Ocular infection can spread through the optic nerve or through the hematogenous route. Approximately 6% of patients with meningoencephalitis have ocular complications, such as papilledema, optic atrophy, chorioretinitis, vitritis, endophthalmitis, neuroretinitis and extraocular muscle paresis. In severe cases, they develop vascular sheathing, mutton-fat keratic precipitates.

Diagnosis is mostly clinical but can be confirmed by demonstrating the organism using India ink stains or culture of the organism from the CNS.

Treatment is with intravenous amphotericin B, oral fluconazole or oral 5-flucytosine.

The prognosis is poor once the optic nerve or the posterior pole is involved.

Aspergillosis

Introduction

Aspergillosis is caused by infection with *Aspergillus flavus* and *fumigatus.* These are filamentous fungi, which are found in soil and decaying vegetation. Like candidiasis, aspergillosis is on the rise because of the increased use of immunosuppressive therapy, hyperalimentation and organ transplants.

Pathogenesis

The spores of the saprophytic spore forming molds become airborne and seed the lung and the paranasal sinuses of humans. Development of infection depends on the virulence of the organism and the immunity of the host. Ocular disease occurs via hematogenous dissemination of the organism to the choroids.

Clinical Features

Symptoms: The patient complains of pain and visual loss.

Signs: A yellowish infiltrate is seen in the macula beginning in the choroid and subretinal space which later develops into a hypopyon. Retinal hemorrhages, vascular occlusions and full thickness retinal necrosis occurs. This infection can spread leading to a dense vitritis and inflammatory reaction in the anterior chamber.

Investigations

- Blood culture
- Gram's and Giemsa stains and culture of the vitreous sample.
- PCR: The aqueous sample or the vitreous sample obtained can be sent for PCR evaluation.

Differential Diagnosis

It can mimic toxoplasmosis, candidiasis, coccidiomycosis, acute retinal necrosis and cytomegalovirus retinitis.

Management

The treatment of choice is intravitreal amphotericin B 5-10 μg. Oral fluconazole has excellent ocular penetration on systemic administration. Systemic corticosteroids can be given 48 hours after starting antifungals. Vitrectomy may be useful in some patients with severe vitritis or endophthalmitis.

Ocular Coccidiomycosis

It is caused by the dimorphic fungi *Coccidioides inmitis.* Ocular involvement is very rare. Ocular manifestations include phlyctenular conjunctival inflammation, iridocyclitis, iris granulomas, choroiditis and chorioretinitis.

It is diagnosed using the Papanicolaou stain. Intravenous amphotericin is the mainstay of treatment.

BACTERIAL UVEITIS

Tuberculosis

Introduction

Tuberculosis is caused by *Mycobacterium tuberculosis,* which is an Acid-fast bacilli. Though, BCG immunization is given to children as part of the immunization program, the incidence of tuberculosis in India is still high.

As there is lack of uniformity in the diagnosis of tubercular uveitis, the exact prevalence is not known. The prevalence of ocular tuberculosis was reported to be 1.39% from one center.

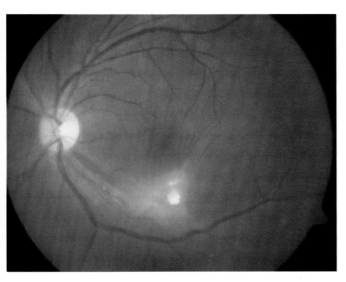

Fig. 22.59: Choroid tubercle: Fundus photograph showing active choroidal tubercle

Pathogenesis

The mycobacteria enters as aerosol droplet and forms a primary focus in the lung called the Ghon's focus. During periods of stress, general illness, immunosuppression, this focus gets activated and the bacilli spread through the blood stream to various tissues.

Clinical Features

Ocular manifestations of TB are varied and include:

- Phlyctenulosis
- Anterior uveitis
- Solitary or multiple tubercles (choroiditis) (Fig. 22.59)
- Tuberculoma
- Vasculitis
- Eales' disease (Fig. 22.60)
- Papillitis
- Adnexal TB of lacrimal gland, muscles and eyelid

Choroiditis (choroidal tubercles): Choroidal tubercles occur primarily in the posterior pole within the vascular arcades. The tubercles are 0.3–3 mm in diameter. They appear yellowish, grayish or whitish in color. Fluorescein angiography shows early hypofluorescence and late hyperfluorescence.

Choroidal tuberculomas/subretinal abscess (Fig. 22.61): Choroidal tuberculomas occur generally in the periphery. They are 2–3 DD in size. They appear grayish white and have indistinct margins. Quite often, they have overlying exudative retinal detachment and intraretinal exudation. Fluorescein angiography shows early hyperfluorescence with leakage around the margins in late phases. USG shows:

- Acoustically dense lesion with no choroidal excavation
- Low internal reflectivity
- High vascularity

Difference between choroidal tubercles and choroidal tuberculomas is shown in Table 22.13.

Table 22.13: Difference between choroidal tubercles and choroidal tuberculomas

Choroidal tubercles	Choroidal tuberculomas
0.3–3 mm in diameter	2–3 DD in diameter
Within the vascular arcade	Periphery
FFA: Early hypofluorescence and late phase hyperfluorescence	FFA: Early hyperfluorescence and late phase leakage around the margins

Investigations

The diagnosis of ocular tuberculosis is presumptive keeping in mind the following points

- Clinical presentation
- Endemicity of the area
- X-ray chest and sputum culture
- Mantoux test
- Isoniazid test
- Definitive test like PCR, culture

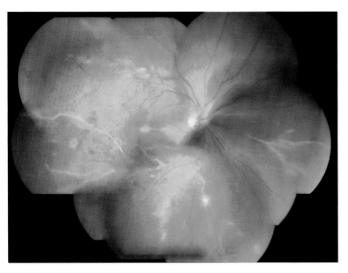

Fig. 22.60: Eales' disease: Montage fundus photograph showing active retinal vasculitis

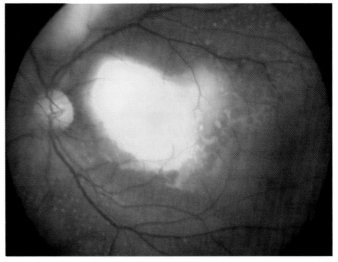

Fig. 22.61: Subretinal abscess: Fundus photograph shows tuberculous subretinal abscess

Endemicity of area: In a country like India where TB is endemic, the diagnosis of TB should be high up on the list, but in a country like United States where it is not so common, it is low down on the list.

X-ray Chest and Sputum Culture

Presence of a Ghon's focus or military tubercles goes in favor of TB.

But the absence of the features does not R/O TB as they are not found in upto 60% of the cases.

Mantoux Test (Fig. 22.11)

Generally in a country like India where TB is endemic, children get exposed to TB bacillus quite early after birth or are immunized against TB. Once, the bacillus enters the body, the person gets sensitized to the bacillus within a period of 2–8 weeks.

This manifests as a positive Mantoux test. The person might not be suffering from TB, but still he gives Mantoux test positive as he is already sensitized to TB. 0.05 mg of purified protein derivative of *Mycobacterium tuberculosis* in 0.1ml aqueous solution equivalent to 2.5 tuberculin units is injected intracutaneously in the forearm.

After 48 hours, the forearm is examined for the presence of induration.

If Induration < 5 mm: Test is negative
5–10 mm: Indicates prior exposure
>10 mm: In a high risk population is highly suggestive of TB
>15 mm: In a low risk population is highly suggestive of TB

False Negatives

If person has been on steroids. Steroids should be stopped minimum for 15 days before taking the test.

If the person has anergy as in sarcoidosis.

QuantiFERON-TB Gold Test

It is the latest test available in the market. It measures the release of interferon gamma from primed macrophages. The test report is available in a day and also it is more specific for *Mycobacterium tuberculosis* compared to the Mantoux test. In this test, macrophages which were primed by the BCG bacilli or most of the atypical mycobacteria will not be picked up. It just gives an idea that the person has the tubercle bacilli, but it does not mean that the patient has active tuberculosis.

Polymerase Chain Reaction, Culture, Biopsy

If it is possible to obtain tissue sample like vitreous, choroids, then the above definitive tests can be done. Though, it is impractical in most cases.

Histopathology

Hematoxylin and eosin stain shows the presence of central caseation surrounded by the presence of Langerhans giant cells.

Culture

Generally, the Lowenstein-Jensen medium is used and then it is checked for growth at the end of 3 weeks.

Management

The treatment is directed against
•   Eradicating the organisms
•   Limiting the effects of inflammation

Eradicating the organisms: The person is given multi-drug treatment depending on the category to which he belongs.

The drugs used in TB are:
•   Isoniazid (H): 5 mg/kg/d
•   Rifampicin (R): 10 mg/kg/d
•   Pyrazinamide (Z): 25 mg/kg/d
•   Ethambutol (E): 15 mg/kg/d
•   Streptomycin (S): 15 mg/kg/d

Various combinations are available in the market. Combination tablets are preferred as it is more likely that the patient will follow the regime.

Concomitant use of steroids is controversial as it may exacerbate the lesion.

But in lesions involving the macula and threatening the sight, the use of steroids helps to reduce the loss of vision by controlling the inflammation.

Syphilis

Introduction

It is a sexually transmitted disease caused by the spirochete *Treponema pallidum*.

Pathogenesis

There are three stages:
1. *Primary syphilis:* It is characterized by an ulcerative lesion called chancre, which occurs at the site where the organism penetrates the skin or mucous membrane. The incubation period is 3 weeks. The stage lasts for 2–8 weeks. The spirochete spreads by lymphatic route.
2. *Secondary syphilis:* It is characterized by fever, malaise, lymphadenopathy and mucocutaneous lesions. This stage lasts for weeks to months. It is seen in 60% to 90% of the patients with syphilis.
3. *Tertiary syphilis:* It is characterized by the presence of focal inflammatory lesions called gummas affecting the heart, vessels and central nervous system.

The CNS involvement is in the form of Tabes dorsalis or general paresis of syphilis.

Quaternary syphilis: Sometimes described for the necrotizing encephalitis that develops in patients with AIDS.

Clinical Features

Conjunctiva: Various clinical features of conjunctiva includes:
Primary: Chancre, i.e. conjunctival ulceration with rolled edges and surrounding conjunctival injection.

Secondary: Nonspecific conjunctivitis with papillary reaction.

Tertiary: Granulomatous conjunctivitis with painful gumma formation.

Episcleritis and scleritis: Occurs in secondary stage in conjunction with conjunctivitis, very rarely alone.

Cornea: Marginal anterior infiltrates are seen. Interstitial keratitis characterized by the presence of stromal vascularization just ahead of the Descemet's membrane and alteration in the Descemet's membrane with the development of ridges, scrolls and webs.

Iris: Nonspecific iritis and iridocyclitis are the most common presentation. It may be granulomatous or nongranulomatous and is characterized by the presence of dilated iris capillaries called 'Roseolae'.

Lens: Cataracts formation can take place.

Pupil

Argyll Robertson pupil: The pupils are unequal and miotic with light reflex absent, but near reflex present. This happens due to the interruption of the fibers from the Edinger-Westphal nucleus to the pretectal nucleus.

Neuro-ophthalmic: 3rd, 4th, 6th cranial nerve palsies can occur. There can be abnormalities of the saccades and the pursuits. Superior orbital fissure syndrome, lateral medullary plate syndrome, Horner's syndrome, internuclear ophthalmoplegia, chiasmal syndrome with bitemporal hemianopia and cortical blindness are some of the other manifestations.

Retina and choroid: Generally, multifocal chorioretinitis is present. Focal chorioretinitis is rare and bilateral with focus near disc or macula.

Pseudoretinitis pigmentosa like picture can be there.

In AIDS patients, there are multiple yellowish-grayish placoid lesions with atrophic centers near the disc and the macula. These are flat atrophic areas with no fluid or hemorrhage. This condition is called acute syphilitic posterior placoid chorioretinitis.

Fluorescein angiography shows early hypofluorescence and late hyperfluorescence. This pattern is called "Leopard Spot" hypofluorescence.

Neuroretinitis can also occur.

Investigations

Screening: Nontreponemal tests like VDRL and RPR tests.

Confirmatory: Treponemal tests like FTA-ABS (fluorescent treponemal antibody absorption test)

Management

Primary, secondary and latent <1 year duration: Single intramuscular injection of 2.4 million units of Benzathine Penicillin G is effective.

Patients who have failed primary treatment: They have syphilis >1 year and there is no CNS involvement. Three injections of Benzathine Penicillin G at weekly intervals are given.

Patients having CNS involvement: Intravenous aqueous Penicillin G 2-4 million units every 4 hours for 10–14 days or daily 2.4 million units of procaine penicillin with probenecid 250 mg qds for 10–14 days.

Lyme's Disease

Introduction

It is caused by spirochaete *Borrelia burgdorferi* and spread by the tick Ixodes damini.

Pathogenesis and Clinical Features (Table 22.14)

Investigation

Definitive diagnosis (Table 22.15)

Management

Early infection without neurological or ocular involvement: Doxycycline 100 mg bd for 14–21 days.

Neurological and/or ocular abnormalities: Ceftriaxone 2 gm IV OD for 14–28 days.

Table 22.14: Pathogenesis and clinical features of Lyme's disease

	Stage 1	*Stage 2*	*Stage 3*
Mechanism	Spirochetemia	Due to immunological reaction	
Systemic	Erythema chronicum migrans Annular spreading rash with central clearing at least 5 cm in size and occurs within one month of the tick bite Flu like symptoms, arthralgia also present	Dissemination of the spirochete to heart, skin, joints and nervous system Neurological manifestations include Meningoencephalitis, cranial neuropathy and peripheral neuropathy Carditis, arthritis, lymphocytoma, i.e. a purplish nodule on the ear-lobe may develop	After months and years Chronic relapsing arthritis Acrodermatitis chronica atrophicans Encephalopathy, demyelination and dementia
Ocular	Conjunctivitis, photophobia and periorbital edema	Iridocyclitis, vitritis, panophthalmitis, exudative RD, retinal vasculitis, macular edema	Stromal keratitis, episcleritis, symblepharon, orbital myositis

Table 22.15: Definitive diagnosis of Lyme's disease

Test type	Method details	Specimens	Diagnostic value
Culture	Barbour-Stoenner-Kelly medium	Plasma, skin lesion, synovial fluid and CSF	100% diagnostic, high yield only in early stage
PCR	Nested PCR	CSF, synovial fluid and vitreous	Highly diagnostic, technically difficult, low yield, useful only in chronic stage
Serology	ELISA, IFA, Western Blot	Serum	High sensitivity, low specificity, negative in stage 1, 90% positive in stages 2 and 3

Endophthalmitis

Endophthalmitis is defined as inflammation within the anterior or posterior segment or both occurring with concurrent partial thickness involvement of adjacent ocular wall, which might be either infectious or noninfectious.

Classification of Endophthalmitis

Infectious

- Exogenous
  1. Surgical
     a. Acute onset
     b. Delayed onset
     c. Bleb associated
  2. Nonsurgical
     a. Posttraumatic
- Endogenous
  1. Infectious: Hematogenous
  2. Noninfectious
     a. Lens induced
     b. Sterile

Classification of Endophthalmitis by Etiology

1. *Acute infectious postoperative endophthalmitis:* It is defined as endophthalmitis occurring within 6 weeks of the surgery. The incidence is 0.07 to 0.13%. The common organisms are coagulase-negative staphylococcus especially *Staphylococcus epidermidis,* gram-negative organisms and anaerobes.

   One study showed that the incidence of positive aqueous culture at the time of surgery was 29%, even then the incidence of endophthalmitis was around 0.1%.

   The factors leading to increased chance of endophthalmitis are:
   - Presence of preoperative ocular or adnexal infection.
   - Intraoperative problems like long duration, PCR, wound dehiscence, contaminated solutions, contaminated instruments, etc.

2. *Chronic/delayed onset endophthalmitis:* It is defined as endophthalmitis occurring after six weeks. It presents with mild anterior chamber reaction with diffuse white plaque behind the lens and presence of fibrin bands in the anterior and mid-vitreous cavity. The causative organisms are *Propionibacterium acnes,* less virulent strains of *Staphylococcus epidermidis* and fungi.

3. *Bleb-associated endophthalmitis:* It occurs following trabeculectomy surgery. The signs range from blebitis to frank purulent discharge. The incidence ranges from 0.06 to 0.3 to 9% when antimetabolites have been used. The causative organisms include Streptococcus and Hemophilus.

4. *Posttraumatic endophthalmitis:* It occurs following open globe trauma. The signs are more severe than in other endophthalmitis either due to the virulent strains of bacteria, multiple organisms and high bacterial load. The incidence ranges from 9 to 30%. The causative organisms include gram-positive cocci and bacillus.

5. *Endogenous endophthalmitis:* It occurs due to hematogenous or direct spread of microorganisms from a site external to the eye. Common conditions include endocarditis and gastrointestinal infections. They occur typically in immunocompromised patients. The causative organisms include *Escherichia coli* and *Staphylococcus.*

Clinical Features

Symptoms:
- Blurring of vision in 94% patients
- Redness of eye in 82% patients
- Pain in 74% patients

Signs:
- Eyelid edema
- Severe conjunctival chemosis
- Scleral dehiscence
- Corneal edema, infiltrates
- AC cells and flare
- Vitritis
- Retinal hemorrhages and periphlebitis
- Hypopyon (86% patients)
- In 79% patients, no view of the retinal vessels was present and in 32% patients, the red reflex was also absent

Investigations

USG B-scan: Presence of echoes in the vitreous along with choroidal thickening is suggestive of endophthalmitis.

Microbiological diagnosis: Aqueous humor 0.1 ml is collected by AC tap. Vitreous humor 0.2 ml is collected by either pars plana vitrectomy or by using a 23-gauge needle inserted into the anterior vitreous cavity 3 mm behind the limbus in pseudo and aphakics and 4 mm behind the limbus in phakics.

The samples are sent for:

Staining:

Gram and Giemsa stain to R/O bacteria

KOH and Calcofluor white to R/O fungi

Culture:

Solid media like blood agar, chocolate agar and Sabouraud dextrose agar.

Liquid media like thioglycollate broth and brain heart infusion.

The vitreous drawn by the needle is inoculated in drops onto the media without streaking.

The vitreous drawn from the cassettes is passed through 0.2 µm thick filters and the filter is cut and the pieces are inoculated into the media.

Confirmed positive growth is characterized by the growth of the same organism on more than one solid media.

Molecular diagnosis: PCR techniques especially the newer ones like the real time PCR against the 16S rDNA gene primers is very sensitive.

Management

Any patient suspected to have endophthalmitis should be:

Started on intravitreal antibiotics immediately.

The idea is to use broad spectrum antibiotics to cover both the gram-positive and gram-negative organisms.

Vancomycin 1mg or 0.1ml (100% sensitivity against Gm + organisms).

Ceftazidime 2.25 mg or 0.1ml (89% sensitivity against Gm–organisms).

Amikacin 400 mg or 0.1ml (Against gram–organisms) was used earlier, but the use is more or less discontinued now due to the macular toxicity caused by the drug.

The EVS did not address the issue of using intravitreal dexamethasone. In a study done by Das and associates, they found that using 400 mg or 0.1 ml reduced the inflammation, but had no impact on the visual acuity six weeks later. So, the use of intravitreal dexamethasone is optional.

Amphotericin 0.5 mg/ml is preferable, if fungus has been detected.

Preparation of the common intravitreal injections is shown in Table 22.16.

Subconjunctival antibiotics:

Vancomycin: 25 mg or 0.5 ml of normal saline

Ceftazidime: 100 mg or 0.5 ml of normal saline

Dexamethasone: 6 mg or 0.25 ml of normal saline

Endophthalmitis Vitrectomy Study (EVS)

Purpose

- To determine the role of initial pars plana vitrectomy in the management of postoperative bacterial endophthalmitis.
- To determine the role of intravenous antibiotics in the management of bacterial endophthalmitis.
- To determine which factors, other than treatment, predict outcome in postoperative bacterial endophthalmitis.

Description

The Endophthalmitis Vitrectomy Study (EVS) patients were randomized to one of two standard treatment strategies for the management of bacterial endophthalmitis.

Eyes received either:

- Initial pars plana vitrectomy with intravitreal antibiotics, followed by retap and reinjection at 36–60 hours for eyes that did poorly as defined in the study or
- Initial anterior chamber and vitreous tap/biopsy with injection of intravitreal antibiotics, followed by vitrectomy and reinjection at 36–60 hours in eyes doing poorly. In addition, all eyes were randomized to either treatment or no treatment with intravenous antibiotics.

Study end points were visual acuity and clarity of ocular media, the latter assessed both clinically and photographically.

Each patient's initial endpoint assessment occurred at three months, after which procedures to improve vision, such as late vitrectomy for nonclearing ocular media, were an option.

The final outcome assessment occurred at nine months. Multiple centers cooperated by enrolling 420 eyes during the 42-month recruitment period.

Patient Eligibility

Inclusion criteria: Patients having clinical signs and symptoms of bacterial endophthalmitis in an eye that had cataract surgery or lens implantation within six weeks of onset of infection are eligible.

The involved eye had to have either:

- Hypopyon or enough clouding of anterior chamber or vitreous media to obscure clear visualization of second-order arterioles,
- Cornea and anterior chamber in the involved eye clear enough to visualize some part of the iris.
- Cornea, clear enough to allow the possibility of pars plana vitrectomy, or

Table 22.16: Preparation of the common intravitreal injections

Antibiotic	Vial size	Amount of initial diluent	Initial concentration	Aliquot	Added to NS of volume	Final concentration	Dose
Vancomycin	500 mg	10 ml	50 mg/ml	0.2 ml	0.8 ml	10 mg/ml	1 mg/0.1 ml
Ceftazidime	250 mg	1 ml	250 mg/ml	0.1 ml	0.9 ml	25 mg/ml	2.25 mg/0.1 ml
Amphotericin	50 mg	10 ml	5 mg/ml	0.2 ml	0.8 ml	1 mg/ml	0.1 mg/0.1 ml

- The eyes had to have a visual acuity of 20/50 or worse and light perception or better.

Exclusion criteria: If the involved eye was known at the time of study entry to have had any preexisting eye disease that limited best-corrected visual acuity to 20/100 or worse before development of cataract.

Any intraocular surgery before presentation (except for cataract extraction or lens implantation).

Any treatment for endophthalmitis before presenting at the study center, or any ocular or systemic condition that would prevent randomization to any of the study groups.

Results

There was no difference in final visual acuity or media clarity with or without systemic antibiotics. If patients presented with hand motions or better acuity, there was no difference in visual outcome with or without an immediate 3 port pars plana vitrectomy.

Vitrectomy

Tripled (33% compared with 11%) the frequency of achieving 20/40 or better.

Doubled (56% compared with 30%) the chance of achieving 20/100 or better.

Decreased by more than one-half (20% compared with 47%) the frequency of severe visual loss in the subgroup of patients who presented with visual acuity of light perception only. These differences were statistically significant.

Conclusions

Initial management for patients who meet EVS entry criteria should include 3 port pars plana vitrectomy, if patients present with vision worse than hand motions.

An initial vitreous tap/biopsy should generally be sufficient if presenting vision is hand motions or better.

Systemic antibiotics were not of benefit in this study, although all patients should receive intravitreal antibiotics.

MISCELLANEOUS UVEAL ABNORMALITIES

Uveal Masquerade Syndromes

Introduction

Masquerade syndromes include conditions, which have the presence of intraocular cells, but are not due to immune mediated entity.

They include neoplastic and nonneoplastic conditions.

Neoplastic masquerade syndromes: These include clinical entities, which might present with cells in the anterior chamber or vitreous or both, but are not due to immune mediated mechanism, but due to tumors.

These include the following malignancies. Of all the malignancies, vast majority of the patients have primary central nervous system lymphoma.

- Primary central nervous system lymphoma
- Systemic lymphoma
- Leukemia
- Uveal lymphoid proliferations
- Uveal melanoma
- Retinoblastoma
- Juvenile xanthogranuloma
- Metastatic tumors
- Bilateral diffuse melanocytic proliferation.

Nonneoplastic masquerade syndromes: Different nonneoplastic masquerade syndromes include the following:

Retinitis pigmentosa: There might be presence of vitreous cells and CME. It can be differentiated from uveitis by the presence of waxy disc pallor, arteriolar attenuation and bone spicules.

Ocular ischemic syndrome: It occurs due to carotid artery obstruction leading to decrease in blood flow in the ophthalmic artery. Patient might have presence of cells and flare in the anterior chamber along with rubeosis. The flare will be characteristically much more than cells. Posterior segment shows presence of disc edema, intraretinal hemorrhages. It can be differentiated from uveitis by doing Fluorescein angiography. There is delayed arteriolar filling, diffuse leakage in the posterior pole and from disc, as well as nonperfusion in the periphery.

Chronic peripheral rhegmatogenous retinal detachment: These patients might have the presence of flare, cells and vitreous cells. On examination with scleral depression, the retinal detachment might get picked up. In some cases, the cells in the anterior chamber might actually be the outer segment of the rod photoreceptors. When these cells block the trabecular meshwork, there is an increase in the intraocular pressure. This condition is called "Schwartz syndrome".

Endogenous endophthalmitis: Nocardia, Candida, Aspergillus and Coccidiomyces might be responsible for endophthalmitis. Patient might just present with the presence of cells in the anterior chamber along with vitreous cells and sometimes a chorioretinal lesion may be detected. A careful history along with a detailed physical examination might give a clue regarding the underlying systemic condition. So, if the patient gives history of exposure, weight loss and on examination any abnormality is picked up, detailed investigations should be done to rule out the above organisms.

Primary Central Nervous System Lymphoma

Introduction

Approximately 98% of primary intraocular lymphomas are extranodal, non-Hodgkin B-cell lymphomas, which are localized to the intraocular structures: vitreous, retina, subretinal and subretinal pigment epithelial spaces. Primary intraocular lymphoma may occur in isolation, without involvement of the CNS. However, since the ocular and the central nervous system components show identical cytologic features and phenotypic expression, many authors lump these two entities under the heading primary central nervous system lymphoma.

There can be secondary involvement of the eye or CNS by nodal lymphoma, in which the uvea is mainly infiltrated by the tumor cells.

Approximately 2% of PCNSL are T-cell lymphomas

Age: Generally affects people in the 6th–7th decade.

Sex: No predilection for any sex.

Incidence: It is said to be around 51 in 10,00,000 immunocompetent patients.

Clinical Features

Symptoms: The most common complaints are decreased vision and floaters.

Signs: There are spill over cells in the anterior chamber. There might be vitritis. There can be presence of yellowish-white subretinal lesions or infiltrates (Fig. 22.62). Many a times, the patients are treated with systemic steroids which decreases the vitritis. But, soon there is a rebound increase in vitritis and when a vitreous tap is done, it is nondiagnostic because of the previous intensive treatment.

CNS signs: The most common CNS sign in these patients include behavioral changes because of the periventricular location of the CNS lesions. Paresis, seizures, cerebellar signs and cranial nerve palsies may also occur.

Investigations

Fluorescein angiography: It shows the presence of hypofluorescent lesions wherever the lesions are present.

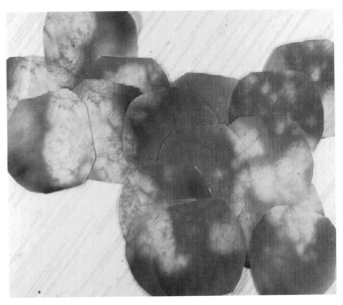

Fig. 22.62: Intraocular lymphoma: Montage fundus photograph shows multiple placoid lesions

USG: It shows the presence of a chorioretinal mass with high surface reflectivity, which is maintained throughout the lesion. Quite often a large serous retinal detachment might be present. There is absence of choroidal excavation and acoustic hallowing.

MRI and CT: They might show the presence of periventricular lesions, which might enhance on the injection of contrast.

CSF analysis: It might show the presence of lymphoma cells.

Histopathology: Specimens obtained from vitreous or subretinal space shows the presence of pleomorphic cells with hyperchromatic nuclei and an elevated nuclear/cytoplasmic ratio. The cytoplasm is very scant and multiple irregular nucleoli may be seen (Figs 22.63A and B).

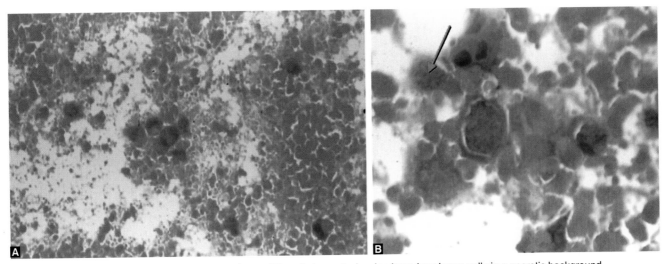

Figs 22.63A and B: Intraocular lymphoma: Microphotograph showing large lymphoma cells in a necrotic background

Cytokine analysis: The IL-10/IL-6 ratio is used to distinguish between vitritis because of lymphoma or vitritis because of other reasons.

Management

Patients < 60 years: Combined radiotherapy and chemotherapy can be tried.

Patients > 60 years: Only chemotherapy is given because of potential CNS toxicity from radiation.

There are anecdotal reports of using intravitreal methotrexate of 400 mg weekly or biweekly. Due to the high chances of CNS involvement (56%), it is advised to use CNS prophylaxis. The drugs used include intravenous and intrathecal methotrexate and intravenous cytarabine.

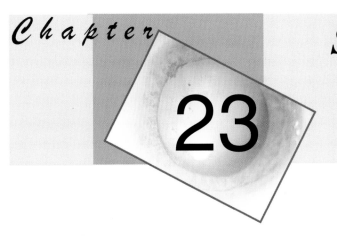

Chapter 23

Surgery in Uveitis: Diagnostic and Therapeutic

Vishali Gupta, Sushmita Kaushik, Amod Gupta

INTRODUCTION

Surgical interventions in uveitis include both diagnostic and therapeutic procedures. Diagnostic interventions include paracentesis or vitreous and/or chorioretinal biopsy that are sometimes required to reach a specific diagnosis. Therapeutic surgical procedures generally include cataract extraction, vitrectomy or glaucoma filtering surgery.

CATARACT SURGERY IN UVEITIS

Cataract occurs commonly in uveitis patients due to the inflammation per se and the concomitant use of corticosteroid as well as antiglaucoma medications (cholinergic agents) in some cases. Corticosteroids are the mainstay of uveitis treatment, and the untoward effects of uncontrolled uveitis far outweigh the development of cataract following corticosteroid therapy. The incidence of cataract approaches nearly 50% in many forms of uveitis, while in conditions like Fuchs' heterochromic uveitis, it is reported to be as high as 77.8% of the cases. Posterior subcapsular cataract is the most common type of cataract seen in uveitis patients.

Modern cataract surgery is reported to be safe even in the patients with a long history of intraocular inflammation. However, despite advances in the microsurgery; cataract extraction still poses a formidable challenge in patients with uveitis. Better understanding of the disease process and the risk factors involved has substantially changed the approach towards these patients. With careful patient selection, the rigorous preoperative and postoperative control of inflammation and meticulous surgery, it now appears possible to obtain a safer and more predictable outcome.

Indications for Cataract Surgery

Visual rehabilitation: The most common indication for cataract surgery is visual rehabilitation, as for any other patient with cataract.

Therapeutic indication: Besides the patient's visual needs, cataract surgery is occasionally indicated to improve visualization of the fundus in patients with uveitis. This is particularly true when the inflammation involves the posterior pole, and the treating ophthalmologist needs to be able to examine the fundus carefully to follow disease activity and/or the efficacy of therapy. In these circumstances, cataract may need to be removed even when the vision is not expected to improve markedly following the procedure.

Preoperative Evaluation

Meticulous preoperative evaluation and careful surgical planning are critical in achieving a successful surgical outcome in these patients. Preoperative factors that influence the surgical plan and outcome include the type and severity of uveitis, its duration, recent activity and associated complications. Preoperative assessment of a uveitis patient includes the following steps:

Establishing the diagnosis: The clinical course, treatment, complications and visual outcome of uveitic cataract are directly related to the type and cause of uveitis. Patients with the certain forms of inflammation respond better to cataract surgery than others. For instance, those with Fuchs' heterochromic uveitis or pars planitis usually respond particularly well to cataract surgery with relatively little postoperative inflammation and little or no tendency for anterior or posterior synechiae formation. These patients usually tolerate primary intraocular lens implantation well, and will require relatively less additional corticosteroid medication perioperatively.

On the other hand, more severe forms of uveitis, such as juvenile idiopathic arthritis (also known as juvenile rheumatoid arthritis and juvenile chronic arthritis); severe HLA-B27-associated uveitis; and granulomatous diseases, such as sarcoidosis and Vogt-Koyanagi-Harada disease tend to predispose these eyes to moderate to severe postoperative inflammation and complications related to synechiae formation. Consequently, patients with these forms of uveitis may not always tolerate an intraocular lens.

Timing of surgery: One of the most important determinants of successful cataract surgery in a patient of uveitis is ability to control the inflammation before surgery. It is important to know how difficult it has been to control uveitis. Patients with severe or more frequent recurrences will have more eventful postoperative course. Conversely, patients who have had only one mild attack of uveitis tend to do better following surgery. In general, cataract surgery in patients with anterior uveitis is more challenging than in patients with intermediate or posterior uveitis.

Most studies agree that longer the intraocular inflammation has been controlled prior to surgery, the better the outcome. The eye should ideally be quiet with no signs of inflammatory activity for six months or at least a minimum of three months prior to the planned procedure. This may involve increasing the dose of topical and/or systemic steroids. One exception to this cardinal rule is that when the cataract itself is the cause of the uveitis, as in traumatic or phacoantigenic uveitis, absolute control of intraocular inflammation is not required prior to cataract surgery.

Predicting the outcome: It is often difficult to predict the post-surgical visual outcome in patients with uveitis. Occasionally, coexisting pathology in the posterior segment like macular scar, cystoid macular edema, choroidal neovascular membrane, vitreous debris or hemorrhage that limit vision prior to surgery will also limit vision following surgery. Other factors that may influence surgical outcome include:

- Age is a major factor as children tend to have more severe inflammation with extensive synechiae, either posterior or anterior both before and after surgery. Cataract surgery in children with uveitis tends to be more challenging than in adults.
- Hypotony usually indicates long-standing and advanced uveitis
- Glaucoma
- A poor outcome of cataract surgery previously performed in the fellow eye.

Besides the patient's visual needs, cataract surgery is occasionally indicated to improve visualization of the fundus in patients with uveitis. This is particularly true when the inflammation involves the posterior pole, and the treating ophthalmologist needs to be able to examine the fundus carefully to follow disease activity and/or the efficacy of therapy. In these circumstances, cataract may need to be removed even when the vision is not expected to improve markedly following the procedure.

Preoperative Management

Once every attempt has been made to establish the cause for the uveitis, the visual potential of the eye with cataract should be assessed. It is beneficial, for example, to know that the eye had a normal visual acuity prior to the development of the cataract. An eye that has had amblyopia since childhood will have

a limited visual outcome even after the most successful cataract surgery. It is also important, whenever possible, to rule out coexisting retinal or optic nerve damage that might limit visual recovery, as mentioned above. When the cataract is so dense that it obscures the fundus, B-scan ultrasound can be used to rule out occult retinal detachment or intraocular tumors.

The intraocular inflammation should have been controlled for 3 to 6 months with corticosteroids or non-corticosteroid immunosuppressive agents, before most patients may undergo cataract surgery if not otherwise contraindicated. It is helpful to treat all uveitis patients with a daily dose of 1.0 mg/kg oral prednisolone 3 to 7 days prior to surgery, in addition to topical prednisolone acetate 1% 6 to 8 times a day.

Surgical Considerations

Phacoemulsification Versus Extracapsular Cataract Extraction

Phacoemulsification is currently the preferred approach to the removal of most cataracts in eyes with uveitis. The small incision, reduction of iris trauma from prolapse into the wound, reduction of iris stretch with nucleus expression, and capsulorhexis favor phacoemulsification. A recent retrospective study reported a lower incidence of cystoid macular edema, epiretinal membranes and posterior synechiae formation in uveitic eyes undergoing phacoemulsification compared to those undergoing extracapsular cataract extractions. However, the eventual visual acuity was comparable in both groups of patients. Two other studies have demonstrated lesser incidence of recurrent inflammation requiring treatment with after phacoemulsification compared to extracapsular cataract extraction. This overall decreased postoperative inflammation is believed to be due to the lesser surgical insult during phacoemulsification surgery (Figs 23.1 and 23.2).

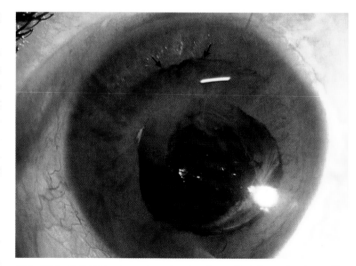

Fig. 23.1: Extracapsular cataract extraction with intraocular lens after Nd:YAG laser capsulotomy. (Patient # 1) Anterior segment photograph following 12 months of surgery. Note the shrink-wrap effect of uveal tissue around the intraocular lens (arrows)

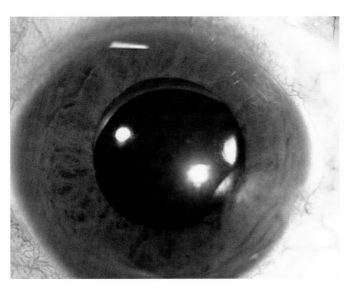

Fig. 23.2: Phacoemulsification with intraocular lens implantation. (Patient # 1) The opposite eye of the same patient 9 months after phacoemulsification with intraocular lens implantation showing round pupil with no capsular opacification

Pars Plana approach

Pars plana lensectomy and vitrectomy is preferable in eyes with extensive preoperative synechiae and the presence of a cyclitic membrane or with concomitant posterior segment disease that needs to be addressed surgically and complete removal of the cataract and capsule is desired. The most common setting for such intervention is in a patient with juvenile rheumatoid arthritis. These eyes often do poorly with intraocular lens implantation and leaving the posterior capsule in place may provide a scaffold for cyclitic membrane formation.

When vision limiting vitreous debris/hemorrhage is present, it may be preferable to perform trans-limbal cataract surgery along with a pars plana vitrectomy.

Problems Specific to the Uveitic Patient and their Management

Regardless of the technique chosen, there are some differences between patients with and without uveitis, and these should be noted while planning for surgery.

- Posterior synechiae are more very common in these eyes that can make pupil small, immobile and irregular. Posterior synechiae can also produce glaucoma by way of pupillary block.
- Less commonly, anterior synechiae may develop, which both damage and occlude the angle, limiting aqueous outflow. While anterior synechiae should seldom be lysed, posterior synechiae in fact need to be released in order to remove the cataract.

Posterior synechiolysis is usually best performed with blunt dissection using either a cannula filled with viscoelastic or a cyclodialysis spatula. Additional viscoelastic can be injected under the iris to help release adhesions and to protect the anterior lens capsule. Once the iris is freed, the pupil may need to be enlarged by stretching it, either by using two instruments, such as a chopper and dialing hook that are commonly found on the surgical tray. Unfortunately this technique works poorly in cases in which iris is fibrotic and firmly adherent and also can result in capsular tear making phacoemulsification difficult.

If simple stretching does not result in adequate pupillary dilatation, self-retaining hooks are required to maintain the configuration of the pupil during surgery. Occasionally, sphincterotomies may also be required.

A new procedure to address this problem has been the description of a carefully performed Nd:YAG laser synechiolysis for release of these synechiae prior to phacoemulsification. This is a viable option with few complications if performed carefully.

Fankhauser, first described Nd:YAG laser synechiolysis in 1985, for three patients. In one patient in that series, the laser procedure was performed prior to contemplated cataract surgery. Despite some damage to the pupil margin in two out of the three patients, pupil contractility was preserved in all three cases. Restoration of pupil mobility in these eyes is important as it normalizes the pupil functions. Another report describes results of Nd:YAG synechiolysis in 15 patients having bound down pupil due to granulomatous uveitis. No significant laser related complications were observed in any of the 15 eyes.

In our experience, preoperative Nd:YAG laser lysis of extensive iridolenticular adhesions in patients with uveitis, followed by phacoemulsification with intraocular lens implantation was found to be a successful strategy in terms of restoration of pupillary mobility and uncomplicated phacoemulsification (Figs 23.3 to 23.6).

Selection of the Intraocular Lens

Although patients with uveitis are at the increased risk of complications following cataract surgery with intraocular lens

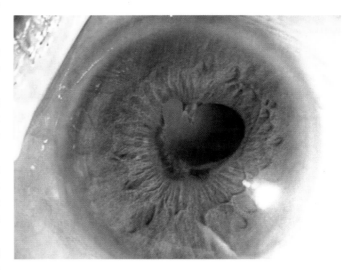

Fig. 23.3: Complicated cataract. (Patient # 2) Preoperative anterior segment photograph showing complicated cataract with posterior synechiae

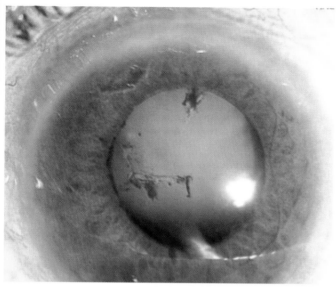

Fig. 23.4: Nd:YAG laser synechiolysis. (Patient # 2) Same eye as in Fig. 23.3 immediately following Nd:YAG posterior synechiolysis

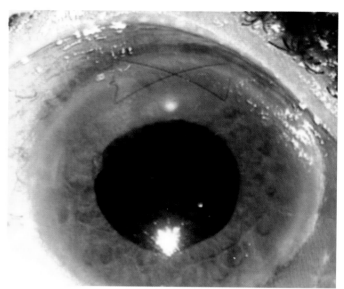

Fig. 23.6: Phacoemulsification with intraocular implantation. (Patient # 2) Same eye one day postoperative following phacoemulsification with intraocular implantation

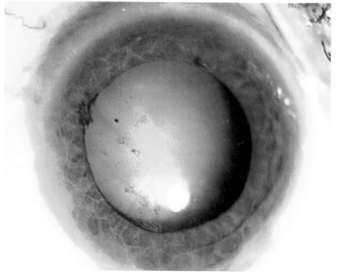

Fig. 23.5: Post Nd:YAG laser synechiolysis (Patient # 2) Same eye one week later, after full pupillary dilatation preoperatively

implantation, due to preexisting inflammation, improvements in technology, materials, and surgical techniques have greatly improved outcomes. State-of-the-art materials and improved intraocular lens designs have helped facilitate these outcomes and encourage ophthalmologists to treat symptomatic cataracts in uveitic patients sooner rather than later.

Patient Selection

Once the cataract is removed, the surgeon must decide whether the patient is a good candidate to receive an intraocular lens implant. Patients with Fuchs' heterochromic uveitis and pars planitis, tend to do well with implants. In contrast, patients with granulomatous disease, such as sarcoidosis or Vogt-Koyanagi-Harada's disease, and children with severe forms of uveitis, such as juvenile idiopathic arthritis, tend to do less well. Similarly,

special care should also be taken with monocular patients, with very young patients, with patients who may have difficulty complying with intensive postoperative medication schedules, and with patients who have had a complicated cataract surgery in the fellow eye.

Intraocular Lens Material and Biocompatibility

Since introducing any foreign object into the eye will lead to additional inflammation and contribute to endothelial cell damage, cystoid macular edema, glaucoma, and the formation of synechiae within the eye, surgeons must carefully consider biocompatibility when selecting an intraocular lens for a uveitic patient.

There are three main determinants of intraocular biocompatibility:

• Effect on the blood-aqueous barrier
• Cellular proliferation on the lens surface
• Opacification of the posterior capsule

Several studies have compared the effects of intraocular lens materials on uveitic eyes. Intraocular lens material is the most important determinant of inflammatory deposits. The single-piece, first-generation silicone plate lenses; three-piece acrylic lenses; and three-piece, second-generation lenses have been compared. Single-piece, first-generation silicone plate lenses show the highest amount of these deposits, with acrylic lenses showing an intermediate amount, and three-piece, second-generation lenses showing the least. This contradicts earlier studies that showed acrylic lenses were less immunogenic due to their surface composition. The three-piece, more modern silicone intraocular lenses may show a smaller inflammatory reaction due to a thinner profile made possible by an increased refractive index.

Performance of hydrophilic acrylic intraocular lenses, hydrophobic acrylic intraocular lenses, and silicone intraocular lenses in uveitic eyes undergoing cataract surgery have been compared with a group of patients without uveitis undergoing phacoemulsification with intraocular lens implantation. Intraocular lens biocompatibility has been assessed by the degree of cellular reaction and capsular opacification. After six months, the uveitic eyes with hydrophobic acrylic intraocular lenses have been found to have a statistically higher number of foreign-body giant cells than either uveitic eyes with other intraocular lenses or control eyes. The rate of posterior capsular opacification is higher in all eyes with uveitis compared with controls, with the hydrophilic acrylic intraocular lens leading to significantly more posterior capsular opacification than the hydrophobic acrylic, or the silicone intraocular lenses in the uveitic eyes.

Amount of anterior chamber cell and flare reaction in uveitic eyes undergoing small-incision phacoemulsification with hydrophilic acrylic intraocular lenses, hydrophobic acrylic intraocular lenses or silicone intraocular lenses have also been compared. At 6 months, there is no significant difference in the amount of anterior chamber reaction.

In general, the newer materials being used in intraocular lenses, such as acrylic and third-generation silicone are more biocompatible within the eye than earlier models. First-generation silicone lenses should be avoided in patients with uveitis, however, as they are less biocompatible.

Current Concept

The general consensus among ophthalmologists is that while uveitic eyes are at higher risk for complications after cataract surgery, with appropriate preoperative control of inflammation and use of more biocompatible intraocular lenses, overall sight improvement can be achieved. Surgeons can decrease the risk of inflammation and other adverse effects with the administration of preoperative topical and/or oral steroids and by minimizing the incision size.

The development of foldable intraocular lenses has improved the success rate of cataract surgery in most patients. Foldable lenses allow incision sizes to be reduced to 2.8 mm, lessening the potential for surgically induced astigmatism and shortening healing times. In addition, foldable intraocular lenses have been shown to minimize the trauma to the corneal endothelium, resulting in less corneal edema. Cataract surgery in uveitic patients has become safer and more successful with improvements in technology, and this will likely continue in the future.

Postoperative Care

Following cataract surgery in patients with uveitis, the oral corticosteroids that were started prior to surgery may be increased if required and should be tapered very slowly. Frequent administration of topical corticosteroids (half hourly to one hourly) is recommended in the early postoperative period. The tapering for both topical and oral corticosteroids usually takes 3 to 6 weeks, but may be even longer in patients with severe or frequently recurrent uveitis. A few patients may require additional immunosuppressive agents, such as methotrexate, azathioprine or cyclosporine, to control their postoperative inflammation, particularly if these agents were required to control their uveitis prior to surgery. In general, if patients were on long-term immunosuppressive therapy prior to surgery, then this should be continued following the procedure.

Postoperative Complications

Excessive Inflammation

Patients with a history of uveitis often have more than usual postoperative inflammation. However, this need to be differentiated from other two potential causes of excessive postoperative inflammation namely infection and retained lens material.

Intraocular Pressure

Following surgery, the intraocular pressure may either be elevated or decreased. Elevated intraocular pressure can usually be controlled with pressure-lowering medication, but may sometimes require glaucoma surgery in very severe and refractory cases. Problems with low pressure after surgery may be due either to an increase in the amount of inflammation, to a wound leak, to a cyclodialysis cleft or to choroidal detachment. Whereas hypotony due to inflammation usually responds to anti-inflammatory medications, such as corticosteroids, wound leaks and cyclodialysis clefts often require additional surgery. Choroidal detachment may settle spontaneously or require drainage.

Cystoid Macular Edema

One of the more common complications for patients with uveitis is cystoid macula edema. It will often respond to topical corticosteroid or nonsteroidal anti-inflammatory drops, but in those patients who do not respond to topical corticosteroids, a periocular corticosteroid injection of triamcinolone acetonide, 40 mg, may be indicated. In some patients, cystoid macular edema may be refractory and require pars plana vitrectomy with removal of posterior hyloid.

Posterior Capsular Opacification

Posterior capsular opacification depends upon the intraocular lens material and design used. In uveitic eyes, the incidence of posterior capsule opacification is directly proportional to the amount of ocular inflammation. It has been reported that in spite of a sharp-edged optic design, hydrophobic acrylic material, capsular bag fixation of intraocular lens, the development of posterior capsule opacification is accelerated in inflamed eyes.

Anterior Capsular Opacification

Anterior capsular opacification of the capsulorhexis rim and between the optic and capsule has been more commonly seen in uveitic eyes than in normal eyes, irrespective of the intraocular lens biocompatibility.

Summary of Present Recommendations for Cataract Surgery in Patients of Uveitis

The following principles are believed to be strongly supported by the medical evidence as published in peer-reviewed journals:

- Control of inflammation for a substantial period of time preoperatively is critical to a good outcome.
- Control of inflammation postoperatively is clearly critical for a good outcome.
- An intraocular lens implant can be part of a reasonable surgical plan for the patient with uveitis and cataract, provided thoughtful considerations are given to patient selection, i.e. not all patients are good candidates for a lens implant.
- Young patients with juvenile rheumatoid arthritis (juvenile idiopathic arthritis) and associated uveitis with cataract should not be routinely implanted with a lens implant.

Vitrectomy for Uveitis

Pars plana vitrectomy in uveitis can be broadly classified into the following categories:

Diagnostic: The diagnostic vitrectomy is indicated in the patients of uveitis with atypical clinical picture, poor response to therapy with suspected infectious or malignant etiology. The main aim is to obtain the vitreous humor sample that can be subsequently microbiology, immunology and molecular genetic methods so as to reach a specific diagnosis. This is estimated that in approximately 8% of cases of uveitis, the clinical presentation is atypical and systemic investigations inconclusive. These types of cases require diagnostic pars plana vitrectomy that is generally done in the acute stage.

Therapeutic: Therapeutic vitrectomy serves two purposes:

- Pars plana vitrectomy helps by physically removing the vitreous with resident inflammatory cells and the mediators of inflammation.
- Managing the secondary effects of uveitis, i.e. nonresolving vitreous hemorrhage, cystoid macular edema, epiretinal membranes, abnormal vitreoretinal tractions, choroidal neovascular membranes and retinal detachments. This is generally done in the chronic inactive stage of uveitis.

Diagnostic-therapeutic: This involves taking the undiluted vitreous humor for laboratory tests and then performing the complete vitrectomy with removal of posterior hyloid membrane to prevent/cure complications associated with severe uveitis. This also allows thorough intraocular distribution of drugs.

Diagnostic Pars Plana Vitrectomy

Diagnostic vitrectomy could involve any of the following:

- Vitreous tap/ aspiration
- Vitreous biopsy
- Chorioretinal biopsy

Indications:

- Atypical clinical presentations

- Nonresponsive to empirical treatment with corticosteroids/immunosuppressant
- Rapidly progressive disease with inconclusive noninvasive work-up
- Strong suspicion of malignancy

Preoperative Preparation

Detailed history, general physical examination, complete ancillary and laboratory investigations should be performed with short listed differential diagnosis and a clear plan of action are must before undertaking diagnostic pars plana vitrectomy. Since the main aim of diagnostic pars plana vitrectomy is to subject the sample for diagnostic tests, it is imperative to inform the microbiologist/molecular biologist/cytologist before taking the vitreous sample so that the laboratory is ready to receive and process the sample. The uveitis expert must have a clear plan as to what tests are to be done so that the concerned laboratories could be informed in advance. Utmost care should be taken to transport the sample to the laboratory, as early as possible, under the optimal conditions as recommended by the cytologist/ molecular biologist so that the cells don't degenerate.

Preoperative Counseling

Since the patients who undergo diagnostic vitrectomy are the ones who are non-responding to the treatment and often difficult to diagnose and manage, it is very important to make them understand that this surgical procedure is mainly for the diagnostic purposes and not a therapeutic intervention. The patient needs to be told that it is also likely that the laboratory tests may not be able to give a definitive report. Informed consent should be taken from all patients.

Surgical Techniques

Anterior Segment Tap/ Paracentesis

This is done translimbally using 26-gauge needle under all aseptic precautions. Approximately 0.2 ml of aqueous humor is withdrawn gently taking care not to touch the lens or corneal endothelium. Anterior chamber should be well formed at the end of procedure. Anterior chamber tap is indicated in various infections, lens-induced uveitis and masquerade syndromes, including retinoblastoma and leukemia (Figs 23.7 and 23.8).

Vitreous Tap/ Aspiration

This procedure is done using a 23-gauge or a 26-gauge needle, directly attached to a syringe via a flexible tube containing balanced salt solution preferably under indirect ophthalmoscopic control. The sample withdrawn is usually 0.2 to 0.5 cc; the cell suspensions resulting from rinsing out of needles should also be added to the sample. The technique is simple and easy to perform and can be done as an outdoor procedure, but may cause traction at the vitreous base, hypotony and retinal detachment. It is the only technique for suspected retinoblastoma, and the sample must be immediately transported to laboratory for processing.

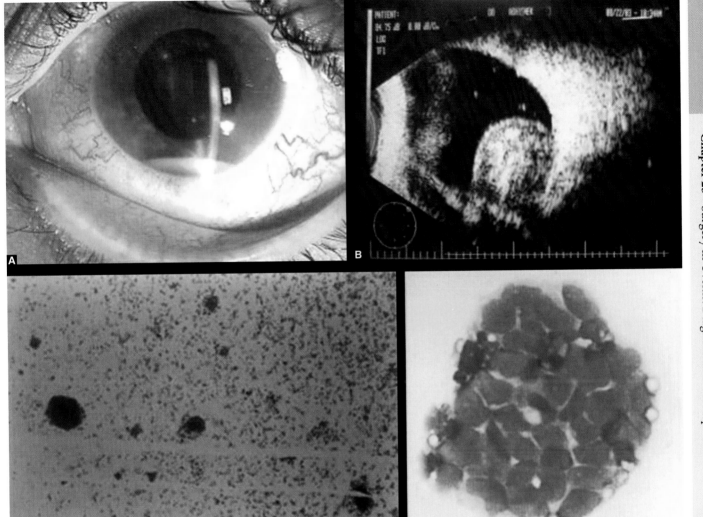

Figs 23.7A to D: Round cell tumor. A 10-year-old boy presented with hypopyon (a), ultrasound B-scan showed a hyperechoeic mass inferiorly (b), Cytology of the aqueous humor from anterior chamber tap showed round cell tumor on MGG (c), and Pap (d) smear. Based on cytology, the child was advised enucleation

Vitreous Biopsy

The procedure can be done under either general or topical anesthesia. Here approximately 1.0 ml of vitreous is obtained directly from the vitrectomy cutter handpiece, with a cutting rate at 1200/minute, through an in-line stopcock and tubing attached to a syringe. For vitreous aspiration the one-port technique can be used. However, in eyes with uveitis, where there can be coexistent media opacities or intraocular inflammation, the three-port technique is preferable once the undiluted sample has been obtained, a complete therapeutic pars plana vitrectomy can also be performed to make it combined diagnostic-therapeutic vitrectomy. Total vitrectomy enhances visualization of the fundus and allows better diffusion of intraocular medications. Finally, approximately 50% of eyes treated with diagnostic pars plana vitrectomy have subsequently improved visual acuity, results comparable with those of therapeutic vitrectomy.

This technique has also an advantage of yielding more samples with enough material available for multiple tests. Also there is more control on vitreous traction and hypotony is avoided. Vitrectomy does not cause cell degradation. The authors find 25-gauge vitrectomy very useful for obtaining the vitreous biopsy and performing therapeutic pars plana vitrectomy.

The vitreous aspirate needs to be shifted to laboratory as early as possible for the preselected tests. The tests could be broadly classified as:

Microbiological tests: The smears and stains are very useful for rapid initial diagnosis of infective organisms. Though the smears have their own limitations with Gram stain positivity only in 66% of culture proven cases. However, positive smears results are available within hours and if positive, the specific therapy could be initiated even before the culture reports are available.

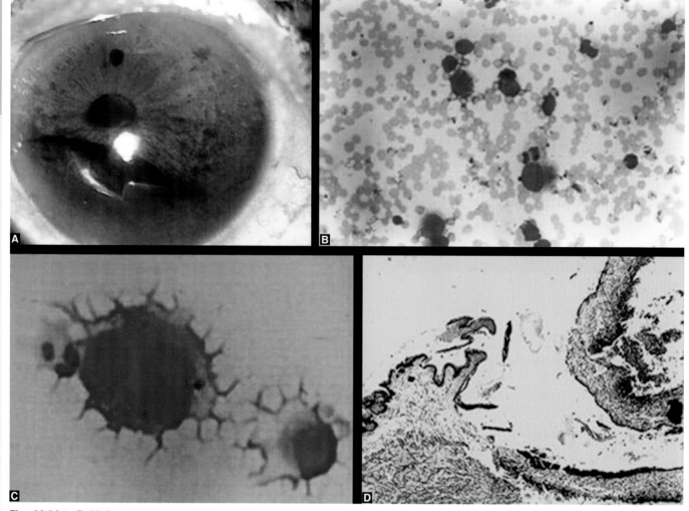

Figs 23.8A to D: Malignant melanoma. A 58-year-old woman was seen with pigmented growth in her left eye that was present since childhood (A), Anterior segment aspirate showed melanin-laden pigment cells on MGG stain (B), Pap smear (40X) showed binucleated pigment containing malignant cells (C), The eye was enucleated and histopathology of the enucleated specimen confirmed malignant melanoma of the ciliary body (D)

Undiluted intraocular fluid samples can be directly inoculated for cultures. In cases of diluted vitreous humor samples, the sample should be first passed through Millipore filters; microorganisms or any cellular elements concentrate on the filter surface. The filter is then cut under sterile conditions and used for culture. Bacterial cultures should be kept 4 to 6 weeks and the microbiologist should be informed not to discard sample early.

Polymerase chain reaction: Polymerase chain reaction is a molecular biologic technique used to amplify the specific region of DNA in order to produce multiple copies of DNA to be adequately tested. To perform polymerase chain reaction one needs a source of DNA and the sequence to be amplified. The sequence being amplified could be a lymphoma gene in the patient's DNA, or a gene from a suspected pathogen, e.g. *Mycobacterium tuberculosis*.

Polymerase chain reaction has a number of advantages; it is rapid, sensitive and can be performed on the small quantities of sample that might be available from the eye. However, one has to be careful about false positive tests. Its use has been increasing for the detection of intraocular infections. It can be used to detect a number of microorganisms:

- *Bacteria*: Pseudomonas , Streptococcus, Staphylococcus, Borrelia, Bartonella, Mycobacterium, Propionibacterium acne
- *Fungi*: Aspergillus, Candida
- *Parasites*: Toxoplasma, Onchocerca
- Viruses: HSV, CMV, VZV, HTLV, Adenovirus

Polymerase chain reaction analysis is also being used for diagnosing intraocular malignancy namely lymphomas, e.g. Bcl-2 gene shows translocation in non-Hodgkin's lymphoma that brings it in proximity to the immunoglobulin (Ig) heavy-chain promoter on chromosome 14 with over expression of Bcl-2. The Ig heavy-chain rearrangement can be detected by the polymerase chain reaction in ocular specimens of patients with intraocular-CNS lymphoma.

Cytopathological analysis of the vitreous: Cytopathology plays an important role for studying the cell morphology that helps to differentiate between infective, noninfective and malignant etiologies. The noninfectious uveitis shows acute and chronic inflammatory cells whereas infective uveitis might show microbes or fungal hyphae along with inflammatory cells.

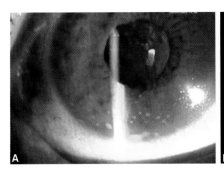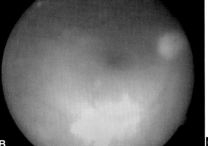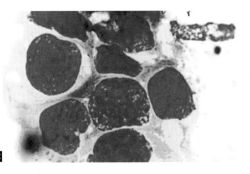

Figs 23.9A to C: Retinoblastoma. An eight-year-old girl was seen with anterior segment inflammation (A), vitreous cells with cellular infiltrates inferiorly (B), Vitreous biopsy with 23-gauge needle showed round cells suggestive of retinoblastoma (C)

Presence of eosinophils is an indicator towards parasitic infections. Malignant cells can be identified and thus cytopathology plays an important role in the diagnosis of masquerade syndromes. Since the technique is based on identifying cell morphology, it is important to take adequate measures to preserve cell morphology and prevent the cells from degenerating. Also it is important that the person who is studying the morphology is an expert cytologist so that the interpretation is correct (Fig. 23.9).

Flow Cytometry and Immunohistochemistry

Both flow cytometery and immunohistochemistry can detect cell- or tissue-bound antigens by using fluorescence-activated cell sorters in flow cytometery and fluorescence-labeled (immunofluorescence) or enzyme-labeled antibodies (immunoperoxidase) in immunohistochemistry. These methods are done after cytopathology report is available and provide additional information regarding the subtypes of the cells. For example, cytology can show T lymphocytes, but it is immunohistochemistry or flow cytometry that will provide information as to whether these lymphocytes represent helper-inducer (CD4+) or suppressor-cytotoxic (CD8+) T-cell populations.

Antibody Production in Vitreous

Local antibody production is a very strong indicator towards the infectious organism within the eye and can be measured by ELISA. However, since blood-ocular barrier is disrupted in the intraocular inflammations, the false positive results need to be eliminated. The Goldmann-Witmer antibody coefficient, which relates vitreous to serum antibodies, can be used to determine local antibody production:

Goldmann-Witmer Antibody Coefficient = [specific vitreous Ig/ total vitreous Ig] / [specific serum Ig/ total serum Ig] A coefficient >3.0 is believed to be diagnostic.

Cytokines in Vitreous

Cytokines are soluble proteins that determine differentiation, migration and activity of T-cells, macrophages and monocyte. Their level determination helps in differentiating inflammatory and malignant diseases. Interleukin-1, -2 and -6 have been found to correlate well with uveitis or infection. IL-10 concentrations have been found to be elevated in intraocular lymphomas.

Chorioretinal Biopsy

It is a highly invasive procedure and is only considered when all other invasive diagnostic techniques like vitreous biopsy fail to provide useful information and the disease is bilateral, rapidly progressive and nonresponding to the best possible therapy. The biopsy is undertaken in an eye with poorer vision with a potential of 20/200 or worse and the contra lateral eye has a vision-threatening disease.

The availability of a competent pathologist experienced in chorioretinal histology is a must for this procedure. The biopsy can be done from outside by making a scleral flap at the site of lesion and getting the chorioretinal tissue using micro blade and scissors. An alternative way is to do an endoretinal biopsy following vitrectomy with the help of intraocular scissors and forceps. The choice of the procedure depends on the type and site of lesion. Endoretinal biopsy is thought to be safer. The biopsy specimen can be divided for culture, histology and immunopathology.

The complications of the procedure include choroidal hemorrhage, retinal detachment, proliferative vitreoretinopathy and infection.

Section

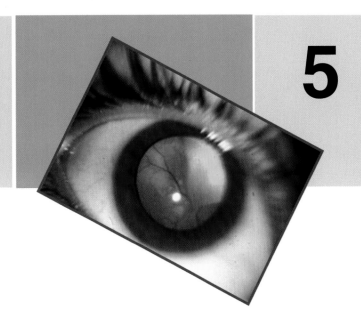

5

Vitreoretinal Diseases

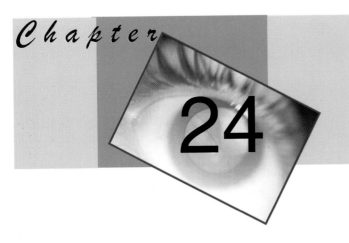

Investigations in Retinal Diseases

Sandeep Saxena

INTRODUCTION

Fluorescein angiography, indocyanine green angiography, optical coherence tomography, B-scan ultrasonography, microperimetry and multifocal electroretinography are the current investigations, which impart useful information regarding the diagnosis, management and follow up in retinal diseases.

FLUORESCEIN ANGIOGRAPHY

Novotny and Alvis performed the first successful fluorescein angiography in humans by using digital imaging technique. Our understanding on fluorescein angiography is still expanding. Sodium fluorescein is yellow-red in color with a molecular weight of 376.67, a spectrum of absorption at 465–490 nm (blue) and excitation at 520–530 nm (yellow-green) wavelengths. Once injected, 80% of the dye binds with plasma proteins, particularly to albumin. It is metabolized by the liver and kidney and within 24–36 hours it gets eliminated through urine, which becomes discolored (bright orange hue). Adverse reactions range from mild to severe.

After rapid injection into the antecubital vein, fluorescein dye enters the short posterior ciliary arteries and is visualized in the choroid and optic nerve head in 10 to 15 seconds. The "choroidal flush" is the hallmark of choroidal filling. The mottled fluorescence of the choriocapillaris is attributed to variable blockage by the retinal pigment epithelium. Patchy filling of the choroid anatomically represents perfusion of choriocapillaris lobules sequentially, rather than simultaneously. In the early angiogram, leakage of the dye from the choriocapillaris and staining of the Bruch's membrane eclipses the choroidal vessel detail. Retinal circulation filling begins at 10 to 15 seconds, approximately 1 to 3 seconds after the onset of choroidal filling. After the dye is seen in the central retinal arteries, the fluorescein travels into the precapillary arterioles, the capillaries, the postcapillary venules and then exits the eye through veins in a laminar pattern. Laminar filling of the veins is caused by a preferential concentration of unbound fluorescein along the vessel walls. This has been attributed to the faster flow of blood, as well as higher concentration of erythrocytes in the central vascular lumen.

The early arteriovenous phase is followed by the late arteriovenous phase, which is characterized by the maximal fluorescence of the arteries and the capillary bed, with early laminar filling of the veins. Juxtafoveal capillary network achieves maximal fluorescence at 20 to 25 seconds. A dark background in the macula, created by blockage of choroidal fluorescence by xanthophyll pigments and a high density of retinal pigment epithelium cells enhances the capillary detail. The normal foveal avascular zone is 300 to 500 μm. At 30 seconds, the first pass of fluorescein dye is complete. This is followed by the recirculation phases, in which there is intermittent mild fluorescence. At 10 minutes both circulations are generally devoid of fluorescein. The last angiogram is characterized by staining of Bruch's membrane, the choroid and sclera, which are more visible in patients with light retinal pigment epithelium. Staining of the disc margin and the optic nerve head, which is independent of the degree of retinal epithelium pigmentation.

Identification of abnormal areas of fluorescence and the identification of hypofluorescence and hyperfluorescence is crucial in interpretation of fluorescein angiograms. Hypofluorescence is the reduction or absence of normal fluorescence, while hyperfluorescence is increased or abnormal fluorescence (Figs 24.1A to 24.3F).

Hypofluorescence can be categorized into blockage or vascular filling defects. Blocked fluorescence can give us clues to the level of the blocking material. Vascular filling of defects cause hypofluorescence, because of decrease or absence of perfusion of tissues.

Hyperfluorescence is caused by an increase in normal fluorescence or abnormal presence of fluorescence. A window defect refers to choroidal fluorescence produced by a relative decrease or absence of pigment in the retinal pigment epithelium. Hyperfluorescence is attributed to the presence of abnormal blood vessels seen in the retina, choroid and the

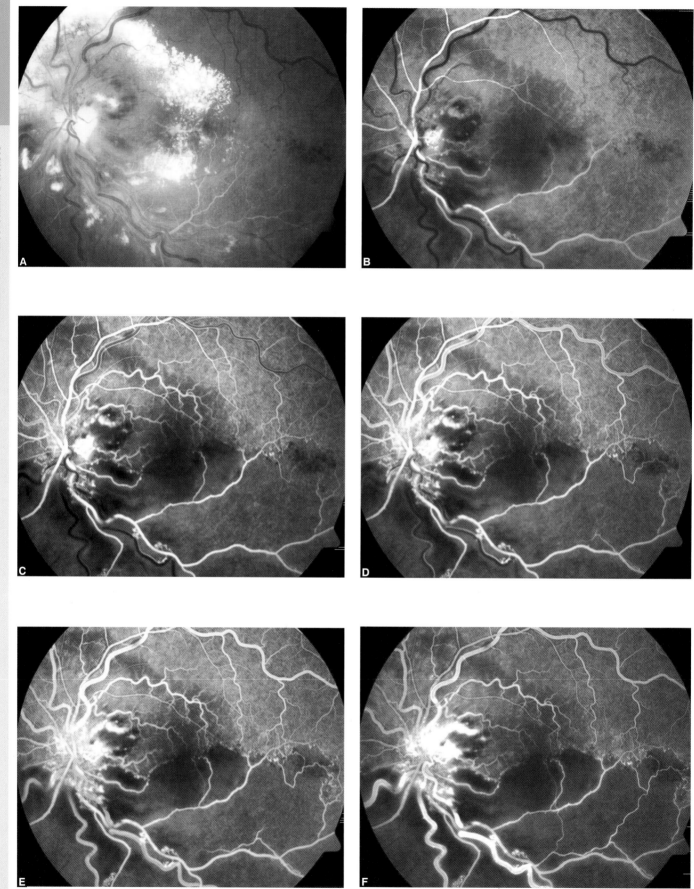

Figs 24.1A to F

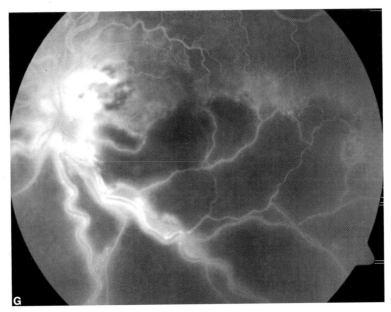

Figs 24.1A to G: Retinal vascular occlusive disease: Color fundus photograph (A). Sequential fluorescein angiography (B to G)

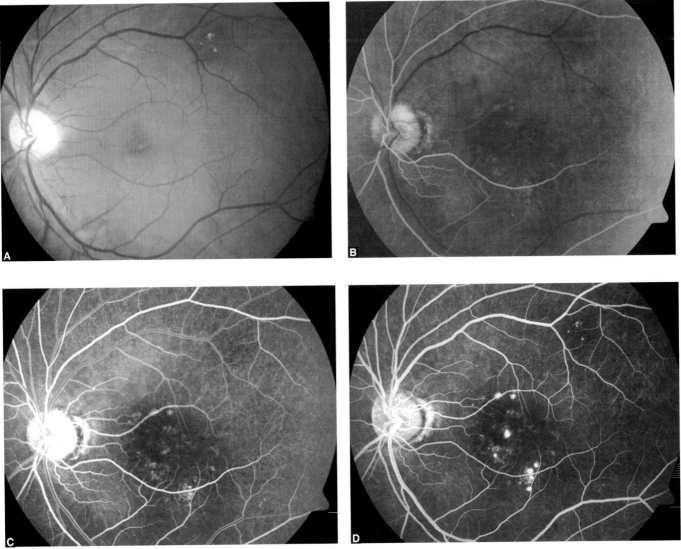

Figs 24.2A to D

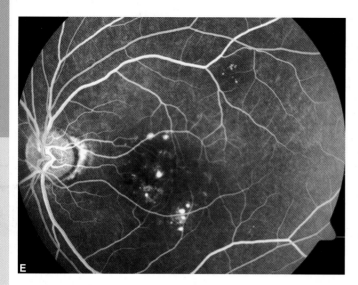

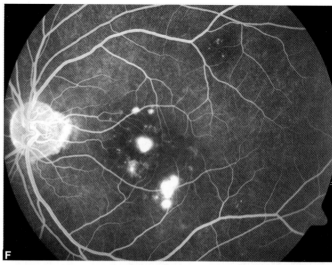

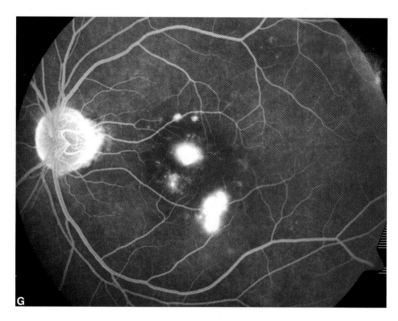

Figs 24.2A to G: Central serous chorioretinopathy: Color fundus photograph (A). Sequential fluorescein angiography (B to G)

optic disc. Leakage of dye into the extravascular space leads to hyperfluorescence.

INDOCYANINE GREEN ANGIOGRAPHY

Digital indocyanine green angiography is useful in imaging the choroid and its associated pathology. Indocyanine green is a tricarbocyanine dye that has several special properties, which gives it an advantage over sodium fluorescein, as a dye for ophthalmic imaging. The dye has a molecular weight of 775 daltons. Eighty percent of the dye is bound to globulins. Indocyanine green is active between 790–805 nm. It is excreted via bile by the liver. The dye is relatively safe. Properties of indocyanine green dye make it useful in imaging occult or poorly defined choroidal neovascularization secondary to age-related macular degeneration.

Three morphological types of choroidal neovascularization may be seen. These lesions include focal spots, plaques and combination lesions, in which both focal spots and plaques are noted. There are three subtypes of combination lesions: Marginal spots (focal spots at the edge of plaques of neovascularization), overlying spots (hot spots overlying plaques of neovascularization) and remote spots (a focal spot remote to from a plaque of neovascularization).

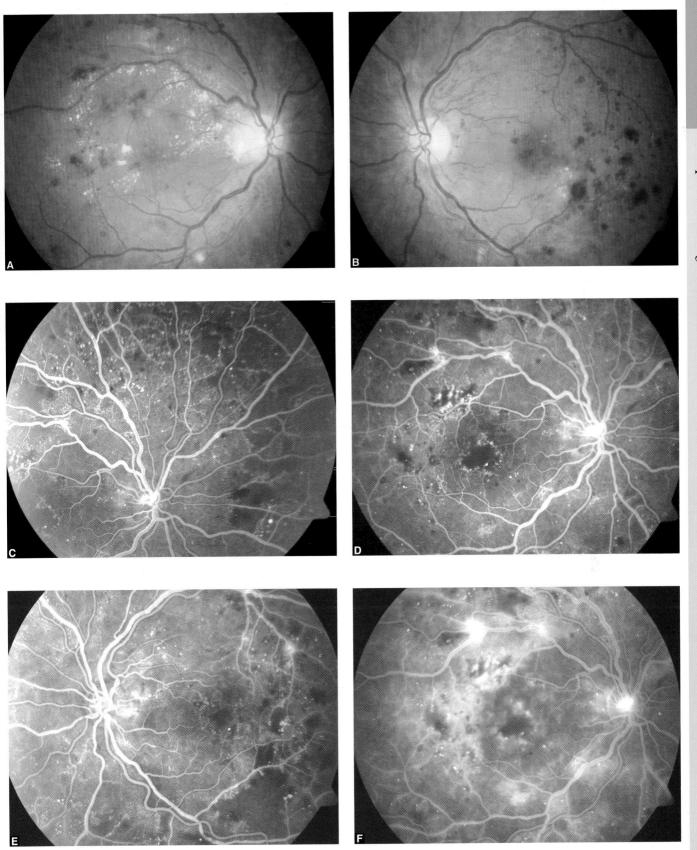

Figs 24.3A to F: Proliferative diabetic retinopathy with clinically significant macular edema: Color fundus photographs (A and B). Sequential fluorescein angiography. Right eye shows enlarged foveal avascular zone, multiple microaneurysms and areas of capillary nonperfusion and leakage of fluorescein dye from the neovascularization at the disc and neovascularization elsewhere. Left eye shows multiple microaneurysms. Areas of capillary nonperfusion and early leakage of fluorescein dye from neovascularization elsewhere (C to F)

SCANNING LASER OPHTHALMOSCOPE-BASED ANGIOGRAPHY

The confocal scanning laser ophthalmoscope has the property of providing optical sections through the use of confocal optics. It utilizes a combination of three lasers at appropriate wavelengths to form a color image, which is analogous to the formation of color television images using red, green and blue phosphors. The lasers used are 790, 820 and 488 nm. Each of the three beams are aimed and detected through the same set of optics. These beams can be used individually or in combination. Main advantages of Heidelberg Retinal Angiography (HRA2), over conventional imaging are its image quality, dynamic capabilities and efficiency. Compared to both the original HRA and fundus cameras, the HRA2 takes higher resolution images, which means better definition and greater detail. With fluorescein, the HRA2 enables physicians to see details just 5 μm in size (three times smaller than the 15 μm details visible with a fundus camera image) and all in an image that is just 1536 × 1536 pixels with a 30° field of view. Fundus cameras with much larger image sizes cannot match this resolution because the HRA2 suppresses scattered light. It can however, resolve to 5 μm per pixel compared to the fundus cameras of 15–18 μm per pixel. Indocyanine green angiography performed with the HRA2 provides greater chorioretinal detail than the ordinary fundus camera's indocyanine green angiography. In terms of the field view, the HRA2 is narrower than the conventional fundus camera. Fundus cameras are generally capable of 45° or 50°, 30° or 35° and 20°, whereas the HRA2's fields of view are 30°, 20° and 15°. One disadvantage of the HRA system is their lack of color imaging, which facilitates angiogram interpretation (Fig. 24.4).

The HRA systems offer still frames and full motion indocyanine green angiography. A significant advantage over the fundus camera's static-only indocyanine green angiography, which is not informative and fast enough. For choroidal studies, the first six seconds are important. Infrared imaging with extremely high resolution and real time video of the vessel filling imparts the detailed information for circulation studies. Simultaneous fluorescein angiography and indocyanine green angiography not only saves time, but also aids diagnosis by helping in correlating with the choroidal pathology on the indocyanine green angiogram with the fluorescein angiogram's retinal landmarks.

OPTICAL COHERENCE TOMOGRAPHY

Optical coherence tomography (OCT) is a new technique for the high resolution, cross-sectional visualization of retinal structure. Optical coherence tomography achieves 2 or 3 dimensional cross-sectional imaging of retina by measuring the echo delay and intensity of back reflected infrared light from internal tissue structures. Optical coherence tomography is based on the principle of Michelson's interferometry.

Using a classic optical measurement technique known as low coherence interferometry in combination with special broad bandwidth light; OCT achieves high resolution, cross-sectional visualization of tissue morphologic characteristics at depths significantly greater than the penetration depth offered by conventional bright field and confocal microscopy.

Imaging with OCT is analogous to ultrasound B-scan in that distance information is extracted from the time delays of reflected signals. However, the use of optical rather than acoustic waves in OCT provides a much higher (≤10 μm) longitudinal resolution in the retina, versus the 100 μm scale of ultrasound. This is due to the fact that the speed of light is nearly a million times faster than the speed of sound. Use of optical waves also allows a noncontact and noninvasive measurement. The ability to evaluate tissue in vivo can have a significant impact on the diagnosis and management of a wide range of diseases.

Time domain detection technique measures the echo time delay of backscattered or back reflected light via an interferometer with a mechanically scanning optically referenced path.

Fourier domain, spectral domain or frequency domain detection technique detects the echo time delays of light, and are measured by Fourier that transforms the interference spectrum of the light signal, which requires no mechanical axial scanning and results in an acquisition speed much higher than that of time domain OCT. Also, this new technology has a higher sensitivity (Figs 24.5A to 24.9).

Three-dimensional optical coherence tomography may be performed using an OCT scanning protocol that achieves high sampling density in all the three dimensions. Volume rendering of the 3-dimensional data generates a 3-dimensional image. Three dimensional OCT data can be used to segment, measure and map intraretinal layer thicknesses.

B-SCAN ULTRASONOGRAPHY

Ultrasound examination is indicated when opacification of the ocular media precludes adequate clinical examination of the

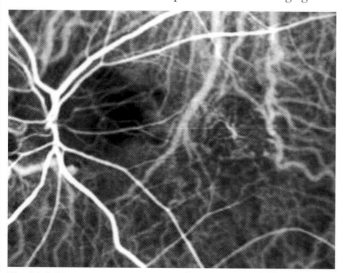

Fig. 24.4: Choroidal neovascularization: Scanning laser ophthalmoscope based indocyanine green angiography (Dr Manish Nagpal)

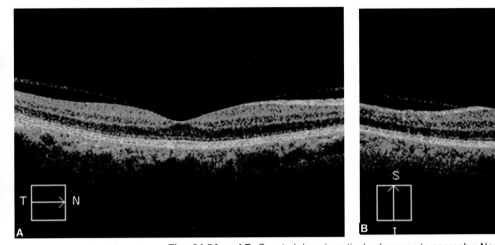

Figs 24.5A and B: Spectral domain optical coherence tomography: Normal scan

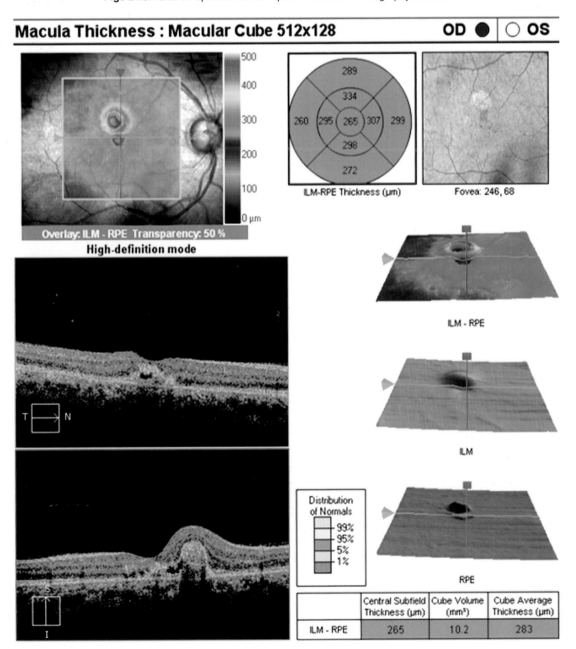

Fig. 24.6: Spectral domain optical coherence tomography: Choroidal neovascularization

Macula Thickness : Macular Cube 512x128   OD ○ | ● OS

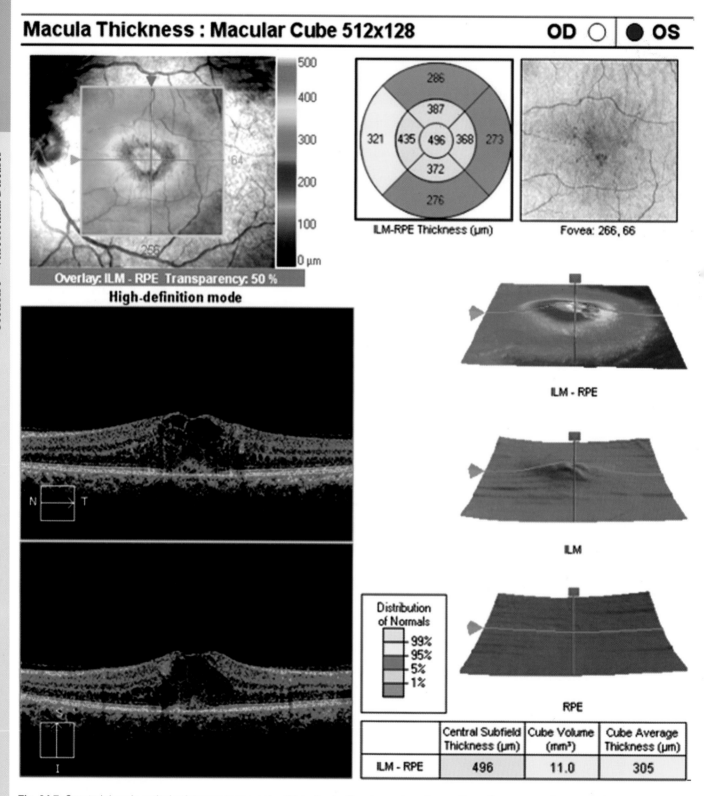

	Central Subfield Thickness (μm)	Cube Volume (mm³)	Cube Average Thickness (μm)
ILM - RPE	496	11.0	305

Fig. 24.7: Spectral domain optical coherence tomography. Clinically significant macular edema with cystic spaces and serous retinal detachment

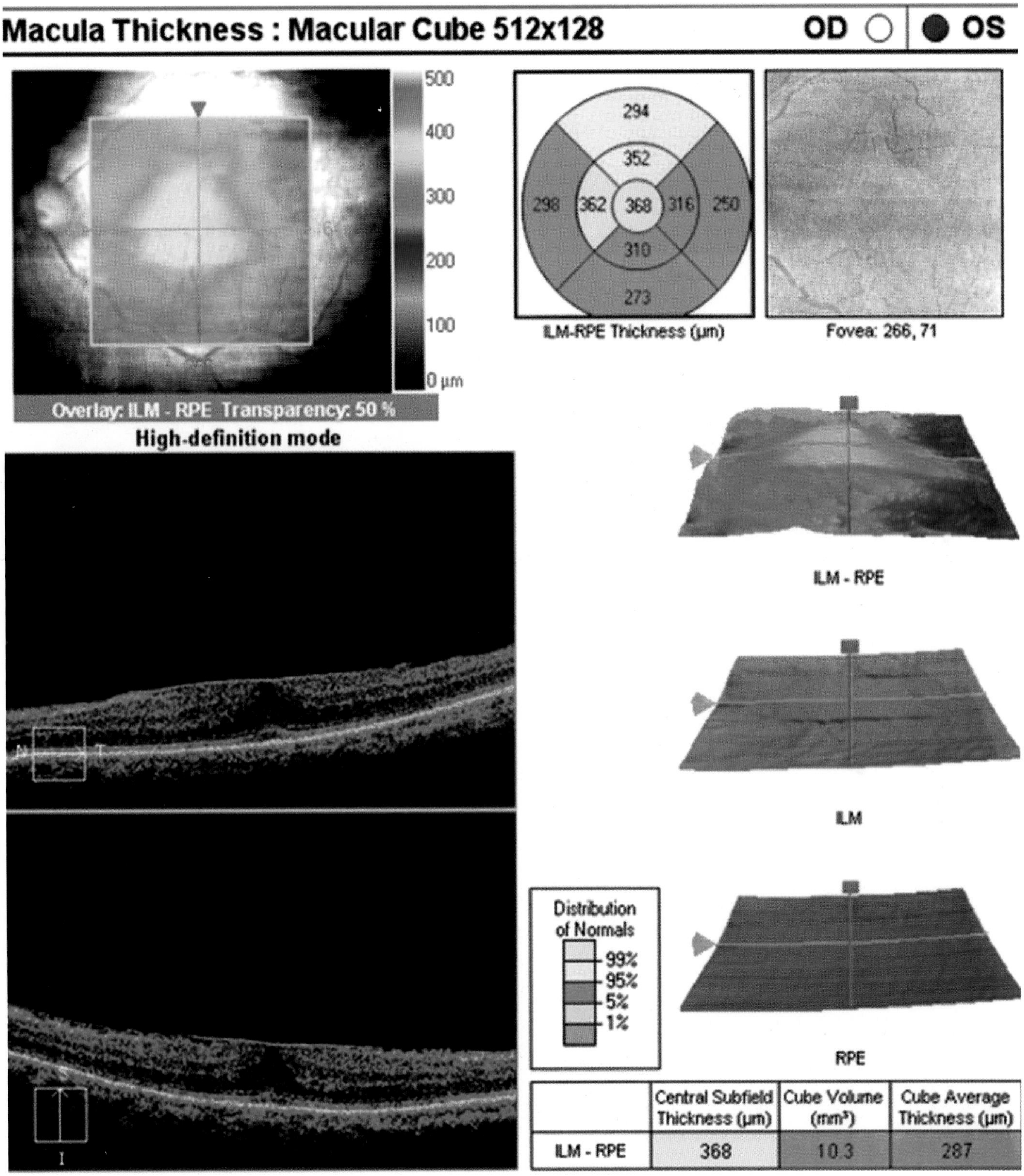

Macula Thickness : Macular Cube 512x128

OD ⃝ | ● OS

500
400
300
200
100
0 µm

Overlay: ILM - RPE Transparency: 50 %

High-definition mode

ILM-RPE Thickness (µm)

294		
352		
298	362 368 316	250
310		
273		

Fovea: 266, 71

ILM - RPE

ILM

Distribution
of Normals
99%
95%
5%
1%

RPE

	Central Subfield Thickness (µm)	Cube Volume (mm³)	Cube Average Thickness (µm)
ILM - RPE	368	10.3	287

Fig. 24.8: Spectral domain optical coherence tomography: Idiopathic epiretinal membrane

Macula Thickness : Macular Cube 512x128   OD ● ○ OS

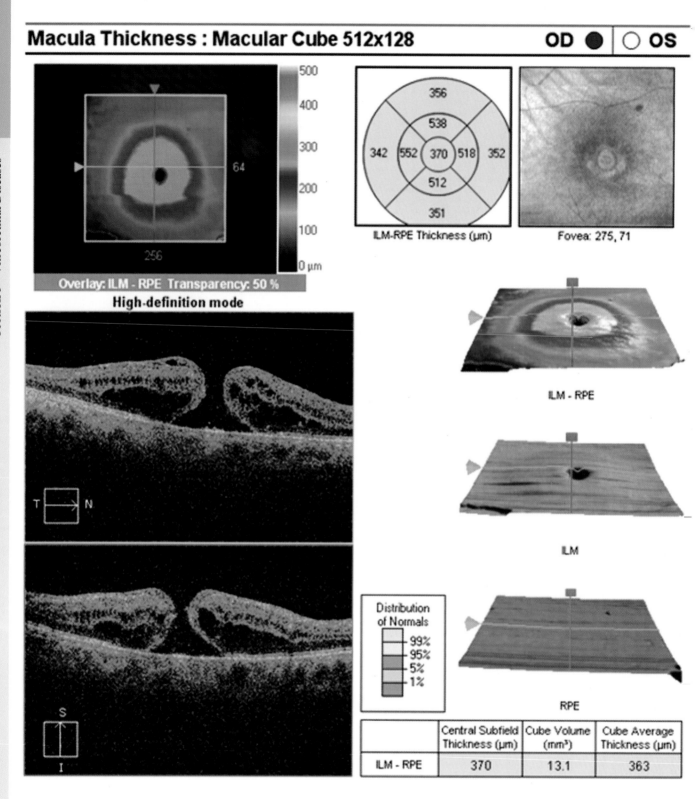

	Central Subfield Thickness (µm)	Cube Volume (mm³)	Cube Average Thickness (µm)
ILM - RPE	370	13.1	363

Fig. 24.9: Spectral domain optical coherence tomography: Idiopathic macular hole

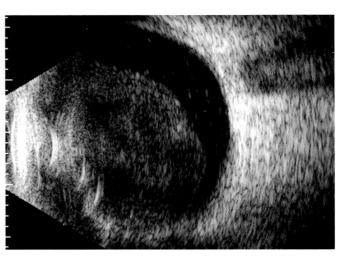

Fig. 24.10: B-scan: Vitreous hemorrhage with posterior vitreous detachment

posterior segment. In the presence of clear media, it is useful for evaluation of the state and position of the vitreous (Figs 24.10 and 24.11). Ultrasound provides a readily accessible means for diagnosing tumors, retinal detachments, hemorrhage and intraocular foreign bodies.

Two useful display modes of ultrasound are:

- *A-scan (time-amplitude)*: In this mode, the echoes appear as amplitude-spikes on a horizontal time axis. Common users for this mode include tissue interpretation and intraocular lens power calculation.
- *B-scan (intensity modulated)*: In this mode, a cross-section display is created from a number of A-scan to produce spots of light on the display screen. The brightness of the spots are a function of this echo amplitude.

There are several concepts that are essential to the understanding of contact B-scan ultrasonography:

Real time: This refers to the quality of motion seen during B-scan imaging. Primary and secondary after movements of the

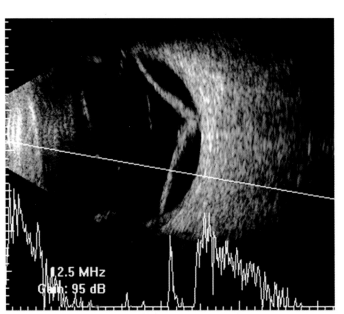

Fig. 24.11: A+B-scan: Retinal detachment

vitreous and retinal detachments are detectable. The quality of movement of intraocular tissue can be used to help differentiate one structure from another. The rapid movement of vitreous hemorrhage differs from the slower and undulating motion of a rhegmatogenous detachment.

Gray scale: The term "gray scale" refers to interpretation of echo amplitudes. In B-scan ultrasound, the brightness of the echo is represented in gray scale. Echoes with higher amplitude (strong reflectors) appear as whiter images and those with lower amplitude (weak reflectors) appear less bright. The gain setting (sensitivity) measured in decibels (dB), is constantly altered to allow interpretation of the echo strength. The object to be studied is placed perpendicular to the examining beam, so that the strongest possible echoes will be recovered by the B-scan transducer.

Interpretation of the B-scan involves creating a composite image of the globe from two-dimension B-scan cross section images. The horizontal dimension on the screen is related to time and distance. The echoes on the left hand side are closer to the probe head. The marker on the probe corresponds to the superior portion of the screen. When the orientation of the probe is held vertically, the top of the screen represents the superior portion of the globe. When the probe is held horizontally with the marker towards the nose, the top of the screen represents the nasal part of the globe. The temporal part of the globe is seen along the bottom of the screen.

In practice, the A- and B-scan are complimentary. B-scan provides the topographic information and the A-scan provides tissue interpretation. Both A and B scans can be performed using water immersion bath or more commonly through a contact method. Immersion techniques are useful in scanning the anterior segment of the globe.

MICROPERIMETRY

Automated full threshold static perimetry has been established in clinical practice to reveal and quantify functional defects of the visual field. It is difficult to obtain adequate evaluation in patients with macular disease because of unstable fixation.

To evaluate correctly the correlation between retinal pathologies and functional defects, microperimetry has been developed for clinical use, providing a simultaneous observation of the fundus and a correction for eye movements during the perimetric examination. Recently, a new instrument named the "Micro Perimeter-1" (NIDEK Technologies, Italy) has been introduced. The Micro Perimeter-1 allows fundus perimetry in a larger field with automated full threshold perimetry software. Furthermore, real color fundus image acquisition is possible and an overlay of the perimetric findings onto the fundus image is also possible (Figs 24.12 A and B).

The Micro Perimeter-1 performs microperimetry using selectable target strategies and programmable parameters by examiners. The Micro Perimeter-1 uses a liquid crystal display to project stimuli. Stimulus intensity can be set on 1step scale

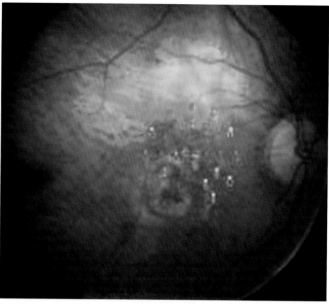

Fig. 24.12A: Microperimetry: Superimposed visual field data and color photograph

Multifocal electrogram consists of positive and negative waveforms that originate from different stages of retinal processing. However, the ERG response to a flash of light is a mass response from retinal photoreceptors, as well as from the other retinal cells. However, it does not provide an insight into localized retinal function.

The multifocal electroretinogram (mfERG) allows for functional retinal field mapping by concomitantly deriving responses from a large number of retinal locations. Recording is done in a light adapted state. This investigation provides local information, which is comparable to cone responses in the full field ERG. An abnormal mfERG indicates that the foveal cones and/or bipolar cell layers are dysfunctional.

Electrical responses from the eye are recorded with a corneal electrode just as in conventional ERG recording, but the special nature of the stimulus and the analysis produces a topographic map of ERG responses.

The display usually contains either 61 or 103 hexagons. The display is scaled so that each hexagon stimulates approximately

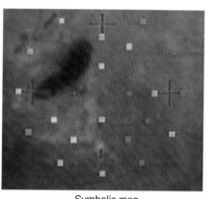

Symbolic map

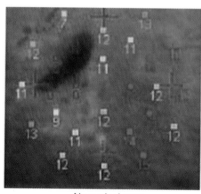

Numerical map

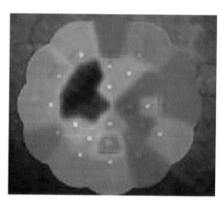

Interpolated color map

Fig. 24.12B: Microperimetry. Map display (Prof Masahito Ohji)

(0.1 log) from 0 to 20 dB, where 0 dB represents the brightest luminance of 400 asb (127 candles/square meter). Stimulus size can be set (from I to V) of Goldmann standard perimeter. The fixation target set at 100 asb can be varied in size and shape (a cross or a ring are commended for patients with central fixation, four crosses or a large ring for patients with paracentral fixation) according to the patient's visual acuity and macular scotoma. The Micro Perimeter-1 accurately overlays data from perimetry and fundus photography. Micro Perimeter-1 makes it possible to combine and cross analyze the visual field defects and visible structural macular pathologies.

MULTIFOCAL ELECTRORETINOGRAM

The electroretinogram (ERG) is an electrical potential generated by the retina in response to a flash of light. It is an excellent tool for studying retinal function independently. It can be recorded noninvasively from the corneal surface.

the same number of receptors. Since the cone density is higher towards the center, the hexagons are smaller.

Although the overall effect is of a randomly flickering screen, each hexagon flashes individually; according to a special pseudorandom sequence known as "m sequence". On an average, only half of them are "on" at any one time. Hence, the overall luminance of the screen over time is relatively equiluminant.

The tracings of the mfERG are not direct electrical responses from a local region of retina. The mfERG waveforms are a mathematical extraction of signals. By correlating the continuous ERG signal with the on or off phases of each stimulus element, the focal ERG signal associated with each element is calculated.

Data can be displayed in various ways such as a topographic 3-D response density plots, group averages or trace arrays. Trace array is the basic mfERG display and forms a part of all standard display protocols. To properly interpret mfERGs, it

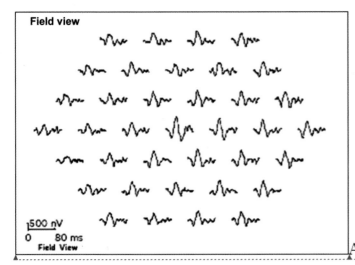

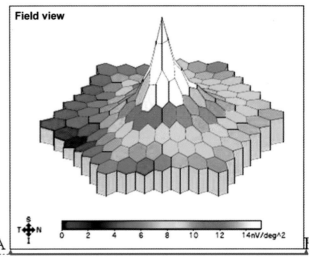

Figs 24.13A and B: Multifocal electroretinogram of a normal subject: (A) Trace array of the mfERG responses of the first order kernel. (B) Three-dimensional plot of the response density of the mfERG response (Dr Parveen Sen)

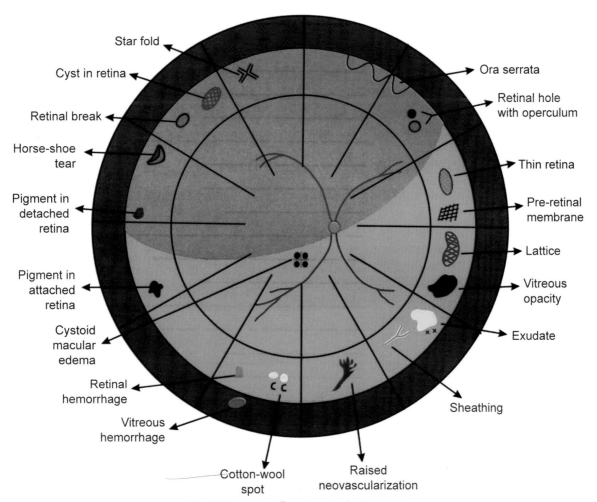

Fig. 24.14: Color coding for various retinal lesions

is imperative to know the response distribution in the normal retina as well as its intersubject variability. The 3-D plots are not to be used by themselves to display mfERG data; they should always be accompanied by a corresponding trace array (Figs 24.13A and B).

COLOR CODING FOR RETINAL LESIONS

Color coding for various retinal lesions is extremely helpful in documentation. Color coding for various retinal lesions is shown in Figure 24.14.

Spectral-Domain Optical Coherence Tomography in Macular Diseases

Sandeep Saxena

INTRODUCTION

Optical coherence tomography (OCT) is an outstanding example of applied physics in medicine. Over the last decade, OCT has become an essential tool in ophthalmology. OCT is a low-coherence, interferometer-based, noninvasive medical imaging modality that can provide noncontact, high-resolution, cross-sectional images of biological tissue.

Optical coherence tomography has become indispensable in the armamentarium of retinal physicians. This imaging technique provides cross-sectional images of the retina, for identifying, monitoring and quantitatively assessing diseases of the macula and the optic nerve head.

Optical coherence tomography can be used to visualize changes in tissue optical scattering properties or refractive index discontinuities, but it cannot distinguish between tissues of similar optical properties. By comparison, histology visualizes tissue according to specific staining properties. Although OCT does not yet enable cellular-level resolution of the retina in vivo, it may be possible to track subtle morphologic changes in intraretinal structure that are altered in retinal disease.

Optical coherence tomography is a field in rapid evolution. Interpretation of OCT images has also advanced, primarily because of improvement in the quality of the images produced, higher resolution and accumulated clinical experience.

SPECTRAL-DOMAIN OPTICAL COHERENCE TOMOGRAPHY AND THREE-DIMENSIONAL RETINAL IMAGING

Spectral-domain optical coherence tomography (SD-OCT) has begun a new era in ocular imaging. New generation of SD-OCT instruments use a low-coherence superluminescent diode, as the light source, with a wavelength in the near infrared at 840 nm and a bandwidth of 50 nm. The axial resolution is 5–6 μm.

Spectral-Domain vs Time-Domain

Spectral-domain technology differs significantly from time-domain technology in that signals returning from the eye are scanned by a spectrometer to analyze alteration of light frequency compared with input frequency. Faster scanning and data collection are possible which result in many improvements, such as less patient-movement artifact and markedly improved image registration. With more data acquired in each scan session, less interpolation between scans is required, making volumetric analysis and 3-D imaging possible. Measurements are reproducible within reasonable tolerances, and registration aids in establishing proper sites for measurement. Several of the spectral-domain devices incorporate overlay software that permits correlation of OCT images with angiographic or autofluorescence photographic studies. A better understanding of the anatomic site represented by the OCT image can be developed and follow-up examinations can closely be correlated with images from previous visits.

The SD-OCT device can produce cross-sectional B-scans, like time-domain OCT with better resolution, and it can also create 3-D area scans by combining B-scans. Its scanning technology takes 20,000 to 26,000 A-scan measurements per second, produces a linear B-scan in less than 0.03 second and combines them to create a 3-D area scan.

3-D Retinal Imaging

The acquisition speed of current SD-OCT instruments allows rapid screening of 3-D volumes of human retinas in clinical settings. To take advantage of this ability requires software used by physicians to be capable of displaying and accessing volumetric data as well as supporting post-processing in order to access important quantitative information such as thickness maps and segmented volumes. Volumetric representations of the retina, as in other medical areas, have become an increasingly useful tool for ophthalmic clinical diagnosis and medical research. Standard OCT (logarithmic scale intensity based) data sets are represented by a 3-D rectilinear grid of scalar values (amount of back-scattered light stored for each voxel). Automated approaches for the classification and segmentation of these data sets aid a practitioner in isolating and examining areas of interest within these volumes.

Since it is possible to acquire high density volumetric data of the macula, the OCT data can be processed to provide comprehensive structural information. With 3-D image reconstruction, the 3-D area scans can be manipulated and viewed from multiple angles. The unprecedented visualization provided by this technology enables determination of specific alterations in retinal anatomy characteristics. Before rendering, the individual cross-sectional OCT images in the 3-D, data set are correlated automatically and aligned by the software to remove axial eye motion artifacts that cause variations in the axial position of the retina between images. Orthogonal slices or an orthoplane rendering of the 3-D OCT data can be obtained. The OCT images can be generated with arbitrary orientations from the 3-D OCT data, but will have varying transverse resolutions depending on the direction of the scan and the density of the initial 3-D OCT data.

The X, Y and Z planes for slicing are defined as follows (Fig. 25.1):

- **X plane** is the horizontal B-scan as it is acquired. The anatomical features as shown in the X plane are real since the eye movement is negligible (Fig. 25.2).
- **Y plane** is the vertical reconstructed B-scan. The eye movement in the reconstructed B-scan is quite noticeable (Fig. 25.3).
- **Z plane** is a reconstructed en-face image. It is also called the coronal scan or C-scan (Fig. 25.4).

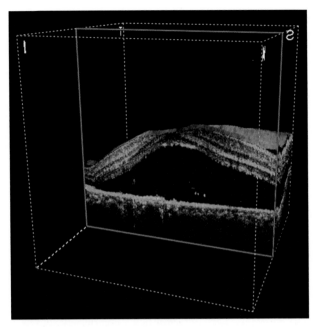

Fig. 25.2: 3-D imaging in X plane showing serous retinal detachment

The relationship among the X, Y and Z plane may exquisitely be observed. In order to visualize the pathology located inside the 3-D-rendered image, cropping of the image may be performed.

Optical coherence tomography images of the individual intraretinal layers can also be generated. Quantitative mapping of retinal layers may be documented in the form of various maps. Peeling and layer separation in 3-D imaging are becoming elegant options. Visualization of separate layers of 3-D images may be utilized to give a novel perspective.

False color coding is used for highlighting thickness of various layers (Figs 25.5 to 25.7).

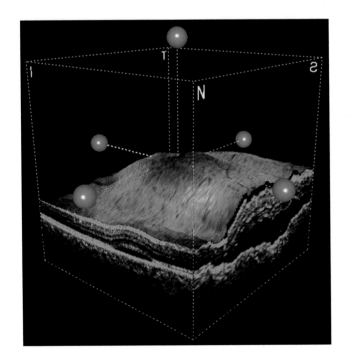

Fig. 25.1: Three-dimensional image showing the X, Y and Z planes

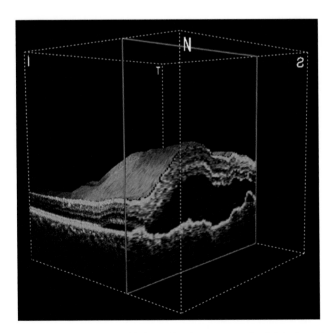

Fig. 25.3: 3-D imaging in Y plane showing serous retinal detachment

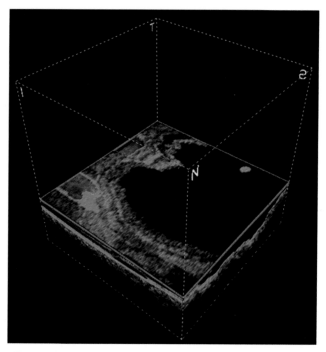

Fig. 25.4: 3-D imaging in Z plane showing serous fluid-filled cavity

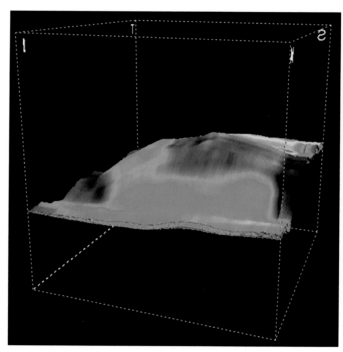

Fig. 25.6: Retinal nerve fiber layer thickness map (false color) on 3-D imaging in X plane

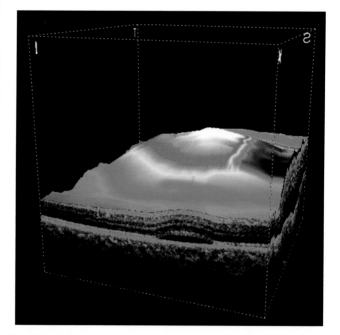

Fig. 25.5: Retinal thickness map (false color) on 3-D imaging in X plane

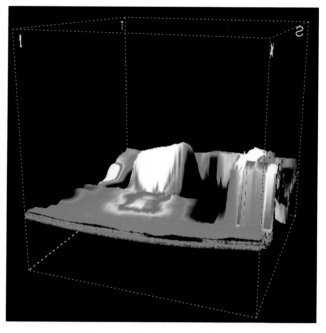

Fig. 25.7: Retinal pigment epithelium deformation map (false color) on 3-D imaging in in X plane

AGE-RELATED MACULAR DEGENERATION

On OCT, classic choroidal neovascular membrane presents as a hyper-reflective area of thickening above and adjacent to the retinal pigment epithelium usually separated by a thin and less reflective band. Active choroidal neovascular membrane discloses direct and indirect signs. The direct signs may not always be clearly defined with regards to the dimension, location, shape and the stage of progression of choroidal neovascular membrane. The indirect signs include increase in retinal thickness and flattening of foveal depression. Detachment and elevation of neurosensory retina may be associated with or without cystic spaces. Retinal pigment epithelium detachment may be present if classic choroidal neovascular membrane is associated with occult choroidal neovascular membrane.

Topographic and volumetric evaluations enable analysis of individual compartments in the entire scanned area. Comparison of the individual slices show improved identification of intraretinal and subretinal structures (Figs 25.8A and B). The raster method decreases the dependence on exploratory methods that have been necessary until now to generate retinal thickness maps. SD-OCT is suitable for monitoring treatment of choroidal neovascular membrane with anti-vascular endothelial growth factor (anti-VEGF) therapy. Development of high-resolution OCT systems in conjunction with development of novel treatment options for exudative diseases offer novel perspectives.

DIABETIC MACULAR EDEMA

In diabetic macular edema, OCT scan allows documentation of intraretinal changes, changes in the shape of the inner boundary of thickened macula, presence of serous retinal detachments and incomplete vitreomacular separation. Intraretinal changes include diffuse swelling, cystoid cavities, foveolar detachment and hard exudates. The posterior hyaloid is only visible on OCT when it is partly detached from the retinal surface. In some cases, the partially detached posterior hyaloid appears much thicker and hyper-reflective (thickened, taut posterior hyaloid).

Optical coherence tomography is very useful to determine whether edema threatens or involves the macular center. In some cases the edges of the macula may be thickened, even though the foveal center retains a normal contour. Macular thickening may be asymmetric, especially in focal edema, and may only involve a sector of the macular area.

Tractional macular edema is strongly suggested upon OCT from the visualization of a combination of hyper-reflective, thick posterior hyaloid adhering to an elevated foveal center and convex slopes of the thickened macula.

Otani, Kishi and Maruyama have described the following patterns of diabetic macular edema:
- Sponge-like thickening of retinal layers
- Large cystoid spaces involving variable depth of the retina with intervening septae
- Subfoveal serous detachment
- Tractional detachment of fovea
- Taut posterior hyaloid

Three-dimensional imaging on SD-OCT shows altered retinal contour and retinal thickness in clinically significant macular edema. Sequential 3-D imaging in X, Y and Z planes and associated color coded changes in retinal thickness maps present novel perspectives (Figs 25.9A and B).

Imaging of the 3-D structures of the proliferative membrane in proliferative diabetic retinopathy is also possible. The 3-D structure of the proliferative membrane can clearly be visualized. The OCT image may show the presence of multiple adhesions between the retina and the proliferative membrane and separation of the proliferative membrane. SD-OCT is suitable for monitoring treatment of clinically significant macular edema with anti-VEGF therapy (Figs 25.10A and B).

RETINAL VEIN OCCLUSION

Branch retinal vein occlusion and central retinal vein occlusion may result in macular edema. On OCT, diffuse retinal

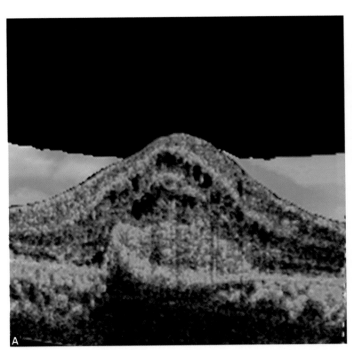
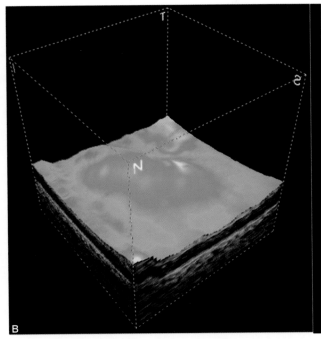

Figs 25.8A and B: Choroidal neovascularization. Optical coherence tomography shows choroidal neovascular membrane with elevation of retina and cystic changes on line scan (A). 3-D image showing altered retinal contour on retinal thickness map (B)

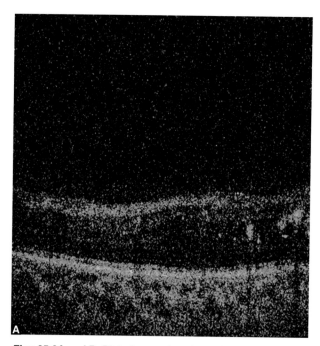

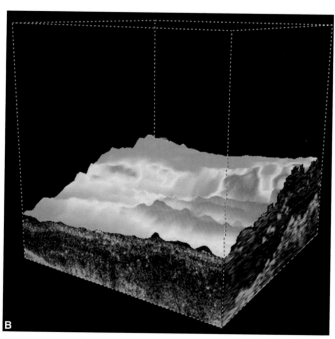

Figs 25.9A and B: Diabetic macular edema. Optical coherence tomography printout shows edematous retina and hard exudates on line scan (A). 3-D image showing retinal thickness map (B)

swelling, cystic changes and serous retinal detachments may be observed. Observation of cystoid macular edema (CME) enables visualization of its spatial extent in each retinal layer and discernment of its relationship to the external limiting membrane. Pathomorphologic features of CME may be visualized. Cystoid spaces are often seen in the inner nuclear layer and outer plexiform layer, but are detected to some extent in all retinal layers. Observation of CME using 3-D OCT enables visualization of its spatial extent in each retinal layer (Figs 25.11 A and B). The use of 3-D OCT thus may improve the monitoring of CME progression and its response to treatment. Optic disc traction may be well recognized on OCT in central retinal vein occlusion.

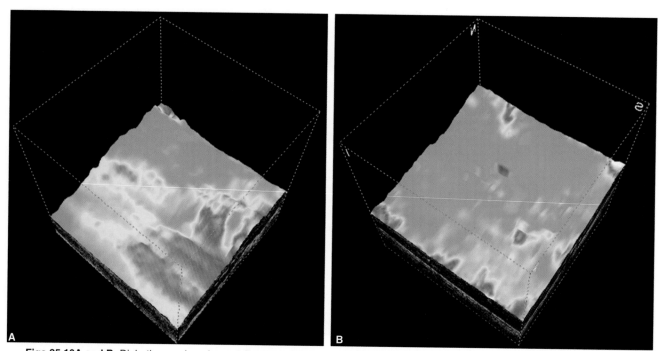

Figs 25.10A and B: Diabetic macular edema. 3-D image shows decrease in retinal thickness following intravitreal bevacizumab: Pre-bevacizumab treatment (A) and Post-bevacizumab treatment (B)

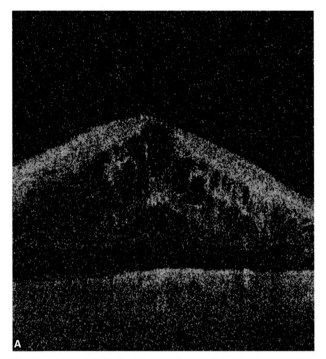
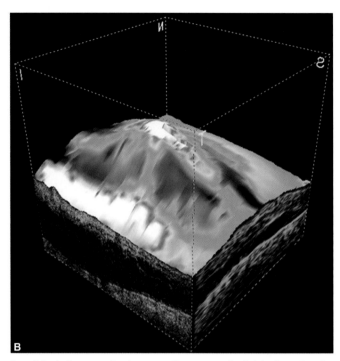

Figs 25.11A and B: Retinal vein occlusion. Optical coherence tomography printout shows cystic changes with serous retinal detachment on line scan (A). 3-D image shows retinal thickness map (B)

RETINAL ARTERY OCCLUSION

Retinal artery occlusion usually results from embolization and thrombosis. On OCT, the affected area demonstrates increased thickness and reflectivity in the inner retina. The marked difference from retinal edema due to other retinal vascular diseases is lack of cystic spaces of low reflectivity due to fluid accumulation. After the resolution of retinal edema, inner retina becomes atrophic and thin, which is characteristic of OCT finding. The extent of macular edema widely differs and does not affect visual prognosis in central retinal artery occlusion eyes. No correlation has been found between the initial macular edema height and the visual improvement. On SD-OCT, topographic evaluations on 3-D imaging show altered retinal contour and retinal thickness (Figs 25.12A and B).

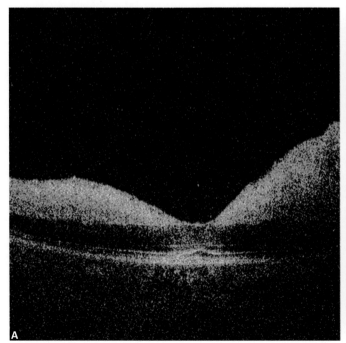
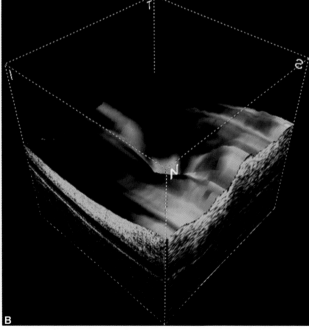

Figs 25.12A and B: Retinal artery occlusion. Optical coherence tomography printout shows retinal atrophy on line scan (A). 3-D image showing retinal thickness map (B)

IDIOPATHIC MACULAR HOLE

Optical coherence tomography has improved the understanding of the pathophysiology and anatomy of idiopathic macular hole. On OCT, idiopathic macular hole can be classified by the following stages:

Stage 1A : Partial thickness pseudocyst with perifoveal posterior vitreous detachment

Stage 1B : Full thickness pseudocyst with roof

Stage 2A : Full thickness macular hole with partial opening of the roof, focal vitreous attachment to flap

Stage 2B : Full thickness operculated macular hole, traction to retina released

Stage 3 : Full thickness operculated macular hole, traction released, ≥ 400 μm diameter

Stage 4 : Full thickness macular hole with complete posterior vitreous detachment, vitreous face may or may not be evident on OCT

Three-dimensional imaging of macular holes with SD-OCT technology offers 3-D overviews that facilitate understanding of the abnormalities in the vitreofoveal interface. It also provides consecutive orthogonal images that allow much more precise and minute observation of three-dimensionally extending intraretinal structural changes associated with a macular hole than conventional OCT imaging, especially in the photoreceptor inner and outer segments (IS/OS) junction (Figs 25.13A and B).

Optical coherence tomography has been successful in staging macular holes and providing a quantitative measure of hole diameter and the amount of surrounding macular edema.

OCT can also detect small separations of the posterior hyaloid from the retina.

Successfully repaired macular holes have been subdivided into the following three patterns based on OCT configuration:
- U-type with normal foveal contour
- V-type with steep foveal contour
- W type with a foveal defect of the neurosensory retina

These patterns have also been shown to correlate with postoperative visual acuity (U > V > W).

A disruption of the IS/OS junction is observed in all eyes with macular holes. The photoreceptor layer appears to be involved for a much larger area than that occupied by the macular hole itself. The abnormality in the IS/OS junction may reflect perturbation of a higher level of retinal organization and not an absolute loss of photoreceptor outer segments. The postoperative IS/OS junction may play an important role in visual recovery after macular hole closure as IS/OS line heals to varying degrees. The visual outcome is significantly better in eyes with a continuous IS/OS line than those with a disrupted IS/OS line. A normal IS/OS line is associated with good visual acuity recovery.

EPIRETINAL MEMBRANE AND VITREOMACULAR TRACTION SYNDROME

Optical coherence tomography demonstrates epiretinal membranes as thin, highly reflective bands anterior to the retina. Based on morphologic characteristics, epiretinal membranes can be classified into two distinct groups; those with focal points of attachment to the retina and those with global adherence to the retina.

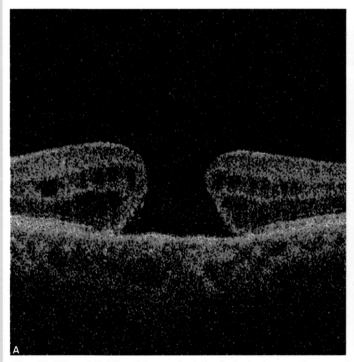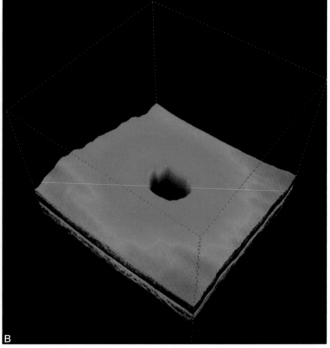

Figs 25.13A and B: Idiopathic macular hole. Optical coherence tomography shows a full thickness macular hole with cystic retina on line scan (A). 3-D image shows altered retinal thickness map with well demarcated macular hole (B)

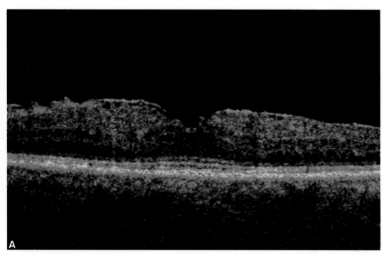
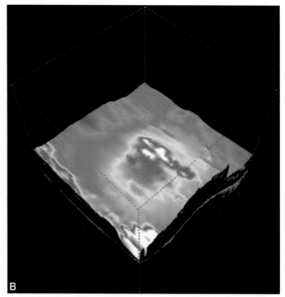

Figs 25.14A and B: Idiopathic epiretinal membrane. Optical coherence tomography shows an epiretinal membrane (A). 3-D image shows retinal thickness map (B)

Majority of epiretinal membranes (approximately 70%) are globally adherent to the retina. The remaining eyes have focally adherent epiretinal membranes (Figs 25.14A and B).

Occasionally, OCT cannot distinguish between the epiretinal membranes and the anterior surface of the retina if the epiretinal membrane is globally adherent to the retina. Discriminating features may be a difference in contrast between the epiretinal membrane (higher reflectivity) and the retina (lower reflectivity), and the appearance of a membrane tuft or edge contiguous with the retinal surface.

Optical coherence tomography provides beneficial information in monitoring surgical removal of ERM and decrease of intraretinal edema after vitreous surgery. The foveal pit reappears occasionally in successful cases.

Preoperative and postoperative mean macular thickness do not correlate with postoperative vision, thus indicating that preoperative macular thickness is not predictive of postoperative visual outcome.

SD-OCT images of eyes with epiretinal membrane are diverse. Morphological changes in the retina, such as edema with cystic spaces, lamellar macular holes, macular pseudoholes and photoreceptor defects, are well defined. Estimation of these changes may be an important prognostic factor.

The SD-OCT with 3-D image reconstruction provided unprecedented visualization of vitreomacular traction and idiopathic epiretinal membrane.

The appearance of the IS/OS junction in the OCT images at the fovea can be graded from 0 to 2:

0: IS/OS line not visible

1: Abnormal (discontinuous) IS/OS line

2: Normal (well preserved) IS/OS line

Eyes in which a normal IS/OS junction is detected after surgery have significantly better visual acuity than those without a normal IS/OS junction. This correlation between the presence of a normal IS/OS junction and the better postoperative visual acuity is probably due to better morphological recovery of the macular photoreceptors.

Optical coherence tomography provides useful information for understanding the pathology of macular pseudoholes. It is beneficial in distinguishing macular pseudoholes from ophthalmoscopically similar-appearing lesions such as macular holes, macular lamellar holes and macular cysts.

Typical OCT configuration of macular pseudohole is the contour of the foveal pit, a thickening of the macular edges, a steeper foveal pit contour and the presence of normally reflective retinal tissue at the base of the pseudohole. The majority of eyes with macular pseudoholes are associated with globally adherent membranes.

Optical coherence tomography enables us to understand vitreomacular tractional force due to membrane adherent to macula with attachment of the posterior hyaloid, inducing significant retinal elevation and edema. OCT is also useful in demonstrating anatomic response after surgery for vitreomacular traction syndrome.

MACULAR DYSTROPHY

Macular dystrophy shows great variability in severity and rate of progression. Cone disease presents with decreased visual acuity and poor color discrimination. OCT, in such cases, reveals foveal atrophy.

Imaging using SD-OCT achieves considerably improved visualization of intraretinal layers, especially the photoreceptor layer. Three-dimensional imaging on SD-OCT shows altered sloping retinal contour and retinal thickness (Figs 25.15A and B).

HEALED TOXOPLASMOSIS

Toxoplasmosis is the most common cause of infectious retinitis in immunocompetent individuals. SD-OCT in active toxoplasmosis

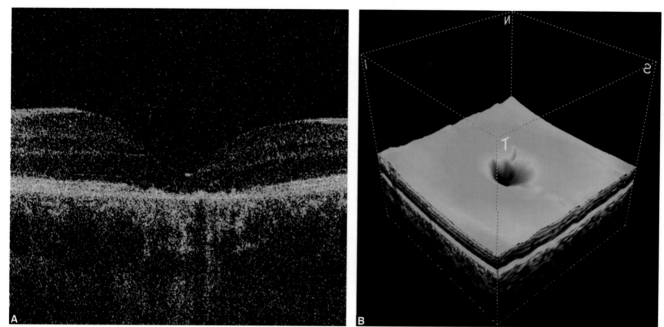

Figs 25.15A and B: Macular dystrophy. Optical coherence tomography shows foveal atrophy with the thinning of photoreceptor layer on line scan (A). 3-D image showing retinal thickness map with altered contour in macular area denoting foveal atrophy (B)

has revealed diffuse macular edema, vitreomacular traction, maculoschisis, focal choriocapillaris/choroidal relative hyper-reflectivity and posterior vitreous detachment. Typical congenital toxoplasmic retinochoroiditis presents as a macular cicatricial lesion.

SD-OCT line scan, at the edge of the lesion, may reveal splitting of retina at the level of the outer nuclear layer. Discontinuation of photoreceptor layer and hyper-reflective retinal pigment epithelium can be observed. In the center of the lesion, break in the continuity of inner retinal layers may be noted. Retinal nerve fiber layer is found to be absent.

Choriocapillaris/choroidal/scleral relative hyper-reflectivity is also observed in the center of lesion. On three-dimensional retinal imaging, an excavated scar is evident. The retinal pigment epithelium deformation map shows increased retinal pigment epithelium thickness at the periphery with loss of retinal pigment epithelium in the center of the lesion. SD-OCT helps in elucidating morphological changes in lesions of healed toxoplasmosis that are not apparent on clinical examination, which may expand the clinical spectrum of the disease (Figs 25.16A and B).

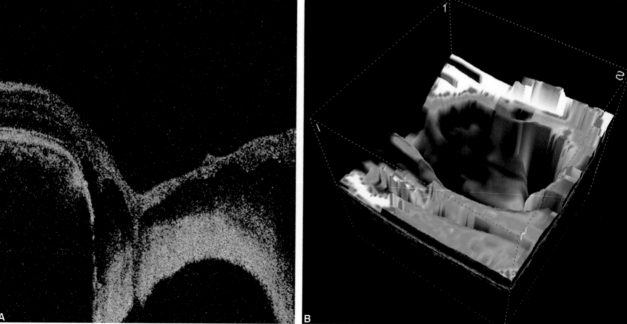

Figs 25.16A and B: Healed toxoplasmosis. At the edge of the lesion, splitting of retina at the level of outer nuclear layer is observed. Discontinuation of photoreceptor layer and hyper-reflective retinal pigment epithelium can be observed. Retinal nerve fiber layer is found to be absent. Choriocapillaris/choroidal/scleral relative hyper-reflectivity is also observed in the center of lesion (A). 3-D image shows grossly altered retinal thickness map with excavated central healed toxoplasmosis scar (B)

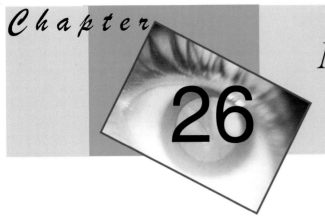

Chapter 26

Macular and Allied Disorders

Pradeep Venkatesh, Lalit Verma, Hem K Tewari

AGE-RELATED MACULAR DEGENERATION

Non-Neovascular Age-Related Macular Degeneration

Introduction

Age-related maculopathy (ARM) is the commonest overall cause of irreversible blindness in the western world and has been categorized into two forms: early and late (Flow chart 26.1). Age-related macular degeneration (AMD) refers to the late form of ARM. Early ARM is characterized by the presence of lesions predisposing to the development of AMD. This includes soft drusen more than 63 μm and areas of hyperpigmentation associated with drusen. Presence of hard drusen, pigment changes and pigment around hard drusen cannot be categorized as ARM. Also, decrease in visual acuity is not a criterion to define ARM. Though presence of soft drusen is a necessity to define ARM; patients with hard drusen alone or pigmentary changes alone may also progress to AMD.

Before ophthalmoscopically visible changes become evident, diffuse changes become evident on pathologic evaluation and are initially confined to modifications on both sides of the retinal pigment epithelium basement membrane. Deposits on the internal side are called basal laminar deposit and those on its external aspect are called basal linear deposit. Basal linear deposits are believed to form soft drusen with the passage of time. Diffuse occurrence of these deposits is the principal feature of ARM (Flow chart 26.1).

Diagnosis

Objective markers (derived from study of postmortem eyes) for the presence of ARM include the presence of at least one drusen larger than 125 μm or an area of pigment clumping more than 500 μm. Pigmentary disturbances suggestive of AMD may occur in the fundus in the absence of visible drusen. Drusen have been categorized into several types based on size, degree of fluorescence (on angiography), density, location and clinicopathologic correlation (Flow chart 26.2). Clinically, non-neovascular ARM may manifest with any of the following patterns:

Flow chart 26.1: Age-related maculopathy

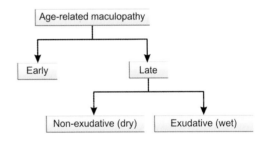

- Stage of drusen and/or hyperpigmentation
- Stage of incipient atrophy (non-geographic atrophy)
- Stage of geographic atrophy

Geographic atrophy by definition must be a hypopigmented or depigmented area larger than 175 u, oval or rounded, with well defined margins and within which the underlying choroidal vasculature is better visible than the surrounding. At this stage there may be no evidence of any drusen and it marks the terminal stage of non-neovascular AMD. Some of these cases may develop choroidal neovascular membrane around its margin and at this stage becomes characterized as neovascular AMD even if geographic atrophy is large and the predominant feature. The evolution of geographic atrophy itself may occur in two variable forms, one commencing in relation to associated drusen and another starting in an area with no drusen. The former is called drusen-associated atrophy and the latter as drusen unrelated atrophy. Another manner in which geographic atrophy may evolve is following the collapse of retinal pigment epithelial detachments. Geographic atrophy may commence as a solitary focus and then spread or as multifocal patches that coalesce with time. Also, spread of geographic atrophy usually tends to spare fixation until its very late stages. An area of ill-defined color change in which the affected region appears pinker than the unaffected area, characterizes incipient atrophy. When associated drusen are present, they appear whiter and harder. The rapidity with which geographic atrophy enlarges is varied. Usually the rate is rapid until all the areas of incipient atrophy coalesce. Subsequent enlargement occurs only gradually. The time interval from onset of geographic atrophy to legal blindness has been reported to be about 9 years. Risk of developing choroidal neovascularization in eyes with initial geographic atrophy (thereby converting to an exudative form of AMD) depends on the status of the fellow eye. If the fellow eye has symmetric geographic atrophy, the risk is only 2% at 2 years and 11% by 4 years. If however the fellow eye has a disciform scar or choroidal neovascularization, the risk increases to 18% and 34% by the end of 2 and 4 years respectively (Flow chart 26.2).

Flow chart 26.2: Drusen: Classification

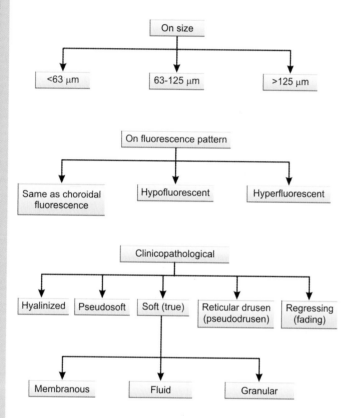

NEOVASCULAR AGE-RELATED MACULAR DEGENERATION

Introduction

In a normal eye, the Bruch's membrane keeps the highly vascular choroid and the highly photosensitive retina away from direct contact with one another and furthermore there is a firm adhesion of the retinal pigment epithelium to this layer. There is hence no potential space beneath the retinal pigment epithelial layer. In contrast to this, a potential space exists between the pigment epithelial layer and the neurosensory retina, although separation along this plane does not occur easily. Sometimes, however, vessels from the choriocapillaris may "grow" into these spaces and when this occurs the condition is known as choroidal neovascularization. Depending on the situation of these vascular networks in relation to the fovea they have been

categorized as extrafoveal, juxtafoveal and subfoveal. By definition, a subfoveal choroidal vascular ingrowth is one that is situated right beneath or has extended (from an initial extrafoveal location) into the center of the fovea. Subfoveal choroidal neovascularization leads to visual loss by causing exudative detachment of the macula, subretinal bleed and disciform scar formation.

Choroidal neovascular ingrowth is known to occur in several conditions, such as age-related macular degeneration, myopia, presumed ocular histoplasmosis syndrome, choroiditis, and angioid streaks and following laser, etc. The single most important cause of choroidal neovascularization in the elderly population is the exudative form of age-related macular degeneration and so it forms the focus of this review. In age-related macular degeneration, choroidal vascular ingrowth accounts for 90% of the severe, irreversible visual loss.

Visual loss due to age-related macular degeneration is a significant cause of posterior segment blindness and is presently not preventable. In North America, it has been reported that choroidal neovascularization is diagnosed in 100,000–200,000 people annually and its incidence in patients with age-related macular degeneration alone as 58%. Since most patients have occult membranes, this incidence is reportedly even higher. Overall incidence of subfoveal choroidal neovascularization however still remains unknown.

Diagnosis

The presenting symptoms in these elderly patients are usually metamorphopsia, central/paracentral scotoma or a rapid decline in vision. Patients who have only soft drusen may be asymptomatic and hence diagnosed during routine fundus evaluation. The disease process is almost always bilateral, but the evolution is frequently asymmetric. The best method to identify choroidal neovascular membranes is fundus biomicroscopy.

On fundus examination, several manifestations of exudative AMD may be seen, either alone or in conjunction. These lesions include confluent soft drusen, subretinal membrane, serous or hemorrhagic retinal pigment epithelial detachment, subretinal hemorrhage or exudation, retinal pigment epithelial tears and disciform scarring. When choroidal neovascular membrane (CNV) arises from the edge of a patch of geographic atrophy, signs of retinal pigment epithelial atrophy are also in evidence.

Clinically, the choroidal neovascular membrane could be identified in some patients by yellow-green discoloration, elevation of the overlying neurosensory retina using a slit beam and by pigment proliferation above the membrane. If the overlying pigment epithelium is atrophic, one may be able to appreciate the subretinal vascular network. Disciform scar appears as a yellow-white fibrovascular tissue that is usually quite irregular appreciably elevated and there is associated distortion of the overlying retinal architecture. When there is an area of bare choriocapillaris with one sharply defined margin and a slightly darker adjacent zone, one must suspect the possibility of a retinal pigment epithelial tear (also called retinal pigment epithelial rip). In a large majority of patients however, the choroidal membrane may not be easily evident on fundus biomicroscopy due to the presence of overlying serous retinal detachment or hemorrhage. In such situations, several techniques like fluorescein angiography, indocyanine angiography and optical coherence tomography could be employed to detect and localize the membrane. Based on the location of CNV in relation to the retinal pigment epithelium Gass has categorized the membranes into three categories, type 1 situated beneath the retinal pigment epithelium, type 2 situated above the retinal pigment epithelium and type 3 having components both above and beneath the retinal pigment epithelium. In patients with CNV secondary to AMD, type 3 membranes predominate.

Fluorescein angiography is an important diagnostic modality in the management of choroidal neovascularization. However, there are certain inherent limitations of this procedure that may be overcome by a simultaneous or sequential indocyanine green angiography. It is emphasized that the angiogram must not be older than 72 hours for planning laser treatment of these membranes. This is because the neovascularization process has a high growth rate (6–10 μm/day) and may rapidly increase in extent. Based on fluorescein angiographic features, choroidal neovascular membranes have been classified into the classic (Fig. 26.1) and occult patterns. The former can be identified in the early phases of the angiogram (may or may not have the characteristic lacy pattern) and there is leakage of dye from the network in the later phases. The margins are well defined except in the late phases when it may become obscured by leakage of the dye. Occult neovascular membranes include two types of hyperfluorescent lesions, fibrovascular pigment epithelial detachments and late leakage of an undetermined source. The former usually shows up as areas of hyperfluorescence 1 to 2 minutes after injection of the dye and may have either well defined or poorly defined margins. On stereoangiography, there is irregular elevation of the overlying retinal pigment epithelium. It corresponds to fibrovascular tissue associated with the choroidal neovascularization. The latter is seen in the late phases of the angiogram as speckled hyperfluorescence with the pooling of dye in the overlying subsensory retinal space. The source of leakage cannot be made out by evaluating the early or mid phases of the angiogram. Other features

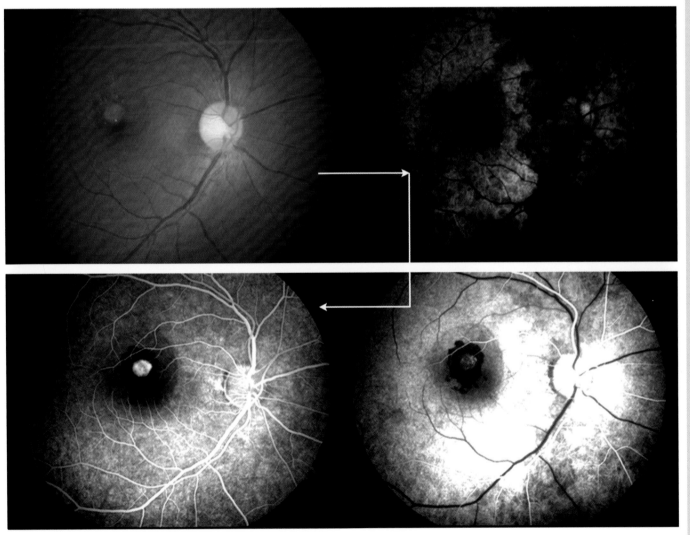

Fig. 26.1: Choroidal neovascularization. Classic choroidal neovascular membrane

that may be evident on fluorescein angiography are blocked fluorescence from subretinal hemorrhage or pigment clumping, fibrovascular or serous pigment epithelial detachments, retinal pigment epithelial tear and drusenoid retinal pigment epithelial detachment. Rarely one may also be able to identify feeder vessels (choroidal vessels unequivocally leading to the neovascular network). Fluorescein angiography is also necessary during follow-up of a patient who has undergone laser photocoagulation for choroidal neovascularization. Lesions are defined as persistent or recurrent based on the angiography features at 6 weeks and subsequent 3 monthly follow-ups.

Indocyanine green angiography may be useful to identify the neovascular membrane in patients showing blocked fluorescence on fluorescein angiography. This procedure is particularly useful in patients with occult CNV and one report has shown that following indocyanine green angiography, 39% of occult CNV could be classified into well defined, classic CNV. Presently three types of morphologic lesions are recognized on indocyanine green angiography in patients with occult CNV on initial fluorescein angiography. There are focal spots, plaques and combination lesions. The most common type of lesion on indocyanine green angiography is the plaque pattern.

Management

Until recently, laser photocoagulation had remained the mainstay in the treatment of patients with subfoveal choroidal neovascularization. This statement may still be true for managing patients with juxtafoveal and extrafoveal CNV secondary to age-related macular degeneration, but not so for the management of subfoveal neovascular membranes. Although the procedure is noninvasive, it has several limitations and disadvantages. The limitations are that it is effective in only a small percentage of cases (10 to 15%) that have a well-defined CNV with distinct margins and wherein the size of the membrane is less than 6.5 MPS (Macular Photocoagulation Study) disc areas. The disadvantages of direct laser treatment are several and include an immediate, significant fall in central vision and the evolution of a dense central scotoma subsequently. The risk of recurrence following treatment of subfoveal choroidal neovascularization by laser photocoagulation is also high. Nevertheless, studies have shown that the beneficial effect of laser treatment becomes appreciable after a 2-year follow-up period. MPS study has reported that while 47% of patients with subfoveal CNV who were not treated with laser lost 6 or more lines of visual acuity from baseline, the corresponding figure in the laser treated group was 22% at the end of 3-year follow-up. A summary of the macular photocoagulation studies undertaken for extrafoveal, juxtafoveal and subfoveal CNV is shown in Tables 26.1 A to C.

Owing to the above mentioned limitations and disadvantages of laser photocoagulation, there has been a constant endeavor to explore the efficacy of alternative modalities for improving the visual outcome in patients with subfoveal choroidal neovascularization, particularly that secondary to age-related macular degeneration.

Alternative therapies to improve the visual outcome in patients with subfoveal choroidal neovascularization presently includes the following modalities (Table 26.2): External beam irradiation (teletherapy), plaque radiotherapy (brachytherapy), pharmacological therapy with anti-angiogenesis factor (anti-vascular endothelial growth factor therapy, interferon alpha-2a) and oral thalidomide, photodynamic therapy, submacular surgery, foveal translocation, gene therapy and retinal pigment epithelial cell transplantation.

Macular Photocoagulation Study (MPS)

Table 26.1A: MPS study for extrafoveal choroidal neovascular membrane ("Argon" Study)

- Study objective was to determine if photocoagulation of extrafoveal CNV was beneficial compared to no treatment
- Study Outcome

SVL*	No Laser Rx	Laser Rx
1 year	41%	24%
3 years	63%	45%
5 years	64%	46%

*SVL= severe visual loss

- Recurrence: 54% by 5 years in laser treated group
- Visual acuity lost at 5 years: 5.2 lines in treated and 7.1 lines in untreated eyes
- Conclusion: Prompt argon laser treatment of extrafoveal CNV reduces the risk of severe visual loss compared with natural course of the disease.

Table 26.1B: MPS study for juxtafoveal choroidal neovascular membrane ("Krypton" Study)

- Study objective was to determine if photocoagulation of juxtafoveal CNV was beneficial compared to no treatment
- Study Outcome

SVL*	No Laser Rx	Laser Rx
1 year	45%	31%
3 years	58%	49%

*SVL= severe visual loss

- Recurrence: ~50% by the end of 2 years in laser treated group
- Maintenance of baseline visual acuity at 5 years: 25% in treated and 15% in untreated eyes
- Treatment benefit doubtful in hypertensive patients, but treatment should still be considered.
- Conclusion: Krypton laser treatment of juxtafoveal CNV reduces the risk of severe visual loss compared to no treatment by approximately 10%.

External Beam Radiation (Teletherapy)

The effects of ionizing radiation and its therapeutic applications has always been an area of interest amongst most medical specialties, including the eye. As the adverse effects of radiation on the eye have become well recognized, it is now clear that radiation retinopathy is unlikely to occur in normal

Table 26.1 C: MPS study for "new" subfoveal choroidal neovascular membrane

- Study Objective was to evaluate effect of laser treatment on vision compared to observation in previously untreated AMD eyes.
- Study Outcome: Indicated by loss of 6 or more lines

	No Laser Rx	Laser Rx
2 year	37%	20%

- Benefit of treatment varied significantly with lesion and baseline visual acuity. Greatest benefit was noted in lesions less than two disc areas in size.
- There is significant initial decrease in visual acuity following treatment (average 3 lines).
- Conclusion: Eyes with smaller (<2.0DA) lesions and poorer visual acuity (< 20/200) benefit most from treatment. Larger lesions (>2.0DA) with relatively good visual acuity (>20/200) have no obvious treatment benefit.

Table 26.2: Alternative treatment approaches for subfoveal choroidal neovascular membrane in age-related macular degeneration

- External beam radiation (Teletherapy)
- Plaque radiotherapy (Brachytherapy)
- Pharmacological therapy:
  - Interferon alpha 2a
  - Oral Thalidomide
  - Anti-vascular endothelial growth factor therapy
- Photodynamic therapy
- Transscleral thermotherapy
- Submacular surgery
- Foveal translocation
- Gene therapy
- Transplantation of retinal pigment epithelium

eyes exposed to 25 Gy or less when delivered at less than 250 cGy daily fractions. However, cataract formation and transient keratoconjunctivitis sicca with epiphora remains a cause for concern. Nevertheless the use of ionizing radiation has been reported in the management of several diseases, including choroidal hemangioma, to close vascular malformations and to stunt neovascular component of wounds. In addition, the potential of external beam radiation to enable regression of subfoveal exudative neovascular networks has been the subject of analysis in several studies. All reported studies have been nonrandomized and the results quite variable. It is difficult to compare these studies because of the lack of standardization in case selection, treatment technique and follow-up criteria for defining regression, etc. Most initial studies showed encouraging results in the 6 to 12 months of follow-up. However, another report containing the largest number of treated patients failed to reproduce results shown by the early reports of teletherapy in subfoveal choroidal neovascularization.

The exact role of radiation therapy, however, still remains highly controversial. In contrast to the several earlier studies showing a beneficial effect, two more recent studies did not find similar results. The exact mechanism by which radiotherapy inhibits neovascularization and scar formation is not yet known. It is thought to affect angiogenesis, by either directly destroying neovascular endothelial cells or cytokine producing macrophages or indirectly by affecting regulatory genes within cells producing endothelial growth regulating cytokines. In human vascular endothelial cell cultures, a single dose of 8.7 to 10.0 Gy radiations has been shown to prevent endothelial cell proliferation. Endothelial cells are the most radiosensitive structures of the vascular wall. This is particularly high for proliferating endothelial cells. Mature, nonproliferating endothelial cells are relatively radioresistant along with the photoreceptors and ganglion cells. Importantly, it has been shown that the crystalline lens is the most radiosensitive tissue in the eye and the chance of developing cataract after a dose of 5.5 Gy is 50%.

External beam radiation therapy has several disadvantages, such as difficulty of targeting the beam exactly at the lesion, need for multiple procedures and the risk of irradiation of other parts of the eye and brain. To overcome these disadvantages clinical evaluation of the effect of plaque radiotherapy on subfoveal choroidal neovascular membranes have been undertaken.

Plaque Radiotherapy (Brachytherapy)

Extensive studies have been performed on the role of plaque radiotherapy in the management of intraocular tumors like choroidal melanoma and retinoblastoma. In comparison there are, at present, only three reports on the effect of brachytherapy on subfoveal choroidal neovascular membranes. This modality of treatment seems promising and helps in avoiding the disadvantages related to external beam radiation therapy, mentioned above. Importantly, the radiation dose reaching the ipsilateral lens is ~3% (versus 50 to 60% during external beam radiation) of the dose prescribed to target volume and so the risk of cataract is significantly decreased.

Radioactive plaques that have been tried for brachytherapy in subfoveal choroidal neovascularization are Ruthenium-106, Palladium-103 and Strontium-90. It has been suggested that Palladium-103 radioactive plaque is probably safer because it delivers less radiation to normal ocular structures, intracranial tissues and health care personnel and also because with low energy photons, the risk of inducing chorioretinal atrophy is also decreased.

Photodynamic Therapy

Conventional laser photocoagulation in the treatment of subfoveal choroidal neovascularization inevitably also causes thermal damage to retinal cells. This is because of the nonspecific nature of laser-tissue interaction and subsequent need to use higher laser energies. Photodynamic treatment in such a situation is considered to have the potential to selectively destroy the neovascular complex without causing any damage to retinal tissue (Fig. 26.2). This modality has been extensively studied in the management of neoplasia and subsequently has been applied to manage choroidal neovascularization.

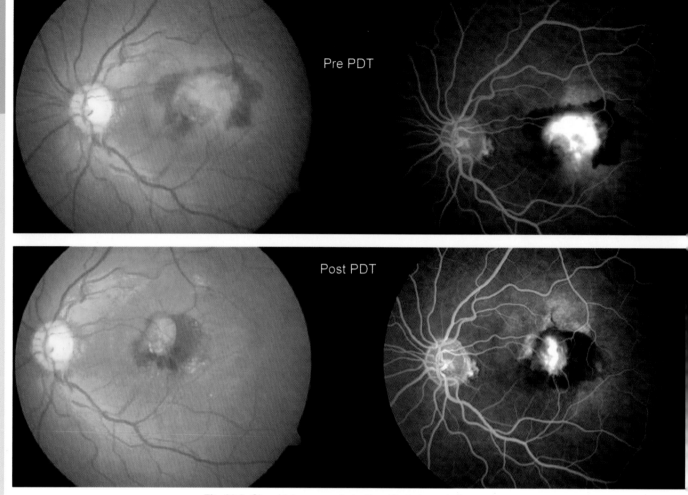

Pre PDT

Post PDT

Fig. 26.2: Choroidal neovascularization. Photodynamic therapy

Photodynamic therapy uses specific photosensitizers that have an affinity for accumulating specially within proliferating vascular tissue despite its distribution into all parts of the body following intravenous administration. These photosensitizers are lipophilic and readily adsorb onto the richly lipophilic membranes of vascular endothelial cells and surface markers, such as lipoprotein receptors are thought to further increase lesion targeting. It has also been shown that pathologic structures, such as proliferating endothelial cells also express more number of membrane lipoprotein receptors. Subsequent exposure of the lesion to light with a wavelength specific for the absorption spectra of the injected dye leads to a photochemical, free radical induced oxidative damage to the endothelium. This is followed by platelet adhesion, degranulation and thrombosis ("photo-thrombosis") of the intralesional vasculature, sparing the surrounding tissues from any thermal damage.

The earliest photosensitizer evaluated for photodynamic therapy was hematoporphyrin. The potential of this could not be applied to therapeutic purposes owing to disadvantages, such as a prolonged half-life within the body. Extensive research has resulted in the synthesis of second-generation photosensitizers, such as Verteporfin (a benzoporphyrin derivative, BPD) and

Purlytin (tin ethyletiopurpurin, SnET2). Unlike first generation photosensitizers, these dyes have a short half-life of five hours and are completely eliminated from the body within 24 hours, thus decreasing the potential for any subsequent systemic photosensitization.

Photodynamic therapy has been advantageous because it combines the noninvasive potential of laser light with the non-thermal effect of a localized chemotoxic reaction.

Transpupillary Thermotherapy

Transpupillary thermotherapy is one of the newer modalities for managing subfoveal CNV (Fig. 26.3) and with which encouraging results were reported a decade ago. Delivery of thermal energy for therapeutic effects has, however, been used earlier in the management of small choroidal melanomas and in these patients sclerosis of the underlying choroidal vessels has been reported on histopathological studies.

In transpupillary thermotherapy, hyperthermic energy is delivered to the region of subfoveal CNV through a dilated pupil using a modified diode laser (810 nm) system incorporated into a slit lamp. This delivery system has apertures measuring 1.2 mm, 2.0 mm and 3.0 mm allowing the laser surgeon to select

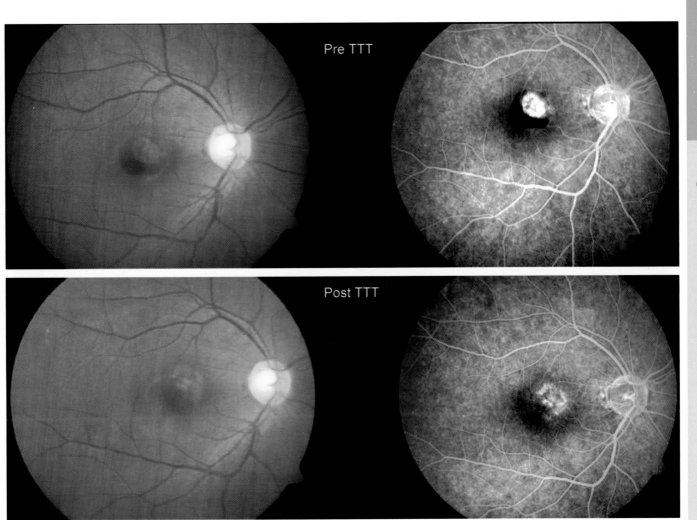

Fig. 26.3: Choroidal neovascularization. Transpupillary thermotherapy

the most appropriate one based on the size of the neovascular membrane. In the ongoing trials, it is planned to initiate treatment with a 3 mm spot for duration of 60 seconds and a power of 800 mW. If a change in the color of the retina is noted at any point during these initial 60 seconds, then the power is reduced in steps of 20% until one identifies the power at which no color change is observed. Now, treatment is restarted at this new power setting to complete the full 60-second treatment. At the end of treatment no color change is detected in most patients, but some may show a mild graying of the lesion.

Initial reports on visual acuity from the several ongoing trials on transpupillary thermotherapy for CNV have shown improvements in 0 to 27% (~20%), stabilization in 43 to 86% and worsening in 14 to 50%. In addition, certain complications like retinal pigment epithelial tear formation after thermotherapy have also been described.

Submacular Surgery

Technical advances in vitreoretinal surgery have made possible submacular surgery for choroidal neovascular membranes. The success of submacular surgery in treating cases of presumed ocular histoplasmosis was reported two decades ago.

Submacular surgery at its inception was stated to have the advantages of being able to treat eyes with not only classic subfoveal neovascular membranes, but also those with occult neovascularization and ill-defined margins and the potential to minimize damage to adjacent structures and to limit central visual loss.

Foveal Translocation

Foveal translocation is an exciting surgical approach to managing subfoveal neovascular membranes. The idea of foveal translocation has been based on anecdotal observations that macular heterotopia can be compatible with good visual recovery, especially in the cases of operated giant retinal tear and in the retinopathy of prematurely. The objective in foveal translocation surgery is to physically shift the foveal neurosensory retina away from the "unhealthy" location above a choroidal neovascular membrane to a location that has "healthy" retinal pigment epithelial cells and Bruch's membrane. The foveal shift achieved in various reports has varied from 300–1,000 μm. To achieve satisfactory results it has been recommended that the surgery should be carried out when the neurosensory retina is relatively less damaged. Two approaches have been tried to obtain foveal translocation, one uses a large retinotomy to induce retinal redundancy and the other uses scleral shortening. Another approach has been to use a scleral buckle in the periphery to induce redundancy and then steamroll the retina and hence the fovea to a position away from the subfoveal neovascular membrane. Foveal translocation has been performed for subfoveal choroidal neovascularization secondary to myopia, presumed ocular histoplasmosis syndrome and age-related macular degeneration.

Pharmacological Therapy

The process of angiogenesis in choroidal neovascularization is complex and involves multiple steps. As in most situations of ocular angiogenesis, the exact trigger and mechanism is still not well understood. It is believed that the endothelial cells are normally in a quiescent state, but have a potential to proliferate in pathologic states or under the stimulus of hypoxia, injury, etc. Although the actual stimulus for choroidal neovascularization is poorly understood several factors have been implicated and these include direct trauma to the Bruch's membrane and inflammatory mediator involvement, loss of scleral elasticity and increase in resistance of the choroidal circulation.

The angiogenesis process is thought to be maintained by a balance of local angiogenic stimulators and inhibitors. It is hence believed that angiogenic inhibitors would probably have a potential in treating subfoveal choroidal neovascularization.

Interferon alfa-2a: Interferon alfa-2a is one of the drugs to have been extensively studied clinically in patients with subfoveal choroidal neovascularization. Interferon alfa-2a has been found to be ineffective for choroidal neovascularization secondary to age-related macular degeneration.

Anti-vascular endothelial growth factor (VEGF) Therapy: Anti-VEGF therapy is the established current mode of treatment for choroidal neovascularization and is discussed separately.

Retinal Pigment Epithelial Transplantation

The role of retinal pigment epithelium in the pathogenesis of age-related macular degeneration remains a matter of speculation. Although the molecular defect in AMD remains unknown, histopathological evidence has revealed that the retinal pigment epithelium is an early target of the disease. Retinal pigment epithelial cells are considered to have a bi-directional effect on the growth of endothelial cells owing to conflicting findings from various studies. One report has shown that these cells can promote endothelial cell proliferation by the production of VEGF under hypoxic conditions. However, there are other studies revealing the ability of retinal pigment epithelial cells to prevent the proliferation of endothelial cells in newly formed choroidal capillaries and also in promoting maturation of aberrant new vessels.

Pathological studies have been carried out on the changes in Bruch's membrane and concomitant changes in the retinal pigment epithelial cells in age-related macular degeneration. These have shown that following progressive severe changes in the Bruch's membrane, the retinal pigment cells begin to cause atrophy of the overlying photoreceptors. Experimental work undertaken on the Royal College of Surgeons (RCS) rats has revealed that this photoreceptor atrophy may be prevented for as long as one year by the transplantation of retinal pigment epithelial cells (both homografts and xenografts) into the sub-retinal space. Efforts have been made to repair the damaged retinal pigment epithelial cells by retinal pigment epithelium transplantation in both exudative and atrophic forms of age-related macular degeneration. Results in exudative form of the disease have not been as encouraging as in the atrophic form.

Retinal pigment epithelial graft survival or rejection is dependent on the status of the blood retinal barrier at the time of transplantation. The risk of rejection has been shown to be higher when the transplant is introduced into the subretinal space after removal of the neovascular membranes than when introduced into an avascular space (when the blood retinal barrier is intact, as in atrophic form of age-related macular degeneration). Studies have shown that graft rejection is likely to occur because retinal pigment epithelial cells express major histocompatibility antigens (particularly class I). However, these studies were performed without immunosuppression.

Gene Therapy

In disease processes, cell death may occur by either apoptosis or necrosis and in a degenerative process it is largely by apoptosis. Apoptosis is also known as programmed cell death or induced cell death and is initiated by endogenous cellular processes triggered off by a gene or set of genes. Programmed cell death is an energy requiring process of self-elimination of cells without production of cellular debris to attract macrophages. Apoptosis is in contrast to necrosis inflicted by noxious stimulus and in which macrophages are attracted and cell death occurs in clusters. Programmed cell death is normally known to occur during embryogenesis and morphogenesis to regulate the size and shape of organs by deletion of selective cells. It is also known to occur physiologically in the normal turnover of intestinal epithelial cells, prostate epithelium, hormone-mediated regression of uterine epithelium, deletion of lymphocyte clones, regression of lactating mammalian gland, atresia of ovarian follicles, etc.

Until recently, the mechanism of cell death in photoreceptors and retinal pigment epithelium was not known. However, studies on RCS rats have now shown that apoptosis is a predominant method. It has also been found that photoreceptor cell death in these rats "is clearly secondary to a genetic defect in the neighboring retinal pigment epithelial cells".

Presently, studies are on to more precisely determine the nature of cell death in age-related macular degeneration and to also evaluate if gene modification of retinal pigment epithelial cells to inhibit this programmed cell death is possible by using material carrying adenovirus E1 and E4 vectors into the subretinal space. So far, most efforts of treatment by controlling apoptosis have been directed at retinal degenerations, such as retinitis pigmentosa. In RCS rats, photoreceptors die as a result of mutation in the neighboring retinal pigment epithelial cells. It has already been demonstrated that in transfected cell cultures and transgenic mouse lines, expression of certain genes can prevent apoptosis. For gene mediated disease, gene therapy would probably be the ultimate approach to its prevention, retardation or may be even cure.

Genes have been experimentally introduced to rescue photoreceptor cells from degeneration and corrective genes have also been introduced into cultured retinal pigment epithelial cells using retrovirus as a vector. As this requires dividing cells for the gene transfer to occur, it cannot be used in the adult retina wherein the cells are not replicating. However, methods have now also been devised to transfer exogenous genes into differentiated living animals with procedures, such as injection of naked DNA or DNA mixed with a highly polar lipid vehicle. Replication deficient adenoviruses used as vectors for gene transfer in post-mitotic cells have not been found to cause any severe tissue damage. Adenovirus has also been tried to transfect post-mitotic photoreceptors and retinal pigment epithelial cells in vivo. Whether they can control gene expression in these cells is not however known.

Although the role and efficacy of both retinal pigment epithelium transplantation and gene therapy is at present very ill-understood, studies and developments in the coming decade or two would probably define the role of these two modalities in age-related macular degeneration more accurately.

Treatment of age-related macular degeneration with subfoveal choroidal neovascular membranes continues to pose a great challenge. Patient education, early diagnosis and management remain the key to preserving vision in patients with age-related macular degeneration.

CENTRAL SEROUS CHORIORETINOPATHY

Introduction

Central serous chorioretinopathy (CSC) is a disorder of the retinal pigment epithelium-choriocapillaris complex that is characterized clinically by a localized serous detachment of the neurosensory retina usually involving the macular region and for which there is no identifiable cause. Concurrent detachment of the retinal pigment epithelium may or may not be present. Choroidal hyperpermeability has been found on indocyanine green angiography.

Diagnosis

Central serous chorioretinopathy affects persons in the 2nd to 5th decade and has a male preponderance (male: female ratio of 8–10:1). It is uncommon in blacks and quite frequent in other races including the Asians. The usual presenting symptoms are blurred vision, decreased vision, metamorphopsia and micropsia due to separation and distortion of visual elements, altered color vision (dyschromatopsia) and recognition of a visually disturbing paracentral scotoma. In some patients there may be migraine like headache. Other associations may also be present, such as Type A personality, hypochondria, hysteria, history of corticosteroids intake, or relation with pregnancy or with dialysis.

Visual acuity in most patients is in the range of 20/20 to 20/400 usually and this may improve with a hyperopic correction. Slit-lamp biomicroscopy is unremarkable and the pupillary reflexes as well as intraocular tension are normal. Ophthalmoscopic features include translucent/grayish, well-defined, ovoid, shallow detachment at the posterior pole (variable size, usually about 2 disc diameters) with a halo of light reflex around the detachment. Yellowish gray retinal pigment epithelial detachment and yellow, grayish-white, dot like, subretinal precipitates may be seen in some cases. Regions of retinal pigment epithelium atrophy may be present, especially in old, recurrent or chronic CSC. The surrounding retina and retinal vessels are normal and there are no retinal/subretinal hemorrhages.

On fluorescein angiography focal, point like hyperfluorescence is seen at the retinal pigment epithelial level in early phases. Hyperfluorescence increases in the later phases to assume inkblot pattern (80 to 90%) or a smoke stack pattern (10 to 20%). Inverse smokestack leak and other irregular patterns have also been described such as pinpoint leak, diffuse leak without leakage point and leaking "scar". The leak is usually unifocal (72%) and infrequently multifocal (2-7) leakage points (Fig. 26.4). Commonest site of leakage is superonasal and less than 1mm from the foveal center; least common site is inferotemporal. Focal blob of hyperfluorescence increasing in intensity in later phases, but constant size is indicative of a retinal pigment epithelial detachment. If no leak is detected on fluorescein angiography, the possibilities are that leak has probably healed and so detachment is likely to resolve soon or there is an extramacular site of leakage, particularly superiorly (sometimes it has been reported that gravity may have caused the leakage point to remain not at the center, but at the margin of the detachment). Also, one must rule out mimics (e.g. inferior retinal detachment). Fluorescein angiography remains an important essential investigation before laser photocoagulation in patients with central serous retinopathy. Fluorescein angiographic prerequisites for laser photocoagulation are the presence of well defined leakage point on fluorescein angiography with the leakage point at least 500 μm away from the center of the foveal avascular zone. On indocyanine green angiography there is diffuse hyperfluorescence in early phases and central hypofluorescence with a surrounding ring of hyperfluorescence in mid and late phases. Location and number of leaking points are the same as in fluorescein angiography. Choroidal staining around the active leaking site is universally seen and additional areas of choroidal hyperpermeability (throughout the posterior pole and peripapillary region) are a common finding. Retinal pigment epithelium detachment is also more commonly detected (75%) on indocyanine green angiography than on fluorescein angiography. The presence of choroidal ischemia

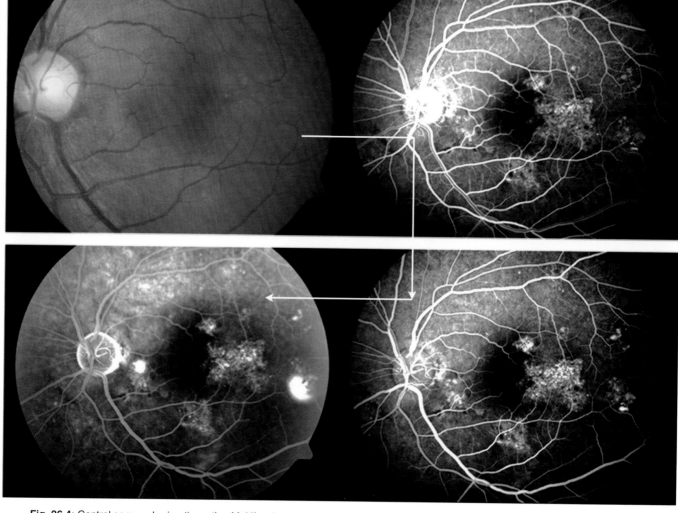

Fig. 26.4: Central serous chorioretinopathy. Multifocal central serous retinopathy with chronic retinal pigment epithelial decompensation

or perfusion defects is, however, controversial. Indocyanine green studies found choroidal capillary and venous congestion in patients with CSC.

Differential Diagnosis

- Macular hole, particularly in high myopes
- Rhegmatogenous retinal detachment with peripheral hole is to be considered particularly if inferior margin is not well defined and no leakage point is identified on fluorescein angiography.
- Kranenburg syndrome, optic nerve pit with serous macular detachment
- Age-related macular degeneration, particularly in those above 50 years. In doubtful cases, repeating the angiogram in the subsequent 2 to 3 weeks is helpful. It is also useful to remember that CSC is almost never associated with any form of hemorrhage in relation to the detachment.
- Tumors: Choroidal melanoma, osteoma, hemangioma, metastasis, leukemic infiltrate. Ocular ultrasonsgraphy is particularly useful in these cases.

- Miscellaneous: Posterior scleritis, uveal effusion syndrome, Harada's disease, collagen vascular disorders and sarcoidosis as well as malignant hypertension may present with serous macular detachments. However, other clinical signs are usually also present in these disorders.

Etiopathogenesis

By definition, there is no detectable etiological agent in the pathogenesis of central serous retinopathy. However, several factors have been blamed so much so that, it may be of multifactorial origin with environmental and genetic factors interacting to a variable extent. Increased catecholamine levels and a psychogenic personality are the most frequently associated factors with CSC. The mechanism of damage is thought to be immune mediated, infectious or a neuronal or circulatory disturbance. The pathogenesis of this disorder has also remained perplexing and highly debatable. It is still not ascertained whether CSC is primarily a choroidal or retinal pigment epithelial disorder. Earlier reports favored the retinal pigment epithelium while more recent studies suggest the possibility of its being a choroidal disorder. Whatever the cause and primary pathology, a disturbance of the retinal pigment epithelium-choroidal pump is thought to be the cause of fluid accumulation. Retinal pigment epithelium pathology may be focal or more widespread. Recent indocyanine green angiography studies favor the latter possibility. The probable events in the pathogenesis of central serous retinopathy are shown in Flow chart 26.3.

Flow chart 26.3: Probable sequence of events in the pathogenesis of central serous retinopathy

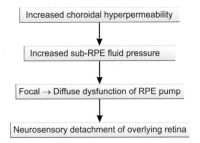

Management

Central serous chorioretinopathy is a relatively benign and self-limited disorder and in most cases the serous detachment resolves spontaneously in about 3–4 months. Recovery of visual acuity is good, but gradual improvement may proceed to normalcy even after 12 months after the initial episode. Other visual complaints (metamorphopsia, dyschromatopsia, relative scotoma) may however persist for a variable period or remain permanently. Recurrences are not infrequent and are reported to occur in nearly one-half of patients. Prognosis decreases with increase in the number of recurrences and some cases may progress to a stage of chronic retinal pigment epithelium decompensation.

Several drugs that have been evaluated in the treatment of central serous retinopathy and some of these are acetazolamide, beta-blockers, tranquilizers, sedatives and barbiturates. Presently, however, medical therapy has no established role in the management of central serous retinopathy. It is stated here with emphasis that corticosteroids in any form are not recommended and may indeed be a contraindication as they risk increase the duration and rate of recurrence of this disorder.

Laser photocoagulation is the only well established treatment modality in patients suffering from central serous retinopathy. Treating the leakage site with laser (argon green, krypton and diode) hastens resolution of the disease, but does not affect the final visual acuity or the recurrence rate. Indeed, laser treatment has been reported to result in suboptimal recovery of contrast sensitivity in comparison to cases that resolve spontaneously. Hence, photocoagulation should be undertaken only in the presence of specific indications. The indications for this treatment are a matter of debate. Some of the recommended indications are:

- Patient prefers treatment following proper explanation. This is usually for occupational reasons or in functionally one-eyed patients wherein the quality of work is disturbed.
- Angiographic leak persists beyond three months (chronic CSC)
- In recurrent CSC to hasten visual recovery and decrease the risk of chronic retinal pigment epithelium decompensation.

POSTSURGICAL CYSTOID MACULAR EDEMA

Introduction

Accumulation of fluid at the macular region, either in the interstitial spaces or within Müller cells of the neurosensory retina, is designated as macular edema. As accumulation of fluid within the parafoveal region assumes the form of cystic spaces, it is often designated cystoid macular edema (CME). It may occur in association with pars planitis, vascular occlusions and diabetic maculopathy or following intraocular surgery. Cystoid macular edema has been reported following cataract surgery, penetrating keratoplasty, glaucoma filtering surgery, retinal detachment surgery and YAG capsulotomy. Cystoid macular edema has also been reported in retinitis pigmentosa, patients on ocular hypotensive lipids, such as latanoprost and also as a dominantly inherited disorder.

Cystoid macular edema was recognized as a "complication" of cataract surgery about half a century ago. Subsequently, characteristic fluorescein angiographic features were reported in this condition and cystoid macular edema occurring after cataract surgery was designated Irvine-Gass syndrome. Postsurgical macular edema may be acute or chronic and clinical or angiographic. Clinically significant CME is defined as the occurrence of angiographic CME accompanied by a decrease in visual acuity of at least two lines on the Snellen visual acuity chart.

The prevalence of angiographic CME is several times more than the prevalence of clinically significant CME. While the reported incidence of angiographic CME ranges from 20 to 60%, the corresponding figure for clinically significant CME is only about 1 to 5%. The risk is higher following ICCE than after ECCE or phacoemulsification. Patients with anterior chamber intraocular lens, iris-fixated intraocular lenses or those undergoing secondary intraocular lens implantation are also at an increased risk. Reported incidence of angiographic and clinically significant CME after various forms of cataract surgery has decreased over the years because of refinement in microsurgical technique and intraocular lens manufacture. Both angiographic and clinically significant macular edema is more common in patients with a history of complicated cataract surgery than in those with uneventful surgery. With regard to cataract surgery, break in the posterior capsule with concurrent vitreous herniation or prolapse increases the risk of postsurgical CME several folds. This risk may, however, be lowered if the complication is appropriately managed. Other factors that have been reported to increase the risk of developing CME following surgery are operating microscope toxicity and a history of diabetes or hypertension. Occurrence of CME in one eye following surgery is known to be associated with an increased risk of its occurrence in the fellow eye.

Diagnosis

In patients with angiographic CME, visual symptoms are absent or mild, but in those with clinically significant CME, visual acuity is appreciably reduced (at least two lines on Snellen visual acuity chart). Symptoms related to CME usually appear within the first several weeks after cataract surgery (frequently between 6–8 weeks). With or without treatment, these symptoms are known to spontaneously abate. The rate of resolution is variable, but nearly 50% of cases do so within 6 months. However, about one in hundred patients develop chronic CME. When clinically significant macular edema persists for more than six months, it is termed chronic CME. Chronic CME results in significant sequelae like formation of epimacular membrane and pseudo or full thickness macular hole. Some patients may have ciliary congestion, photophobia, anterior chamber cells and flare, ciliary tenderness and some degree of hypotony. Signs of complicated surgery like iris incarceration, posterior capsular tear, vitreous incarceration or herniation and intraocular lens malposition may also be evidence.

Ophthalmoscopically, macular edema is suspected whenever there is a loss of foveolar reflex along with a grayish color and thickening of the macular region. The characteristic cystoid or "honeycomb" pattern is not an infrequent finding on ophthalmoscopy. A more common form of macular edema is noncystoid macular edema. Few perifoveal and/or peripapillary splinter hemorrhages may also be present. Concurrent edema of the optic nerve head is also not an uncommon finding. In the presence of hemorrhages there is a possibility of vitreomacular traction being the cause of CME. The best method to identify macular edema is probably contact fundus biomicroscopy or a plus 90 D examination. The presence of petechial hemorrhages is probably indicative of some vitreomacular traction as the probable cause of the edema.

Fluorescein angiography is invaluable in establishing a firm diagnosis of macular edema and it is important to study the late phase angiograms. The characteristic angiographic features in CME are the visualization of perifoveal telangiectatic capillaries in the early phases, leakage from these vessels in the mid and later phases followed by a rosette or petalloid pattern of pooling in the late phases (~ 5–10 minutes). Concurrent leakage of dye from the optic disc vessels is also seen in a large number of patients with postsurgical macular edema (Fig. 26.5). Macular edema has graded on fluorescein angiography into 5 grades, grade 0 indicating absence of any leak and grade 5, severe

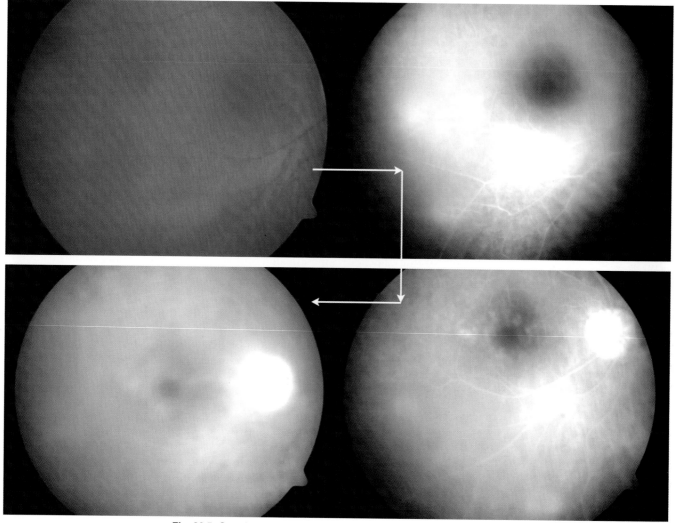

Fig. 26.5: Cystoid macular edema. Postsurgical cystoid macular edema

perifoveal edema greater than 1 disc diameter. It is important to emphasize here that the severity of angiographic leakage may have no direct correlation with the degree of macular thickening or visual loss. Retinal thickness analyzer and optical coherence tomography may aid in quantifying the degree of macular thickening in future.

Differential Diagnosis

Conditions that may be mistaken for macular edema are macular schisis, incipient macular hole and serous detachment of the macula. When the condition occurs in young individuals and is bilateral one must consider the possibility of dominant cystoid macular dystrophy.

Etiopathogenesis

The exact pathogenesis of cystoid macular edema is poorly understood. Common to its appearance is a breakdown of the inner and/or the outer blood retinal barrier. Whether the fluid accumulates within the interstitial spaces or within the Müller cell bodies has been a matter of debate. Probably both processes are involved depending on which of the two blood-retinal barriers is mainly affected. The accumulated fluid is almost always transudative in nature and so no exudates are seen in patients with postsurgical cystoid macular edema. A multitude of factors makes the macular region prone to the development of cystoid macular edema. Some of these factors are increased thickness of the outer plexiform layer (layer of Henle), increased capillary density, thinner internal limiting membrane and metabolically the most active region of the retina.
The ultimate trigger in the genesis of CME seems to be the release of prostaglandins following breakdown of the blood-ocular barrier.

Management

Before considering any treatment option in patients with postsurgical CME, it is important to ascertain its cause and nature. As indicated earlier, angiographic CME does not need any treatment. In patients with clinically significant CME, medical, laser and surgical interventions become necessary depending on the cause and initial response to medical treatment alone. Topical nonsteroidal anti-inflammatory drugs (NSAIDs) and topical or periocular corticosteroids form the mainstay in medical management. Ketorolac tromethamine 0.5% given four times daily for three months has been found to be effective in bringing about a resolution of the macular edema. Bromfenac and nepafenac have also been introduced. It has been shown that a dual therapy with NSAIDs and topical corticosteroids is superior to either of the drugs prescribed alone. Some authors recommend the concurrent use of oral indomethacin 25 mg thrice daily for 10 days at this stage. If no response is seen following topical therapy, one must consider injection of corticosteroids into the periocular space. The usual drugs are triamcinolone or methylprednisolone 20 mg in 0.5 mL. If no response is seen

following one injection, the rationale for giving repeat injections is questionable. The next consideration should be prescription of oral corticosteroids at a dosage of 1–1.5 mg/kg/day, followed by a gradual taper. Although corticosteroids are prescribed, most reported studies have not shown any benefit in the terms of improvement in visual acuity. The role of carbonic anhydrase inhibitors and hyperbaric oxygen is controversial and they are yet to gain widespread acceptance. Carbonic anhydrase inhibitors may be useful in situations wherein macular edema is present in the absence of inflammation (e.g. in retinitis pigmentosa).

When obvious aggravating factors are evident, like vitreous incarceration in the wound or intraocular lens malposition, the same should be managed early (if initial medical therapy fails or there are relapses) to prevent the edema from becoming chronic. YAG laser vitreolysis has been used successfully, by some authors, to manage fine vitreous strands adherent to the wound. This modality of treatment has the risk of producing retinal detachment and elevation of intraocular pressure. In many cases, it is probably more prudent to undertake pars plana vitrectomy as vitreous adherent to the iris can also be removed.

MYOPIA

Introduction

Optically, myopia is that refractive state of the eye at rest wherein parallel rays of light are brought to a focus in front of the neurosensory retina. In other words, the myopic eye has excessive plus power and its far point is less than at infinity. The term "myopia" is derived from the Greek words "myein", which means "to close" and "ops" meaning "eye". The term in fact describes the tendency of these individuals to habitually bring the eyelids close to form a stenopaeic slit to see better. Before discussing the etiopathogenesis, classification and natural progression of myopia and the causes for the visual handicap induced by it, it is necessary to briefly review the development of the refractive apparatus of the eye and the process of its emmetropization.

The major variables whose interplay is responsible for the emmetropization of refraction are the corneal power and axial length. Lenticular power and anterior chamber depth play a minimal role in the process. A defective correlation among these factors during development leads to a correlation ametropia. However, a gross abnormality in any of these components leads to a breakdown of the correlation and results in component ametropia. During embryological development, it is believed that expansion of the globe is dependent upon vitreous accumulation and the increasing intraocular pressure produced by an expanding vitreous body. The neural ectoderm by virtue of its control of vitreous formation and choroidal development is the basic determinant of ocular growth. The fact that both scleral and choroidal growths are believed to be induced and controlled by the retinal pigment epithelium may also influence the development of myopia. Scleral development begins at the limbus and proceeds slowly towards the posterior pole. It is felt that most of the sclera is derived from ectodermal neural crest except, posterior sclera that is derived from mesoderm. Postnatal ocular growth occurs in two stages: An early or infantile state (ends at 3 years of age) and a juvenile stage (ends at 14 years of age; the study extended only up to 14 years of age). By the early stage, i.e. 3 years, the human eye is for the most part, fully developed. The remaining growth, however, is crucial in determining the refractive state.

The mean corneal power of a full-term infant is 55.2 D. This decreases to about 43 D at 3 years of age. Axial growth from 3 years to 14 years of age is about 1 mm or 2.5 D of myopia if this remains uncompensated by a decrease in lens power (corneal changes play a lesser role in compensating for the increase in myopia in the juvenile stage). As axial lengthening becomes excessive, the ability to compensate decreases and a consequent increase in the degree of myopia occurs. At birth, in term infants, the average sagittal diameter of the eyeball is about 18 mm. This increases by 3.8 mm in the first year of life and then at a progressively slower rate until puberty. Corneal radius of curvature probably increases because of an increase in scleral dimensions. Lens power decreases because the diameter of the ciliary ring increases and consequently the zonular tension.

Ocular refraction at birth is 2.3 D of hyperopia. A normal correlation of the various components, which modulate the refractive status, leads to emmetropia. A moderate breakdown of this correlation leads to +/- 4 D of refractive error. In myopia, the mean corneal power is 1 D greater than in emmetropes and hyperopes (range: 39–47 D); the mean chamber depth is 3.67 mm (range: 2.8–4.55 mm), mean lens power, 17–35 D (range: 12.5 D) and the range of axial length, 21.62 to 26.37 mm in low myopia and 21.88 to 34.77 mm in high myopia.

Diagnosis

Myopia is a very common ocular abnormality with a female preponderance and peak prevalence at 20 years of age. Myopia occurs least commonly in blacks and is comparatively more common in the Asians. The incidence of myopia is higher in the upper economic classes and those with academic training. The clinical features in myopia depend on the type and severity of myopia. The current terminology and classification seems inadequate and a differential diagnosis of myopia based on the use of axial length measurements or degree of refractive error is often difficult. The only reliable method of classification presently available is probably fundus examination. Pathologic myopia is defined as that ocular disease in which a number of serious complications are associated with an excessive axial elongation of the eye. Degenerative myopia as a synonymous term for pathologic myopia is not acceptable because it actually describes a stage in the disease process. It cannot be applied to the younger patients with pathologic myopia, since true

degenerative changes are rarely seen under the age of 20. The term malignant myopia should also be avoided.

Simple myopia (Low myopia): The development of these eyes is normal. All components of refraction lie on their normal distribution curve. Myopia occurs because there is a correlation failure between total refractive power (of the lens and cornea) and the normal axial length. The cause for non-correlation is multifactorial. Most eyes have myopia of less than 3 diopters, some between 3–5 D. Crescent formation is absent as are other fundus changes. The axial length in these patients is between 22.0 mm and 25.5 mm.

Intermediate myopia (Medium, moderate myopia): The term intermediate myopia was introduced about two decades ago, by Otsuka. In these cases, postnatal posterior segment expansion is in excess of normal. There is probably an exaggerated enlargement of the normal postnatal distention of the oro-equatorial zone. If it involves the entire posterior pole, generalized spreading and thinning of retinal pigment epithelium can lead to tessellation. Hereditary and environmental factors interact to produce this abnormality. This is a form of component myopia, with the axial length being abnormal. Patients with intermediate myopia have an axial length of 25.5–32.5 mm. This form of myopia is most commonly found in eyes with 3–8 D of myopia, but rarely also in eyes below 3 D of refractive error. The prevalence of white without pressure, lattice, pigmentary and paving stone degeneration increases in these cases. The incidence of glaucoma and retinal detachment is also increased. Unlike patients with pathological myopia, these eyes, however, do not have posterior staphyloma.

Pathological myopia: Pathological myopia accounts for the most cases of myopia-related blindness and is essentially a hereditary disease. Its sine qua non is the presence of a posterior staphyloma. It is generally transmitted as an autosomal recessive trait. Decreased scleral resistance combined with an increased expansion force is the probable cause of staphyloma formation. These patients have a high incidence of peripheral retinal degeneration, retinal breaks and detachment. The refractive error is usually above 6–8 D and the axial length is over 32.5 mm in most cases. In high myopia, all diameters of the globe are grossly increased, but the maximum increase occurs in the anteroposterior diameter. The overall area of the retroequatorial zone of the eye increases from 9 sq.cm. to 13–15 sq. cm. Anterior segment changes may include corneal thinning, anterior iris insertion, greater frequency of iris processes and increased anterior chamber depth. The sclera is defective qualitatively and quantitatively. The fibers are of smaller dimensions and their interweaving is defective. Choroidal vascular occlusions are a prominent feature of the disease and smaller diameter vessels are affected initially. Retinal pigment epithelium shows both hyper and hypopigmentation with multilayered pigment clumping. Migration of pigment into the inner retina also occurs. The lamina vitrea shows thinning, splitting and ruptures. The ruptures are seen clinically "as lacquer cracks". The macula shows thinning of the ganglion cell layer, cystic degeneration and later, atrophy which might lead to hole formation. In the peripheral retina there are accentuated cystoid changes with formation of Blessing-Iwanoff cysts. The prevalence of paving stone degeneration and lattice degeneration also increases. The optic nerve is vertically oval and in moderate degrees of myopia, the cup-disc ratio is increased due to the enlarged cross-sectional area of the nerve.

Childhood myopia (School myopia): Most cases develop this type of myopia between 5–12 years of age and most are physiologic variety. Myopia with an earlier onset tends to demonstrate earlier progression that may continue up to the third decade. Depending on the clinical course, Donders recognized two forms of childhood myopia: the stationary type, which was characterized by slight increase between 10 years and 26 years of age and the temporally progressive type, which is characterized by a fairly rapid increase between 18 years and 25 years of age. No further changes are seen after 25 years of age.

Clinical Features

Blurring of distant vision with good near vision is the commonest presentation. Asthenopic headaches occur due to an increase in accommodative convergence/accommodation ratio (AC/A ratio) and a reduced range of accommodation between the far and near points. Other causes of asthenopia are fatigue of accommodation; excessive convergence required owing to a short focal length and induced aniseikonia and prism-related phorias. The patient may also be present with irritation and itching with vigorous rubbing of the eyes, which is to be discouraged. In a child, the parent may complain about the nearsighted attitudes adopted by the child. Gradual reduction of vision may be due to progression of refractive error or due to degenerative change involving the macula, cataract and glaucoma. Causes of rapid loss of vision include vitreous hemorrhage due to posterior vitreous detachment with or without retinal detachment and macular hemorrhage. Floaters have an earlier age of onset due to vitreous synchysis, syneresis and detachment. Patients may also present with complaints of metamorphopsia that may be indicative of a choroidal neovascular membrane or Fuchs spot.

Visual acuity is normal with optical correction in low myopia. In higher grades of intermediate myopia, minification may cause a slight reduction in visual acuity. This becomes normal on using contact lenses. In high myopia, there may not be any ophthalmoscopic cause for subnormal vision. In such cases, the probable cause is a Stiles-Crawford effect (directional sensitivity of the retinal receptors) and a reduction of photoreceptor cells in the highly myopia macula.

A pseudoconvergent squint may be evident owing to a negative angle kappa. This occurs because the visual axis has a tendency to shift to the temporal side from the pupillary axis. In myopia, there is a reduced accommodative demand that results in decreased accommodative convergence. As a result, exophoria or exotropia may also occur. Since the accommodative convergence/accommodation ratio is higher in myopic patients, correction of myopia may result in an increase in accommodative convergence with resultant esophoria or esotropia during near work. In general, the younger the myope and the more constant the use of optical correction, the more likely it is that the defect will be convergent rather than divergent. Esotropia is more common in patients with unilateral or anisometropic myopia probably because the onset of strabismus is earlier in life owing to a hindrance to fusion. Other specific motility disturbances include congenital esotropia, adult onset esotropia and lateral rectus underaction. Tonic esotropia in infants results from constant use of their eyes at the near point. Adult onset esotropia results from an uncorrected high AC/A ratio and functional divergence insufficiency.

In physiologic myopia, the anterior segment is unremarkable. In high myopia, anterior segment findings may include corneal thinning, anterior insertion of the iris, a deep anterior chamber, prominent iris processes and increased trabecular pigmentation. The lens shows increased prevalence of nuclear and posterior subcapsular cataract. The vitreous undergoes lacunar degeneration that is characterized by formation of pockets of fluid vitreous. This is later followed by microfibrillary degeneration and vitreous detachment from the internal limiting membrane. Vitreous detachment may lead to retinal or vitreous hemorrhage with or without formation of a retinal tear.

Until the maturation and cross linkage of scleral collagen, the eye responds to higher levels of intraocular pressure by increasing its size with the consequent evolution and progression of myopia. Mean intraocular tension in myopia is distinctly higher than in emmetropes. Ocular rigidity is decreased because of an increase in ocular volume and an increased ability of the sclera to distend. However, no correlation exists between the degree of myopia and ocular rigidity. Due to an increase in the area of the scleral foramen, there is an increased risk of optic nerve damage. In high myopia, cupping is limited to a large extent because the lamina cribrosa gets displaced forwards and super traction tends to limit excavation. One-third of myopic eyes with ocular hypertension develop visual field defect. Corresponding figures in an emmetrope and hyperope are 1/20 and 1/40 respectively. The overall prevalence of glaucoma in myopia is 7.5 to 12.5% and of myopia in glaucoma is 14.5 to 31%. There is a higher prevalence of pigmentary and low-tension glaucoma in myopic eyes and in most of these cases, myopia is of a low grade. The outflow facility is decreased in many patients of high myopia.

Evaluation of the fundus changes is the most reliable method of distinguishing pathologic from physiologic myopia. It also forms the most reliable basis for deciding the prognosis of pathological myopia. Direct ophthalmoscopy is of limited value in high myopia. Stereoscopic examination is essential and binocular indirect ophthalmoscopy is the ideal method of examination of these patients. Ophthalmoscopically, four signs are indicative of excess axial expansion of the eyeball. These are crescent formation, super traction, tessellation with pallor and posterior staphyloma formation. The last is pathognomonic of pathological myopia and was first described by Scarpa.

Generalized tessellation with pallor results from under pigmentation of the retinal pigment epithelial cells. It is considered abnormal only when it is observed in eyes previously known to have had moderate to heavy pigmentation. Crescent formation occurs as a result of a disparity in area between the scleral shell and the retinal pigment epithelium-choriocapillaris complex (Fig. 26.6). That the crescent is most frequently located temporally is attributable to the fact that a greater degree of postnatal expansion of the globe occurs on the temporal side. The location of the crescent in one study was temporal (69%) and less commonly annular (9.6%), inferior (5%) or superior (3.5%). Crescents may be of three kinds: Scleral crescent that is white in color and is seen in fair complexioned individuals; choroidal crescent has mottled pigmentation and is seen in moderate to dark complexioned individuals; and mixed crescent that have both scleral and choroidal crescentric patterns. Crescents in low myopia are rarely greater than one-third disc diameter and the optic nerve surface is flat. Crescents of less than 1/10th disc diameter may be normal even if they are temporal. Unlike myopic crescents, congenital crescents are usually found on the lower aspect of the disc margin, are devoid of pigment mottling and do not change in size. Supertraction results from an apparent dragging of retinal and choroidal tissue nasally over the surface of the optic nerve. Supertraction gives rise to light reflex that are best seen by direct ophthalmoscopy. These appear as thin streaks with the concavity towards the disc and are called "Weiss Streaks". With advancing myopia and expansion of the posterior funds, there is a flattening of the supertraction mound and the reflexes disappear.

The presence of a posterior staphyloma (Scarpa's Staphyloma) is pathognomonic of pathologic myopia. By the fifth decade, almost half the eyes with staphylomas are legally blind. Direct ophthalmoscopy is of limited value for detection of a posterior staphyloma. On stereoscopic examination by binocular indirect ophthalmoscopy, one should look for a dark crescentric nasal reflex, bending of the vessel at the staphyloma

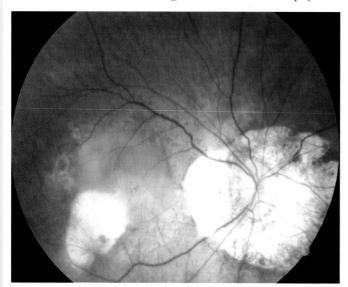

Fig. 26.6: Myopia. Peripapillary crescent with macular degeneration

margin and dioptric changes between normal and ectatic fundus areas.

Posterior staphylomas could be primary (types I–V) or compound (types VI–X). The prevalence of posterior staphyloma increases with an increase in the axial diameter of the globe. In general, only primary types I and III can eventually develop into large ectatic areas. Compound staphylomas are rarely seen during the first three decades. In the staphylomatous region, the blood vessels straighten in their course. In addition, expansion of the staphyloma also produces an eversion of the inner aspect of the optic nerve and a forward movement of the lamina cribrosa. This causes exposure of the central retinal artery and vein for a variable distance posterior to their primary bifurcation and they assume the configuration of a horizontal T or Y. Peripapillary atrophy is also a frequently evident change. The margin of the crescent is involved first. The previously sharp margin becomes irregular and fragmented. This causes an enlargement of the blind spot, but has no effect on central vision. Patients with bilateral nasal posterior staphyloma may show on visual field testing, incongruous bitemporal hemianopic field defects. This should not be interpreted as a chiasmal pathology and the patient should not be subjected to unwarranted neurological evaluation.

At the macula, the earliest change is an unusual degree of hyperpigmentation. Fuchs spot may also occur in the absence of myopia. In myopic eyes, the prevalence of these lesions is greater with increasing age. This is possibly a consequence of retinal pigment hyperplasia in this region and pallor of the surrounding fundus accentuates this appearance. Staphyloma formation further accentuates the process of spreading out of the retinal pigment epithelial cells and gives the macular a granular appearance. In the late stages, chorioretinal degeneration may involve the macula. The foveal reflex becomes difficult to discern because of retinal thinning and flattening. Macular degeneration in myopia usually occurs earlier than in patients with senile macular degeneration (on an average about 16 years earlier). It is often bilateral and females are more frequently affected. Macular holes are more frequent in myopic eyes, but before considering them as the cause of a detachment; it is first essential to rule out the presence of a peripheral retinal break.

In the early stages, lacquer cracks, retinal hemorrhages and small focal areas of chorioretinal atrophy characterize chorioretinal changes. Lacquer cracks are seen as yellow-white irregular lines that course across the posterior pole. They have a slight male predilection and are associated with the presence of posterior pole staphyloma. Lacquer cracks are usually multiple and horizontally oriented. They may also form a reticular pattern. Lacquer cracks are fissures in the retinal pigment epithelium—lamina vitrea choriocapillaris complex and are thought to originate as mechanical tears. On fluorescein angiography, lacquer cracks appear as pseudofluorescent tracks with no subretinal dye leakage. The prevalence of lacquer cracks decreases with age probably because the fundus areas in which they occur are extremely prone to extensive degeneration. When lacquer cracks involve the macular region, the visual prognosis is always guarded.

Focal areas of chorioretinal atrophy may occur in association with lacquer cracks or independent of them. They appear as white to yellow round lesions with or without pigment clumping at their margins. Initially these areas are not confluent. In the late stages, the regions of chorioretinal atrophy enlarge and tend to become confluent. The margins become pigmented and may no longer be sharply defined. The cause of these atrophic zones is probably choroidal vascular occlusion and abiotrophic degeneration. Another unproven cause is involution of choroidal neovascular membranes.

Subretinal neovascularization most commonly involves the macular and peripapillary region and may give rise to transudates or to frank hemorrhages. The hemorrhage per se or hyperplasia of retinal pigment epithelial cells or both may give rise to a dark spot called the Foster-Fuch's spot (Fig. 26.7). If it turns gray, the possibility of overlying epithelial detachment exists. Over time, these spots disintegrate and become surrounded by a halo of fundus atrophy. These lesions occur earlier in patients with higher myopic errors and affects 5 to 10% of the myopic population. The lesion is seen more commonly in females. The visual prognosis remains guarded in eyes with a Fuchs spot.

The normal postnatal expansion of the globe occurs in the oro-equatorial region. This is true even in the presence of a deep posterior staphyloma. This expansion leads to peripheral retinal changes that can lead to retinal breaks and detachment. The yearly incidence of retinal detachment in the phakic population is 5 to 10 persons per 1,00,000 population (0.005% to 0.01%). This amounts to a lifetime risk of retinal detachment in these patients of 0.30 to 0.60%. On the other hand, the lifetime risk of detachment in a person with myopia of more than –5.0 D living up to 60 years of age is 2.4%. It is generally agreed that, higher the myopia, greater is the possibility of retinal detachment. In myopes, the detachment is bilateral in 8 to 32% of patients in hospital-based statistics. Most eyes with detachment have an increased equatorial diameter. Myopic eyes are more prone to retinal detachment because of the earlier onset of posterior vitreous detachment, increased prevalence of lattice degeneration, thinned retina and areas of abnormal vitreoretinal adhesions.

Four types of peripheral fundus abnormalities are found in association with axial elongation of the eye. These abnormalities are white without pressure, lattice degeneration, pigmentary degeneration and paving stone degeneration. White without pressure represents areas of grayness or whiteness running circumferentially about the retinal periphery. The regions may appear flat or elevated and can have a bizarre distribution. They are found frequently in the region of the vitreous base and ora serrata. The inferotemporal quadrant is most frequently involved. Flat areas of white without pressure may even reach the retinal vascular arcades. White without pressure is considered as an advanced form of white with pressure and Schepens first described it. These areas are usually an isolated finding, but are more frequently found in association with lattice degeneration. White without pressure lesions have an increased prevalence in blacks and prematures and they are considered to be essentially benign except in patients with a giant retinal tear in the fellow eye.

Lattice degeneration is most closely associated with the occurrence of retinal breaks and detachments. These are linear or cigar-shaped ora parallel lesions in single or multiple rows with variable size and number. They have well defined margins and may or may not be pigmented. In relation to the vitreous base, they may be intrabasal, juxtabasal or extrabasal. In the region of the lattice, retina is thinned, the internal limiting membrane is absent, overlying vitreous is liquefied and there are strong vitreous adhesions along the edges. They have white interlacing lines when typical. These represent hyalinized vessels and constitute the lattice wicker. Lattice degeneration has no sex predilection and shows no increase in prevalence with age. Lattice tends to be bilateral in 34 to 63% of cases and is commonest in the superotemporal quadrant. Snail-track degeneration is considered a variant of lattice in that it lacks pigmentation and white lines typical of a lattice. They are less common than lattice, but pose a greater risk of causing retinal detachment. Some consider snail-track degeneration as an early stage of lattice. Lattice lesions are prone to hole formation within and tears at the posterior margin and ends of the lesion. Lattice degeneration with holes is less likely to cause detachment (45%) than those with tears (55%).

Lattice is present in 6 to 8% of the normal population. The risk of detachment in patients with lattice with holes is 1 in 92. Detachment secondary to holes is commonly seen in the younger, high myope, whereas detachments due to tears occur more frequently in the older, less myopic patient. Retinal detachments due to atrophic holes usually show an insidious progression of shallow detachment. In early life, lattice is most commonly associated with white without pressure, in middle

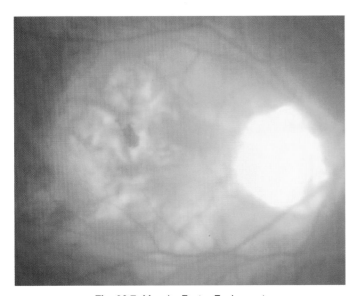

Fig. 26.7: Myopia. Foster-Fuchs spot

life with pigmentary degeneration and in those above 40 years of age with paving stone degeneration. Except paving-stone degeneration, the others have been reported to cause retinal breaks and detachment.

Differential Diagnosis

Transient or prolonged myopia can result from ciliary muscle contraction (spasm) or edema involving the ciliary body. The causes could be prolonged use of the eyes, especially at short focal distances; posttraumatic; drug induced, e.g. sulphonamides, miotics; and systemic disease, e.g. diabetes. Nocturnal myopia, empty field myopia and instrument myopia are related to a critical loss of target illuminance and loss of either contrast or size and reduced accommodation needed respectively.

Etiopathogenesis

Retinal photoreceptors are phototropic and the retina is a dynamic, image seeking tissue. Anomalous visual experience due to both hereditary and environmental factors during development appears to disrupt the emmetropization process. There probably exists a myopia gene that has poor penetrance and expressivity. Low myopia is usually inherited as dominant trait while high myopia is inherited as a recessive one. Attempts have been made to explain the changes in pathological myopia by different hypotheses. The mesodermal theory postulates that the abnormal qualitative and quantitative induction of scleral growth at the posterior pole is responsible for the occurrence of myopia. According to the ectodermal theory, abnormal pigment epithelium is responsible for induction of defective development of the choroid and sclera. The theory of ectodermal-mesodermal growth disparity states that overgrowth of the retina consequently leads to overgrowth of the choroid and sclera. Retinal overgrowth probably results from an excessive formation of vitreous or vitreous like substances. A fourth hypothesis considers the ciliary muscle as a pivotal mechanism in controlling ocular growth by acting as a counterforce to excessive ocular expansion. According to this hypothesis, underdevelopment of the ciliary muscle leads to excessive axial growth due to a decrease in the inhibitory activity of the ciliary body on ocular growth. There are however few supporters of this theory. Factors that have been blamed as being myopigenic in the past are increased scleral stress caused by extraocular muscle tension, convergence (i.e. near work) and stooping posture at near work. Accommodation is now viewed as an anti-myopia factor because ciliary muscle contraction decreases ocular tension and increases facility of outflow. Contrarily, fatigue of accommodation results in formation of a blurred image on the retina and this may act as a myopigenic stimulus. There is a strong suggestion that the near work hypothesis does play a role in the development of myopia in childhood.

Management

The aims in management would be prevention of myopia from developing (primary level), prevention of myopia progression

and management of complications and visual rehabilitation. Myopia per se cannot be prevented by any known treatment. It is advisable to forewarn a couple with high myopia about a strong possibility of their children also being affected.

Proper ophthalmologic examination is mandatory before an optical aid is prescribed to visually rehabilitate a myopic patient. Of particular importance is the evaluation of ocular motility, intraocular pressure and the fundus. Optical and laser correction of myopia is not discussed herein. Complications associated with myopia include motility problems, cataract, glaucoma, retinal detachment and chorioretinal degeneration.

In myopia, the intraocular pressure is particularly labile and so frequent measurement of the intraocular pressure by an applanation tonometer is essential. The intraocular pressure should be maintained below 20 mm Hg. This probably enhances the choroidal circulation and reduces stress on the defective posterior sclera. Glaucoma may remain undiagnosed in myopes because indentation tonometers are likely to record a false low intraocular pressure due to the low scleral rigidity in myopes. Secondly, optic nerve cupping my not be seen. Also, the visual field defects tend to be atypical in myopes.

The role of prophylactic treatment of retinal breaks in the management of myopic eyes is a controversial subject. Breaks that need to be treated are those that have a propensity to cause a detachment, such as breaks in the superior quadrants, horseshoe tears, breaks with contiguous subretinal fluid, breaks seen prior to cataract surgery and fellow eyes with retinal breaks. Some believe that all retinal breaks in myopia need treatment irrespective of any other factor. This, however, is not accepted universally. Either cryotherapy or photocoagulation can be used.

Chorioretinal degeneration forms the most important complication of pathological myopia. Focal atrophy appears to be ischemic in nature to some extent and it has been suggested that lowering the intraocular pressure may be protective. In the presence of well-defined choroidal neovascular membranes, photocoagulation is the treatment of choice. However, the long-term visual prognosis is these patients remain poor.

PARAFOVEAL TELANGIECTASIS

Introduction

Telangiectasia is thinning and dilation of the capillary walls. In the retina this abnormality may occur in the macular region or in the periphery. Parafoveal telangiectasis is dilation of the capillary bed confined predominantly to the parafoveal region and that is congenital/developmental or acquired in origin.

Diagnosis

Age at presentation and unilateral or bilateral involvement depends on the type of parafoveal telangiectasis. Most patients do not have any other concurrent ocular or systemic pathology. However, there are reports for and against an association between type-2 telangiectasis and diabetic retinopathy. Also, abnormalities on central nervous system examination are a feature in patients with type-3b telangiectasis.

The most recent classification of parafoveal telangiectasis is that by Gass and Blodi. Primary retinal telangiectasias involving the macular region has been classified into the categories as shown in the Flow chart 26.4. The most common type of parafoveal telangiectasis belongs to group 2 (bilateral and acquired). Almost all patients, present between the 4th–6th decade, with blurring or distortion of vision secondary to serous exudation involving the macula, some may develop subretinal neovascularization. Fundus examination reveals subtle to mild dilation of the involved capillaries. The area of involvement may vary from just one clock hour (as in group 1b) to as large as 1-2 disc areas. Right-angled venules draining the area may be present along with hyperplasia of the adjacent retinal pigment epithelium (as in group 2). A few small refractile deposits also may be present. Fluorescein angiography more clearly delineates the involved vessels (Fig. 26.8). They appear as dilated and ectatic vessels with no or minimal leakage in the late phases. Associated findings may include those suggestive of subretinal neovascularization or blocked fluorescence due to retinal pigment epithelium hyperplasia.

Flow chart 26.4: Classification of parafoveal telangiectasis

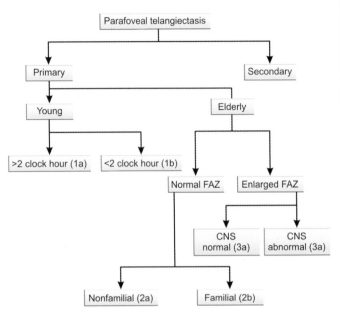

FAZ: Foveal avascular zone

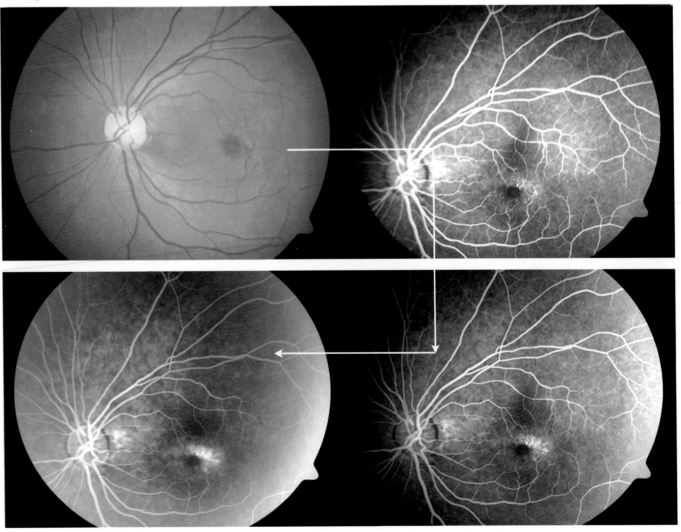

Fig. 26.8: Parafoveal telangiectasia. Type 2 parafoveal telangiectasia

Differential Diagnosis

Primary retinal telangiectasias should be differentiated from secondary telangiectatic changes seen in conditions, such as branch retinal vein occlusion, radiation retinopathy, etc.

Management

Laser photocoagulation is indicated only in a limited number of patients (those who have serous detachment or subfoveal neovascularization) as most telangiectasias are situated close to or within the foveal avascular zone. Prophylactic treatment is not recommended, as they are also known to undergo spontaneous regression.

RETINAL ARTERY MACROANEURYSM

Introduction

Cousins and associates have classified macroaneurysms involving the retinal vasculature into four types. These are typical retinal artery macroaneurysm, retinal venous aneurysms, retinal capillary macroaneurysm and collateral associated macroaneurysm. The last three types of macroaneurysms are more common and may be encountered in diabetic retinopathy, venous occlusive disease, radiation retinopathy, sickle cell disease, etc.

Diagnosis

Retinal artery macroaneurysm is usually an isolated finding with characteristic features. By definition, they are saccular or fusiform dilation of the retinal arteriole involving usually, the first three divisions. Their diameter is more than 100 μm (the upper limit for microaneurysm), but less than 250 μm. They are usually solitary and unilateral, but may be multiple in 20% and bilateral in 10%. They usually involve the temporal vessels and are often located at the bifurcations.

Retinal artery macroaneurysms generally occur in elderly women (6th decade) and about 75% of patients have associated systemic hypertension. Clinically two forms of presentation are seen, the acute type and the chronic type. In the acute form, patient presents with a sudden loss of vision (due to retinal or vitreous hemorrhage) while in the chronic form they present with a gradual loss of vision due to leakage and exudation into the macular area. The latter is usually diagnosed easily while the former is difficult to diagnose because of two reasons. Firstly, associated hemorrhage during the acute stage obscures visibility of the macroaneurysm and secondly, most resolve spontaneously after the hemorrhage and so may not be easily evident by the time the retinal or vitreous hemorrhage clears. The only characteristic feature during the acute stage is the presence of an "hourglass" shaped hemorrhage due to simultaneous preretinal and subretinal collection of blood (Fig. 26.9). This type of hemorrhage is not seen in all patients however. Fluorescein angiography may be helpful in identifying

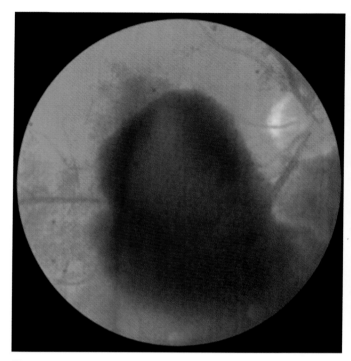

Fig. 26.9: Retinal macroaneurysm. Preretinal hemorrhage from a retinal macroaneurysm

retinal artery macroaneurysms. Some authors have considered pulsatility of a macroaneurysm as an imminent sign of rupture. Branch retinal artery occlusion as a complication of retinal artery macroaneurysm with and without laser photocoagulation has also been reported.

Management

No treatment is recommended for a macroaneurysm with the acute form of presentation, as recurrent hemorrhages are not known to occur and the visual recovery is good in most patients without treatment. Occasionally, pars plana vitrectomy may be necessary in patients with nonclearing vitreous hemorrhage. There is, however, no established role of submacular surgery to remove submacular hemorrhage. For those presenting with exudation into the macular area one may consider direct or indirect laser photocoagulation of the macroaneurysm if exudation is tending to progress towards the fovea and there is associated decrease in vision.

PHOTIC RETINOPATHY

Introduction

Photic retinopathy may be defined as manifestations of the toxic effects resulting from photochemical, photothermal and mechanical interaction between light and retinal tissue. The source of light may be natural, industrial, or that used for diagnostic and therapeutic interventions in medicine. Causes of photic retinopathy other than that caused by viewing of solar eclipse include exposure to operating microscope light, welding arc, light in neonatal intensive care unit and in those using tanning bed. Photic maculopathy may take several forms, such as solar retinitis, intraoperative light damage, laser retinal burn and probably cystoid macular edema and age-related macular degeneration.

Possibility of retinal phototoxicity from artificial light under experimental conditions in rhesus monkey eyes was reported several decades ago. Several cases have been reported following various forms of ophthalmic surgery. These procedures include cataract extraction, epikeratophakia, triple procedure, vitreous surgery, Molteno implant and pterygium surgery. The actual incidence from operating microscope induced macular phototoxicity is not well established. Some retrospective studies have shown an incidence of 3% and 7% and some prospective studies, an incidence of 28%.

Diagnosis

Clinically, photic maculopathy is usually not visible for one or two days. The shape and size depend on the light source. Operating light-induced lesions are sharply defined and are rarely more than 1–2 disc areas while endoilluminator lesions are larger and have less distinct margins. The location of the lesion in operation microscope induced photic maculopathy is typically superior or inferior to the fovea. This is determined by the effect of the bridle suture and also because the coaxial light is normally 1.5 to 6 degree off normal. While using the endoilluminator, damage is said to occur more often while using a 19-gauge continuous fiber endoilluminator with a 150W light bulb at maximum output for videotaping and surgeries like membrane peeling.

Clinical features depend on the severity and stage of phototoxicity (early or late). The threshold for functional damage has been reported to be lesser than that needed to produce clinically and histopathologically evident lesions. When the degree of photochemical damage is mild, it may not be evident on ophthalmoscopic examination. In the early stages, there is well-circumscribed outer retinal whitening. Within a few days, mild pigmentary disturbances become evident and in the subsequent 1 to 2 weeks the pigmentation becomes coarse and may also take on a targetoid appearance. After a period of about 4 weeks, the lesion appears smaller and epiretinal membrane formation may occur. At three to six months, the only remnant may be a yellow-white plaque. On fluorescein angiography there is early mottled hyperfluorescence and late staining. Dye leakage is not a characteristic feature of operating light microscope induced retinal damage. Fluorescein angiography may also reveal the presence of complications, such as choroidal neovascular membrane formation and probably cystoid macular edema. A correlation between retinal phototoxicity and CME has also been reported in literature.

Etiopathogenesis

Light is a form of electromagnetic energy of which three major components are recognized, the ultraviolet range, visible range

and infrared range. Ultraviolet radiation occupies the region between visible blue light and X-rays, visible radiation between 400 nm and 760 nm while infrared radiation extends beyond this. Ultraviolet radiation has been further sub-classified into three categories, UV-A, UV-B and UV-C. UV-A occupies the region between 400 nm and 320 nm and this range is also known as "black light". The region between 320 nm and 280 nm is called UV-B while that between 280 nm and 220 nm as UV-C radiation. Cumulative damage from UV exposure is thought to contribute to the formation of cataract and age-related macular degeneration. Solar retinitis also results from irradiation of the retina by high-energy wavelengths of visible blue light (around 400 nm) and lower levels of UV-A radiation. With regard to iatrogenic light-induced maculopathy, the percentage contribution by each component of the electromagnetic radiation is not known. Most reports consider visible blue light and UV-A as the most significant contributors while others believe that the near infrared radiation also carries great potential to produce light-induced maculopathy.

Forms of light-tissue interaction that can cause photic retinopathy are threefold. These mechanisms are photochemical, photothermal and mechanical. The latter two mechanisms come into play when there is an intense exposure to a light source over a focal area even when the duration of exposure is brief. On the other hand, photochemical damage results from prolonged exposure (minutes to hours) to a light source that would normally be well tolerated if the limits were below the threshold for retinal damage. Threshold for visible retinal damage has been defined as the time it takes for ophthalmoscopically detectable damage to occur in 50% of the subjects. Light in the shorter wavelength range is reportedly most efficient in producing photochemical damage.

Retinal irradiance (mWatts/cm^2) and safe exposure for common ophthalmic instruments that have been reported in literature are, operating microscope (970; 3 seconds); fiberoptic probe (220; 14 seconds); indirect ophthalmoscopy (100; 35 seconds); biomicroscopy (225; 15 seconds) and overhead lamps (20; 175 seconds). For practical purposes this translates in terms of duration of exposure to 4.0 to 7.5 minutes for a 30W operating microscope, 15 minutes for the indirect ophthalmoscope, 60 minutes for direct ophthalmoscope and 40 minutes for the slit lamp. Retinal irradiance from endoilluminators used during vitrectomy has been detailed by Meyers and Bonners.

Absorption and scattering of light by the crystalline lens decreases the ocular transmittance drastically in the 400 nm to 440 nm range. The cornea absorbs wavelengths below 400 nm (UV range). Since the retina is most sensitive to the blue end of the visible spectrum, in the presence of the crystalline lens very minimal exposure to this wavelength occurs. Ham et al have reported that melanin possesses preferential absorption for short wavelengths and thereby photochemical rather than thermal damage to the retina is more likely.

To a large extent, wavelength, power density and duration of exposure are the most significant factors in the genesis of photic retinal damage. Not all patients develop phototoxic reactions because the above factors are highly variable and also because of inherent protective mechanisms. Inherent factors that protect from the risk of photic retinopathy are photoreceptor shedding, quenching of singlet oxygen radical damage by xanthophyll, absorption by melanin and the presence of antioxidant enzymes, vitamin E, zinc and selenium. Aging is thought to enhance susceptibility to photic retinal damage as there is increasing lipofuscin and decreasing retinal pigment epithelial defense mechanisms. Ingestion of photosensitizing drugs preoperatively is also reported to increase the risk of ocular phototoxicity.

Management

Visual prognosis is variable and most reports show a favorable outcome. There is no known effective treatment for photic retinopathy. There is a protective effect of dexamethasone against retinal phototoxicity. In an experimental study, amelioration of retinal photic injury using a combination of flunarizine and dimethylthiourea has been reported. Protective effect of ascorbate against light-induced retinal damage in rats has also been reported. Patients taking photosensitizing drugs like hydroxychloroquine, allopurinol, retinoic acid, phenothiazines and psoralen compounds must be asked to discontinue them several days before any surgical procedure under the operating microscope.

The most effective measure to avoid iatrogenic light-induced retinal damage is protection of the retina from exposure to wavelengths that have the greatest potential to produce such damage. Mainly decreasing corneal and foveal irradiance and implanting intraocular lenses with UV chromophores following cataract surgery can achieve this. Some have suggested use of prophylactic dexamethasone and use of mildly cool infusion fluid.

However, it has been found that light-induced retinal damage may be produced despite use of UV and infrared filters. Hence, filters blocking these wavelengths alone are not necessarily protective. Studies on the role of UV absorbing intraocular implants in protecting against the occurrence of cystoid macular edema have shown conflicting results. Other protective measures that have been described to decrease foveal irradiance are use of an eclipse filter, injecting an air bubble temporarily into the anterior chamber and avoiding direct foveal exposure by tilting the microscope about 10 degrees and infraduction of the globe. The eclipse filter consists of an opaque disc placed at an appropriate plane along the illumination path of the operating microscope so as to project a sharply focused opaque spot of 11 mm on the cornea to decrease retinal irradiance. Use of corneal covers, such as gelfoam and opaque soft contact lenses has also been described. In conclusion, it may be said that, as phototoxicity has a cumulative effect, the most effective modality to prevent retinal damage is to decrease total energy delivered.

RADIATION RETINOPATHY

Introduction

Radiation retinopathy is a delayed manifestation of the effect of ionizing radiation on the vascular and cellular elements of the retina. The source of radiation may be iatrogenic or accidental. Iatrogenic causes result from inclusion of the eye within the radiation field while managing ocular or head and neck tumors using teletherapy or by direct involvement during the management of ocular tumors using brachytherapy. Radiation retinopathy usually manifests one to several years after exposure to the radiation source. Though, posterior segment findings have been reported in survivors of the atomic explosion at Nagasaki and Hiroshima during World War II, these are not thought to be a manifestation of the acute effects of radiation. Contrarily, most cases of radiation retinopathy result from recurrent exposure over a short or prolonged period of time.

Diagnosis

A history of being treated with an ionizing radiation source in the past is present in all patients. As susceptibility to its effects is variable, the amount of radiation the patient received does not always dictate the time of onset and the severity and rapidity of disease progression. The presenting feature is usually decreased in vision secondary to hemorrhages or exudation within the macular region. Radiation retinopathy may manifest with a multitude of ocular features like macular edema, optic disc edema, optic atrophy, telangiectasia of the capillaries and microaneurysmal dilation, nerve fiber layer infarcts (soft exudates), retinal hemorrhages and exudation, areas of capillary nonperfusion and disc and retinal proliferation (NVD and NVE) (Fig. 26.10). Neovascularization is believed to be more common after external beam radiation than following brachytherapy because of a larger area exposed to the radiation. Although radiation retinopathy is primarily a microangiopathy, occlusion of the central retinal artery and central retinal vein has also been reported.

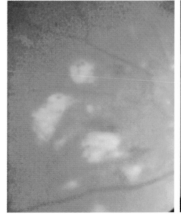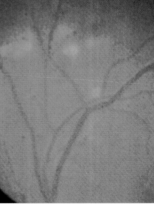

Fig. 26.10: Radiation retinopathy. Nerve fiber layer infarcts (soft exudates)

Macular edema is reported to be an early and common sign of radiation retinopathy. The condition usually is inexorably progressive in most patients and with passage of time a number of other ocular features become evident. In very late stages visual loss results from macular nonperfusion, vitreous hemorrhage, neovascular glaucoma and retinal detachment.

Etiopathogenesis

Radiation retinopathy is essentially an occlusive vasculopathy and changes in the neural retina are secondary to vascular damage. The inner retina is more prone to damage and the photoreceptors are relatively resistant. In radiation retinopathy endothelial cell loss predominates unlike in diabetic retinopathy. The incidence depends on both the total radiation source and the fraction size with reported showing that minimal of 30–35 Gy is necessary to induce pathologic changes. The risk is increased in patients with diabetes and in those receiving concurrent chemotherapy.

Management

Macular grid photocoagulation and panretinal photocoagulation in patients with macular edema and extensive areas of capillary nonperfusion and/or neovascularization respectively have been reported to be beneficial in retarding visual loss. Despite lack of conclusive evidence, in the absence of randomized studies it is recommended that laser photocoagulation be undertaken to reduce the rate of progression to macular nonperfusion and neovascular glaucoma. Visual loss from macular nonperfusion cannot however be reversed.

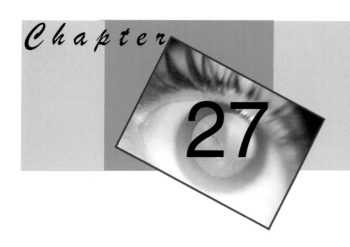

Retinal Vascular Disorders

*Taraprasad Das, Subhadra Jalali,
Vasumathy Vedantham, Ajit B Majji*

INTRODUCTION

Retinal vascular disorders are the commonest retinal lesions. Most of these disorders are closely associated with systemic disease, such as diabetes and hypertension directly or indirectly. Common vasculopathies with proven treatment modalities will be discussed. They include diabetic and hypertensive retinopathy, retinal vein and artery occlusion and Eales' disease. Many randomized clinical trials have been conducted in several retinal vasculopathies. Today they govern the management principles.

DIABETIC RETINOPATHY

Diabetic retinopathy is the commonest cause of moderate to severe retinal blindness. It is a complex multifactorial disease. Approximately 8% of legally blind individuals are reported to have diabetes and approximately 12% of new blindness is due to diabetic retinopathy. Insulin-dependent diabetic patients with retinopathy are 29 times more likely to become blind than nondiabetic individuals. In India, the estimated incidence of diabetic retinopathy in tertiary care diabetes center is estimated 34.1%. The diabetic retinal disease typically progresses (Fig. 27.1) through a succession of recognizable stages from early nonproliferative to advanced proliferative retinopathy (Table 27.1).

Nonproliferative Diabetic Retinopathy

Clinical signs: Nonproliferative diabetic retinopathy (NPDR) (Figs 27.2 to 27.4) is characterized by microaneurysms, intra-retinal hemorrhages, cotton-wool spots, hard exudates, venous beading and intraretinal microvascular abnormalities (IRMA).

Microaneurysms represent a localized endothelial cell proliferative response to small areas of capillary nonperfusion. They are visible ophthalmoscopically as red, round intraretinal lesion mostly in the posterior pole. Fluorescein angiography usually demonstrates the microaneurysms as hyperfluorescent spots and the smaller ones are easily identified by angiography than ophthalmoscopy. Dye may leak from them to the surrounding retina. Microaneurysm count appears to be an important predictor of the risk of progression to proliferative retinopathy.

Intraretinal exudates are visible as creamy yellow plaques, flecks or dots. This represents deposition of lipoprotein at the junction between thickened retina (adjacent to microvascular

Preretinopathy	Mild NPDR	Moderate to severe NPDR	PDR	Advanced Diabetic Eye Disease
Abnormalities of:	Microaneurysms	Venous beading	NVE, NVD	NVI
Electrophysiology	Intraretinal hges	Venous loop	Fibrovascular	NVG
Psychophysics	Cotton wool spots	IRMA	proliferation	Vitreous hge
Retinal blood flow	Venous dilatation	Cotton wool spots		TRD
Vascular permeability	Exudates	Cluster hges		

NPDR: Nonproliferative diabetic retinopathy

IRMA- Intraretinal microvascular abnormalities

NVD- New vessels on disc

NVE- New vessels elsewhere in retina

NVG- Neovascular glaucoma

NVI- New vessels in iris

TRD- Traction retinal detachment

Hge-Hemorrhage

Fig. 27.1: Diabetic retinopathy: Ophthalmic progression of diabetic retinopathy

Table 27.1: Diabetic retinopathy stages

Stage of diabetic retinopathy	Symptoms	Clinical Signs	Abnormal test results
Preclinical	None	None	Color perception: decreased ERG: decreased OP
Nonproliferative	Blurred vision	Retinal vasodilation	FFA: leaking aneurysms
		Microaneurysms	
		Intraretinal hemorrhages	
		Cotton-wool spots	
		Hard exudates	
		Venous beading	
		IRMAs	
Proliferative	Reduced vision	NVE / NVD	FFA; capillary dropouts
		Partial PVD	USG: vitreous hemorrhage / TRD
		Vitreous hemorrhage	
		Traction RD	

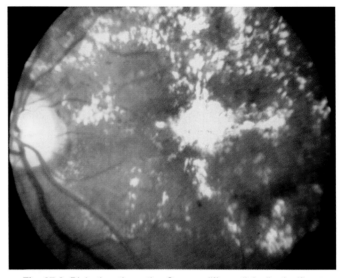

Fig. 27.3: Diabetic retinopathy. Severe, diffuse clinically significant macular edema in a patient having concurrent nephropathy

leakage) and the surrounding non-thickened retina. They are closely associated with diabetic maculopathy and very extensive posterior pole exudation is invariably associated with renal failure.

Intraretinal hemorrhages are seen throughout the fundus in NPDR, mostly confined posterior to equator. Flame shaped hemorrhages occur within the retinal nerve fiber layer, the long axis of the hemorrhage aligned with the nerve fibers. Deeper retinal layer hemorrhages assume punctate dot or large blot configuration. On fluorescein angiography all retinal hemorrhages block fluorescence.

Venous abnormalities, including venous beading, segmentation and loops are predictors of capillary nonperfusion and in general with increased venous irregularities the risk of progression from nonproliferative to proliferative retinopathy increases.

Intraretinal microvascular abnormalites (IRMA) consists of vascular elements within the retina. Unlike normal retinal vessels they branch frequently. Similar branching patterns occur in retinal new vessels too, but unlike the retinal new vessels, the IRMAs lie in the retinal tissue only and on fluorescein angiography, they stain but not leak. The IRMAs are associated with capillary nonperfusion; hence with increasingly widespread IRMAs the risk of development of proliferative retinopathy within a year increases four fold.

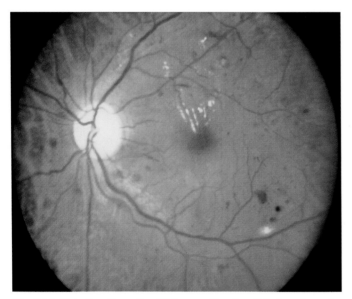

Fig. 27.2: Diabetic retinopathy. Mild nonproliferative diabetic retinopathy with focal clinically significant macular edema

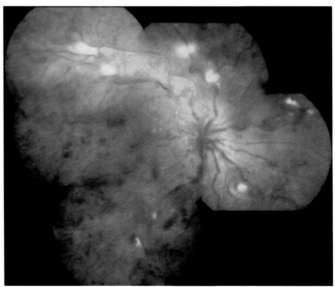

Fig. 27.4: Diabetic retinopathy. Severe nonproliferative diabetic retinopathy, showing extensive retinal hemorrhages, soft exudates and dilated tortuous retinal veins

Proliferative Diabetic Retinopathy

Clinical signs: Proliferative diabetic retinopathy (PDR) is characterized, primarily by retinal or disc new vessels and their sequelae. As the area of retinal capillary nonperfusion increases, neovascularization typically occurs, first on the retinal vessels and then at the optic disc and finally on the iris. The interaction between proliferating endothelial cells and the vitreous gel collagen produces contraction of the vitreous gel and a partial posterior detachment. The resulting traction on the optic disc or the retinal new vessels may precipitate hemorrhage and later traction retinal detachment.

Retinal new vessels elsewhere (NVE) typically takes spider-like form of multiple radial loops arising from a central feeding vessel derived from a vein. They commonly arise posterior to equator at margins of capillary nonperfusion. Fluorescein angiography shows retinal new vessels as the foci of increasing fluorescence, with dye leakage occurring most prominently at the growing tips of the vessels. One-fifth to one-third of eyes with NVE progress to optic disc new vessels and carry a 30% risk of severe visual loss over two years.

New vessel on disc (NVD) appears as an abnormally branching vascular network arising from the optic disc. Preretinal and vitreous hemorrhage may be present, along with signs of severe retinal ischemia. NVD leaks the dye in fluorescein angiography (Fig. 27.5) and thus is differentiated from collaterals on the optic disc. The risk of severe visual loss over 2-year period in eyes with NVD is 26 to 37%.

Visual Loss in Diabetic Retinopathy

The causes of moderate to severe reduction of vision in diabetic retinopathy could occur in several stages of the disease and for a variety of reasons (Table 27.2). The most common retinal lesions are diabetic maculopathy and the advanced diabetic retinal diseases.

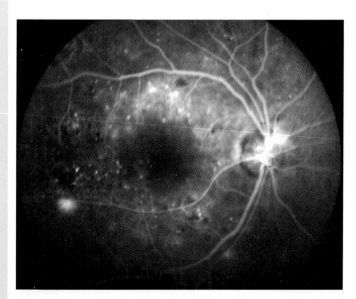

Fig. 27.5: Proliferative diabetic retinopathy. Fluorescein angiography showing < ¼ DD NVD and single NVE, illustrating proliferative diabetic retinopathy without high risk characteristics

Table 27.2: Visual loss in diabetes

Tissue	Pathology
Cornea	Epithelial erosions, Infectious keratitis
Iris	New vessels and Neovascular glaucoma
Retinal vessels	Venous occlusion, Arterial occlusion, Ocular ischemic syndrome
Vitreous	Vitreous hemorrhage
Retina	Macular edema, Macular ischemia, Macular traction, Exudates over macula center, Macular detachment, Traction and rhegmatogenous retinal detachment
Optic nerve	Diabetic papillopathy, Anterior ischemic optic neuropathy (AION)

Diabetic maculopathy is the commonest cause of moderate to severe central visual loss in diabetic individuals. The common lesions are macular edema and macular ischemia. Macular edema could be focal or diffuse (Figs 27.2 and 27.3). Focal leakage from microaneurysms or dilated capillaries results in localized retinal thickening. Fluid absorption in the surrounding retina results in the deposition of insoluble lipoprotein as hard exudate, at the interface between the thickened and non-thickened retina. Ophthalmoscopically the leaking microaneurysms are visible in the center of a ring of exudates. More widespread microvascular leakage causes diffuse macular edema. Deposition of lipoprotein is less prominent, macula is diffusely thickened and there is severe visual loss. Fluorescein angiography can differentiate focal from diffuse macular edema. Clinically significant macular edema (CSME) is vision threatening (Fig. 27.2).

The early treatment diabetic retinopathy study (ETDRS) has defined the CSME as any one of the following in decreasing order of severity:

- Retinal thickening or hard exudates associated with retinal thickening involving the center of fovea
- Any retinal thickening or hard exudates adjacent to retinal thickening extending within 500 μm of center of fovea
- Retinal thickening involving one disc area or more of retina, part of which is within one disc diameter of center of macula.

Ischemic maculopathy is characterized by macular microvascular occlusion and severe visual loss (Figs 27.6A and B). In acute stage of capillary closure, a cloudy swelling may occur and may mimic retinal edema; but with chronic ischemia, retinal thinning and pigment epithelial disturbance ensues. Fluorescein angiography is very characteristic-enlargement and irregularity of the foveal avascular zone and dry leakage from the dilated vessels surrounding the fovea.

Advanced diabetic eye disease describes a collection of processes, which complicate proliferative diabetic retinopathy and threatens the vision. Proliferation in the retina and the optic disc is the initiating event, but complications occur with incomplete vitreous detachment and vitreous contraction. These pathological events provide the necessary scaffold for the retinal vessels to grow; this causes progressive traction on the retinal vessels and/or the retina. As a consequence there is avulsion of thin retinal vessels causing preretinal or vitreous hemorrhage, or cause traction retinal detachment. The neovascular glaucoma is the end stage of the disease process.

Management

The key to successful long-term preservation of vision in diabetes includes the prevention of retinopathy, early detection, prompt treatment and regular follow-up. We will discuss the various management strategies, such as medical management, photocoagulation and surgery.

Medical Management

Medical management is largely aimed at prevention. Controlled clinical trials have demonstrated that aggressive control of blood sugar, blood pressure and dyslipidemia reduces the risk of retinopathy and its progression.

Glycemic control: The Wisconsin Epidemiologic Study of Diabetic Retinopathy (WESDR), the Diabetes Control and Complications Trial (DCCT) and the United Kingdom Prospective Diabetes Study (UKPDS) have suggested strict diabetes and glycemic control helps control diabetic retinopathy and possibly also helps retain good visual acuity. The current recommendation is to aim for fasting plasma glucose < 110 mg/dL (normal: 60–90 mg/dL) and HbA_{1C} < 7% (normal: 3 to 6%). Unacceptable glycemic control are fasting plasma glucose > 140 mg/dL and HbA_{1C} > 8%.

Hypertension control: In the WESDR diabetic subjects with elevated blood pressure (both systolic and diastolic) had two-fold increase in risk of developing or progressing to PDR. The Hypertension in Diabetes Study (HDS), an off shoot of the UKPDS done in subjects with type II diabetes, demonstrated that tight control of hypertension (BP < 150/85 mm Hg) had

a 37% reduction of risk of microvascular abnormalities. The current recommendation is to keep the blood pressure under 130/85 mm Hg.

Dyslipidemic control: In patients with poor glycemic control, the diabetic dislipidemia is characterized by the increased levels of total cholesterol, low-density lipoproteins (LDLs) and triglycerides and by decreased levels of high-density lipoproteins (HDLs). Control data from WESDR have shown that there was a significant trend for increasing severity of diabetic retinopathy and retinal hard exudate with increasing cholesterol in insulin-using persons. Data from the Early Treatment Diabetic Retinopathy Study (ETDRS) has shown that elevated total serum cholesterol and LDL is associated with a significant increase in presence of retinal lipid exudates and that treatment of hyperlipidemia is likely to stabilize the retinal status. But the current data is not convincing to suggest that the control could also improve the visual acuity.

Platelet Inhibitors: The platelet inhibitors, aspirin and dipyridamole have been evaluated either alone or in combination. The USA clinical trial, ETDRS and the European clinical trial, the Dipyridamole and Aspirin Microangiopathy of Diabetes (DAMAD) evaluated aspirin alone or in combination with dipyridamole. Both the studies did not demonstrate any clear benefit of aspirin and/or dipyridamole in diabetic retinopathy.

Laser Photocoagulation

Laser treatment is effective for both diabetic macular edema and proliferative diabetic retinopathy.

Macular edema: The ETDRS proved that laser treatment reduces moderate visual loss in patients with CSME. Patients with hard exudates in the fovea have poor prognosis, but are still considered for treatment when the exudates are associated with diabetic macular edema. Patients with marked capillary

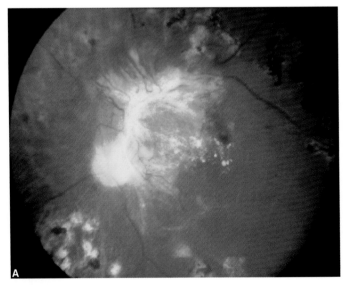
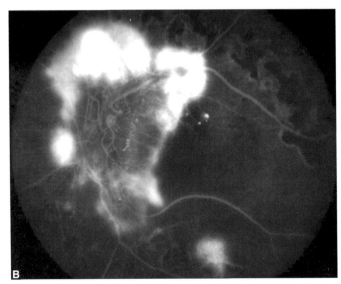

Figs 27.6A and B: Proliferative diabetic retinopathy. (A) Partially regressed proliferative diabetic retinopathy with NVD, but poor vision due to severe macular ischemia. Note white thread-like arterioles at posterior pole, (B) Corresponding fluorescein angiogram showing complete nonperfusion of macular area

nonperfusion involving macula are likely to have reduced visual acuity and are unlikely to respond to laser treatment.

The mechanism of action for laser treatment is uncertain. On fluorescein angiography, most of the leakage in eyes with focal diabetic macular edema appears to be caused by microaneurysms or the retinal vessels in the inner and middle retina. Focal burns appear to coagulate these microaneurysms; consequently the leaking microaneurysms stop leaking and may result in reduction in macular edema. In eyes with diffuse edema, fluorescein angiography demonstrates diffuse leakage from retinal vessels, suggesting that leakage from microaneurysms may not be the only cause of diabetic macular edema. Hence, direct coagulation of microaneurysms may not be the only mechanism of decreasing macular edema.

Proliferative diabetic retinopathy: The DRS showed that scatter laser treatment reduced visual loss by 50% or more in patients with PDR with high-risk characteristics (HRC). The ETDRS results suggest that, because 50% of patients with early PDR or very severe NPDR developed HRC during first year follow-up, clinicians may consider scatter laser treatment before the onset of high-risk PDR.

The mechanism of scatter laser treatment is considered to be the destruction of the larger portion of ischemic retina, thereby reducing retina's oxygen demand and allowing more oxygen from the choroid to diffuse into the retinal tissue by inducing retinal thinning.

Many factors influence the decision for photocoagulation. Although the results of DRS are well documented, clinical judgement must still be used when deciding whether to treat. Patients with iris and angle neovascularization should be considered for early scatter treatment.

Laser lenses: A variety of lenses are available for delivering laser photocoagulation. Some of the lenses provide upright view and others inverted. The field of view and magnification varies. Choice of appropriate lens and good knowledge of the lens optics are important for effective laser treatment. The plano concave contact lens is the most commonly used lens for the treatment of diabetic macular edema. Indirect lenses also can be used, as long as one does not forget that the retinal images are inverted similar to binocular indirect ophthalmoscope. Goldmann lenses have been used for many years for scatter treatment of retina. Several newer indirect lenses are currently available thus enlarging the choice (Table 27.3).

The magnification is in relation to Goldmann lens.

Spot magnification is the spot size in the retina versus laser spot size setting. For example, if the laser spot size is set at 100 μm, the spot size on retina will be 108 μm with Goldmann lens, 141 μm with Panfundoscope, 105 μm with Mainster Standard, 147 μm with Mainster Wide Field and 182 μm with Volk QuadAspheric lens.

Laser wavelengths: Argon green is the most commonly used wavelength for the treatment of diabetic macular edema. Krypton red, diode green and diode infrared lasers are also effective. In treatment of diabetic macular edema green or yellow wavelengths are more commonly used because they do not penetrate the choroid as much as the red or diode infrareds do. The red and diode infrared wavelengths penetrate vitreous hemorrhage and yellow lens nucleus better than the green wavelengths. Despite these theoretical advantages of the laser wavelengths and retinal tissue reactions, no study has clearly demonstrated significant advantage of one over the others. The choice therefore is directed more by the availability, media opacity and physician preference.

Laser Treatment Techniques

Focal/grid laser treatment is advocated in diabetic macular edema and panretinal photocoagulation (PRP) for proliferative diabetic retinopathy. The patient is seated comfortably at the laser slit lamp, patient is asked to fixate the eye with the fixation light and target, the desired laser lens is placed over the cornea after topical anesthesia and a coupling solution. The laser parameter is chosen for appropriate treatment. It is important to study the fluorescein angiogram before treatment, particularly in diabetic macular edema. The fluorescein viewer or digital enhancement of the fluorescein picture is important for precise treatment (Table 27.4).

Focal/grid laser treatment: Laser parameters are: spot size, 50 to 100 μm size and duration, 0.05 to 0.1 second. Focal treatment

Table 27.3: Contact lenses for retinal photocoagulation

Contact lens	Uses	Image	Relative magnification	Spot magnification	Field of view
Goldmann	Macula, equator, periphery	Virtual, erect	1.00	1.08	36°
Panfundoscope	Equator, periphery	Real, inverted	0.76	1.41	120°
Mainster Standard	Macula, equator	Real, inverted	1.03	1.05	90°
Mainster High Mag	Macula	Real, inverted	1.34	0.81	75°
Mainster Wide Field	Equator, periphery	Real, inverted	0.73	1.47	125°
Mainster Ultrawide	Equator	Real, inverted	0.57	1.89	140°
Volk Area Centralis	Macula, equator	Real, inverted	1.13	0.95	82°
Volk QuadrAspheric	Equator, periphery	Real, inverted	0.56	1.92	130°
Volk SuperQuad	Equator, periphery	Real	0.56	1.92	160°

Table 27.4: Recommended techniques for laser treatment

Argon/ Diode green	Spot size (µm)	Duration (sec)	Power (mW)	Intensity	Number	Placement
Diabetic Macular Edema						
Focal / Direct	50–100	0.05–0.1	50–100	whiten/darken microaneurysms	target all leaking microaneurysms	500–3,000 µm from center of macula
Focal / Grid	50–200	0.05–0.1	100–150	mild, light	cover areas of diffuse macular edema	spaced >1 burn apart 500–3,000 µm from macula
Proliferative Diabetic Retinopathy						
Scatter (PRP)	500	0.1	200–300	moderate	1,200–1,600	1/2 burn width apart > 2 DD from center of macula; 1/3 DD from disc

is advised for focal macular edema and grid laser treatment for diffuse macular edema.

Panretinal photocoagulation (PRP): The DRS treatment protocol consists of 1,200 burns, spaced at half burn width apart from posterior pole to the equator. Laser parameters are: spot size, 500 µm; time, 0.1–0.2 second and power, 200–300 mW. Treatment borders are 1 DD nasal to disc, just outside the temporal arcade and 4 DD temporal to fovea. Evenly placed scatter treatment in a uniform pattern through out the retina usually induces involution of the NVD and NVE. Larger areas of NVE with vitreous traction or retinal detachment are not usually treated directly; treatment is placed right up to, but not over these areas. Most clinicians apply scatter treatment in multiple sessions to reduce posttreatment pain and laser treatment complications, such as iritis, choroidal detachment, angle-closure glaucoma, worsened macular edema and serous retinal detachment. Repeat treatment is needed if the retinal or the disc new vessels do not regress in 12 weeks following PRP (Fig. 27.7). In several occasions, the number of laser spots could far exceed the recommendations of DRS.

Surgery

Vitrectomy: Vitrectomy for diabetic retinopathy is needed in substantial number of patients despite timely laser treatment in proliferative diabetic retinopathy. Historically, the first indication for vitrectomy was severe, non-clearing vitreous hemorrhage. As timely application of PRP has become widespread, the incidence of profound visual loss from dense vitreous hemorrhage has lessened. At the same time, with the development of refined instruments the indications of vitreous surgery in advanced diabetic have expanded. The new indications are persistent subhyaloid hemorrhage over macula, taut posterior hyaloid causing macular edema, recurrent vitreous hemorrhage and anterior hyaloid vitreous hemorrhage (Table 27.5).

Non-clearing vitreous hemorrhage: Several clinical features may influence the decision on the timing of vitrectomy. Earlier surgery is generally recommended when previous laser treatment has not been performed, when the fibrovascular complexes are

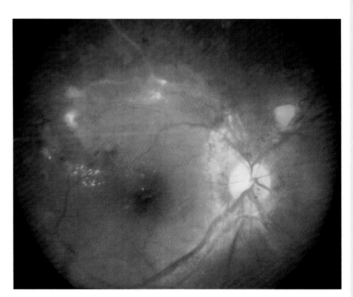

Fig. 27.7: Proliferative diabetic retinopathy. Residual new vessels after initial panretinal photocoagulation

Table 27.5: Indications for vitrectomy in severe complications of diabetic retinopathy

I. Media Opacities

    Non-clearing vitreous hemorrhage

    Subhyaloid premacular hemorrhage

II. Tractions

    Progressive fibrovascular proliferation

    Traction retinal detachment involving macula

    Combined traction-rhegmatogenous retinal detachment

    Macular edema associated with taut posterior hyaloid membrane

III. Other Indications

    Recurrent vitreous hemorrhage

    Anterior hyaloid fibrovascular proliferation

extensive, or when the fellow eye is blind. The surgical decision can be appropriately deferred when there is posterior vitreous detachment, when extensive prior PRP has been delivered and when other labile medical conditions coexist. Patients with elevated blood pressure or uncontrolled diabetes should receive appropriate medical attention before scheduling for surgery. Serial ultrasonography is important to evaluate the extent of vitreous hemorrhage, the state of posterior vitreous and to identify any retinal traction.

The surgery consists of a standard three-port vitrectomy. After the initial core vitrectomy, the posterior hyaloid is identified. A midperipheral rent is created in the posterior hyaloid with the vitreous cutter and extended circumferentially. Often unaltered red blood will be present in the subhyaloid space; this is aspirated by passive or active suction. The vitrectomy is completed with complete excision of posterior hyaloid, peripheral vitrectomy, endolaser application and internal tamponade with long-acting gas or silicone oil. Over past two decades, the results of vitrectomy for non-clearing vitreous hemorrhage have been reviewed extensively. The Diabetic Retinopathy Vitrectomy Study (DRVS) demonstrated that early vitrectomy (1–4 months after onset of severe vitreous hemorrhage) for type I diabetes yields visual acuity of 6/12 or better at 2 years in 36% of this subgroup, compared to only 12% with conventional management.

Vitreoretinal tractions: The elimination of traction involves removal of anteroposterior and tangential vitreoretinal traction, as well as removal of membrane-induced surface traction. The described techniques include segmentation, delamination and en bloc dissection of membrane.

In the segmentation technique, the traction is sequentially dissected by removal of the anterior posterior traction, vertical scissors-dissection of bridging epiretinal traction and finally removal of the residual traction including the epiretinal membrane.

In the delamination technique, the anteroposterior traction is commonly removed first using the segmentation technique. With the horizontal or vertical scissors, the preretinal tissue is removed at the retinal plane as one or more large pieces. The remaining fibrovascular stalk from the optic disc can be removed to complete the surgery.

In the en bloc technique, the surface traction is removed with the horizontal scissors using the anteroposterior traction for the counter traction on the epiretinal proliferation. The theoretical advantage of this technique is that the anteroposterior traction serves as a "third-hand function" by retracting the surface retinal tissue so that subsequent surface dissection is facilitated. The anteroposterior traction and vitreous are removed as the last step.

Despite the description of the three separate techniques, hybrid of all three techniques is usually used in most surgeries. Belt buckling is sometimes recommended to relieve peripheral retinal traction from unreachable or undissectable membranes. A host of multifunctional intraocular instruments have been developed to facilitate the surgical objectives. They include three-port vitrectomy, intravitreal instruments, illuminated instruments, multifunction instruments, endolaser system, wide-angle viewing system and finally longer tamponading agents, such as long-acting gas (sulfur hexafluoride/ perfluoropropane) and silicone oil. All these new and finer instruments have certainly improved the outcome of diabetic vitrectomy. In general the visual outcome is better in eyes with non-clearing vitreous hemorrhage uncomplicated with macular exudation and ischemia or diabetic optic neuropathy. The principal complications of vitrectomy in diabetic patients include recurrent vitreous hemorrhage, anterior hyaloid proliferation, retinal detachment and rubeosis iridis. Vitreous base surgery and endolaser photocoagulation and perioperative meticulous care help reduce some of the complications.

New Management Strategies

These strategies are directed to the use of novel diagnostic and therapeutic agents. They include the use of optical coherence tomography (OCT) (Fig. 27.8) in management of and monitoring to response to treatment in diabetic maculopathy; intravitreal triamcinolone and antivascular endothelial growth factors and intravitreal insert of fluocinolone acetonide in chronic macular edema and finally use of antiangiogenesis agents. The promising antiangiogenic molecules currently under trial are vascular endothelial growth factor (VEGF) and protein kinase C-β (PKC-β) inhibitor.

Enzymatic Manipulation of the Posterior Hyaloid in Diabetic Retinopathy

The occurrence of a posterior vitreous detachment (PVD) is a physiologic condition. Complete PVD has been associated with less neovascularization in diabetic retinopathy. A PVD may protect diabetic eyes from neovascularization. Experimental studies using hyaluronidase, collagenase, alpha- chymotrypsin and chondroitinase have confirmed the possibility of chemically modulating the vitreous structure and inducing PVD in rabbits. The vitreous in diabetic patients may have early aging changes that would facilitate its manipulation by enzymes or gas. In the vitreous of diabetic eyes, the gas bubble may remain in the vitreous body rather than in the space between the posterior hyaloid and the retina, as opposed to eyes with a rhegmatogenous retinal detachment (that already have a PVD). The induction of PVD may have a therapeutic value in NPDR. This therapy could avoid laser treatment or ameliorate it if needed.

With the discovery and use of insulin in 1922 there has been an excellent appreciation of the fundamental process underlying diabetes. The ocular complications are long since recognized. In last three decades, excellent scientific data accumulated with several prospective randomized studies have provided a standardized classification of retinopathy and the evidence-based treatment protocols. Current work to understand the genetic clues and the molecular basis of retinopathy

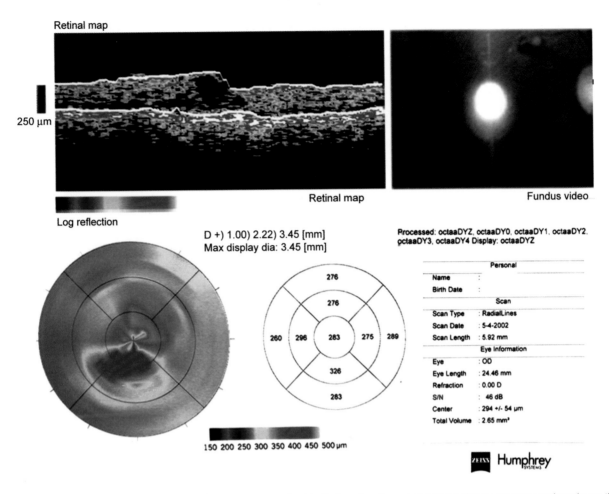

Fig. 27.8: Diabetic retinopathy. Optical coherence tomography: Vertical section through the fovea shows spongy macular edema; the retinal map shows the edema mostly confined inferior to the fovea (326 μ). The fovea is 283 μ (normal is ≤ 200 μ)

could provide further insights. These new information and intervention strategies, to our belief, hold greater promise for the care of diabetes in general and the retinopathy in particular. However, ophthalmoscopy will continue as the principal tool in the diagnosis of diabetic retinopathy. This is of value both in primary and secondary care where the fundus signs can be used to determine the urgency of review, referral and treatment.

HYPERTENSIVE RETINOPATHY

Systemic hypertension affects the retinal vessels (hypertensive retinopathy), choroid (hypertensive choroidopathy) and the optic nerve (hypertensive optic neuropathy). They have specific and occasionally unrelated manifestation. In this chapter we will mostly confine to hypertensive retinopathy and give a brief description of hypertensive choroidopathy and optic neuropathy. Essential hypertension is the commonest cause of systemic hypertension. Systemic hypertension is defined as a state of persistent elevated blood pressure above 140/90 mm Hg. Based on the blood pressure value this American classification (Table 27.6) categorizes into several grades of severity. Essential hypertension is the commonest cause of systemic hypertension.

Table 27.6: Fifth Joint Committee Classification of blood pressure

Category	Systolic BP (mm Hg)	Diastolic BP| (mm Hg)
Normal	< 130*	< 85
High Normal	130–139	85–89
Hypertension **		
Stage I (mild)	140–159	90–99
Stage II (moderate)	160–179	100–109
Stage III (severe)	180–209	110–119
Stage IV (very severe)	> 210	> 120

* Not taking any antihypertensive drugs and not actually ill
** Based on the average of two or more blood pressure readings taken at each of two or more visits following an initial screening.

Pathogenesis of Ocular Changes

Elevated systemic blood pressure causes both focal and generalized constriction of the retinal arterioles mediated by autoregulation and is commonly seen in long-standing benign hypertension. A prolonged duration of hypertension can lead to a breakdown of the inner blood-retinal barrier. Retinal hemorrhages, cotton-wool spots, intraretinal lipid and in severe cases macular star formation occurs (Fig. 27.9). In severe hypertension, closure of the retinal capillaries can be seen. With increased severity and duration of hypertension, the arterioles show progressive arteriosclerotic changes.

These changes are classified into the following five grades.

Grade 0 - Normal

Grade I - Increased light reflex, with mild arteriovenous crossing defects

Grade II - Copper wire appearance

Grade III- Silver wire appearance, with marked arteriovenous crossing defects

Grade IV- Fibrous cord.

Grading

The classification of hypertensive retinopathy is complex owing to the inter-relationship of the arteriosclerotic and hypertensive changes. The Scheie classification is a very practical one and a simplified modification by Hayreh and associates has several prognostic importance (Table 27.7).

Table 27.7: Classification of hypertensive retinopathy

Grade I	Generalized arteriolar attenuation
	Broadening of arteriolar light reflex
	Concealment of vein at arteriovenous crossing
Grade II	Severe generalized and focal arteriolar constriction
	Arteriovenous crossing changes (Salus' sign)
Grade III	Copper wiring of arterioles
	Venous tapering on either side of the crossing (Gunn's sign)
	Right-angled deflection of veins
	Flame-shaped hemorrhages, cotton-wool spots, hard exudates
Grade IV	All changes of Grade III, with silver wiring of arterioles
	Disc edema

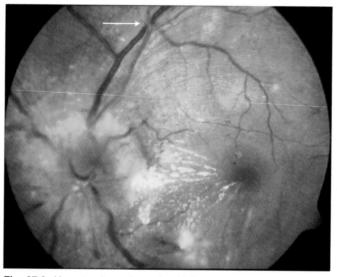

Fig. 27.9: Hypertensive retinopathy. Malignant hypertension with disc edema, macular star and arteriovenous nicking with copper wiring of arterioles (arrow)

Clinical Features

The hypertensive retinopathy can be divided into four phases:
- Vasoconstrictive phase
- Sclerotic phase
- Exudative phase
- Complications of the sclerotic phase

While each phase may have distinctive clinical feature, they often merge with each other and the changes may not be sequential. The vasoconstrictive and sclerotic phases are relatively asymptomatic. Complications of sclerotic phase and occasionally that of exudative phase cause loss of vision.

Vasoconstrictive phase manifests in focal and diffuse constriction of arteries. Clinically, the vasoconstriction occurs in the second and third order arteries and is most commonly seen in young patients.

Sclerotic phase sets in when the blood pressure remains elevated for a long period of time. The clinical features include narrowing of arteries, arteriovenous crossing changes, sclerosis of vessel wall (copper/silver wiring), vascular tortuosity and increased angle of branching of the arteries and arterioles. The arteriovenous crossing changes could vary from mild to severe form; many of them carry specific names of scientists who described them first (vide infra).

Exudative phase manifests as flame-shaped hemorrhage (early sign) and both cotton-wool spots (soft exudates) and hard waxy exudates. The retinal hemorrhages assume the flame-shaped appearance since the bleeding occurs in the nerve fiber layer. Cotton-wool spots are whitish gray or yellow patches in the retinal nerve fiber layer. The hard exudates represent extravasated plasma lipoproteins, phospholipids, cholesterol and triglycerides. The exudates could arrange in a specific fashion, such as in a star-shaped configuration radiating from the macular area along the nerve fiber layer, or in a circular fashion (circinate retinopathy) around one or a cluster of leaking microaneurysms.

Complications of the sclerotic phase include central or branch retinal vein occlusion. This could follow with macular edema, retinal neovascularization, vitreous hemorrhage, traction or combined traction-rhegmatogenous retinal detachment. When the blood pressure is controlled subsequently, vascular remodeling often occurs. Despite the anatomic remodeling, the visual functions in many occasions do not return because of earlier ischemic necrosis in the acute phase of the disease.

The central vision in hypertensive retinopathy is affected when the macula is involved (Fig. 27.9). The macula gets involved in vascular occlusions, macular hemorrhages and exudates, in macular ischemia, occurrence of macular epiretinal membrane and traction/rhegmatogenous retinal detachment that involves the macula.

Pathophysiology

A sharp rise in systemic blood pressure (vasoconstrictive phase) stimulates the vascular tone of the retinal muscular arteries by myogenic autoregulation. In the event of persistently elevated blood pressure, the vascular tone increases further and results in a reduction in the lumen of the precapillary arteriole. Disruption of blood retinal barrier leads to the exudative retinopathy phase. With damage to the vessel wall, reduction in blood flow occurs and ischemia develops. Cotton-wool spots are one of the signs of ischemia. Cotton-wool spots are an accumulation of axoplasmic components in the nerve fiber layer, consisting of mitochondria, lamellated dense bodies and axoplasmic ground substances in the proximal or distal ends of the axons in the ischemic area. Disturbance of both retrograde and orthograde axoplasmic transport occurs. With continued hypertension, hyaline degeneration of retinal vessels occurs, accompanied by the loss of muscle cells in the vessel wall. In the reparative phase vascular remodeling takes place when the nonperfused arteries become recanalized. However, the retinal functions do not return.

Management

Control of hypertension is essential for good visual function and the long-term survival of the patient. If and when the blood pressure is severely elevated, it should be lowered slowly and cautiously to avoid irreversible tissue damage and blindness. The general measures include weight control, sodium restriction and exercise.

HYPERTENSIVE CHOROIDOPATHY AND OPTIC NEUROPATHY

Hypertensive choroidopathy occurs in relatively young individuals with acute hypertension (malignant hypertension). The associated clinical conditions include eclampsia and pre-eclampsia, renal disease, pheochromocytoma and accelerated hypertension. In early phase of choroidopathy, the fundus develops outer retina pale white or reddish patches (Elschnig's spots) corresponding to areas of underlying choriocapillaries hypoperfusion. The late phase of choroidopathy develops focal posterior pole serous retinal detachment and macular star due to the accumulation of hard exudates in the Henle's nerve fiber layer.

Hypertensive optic neuropathy causes a variety of optic nerve and retinal changes. The three common manifestations include optic disc edema, optic atrophy and ischemic optic neuropathy.

Detailed description of these conditions are beyond the scope of this book and the readers are advised to refer to other textbooks. Systemic vascular accidents (stroke/myocardial infarction) may occur if they miss the dose of anti-hypertensive drugs. Hence, the need for strictly following the medications is prescribed.

ARTERIAL OCCLUSIONS

Retinal vascular occlusion occurs from a compromise of the retinal perfusion and could occur anywhere from the internal carotid artery up to the small retinal arterioles. The manifestation of such an occlusion could be as benign as the cotton-wool spots or as grave as the central artery occlusion (Table 27.8).

Table 27.8: Clinical manifestation of artery occlusion

a. Cotton-wool spots
b. Branch retinal artery occlusion (BRAO)
c. Central retinal artery obstruction (CRAO)
d. Ophthalmic artery occlusion
e. Cilioretinal artery obstruction
f. Combined central retinal artery and vein obstruction
g. Ocular ischemic syndrome

Cotton-Wool Spots

Cotton-wool spots (soft exudates) are transient, small yellow-white lesions with feathery edges in the superficial retina. They occur either singly or in multiple numbers and are most commonly located around the optic disc and posterior retina (Fig. 27.10). They are usually asymptomatic. Fluorescein angiography shows hypofluorescence, secondary to both arteriolar hypoperfusion and blocked fluorescence by this cellular debris. Clinical resolution occurs over a period of weeks to several months. Cotton-wool spots represent microinfarctions of small retinal arterioles and are a marker for an underlying systemic vascular disease. The common associated systemic vascular diseases are diabetes mellitus, hypertension and collagen vascular disorders. The other associations are hematological (leukemia and anemia), gastrointestinal (pancreatitis) and AIDS-associated retinopathy.

Branch Retinal Artery Obstruction

The branch retinal artery occlusion (BRAO) accounts for 38% of all cases of retinal arterial obstructions, and in three-fourth of the patients it is due to carotid occlusive disease or systemic hypertension. Branch retinal artery occlusion usually

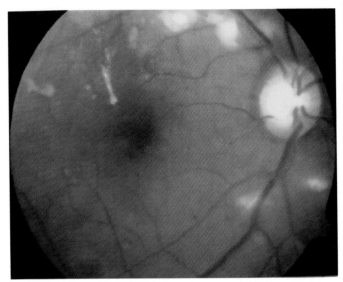

Fig. 27.10: Cotton-wool spots. Transient, small yellow-white lesions with feathery edges in the superficial retina

occurs in patients beyond fifth decade of life. Less frequently, younger patients (less than 30 years) are affected and underlying conditions include cardiac diseases, vasculopathies, thrombosis, vasculitis and vasospasm (migraine). The emboli causing occlusion of the branch retinal are usually of cardiac origin with or without cholesterol emboli (Hollenhorst's plaques) (Fig. 27.11).

Clinical Features

Branch retinal artery occlusion presents with a sudden unilateral, painless partial loss of vision with a corresponding visual field defect. Ophthalmoscopically, it is seen as a zone of segmental retinal whitening. In the acute phase, fluorescein angiography shows hypofluorescence due to delayed or non-filling of the involved arteriole. Following resolution, the involved artery remains narrow or sclerotic despite restoration of the blood flow. The normal retinal transparency returns after several weeks. The visual acuity could restore partially mainly due to the formation of artery-artery collaterals though some degree of permanent visual loss persists in nearly all cases. Other rare sequelae are optic atrophy and rubeosis iridis, often seen in patients with diabetes mellitus.

Treatment

No therapeutic intervention is warranted, because the majority of patients regain some vision and have a similar outcome irrespective of whether treated or not. However, in cases where most of the perifoveolar capillaries are involved, treatment similar to that for the central retinal artery occlusion (CRAO) (vide infra) may be attempted.

Central Retinal Artery Occlusion

Central retinal artery occlusion (CRAO) is one of the true ophthalmic emergencies. It accounts for about 57% of all retinal arterial obstructions.

Clinical Features

The mean age of presentation is in the early sixties, though occasionally the disorder may be seen in young adults. Men are more commonly affected and sometimes (1 to 2%) both eyes are involved. Patient presents with a sudden, profound, unilateral and painless loss of vision. The vision is invariably reduced to counting fingers, or to only perception of light. There may not be a previous history of amaurosis fugax.

The earliest sign of CRAO seen within a few seconds is a relative afferent pupillary defect (RAPD). Ophthalmoscopically visible thread-like narrow arterioles, with segmentation appear within next few minutes and over the next few hours, there is an opacification of the ischemic retinal tissue due to the intracellular edema, cellular necrosis and accumulation of cellular debris outside the fovea. The retinal pigment epithelium and choroidal circulation, behind the thin foveola, shines through to present the characteristic cherry-red spot (Fig. 27.12), which is nearly pathognomonic of the CRAO. In 20% of eyes with CRAO, emboli can be seen. The mortality rate in patients with retinal emboli is 56% over 9 years vs 27% in age-matched controls. Retinal opacification usually fades with the restoration of circulation. The diffuse arteriolar narrowing and RAPD persist and consecutive optic atrophy with associated macular pigmentary changes ensues. Secondary complications like rubeosis iridis and disc neovascularization are reported to occur in the one-fifth of patients. Many times the patients with ocular neovascularization also have concomitant ipsilateral carotid artery obstruction. In quarter cases the cilioretinal artery is spared and if the fovea also is spared useful vision is likely to return.

Ancilliary Tests

Ancilliary tests to confirm diagnosis in atypical cases include fundus fluorescein angiography (FFA), electroretinography

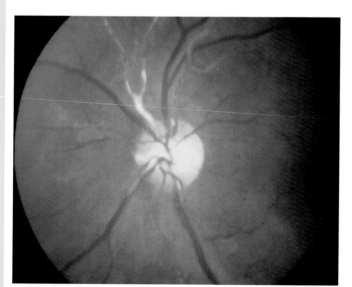

Fig. 27.11: Retinal artery occlusion. Hollenhorst's plaques in retinal vessels

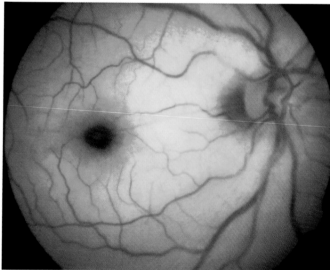

Fig. 27.12: Central retinal artery occlusion. Complete posterior pole opacification and cherry-red spot in central retinal artery occlusion (VA:CF)

Table 27.9: Work-up in central retinal artery obstruction

History

Physical examination especially blood pressure and carotid bruit

Laboratory investigations

Hematological:	Hemoglobin (Hb), total and differential leukocyte count, Peripheral blood smear, Blood sugar (fasting and post prandial), Platelet count, Erythrocyte sedimentation rate (ESR), Lipid profile, Hb electrophoresis, C_3 total complement, Partial thromboplastin time, Prothrombin time, Bleeding and clotting times.
Immunological:	FTA-Abs , ANA, LE cell, anti-cardiolipin antibodies, Homocysteine levels, Rheumatoid factor.
Cardiac:	ECG, Echocardiogram, including transesophageal and transthoracic if needed, Chest X-ray
Carotid artery:	Transcranial Doppler and if needed, Magnetic resonance angiography.

(ERG) and visual field testing. The commonest anomaly in FFA is delayed arteriovenous transit time with normal choroidal filling. On ERG there is a decrease in the *b* wave due to ischemia affecting the inner retinal layers. The *a* wave (corresponding to the photoreceptor function) is normal. Visual field evaluation shows often retention of the temporal island of vision. In cases of patent cilioretinal artery, small areas of the central field may also be spared. The work-up in cases of CRAO is listed in Table 27.9.

Systemic Association

Embolus is the commonest cause of CRAO. Other causes include intraluminal thrombosis, hemorrhage under atherosclerotic plaque, vasculitis, spasm and circulatory collapse. Systemic associations include hypertension in 60%, diabetes mellitus in 25%, cardiac valvular disease in 25% and carotid atherosclerosis (ipsilateral stenosis or plaque) in 45% of cases.

Management

The crucial factor for successful treatment is the time. Although irreversible cell injury is known to occur by 90 minutes after a total central retinal artery occlusion, most authorities recommend attempting treatment even up to the first 24 hours following acute visual loss. Currently, all the treatment modalities aim to increase the perfusion, by lowering the intraocular pressure in the hope that the perfusion pressure behind the obstruction would push on an obstructing embolus. Treatment modalities include anterior chamber paracentesis, ocular massage, intravenous acetazolamide, inhalation of carbogen (a mixture of 95% O_2 and 5% CO_2), fibrinolytic agents injection through the supraorbital artery and corticosteroid therapy.

Ocular massage followed by paracentesis is the most commonly employed immediate intervention. Ocular massage consists of applying pressure over the closed eyelids for 10 to 15 seconds, followed by sudden release of pressure and is continued for 15 minutes or till the artery is dilated. The arterial dilatation is likely to increase the perfusion. While the ocular massage can be done digitally, applying pressure with a Goldmann contact lens is more convenient; the patient need not be shifted from the slit lamp for the optic disc and retinal examination.

Paracentesis is done under topical anesthesia, under strict aseptic conditions.

Corticosteroid therapy is indicated in bilateral cases and in elderly patients. Corticosteroid use is mandatory in giant cell arteritis to avoid involvement of the second eye.

Ophthalmic Artery Obstruction

The clinical picture of ophthalmic artery obstruction (OAO) is so much similar to CRAO, that 5% of patients initially labeled CRAO, actually had OAO. Eyes with OAO have extensive superficial retinal whitening, suffer severe visual loss (often no light perception), the IOP is usually lower by 4 mm Hg than the contra lateral normal eye and finally the ERG demonstrates both inner and outer retinal ischemia, yet without ocular neovascularization (Table 27.10). The systemic associations and work-up is similar to CRAO. Markedly delayed choroidal filling in the presence of a cherry-red spot and an abnormal *a* wave signifies an ophthalmic artery occlusion.

Cilioretinal Artery Obstruction

An obstruction in the cilioretinal artery, arising from the short posterior ciliary artery, presents as a localized area of retinal whitening temporal to the disc, in the papillomacular bundle area. The extent of involvement varies with extent of area of supply by the cilioretinal artery. Brown and associates have described three varieties of such occlusion: (1) isolated in 40%, (2) associated with CRVO in 40% (Fig. 27.13) and (3) along with anterior ischemic optic neuropathy (AION) in 20% cases. No treatment is needed. Causes and systemic work-up is also similar to CRAO. In eyes with AION, giant cell arteritis should be ruled out.

Table 27.10: Differentiation of central retinal artery occlusion (CRAO) and ophthalmic artery obstruction (OAO)

	Sign	CRAO	OAO
1.	Visual acuity	CF to HM	NLP
2.	Fundus, acute phase		
	Cherry-red spot	Present	Absent to present
	Retinal opacification	Mild to moderate	Moderate to severe
3.	Fundus, late phase		
	Pigment disturbances	Absent	Present
	Optic Atrophy	Mild to moderate	Severe
4.	FFA	Compromised retinal blood flow	Compromised retinal and choroidal blood flow
5.	ERG	Reduced *b* wave	Reduced *a* and *b* waves

CF-Counting finger close to face; ERG-Electroretinogram; FFA-Fundus fluorescein angiography; HM-Hand motions close to face; NLP-No light perception

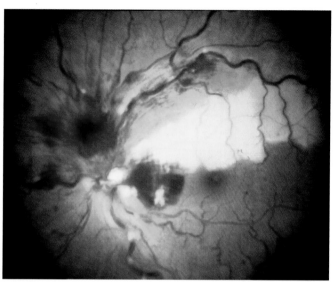

Fig. 27.13: Central retinal artery occlusion. Cilioretinal artery occlusion combined with nonischemic central retinal vein occlusion and macular sparing. VA 20/30 with inferior sectoral field loss. Note localized retinal opacification

Ocular Ischemic Syndrome

The ocular changes associated with severe carotid artery disorder manifest as ocular ischemic syndrome (OIS). The commonest symptom is a gradual loss of vision, often with dull pain. Rarely visual loss is sudden and can be associated with amaurosis fugax. Visual acuity could vary widely, from normal to no light perception. Signs include few cells and flare or keratic precipitates in the anterior chamber, cataract, variable IOP (from hypotony to severe glaucoma), rubeosis, retinal arterial narrowing, scattered retinal hemorrhages, microaneurysms and retinal or optic disc neovascularization, often with pale disc (Fig. 27.14A) and retinal pigment epithelium atrophy. Fundus fluorescein angiography and ERG can demonstrate retinal ischemia and poor perfusion similar to seen in the

CRAO, besides areas of new vessels. Carotid artery evaluation is essential to confirm diagnosis and plan the management. Treatment (medical/surgical) is as per the assessment of the neurophysician and neurosurgeon. Eyes with rubeosis and/ or glaucoma need extensive panretinal photocoagulation and medial/surgical therapy to control the intraocular pressure (Fig. 27.14B).

VENOUS OCCLUSIVE DISEASES OF RETINA

Retinal vein occlusion is the second common vascular retinopathy, after diabetic retinopathy. Depending on the site of involvement, the vein occlusion could be central, branch or hemicentral type. Each one again could be ischemic or nonischemic variety.

Central Retinal Vein Occlusion

Central retinal vein occlusion (CRVO) usually occurs in elderly individuals and males are more commonly affected. In the evaluation and management of CRVO, the most critical factor is to differentiate ischemic from the nonischemic variety. There is a significantly higher proportion of the ischemic type in the elderly patients (67% vs 44%) and nonischemic variety in younger patients (18% vs 7%).

Pathogenesis

Pathogenesis of CRVO is multifactorial–local, systemic and hematologic.

Local risk factors include the following: (1) occlusion of the vein by external compression by the sclerotic adjacent structures, such as the central retinal artery and the fibrous tissue envelope; (2) occlusion by primary venous wall disease (degenerative or inflammatory in nature); and (3) hemodynamic disturbances (produced by subendothelial atheromatous lesions in the central retinal artery, arterial spasm, sudden decrease in blood

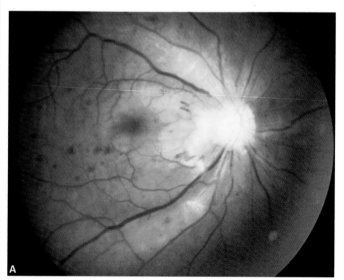

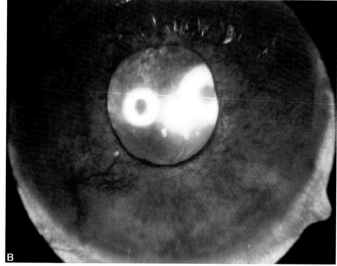

Figs 27.14A and B: Ocular ischemic syndrome. (A) Fundus photo showing minimal retinopathy with few hemorrhages and gliosis on disc, (B) Extensive rubeosis iridis, ectropion uveae and early cataract in same eye suggestive of ocular ischemic syndrome

pressure, blood dyscrasias, etc.). Central retinal vein occlusion is significantly more common in patients with raised intraocular pressure and glaucoma. This is due to increased resistance to blood flow in eyes with raised intraocular pressure.

Systemic risk factors include arterial hypertension, diabetes and cardiovascular disease in ischemic CRVO and arterial hypertension and increased fibrinogen levels in nonischemic CRVO.

Regarding hematologic risk factors, there are anecdotal case reports of CRVO due to alteration in the coagulation cascade following abnormalities in the anticoagulation factors. The systemic blood pressure is shown to fall significantly during sleep and is likely to convert a partial central retinal vein thrombus to a complete occlusion during sleep, due to sluggish circulation.

In 7 to 12% of the eyes, nonischemic CRVO gets converted to the ischemic type either due to nocturnal hypotension or due to a gradual extension of the thrombotic process in the central retinal vein towards the lamina cribrosa.

Clinical Features

The commonest presenting complaint is a sudden decrease in central vision, usually on awakening. Ophthalmoscopically, there is extensive superficial flame-shaped retinal hemorrhages, involving all four quadrants of the retina, or few limited superficial hemorrhages confined to the retinal periphery associated with a variable degree of disc edema (Fig. 27.15A). The management strategy in CRVO lies in the differentiation of ischemic and nonischemic variety. In our opinion the time spent in understanding these differences is very rewarding. Several factors help (Table 27.11).

Fluorescein angiography is useful only after 4–6 weeks when some of the retinal hemorrhages are cleared (Fig. 27.15B). A recent multicentric study has shown that a capillary nonperfusion area of 7.5 DD areas could lead to retinal neovascularization. Ocular neovascularization does not occur

Table 27.11: Differentiating feature between ischemic and nonischemic central retinal vein occlusion (CRVO)

Symptom/Sign	Ischemic CRVO	Nonischemic CRVO
Visual acuity	< 6/60	> 6/60 The visual acuity could be low due to macular edema and hemorrhages (hges)
Visual field defect (Goldmann)	All eyes	54–78% eyes
RAPD	Affected	Affected
ERG b wave	Reduced ≤ 60%	
Implicit time	Increased	Increased
Ophthalmoscopy	Extensive sup retinal hemorrhages	Less extensive retinal hemorrhages
Fluorescein angiography	Retinal ischemia > 10 DD	Ischemia absent / minimal
Ocular neovascularization	Usually present/ develop	Never present

in the one-third of ischemic CRVO and if it occurs one should strongly suspect associated diabetic retinopathy, carotid artery disease and other conditions that might cause retinal ischemia.

Natural Course and Complications

The CRVO could be self-limiting, but the resolution occurs over a period of weeks to years. Some eyes develop one of the complications, alone or in combination—macular edema, ocular neovascularization and vitreous hemorrhage.

Macular edema in CRVO is typically due to leakage from perifoveal capillaries, secondary to hydrostatic stress and ischemia. It has the clinical and angiographic picture of cystoid macular edema (CME).

Ocular neovascularization common sites are iris and the angle of anterior chamber. Curiously, the retina is less often involved. The greatest risk is seen in the first 7 months of the

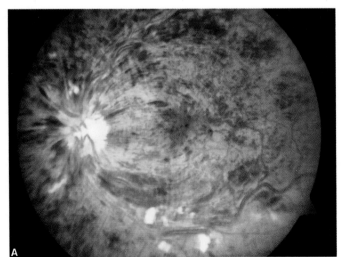

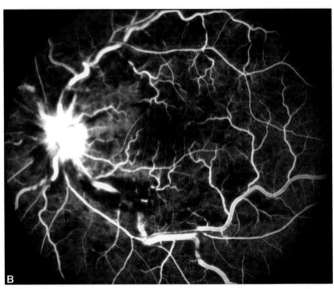

Figs 27.15A and B: Central retinal vein occlusion. (A) Classical retinal features of central retinal vein occlusion. (B) Corresponding fluorescein angiogram showing well perfused retina, suggestive of nonischemic central retinal vein occlusion. Note arterial narrowing and significant arteriovenous crossing changes along upper temporal and inferotemporal veins, increasing possibility of conversion to ischemic type

disease. The overall incidence of rubeosis iridis in all cases of CRVO is 20% and is higher (45 to 80%) in the ischemic CRVO eyes. One-third of eyes with iris neovascularization (NVI) and one-fourth of eyes with both iris and angle neovascularization never develop neovascular glaucoma. Unfortunately, none of the currently used tests can reliably predict neovascularization in ischemic CRVO. Some patients may present with severe pain and neovascular glaucoma (NVG), with a history of visual loss of 3 to 4 months duration. This condition is called 100-day glaucoma.

Vitreous hemorrhage occurs in late stages of ischemic CRVO, secondary to NVE or NVD.

Management

Management of CRVO includes a detailed history and systemic work-up. Hematological work-up is more important for patients with bilateral or recurrent venous occlusions and in younger patients (Table 27.12).

Table 27.12: Systemic work-up in central retinal vein occlusion

All patients

Hypertension

Diabetes

Cardiovascular risk factors: Cardiac evaluation, ERG, Lipid profile, Echocardiography

Younger patients (< 50 years)

History (oral contraceptive use in women, repeated episodes of bleeding)

Hematology: Hematocrit, ESR, Plasma viscosity, Lipid profile

(Including Lipoproteins, Protein C &S and Antithrombin III levels, presence of Lupus anticoagulant, antiphospholipid antibody).

Medical Therapy

Due to the self-limiting nature of nonischemic CRVO, it is difficult to assess the beneficial effect of any treatment modality in this disease. Anticoagulants, antiplatelet agents, systemic acetozolamide, fibrinolytic and thrombolytic agents have no proven efficacy. Topical antiglaucoma medications are indicated only when the intraocular pressure is raised.

Systemic Corticosteroids

These could be tried in tapering doses of 1 to 1.5 mg/kg body weight, in patients with nonischemic CRVO with visual loss due to unresolving macular edema. They are, however, not effective in every patient. Improvement if any is usually seen within two weeks. The corticosteroids could be beneficial in young patients where CRVO may be due to periphlebitis.

Laser Photocoagulation

Panretinal photocoagulation (PRP) does not have any role in nonischemic CRVO. It has traditionally been considered the treatment of choice for ischemic CRVO. But a ten-year prospective study of argon laser PRP in ischemic CRVO did not find statistically significant difference between lasered and non-lasered eyes in the incidence of development of neovascular complications of CRVO. The incidence of NVI was less in the lasered eyes provided the PRP was done within 90 days of onset of CRVO. It has been suggested that investigation and treatment of the associated systemic conditions are as important and should always precede PRP.

Grid laser as a treatment modality for unresolving macular edema was evaluated in a multicentric clinical trial. There was no difference between the treated and untreated eyes.

Laser-induced chorioretinal venous anastomosis was proposed by McAllister is believed to act by rerouting the blood from retinal to choroidal veins. The technique consists of applying multiple overlapping blue-green argon laser of 1.5 W power, 0.1 second duration and 50 μm spot size, over the vein in the lower part of the fundus at least 3 DD from the optic disc. The laser is applied till a deep white burn is obtained (Figs 27.16A and B). The reported complications include vitreous hemorrhage, subretinal hemorrhage, preretinal and subretinal fibrosis and potential for choroidal, intraretinal and intravitreal neovascularization. Successful anastomosis can often be elusive. In our unpublished series, functional chorioretinal anastomosis was obtained in 60% (18 of 24) eyes and choroidovitreal neovascularization was seen in 12% (3 of 24) eyes.

Surgery

Surgical chorioretinal anastomosis, intravitreal tissue plasminogen activator (tPA), intraretinal vein injection of tPA, optic nerve sheath decompression, and optic nerve hemineurotomy have been described for nonischemic CRVO with a variable success. Currently all the surgeries lack popularity in the absence of large randomized trials.

Branch Retinal Vein Occlusion

Branch retinal vein occlusion (BRVO) is an occlusive retinopathy involving a portion of the retina that is drained by the occluded vein. BRVO is more commonly seen in the fifth and sixth decades of life. Patients usually present with painless, reduction of vision and field defect. In 10% of cases, BRVO develops in the fellow eye. Reported associations include, hypertension, diabetes and open-angle glaucoma. In our study hyperopia was seen in 70.7% eyes; the odds ratio of developing BRVO amongst patients with hyperopia was 3.42 as compared to emmetropes and 5.3 as compared to myopes. In 50 to 64% of the eyes with BRVO, the visual acuity remains at 20/40, in 25% of the eyes it is between 20/15–20/100 and in the remaining the vision is ≤20/200.

Clinical Features

A classic acute BRVO occurs at an arteriovenous (AV) crossing, with the apex sof the involved segment at the crossing that usually shows some AV nicking (Fig. 27.17A). It is associated

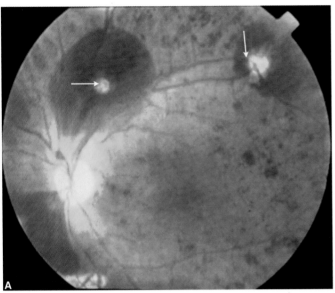

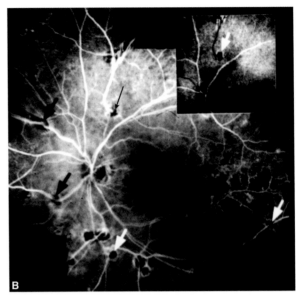

Figs 27.16A and B: Central retinal vein occlusion. (A) Fundus picture and (B) corresponding fluorescein angiogram showing resolved central retinal vein occlusion after successful (white arrows) chorioretinal anastomosis. Black arrows show site of failed chorioretinal anastomosis

with dilated and tortuous veins, superficial retinal hemorrhages and retinal edema and cotton-wool spots. Depending on the site of occlusion, the BRVO could be of the (a) major type (the occlusion at the optic disc or farther away), (b) macular branch occlusion, or (c) small tributary occlusion. In chronic cases, the typical distribution of microvascular abnormalities and intraretinal collaterals draining across the median raphe with sclerosis and sheathing of the retinal veins and arteries in the distribution of the occlusion are found. Fundus Fluorescein Angiography is useful in assessing the presence and degree of macular edema and retinal ischemia (Fig. 27.17B). It is best done after couple of months, when the hemorrhages are relatively cleared.

Complications

Macular changes are the commonest complication and cause of decreased vision in BRVO. Persistent CME is seen in 48% of cases of BRVO, with one-third showing spontaneous recovery of some vision. Macular nonperfusion results in a poor, usually non-improving, visual acuity. Intact perifoveal nets are reportedly better predictor of better vision. Other macular changes seen occasionally include epimacular membrane, macular hole and pigment clumping.

Retinal neovascularization is the most serious complication in BRVO. It is seen when there are more than 5 DD of capillary nonperfusion areas. It usually occurs in the first 6–12 months of occlusion.

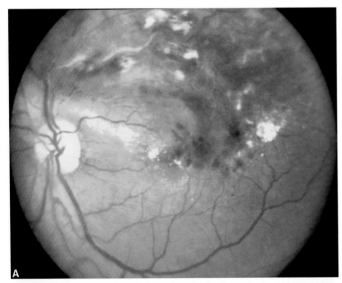

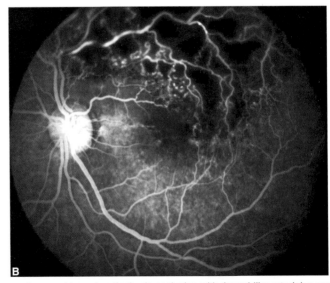

Figs 27.17A and B: Ischemic branch retinal vein occlusion. (A) Resolving upper temporal branch retinal vein occlusion with thread-like arterioles and macular exudates, (B) Corresponding fluorescein angiogram shows areas of capillary non-perfusion, few collaterals and distorted foveal avascular zone suggestive of ischemic branch retinal vein occlusion. Follow-up is required for any new vessels formation

Vitreous hemorrhage occurs in about 60% of the eyes with untreated new vessels. Traction retinal detachment occurs secondary to vitreous hemorrhage and fibrous proliferation and traction tears lead to combined retinal detachment.

Management

A detailed history, evaluation of systemic factors like blood pressure and ocular factors like the intraocular pressure, are necessary in every patient.

Laser Photocoagulation

Guidelines have been established as per the Collaborative Branch Vein Occlusion Study. Macular edema responds well to grid photocoagulation. The eligibility criteria include the BRVO of recent origin and fluorescein angiographic evidence of foveal edema and absence of macular ischemia. The laser parameters include application of medium intensity burns of 100 μm spot size. If the foveal area is not clearly visualized, then one should treat initially well away from the foveal area and re-treat the area after two months. In nonresponders also, repeat treatment is advised after 2–4 months. 63% of the treated eyes in the Collaborative BVO study gained ≥2 lines of visual acuity, as compared with 36% of the untreated or control patients. In patients with BRVO and evident neovascularization, peripheral scatter photocoagulation should be done with 200 to 500 μm spot size, 0.1 to 0.2 sec duration burns, one burn width apart, avoiding the collaterals and not closer than 2 DD from the foveola. The scatter laser application should be confined to the quadrant of BRVO.

Surgery

The surgical intervention in BRVO includes arteriovenous sheathotomy and vitrectomy.

Arteriovenous sheathotomy: This surgery aims at separating the artery and the vein from the common sheath at the site of occlusion. A randomized clinical trial is underway to assess the efficacy of this technique.

Vitrectomy: It is also been demonstrated that BRVO patients who received pars plana vitrectomy and a surgical posterior vitreous detachment had a significantly lower rate of macular edema and neovascularization. Surgery is also indicated in cases of non-clearing vitreous hemorrhage, traction retinal detachment and combined traction-rhegmatogenous retinal detachment.

Hemicentral Retinal Vein Occlusion

In 20.5% of the eyes, a dual trunked central retinal vein that usually disappears at birth persists as a congenital anomaly. When the pathologic events that typically cause a CRVO, affect only one of these veins, a picture of hemicentral retinal vein occlusion (HCRVO) results. In HCRVO the superior or the inferior part of the fundus is affected. HCRVO is a variation of CRVO. It is of two types: nonischemic (2/3 of the cases) and ischemic (1/3 of the cases). The risk factors for the development of HCRVO are similar to that of CRVO, but different from that of BRVO.

Clinical Features

One-half to two-third of the fundus is involved by the retinopathy. The ophthalmoscopic picture consists of superficial hemorrhages and cotton-wool spots (Fig. 27.18). There is nearly no risk of neovascularization in cases of nonischemic HCRVO. The sequelae and complications in ischemic HCRVO are similar to ischemic CRVO.

Management

The utility of photocoagulation has not been studied in HCRVO. But since the rate of neovascular complications are high in ischemic HCRVO, prophylactic scatter laser photocoagulation to the affected hemisphere is recommended. Macular edema, if associated, could also be treated with grid photocoagulation, using the guidelines of the Colloborative Branch Vein Occlusion Study.

EALES' DISEASE

Eales' disease is an idiopathic obliterative vasculopathy, primarily affecting the peripheral retina. It is characterized by perivascular inflammation, peripheral nonperfusion and neovascularization. Visual loss is usually due to unilateral or bilateral recurrent vitreous hemorrhage and its sequelae. The four stages of Eales' disease are: Periphlebitis of small retinal capillaries (Stage I), widespread perivasculitis of the venous capillary system affecting the larger veins (Stage II), retinal new vessel formation and vitreous hemorrhage (Stage III) and finally retinitis proliferans and tractional retinal detachment (Stage IV). Though initially described from England, Eales' disease is commonly seen in the Southeast Asian subcontinent. It affects 1 in 200–250 ophthalmic patients in India and the peak age of onset is 20–30 years. Males are more affected than females.

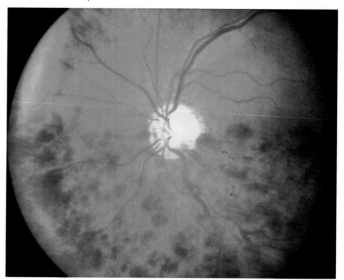

Fig. 27.18: Inferior hemicentral retinal vein occlusion. The inferior part of the fundus is affected

Clinical Features

The initial visual symptom could be floaters, due to mild vitreous hemorrhage. Retinal vasculitis and secondary vitritis leads to reduced vision. Usually the patients complain of involvement of one eye only, but careful examination of the fellow eye could show peripheral retinal vasculitis. The condition is bilateral in 50 to 90% of the patients.

The fundus examination in the early stages shows varying amounts of inflammatory venous dilatation in the periphery, with accompanying tortuosity and perivascular exudates (Fig. 27.19). Vascular sheathing can range from thin white lines, limiting the blood column on either side, to heavy exudative sheathing, often with superficial retinal hemorrhages. The peripheral arteries subsequently get attenuated. Recurrent vitreous hemorrhage is the hallmark of Eales' disease. It is due to retinal neovascularization and/or retinal vasculitis. The degree of vitreous hemorrhage depends on the degree and nature of vascular occlusion. In the active stage, fluorescein angiography demonstrates extravasation of the dye from the inflamed vessels (seen clinically as sheathing) and in the later stages, the vessels are only stained without dye leakage. Areas of capillary nonperfusion and retinal new vessels are delineated by angiography.

Natural course in Eales' disease is quite variable. There is temporary or even permanent remission in some patients and relentless progression with the episodes of recurrent vitreous hemorrhage in others.

Etiopathogenesis

The etiopathogenesis of Eales' disease has remained ill understood, till date. Retinal vasculitis and peripheral retinal

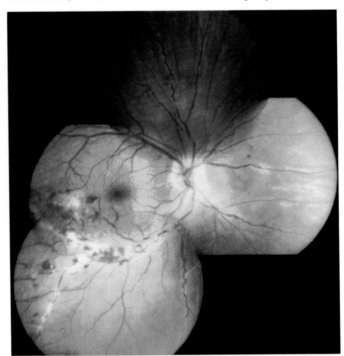

Fig. 27.19: Eales' disease. Inflammatory stage of Eales' disease showed peripheral retinal periphlebitis with macular sparing

Table 27.13: Disorders with peripheral retinal neovascularization in young adults

Systemic	Ocular
Diabetes mellitus	Eales' disease
Sickle cell disease	Branch retinal vein occlusion
Sarcoidosis	Central retinal vein occlusion
Behcet's disease	Pars planitis
Leukemia	Familial exudative vitreoretinopathy

Table 27.14: Disorders with retinal vasculitis as a common finding in young adults*

Systemic	Infectious	Ocular
Behçet's disease	Tuberculosis	Eales' disease
Sarcoidosis	Syphilis	Pars planitis
Systemic lupus erythematosus	Toxoplasmosis	Birdshot retinopathy
Multiple sclerosis		
Wegener's granulomatosis		

*Modified from Das and Namperumalsamy

neovascularization in young adults could also occur in various other systemic and ocular diseases (Tables 27.13 and 27.14). Hence, it is mandatory to investigate and rule out all other causes of retinal vasculitis and retinal neovascularization. Of many systemic associations, tuberculosis and allergy to tuberculoprotein have been strongly emphasized in India.

The assumption of tubercular etiology is based on the observations of active or healed tuberculosis in some patients of Eales' disease. This is universally accepted or proved. Recently association of tuberculosis in Eales' disease is reemphasized following PCR studies of the epiretinal and subretinal membranes. The credence to hypersensitivity to tuberculoprotein comes from the observation of a positive Mantoux reaction in patients with Eales' disease. It is hypothesized that the retina of patients with Eales' disease could be selectively sensitized against tuberculoprotein. Reexposure to this antigen could result in allergic retinal vasculitis. However, Eales' disease has also been reported in Mantoux-negative patients. The hypothesis further fails to convince since the incidence of Mantoux-positivity in healthy adults in India is very high. Eales' disease is an immunologic reaction that may be triggered by an exogenous exposure. Retinal S-antigen and interphotoreceptor retinoid binding protein (IRBP) play an important role in the etiopathogenesis of this condition.

Report of significantly higher frequencies of HLA B5 (B51), DR1 and DR4 in Eales' disease patients could not be confirmed by another study. Light microscopic and immunohistochemical studies have demonstrated predominant T-cell involvement in the epiretinal and subretinal membranes of patients with Eales' disease. This probably indicates that cell-mediated immune mechanisms might be playing a role in the proliferative phase of the disease. Hence, treatment could be directed to the down-regulation of the activated T-cells. A distinct protein band (at isoelectric point 5.9; molecular weight 23 kD) has been found in the serum of Eales' patients; but the clinical implication of this is not established.

Management

Treatment of Eales' disease is mainly symptomatic. This is aimed at (a) reducing retinal perivasculitis and vitritis (corticosteroids and antituberculosis drugs); (b) at reducing the risks of vitreous hemorrhage from new vessels (photocoagulation and cryotherapy) and surgical removal of nonresolving vitreous hemorrhage and/or traction membranes (vitrectomy).

Oral corticosteroids form the mainstay of treatment for cases with active perivasculitis. High doses of oral prednisolone (2 mg/kg body weight) are given initially and then gradually tapered as the vasculitis begins to subside. Periocular depot preparations can be given in florid cases.

Vasculitis has been found to be a good target for immunotherapy. Saxena and associates have highlighted the efficacy of oral methotrexate pulsed therapy in Eales' disease. Methotrexate, a folic acid antagonist, has a marked effect on rapidly proliferating cells and causes B- and T-cell suppression. A "pulse" differs from chronic-moderate therapy in its ability to reset an aberrant immune response. Weekly oral dose of 7.5 to 12.5 mg, for 3 months, has been found to be safe.

Photocoagulation remains the mainstay of treatment in the proliferative stage of the disease. Beneficial effect of combined postequatorial xenon arc photocoagulation and peripheral cryoablation has been demonstrated. Laser photocoagulation alone similarly benefits the patients in proliferative stage, but is not useful (actually could be harmful) after severe retinal traction sets in. Moderate intensity focal treatment of flat retinal new vessels, sectoral scatter photocoagulation of areas of capillary dropouts and the direct treatment of retinal neovascular frond

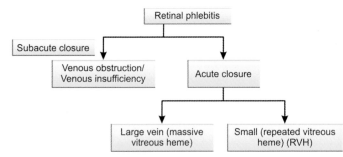
Fig. 27.20: Eales' disease. Pathogenesis of Eales' disease

is beneficial in proliferative Eales' retinopathy. An anchor photocoagulation is suggested to avoid the development of traction retinal tears in eyes with evident retinal traction.

Anterior retinal cryoablation is generally reserved as an adjunct to photocoagulation in Eales' disease.

Pars plana vitreous surgery as in other proliferative retinopathies helps restoring vision by clearing the media (removal of the unabsorbed blood) and relieving the retinal tractions (vitreoretinal membranes). The prognosis of vitreous surgery in Eales' disease is usually good due to the early and complete posterior vitreous detachment. Patients with fewer episodes and shorter duration of vitreous hemorrhage do better.

The pathogenesis (Fig. 27.20) and treatment of Eales' disease is well understood. But the etiology is still obscure. With the emphasis on possible exclusion of systemic and ocular diseases where retinal vasculitis and peripheral retinal neovascularization are prominent clinical features, it is rather a disease of exclusion. It is often debated that Eales' disease is not a single disease entity, but a combination of a variety of diseases where both retinal vasculitis and peripheral retinal neovascularization are the common denominators. Obviously further research is necessary to understand more clearly.

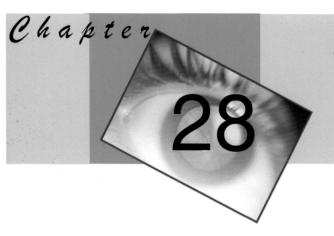
Laser Treatment in Posterior Segment Disorders

Pradeep Venkatesh, Satpal Garg

INTRODUCTION

Laser treatment has become an important therapeutic modality in the treatment of most retinal disorders.

LASER TREATMENT IN CHOROIDAL NEOVASCULAR MEMBRANES

Abnormal ingrowth of choroidal vessels between the Bruch's membrane and the retinal pigment epithelium or between the retinal pigment epithelium and neurosensory retina is known as choroidal neovascularization (Figs 28.1 and 28.2). This ingrowth may occur in extrafoveal, juxtafoveal or subfoveal location. Subfoveal choroidal neovascularization leads to visual loss by causing exudative detachment of the macula, subretinal bleed and disciform scar formation. When the posterior edge of a choroidal membrane lies beneath the foveal center it is designated subfoveal, when it is between 1 μm and 199 μm as juxtafoveal and between 200 μm and 2,500 μm as extrafoveal membrane. Results of focal laser treatment of choroidal neovascular membrane in age-related macular degeneration are shown in Table 28.1.

Apart from age-related macular degeneration there are other conditions in which choroidal neovascular ingrowth may occur. These include pathological myopia, angioid streaks, chorioretinal scar (after choroiditis, laser burn and cryotherapy), presumed ocular histoplasmosis syndrome and idiopathic choroidal neovascularization.

Choroidal Neovascularization in Age-Related Macular Degeneration

The ideal treatment in choroidal neovascular membranes would be one that selectively and permanently eradicates the "ingrowth" without causing any collateral damage to the surrounding normal retina. Modalities that destroy the membrane more effectively cause significant collateral damage while those that decrease this damage, result in only transient regression of

Table 28.1: Results of focal laser treatment of choroidal neovascular membrane in age-related macular degeneration

Extrafoveal CNV		
SVL	*No Laser*	*With Laser*
1 year	41%	24 %
3 years	63%	45 %
5 years	64%	46 %
Recurrence at 1 year 75%		
Juxtafoveal CNV: Severe visual loss at 1 Year		
No Laser	45%	
With Laser	31%	
Recurrence at 1 Year 22 %		
Subfoveal CNV: At 2 years (> 6 line loss)		
No laser	37%	
With laser	20%	

the membrane. Hence, all available laser modalities have advantages and disadvantages and help in preventing severe visual loss to varying extent.

The goal of treatment has been only to reduce the risk of additional visual loss. Restoration of vision occurs only rarely with all modalities of treatment. Hence success is usually defined in terms of stabilization of vision. With the advent of anti-vascular endothelial growth factor therapies, laser treatment is not the current modality of management in age-related macular degeneration.

Conventional (Direct) Laser Treatment

Direct treatment using conventional laser systems may still be a modality of choice for treating patients with extrafoveal choroidal neovascular membranes.

Procedure: Pretreatment evaluation constitutes slit-lamp biomicroscopy, fundus photography, and a good quality fluorescein angiography, not more than 72–96 hours old. The desired result of focal direct photocoagulation is total obliteration of

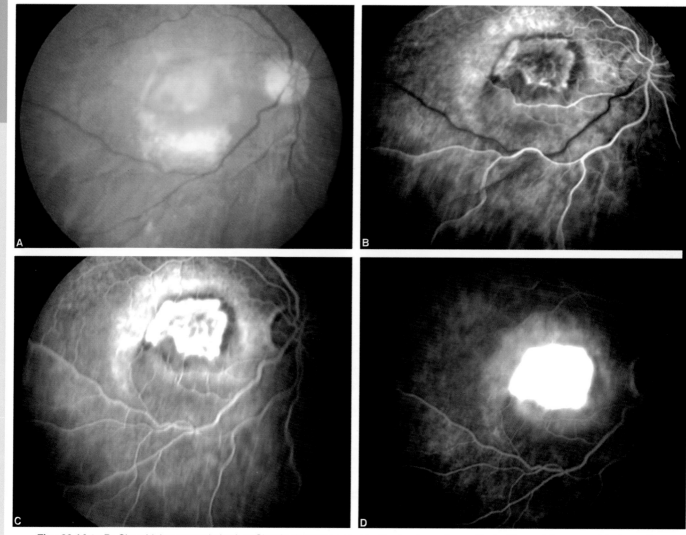

Figs 28.1A to D: Choroidal neovascularization: Classic choroidal neovascular membrane in a patient with exudative age-related macular degeneration. Well-defined neovascular net is clearly visible in the early angiographic frame

the neovascular membrane. The membrane is first delimited by moderate intensity non-confluent laser spots extending to at least 100 μm of the surrounding normal retina. Subsequently, intense confluent burns are applied to the membrane per se until uniform whitening is observed (Figs 28.3A and B and 28.4A to C). A 532 nm frequency doubled-YAG laser is used. A feeder vessel, if present, is also treated. Most of the patients can be treated under topical anesthesia. Pressure on the globe during treatment may improve results and also decrease the risk of laser-induced bleeding. Summary of the treatment parameters for direct treatment of choroidal neovascular membranes is depicted in Table 28.2.

Follow-up is done every 2–3 months at least until a year. Avoiding aspirin and lifting of heavy objects until regression of new vessels occur, has been advised by Macular photocoagulation study, as these are thought to increase the risk of bleeding.

Table 28.2: Treatment parameters for focal laser of choroidal neovascular membrane in age-related macular degeneration.

Type of CNV	Characteristics	Border	Membrane	Treatment area
Extrafoveal	Spot-size Time Intensity	100-200 μm 0.1-0.2 sec Moderate	200 μm 0.2-0.5 sec Intense	100 μm beyond hyperfluorescence on FA
Juxtafoveal	Spot-size Time Intensity	200 μm 0.2-0.5 sec Moderate	200 μm 0.2-0.5 sec Intense	Confined to hyperfluorescence on FA
Subfoveal	Spot-size Time Intensity	200 μm 0.2 sec Intense	200 μm 0.2-0.5 sec Intense	Confined to hyperfluorescence on FA

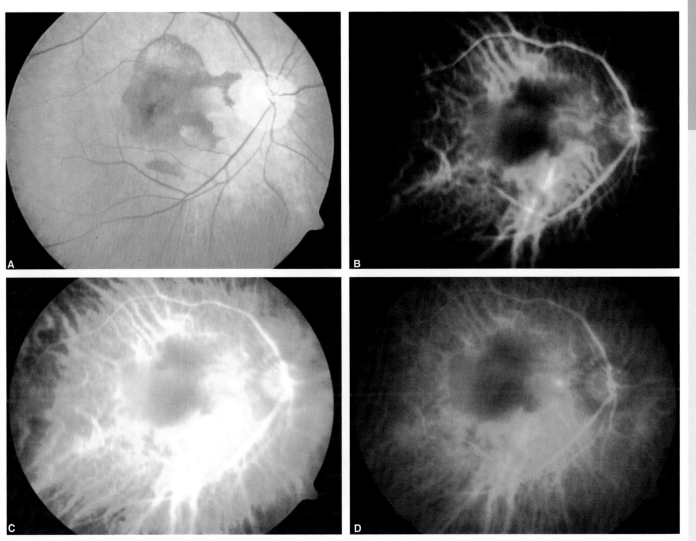

Figs 28.2A to D: Choroidal neovascularization: Indocyanine green angiography showing "hot-spot" in a patient with choroidal neovascularization and subretinal hemorrhage

Follow-up angiograms have been advised at 1, 3 and 6 weeks to identify incomplete treatment, persistence and new recurrent lesions.

Photodynamic Therapy

Photodynamic treatment is considered to have the potential to selectively destroy the neovascular complex without causing any damage to retinal tissue. This modality has been extensively studied in the management of neoplasia and has also been applied to manage choroidal neovascularization.

Principle: Photodynamic therapy uses specific photosensitizers that have an affinity for accumulating within proliferating vascular tissue despite its distribution into all parts of the body following intravenous administration. These photosensitizers are lipophilic and readily adsorb onto the richly lipophilic membranes of vascular endothelial cells and surface markers, such as lipoprotein receptors are thought to further increase lesion targeting. It has also been shown that pathologic structures, such as proliferating endothelial cells also express more number of membrane lipoprotein receptors. Subsequent exposure of the lesion to light with a wavelength specific for the absorption spectra of the injected dye leads to a photochemical, free radical-induced oxidative damage to the endothelium. This is followed by platelet adhesion, degranulation and thrombosis (photo-thrombosis) of the intralesional vasculature, sparing the surrounding tissues from any thermal damage.

For clinical ocular photodynamic therapy, verteporfin (Visudyne) is still the only approved dye.

Procedure: The dosage of verteporfin to be infused intravenously is determined by the body surface area (6 mg/m^2). The amount of dye calculated is given over 10 minutes (infusion phase) and then a further 5 minutes are allowed for the dye to accumulate (accumulation phase). After this 15 minute interval, the choroidal membrane complex is exposed to low energy diode laser light (689 nm) for 83 seconds. This activates the dye accumulated with the neovascular complex and results in its closure. The treatment spot size is 1000μ more than the greatest linear dimension of the choroidal membrane identified in the early

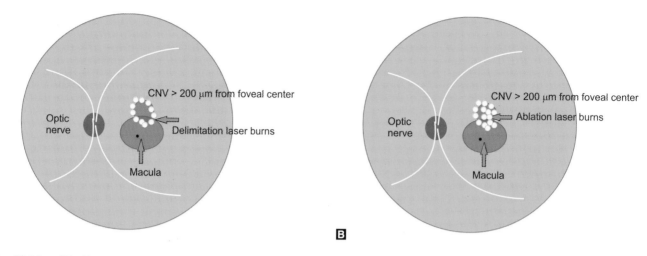

Figs 28.3A and B: Choroidal neovascularization: Diagrammatic representation of treatment technique for managing choroidal neovascularization using conventional laser. The perimeter of the membrane is first demarcated (A) followed by direct laser of the entire membrane (B)

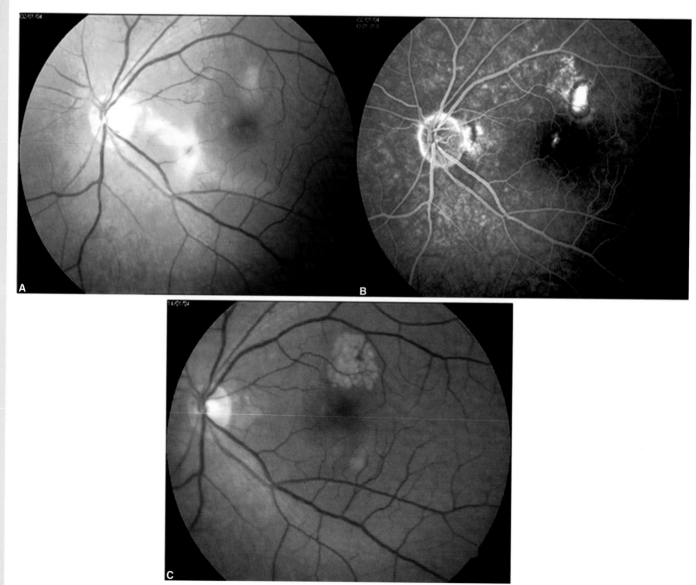

Figs 28.4A to C: Choroidal neovascularization: Pre-laser clinical photograph, late phase angiographic frame and immediate post-laser photograph of a treated extrafoveal choroidal neovascularization using the conventional technique

angiographic frame (for classic membranes) using digital systems. Patient is educated about protective body and eye wear and asked to avoid exposure to direct sunlight or bright illumination for five days to prevent photosensitization (Figs 28.5A and B).

Overdosage and excessive light activation may cause macular infarction and are to be avoided. Other adverse events include variable visual disturbances (mild to severe), extravasation of the dye, backache and allergic reaction.

Verteporfin has undergone several randomized trials, including the TAP (Treatment of age-related macular degeneration with photodynamic therapy) and VIP (Verteporfin in photodynamic therapy) studies.

Transpupillary Thermotherapy

Transpupillary thermotherapy is one of the modalities for managing subfoveal choroidal neovascular membrane. Encouraging results in occult choroidal membranes were reported in 1999.

Principle: Delivery of thermal energy for therapeutic effects has been used earlier in the management of small choroidal melanomas. In these patients sclerosis of the underlying choroidal vessels has been reported on histopathological studies. Compared to the 40° temperature elevation with conventional laser photocoagulation, transpupillary thermotherapy is reported to produce only a 10° rise of temperature, so minimizing collateral damage.

Procedure: A long duration, large spot, subthreshold laser energy is delivered to the region of subfoveal choroidal neovascular membrane through a dilated pupil using a modified diode laser (810 nm) system incorporated into a slit lamp. This delivery system has apertures measuring 0.5 mm, 0.8 mm, 1.2 mm, 2.0 mm and 3.0 mm allowing the laser surgeon to select the most appropriate one based on the size of the neovascular membrane.

It is planned to initiate treatment with a 3 mm spot for duration of 60 seconds and a power of 800 mW. If a change in the color of the retina is noted at any point during these initial 60 seconds, then the power is reduced in steps of 20% until one identifies the power at which no color change is observed. Now, treatment is restarted at this new power setting to complete the full 60 second treatment. At the end of the treatment no color change is detected in most patients, but some may show a mild graying of the lesion (Figs 28.6A and B).

Feeder Vessel Treatment

Feeder vessel treatment was advocated by the macular photocoagulation study report. However, identification of such vessels was very rare due to technical limitations inherent in the fluorescein angiographic systems available in the last decade and earlier. With the advent of high-speed indocyanine green angiography and good resolution digital monitors, identification of feeder vessels has been reported to become easier.

A feeder vessel is an afferent choroidal arteriole that directly supplies the choroidal neovascular net. Most feeder vessels are about a hundred to 100,000 µm long. Some neovascular nets may have more than one feeder vessel. It is usually visible only for a second or so during circulation of the dye in the initial phases. High-speed indocyanine green angiography allows visualization of these vessels as images can be captured at a rate of 30–40 frames per second. There is a learning curve for capture and detection of these vessels.

Procedure: Multi-pulse 810 nm diode laser and microburst yellow laser is used.

After superimposing the feeder vessel image onto a good quality retinal image, a 75–200 µm laser spot is placed on an extrafoveal path of the feeder vessel. Multiple pulses are applied for a total of 400 to 1,200 pulses. The duration of each

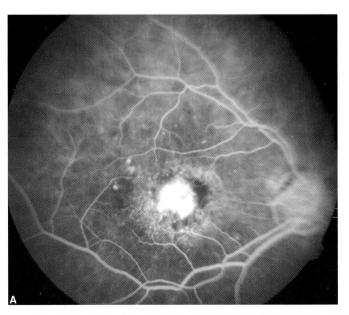
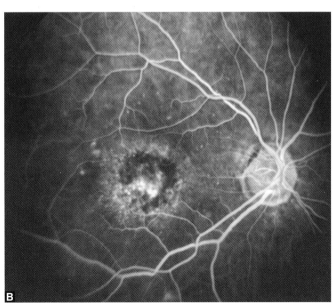

Figs 28.5A and B: Choroidal neovascularization: Pretreatment and posttreatment images of a patient with exudative age-related macular degeneration treated by photodynamic therapy

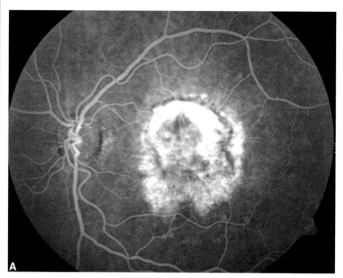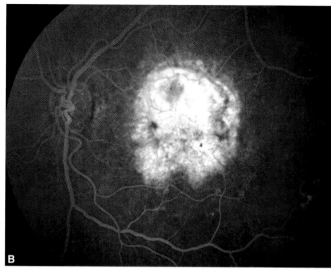

Figs 28.6A and B: Choroidal neovascularization: Pretreatment and posttreatment images of a patient with exudative age-related macular degeneration treated by transpupillary thermotherapy

pulse is 100 ms and inter-pulse interval is 100–200 ms. The laser power varies from 150–1000 mW. Repeat high-speed indocyanine green angiography is performed within 72 hours in case of classic membranes and retreatment is done if complete closure is not detected.

Limitations of this method other than the difficulty in detecting feeder vessels are the risk of reperfusion and occurrence of hemorrhages following laser.

Transscleral Diode Laser Photocoagulation

It is well established that the laser-tissue interaction during photocoagulation is largely pigment dependent and this is true even in the treatment of choroidal neovascular membranes. The transscleral route does not cause direct and intense absorption of laser energy by the retinal pigment epithelial cells. Hence, the outer retinal elements are preserved and there would be no immediate and sustained decrease in visual acuity.

Procedure: All patients were treated within 72 hours of obtaining the fluorescein angiogram. Laser photocoagulation is performed in the operating room under aseptic conditions and peribulbar anesthesia. Lateral rectus muscle is bridled after doing a limited peritomy temporally. Intermusuclar septa on either side are dissected and then the diopexy probe is introduced. With the laser set to continuous mode a test burn is applied to the temporal retina and the time taken to obtain a visible burn is noted. The probe was then gently guided to the submacular area under indirect ophthalmoscopy control. After this treatment, burn is applied to the region of the membrane as determined by site of leakage seen on early phase of fluorescein angiography. End point is taken as either appearance of a visible reaction or four times the time taken to obtain the test burn. Accuracy of the spot is established by indirect opthalmoscopic visualization throughout the treatment period. Conjunctiva is closed with 6-0 vicryl interrupted sutures and subconjunctival gentamicin and dexamethasone injection is given (Fig. 28.7).

Choroidal Neovascularization from Non-Age-Related Macular Degeneration

Etiology

Most of these lesions, unlike in age-related macular degeneration, are usually subfoveal and well defined. The same topographic and angiographic patterns probably apply to choroidal membranes in this group of patients as well.

Parafoveal telangiectasis is dilation of the capillary bed confined predominantly to the parafoveal region and that is congenital/developmental or acquired in origin. Age at presentation and unilateral or bilateral involvement depends on the type of parafoveal telangiectasis.

Laser photocoagulation for parafoveal telangiectasis is indicated only in a limited number of patients who develop serous detachment or subfoveal neovascularization as most

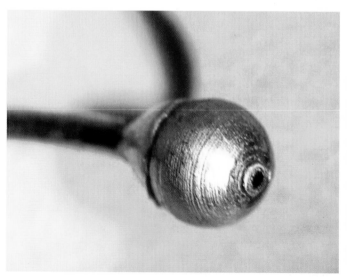

Fig. 28.7: Choroidal neovascularization: Diopexy probe used for transscleral diode laser photocoagulation of exudative age-related macular degeneration

telangiectasias are situated close to or within the foveal avascular zone. Rarely, patients with type 1 telangiectasis and associated macular edema or lipid exudation may also benefit from grid laser photocoagulation. Prophylactic treatment is not recommended, as they are also known to undergo spontaneous regression. Successful treatment of choroidal neovascular membrane using transpupillary thermotherapy in a patient with parafoveal telangiectasis is shown in Figures 28.8A to 28.9D shows resolution of exudates in a patient with type 1 telangiectasis and 20/40 vision following grid laser photocoagulation.

Osseous choristoma of the choroid, also called choroidal osteoma, is a very rare and unusual form of intraocular ossification. Histopathologically a plaque like bony lesion replaces the choroid in a focal area. The bone is mature and cancellous in nature with a hypocellular marrow lacking hemopoietic tissue. Because of thinning and degeneration of the overlying retinal pigment epithelium treating such choroidal neovascular membranes might require multiple sessions. Successful treatment of a juxtafoveal choroidal neovascular membrane in a patient with choroidal osteoma is shown in Figures 28.10A to D. The patient was treated using 532 nm laser and has maintained a vision of 20/40 at 18 months of the follow up.

Myopia may be associated with choroidal neovascularization most commonly involving the macular and peripapillary region and may result in transudates or frank hemorrhages. The hemorrhage per se or hyperplasia of retinal pigment epithelial cells or both may give rise to a dark spot called the Foster-Fuchs spot.

Laser photocoagulation for choroidal membranes in highly myopic eyes has remained ill defined. Both photodynamic therapy and transpupillary thermotherapy have been used to treat choroidal membranes in patients with high myopia. Successful treatment of myopic choroidal neovascular membrane with transpupillary thermotherapy is shown in Figures 28.11A to 28.12D.

Choroidal rupture is a manifestation of blunt trauma to the eye. Only the choroid ruptures and not the retina or sclera because of the following biomechanical characteristics of the three tissues: the retina has a degree of elasticity that prevents it from tearing; the sclera, though inelastic has the ability to withstand a greater degree of force; the Bruch's membrane (to which the choroid and retinal pigment epithelium) is neither elastic and nor does it have a great degree of resistance to withstand concussional forces. Choroidal neovascularization is a component of the healing process, but usually regresses spontaneously without any sequelae. Sometimes however, laser photocoagulation may become necessary.

Angioid streaks are ophthalmoscopically visible cracks in the Bruch's membrane. It may be an incidental finding or may be a manifestation of a systemic disease, such as pseudoxanthoma elasticum, Ehlers-Danlos syndrome, Paget's disease, senile elastosis and sickle cell disease. Choroidal neovascularization is reported to occur in 70% of patients with angioid streaks. Successful treatment of choroidal neovascular membrane in patients with angioid streaks has been reported with conventional laser and photodynamic therapy. Appearance of "new" choroidal neovascular membrane in a patient of angioid streaks treated with transpupillary thermotherapy is shown in Figures 28.13A to D. Immediate post-laser photograph of another patient treated with conventional laser is depicted in Figures 28.14A to 28.15D shows resolution of choroidal neovascular membrane associated with angioid streaks following conventional laser.

Idiopathic choroidal neovascular membranes have clearly documented the role of laser photocoagulation in the treatment. Regression of choroidal neovascular membrane following transpupillary thermotherapy is shown in Figures 28.16A to D.

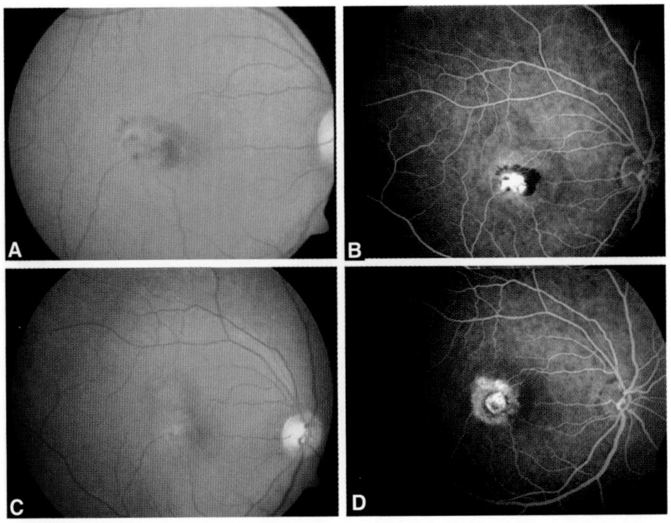

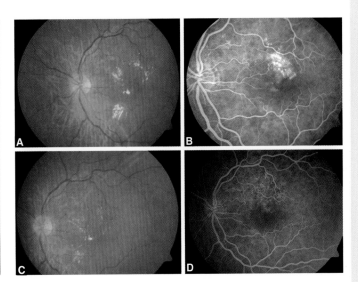

Figs 28.8A to D: Choroidal neovascularization: Pretreatment and posttreatment images of a patient with subfoveal choroidal neovascular membrane secondary to idiopathic parafoveal telangiecatasis type 2b. Pre transpupillary thermotherapy vision was counting finger at 1 meter; posttreatment vision has remained 20/60 at 12 months follow-up. No recurrence was observed

Figs 28.9A to D Choroidal neovascularization: Pretreatment and posttreatment images of a patient with parafoveal telangiecatasis, type 1b. Decrease in exudation and angiographic leakage is evident post laser. Vision has stayed 20/30

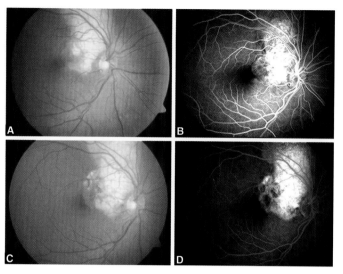

Figs 28.10A to D: Choroidal neovascularization: Pretreatment and posttreatment images of choroidal neovascularization along the foveal margin of a lady in the fourth decade with choroidal osteoma. Treatment of this juxtafoveal membrane was with conventional 532 nm laser. Pretreatment vision was 20/30. Posttreatment vision has remained 20/40 at 18 months of the follow up. No recurrence has been observed

Inflammatory disorders, such as sarcoidosis, toxoplasmosis, syphilis, serpiginous choroidopathy, Vogt Koyanagi Harada's disease and presumed ocular histoplasmosis syndrome may result in choroidal neovascularization. Success with conventional laser has been reported. Adjunctive use of systemic corticosteroids is poorly defined in the management of postinflammatory choroidal neovascular membranes.

Idiopathic polypoidal choroidal vasculopathy is now being recognized following superior imaging provided by indocyanine green angiography. Laser photocoagulation is reported to decrease the exudation and risk of hemorrhage. The overall role of laser is however still poorly defined.

PROPHYLACTIC LASER FOR DRUSEN

Drusen are considered predisposing lesions for the evolution of visually threatening complications in elderly patients. This is more so in patients with large and confluent drusen. Since the advent of laser therapy it has been observed that laser burns applied to the macula cause a decrease in the number and size of drusen. However, the actual benefit of such treatment in reducing the risk of later stages of age-related macular degeneration is still not clear. Some reports have shown definite decrease in the size of drusen, but have also cautioned that such treatment may increase the risk of developing choroidal neovascularization. Two randomized trials have evaluated prophylactic treatment outcomes with argon green laser and diode laser in patients with drusen. While both these trials showed drusen reduction, the argon laser study cautioned against the possibility of increased risk of choroidal neovascular membrane development in treated patients at 3 years of the follow up.

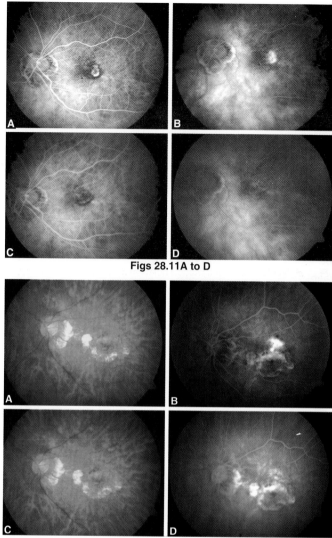

Figs 28.11A to D

Figs 28.11A to D and Figs 2812A to D: Choroidal neovascularization: Pretreatment images and post-laser photograph of two patients with choroidal neovascular membrane secondary to myopia. Resolution of choroidal neovascularization following transpupillary thermotherapy is evident

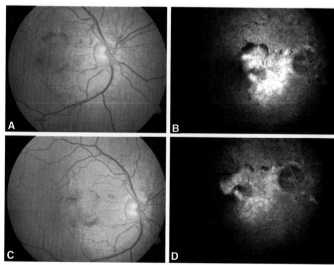

Figs 28.13A to D: Choroidal neovascularization: Development of new choroidal neovascular membrane is evident 6 months after this patient with subfoveal choroidal neovascular membrane secondary to angioid streaks was treated with transpupillary thermotherapy

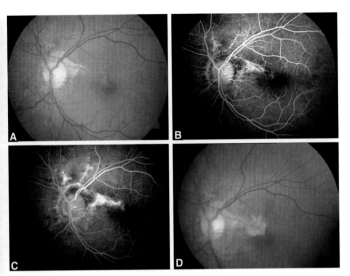

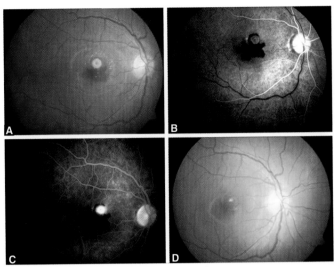

Figs 28.14A to D: Choroidal neovascularization: Pretreatment images and immediate post-laser photograph of a patient with juxtafoveal choroidal neovascular membrane secondary to angioid streaks

Figs 28.16A to D: Choroidal neovascularization: Resolution of choroidal neovascular membrane following transpupillary thermotherapy can be appreciated in these pretreatment and posttreatment images of a young patient with idiopathic choroidal neovascular membrane

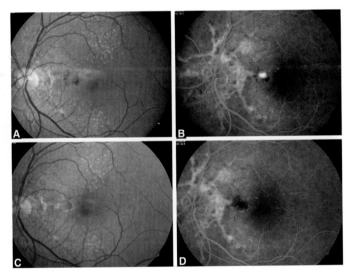

Figs 28.15A to D: Choroidal neovascularization: Resolution of extrafoveal choroidal neovascular membrane is evident in these pre- and post-laser images of another patient with angioid streaks treated with conventional laser

LASERS IN DIABETIC RETINOPATHY

Introduction

Diabetic maculopathy is today the commonest cause of visual loss in diabetics. Visual loss due to macular edema is five times the visual loss due to the complications of proliferative diabetic retinopathy. Diabetic maculopathy has been subdivided for the purposes of management into two broad categories by the early treatment diabetic retinopathy study (ETDRS). Those that are clinically significant and those that are not. The hallmark of clinically significant macular edema is thickening of the retina. Similarly, the diabetic retinopathy study (DRS) has identified

certain high-risk characteristics, the presence of which predisposes to the risk of severe visual loss in the stage of proliferation of abnormal, new vessels on the retinal surface and optic nerve head. In the presence of these high-risk characteristics, it becomes necessary to initiate treatment without any further delay so as to reduce the risk of severe visual loss.

Before undertaking laser treatment the patient must be told about the nature of his disease and the aims of treatment. An informed consent should also be obtained. The patient must be informed that:

- Laser photocoagulation may cause an initial fall in vision for a few weeks.
- Three-four sessions might be required for complete treatment.
- In most cases laser does not improve vision.
- Laser can cause alteration in contrast sensitivity, color perception, dark adaptation and can result in visual field defects.
- Even after laser life-long evaluation is essential, again with the aim of detecting recurrence early and augmenting the laser treatment.
- Response to laser is best when blood sugar levels and other risk factors, such as hypertension, nephropathy and lipid profile are well controlled.
- The retinopathy may progress even after laser photocoagulation.

As in other laser procedures for posterior segment diseases, adequate pupillary dilation must be obtained. In some diabetics, pupillary dilation may be difficult and laser photomydriasis may be useful. Laser photomydriasis can dilate the pupil a few extra millimeters to aid laser delivery in the peripheral retina. This can be achieved by placing 2–3 rows of argon or double frequency-YAG laser burns circumferentially around the pupillary margin.

The first row must be 1 mm away from the pupillary margin. A spot size of 200–400 μm, power of 200–500 mW is usually adequate. Two drops of topical paracaine suffice to obtain surface anesthesia. Retrobulbar anesthesia is almost never necessary.

The mainstay in the treatment of diabetic maculopathy and proliferative retinopathy is laser photocoagulation. The aim is not to recover lost vision, but to prevent or retard the risk of further moderate to severe visual loss. The maximum beneficial effect of laser treatment in diabetic maculopathy is seen in eyes treated early. The first conclusive evidence that laser treatment decreases the risk of severe visual loss and moderate visual loss by almost 50% in patients with proliferative retinopathy and high-risk characteristics and diabetic maculopathy respectively was shown by the DRS and ETDRS study (Table 28.3).

Focal and Grid Laser in Diabetic Maculopathy

Diabetic maculopathy is the leading cause of moderate visual loss in diabetics. The prevalence of diabetic maculopathy is more in older onset insulin-dependent patients, i.e. NIDDM patients requiring insulin. Diabetic maculopathy can be exudative, ischemic or of a combined nature. The exudative component of maculopathy is amenable to treatment by laser. According to ETDRS all patients with clinically significant macular edema should undergo laser treatment as this reduces the risk of moderate visual loss by around 50%. Moderate visual loss was defined (by ETDRS) as doubling of visual angle, i.e. drop of 15 or more letters on ETDRS charts or drop of 3 or more lines of Snellen equivalent. Clinically significant macular edema was defined as (based on slit-lamp biomicroscopy and regardless of visual acuity) the presence of any of the following:

- Retinal thickening at or within 500 μm of the foveal center
- Retinal thickening 1,500 μm or larger in size any part of which is within 1,500 μm of the foveal center
- Hard exudates at or within 500 μm of the foveal center if associated with thickening of the adjacent retina.

Diagrammatic representation of what constitutes clinically significant macular edema is shown in Figures 28.17A to C.

The treatment strategy of macular laser photocoagulation was proposed by ETDRS, and has been followed by the ophthalmologists worldwide with few minor alterations. The basic guidelines are:

- All areas of macular thickening must be treated.
- Once a decision to treat has been made, a good fundus fluorescein angiography is done to look for the points of leakage.
- In case of a focal leak, focal laser photocoagulation is done. If fluorescein angiography shows a diffuse leak, grid photocoagulation is recommended.
- Laser parameters: 50–100 μm spot size, 0.1–0.2 second duration, least power to create a mild intensity burn (80–180 mW). Spots must be one burn width apart.

Table 28.3: Diabetic retinopathy study and early treatment diabetic retinopathy study

Diabetic Retinopathy Study (DRS)
- Enrolled 1,758 patients between 1972–1975
- Study Objective was to determine:
  - If photocoagulation helps to prevent severe visual loss in PDR
  - If extensive scatter and focal laser for flat NVE (Xenon arc) and elevated NVE (argon laser) has any efficacy and safety
  - At what stage of retinopathy is laser most beneficial?
- Study Outcome
  - Defined high-risk characteristics (HRC) for developing severe visual loss
  - Defined severe visual loss (SVL) as a visual acuity of less than 20/500 at two consecutive 4 monthly visits
  - Scatter photocoagulation decreases the risk of SVL in patients with HRC by 50%
  - Did not provide clear guidelines for laser treatment in eyes with less severe retinopathy (without HRC).

Early Treatment Diabetic Retinopathy Study (ETDRS)
- Enrolled 3,700 patients with bilateral NPDR (mild-severe) or early PDR with or without macular edema between 1980–1985
- Study Objective was to determine:
  - If photocoagulation is effective in macular edema
  - If aspirin is effective in altering the course of diabetic retinopathy
  - When in the course of diabetic retinopathy should scatter photocoagulation be initiated so as to be most effective?
- Study Outcome
  - Defined clinically significant macular edema (CSME)
  - Defined moderate visual loss (MVL): Doubling of visual angle or decrease in 3 or more lines on ETDRS chart at two consecutive 4 monthly follow-up. (e.g. 20/20 to 20/40)
  - Concluded that:
    1. Focal laser decreases risk of MVL by ~50% in eyes with CSME
    2. Aspirin (650 mg) does not have any overall effect on the progression of retinopathy
    3. Risk of SVL for all groups was not significant (even in those with deferral of laser treatment). However, immediate full scatter reduces the risk of progression to HRC by 50% and immediate mild scatter by 25%.

Laser Management: Guidelines
- Macular edema (CSME) has to be treated irrespective of grade of retinopathy
- Treat one eye if severe/very severe NPDR with full scatter (but manage CSME appropriately)
- In special situations treat both eyes even if severe NPDR only
- If HRC is present, then do not delay laser

Technique

(i) *Focal laser photocoagulation:*

- All focal leaks located between 500 μm and two disc diameters (=3000 μm) are treated directly.
- Initially, 50–100 μm spots at 0.1 second duration are used to produce a whitening of the microaneurysm. Repeat burns may sometimes be necessary.
- Focal lesions located 300–500 μm from the center of the macula are treated if the visual acuity was ≤ 20/40 and the clinician believes that the laser photocoagulation of these areas will not damage the remaining foveal capillary network.

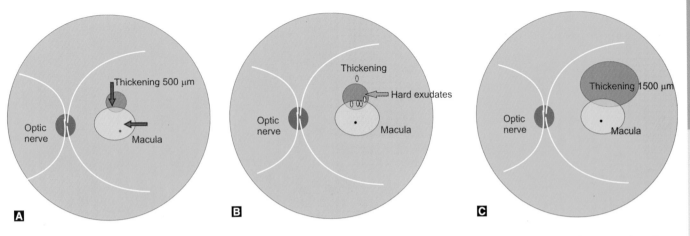

Figs 28.17A to C: Clinically significant macular edema. Diagrammatic representation of the three categories of clinically significant macular edema

(ii) Grid laser photocoagulation:

- Areas of diffuse leakage are treated. A diffuse leakage is one that extends from arcade to arcade, is deep in location and may or may not have concurrent cystoid macular edema.
- 50–200 μm spot size burns placed one burn width apart, at 0.1 second duration.
- Laser is done in a C-shaped manner within the vascular arcades and avoiding the area of the papillomacular bundle. Also the burns must be at least 500 μm away from the foveal center and 500 μm away from the disc margins. About 90–200 spots may be necessary.

Pattern for grid laser is shown in Figures 28.18. Resolution of macular edema following focal and grid laser in patients with diabetic retinopathy is shown in Figures 28.19A to 28.20D.

A repeat fluorescein angiography is to be done four months later. Laser for any persisting focal or diffuse leak is to be augmented accordingly. Most patients require 1–3 sessions. In case the macular edema still persists one should contemplate other treatment modalities, such as intravitreal steroid injection or vitrectomy. Some authors suggest grid laser photocoagulation once the edema subsides with intravitreal steroid injection.

Subthreshold Diode Laser in Diabetic Macular Edema

Olk and associates have shown that subthreshold diode laser burns are as effective as creating visible burns in the treatment of macular edema in diabetic maculopathy. In this method, the authors first noted the amount of power needed to produce a visible burn on the nasal retina with the spot size and duration constant at 125 μm and 200 msec respectively. Subsequently, the duration was reduced to 100 msec and it was then used as the treatment burn parameter. The only disadvantage that they found with this approach is that the macular edema needed a longer duration to resolve.

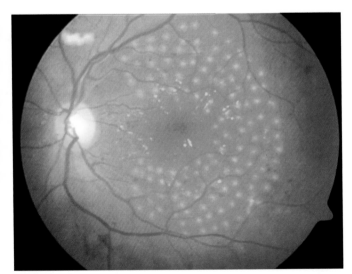

Fig. 28.18: Macular grid laser photocoagulation: Immediate post-laser photograph of a patient subjected to grid laser photocoagulation for clinically significant macular edema

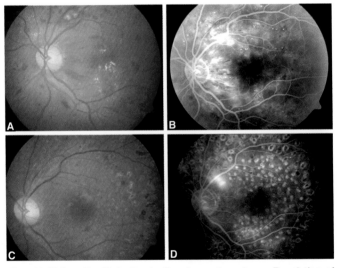

Figs 28.19A to D: Clinically significant macular edema: Resolution of clinically significant macular edema is evident in a patient subjected to grid laser and panretinal photocoagulation for concurrent early proliferative diabetic retinopathy. However, there is persistence of new vessels

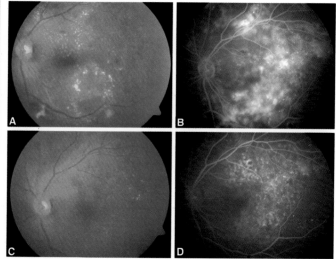

Figs 28.20A to D: Clinically significant macular edema. Complete resolution of clinically significant macular edema following two sessions of grid laser can be appreciated in these pretreatment and posttreatment images

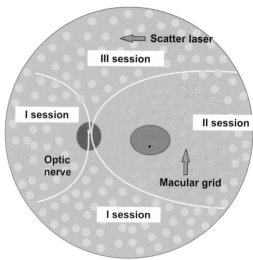

Fig. 28.21: Laser photocoagulation: Diagrammatic representation of combined macular grid and scatter laser in diabetic retinopathy

Scatter Laser in Diabetic Retinopathy

Diabetic retinopathy study recommends prompt panretinal photocoagulation in all patients meeting the high-risk criteria as laser reduces the risk of severe visual loss (defined as visual acuity <5/200 on two consecutive follow-up examinations 4 months apart) by more than 50%. The progression to severe visual loss at 5 years was 50% in those not lasered and only 20% in those lasered. High-risk characteristics was defined as:

- Neovascularization of disc (NVD) that is atleast 1/4th–1/3rd disc area or larger
- Milder neovascularization of disc associated with preretinal or vitreous hemorrhage
- Neovascularization elsewhere (NVE) atleast ½ disc area or larger and associated with preretinal or vitreous hemorrhage

Scatter laser is also urgently indicated in patients with anterior neovascularization or rubeosis iridis. Panretinal photocoagulation can be considered prior to development of high-risk characteristics in cases of very severe or severe non-proliferative diabetic retinopathy in special situations such as patients who cannot maintain a regular follow-up, pregnancy, patients with severe nephropathy and whenever the fellow eye has had a bad visual outcome due to some complication of proliferative retinopathy (Fig. 28.21).

Technique

- Topical anesthesia is usually sufficient although, some prefers peribulbar/ retrobulbar anesthesia.
- Goldmann/Rodenstock pan fundoscopic lenses can be used, the latter allows a spot size magnification of 1.3–1.6. Newer lenses, such as the Volk TransEquator and Volk SuperQuad 160 lens are now more often preferred than the older lenses for scatter laser.
- The whole of the retina other than the posterior pole within 3000 μm (vascular arcade) from the foveal center and 500 μm from the disc margin are treated.

- Treatment is completed in 2 to 4 sessions at intervals of 7 to 14 days. No more than 1,000 spots are recommended at each sitting.
- Laser parameters: 300 – 500 μm spot size, 0.2–0.5 second duration, burn intensity must be of moderate degree (150–400 mW) and the burns must be ½ to 1 burn width apart. Generally 1,800–2,200 burns are given for a complete treatment. Some patients may need as many as 4,000 spots.
- Initially, the inferior and the nasal areas are treated, so that if vitreous hemorrhage were to occur between the sessions, it would settle inferiorly, allowing superior retinal treatment.
- Treatment of major vessels, chorioretinal scars, areas of preretinal blood, and elevated NVE is not recommended.
- Progression of retinopathy, tractional retinal detachment, or increase in vitreous hemorrhage is not influenced by the number of sessions employed for photocoagulation. However, choroidal effusion, exudative retinal detachment and angle closure may be less frequent when photocoagulation is performed in multiple sessions.
- The patient is evaluated after 6–8 weeks to assess requirement for supplemental treatment, which is the case in at least 75 to 80% of the cases.
- The indications for supplemental treatment are eyes with absent or minimal clinical improvement, progressive retinopathy, rubeosis of the iris and new vitreous or preretinal hemorrhage.

Complete regression of NVE following scatter laser is evident in Figures 28.22A to 28.23D.

LASERS IN RETINAL VEIN OCCLUSION

Introduction

Occlusion of the retinal venous system occurs more commonly than arterial occlusions. Systemic hypertension is the commonest association and thrombus formation the most likely

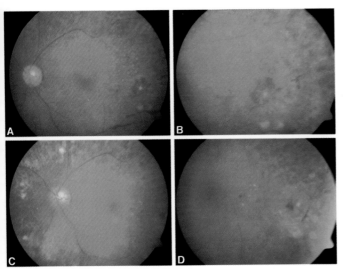

Figs 28.22A to D: Proliferative diabetic retinopathy. Regression of neovascularization elsewhere following focal strengthening of scatter laser is evident 3 months following the procedure in a diabetic patient

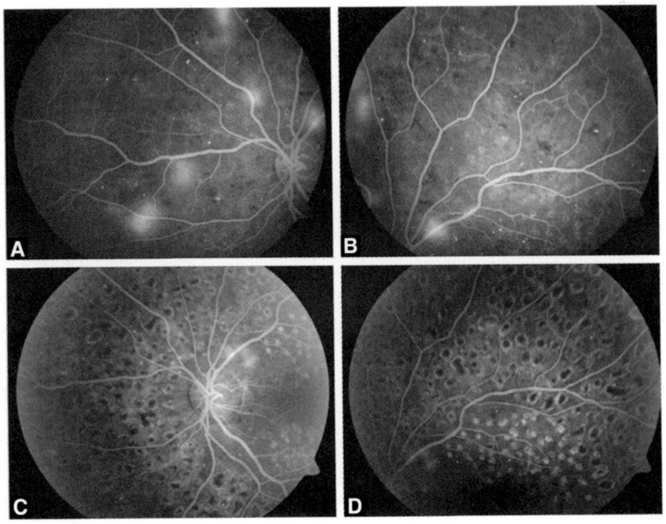

Figs 28.23A to D: Proliferative diabetic retinopathy: Pre- and post-laser fluorescein angiograms show regression of multiple neovascularization elsewhere following panretinal photocoagulation in a patient with proliferative diabetic retinopathy

mechanism. Other factors include compression of the vein by extra-luminal factors and inflammation of the vessel wall. Retinal vein occlusions may occur in the elderly (common) as well as in young individuals. Apart from hypertension, other risk factors for retinal venous occlusion are open-angle glaucoma, male gender and hyperopic refractive error. Diabetes mellitus does not seem to be an independent risk factor although these occlusions are seen frequently in diabetics. Some of the other associations are cardiovascular and peripheral vascular disease, elevated serum cholesterol and lipids, lupus anticoagulant factor and hyperviscosity syndromes.

Venous occlusion of the retina may be incidentally detected or the patient may present with features of a sudden/rapid loss of vision (due to macular hemorrhage, vitreous hemorrhage) or a gradual blurring of vision (macular edema, macular ischemia, tractional detachment of the macula). The ophthalmoscopic appearance is dependent on the severity of occlusion and the size of vessel involved. Common to all is dilation and tortuosity of the vessels and intraretinal hemorrhages in the corresponding quadrant. Rarely, cotton-wool spots and arteriolar narrowing may be seen in severe occlusion of the central retinal vein. Optic disc edema is a common feature in central retinal vein occlusion. In later stages, one may find disc and iris neovascularization, neovascularization elsewhere, venous-venous collaterals, opto-ciliary vessels at the disc, fibrous proliferation and traction on the retina.

Although there are several clinical features that help to distinguish ischemic from nonischemic central retinal vein occlusion (Table 28.4), one criterion for making such a differentiation is fluorescein angiography. The ischemic index is calculated based on the extent of capillary nonperfusion evident on fluorescein angiography. Based on the ischemic index, central retinal vein occlusion (CRVO) into three types, well perfused (42%), very ischemic (43%) and intermediate (15%). An eye is considered to be very ischemic if the ischemic index is more than or equal to 50%. Even initially well-perfused eyes should be watched carefully during follow up as some of these have been reported to become ischemic later on. The patients presenting with recent onset CRVO are classified as ischemic or nonischemic variety so as to prognosticate and advice regarding follow-up.

Management of Branch Retinal Vein Occlusion (Branch Vein Occlusion Study Recommendations)

1. A high quality fluorescein angiogram depicting the retinal vascular characteristics is obtained after the intraretinal hemorrhages have cleared (3–6 months).
2. The capillary abnormalities, such as macular edema, macular nonperfusion, and large segments of capillary nonperfusion (>5 disc diameters) are defined.

Table 28.4: Differences between ischemic and nonischemic central retinal vein occlusion

	Nonischemic	*Ischemic*
Visual acuity	> 6/60	< 6/60
Afferent pupillary defect	< 0.3 log units	> 1.2 log units
Severity of hemorrhage	Not extensive	Extensive
Ischemic index	< 50%	> 50%
Electroretinography (b/a ratio)	> 1.0	< 1.0
Complications (NVI / NVG)	Rare	Common

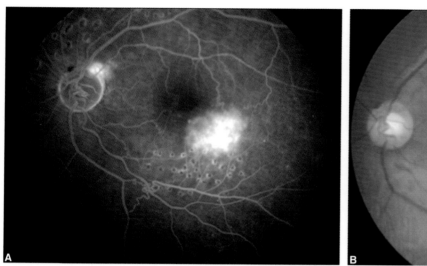
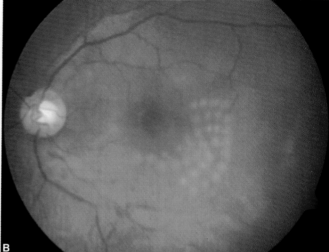

Figs 28.24A and B: Branch retinal vein occlusion: Immediate post-laser color photograph depicting strengthening of grid laser photocoagulation for persisting macular edema in an elderly patient with branch retinal vein occlusion

3. Treatment of macular edema
a. Fluorescein angiography demonstration of cystoid macular leakage without capillary nonperfusion suggests that macular edema is the cause of visual loss.
b. If the visual acuity is < 20/40 even after 3 months in such patients, which precludes spontaneous improvement seen in a sizeable number of patients, grid laser photocoagulation is advocated. The grid laser is done in the areas of capillary leakage essentially in the same way as that of a diabetic grid laser and is confined only to the area of angiographic leakage (Figs 28.24A and B).
c. If macular ischemia explains the visual loss, there is no treatment.
4. Treatment of neovascularization
a. Patients showing >5 disc areas of capillary nonperfusion are followed at 4-monthly intervals for development of neovascularization.
b. If confirmed new vessels are seen, laser photocoagulation in the involved quadrant will suffice.
c. Medium white burns, 200–500 µm in diameter spaced one burn width apart, covering the entire area of nonperfusion, beyond two disc diameters from the center of the macula and extending peripherally to the equator.

Regression of NVE and NVD is seen in two different patients with branch retinal vein occlusion which are shown in Figs 28.25A to 28.26C. The patient with NVD needed panretinal photocoagulation augmentation to achieve regression of NVD.

Management of Central Retinal Vein Occlusion (Central Vein Occlusion Study Recommendations)

- Perform fluorescein angiography for macular edema and retinal nonperfusion at four monthly intervals. Perform

gonioscopy and slit-lamp biomicroscopy (in undilated pupil) for angle and iris neovascularization every one month.
- Perform panretinal photocoagulation only if iris or angle new vessels more than two clock hours develop. The technique and parameters for scatter laser are as for proliferative diabetic retinopathy.
- Macular grid for macular edema may not improve central visual acuity although angiographic resolution can be obtained. Patients below 50 years of age and non-hypertensives however may show some benefit. The technique of grid laser is as described for diabetic macular edema.

Angiographic resolution of cystoid macular edema is evident in Figures 28.27A to D following grid laser in a patient with central retinal vein occlusion. Visual acuity however remained unchanged at 20/400.

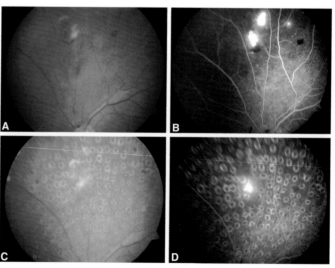

Figs 28.25A to D: Branch retinal vein occlusion: Pre- and post-laser images of a patient with branch retinal vein occlusion show regression of new vessels following one session of scatter laser

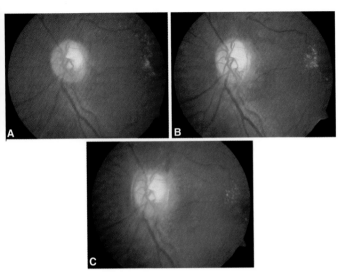

Figs 28.26A to C: Branch retinal vein occlusion: Neovascularization of the disc in a patient with branch retinal vein occlusion and hypertension (A) Increasing proliferation is evident 3 months after panretinal photocoagulation (B) Signs of regression become evident at the 6-month follow-up after panretinal photocoagulation augmentation (C)

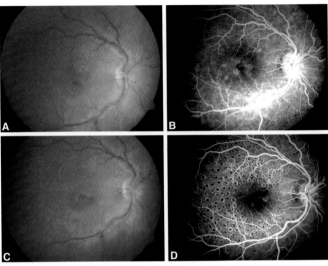

Figs 28.27A to D: Central retinal vein occlusion: Resolution of macular edema is visible in these pre- and post-laser images of a young, non-hypertensive patient with central retinal vein occlusion. Visual acuity however remained at the pre-laser value of 20/200

Laser-Induced Chorioretinal Anastomosis

Earlier experiments had demonstrated the feasibility of creating an anastomosis between a retinal vein and the choroidal circulation. Subsequently, role of laser-induced chorioretinal anastomosis in patients with the nonischemic form of central retinal vein occlusion was highlighted. In all 29 patients whom they studied the indication was progressing loss of vision from macular edema. A successful arrest of this progression with subsequent improvement was seen in 33% of cases following chorioretinal anastomosis. The laser used was argon green laser (50 μm spot size, 1.5–2.5 W power, 100 msec. duration), delivered to a focal spot on a retinal vein located atleast 3 disc diameters away from the disc in the inferotemporal or inferonasal quadrant (to avoid the posterior ciliary arteries and the long ciliary arteries along the horizontal meridian). A small intraretinal or subretinal hemorrhage was observed in all patients (the bleed being controlled by pressure on the contact lens). On an average each patient needed 1.8 sittings and the time for formation of the anastomosis varied from 3 to 7 weeks. They called for larger, randomized controlled trials to further demonstrate the efficacy or otherwise of this treatment option in patients with nonischemic central retinal vein occlusion.

Successful creation of a chorioretinal anastomosis has been observed in 38% patients. Patients in whom successful anastomosis is created are said to improve by an average of four lines. A serious complication of this procedure is said to be the development of choroidal neovascularization, this risk being greater in more ischemic eyes. It has been suggested that ideal candidates for laser-induced anastomosis procedure are those with vision below 10/200 and have perfused macular edema that does not resolve within 4 months. Patients with long standing vascular occlusion (more than three months) are said to be poor candidates.

LASER IN CENTRAL SEROUS CHORIORETINOPATHY

Introduction

Central serous chorioretinopathy is a relatively benign and self-limited disorder and in most cases the serous detachment resolves spontaneously in about 3–4 months. Recovery of visual acuity is good, but gradual improvement may proceed to normalcy even after 12 months after the initial episode. Other visual complaints (metamorphopsia, dyschromatopsia, relative scotoma) may however persist for a variable period or remain permanently. Recurrences are not infrequent and are reported to occur in nearly one-half of patients. Prognosis decreases with increase in the number of recurrences and some cases may progress to a stage of chronic retinal pigment epithelial decompensation.

Laser Photocoagulation

Laser photocoagulation is the only well established treatment modality in patients suffering from central serous chorioretinopathy. Treating the leakage site directly with laser (argon green, krypton, diode or frequency doubled YAG laser) hastens resolution of the disease, but does not affect the final visual acuity or the recurrence rate. Laser photocoagulation has also been reported to be beneficial in patients with multifocal leaks and large detachments and also in some patients with retinal pigment epithelial decompensation. For the latter, grid laser photocoagulation, as used for the management of diabetic macular edema has been found to be useful.

Laser treatment has however been reported to result in sub-optimal recovery of contrast sensitivity in comparison to cases that resolve spontaneously. Hence, photocoagulation should be undertaken only in the presence of specific indications. The indications for this treatment are a matter of debate. Some of the recommended indications are:

- Patient prefers treatment following proper explanation. This is usually for occupational reasons or in functionally one-eyed patients wherein the quality of work is disturbed.
- Angiographic leak persists beyond three months (chronic central serous retinopathy).
- In recurrent central serous retinopathy to hasten visual recovery and to decrease the risk of chronic retinal pigment epithelial decompensation.

Prerequisites: Before proceeding with laser photocoagulation, the following prerequisites should be taken into consideration. The visual acuity must be less than 20/40 and there should be a well-defined leakage point on fluorescein angiography that is atleast 500 μm away from the center of the foveal avascular zone.

Technique: The preferred technique is direct treatment to the leakage point using 100–200 μm spot size, 0.1–0.2 second duration, 100–200 mW energy. Not more than 3–5 spots are generally required and the end point is mild whitening. Some of the complications that are known to occur following laser photocoagulation are foveal burn, traction lines, retinal pigment epithelial tear and secondary choroidal neovascularization when high energy is used. Resolution of leakage in central serous retinopathy following laser photocoagulation is seen in Figs 28.28A to 28.29F).

Currently, successful treatment of persistent leaks in central serous chorioretinopathy has also been reported using photodynamic therapy and micropulse laser.

LASERS IN RETINAL LESIONS PREDISPOSING TO DETACHMENT AND RETINAL TEARS

Introduction

Gonin, the father of retinal detachment surgery, proved beyond doubt, that the cause of rhegmatogenous retinal detachment was the development of a retinal break. However, it was soon noticed that a retinal break is not an infrequent occurrence in the general population, being seen in nearly 8 to 10% of "normal" cases. In contrast, the frequency of retinal detachment in any given population was only about 0.01% each year. Thus it became evident that not all retinal breaks necessarily progress to a retinal detachment. Moreover, it was also observed that there were several peripheral lesions, some of which predisposed an eye to the formation of a retinal break and hence, to a retinal detachment and several that were relatively benign. Some of these benign lesions were also observed to closely mimic a retinal break if the examination was cursory or when the surgeon was unaware. These observations lead to a raging debate on the role of prophylactic treatment of retinal breaks in decreasing the incidence of retinal detachment. In addition, surgeons who propagated prophylaxis were unsure of which breaks to treat and which not to treat. The debate continues unabated even today regarding the above issues. No well-established statistical data exists to prove or disprove the two schools. This is possibly because of the small numbers involved in the general population. If there is one report showing no significant decrease in the incidence of retinal detachment in a given population following prophylactic treatment, there is another showing a decrease. Presently, two factors that determine the approach to treatment of peripheral retinal lesions are the surgeon's experience and the kind of population one is catering to.

Why Should We Aim at Treating Peripheral Retinal Lesions Predisposing to Retinal Detachment?

There are three reasons attributed. Firstly, even now about 5 to 10% of retinal detachment surgeries are a failure. Secondly, among those cases that succeed, only 50% regain a vision of 20/50. Lastly, the risks of retinal detachment surgery are several times higher than the risks associated with prophylactic treatment. Restraint has to be shown and prophylaxis undertaken only in selected cases wherein the risk of progression to retinal detachment far outweighs the risk of inducing epiretinal membrane formation by the prophylactic measure itself.

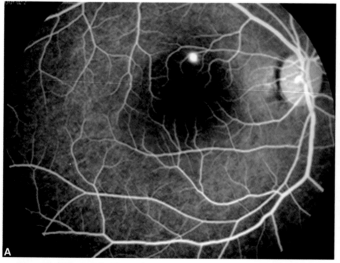
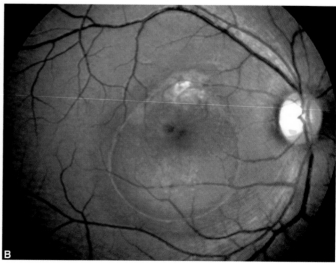

Figs 28.28A and B: Central serous chorioretinopathy: Fluorescein angiographic image and immediate post-laser photograph in a patient with central serous chorioretinopathy

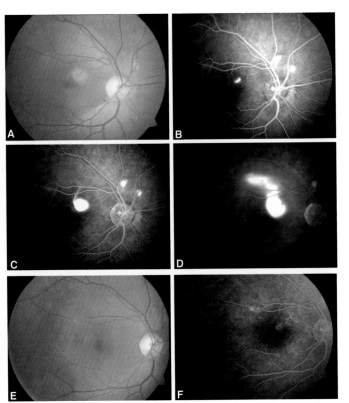

Figs 28.29A to F: Central serous chorioretinopathy: Pre- (A–D) and post-laser (E, F) images showing resolution of active leak following direct laser in a patient with recurrent central serous retinopathy

What Are the High-Risk Characteristics One Has to Look for Before Contemplating Treatment in Cases of Peripheral Retinal Lesions?

These features are:

- *Clinical background of involved eye*: Presence of acute onset of symptoms, such as a shower of floaters and flashes; blurring of vision due to a retinal tear-induced vitreous hemorrhage and the presence of Shafer's sign (in a eye that has not undergone surgery or has not had any inflammation) and the absence of a complete posterior vitreous detachment or focal vitreoretinal adhesion on dynamic scleral indentation are indicators that the break risks progression to a retinal detachment. Other high-risk factors include moderate to high myopia, aphakia and pseudophakia. Presence of a vitreoretinal degenerative condition is also considered as a risk factor.
- *Clinical background of fellow eye*: The presence of a non-trauma-related retinal detachment in the fellow eye is indicative that the fellow eye also risks a similar fate. Peripheral retinal lesions have to be treated without exception (even if asymptomatic). Some of them however may prefer to only observe these patients periodically in the absence of other high-risk characteristics provided the patient has access to an appropriate center and is complaint.
- *Clinical background of patient's family*: History of retinal detachment in the family is considered a high-risk characteristic for a peripheral retinal lesion to progress to retinal detachment.

- *Clinical characteristics of the tear*: Risk factors for the involved eye include a large tear (>2 disc diameter), a posterior tear, a superior tear and a U-shaped or flap tear. Presence of an atraumatic giant retinal tear is a high-risk characteristic that the fellow eye is also likely to follow suit and so needs to be treated prophylactically even in the absence of any abnormal lesion.
- *Clinical nature of the peripheral retinal lesion.* Predisposing lesions for a retinal detachment include lattice degeneration, including associated pigment "clumps" and snail track degeneration, cystic retinal tufts and meridional folds. While intrabasal lesions almost never lead to a detachment, juxtabasal and oral tears are at high risk.
- *Clinical status of the retina.* All peripheral lesions associated with a subclinical retinal detachment obviously constitute a high risk and need to be promptly treated. One should avoid treating patients with a retinoschisis, as there is a risk of creating a hole in the outer layer and hence full thicknesses break.

All of the above factors must be collectively taken into consideration in the final decision-making. Once a surgeon has decided on undertaking a prophylactic treatment, the next question that needs to be addressed is what the mode of treatment is to be adopted is. There are several options available in the form of cryotherapy, which is the commonest treatment, and laser photocoagulation, which is now more commonly being preferred by several surgeons. The purpose of cryo or laser treatment is to induce a sterile inflammation so as to stimulate proliferation of the retinal pigment epithelium. This indirectly improves adhesion between the retinal pigment epithelium and the neurosensory retina. As a working guide, cryotherapy is indicated when the lesion is anterior, the media is hazy for laser delivery and if laser facility is not available. In most cases topical anesthesia alone is adequate. However some cases may need a subconjunctival, peribulbar or retrobulbar block. In the presence of slightly posterior breaks, a limited peritomy allows easier access during cryotherapy.

Laser Photocoagulation

Laser can be delivered by the transpupillary approach with the aid of contact lenses or directly using the laser indirect ophthalmoscope and also transsclerally. Laser treatment is definitely more patient friendly, as it is almost a painless procedure. While it can be used to treat peripheral lesions also using the laser indirect ophthalmoscope or with a degree of difficulty using the Goldmann three-mirror contact lens, it is largely used to treat more posterior lesions when the media is clear.

The principles of laser treatment to decrease the risk of failure and preventing complications are:

- Surround the entire perimeter of the break by laser application.
- During laser therapy: Two-three rows of confluent burns; 200–500 μm in size and of mild to moderate intensity.

- In the presence of a rim of fluid or in subclinical detachment apply laser to the attached retina immediately around the detachment. If applied to the area of detachment, not only is the treatment futile, in addition it risks further progression of the detachment.
- Laser treatment of an inflamed retina is avoided (even if the inflammation is induced by cryotherapy a few days earlier) as there is a risk of producing a retinal break).

Prophylactic treatment of retinal tears is shown diagrammatically in Figure 28.30. Laser photocoagulation for the treatment of retinal tear is shown in Figures 28.31A and B.

LASERS IN RETINAL DETACHMENT: PROPHYLACTIC/DELIMITING

Introduction

Complete anatomical reattachment of the retina is the objective while managing rhegmatogenous retinal detachments. In certain situations however, the surgeon may choose to confine a detachment by conventional laser or laser indirect ophthalmoscope, to its peripheral/non-macular location.

Technique

For delimiting laser several rows of 300–500 μm, mild-moderate intensity spots are applied to attached retina along the posterior extent of the detachment and extending it up to the ora. Such an approach may be considered in patients with subclinical retinal detachments, near total cupping of the optic disc and concurrent detachment not involving the macula and in patients following buckling or vitreoretinal surgery. The latter group of patients would be categorized as partial success of surgery. This approach could be very useful in retaining central vision in one-eyed patients at least by avoiding the risks involved with multiple surgeries. Delimiting laser is unlikely to have long-term results

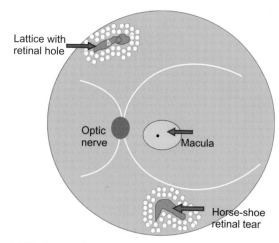

Fig. 28.30: Laser photocoagulation for retinal tear: Diagrammatic representation of prophylactic laser for lattice degeneration and retinal tear

in the presence of significant proliferative vitreoretinopathy. Another group of patients wherein laser may be beneficial even in the absence of a retinal detachment or evident predisposing lesion is in patients with choroidal colobomas (Fig. 28.32).

Prophylactic peripheral confluent laser photocoagulation has also been useful in decreasing the risk of retinal detachment or in preventing its spread to the macula in patients with infectious retinitis, such as acute retinal necrosis and progressive outer retinal necrosis.

LASERS IN INFLAMMATORY DISEASES

Post-vasculitis Retinal Proliferation

Eales' disease is an idiopathic, noninfective, inflammatory vasculitis of the retinal vasculature that is usually seen in males in their second and third decade. In about 90% of the patients, the disease becomes bilateral within a few years. Eales' disease is characterized by retinal periphlebitis and capillary nonperfusion

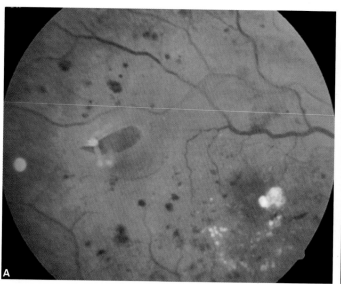
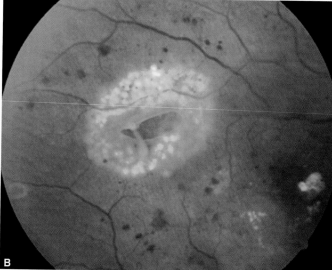

Figs 28.31A and B: Laser photocoagulation: Pre and immediate post-laser photograph of a patient following treatment for a posterior retinal tear

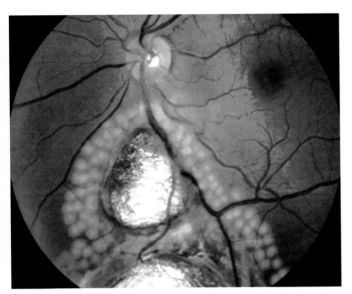

Fig. 28.32: Choroidal coloboma: Immediate post-laser photograph following prophylactic laser in a patient with choroidal coloboma

that results in hypoxia. Retinal hypoxia leads to neovascularization either on the retinal surface or on the optic nerve head. These new vessels being extremely fragile have a propensity to bleed into the vitreous. In some cases, this can lead to tractional or secondary rhegmatogenous retinal detachment and an irreversible visual loss. Laser photocoagulation is helpful in causing regression of neovascularization secondary to Eales' disease.

It is advisable to do a fluorescein angiography/scopy after the active vasculitis subsides to ascertain the presence of neovascularization elsewhere or neovascularization of the disc and the extent of capillary nonperfusion areas. In presence of NVD a panretinal photocoagulation is indicated. In presence of a single NVE a sectoral scatter photocoagulation, i.e. only 45° on either side of the NVE is done. Anchoring laser around fibrovascular fronds and around the posterior pole has also been described in cases of Eales' disease. Whether capillary nonperfusion areas alone should be lasered is controversial. We believe that this should only be undertaken if the capillary nonperfusion areas are extensive and the patient has lost one eye due to Eales' disease or is one eyed or cannot come for regular follow-up. Else such cases should undergo periodic follow-up. Few cases of Eales' disease that develop neovascularization of the iris should also be treated with panretinal photocoagulation.

The technique of scatter laser is as described for proliferative diabetic retinopathy. Regression of new vessels following scatter photocoagulation in a patient with vasculitis is shown in Figures 28.33A to D.

Laser in Intermediate Uveitis

Peripheral retinal neovascularization and rarely disc neovascularization have been reported in some patients with long standing intermediate uveitis. This can lead to vitreous hemorrhage. Unlike in other conditions leading to retinal and disc neovascularization, in intermediate uveitis there is no demonstrable

capillary nonperfusion. Park and associates found regression of new vessels, stabilization of inflammation and resolution of macular edema following peripheral scatter laser in 10 patients who were resistant to treatment with steroids. They used three rows of argon green or diode laser posterior to the region of exudation and new vessel formation. The treatment was extended one clock hour on either side of the lateral margins of neovascularization. In another retrospective study found that peripheral laser photocoagulation in patients with pars planitis may help in reducing the steroid dose and also in decreasing vitreous inflammation. Peripheral laser should be considered in patients who are intolerant to steroids or in those who develop steroid-related adverse effects. Regression of retinal new vessels in chronic uveitis has also been reported in other studies.

Laser in Idiopathic Retinal Vasculitis, Aneurysms and Neuroretinitis

Idiopathic retinal vasculitis, aneurysms and neuroretinitis (IRVAN) is presumed to be an inflammatory disease of the retinal arterioles affecting young individuals. Its characteristic feature is the presence of aneurysmal dilations along the arterioles; usually at the bifurcations. Aneurysmal dilations may also be evident on the epipapillary vessels. The etiology remains unknown. The natural course is varied and poor vision may result in this condition from macular exudation, new vessel formation and vitreous hemorrhage.

Laser photocoagulation is definitely indicated in the presence of new vessels. However, its role for nonperfusion of the retina alone is controversial. Direct laser treatment of the aneurysmal dilation has also been reported, including arteriolar occlusion as a complication following such treatment. We also caution against such direct treatment as we have seen a child with IRVAN in whom spontaneous resolution of macular

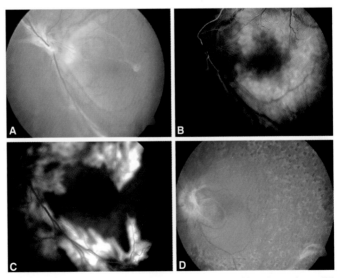

Figs 28.33A to D: Retinal vasculitis: Pre-laser (A–C) and post-laser (D) images showing regression of extensive neovascularization in a young adult with retinal vasculitis. Multiple panretinal photocoagulation sessions were needed to achieve satisfactory response

exudation and good visual recovery was seen almost one year after initial presentation. This child underwent vitrectomy for vitreous hemorrhage and absence of macular exudes was noted intraoperatively.

Laser in Diffuse Unilateral Subacute Neuroretinitis

Diffuse unilateral subacute neuroretinitis is a disease of young adults. The disease results from the presence and migration of nematodes within the subretinal space. It is usually unilateral and the implicated nematodes include the ascarid (Baylisascaris procyonis). Restoration for visual acuity has been reported in three of four patients by early recognition and direct treatment with laser. Unlike in photocoagulation for cysticercosis, laser for other intraocular worms like toxocara, trematodes, fly larva and including that in diffuse unilateral subacute neuroretinitis, does not incite any intraocular inflammation.

LASER IN RETINAL VASCULAR ANOMALIES

Retinal Artery Macroaneurysm

Cousins and associates have classified acquired macroaneurysms involving the retinal vasculature into four types. These are typical retinal artery macroaneurysm, retinal venous aneurysms, retinal capillary macroaneurysm and collateral associated macroaneurysm. The last three types of macroaneurysms are more common and may be encountered in diabetic retinopathy, venous occlusive disease, radiation retinopathy, sickle cell disease etc. Retinal artery macroaneurysm is usually an isolated finding with characteristic features. By definition, they are saccular or fusiform dilation of the retinal arteriole involving usually, the first three divisions. Their diameter is more than 125 μm (the upper limit for microaneurysm), but less than 250 μm. They are usually solitary and unilateral, but may be multiple in 20% and bilateral in 10%. They usually involve the temporal vessels and are often located at the bifurcations.

Retinal artery macroaneurysms generally occur in elderly women (6th decade) and about 75% of patients have associated systemic hypertension. Clinically two forms of presentation are seen, the acute type and the chronic type. In the acute form, patient presents with a sudden loss of vision (due to retinal or vitreous hemorrhage) while in the chronic form they present with a gradual loss of vision due to leakage and exudation into the macular area. The latter is usually diagnosed easily while the former is difficult to diagnose because of two reasons. Firstly, associated hemorrhage during the acute stage obscures visibility of the macroaneurysm and secondly, most resolve spontaneously after the hemorrhage and so may not be easily evident by the time the retinal or vitreous hemorrhage clears. The only characteristic feature during the acute stage is the presence of hour-glass-shaped hemorrhage due to simultaneous preretinal and subretinal collection of blood. This type of hemorrhage is not seen in all patients however. Fluorescein angiography may be helpful in identifying retinal artery macroaneurysms.

No treatment is recommended for a macroaneurysm with the acute form of presentation as recurrent hemorrhages are not known to occur and the visual recovery is good in most patients without treatment. Occasionally, pars plana vitrectomy may be necessary in patients with non-clearing vitreous hemorrhage. For those presenting with exudation into the macular area one may consider direct or indirect laser photocoagulation of the macroaneurysm if exudation is tending to progress towards the fovea and there is associated decrease in vision. *Technique*: In direct treatment a spot size of 200–300 μm is chosen, power of about 200 mW and duration of 0.2–0.5 sec. is set. The laser is focused directly on the macroaneurysm so as to obtain slow and gentle whitening. In indirect treatment, the laser burns are placed around the aneurysm. Branch retinal artery occlusion has been reported as a complication of direct treatment.

Coats' Disease

Congenital aneurysmal dilations involving the retinal vascular system may be classified into the following categories:

* *Leber's multiple miliary aneurysms*: Aneurysmal dilations without any subretinal exudation. They are probably a nonprogressive or early form of Coats' disease.
* *Coats' disease*: Multiple aneurysmal dilations with massive subretinal exudation and intraretinal hemorrhages.
* *von- Hippel's syndrome*: Frank retinal arteriovenous malformations with massive subretinal exudation.

All of the above have been collectively designated as the exudative vasculopathies. Whether the term Coats' disease should be referred to include only those cases encountered in childhood (and adolescence) or also those encountered in adults is controversial (adult onset disease: diagnosis after 16 years of age). Analysis of the subretinal fluid in Coats' disease shows the presence of cholesterol crystals.

Ophthalmoscopic examination in Coats' disease reveals varying degree of subretinal exudation and varying forms of vascular anomalies (aneurysmal dilations, telangiectasias, sheathing, tortuosity, neovascular tufts). In severe cases there is an extensive exudative retinal detachment. The vascular anomalies may be missed either because they are very subtle or because they are obscured by the retinal exudation and hemorrhages. Not infrequently, the vascular anomalies are situated peripherally while the exudation is predominantly in the macular region or posterior pole. The disease is usually progressive with periods of quiescence and exacerbations. Pain is a feature only when neovascular glaucoma develops in the end stage of very severe disease. Fluorescein angiography reveals more number of vascular anomalies than that seen by fundus examination and may also demonstrate other signs of a more generalized blood retinal barrier defect, such as perivascular leakage, areas of capillary nonperfusion around the areas of vascular anomalies and vascular communicating channels.

Treatment should be considered early as prospective studies have shown that even small lesions tend to increase in size and severity with time. This increases the risk of visual loss from macular exudation or exudative retinal detachment. Precede treatment by fluorescein angiography to identify all areas of vascular anomalies. If the vascular anomalies are posterior to the equator and there is no exudative detachment direct laser photocoagulation is performed (slit-lamp/laser indirect ophthalmoscope). If the vascular anomalies are anterior to the equator and there is no exudative detachment cryotherapy (freeze-refreeze cycle) or laser indirect ophthalmoscope may be effective. If there is an exudative detachment drain subretinal fluid externally (may need to reform the globe) and treat the vascular anomalies using laser photocoagulation or cryotherapy. Single session of laser is rarely successful and most patients need multiple sessions.

Technique: Laser is performed by directly treating all aneurysmal dilations. Whitening of the lesions should be the end point. A spot size of 200–500 μm is chosen with power setting of about 200 mW and duration of 0.2–0.5 sec. Excessive energy use must be avoided as it can increase the exudation. Some authors have also advocated a grid pattern of laser photocoagulation. Successful treatment allows preservation of vision and prevents complications like neovascular glaucoma.

Retinal Capillary Hemangioma

Capillary hemangioma of the retina is a vascular hamartoma with distinct clinical and angiographic features. These tumors may be situated in the peripapillary region or in the periphery. Peripheral retinal capillary hemangiomas are also called as the von Hippel tumor. The peripapillary tumors may be endophytic or intraretinal. These tumors are progressive, have feeder vessels, and lead to varying degrees of retinal exudation (circinate retinopathy to exudative retinal detachment). The peripheral tumors are said to be minuscule in the early stages (as small as a microaneurysm) with no obvious feeder vessels. They are also said to resemble grayish nubbins or telangiectatic vessels in the early stages. With time, the capillary channels proliferate; begin to function as arteriovenous shunts with subsequent formation and dilation of afferent and efferent feeder vessels. Ophthalmoscopically they appear as an orange mass with dilated feeder vessels.

von Hippel-Lindau syndrome is considered as one of the neurocristopathies or phakomatoses with an autosomal dominant inheritance. It is characterized by retinal capillary hemangiomas (the most frequent manifestation), infratentorial (cerebellar, brainstem, spinal cord) hemangioblastomas, renal cell carcinoma and pheochromocytoma. One fourth of patients with von Hippel tumor are said to harbor this syndrome; the risk is said to be higher if the tumor is bilateral or multiple.

Capillary peripheral hemangiomas may lead to visual loss by the ability of the exudates to accumulate preferentially in the macula or by breaching the internal limiting membrane and growing into the vitreous (may simulate neovascularization) and causing subsequent tractional effects and vitreous hemorrhage. These tumors should be treated early (at the time of detection)

even in the absence of exudation or large size because they invariably progress and when large is more resistant to treatment. Observation alone is only recommended for those touching the optic nerve head. The treatment of choice is laser photocoagulation, cryotherapy or a combination of the two. Recent reports on the use of transpupillary thermotherapy are also available. Tumors larger than 2.5 disc diameters are extremely resistant to any mode of treatment and carry a poor prognosis.

Technique: Direct treatment is employed for small lesions while feeder vessel treatment is indicated for larger lesions. For direct treatment argon green or frequency-doubled YAG laser may be used. A large spot (200–500 μm) and long duration (0.2–1.0 seconds) is chosen and power is set so as to obtain mild-moderate whitening of the lesion. Here again, multiple sessions at 1–2 week intervals are usually necessary to achieve complete closure. Excessive treatment at one sitting may lead to secondary exudative detachment. For feeder vessel treatment, the afferent vessel is treated with confluent, moderately intense burns (with parameters mentioned above) until there is no spontaneous reopening. Repeat sessions are performed at 2–8 weekly intervals until the angioma is non-perfused.

Regression of retinal angioma following laser photocoagulation is shown in Figures 28.34A to C.

LASER IN CHOROIDAL TUMORS

Choroidal Hemangioma

Hemangioma is a benign vascular malformation formed by an abnormal profusion of vessels relative to the anatomical site (i.e. they are vascular hamartomas). Hemangiomas involving the choroid occur in two forms: Diffuse choroidal hemangioma and circumscribed choroidal hemangioma. The former usually occurs in patients with the Sturge-Weber syndrome while the latter is commonly an isolated finding without any other systemic or ocular association.

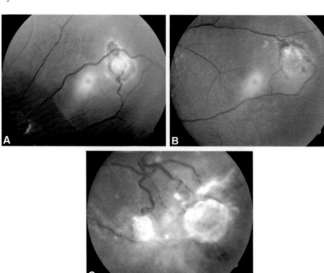

Figs 28.34A to C: von Hippel-Lindau disease: Appearance of scarring and atrophic changes around the multiple retinal angiomas following laser

Though congenital, they come to notice only when they begin to produce symptoms, such as decrease in vision (due to serous retinal detachment involving the macula). Choroidal hemangiomas are usually solitary and variable in size (both basal diameter and height), but are relatively flatter than choroidal melanomas. They are most commonly situated in the posterior pole and have orange-red color with ill-defined round to oval margins. The tumor surface may have few pigment clumps. Other associated fundus changes may include the dilation of adjacent retinal and choroidal vessels, hard exudates in the macula, epiretinal membrane, cystic macular degeneration and atrophy of the overlying retinal pigment epithelium.

These tumors usually need no treatment. The only accepted indication to treat these tumors is when they cause a serous retinal detachment and the most accepted treatment modality is laser photocoagulation. If serous detachment is extensive and prevents laser take then cryotherapy may be considered. The aim of treatment is to achieve resolution of the serous retinal detachment and not tumor obliteration. Most serous detachments resolve only after two laser sittings and take 4–8 weeks to do so after the second treatment session. More recently these tumors have also been treated with transpupillary thermotherapy and photodynamic therapy.

During treatment with conventional laser the entire tumor surface is covered with laser spots. In cases of subfoveal lesions the central avascular area is spared. Success in terms of resolution of subretinal fluid has been shown in up to 80% cases. Recurrences are re-treated in a similar manner.

For treatment with photodynamic therapy, the diameter of the treatment spot is calculated on the early frames of pretreatment indocyanine green angiography (ICGA). Verteporfin at a dose of 6 mg/m^2 body surface area is administered intravenously prior to laser (689 nm) application. The maximum treatment spot diameter at present available is 6000 μm using a Mainster wide-field lens. In the case of peripapillary choroidal hemangiomas, the laser spot is applied at a distance of 200 μm from the optic disc edge. The laser beam is applied to the retina 15 minutes after the start of the infusion. Two different treatment procedures have been described according to the height of the lesion. A radiant exposure of 100 J/cm^2 with an exposure time of 186 seconds is applied to lesions larger than 2 mm. For lesions smaller than 2 mm, a radiant exposure of 75 J/cm^2 with an exposure time of 125 seconds is used. Reduction in tumor height to complete resolution, resolution of exudative detachment and cystoid macular edema has been observed after 1–3 treatment sessions.

Resolution of retinal detachment and decrease in leakage from choroidal hemangioma following laser photocoagulation is seen in Figures 28.35A to D.

Laser Photocoagulation for Choroidal Melanomas

Choroidal melanomas are the commonest primary malignant intraocular tumors. It is said to be common in the elderly and

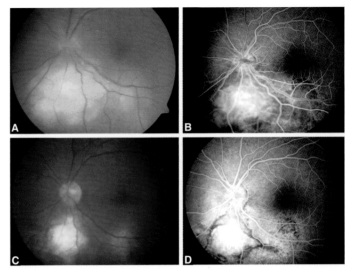

Figs 28.35A to D: Choroidal hemangioma. Pre- and post-transpupillary thermotherapy images of a patient with choroidal hemangioma. Decrease in tumor leakage and resolution of retinal detachment is observed

in the white population. They arise from choroidal melanocytes and have a great propensity for local and systemic spread (the liver being the most common site of metastasis). Hence they are a threat to both the patient's vision as well as life.

Histopathologically four types of choroidal melanomas are recognized based on the cell type: spindle cell, epithelioid cell, mixed type and necrotic type. Important prognostic factors include cell type, presence of extrascleral extension, size of tumor and anterior extent of tumor. These tumors have been classified based on size into small, medium and large. Laser photocoagulation has been used to treat only small melanomas.

The natural history of small choroidal melanoma is poorly understood. The collaborative ocular melanoma study reported 2-year and 5-year tumor growth rates of 21% and 31%, respectively. Clinical risk factors associated with tumor growth included increased tumor thickness, presence of subretinal fluid, orange pigmentation, absence of drusen, absence of retinal pigment, margin at the optic disc and epithelial changes surrounding the tumor. The 5-year melanoma-related mortality rate in patients treated for small choroidal melanomas has been reported as high as 12%.

One of the options for treating a small choroidal melanoma in the posterior fundus is laser photocoagulation alone or laser photocoagulation in combination with plaque radiotherapy. Laser photocoagulation using the argon laser has been described as being useful for tumors having up to 15 mm basal diameter and thickness up to 5 mm. However some authors have also reported laser photocoagulation as not being effective. Laser photocoagulation of melanomas can also lead to many complications like cystoid macular edema, branch vein occlusion, vitreous hemorrhage, optic atrophy, choroidal neovascularization and thrombotic glaucoma.

LASER IN RETINOPATHY OF PREMATURITY

Retinopathy of prematurity (ROP) is a vasoproliferative condition of the eye that occurs in premature infants. Risk factors include degree of prematurity, birth weight, supplemental oxygen therapy, systemic infections in the early weeks of delivery, etc. The disease occurs from abnormal maturation of the immature and incomplete retinal vasculature present at birth in babies born prematurely. The disease is potentially blinding and so screening of such children is a must for all countries in order to enable early detection and treatment, whenever indicated. Children with very early stages of retinopathy of prematurity do no need treatment because spontaneous regression is known to occur in a large majority.

The earlier recommendation on treating retinopathy of prematurity only when it approached the threshold stage was based on the disease having progressed enough that the risk of retinal detachment approached 50%. Using computer generated risk analysis; the early treatment of retinopathy of prematurity study (ETROP) has however indicated that treatment of early retinopathy of prematurity (even before development of threshold disease) may also have a beneficial effect in preventing later blindness from retinopathy of prematurity. Early treatment in ETROP study was defined as retinal ablation administered to the avascular retina when an eye reaches high-risk prethreshold retinopathy of prematurity. Prethreshold indicates any Zone I retinopathy of prematurity; or Zone II stage 2 with plus disease, or stage 3; or Zone II with less than 5 contiguous or 8 cumulative clock hours of stage 3 retinopathy of prematurity with plus disease.

The cryo-ROP study has very clearly identified the beneficial effect of ablating the retina in retinopathy of prematurity when the eye reaches the threshold stage. However, this form of treatment with cryo is known to be painful, results in greater lid edema and may lead to more respiratory distress (requiring temporary respirator facilities). Follow-up analysis has shown that cryo may also contribute to the myopic shift seen in a significant number of treated children. Cryo was possibly chosen in this study because laser indirect ophthalmoscopic delivery systems were not well developed and also because portable lasers were not readily available.

Currently, with the availability of portable lasers and laser indirect ophthalmoscopic delivery systems, laser has become the recommended treatment modality for infants with retinopathy of prematurity. In the available reports and studies, laser has been found to be at least as effective as cryotherapy. With regard to safety, it is considered superior to cryo as it is relatively painless, causes absent/minimal lid edema and risk of respiratory distress is marginal. Laser is also thought to decrease the risk of myopic shift. Retreatments are also reported to be easier with laser than with cryotherapy. Laser treated children have also been found to have better visual and anatomical results. Moreover, laser has been reported to be more cost effective.

Argon, diode laser and frequency-doubled YAG laser have all been used to treat retinopathy of prematurity. In one study using diode laser, 80% success was achieved with two sessions of laser with the disease usually regressing around the 39th week. During the first session about 900 laser spots were applied using a power of 200–1000 mW. About 40% eyes needed retreatment and the average number of spots applied at the second session averaged about 700.

MISCELLANEOUS PROCEDURES

YAG Laser Hyaloidotomy

Hemorrhage into the subhyaloid space overlying the macula can result in sudden and gross decrease of vision. Though the hemorrhage tends to layer over a period of time, its resolution and hence restoration of vision may be inordinately delayed. Apart from delayed visual recovery, premacular hemorrhage is also reported to induce late macular traction and iron toxicity. Significant premacular hemorrhage is usually unilateral and may result in conditions, such as diabetic retinopathy, aplastic anemia, Terson's syndrome, Valsalva retinopathy, vasculitis, ruptured retinal artery macroaneurysm, retinal vascular occlusions, etc.

Laser treatment to create a defect in the hyaloid under which the bleed is accumulated has been used to enhance resorption of premacular hemorrhage. Through the defect so created, blood escapes into the vitreous gel and is subsequently eliminated from the eye. Comparative studies have shown the procedure to be safe and effective.

Laser is delivered through the transpupillary route using a slit-lamp delivery system. Having obtained an informed consent, pupil is adequately dilated using cycloplegic-mydriatic drops. The cone angle is set at 10 degrees and laser energy is focused above the inferior extent of the hemorrhage to facilitate gravity-aided drainage of blood into the vitreous cavity. Begin with an energy of 1.5 mJ using single pulse. About 5–6 spots may be needed to create a dehiscence and a further 8–10 spots of lower energy to achieve drainage of the blood.

Recommendations while deciding on the suitability of a patient with premacular hemorrhage for YAG laser hyaloidotomy include:

1. *Duration of hemorrhage*: Premacular hemorrhage that has persisted beyond 4 weeks may be difficult to drain.
2. *Size of hemorrhage*: Usually more than 3 disc diameters. Smaller hemorrhages may risk formation of retinal holes.
3. *Absence of retinal proliferation*: If present do a full scatter first. Scatter laser may not be possible if vitreous hemorrhage remains for an extended period following hyaloidotomy.

Most patients are said to recover significant vision within the four weeks of the procedure if there is no underlying macular pathology. About 1 in 4 patients may develop non-resolving vitreous hemorrhage necessitating later vitreous surgery. Potential complications include the creation of retinal hole and retinal detachment. These complications are considered infrequent when compared to the risks of undertaking vitreous surgery in these eyes. Even if the laser procedure fails it is reported not to alter the outcome of subsequent vitreous surgery. Patients with underlying choroidal/retinal proliferation fare poorly with this procedure.

PROCEDURES TO IMPROVE POSTERIOR SEGMENT VISUALIZATION

YAG Laser Capsulotomy

After cataract or posterior capsular opacification is a common occurrence following cataract extraction and is reported to occur in 16 to 50% of patients. The prevalence of this complication depends primarily on the age of the patient at surgery, senile or complicated cataract, completeness of removal of the lens matter and type of intraocular lens implanted. When an after cataract evolves following cataract extraction, it leads to the same symptoms of a cataract, such as a decrease or blurring of vision and glare. The severity of these symptoms depends on the density of the after cataract. After cataract needs to be managed in order to treat concurrent posterior segment diseases with laser (e.g. diabetic retinopathy). This procedure is hence included herein.

Today, the most widely practiced procedure for the management of symptomatic after cataract is Neodymium:YAG laser capsulotomy. Before YAG laser capsulotomy, the risk-benefit ratio must be assessed by a complete clinical evaluation of the eye to be treated. This is necessary because the procedure is not always free of complications and these complications occur more often in a predisposed eye. Several complications have been reported following YAG laser capsulotomy and these include cystoid macular edema (< 1%), retinal detachment (total population 1.4% vs 2.8% after YAG capsulotomy), elevated intraocular pressure (< 3%), neovascularization of the iris in diabetics (< 1%) and rarely late onset endophthalmitis (< 1%). Patients with preoperative intraocular pressure more than 20 mm Hg, known glaucoma and prior filtering surgery, are at a higher risk of post-YAG capsulotomy elevation of intraocular pressure. In addition to these vision-threatening complications, a large number of patients develop pitting of the lens implant (in pseudophakic patients) or rupture of the anterior hyaloid face in aphakic patients. Hence, the following conditions must be considered as contraindications for undertaking this procedure if the patient's vision is not unduly reduced: One-eyed individuals, history of retinal detachment surgery/presence of predisposing lesions in the retinal periphery, active intraocular inflammation and pre-existing cystoid macular edema. If preoperative selection of patients is not proper, 2 to 7% of patients may experience a reduction in visual acuity following the procedure. This procedure is absolutely contraindicated in the presence of a glass intraocular lens as the implant may shatter.

The risk of some of the complications is strongly related to the following factors: Total energy delivered to the eye during the procedure and presence of predisposing lesions. The latter can be identified by a proper pre-laser work-up, including an indirect ophthalmoscopic evaluation. Total energy delivered depends to a large degree on the focusing technique as well as the density of the after cataract. The following procedure is recommended to achieve appropriate focusing during Nd:YAG capsulotomy:

- Adjust the eyepiece and then move the microscope towards the target so as to obtain good visibility of the after cataract.
- Fine tune the focus using the joystick such that the aiming beams of the laser (usually appear as red dots) are coincident on the membrane.
- Decrease the intensity of the aiming beam to a obtain good spot contrast with respect to the membrane.
- Adjust the posterior YAG offset wheel/lever to the recommended position. With energy of 1.2–1.5 mJ, the posterior YAG offset recommended is 150 μm. With higher energies, a greater posterior YAG offset must be used (250 μm) since in such circumstances, the plasma elongates anteriorly along the axis of the laser beam increasing the risk of intraocular lens pitting. An offset closer to zero also increases the risk of intraocular lens pitting.
- Use of an appropriate contact lens helps in achieving better focus and hence in achieving the desired photodisruptive effect with lesser energy.

For routine use, discission of the membrane must first be attempted using the lowest possible energy (0.5–1.5 mJ) and then increasing it at 0.5–1.0 mJ steps if necessary. The burst mode must be avoided for all practical purposes. It may be considered as a last resort in cases with very thick after cataract. Reported mean energy needed in most patients has been 2.5–3.0 mJ and discission could be achieved in 97% of cases with less than 5 mJ of energy. Also, the minimum number of pulses must be used.

The procedure must be undertaken without pupillary dilation when the procedure is performed to restore visual acuity (whenever the pupillary aperture before treatment is normal). This ensures that the opening created corresponds to the pupillary aperture and is not excessive. If the procedure is done to improve posterior segment visualization, prior pupillary dilation may be of greater value.

As some patients may develop significant elevation of the intraocular pressure, the intraocular pressure must be monitored during the initial 24 hours (more so in the first 2–5 hours). Using one drop of apraclonidine one hour before the procedure and one drop after can decrease increase in intraocular pressure. If apraclonidine is not available one may use timolol eyedrops. In addition, patients must be treated with topical corticosteroid eyedrops four times daily for atleast 3 days following the procedure.

Neodymium:YAG Sweeping

Not uncommonly, it is seen that following cataract surgery patients develop significant intraocular inflammation followed by deposition of variable amounts of inflammatory debris and pigment on the anterior surface of the intraocular lens. These deposits may not resolve despite treatment with topical corticosteroids for an adequate period of time and may also lead to blurred vision. In such situations, the technique of Nd:YAG sweeping has been reported to be safe and effective in clearing the deposits over the anterior surface of the implant.

The recommended technique is as follows:

- Pupil must preferably be in the mid-dilated position and no contact lens is necessary.
- Move the microscope to obtain good visibility of the anterior surface of intraocular lens.
- Using the joystick, fine focus the aiming beams to achieve a point focus on the anterior surface of intraocular.
- Now, slightly defocus the beam anteriorly by moving the joystick or using the anterior defocus lever (if available in the machine).
- Deliver the laser pulse (single) using an energy level of 0.5–1.0 mJ.
- The usual number of spots required to obtain adequate clearing of the deposits have ranged from 6–16. Post-laser treatment is with topical corticosteroids and timolol maleate for 3 days. Authors following this procedure have reported minimal post-laser inflammation and no intraocular pressure elevation.

Nd:YAG sweeping is said to achieve its effect by generating an acoustic shock wave within the aqueous that while sweeping over the anterior IOL surface of intraocular lens dislodges any uncoalesced inflammatory deposits or pigment.

Coreoplasty

This is the technique of enlarging the pupil (photomydriasis) or changing its contour (pupilloplasty) by application of laser energy.

Technique

- Anesthetize and insert appropriate contact lens (e.g. Abraham lens)
- Set following laser parameters: single pulse, 200–500 μm spot size, 0.2 second duration and a power of 200–500 mW.
- For photomydriasis: Place 2–3 rows of burns circumferentially around the pupillary margin. The first row must be 1 mm away from the margin of the pupil. The innermost row has about 8 spots and is created using a spot size of 200 μm and power of 200–400 mW. The outer rows consist of 10–12 spots formed by a laser spot size of 400 μm and power of 300–500 mW.
- For stretching an up drawn pupil: The laser parameters are as for photomydriasis, but the laser burns are placed only along the inferior margin of the up drawn pupil. Also, the innermost row of burns must be about 2 mm from the pupillary margin.

Diagrammatic representation of Coreoplasty is shown in Figure 28.36.

Nd:YAG Vitreolysis

Before considering any treatment option in patients with postsurgical cystoid macular edema, it is important to ascertain its cause and nature. Angiographic cystoid macular edema alone does not warrant any treatment. In patients with clinically significant cystoid macular edema, medical, laser and surgical interventions become necessary depending on the cause and initial response to medical treatment alone. Topical nonsteroidal anti-inflammatory drugs and topical or periocular corticosteroids form the mainstay in medical management. Ketorolac tromethamine 0.5% given four times daily for three months has been found to be effective in bringing about a resolution of the macular edema. A more recent report has shown however that a dual therapy with nonsteroidal anti-inflammatory drugs and topical corticosteroids is superior to either of the drugs prescribed alone. Some authors recommend the concurrent use of oral indomethacin 25 mg thrice daily for 10 days at this stage. If no response is seen following topical therapy, one must consider injection of corticosteroids into the periocular space. The usual drugs are triamcinolone or methylprednisolone 20 mg in 0.5 mL. If no response is seen following one injection, the rationale for giving repeat injections is questionable. The next consideration should be prescription of oral corticosteroids at a dosage of 1–1.5 mg/kg/day, followed by a gradual taper. Although corticosteroids are prescribed, most reported studies have not shown any benefit in terms of improvement in visual acuity.

When obvious aggravating factors are evident, like vitreous incarceration in the wound or intraocular lens malposition, the same should be managed early (if initial medical therapy fails or there are relapses) to prevent the edema from becoming chronic. Some authors to manage fine vitreous strands adherent

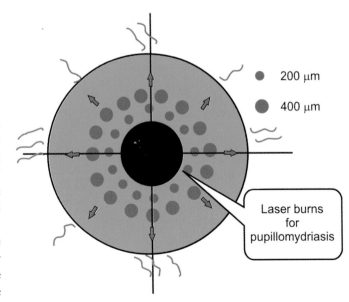

Fig. 28.36: Diagrammatic representation of laser technique for achieving pupillomydriasis

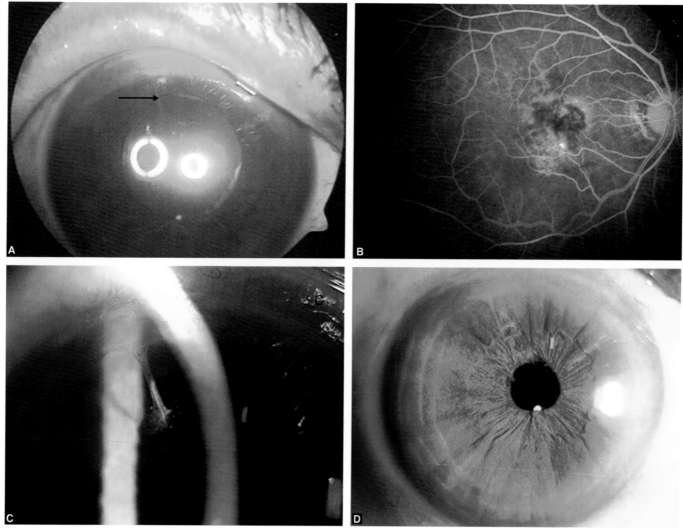

Figs 28.37A to D: Pre (A) and post (C, D) YAG vitreolysis photographs in a patient with post-cataract surgery cystoid macular edema (B) and vitreous incarceration into the wound (see arrow in Fig. 28.37A).

to the wound have used YAG laser vitreolysis successfully. This modality of treatment has the risk of producing retinal detachment and elevation of intraocular pressure. In many cases, it is probably more prudent to undertake pars plana vitrectomy as vitreous adherent to the iris can also be removed.

Successful sectioning of vitreous strand going into the cataract wound in a patient with concurrent and macular edema resistant to medical therapy is shown in Figures 28.37 A to D. This patient had a visual improvement of one line (from 20/60 to 20/40) following the procedure.

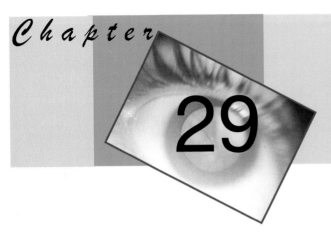

29

Anti-Vascular Endothelial Growth Factor Therapy

Atul Kumar, Subijoy Sinha

INTRODUCTION

Michaelson first suggested that a diffusible "Factor X" from the retina stimulated the retinal and iris neovascularization seen in diabetic retinopathy. Two decades ago, a molecule was identified in the conditioned media from bovine pituitary follicular cells that promoted the proliferation of endothelial cells and was called vascular endothelial growth factor (VEGF). In 1992, it was demonstrated that hypoxia could up-regulate VEGF expression. It had long been appreciated that neovascularization of the retina and iris is related to retinal ischemia due to various etiologies, and the property of hypoxia inducibility made VEGF a plausible candidate for the "Factor X," proposed by Michaelson, as the mediator of abnormal blood vessel growth in the eye. Evidence from both clinical and animal studies accumulated in the next several years to support the critical role of VEGF in ocular neovascularization.

Angiogenesis

The development of new blood vessels from preexisting ones, a process known as angiogenesis, is a physiological process that is fundamental to normal healing, reproduction and embryonic development. Angiogenesis plays an important role in a variety of pathologic processes, including tumors, proliferative retinopathies and wet age-related macular degeneration (AMD) (Figs 29.1 and 29.2).

Vascular Endothelial Growth Factor

Over the past decade, our understanding of the complex processes involved in new vessel development has led to the isolation of a family of angiogenic stimulators known collectively as vascular endothelial growth factor (VEGF). Of the various members of the VEGF family namely-VEGF-A, VEGF-B, VEGF-C, VEGF-D and VEGF-E, VEGF-A (Fig. 29.3) plays the pivotal angiogenic stimulator that binds to VEGF receptors promoting endothelial cell migration, proliferation and increasing vascular permeability. VEGF exerts its action on endothelial cells through the VEGFR-1 and VEGFR-2 receptors (Fig. 29.4).

Measurements of vitreous VEGF levels demonstrated significantly higher VEGF concentrations in patients with active proliferative diabetic retinopathy compared to patients

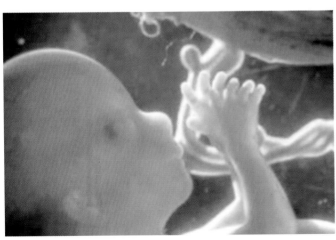

Fig. 29.1: Angiogenesis: Normal angiogenesis

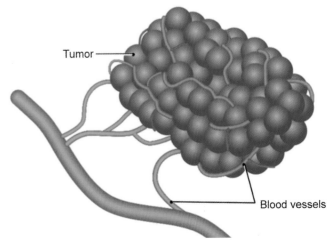

Tumor

Blood vessels

Fig. 29.2: Angiogenesis: Abnormal angiogenesis

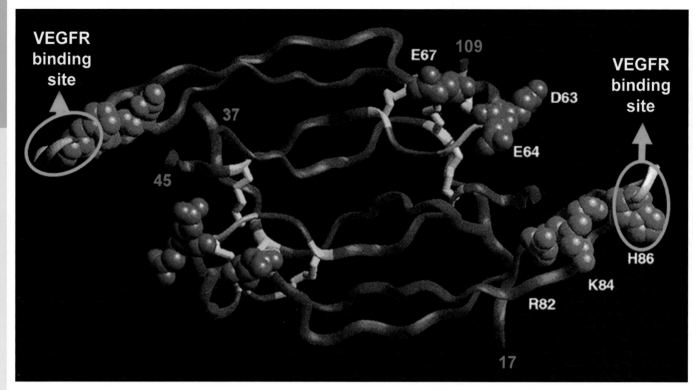

Fig. 29.3: Vascular endothelial growth factor: The VEGF-A molecule

other retinal disorders not characterized by abnormal blood vessel growth.

Role of Vascular Endothelial Growth Factor in Angiogenesis

Following are the significant roles of VEGF in angiogenesis:
- Stimulates cell migration and inhibits apoptosis
- Stimulates endothelial cell growth
- Survival factor for newly formed vessels
- Chemotactic factor for inflammatory cells
- Primary driver of angiogenesis
- Inflammatory processes are involved in the formation of choroidal neovascular membrane and interact with VEGF-A expression.

The exact trigger that starts the VEGF cascade and results in neovascularization is not known. However, there are many stimuli that cause over-expression of VEGF, including reduction in the choriocapillaris blood flow, accumulation of lipid metabolic byproducts, oxidative stress and alterations in Bruch's membrane. Clearly the VEGF cascade is a cyclic process that is self perpetuating once set in motion. Along different pathways, the VEGF cascade leads to choroidal neovascularization with the breakdown of the blood-retinal barrier—the hallmarks of neovascular AMD (Fig. 29.5).

The strong supportive evidence from animal studies defined VEGF as an optimal therapeutic target for the treatment of

Fig. 29.4: Vascular endothelial growth factor. Binding of VEGF to its receptor leads to angiogenesis and increase in vascular permeability

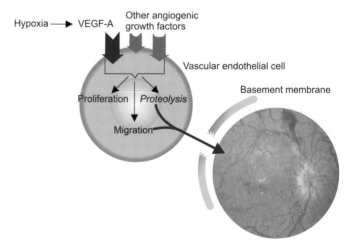

Fig. 29.5: Vascular endothelial growth factor: The VEGF cascade leading to angiogenesis

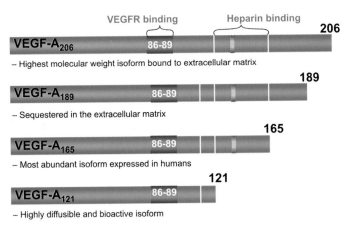

Fig. 29.6: Vascular endothelial growth factor: The different VEGF-A isoforms

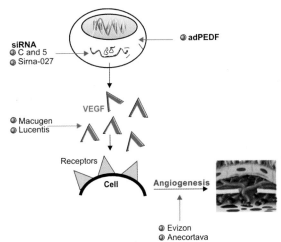

Fig. 29.7: Anti-VEGF therapy: Mechanism of action of anti-VEGF therapy in wet age-related macular degeneration

ocular diseases in which neovascularization leads to blindness. The need for better treatments for neovascular AMD, leading cause of blindness in individuals over the age of 55, provided the opportunity to develop anti-VEGF agents for clinical use. While regression of retinal neovascularization due to proliferative diabetic retinopathy and ischemic retinal vein occlusion can, in most cases, be successfully achieved with laser photocoagulation, laser treatment for subfoveal choroidal neovascularization due to AMD is suboptimal due to the inevitable destruction of the foveal retina. Choroidal neovascular membranes have demonstrated both VEGF and VEGF receptors as seen histopathologically in choroidal neovascular lesions that have been excised from surgical patients and also from autopsy eyes.

There are five different isoforms of VEGF-A with varying numbers of amino acids due to alternative splicing of the VEGF mRNA (Fig. 29.6). The VEGF-165 isoform is the most potent and responsible for angiogenesis.

ANTI-VEGF THERAPY IN WET AGE-RELATED MACULAR DEGENERATION

The strong supportive evidence from animal studies defined VEGF as an optimal therapeutic target for the treatment of ocular diseases in which neovascularization leads to blindness (Fig. 29.7). The need for better treatments for neovascular AMD, a leading cause of blindness in individuals over the age of 50, provided the opportunity to develop anti-VEGF agents for clinical use. While regression of retinal neovascularization due to proliferative diabetic retinopathy and ischemic retinal vein occlusion can, in most cases, be successfully achieved with laser photocoagulation, laser treatment for subfoveal choroidal neovascularization due to AMD is suboptimal due to the inevitable destruction of the foveal retina. The introduction of photodynamic therapy in 2,000 offered the first selective treatment for choroidal neovascular membrane, allowing for the closure of choroidal neovascular membranes with relative sparing of the overlying retina. However, the visual results left room for improvement.

Pegaptanib emerged as the first antiangiogenic agent with proven efficacy in clinical trials for neovascular AMD. It is a modified 28-base RNA aptamer that selectively binds VEGF.

Anti-VEGF drugs being used or being investigated in wet age-related macular degeneration:

- Pegaptanib (Macugen)
- Ranibizumab (Lucentis)
- Bevacizumab (Avastin)
- Anecortave acetae (Retaane)
- VEGF-trap
- Squalamine Lactate (Evizon)
- Combretastatin-A4 Prodrug (CA4P)
- AdPEDF
- siRNA
- C and 5
- TG100801

Pegaptanib

Pegaptanib (Macugen) is a synthetic oligonucleotide that binds to the pathologic isoform of VEGF, which is VEGF 165 and this binding, happens in the extracellular space. The molecule is then prevented from interacting with the VEGF receptor (Fig. 29.8).

The FDA approved it in December 2004, with a brand label for indication and usage that included treatment of all neovascular or wet age-related macular degeneration; however the drug results have been largely equivocal.

Ranibizumab

Ranibizumab (Lucentis) was genetically manipulated from bevacizumab and is presently FDA approved for usage. Vascular endothelial growth factor has multiple isomers, isoforms that are formed by different splicing of the original messenger RNA. Ranibizumab binds in such a region so that all the

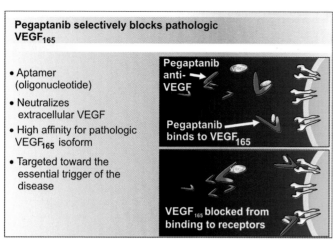

Pegaptanib selectively blocks pathologic VEGF₁₆₅

- Aptamer (oligonucleotide)
- Neutralizes extracellular VEGF
- High affinity for pathologic VEGF₁₆₅ isoform
- Targeted toward the essential trigger of the disease

Pegaptanib anti-VEGF

Pegaptanib binds to VEGF₁₆₅

VEGF₁₆₅ blocked from binding to receptors

Fig. 29.8: Anti-VEGF therapy: Mechanism of action of pegaptanib

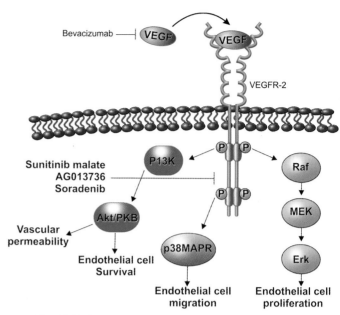

Fig. 29.10: Bevacizumab: Site of the action of bevacizumab

isoforms are bound, including VEGF-110, a plasmin cleaved form of VEGF-165. Following treatment, optical coherence tomography reveals reduced intraretinal and subretinal fluid (Figs 29.9A and B). Currently a number of large randomized double masked trials are underway, which are investigating these drugs either as monotherapy or as combination therapy.

Currently a number of large randomized double-masked trials are underway, which are investigating these drugs either as a monotherapy or as a combination therapy.

- *FOCUS trial-phase 1/2 trial:* Ranibizumab + photodynamic therapy versus photodynamic therapy in predominantly classic lesions.

- *MARINA trial-phase 3 trial:* Ranibizumab vs sham injection in minimally classic or occult with no classic lesions.

  Both FOCUS and MARINA year 1 results showed favorable outcome with ranibizumab in terms of loss of fewer than 15 letters and other visual outcomes also favored ranibizumab. Adverse effects were also very few.

- *PIER trial- phase 3b:* Ranibizumab vs sham injection.

- *ANCHOR Trial-Phase 3 trial:* Ranibizumab vs photodynamic therapy in predominantly classic lesions.

- *PROTECT study:* Combination therapy of intravitreal ranibizumab injection and photodynamic therapy.

Bevacizumab

The anti-VEGF drug, which has opened up new vistas in the management of choroidal neovascular membranes secondary to wet AMD is bevacizumab (Avastin). Bevacizumab is a humanized monoclonal antibody that inhibits all active isoforms of VEGF (Fig. 29.10) and is approved by the United States Food and Drug Administration (USFDA), since February 2004, for the treatment of metastatic colorectal cancer. It was developed as an intravenous therapy for cancer patients because VEGF is one of the major angiogenic stimuli responsible for neovascularization in tumors. Ranibizumab, a humanized monoclonal antibody fragment against VEGF highly related in structure to bevacizumab, has also proven efficacious in the treatment of subfoveal choroidal neovascularization due to AMD. A number of studies have shown encouraging results after using ranibizumab in wet AMD and currently is in the process of review by the USFDA.

Bevacizumab, which is FDA approved for use in metastatic colorectal cancer came to the attention of ophthalmologists as an anti-VEGF antibody (although not a fragment like

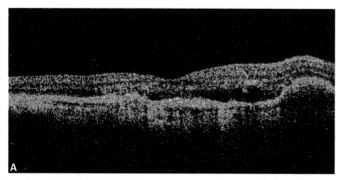

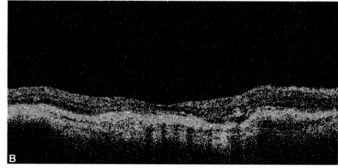

Figs 29.9A and B: Ranibizumab for classic choroidal neovascular membrane. (A) Optical coherence tomography shows a classic choroidal neovascular membrane with subretinal fluid. (B) Resolution of fluid one month following 0.3 mg intravitreal ranifizumab injection

ranibizumab, a VEGF antibody fragment that was specifically developed for intraocular use).

Treatment of wet AMD was started with the off-label use of intravitreal bevacizumab and a dramatic therapeutic response was noted. Initially, it was deemed unlikely that this big molecule (it is a humanized monoclonal antibody) would penetrate the full thickness of the retina when given intravitreally. Intravitreal use of bevacizumab involves both, an off-label application of the drug and an alternative route of drug delivery. Improvement in visual acuity and a decrease in retinal thickness have led the retinal community to embrace this new treatment. As a result, the use of intravitreal bevacizumab has increased exponentially in the past several months. The main force driving intravitreal bevacizumab usage is the high percentage of patients who experience symptomatic relief from active subfoveal choroidal neovascularization (Fig. 29.11).

There are a number of factors surrounding intraocular use of bevacizumab. These include:

- High efficacy
- Longer half-life thus reducing the number of injections
- Potential antigenicity of the full antibody
- Lack of preservatives is a potential benefit with bevacizumab
- Potential retinal toxicity in higher doses (>3.5 mg), we currently use 1.25 mg, which is extremely safe
- Low cost of bevacizumab versus ranibizumab or pegaptanib

- Bevacizumab is a full-sized antibody, unlike the ranibizumab fragment and has a longer half-life (up to 20 days) and thus longer anti-VEGF action (in contrast, the half-life of ranibizumab was targeted for four hours).

Reasons to use bevacizumab center on this one fact: fast onset of improved retinal morphology and visual acuity. Indeed, the reports show dramatic improvement in optical coherence tomography appearance and corresponding improvement in visual acuity. Other reasons to use it include its low cost and wide availability, with no experimentally proven toxicity shown till date.

For patients who have failed therapy with approved drugs and have not yet evolved to disciform scars, off-label bevacizumab could be recommended as a salvage therapy. Among these reasons, the overwhelming reason to use it is of course, efficacy.

ANTI-VEGF THERAPY IN DIABETIC RETINOPATHY

The discovery and cloning of VEGF and the subsequent development of antibodies to it allowed for the identification of VEGF's key role in the development of retinal neovascularization. Studies have demonstrated not only a correlation of VEGF levels with the severity of proliferative diabetic retinopathy (PDR), but also a reduction in levels after successful laser

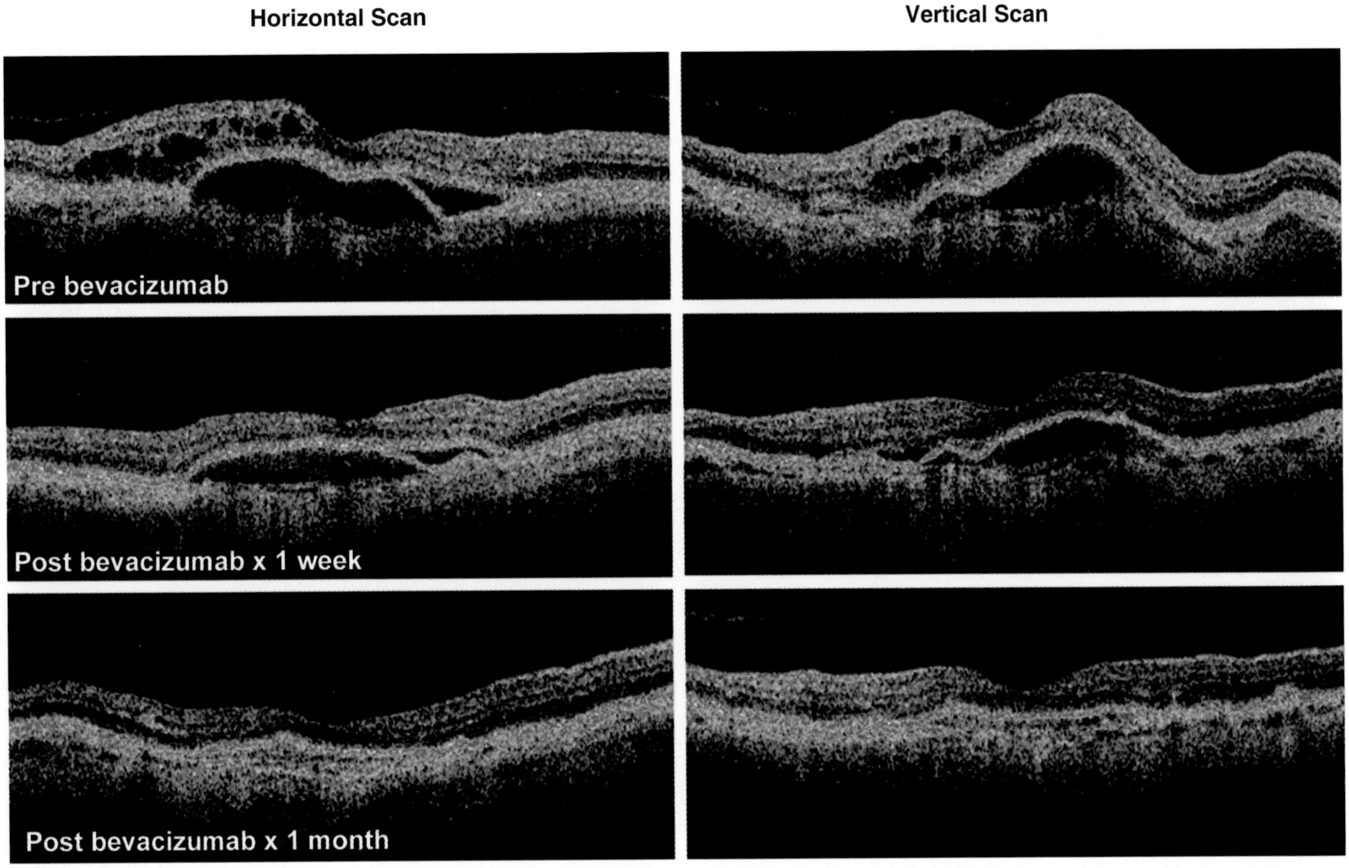

Horizontal Scan	Vertical Scan

Fig. 29.11: Bevacizumab for occult choroidal neovascular membrane: Serial optical coherence tomography scans show resolution of pigment epithelial detachment after intravitreal 1.25 mg bevacizumab

treatment of PDR. Injection of VEGF in primates can produce a retinopathy similar to diabetic retinopathy and even produce iris neovascularization. Furthermore, inhibition of VEGF can prevent iris neovascularization in primates. In addition, VEGF is a potent inducer of vascular permeability and has a role to play in diabetic macular edema.

ANTI-VEGF THERAPY IN DIABETIC MACULAR EDEMA

Diabetic macular edema is the swelling of the retina resulting from the exudation and accumulation of extracellular fluid and proteins in the macula. Exudation arises from structural changes in the endothelium of retinal vasculature that lead to the breakdown of the blood-retina barrier and an increase in vascular permeability. Nearly half of the world's diabetic population has some degree of diabetic retinopathy and diabetic macular edema is a leading cause of blindness in these patients. The prevalence of diabetic macular edema in the diabetic population is 10%, but the prevalence is dramatically increased in eyes with more severe retinopathy.

Vascular endothelial growth factor (VEGF-A) has been implicated as an important factor in the occurrence of vascular permeability in ocular disease, such as diabetic macular edema. Vascular endothelial growth factor was originally described as "tumor vascular permeability factor" for its ability to induce vascular leakage in an animal model. In diabetic macular edema, the development of retinal ischemia leads to an increase in the production of VEGF-A, which increases vascular permeability by affecting endothelial tight junction proteins. In patients with diabetic macular edema, VEGF-A levels are significantly elevated relative to patients with nondiabetic ocular disease, including macular holes and epiretinal membranes. In addition, VEGF-A levels are significantly higher in diabetic macular edema patients showing extensive leakage in the macular region than in patients showing minimal leakage. These observations have implicated VEGF-A as an important therapeutic target in the treatment of ocular diseases characterized by excess vascularization and permeability.

Currently, there are 2 main anti-VEGF therapies for the treatment of ocular disorders, each of which targets a distinct set of VEGF-A isoforms. Human VEGF-A is found in at least 9 isoforms derived from alternate exon splicing of the VEGF-A gene: VEGF121, VEGF 145, VEGF148, VEGF 162, VEGF 165, VEGF 183, VEGF 189 and VEGF 206. All isoforms carry the plasmin cleavage site and have the potential to be cleaved by plasmin to generate a smaller form, VEGF. Pegaptanib is a ribonucleic acid aptamer that targets only the VEGF 165 isoform, and it is currently approved for the treatment of neovascular AMD. Ranibizumab which is a fully humanized monoclonal anti-VEGF-A Fab fragment was designed to bind all biologically active forms of VEGF-A. Ranibizumab which is approved for treatment of neovascular AMD has also been tried in the treatment of diabetic macular edema. Bevacizumab has also recently been shown to be effective in persistent diffuse diabetic macular edema. Figures 29.12A and B shows resolution of cystoid macular edema after intravitreal bevacizumab.

ANTI-VEGF TREATMENT FOR PROLIFERATIVE DIABETIC RETINOPATHY

Since the diabetic retinopathy study, panretinal photocoagulation has been the treatment of choice for PDR. It has proven to be remarkably effective and has saved vision in countless patients over the past several decades. However, it is a destructive therapy with adverse effects, such as loss of peripheral visual field and night vision as well as the exacerbation of macular edema and subsequent reduction of central vision. In patients with media opacity, such as vitreous hemorrhage or cataract, it is not always possible to administer complete panretinal photocoagulation. Furthermore, patients with iris neovascularization and neovascular glaucoma often present with hyphema and corneal edema, which prevent full laser treatment, and there are case that, despite extensive panretinal photocoagulation, continues to demonstrate progressive retinal anterior hyaloidal proliferation and iris neovascularization. Therefore there has existed an urgent need for an alternative or adjunctive therapy for PDR.

There are a large number of initial encouraging reports of intravitreal bevacizumab in cases of proliferative diabetic retinopathy. In most of the cases there has been a dramatic and rapid response to the injection, with complete resolution of the vascular leakage (Figs 29.13A to 29.14B). This rapid biologic effect is not surprising, as previous animal studies have demonstrated that intravitreal VEGF antibodies can produce a similar effect on iris neovascularization induced by vein occlusions in primates. Both pegaptanib and bevacizumab have

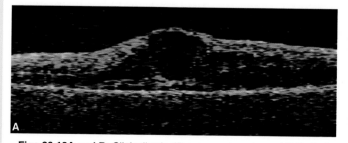
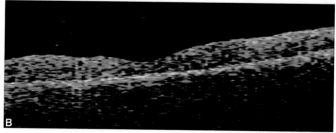

Figs 29.12A and B: Clinically significant macular edema. (A) Optical coherence tomography shows cystic macula and serous retinal detachment (B) Resolution of cystic spaces and serous retinal detachment at 6 weeks following 1.25 mg intravitreal bevacizumab

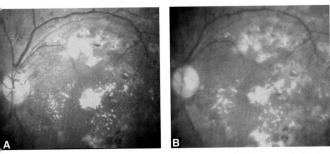

Figs 29.13A and B: Proliferative diabetic retinopathy. (A) Neovascularization at the disc (B) Regression of neovascularization following intravitreal bevacizumab

been shown to be effective in inducing regression of retinal neovascularization secondary to PDR.

There is, however, also the possibility that the pan-isoform inhibition of bevacizumab may increase its toxicity. However till date there are no reports of any toxicity with the dose of bevacizumab used in intravitreal injection (1.25 mg in 0.05 ml), which is about 300 to 400 fold lower than that administered intravenous in colorectal cancer patients.

Bevacizumab's role in the treatment of PDR will likely be limited by the duration of its effect. Panretinal photocoagulation, despite its shortcomings, has remarkable durability in the vast majority of patients treated. In many of the patients of PDR treated with intravitreal bevacizumab recurrence has been noted as early as 3–4 weeks after injection. It remains unclear how frequently repeat anti-VEGF therapy would be necessary to ensure the regression of neovascularization and panretinal photocoagulation may seem to be advantageous. However, even a transient effect of intravitreal bevacizumab may prove to be of benefit in a variety of clinical settings, such as when media opacity prevents the placement of panretinal photocoagulation, or in cases of severe PDR with concurrent macular edema, in which injection of bevacizumab in conjunction with gentle panretinal photocoagulation may minimize the exacerbation of macular edema, which can sometimes be caused by panretinal photocoagulation.

Adjunct Role of Intravitreal Bevacizumab in Surgery for Proliferative Diabetic Retinopathy

Intravitreal bevacizumab may have an adjunctive role in the surgical treatment of PDR and tractional retinal detachment, as preoperative administration may allow less intraoperative bleeding when cutting fibrovascular tissue. Less bleeding could facilitate surgery and, in theory, also make it safer by reducing the need to elevate intraocular pressure for homeostasis in these patients with impaired retinovascular perfusion.

ANTI-VEGF THERAPY IN RETINAL VEIN OCCLUSION

Retinal vein occlusion, including both central retinal vein occlusion (CRVO) and branch retinal vein occlusion (BRVO) represents the largest group of vascular retinal affections after arteriosclerotic hypertensive changes and diabetic retinopathy. Retinal venous occlusive disease can involve the central trunk or branches of the venous circulation.

Anti-VEGF Therapy in Central Retinal Vein Occlusion

The main risk factors for central retina vein occlusion include age, hypertension, arteriosclerosis, diabetes, hypercholesterolemia and elevated serum homocysteine levels. Visual loss associated with retinal vein occlusion can be a result of macular edema, macular ischemia, and other complications associated with anterior and posterior segment neovascularization. The main strategy to reduce visual loss in these patients has been the treatment of macular edema.

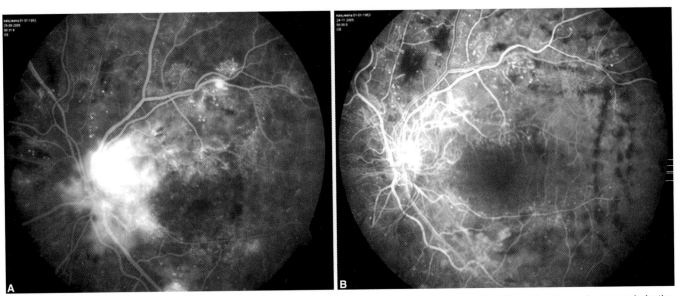

Figs 29.14A and B: Proliferative diabetic retinopathy: (A) Fluorescein angiography shows gross neovascularization of the disc and neovascularization elsewhere, (B) Regression of neovascularization at the disc and neovascularization elsewhere 2 weeks following intravitreal bevacizumab (1.25 mg)

Pathogenesis can be represented in three stages:
1) Triggering of the venous outflow reduction;
2) Development of the retinopathy; and
3) Transition into severe neovascular disease.

The goal of central retinal vein occlusion therapy is to prevent: (1) chronic macular edema and macular scarring and (2) neovascular complications.

Anti-VEGF Therapy for Macular Edema

The rationale for the use of VEGF inhibitors is to reduce macular edema, an important cause of visual loss in these patients (Figs 29.15A to 29.17B). The off-label use of anti-VEGF agents in patients with retinal vein occlusion has been impressive in some cases, although it is well recognized that the natural history is variable in patients with retinal vein occlusion. Controlled clinical trials are needed to determine and quantify the safety and benefit of treating macular edema with anti-VEGF therapy versus current standard therapies or observation.

A number of pilot trials and two larger multicenter trials are currently evaluating whether inhibition of VEGF by ranibizumab may be an effective treatment for macular edema associated with retinal vein occlusion. A phase 3 multicenter, prospective clinical trials is currently underway, assessing the safety, tolerability, and efficacy of intravitreal ranibizumab injection in the treatment of macular edema secondary to central retinal

vein occlusion. CRUISE is a phase 3, multicenter, randomized, sham injection-controlled study of the efficacy and safety of ranibizumab injection compared with sham in patients with macular edema secondary to central retinal vein occlusion. This Genentech-sponsored trial was designed in conjunction with the US Food and Drug Administration (FDA), potentially to allow approval of the drug for the treatment of retinal vein occlusion.

Besides ranibizumab there are several reports (nonrandomized uncontrolled) of beneficial effects of bevacizumab in macular edema secondary to retinal vein occlusion. Though the advent of anti-VEGF injections has opened a new frontier towards treating patients with macular edema, one area of concern may be the reports of rebound macular edema following intravitreal bevacizumab injections. In the eyes where the macular edema recurred, it was more pronounced than at the initial presentation. This evolution may actually represent a rebound phenomenon. Specifically, molecular processes in the VEGF cascade may be inhibited and/or stimulated resulting in an increase in edema.

Anti-VEGF Therapy for Neovascular Complications

Neovascular complications usually start with iris/angle neovascularization and culminate in secondary neovascular glaucoma. Currently, panretinal photocoagulation is the only standard

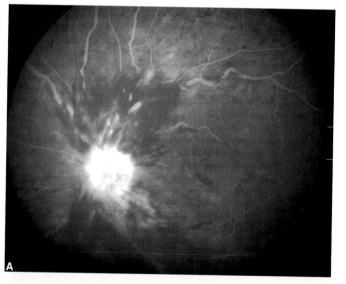
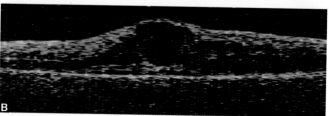

Figs 29.15A and B: Central retinal vein occlusion. (A) Fluorescein angiography shows macular edema. (B) Optical coherence tomography shows cystoid macular edema

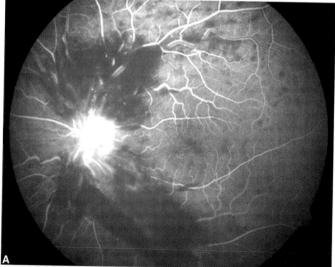
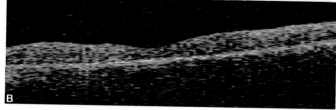

Figs 29.16A and B: Central retinal vein occlusion. (A) Six months after monthly treatment with 1.25 mg intravitreal bevacizumab, resolution of the macular edema is visible. (B) Optical coherence tomography shows resolution of the cystoid macular edema

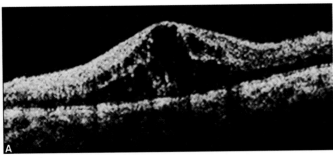
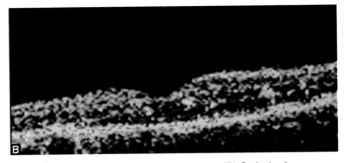

Figs 29.17A and B : Central retinal vein occlusion: (A) Optical coherence tomography shows cystoid macular edema. (B) Optical coherence tomography shows marked reduction of the macular edema three months after treatment with monthly dosing with intravitreal ranibizumab

treatment of choice. Vascular endothelial growth factor levels in patients with ischemic retinal pathologic features are reduced indirectly after laser photocoagulation.

Direct targeting of VEGF with anti-VEGF therapy may be another possible therapeutic strategy to treat ocular neovascularization. Recent encouraging results from several small case studies of intravitreal bevacizumab in the treatment of iris neovascularization, neovascular glaucoma or both promoted the authors to consider the drug as the first treatment of choice not only for iris neovascularization, but also for more severe neovascular glaucoma secondary to ischemic retinal disorders. The rapid biologic effect of bevacizumab is favorable and is not surprising. However, the effect of bevacizumab on regression of iris neovascularization may be transient because of the drug's short half life. Another concern is that the pan-isoform inhibition of VEGF may increase its side effects in normal retinal tissue and circulation. The RAVE (Rubeosis Anti-VEGF) trial, utilizes monthly intravitreal ranibizumab injections for nine months to see if total VEGF blockade will prevent neovascular glaucoma and eliminate the need for panretinal photocoagulation in patients with ischemic central retinal vein occlusion.

Anti-VEGF Therapy in Branch Retinal Vein Occlusion

The pathological process at the site of branch retinal vein occlusion consists of degenerative changes in the vessel walls, abnormal blood constituents and blood flow (stasis). These three classical components, known as Virchow's triad, that play a role in thrombogenesis are interrelated.

The fact that branch retinal vein occlusion is typically located at arterial overcrossings suggests a hemodynamic difference between arterial and venous overcrossings.

Treatment of branch retinal vein occlusion has two aims: To reduce macular edema and to prevent neovascularization caused by retinal ischemia.

Currently anti-VEGF injections in the form of bevacizumab and ranibizumab are being used very commonly for the management of macular edema (Figs 29.18A to C). Application of VEGF inhibitors represents a treatment option that targets the disease at the causal molecular level. Increased VEGF levels were measured in patients with vein occlusion and correlated with the extent of macular edema. Anti-VEGF is a potent anti-edematous agent, possibly specifically reducing the permeability of retinal capillaries or even down regulating VEGF, but they

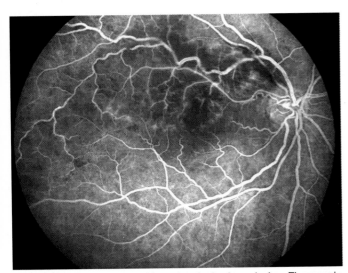

Fig. 29.18A: Superotemporal branch retinal vein occlusion. Fluorescein angiography shows macular edema

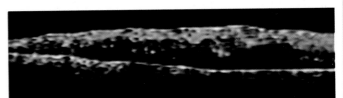

Fig. 29.18B: Superotemporal branch retinal vein occlusion: Optical coherence tomography shows macular edema with cystoid spaces

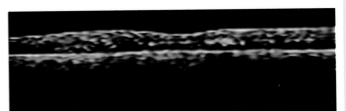

Fig. 29.18C: Superotemporal branch retinal vein occlusion: Optical coherence tomography shows reduction of macular edema three months after treatment with two doses of 1.25 mg bevacizumab given six weeks apart

do not eliminate the cause of the disease. The exact duration of therapeutic effect is as yet unknown and seems to decrease within a few weeks. The need for repeat injections has been reported after four weeks.

BRAVO is a phase 3, multicenter, randomized, sham injection-controlled study of the efficacy and safety of ranibizumab injection compared with sham in patients with macular edema secondary to branch retinal vein occlusion.

Spectrum of the use of anti-VEGF therapy is expanding with good results in Eales' disease and refractory postsurgical cystoid macular edema.

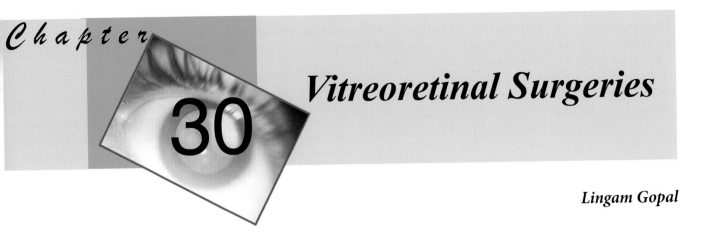

Management of posterior segment diseases has undergone a sea of change with the introduction of vitrectomy. Many diseases considered inoperable have become amenable to treatment. This chapter deals with the current management strategies of some selected important posterior segment disorders, wherein surgery is the mainstay of management—namely rhegmatogenous retinal detachment; proliferative vitreoretinopathy (PVR); giant retinal tear; dislocated lens and intraocular lens; endophthalmitis; retinopathy of prematurity, diabetic retinopathy, vein occlusions and intraocular foreign body.

RHEGMATOGENOUS RETINAL DETACHMENT

Introduction

Rhegmatogenous retinal detachment by definition is the separation of the neurosensory retina from the underlying retinal pigment epithelium caused by the presence of a retinal break. Although the occurrence of retinal detachment was known for a long time, the relation of the same with retinal break was identified first by Jules Gonin. With the widespread use of indirect ophthalmoscope popularized by Charles Schepens, the management of rhegmatogenous retinal detachment has undergone a dramatic change. The advent of vitreous surgery due to the pioneering efforts of Robert Machemer has increased the scope of surgical correction of different types of retinal detachment. Other important contribution in the management of relatively simple retinal detachments is of George Hilton in the form of pneumatic retinopexy.

Normal retina remains attached due to the multitude of factors, such as adhesion caused by interdigitations between retinal pigment epithelium and photoreceptors, presence of viscous matrix that binds the photoreceptors to retinal pigment epithelium, the metabolic pump of the retinal pigment epithelium, and the mechanical action of the vitreous gel. When the balance of forces is disrupted, retinal detachment results. Hence, the presence of retinal hole alone does not suffice to cause retinal detachment, but needs additional vitreous traction along with fluid currents that lift up the retina around the hole to initiate retinal detachment. Treatment modalities aim at altering the physical forces, such as:

a. Cutting of the access to subretinal space,
b. Altering the net balance of forces by relieving vitreous traction by placing a scleral buckle or removing the offending vitreous, and
c. Increasing the adhesive force between the retinal pigment epithelium/choroid and the neurosensory retina around the retinal hole by creating inflammatory reaction using cryo or photocoagulation or diathermy.

Symptomatology

The patients may present with symptoms, such as floaters, flashes, and vision loss or field loss. On occasions, the diagnosis may be picked up on routine evaluation. This is likely in the cases of extramacular retinal detachments, chronic retinal detachments leading to insidious loss of vision, retinal detachments in densely amblyopic eyes and retinal detachments occurring in preverbal children. The symptoms of flashes and floaters are more related to the preceding event of retinal break formation and hence can antedate the onset of retinal detachment by several days to weeks. Not all the retinal detachments have the preceding history of flashes and floaters. Vision loss obviously occurs only when the macula is detached while field loss can be detected when the detachment spreads posterior to the equator.

Clinical Features

The anterior segment can be normal in fresh detachments while depending upon the type of detachment and chronicity, one can find variable amounts of anterior segment inflammation in the form of anterior chamber flare and cells, posterior synechiae and complicated cataract. The intraocular pressure (IOP) is usually low; hence, normal pressure in the presence of gross rhegmatogenous retinal detachment should make one think about the possibility of preexisting chronic simple glaucoma.

The presence of raised pressure in the presence of retinal detachment is rare and should raise the suspicion of secondary retinal detachment. Profuse hypotony is characteristically associated with choroidal detachment and is often seen in eyes with giant retinal tear. The presence of pigment dusting is characteristic of rhegmatogenous retinal detachment; but in addition, the vitreous can be hazy to a variable extent due to inflammatory reaction as well as preexisting vitreous membranes associated with vitreous degeneration. In addition, variable amounts of vitreous hemorrhage can be present as a result of traction on blood vessels that may be bridging the retinal tear. Posterior vitreous detachment is almost always present in the presence of tractional retinal tears, while atrophic holes within lattice degeneration leading to retinal detachment can be associated with the lack of posterior vitreous detachment. Traumatic retinal dialysis is characteristically an intrabasal split at the level of ora serrata and does not have posterior vitreous detachment. Eyes with retinal detachments associated with choroidal coloboma also often do not have vitreous detachment.

Retinal Break

Retinal break is a dehiscence in the neurosensory retina through which the liquefied vitreous finds its way into the subretinal space.

Traction–Related Tears

Traction-related tears could be:

- Horseshoe tears that characteristically have a 'V' shape with the apex facing the optic disc. The apex of the retinal flap has the vitreous attachment.
- Operculated tears that have a free floating operculum in the vitreous cavity with a round or oval hole in the retina. There is no persistent vitreous traction once the operculum is free.
- Giant retinal tears that may form along the posterior border of the vitreous base; along posterior border of long patches of lattice degeneration; or along areas of white with pressure.
- Breaks can also form at the sites of abnormal vitreoretinal traction, such as pigment clumps, granular tags, meridional folds and rarely chorioretinal scars. Retinal breaks not caused by vitreous traction include those caused by atrophic holes and retinal dialysis. Atrophic holes are usually located in the patches of lattice degeneration. Atrophic holes can also be found in the patches of chorioretinal atrophy associated with high myopia located in the posterior pole. Such holes can be hidden in posterior staphylomata. Macular holes are unique and are only rarely the cause of rhegmatogenous retinal detachment. Atrophic holes are also seen in the intercalary membrane of eyes with choroidal coloboma. The number of breaks that can be found in a given eye is highly variable and it is important that all the breaks are identified for proper management. The upper temporal quadrant is the commonest site for retinal breaks.

Other Features

Secondary changes can occur due to the retinal detachment and these can have a bearing on the management and outcome. Occurrence of choroidal detachment is an important complication that is considered a poor prognostic indicator. Other changes due to chronicity include demarcation lines, and retinal cystic changes. Demarcation lines tend to be concave towards the ora serrata and can be a guide to the location of the break. More than one demarcation line can be present indicating the intermittent progression of detachment. Presence of demarcation line does not necessarily offer protection against progression of the detachment unless there is gross chorioretinal atrophy with pigmentation surrounding the detachment. Retinal cysts are not true cysts in the sense that they are not lined by epithelium, but their presence indicates chronicity of the detachment. Proliferative vitreoretinopathy is a well-recognized entity that will be discussed in the subsequent chapters.

Evaluation

The evaluation of a patient with retinal detachment has several goals in mind:

- Identify the causative retinal break(s).
- To plan the surgical procedure that can produce retinal reattachment with least morbidity.
- Valuate fellow eye and plan for any prophylaxis.
- General medical evaluation for the administration of anesthesia and medications.

Ocular examination includes record of history regarding the duration of symptoms, refractory error, previous visual acuity (for prognosis), record of best-corrected visual acuity (BCVA), slit-lamp examination of anterior segment, applanation tonometry and fundus evaluation. Fundus evaluation is done by indirect ophthalmoscopy and slit-lamp biomicroscopy after pupillary dilatation. It is outside the scope of this chapter to discuss the nuances of indirect ophthalmoscopy. The evaluation of the retinal detachment includes the performance of detailed retinal drawing, wherein the lesions are drawn in relation to the blood vessels, which serve as good landmarks during surgery. The details that should be drawn are the extent of retinal detachment, location of retinal breaks with respect to their clock meridian and anteroposterior extent, size of retinal breaks and other lesions, such as lattice patches, etc. Scleral indentation is a must in the evaluation of retinal detachment. It not only confirms lesions noted, but also permits the periphery to be better visualized. The importance of examining the periphery in detail cannot be overemphasized. Suspected posterior breaks are best evaluated using the slit-lamp biomicroscopy with +78 D or other precorneal lens.

Identifying the Retinal Break

Impediments in this vital step could be the presence of medial opacities, poor pupillary dilatation, presence of tiny retinal holes, lack of proper contrast (holes in chorioretinal atrophic patches and colobomata) and poor patient cooperation. In most cases, however, a careful indirect ophthalmoscopy with scleral indentation helps identify all the causative lesions. In those cases with difficulty in identifying the same, help can be taken from Lincoff's rules so that the search can be focused to a more likely location.

Rules

The rules are (Fig. 30.1):

- Eyes with partial retinal detachment extending to different heights nasally and temporally are likely to have a break within 1 to 2 clock hours of the highest limit of the detachment.
- Eyes with partial retinal detachments extending equally on both sides are likely to have a break in the vicinity of 6 o'clock meridian. However, breaks in the 12 o'clock meridian can also produce similar pattern with a track of fluid in the periphery connecting the break to the detachment.
- Total retinal detachments can be caused by breaks anywhere, but more likely to be due to break in the 12 o'clock meridian.

One should understand that when there is more than one break existing, these rules do not apply.

Diagnosis

The diagnosis of rhegmatogenous retinal detachment is relatively straightforward in most cases. The typical feature of mobile undulating folds of retina with wrinkles is rather diagnostic. However, there are occasions when the diagnosis may not be that obvious and one may have to use other clues.

Differential Diagnosis

The important differential diagnosis includes the following:

1. *Secondary retinal detachment*: The typical signs are the presence of shifting fluid, causative lesion, such as intraocular tumor, presence of inflammatory signs, absence of pigment in the vitreous, absence of retinal break, etc. Other investigations, such as fluorescein angiography, ultrasonography may be needed to diagnose the condition.
2. *Retinoschisis*: The location of these lesions is typically infero-temporal and bilateral. The lesions are immobile and dome-shaped and cause absolute scotoma on field charting. In contrast to retinal detachment, test photocoagulation of the lesion produces burn at the outer layer. However, one should realize that rhegmatogenous retinal detachment could supervene on retinoschisis.
3. *Choroidal detachment*: This presents as multiple brown smooth elevations usually anterior to vortex veins. However, choroidal detachment is a known complication of retinal detachment.
4. *Vitreous changes that can be mistaken for retinal detachment*: Old vitreous hemorrhage and vascularized vitreous membranes may on occasions be mistaken for retinal detachment.

Management

The principles of management revolve around the sealing of the retinal breaks as enunciated by Jules Gonin. Scleral buckling remains the most common method of retinal reattachment surgery performed all over the world despite the advent of other methods. Alternate methods that are in vogue now are the use of pneumatic retinopexy and primary vitrectomy. Other methods that have been tried and largely given up are the use of implant in suprachoroidal space, etc. Balloon temporary buckle has been popularized by Lincoff, but remained in use by only a small group of surgeons.

Common Method of Retinal Reattachment

Scleral Buckling

The commonest modality of retinal reattachment surgery is scleral buckling and involves basically three steps—the treatment of the retinal break with cryo or diathermy, the placement of

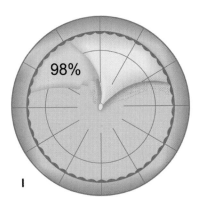
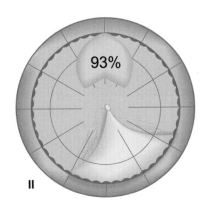
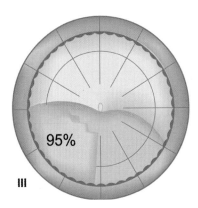

Fig. 30.1: Lincoff's Rules for finding the primary break in rhegmatogenous retinal detachment
I. Superior temporal or nasal detachments: In 98% the primary break lies within 1½ clock hours of the highest border.
II. Total or superior detachments that cross the 12 o'clock meridian: In 93% the primary break is at 12 o'clock or in a triangle, the apex of which is at the ora serrata and the sides intersect the equator 1 hour to either side of 12 o'clock.
III. Inferior detachments: In 95% the higher side of the detachment indicates on which side of the 6 o'clock radian an inferior break lies.
When an inferior detachment is bullous the primary break lies above the horizontal meridian

a buckle to indent the eye at the site of the break and to drain the subretinal fluid if necessary. There are variations in the theme depending on individual case and different practices. The individual steps will be described along with the variations.

1. *Conjunctival opening:* The conjunctiva can be opened either at the limbus or 3 mm away from limbus. Limbal incisions would need two relaxing incisions at diagonally opposite meridians.

2. *Tagging the muscles:* The extraocular muscles are tagged to enable exposure of the sclera (Figs 30.2 and 30.3). The hooking is done with use of fenestrated muscle hooks with relatively thick cotton sutures (4-0). Alternately, one can use curved needles loaded with the suture, but the needle is introduced under the muscle with the blunt end leading. The number of muscles tagged will depend upon the extent of scleral exposure required.

3. *Inspection of the sclera:* The surface of the sclera is inspected to specifically look for sites of scleral dehiscences, thinning and staphylomata, which can alter the surgical plan.

Localization of the Retinal Break

This is perhaps the most crucial step that dictates the size and location of the buckle and the final success of the surgery (Fig. 30.4).

The points to be localized are as follows:

- If the break is single, the posterior most point of the break is localized.

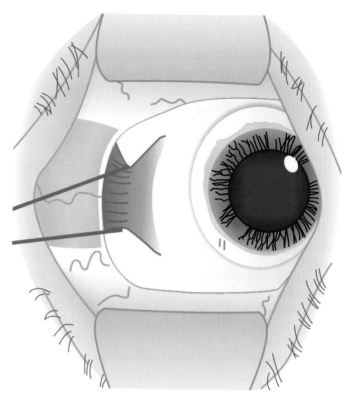

Fig. 30.3: Schematic diagram showing the tagged muscle (Modified with permission from Travis A Meredith, MD)

- If there are multiple breaks in the near vicinity of each other and one estimates the need for only one continuous buckle, the posterior most point of the posterior most break is localized to define the posterior extent. The lateral limits as defined by the breaks at the two extremes of the proposed buckle are also localized.

- If the breaks are multiple, but one envisages the use of more than one buckle, the same principles are used as above

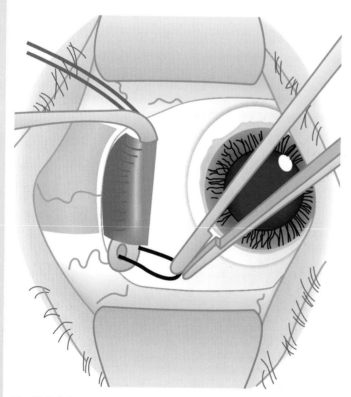

Fig. 30.2: Schematic diagram of rectus muscle being hooked by a muscle hook with eyelet. (Modified with permission from Travis A Meredith, MD)

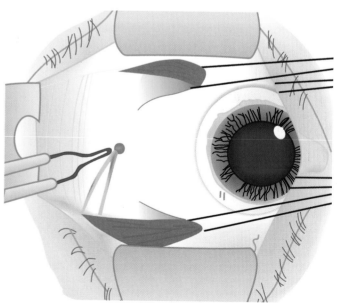

Fig. 30.4: Schematic diagram showing localization of the retinal break. (Modified with permission from Travis A Meredith, MD)

to localize one or a group of breaks that will be covered by the buckle elements.

- If 360° buckling is required, only the posterior most break needs to be localized.

Technique of localization: One can use custom-made localizers or closed blades of a toothed forceps to indent the sclera while doing indirect ophthalmoscopy. The point needing localization is identified by trial and error and the indentation mark left behind on the sclera can be made permanent with cautery or other markers. Schepens uses diathermy to mark the localization point and the procedure involves active participation of the assistant who will be holding the diathermy.

Difficulties in localization: Bullous retinal detachments can pose difficulties in the localization of retinal breaks. Approximate localization is possible by localizing anterior to the break where indentation is better visualized and then sliding the localizer posteriorly to the expected point. Alternately, one may have to drain first and then localize (Table 30.1). One can also take guidance from the presence of pigment changes at the retinal pigment epithelium level that sometimes correspond to the lesions, such as lattice. It is expected that the lattice will fall on this point once the retina is settled.

Retinopexy: The most common modality of creating permanent adhesion between retinal pigment epithelium/choroid and the neurosensory retina is by the use of cryo (Fig. 30.5). Diathermy is not commonly used at the present time. Diathermy involves the mandatory performance of lamellar scleral dissection to avoid scleral damage. It involves use of discrete non-confluent burns, one burn apart throughout the dissected bed. Photocoagulation can also be used for this purpose, but is possible only after the retina is settled. Cryo involves the use of Joule-Thomson effect. Carbon dioxide gas is used to produce –79.5°C at the tip of the probe. The adhesion formed per square cm is strongest with diathermy and weakest with cryo.

Table 30.1: Tips to use cryo

1. Attempt is made to freeze just up to the retina if possible. However, if the retina is highly elevated, freezing is done only up to the retinal pigment epithelium. Vitreous is never frozen.

2. The probe is never moved while frozen.

3. Temporary mark left by the cryo probe can sometimes serve to confirm the localization mark.

4. Attempts are made to avoid freezing the bare choroid within the open part of the break to avoid unnecessary liberation of the retinal pigment epithelial cells.

5. Small breaks may be covered all round by placing the probe tip under the center of the lesion.

6. Larger lesions are surrounded with contiguous burns with least overlap.

7. Beginners can confuse between indentation caused by tip and the shaft of the cryo probe with disaster results. Movement of the probe in its axis leads to movement of the indentation caused by the tip and not by the shaft. Failure to recognize the true location of the tip vis-à-vis the indentation seen with the ophthalmoscope can lead to freezing very posterior locations, such as macula inadvertently.

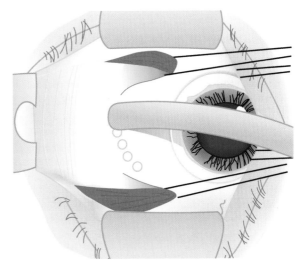

Fig. 30.5: Schematic diagram showing cryopexy being performed to the lesions. (Modified with permission from Travis A Meredith, MD)

The Buckle

Buckling materials: Most materials used now are silicone based. Historically, people have used materials, such as polyethylene tube, Arruga's string, etc. Either solid silicone or silicone sponge can be used. Solid silicone is available as tires of different widths and thickness (with a groove for the band); as strips; or as bands. Silicone sponge is available in strips with round or oval cross-section. In addition, buckle elements are available for special purposes, such as meridional buckle for extending the buckle effect posteriorly in a localized area; silicone boat to place under the tantalum clips that are used to tie the band ends together. The encircling bands are narrow strips of 2 to 2.5 mm width that are usually used along with the circumferentially placed tires. The ends of the bands are held together by a cow hitch knot or tantalum clips or Watzke's sleeve.

Choice of buckle: Most surgeons use the circumferential silicone tires for most cases. However, a radially placed silicone sponge is useful for isolated large horseshoe tears and avoids fish mouthing (Table 30.2). Circumferential buckle has the advantage of being able to cover many lesions. An encircling band is usually added to the tire to give permanency to the buckle as well as to relieve vitreous traction all round near the vitreous base. The buckle size should be chosen to indent the area of the lesion and a 2 mm margin all round. Anterior coverage of the lesion is as important as the posterior coverage. There is no necessity to buckle all the way up to the ora serrata in case of posteriorly located breaks.

Implant versus exoplant: Traditional Schepens' buckle (implant) involved the dissection of a scleral bed slightly larger than the buckle and burying the buckle between the flaps using mattress sutures (Figs 30.6 to 30.9). This technique is best suited along with the use of diathermy although it can be used with cryo as well. The perceived advantages of this technique are: (a) the ability to get good indentation with less rise in IOP caused thereof, since only partial-thickness eye wall is indented,

Table 30.2: Tips in placement of buckle

1. Posterior bite should be circumferentially placed for exoplant. Anterior bite can be either circumferential or two radial bites can be taken.

2. The width of the intrascleral passage of needle should be as long as possible since there is a tendency for this to shorten while tightening.

3. At least two mattress sutures should be taken per quadrant.

4. The width between the sutures should give 2 mm clearance from the edge of the buckle on both sides. For a thicker buckle, such as no. 281 (MIRA)—one has to give more clearance to give more space to imbricate the thickness of the buckle.

5. Spatulated needle with 5-0 green-colored mersilene suture is ideal. The green color helps identify it in case of revision surgery.

6. Avoid unnecessary large buckles.

7. If the posterior bite placement is close to the vortex vein exit, the mattress suture can be passed in two segments avoiding the vortex vein in between.

8. If the posterior bite placement is significantly posterior to the exit of vortex vein exit, one can take a continuous bite by lifting the vortex vein. The vein will be compressed by the buckle, but is still likely to be patent partly.

9. Unnecessary sacrifice of vortex vein should be avoided.

10. Avoid placement of radial sponge underneath a muscle.

11. Radial sponge is placed by taking radial mattress sutures. For posterior sponges, the passage of posteroanterior bite may be technically difficult. This is countered by passing both bites antero-posteriorly resulting in a figure of 8 suture. This is converted to mattress suture by cutting in the center and tying the posterior ends together. In effect, this produces a mattress suture with 2 knots across both loops.

12. Disinserting a muscle is seldom required today. Most such cases with posterior lesions are handled by vitreous surgery.

13. If oblique muscles come in the way of passing mattress sutures, partial disinsertion of these can be done. This problem is frequently encountered with superior oblique.

14. While placing an encircling band over a scleral buckle, the band should be anchored in the quadrants other than those with the buckle; the anchorage is done along the greatest circle of the eye. This prevents the tendency for shifting of the band.

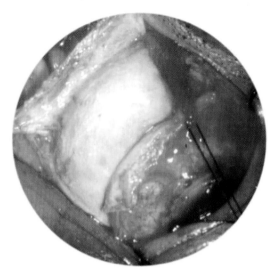

Fig. 30.7: Scleral bed is completed. Note uniform thickness of the bed

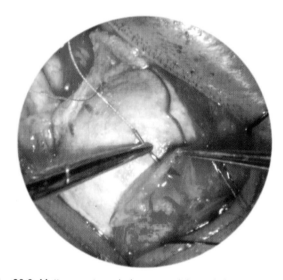

Fig. 30.8: Mattress sutures being passed through the scleral flaps. A spatulated needle is preferred

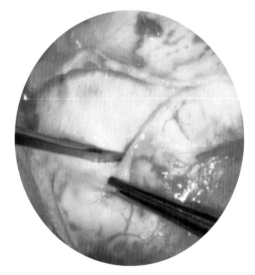

Fig. 30.6: Dissection of scleral bed in progress. Note that the knife cuts the junctional tissue between elevated flap and the scleral bed

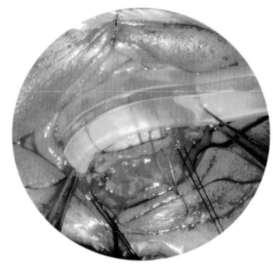

Fig. 30.9: The implant is measured for placement. The bed should be wide enough to accommodate the width and thickness of the buckle element

Table 30.3: Tips in performing subretinal fluid drainage

1. Inspection of choroidal knuckle under operating microscope will show any large choroidal vessels traversing the site. In such a circumstance, one may have to abandon that site and choose an alternate one.

2. At the time of actual puncture of the choroids, the assistant must be told to relax the traction sutures to avoid precipitous drainage.

3. Continued flow of subretinal fluid can occur only if IOP is maintained by pressure on the eye.

4. Edematous choroid may not permit free flow of subretinal fluid.

5. Pigment in the subretinal fluid can indicate near completion of drainage.

6. Long-standing detachments are associated with drainage of thick subretinal fluid.

7. If drainage is profuse, the drainage site can be temporarily closed; the mattress sutures tied up temporarily in other quadrants and drainage is resumed.

8. Sudden cessation of fluid flow could mean retinal incarceration.

9. Never try to make up the IOP by tightening the buckle or band. Normalization of IOP should be by intraocular injection of BSS or air if needed.

10. Avoid intraocular injection of fluid or air unless really indicated.

and (b) better coverage of the buckle material. The exoplant technique is more commonly practiced and involves direct placement of the mattress sutures in full-thickness sclera to imbricate the buckle (Figs 30.10 and 30.11).

Subretinal Fluid Drainage

To drain or not to drain: Although the decision to drain is based on individual practices, most surgeons drain most of the times. There are, however, certain definite indications and contraindications leaving a significant chunk for option of draining or otherwise (Table 30.3).

Indications for drainage:

• Bullous detachment—placement of buckle can be checked accurately only after drainage.

• Preexisting glaucoma.

• Extensive buckle—drainage provides space for indenting the large buckle.

• Presence of significant vitreous traction—drainage helps to gauge the behavior of the retina and provide adequate buckle to relieve traction.

• Chronic retinal detachment—absorption of fluid likely to be very slow.

• Eyes with sick retinal pigment epithelium—fluid absorption likely to be slow.

Contraindication: The main contraindication for drainage is the presence of only shallow retinal detachment where the risk of iatrogenic complications will be high.

Choosing the site for drainage: The ideal site would be under the site of maximum fluid and farthest from vertical meridians in order to avoid potentially vascular choroid. Given the option, nasal quadrants may be preferable since any subretinal bleed may not migrate under the macula. A relatively posterior drainage site allows more complete drainage with more safety since the retina is likely to be maximally separated posteriorly.

Drainage inside versus outside the bed of the buckle: Obvious advantage of draining within the bed of the buckle is that any complication, such as iatrogenic break and incarceration are more easily managed without need for modifying the buckle. However, the area of the buckle is most likely to have been treated with cryo and so would be having engorged choroidal vasculature thus increasing the risk of hemorrhage. In addition, the site may be close to the break. In the case of large break, this can lead to the drainage of liquid vitreous through the break. Drainage posterior to the buckle obviates these two problems (Fig. 30.12).

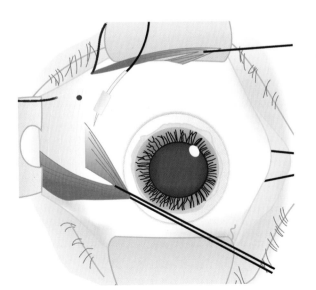

Fig. 30.10: Schematic diagram of exoplant suture being passed. (Modified with permission from Travis A Meredith, MD)

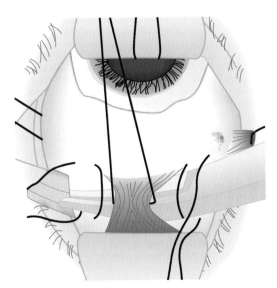

Fig. 30.11: Schematic diagram of exoplant being placed in position under the rectus muscle. (Modified with permission from Travis A Meredith, MD)

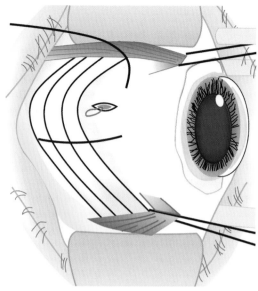

Fig. 30.12: Schematic diagram showing drainage of subretinal fluid in the area of buckle. (Modified with permission from Travis A Meredith, MD)

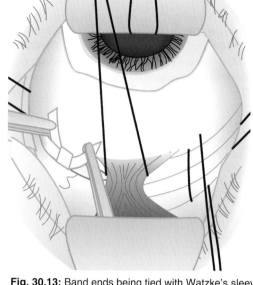

Fig. 30.13: Band ends being tied with Watzke's sleeve

Technique of drainage: It is imperative to inspect the fundus just before drainage, since the fluid could have shifted. The drainage site selection should never be based on preoperative examination. Several techniques are available to drain the fluid.

a. The commonest technique involves performing a sclerotomy and perforating the choroidal knuckle. A sclerotomy (commonly vertical) is made at the intended site until the choroidal knuckle is exposed. Light cautery to lips of the sclerotomy helps in exposing the choroidal knuckle better. The choroid itself can also be lightly cauterized. A fine needle (needle of 10-0 suture) can be used to puncture the knuckle of choroid. Pressure is applied on the eye to maintain the flow of fluid. The pressure is meant to maintain the normal IOP and not to squeeze the fluid out. A pre-placed suture is placed around the drainage site if it is outside the buckle bed. This suture is used to close the drainage site before tightening the mattress suture.

b. Some surgeons penetrate the full-thickness eye wall without exposing the choroid. A relatively thicker needle is used for this.

c. Alternate method of performing the choroidotomy was to apply laser on the surface of the choroidal knuckle using the endolaser probe. The perceived advantages with this technique are that chances of occurrence of choroidal hemorrhage and iatrogenic retinal break are reduced since the laser cauterizes the blood vessels and there is no actual entry of instrument into the eyeball. In a study by Ailward, the incidence of subretinal hemorrhage was 4.3% with use of laser probe compared to 28.3% with needle drainage.

d. Pitts and associates have used indirect delivery system of argon laser to the exposed choroidal knuckle for the perforation of the same.

Intraocular injection: In most cases, intraocular injection of fluid or air is not required or desirable. If the fluid was extensive leading to profuse hypotony on drainage, one may have to inject balanced salt solution (BSS) through the pars plana. Air is chosen when there is fish mouthing of a horseshoe tear. A 30-gauge needle is used to inject air.

Role of paracentesis: In case of non-drainage cases, one may have to perform paracentesis to accommodate the buckle. Paracentesis is done using 30-gauge needle. Controlled drainage of aqueous is possible by having a long intracorneal track so that continued leak of aqueous will not occur after withdrawal of the needle. In aphakic eyes with vitreous in anterior chamber, it is preferable to approach the aqueous pocket via pars plana to avoid vitreous incarceration in the paracentesis wound. Concluding steps: After the mattress sutures are temporarily tied, the fundus is inspected to look for perfusion of the disc, the drainage site complications, and status of the retina. The relationship of the break to the buckle is also noted. Any adjustments of the position of the buckle may be done if needed. Final knots are tied. The ends of the encircling band are tied using either clove hitch knot or Watzke's sleeve (Fig. 30.13). The orbit is irrigated with antibiotic solution and the conjunctiva is closed with absorbable suture. The Tenon's capsule is preferably closed as a separate layer before the conjunctival closure.

Complications of Scleral Buckling

Briefly, this subject can be discussed as preoperative, intraoperative and postoperative complications.

Preoperative complications: Conditions that can make the evaluation and management difficult would be listed under preoperative complications. The evaluation can be made difficult by the presence of medial opacities, such as corneal opacities, cataract and vitreous opacities. Non-dilating pupil can also make it difficult to evaluate the fundus properly.

The presence of IOL can pose problems in visualizing because of the after-cataract and IOL deposits. Associated choroidal detachment can make the management difficult due to the difficulty in localizing and treating of the retinal break, difficulty in producing a buckle effect and the increased risk of proliferative vitreoretinopathy. Most cases of retinal detachment with choroidal detachment are best managed by vitrectomy with or without buckling procedure. Significant medial opacities will need to be cleared for proper management of retinal detachment. This may involve removal of cataract, removal of IOL, vitreous surgery to remove the vitreous opacities and rarely combined penetrating keratoplasty in the case of significant corneal opacities.

Intraoperative complications:

1. *Complications during anesthesia*: These are common to any surgery. However, patients needing retinal reattachment surgery are more likely to be highly myopic than other group of ophthalmic patients and this factor should be kept in mind while administering local anesthesia.

2. *Complications during initial steps*: During hooking of the extraocular muscles, one can potentially damage the muscles and vortex veins. Globe rupture during this step is extremely unlikely except in the cases of revision buckling procedure.

3. *Difficult visualization:* This problem has been partly covered in the preoperative complications. However, there are some cases where the problem is faced only during surgery and not anticipated before hand.
   a. *Corneal edema*: During prolonged cryopexy, corneal edema can occur. Waiting for a few seconds will restore clarity. Only rarely should it be required to remove the corneal epithelium.
   b. *Pupillary constriction*: Pupil can constrict due to rough handling of the eye and hypotony. If the pupil becomes small during the last steps of surgery, it may not be needed to address this problem. If it occurs during the initial steps, one can inject intracameral adrenaline (1:10000) to produce dilatation of pupil. Alternatively, one can apply temporary iris hooks. The importance of a detailed preoperative drawing cannot be overstressed under conditions of compromised visualization to enable localization and treatment of all retinal breaks.
   c. On occasions, minimal hyphema can occur coating the lens or IOL leading to hampered visibility. The layered blood can be washed off through a self-sealing stab incision.

4. *Complications during localization*: This can involve wrong localization due to wrong technique, bullous retinal detachment, etc; vortex vein damage; and on occasions, scleral perforation if the point of localization has thinned sclera.

5. Complications during subretinal fluid drainage:
   a. *Dry tap*: Inability to drain fluid could be due to wrong selection of site (less or no fluid or shifting fluid) or incomplete perforation (common in suffused choroid).
   b. *Subretinal hemorrhage*: Bleeding from drainage site can occur to a variable degree and can migrate under the macula in temporal drainage sites in eyes with macular detachment. Significant hemorrhage can have deleterious effect on the visual improvement.
   c. *Retinal incarceration*: One of the dreaded complications is the occurrence of retinal incarceration. Sudden cessation of fluid is an indicator of such an occurrence. One should immediately stop further attempts at drainage and examine the fundus after tying up the mattress suture. Early incarceration is indicated by the presence of star-like fold at the drainage site, while more extensive incarceration can lead to prolapse of white translucent retina through the choroidotomy. Retinal break formation can accompany this complication. In most cases, buckling the site of perforation along with cryopexy should suffice.
   d. *Retinal perforation*: Retinal break can occur secondary to incarceration. It can also occur during the perforation itself if the fluid is not sufficient in amount. It can be accompanied by vitreous prolapse. Presentation of vitreous has serious consequences.
   e. *Drainage of liquid vitreous*: In cases with large retinal breaks where the drainage site is close to the open break, liquid vitreous can find its way through the choroidotomy. The indication for this happening is by the observation of profuse drainage, hypotony and lack of settlement of the retina. To some extent, one can limit this by trying to approximate the retina in the area of the break using the cotton-tipped applicator. Alternately, other drainage sites may have to be chosen.
   f. *Choroidal detachment*: Serous choroidal detachment is usually sequelae of prolonged hypotony. Aphakic eyes and eyes with high myopia are especially prone to this complication. Hypotony should be kept to a minimum duration by quickly tying up the mattress sutures. Residual hypotony should be made up by intraocular injection if it is significant. Hemorrhagic choroidal detachment is a more significant complication in terms of its effect on the overall outcome. Elderly patients and patients with high myopia are at the special risk of this complication. Although hypotony can precipitate this complication, it can occur at any stage of the surgery unrelated to hypotony also. The first indication is a hardening eyeball. One may visualize mounds of choroidal detachment appearing. Sclerotomy at these sites may provide an alternate route for the blood. One should avoid creating hypotony by this procedure since it can perpetuate the cycle. Small mounds do not influence the success of the surgery. But large hemorrhagic choroidals can be disastrous. One may have to reoperate after 5 to 6 days to try and drain the blood once it is liquefied.

6. *Complication of paracentesis*: Paracentesis can potentially lead to damage to the crystalline lens, corneal touch in case of iris-supported lens, and vitreous incarceration in case of aphakic eyes with vitreous in anterior chamber.

Early Postoperative Complications

1. *Lid edema*: Mild reaction in the form of lid edema and orbital reaction is fairly common and is proportional to the extent of the buckling done. Excessive edema with severe pain should make one suspect early infection.

2. *Anterior segment ischemia*: This is a relatively rare complication. It is more common with encircling buckles and in patients with hemoglobinopathies. Disinsertion of three extraocular muscles can potentially lead to this complication. However, disinsertion of muscles to place posterior buckles is no longer practiced since the advent of vitreous surgery to manage these cases. Anterior segment ischemia is characterized by pain, glaucoma or hypotony, corneal edema, hyphema, iris atrophy, rapid onset cataract, vitreous haze and hemorrhage. The severity of the ischemia can vary. Treatment with steroids does not alter the prognosis.

3. *Secondary glaucoma*: Raised IOP sure can be caused by angle closure due to forward movement of iris lens diaphragm as in choroidal detachment. Predisposed eyes can also develop the same due to atropinization of the eye. Open-angle glaucoma can be due to preexisting glaucoma that has become obvious once the retinal detachment has been corrected, or could be due to steroids. Other cause of glaucoma could be hemorrhagic choroidal detachment.

4. *Recurrent retinal detachment*: Recurrent retinal detachment should be differentiated from persistent fluid. Persistent fluid could be because of chronic retinal detachment, wherein the fluid is thick and takes a long time to absorb. If the retinal breaks are closed and there is no increase in the retinal detachment, one can safely watch these eyes.

   Persistent fluid could be also due to the break remaining open. Recurrent retinal detachment, strictly speaking, describes a condition, wherein the retina was attached to start with and followed by reoccurrence of retinal detachment. The causes of persistent/recurrent retinal detachment are discussed below:

   a. *Inappropriate buckle*: The buckle may be too anterior, too posterior, or may not be adequate circumferentially. It is wrong to think that good posterior coverage is enough for surgical success. Fluid can seep from an inadequately covered anterior edge of retinal break and track down inferiorly.

   b. *Inadequate height of buckle*: In most cases, a mild-to-moderate buckle height is enough to ensure closure of retinal breaks. Eyes requiring high buckles are best managed by vitreous surgery rather than distorting the eye with high buckles. However, very shallow buckles can lead to problems even with mild traction. This problem can occur when breaks are located under the muscles and the mattress sutures are on either side of the break and not over the same. If care is not taken to remove the laxity of the buckle in between the sutures, the external hump can lead to the lack of buckling effect under the break.

   c. *Fish mouthing*: This is a phenomenon unique to traction-related tears and circumferential buckles. The larger the tear, the more likelihood of this happening. Measures to circumvent the problem include the use of radial buckle, injection of air or gas, and using a broader and shallower buckle.

   d. *Retinal folds*: These assume significance if they communicate with a retinal break and keep it open. Air injection can help cut off this communication.

   e. *Inadequate retinopexy*: If the tear is not adequately surrounded by the cryo, the break can leak later on, especially if the vitreous traction increases. Removal of the buckle or shallowing of the buckle effect as is common with radial buckles, can lead to recurrent retinal detachment if the tear is not well-surrounded by chorioretinal adhesion.

   f. *Vitreous traction*: Significant vitreous traction can lift up a break from a good buckle also and lead to recurrent retinal detachment.

   g. Missed retinal breaks.

   h. *New retinal breaks*: New breaks can be iatrogenic (discussed above) or due to vitreous traction. Theoretically, the presence of encircling band in addition to the buckle is expected to reduce the risk of new traction-related breaks.

   i. *Proliferative vitreoretinopathy*: This is by far the most important cause of failure of retinal reattachment surgery.

5. *Corneal complications*: Minor problems, such as corneal epithelial defects, can occur in the first few days after surgery, especially if the epithelium was removed on the table. Corneal edema can be an indicator of secondary glaucoma. Rarely one may get Dellen.

Late Postoperative Complications

1. *Changes in refractory error*: Most circumferential buckles produce increase in myopia due to the increase in the anteroposterior diameter of the eyeball. However, if the indentation is too high, one may end up with a hypermetropic shift due to shortening of the eyeball.

2. *Infected buckle*: Buckle infection can occur even years after the surgery. Initial manifestation can be in the form of subconjunctival hemorrhage, which can be surprisingly severe sometimes. These hemorrhages emanate from the fine blood vessels in the granuloma. More advanced changes include conjunctival granulomas, exposed buckle and scleral necrosis. Intraocular abscess has also been seen in association with buckle infection and can be sterile in nature. This usually resolves with the removal of the buckle. Infected buckle needs the removal of all alloplastic materials, including the buckle, encircling band (if placed) and the sutures.

3. *Intrusion of the buckle*: Buckle intrusion was a common complication when polyethylene tube and Arruga's string

were used for circumferential buckling. With the silicone bands, it is less common. It is more commonly seen at the site of the band rather than the buckle due to the smaller width of the band. This is especially possible when one tries to build up the IOP after the drainage of subretinal fluid by tightening the band. The unnecessarily high buckle coupled with the areas of thin sclera lead to progressive erosion of the walls of the eye leading to intrusion of the buckle. The process is chronic and never leads to spontaneous rupture of the eye, since as the buckle intrudes, there is fibrous tissue cover over the same. Early intrusion is indicated by occurrence of hemorrhages along the buckle and later by the visibility of the silicone material through the retina. Removal of the buckle with actual intrusion of the same is a risky proposition with the high-risk of globe rupture at the site of intrusion. Since it is the band that intrudes more often than the broader buckle, it may be possible to cut the band at a site other than the site of intrusion and limit further damage.

4. *Migration of the buckle*: Anterior migration of the buckle is more common than posterior migration. The most common reason is the presence of the buckle/band anterior to the greater circle of the eye in one or more quadrants. There is natural tendency of the buckle to migrate anteriorly. Migration occurs very slowly and cuts through the muscle insertion and can lie next to the limbus as well. However, the muscle does not get disinserted due to the chronicity of the process. Anterior migration is not a major problem unless it is a cause of recurrent retinal detachment due to removal of the buckle effect under the break or the buckle is protruding out at the limbus. Posterior migration can be dangerous if the band/buckle slips close to the optic nerve.

5. *Extraocular muscle imbalance*: This is a potential problem when an alloplastic element is placed on the sclera under the extraocular muscles. The unpredictable adhesion that occurs between the muscle and the sclera leads to variable restriction of the eye movements and could result in troublesome diplopia. Radial sponges placed under the muscles are especially prone to this problem. Minor degrees can be corrected by prism correction. In most cases, surgical correction of the strabismus is done on the fellow eye since the adhesions make it difficult to perform the surgery on the same eye. Removal of the buckle does not necessarily correct the strabismus nor improve the motility.

ALTERNATE METHODS OF RETINAL REATTACHMENT

Pneumatic Retinopexy

Although air was used in the management of retinal detachment as far back as 1911 by Ohm, it was Hilton and Grizzard who in 1984–85 popularized the technique of using gas to reattach selected cases of retinal detachment.

Principle

The buoyancy of the air/gas injected allows it to float up and provides the force needed to press against the retinal break when a patient is properly positioned. The surface tension of the gas bubble effectively closes the break and permits the subretinal fluid to absorb (Table 30.4).

Table 30.4: Tips in performance of pneumatic retinopexy

1. Careful case selection—by preoperative evaluation including detailed retinal drawing to exclude other retinal breaks.
2. Needle to be pushed deep to clear the vitreous base—otherwise, gas may be injected in the potential space between the lens and the anterior hyaloid face creating a trapped bubble that is ineffective.
3. Needle to be withdrawn to some extent so that the tip of the needle is located just internal to the pars plana. This permits the injection of the gas into the initial bubble leading to a single bubble.
4. Brisk injection also ensures a single bubble.
5. Steamroller technique: In case of macula-attached retinal detachment, there is a risk of the retinal detachment dissecting to involve the macula due to the gas injection. To avoid the same, the patient is made to lie prone as soon as the gas is injected. After about 10 to 15 minutes, the head position is changed in stages until the desired position is achieved. This permits the gas bubble to initially collect near the disc and then slowly displace the subretinal fluid through the retinal break into the vitreous cavity thus eliminating the possibility of inducing macular retinal detachment.

Indications

A retinal break or group of retinal breaks occupying one clock hour or less of circumferential extent and located between 8 and 4 o'clock of the superior fundus would be amenable for treatment by pneumatic retinopexy. Some have used pneumatic retinopexy for breaks separated by more than 1 clock hour and used alternate positioning to tamponade the breaks. Irvine and Lahey have used pneumatic retinopexy along with repeated paracentesis to manage five cases of giant retinal tear of less than 180°. Pneumatic retinopexy has also been used to treat selected cases of recurrent retinal detachment. A clear media is of paramount importance to evaluate the fundus properly so that there is no possibility of missed breaks. The patient should be able to adopt the posture required postoperatively.

Contraindications

Proliferative vitreoretinopathy of grade greater than B is a contraindication. If there is glaucoma that is medically uncontrolled or wherein there is already evidence of a significant glaucomatous disc damage, it is not advisable to perform pneumatic retinopexy. The most important contraindication is the inability to be certain of absence of any other breaks.

Surgical Technique

The two major components of the treatment are the treatment of the retinal break and the injection of gas.
Anesthesia and asepsis: It is usually performed under peribulbar anesthesia. The digital massage helps in lowering the IOP. Local

asepsis is a must like any surgical procedure. Povidone-iodine is instilled before the surgery and the area is prepped.

Retinopexy: When cryopexy is used, this is the first step in the procedure. However, if laser is planned, one has to wait for the retinal reattachment to take place before performing the laser. Performing the cryopexy also helps in softening the eye to some more extent.

Injection of gas: Expansile gas, such as SF_6 or C_3F_8 is used, although air has also been tried. If air is used, usually repeated injections are required since it is absorbed fast 0.3 cc of C_3F_8 or 0.5 cc of SF_6 is used for the purpose of pneumatic retinopexy. The required quantity of gas is taken in a 1 cc syringe and a 30-gauge needle is attached to it. Brisk injection of the gas is done and the perforation site is closed with a cotton-tipped applicator while the needle is withdrawn. Simultaneously, the head is turned to one side to permit the gas bubble to slide away from the needle track. The fundus is examined to look for retinal perfusion. If need be, a paracentesis is done to normalize the IOP. The patient is returned to the room where he/she is positioned so that the break will be occupying the topmost position. Guidance can be given by placing an arrow on the eye pad in the direction of the retinal break so that the patient aims at keeping the arrow always straight.

Follow-Up

Usually, by the next day, the retinal break is flattened and the fluid resolves either partly or totally. On occasions, residual fluid may remain for a long time, especially if the retinal detachment is of long-standing duration. If retinal break is flat and is sealed by the retinopexy, residual fluid can be observed. Review examination should involve careful inspection of the peripheral fundus for any new breaks in the retina, especially inferiorly.

Complications

In addition to the complications of local anesthesia, one can have rarely injury to the lens in phakic eyes. The gas can be injected into the space between lens and the anterior hyaloid face. Small bubbles (frog eggs) can be troublesome and lead to subretinal gas by migrating through a relatively large break. If one sees small gas bubbles immediately after injection, it is best to position the patient so that the gas is away from the break for the first 24 hours followed by the correct positioning once the bubbles have coalesced. The other most important complication is the occurrence of new retinal break. Because of the buoyancy of the gas, there is traction on the inferior vitreous base, which can result in inferior retinal breaks. New or missed breaks were seen in 23% of pneumatic retinopexy group versus 13% in the scleral buckle group in a multicentric trial. Other complications can be endophthalmitis very rarely.

Balloon Buckle

Lincoff introduced the concept of temporary buckle for cases similar in indication to pneumatic retinopexy, i.e. break or breaks within one clock hour. The procedure involves retinopexy intraoperatively with cryo or postoperatively with laser. A balloon catheter made of siliconized latex is positioned under the break and fluid is injected to inflate the same. Over the next two days, more fluid is injected depending upon the closure of the break or otherwise. Up to 2 ml of fluid can be injected. No suture is required since the balloon remains in position in between the eyeball and the orbital tissues. The balloon is deflated partly on the fifth day. On seventh day, the balloon is totally deflated and removed. Lincoff and Kreissig reported 82% success with this procedure. Failure was noted to be either due to the break being larger than the balloon indentation or due to missed breaks. Traction-induced recurrent retinal detachment on removing the balloon was seen in 6% cases.

The advantages of this technique are the absence of a permanent buckle with the attendant risk of infection and limitations to extraocular movements. Placement of balloon buckle even under the extraocular muscles does not leave behind any residual muscle imbalance once the balloon is removed. The advantage over pneumatic retinopexy is its usefulness in inferior breaks as well. However, the technique has not caught the imagination of a majority of retinal surgeons.

Absorbable Buckling Materials

1. *Gelatin*: A dehydrated sheet of gelatin swells if soaked in fluid. Multiple layers can be used depending upon the height of buckle needed. It is used as an episcleral implant. Since the materials are absorbable, a synthetic absorbable suture may be used with it.

2. Suprachoroidal implantation of sodium hyaluronate was also attempted through an external sclerotomy. A pocket is created using the cyclodialysis spatula. However, the risk of choroidal hemorrhage is significant.

3. The advantages of pneumatic retinopexy and conventional operation have been combined by some surgeons, wherein subretinal fluid was drained along with injection of gas. Specific indications for this technique may be in cases with thin sclera.

4. *Nd:YAG vitreolysis*: In selected cases, with focal vitreous traction on the flap of retinal tear, one may be able to break the tractional band using the YAG laser and follow it up with gas tamponade. Berglin and associates performed this procedure in 21 cases and had 73% success in primary detachment surgeries and 80% in eyes buckled previously.

5. *Combinations of procedures*: Combinations, such as scleral buckle with air injection, pneumatic retinopexy with orbital balloon and pneumatic retinopexy with absorbable scleral buckle materials have also been tried. Van Effenterre performed aspiration of liquid vitreous and injection of gas with a success rate of 85% in 60 eyes. This technique may permit better control of IOP with gas injection, but involves aspiration of liquid vitreous with risk of exaggerated traction on the retina.

Primary Vitrectomy for Rhegmatogenous Retinal Detachment

Ever since the introduction of pars plana vitrectomy by Machemer in 1970s, this approach has been used for the complicated retinal detachments, such as retinal detachments with proliferative vitreoretinopathy, macular holes, giant retinal tears, etc. However, surgeons have used this approach for conditions considered simple retinal detachments also based on individual perceptions. These included cases of medial opacities that did not offer clear view, relatively posterior breaks, radially or obliquely located lattice patches, cases with unidentified breaks, need to buckle extensive areas, etc. However, mostly, the vitrectomy has been combined with scleral buckling. There have been reports of primary vitrectomy without scleral buckling. The presumed advantages of this technique are the lack of muscle imbalance, direct relief of vitreous traction on the break rather than indirectly through indentation and a definite identification of the retinal break. However, vitrectomy has its share of complications. The uncut peripheral vitreous can produce traction and induce new breaks. Occurrence of cataract to some extent is universal. Supporting the inferior break with internal tamponade is also practically difficult, as the patient has to assume a Trendelenburg position, which is most uncomfortable for a long duration. In the study by Escoffery and associates, vitrectomy without scleral buckling has been done for a variety of cases in which scleral buckling would have been the procedure of choice. The authors had 79% successful retinal reattachment rate, which was achieved after one operation that improved to 93% with a second surgery. The authors quote the advantages of avoiding a buckle-reduced risk of anterior segment ischemia (especially in patients with hemoglobinopathies), absence of changes in refractory error and reduced risk of postoperative CME. Primary pars plana vitrectomy can be considered as an alternative to scleral buckling in selected cases.

Revision Surgery

Revision surgery for recurrent retinal detachment can be approached in different ways (Table 30.5).

First a decision needs to be taken whether one can wait for some time or there is a decided need for the reintervention. With time, the buckle effect tends to increase due to the tonographic effect of the buckle; and very often, a retinal break gets closed provided the buckle placement is accurate. Residual fluid after successful closure of retinal break can also take a long time to absorb in case of chronic retinal detachments. These should not be mistaken as cases of recurrent retinal detachments.

Approach to Management of Recurrent/Persistent Retinal Detachment

The most important thing to be evaluated is the cause of the problem. One should carefully evaluate the relationship of the break to the buckle. The connection between the fluid and the

Table 30.5: Tips for the performance of revision buckling

1. It is easiest to open the eye for revision buckling in the first 10 days time when the adhesions are not well-formed and the surgery is less bloody.

2. It is not necessary to open all round and hook all the 4 recti. Limited opening can be done to open one or more quadrants as the case may be.

3. If one quadrant exposure is needed, it is usually necessary to open the conjunctiva at least one clock hour beyond the insertion of the recti to give space for tagging of the recti.

4. For tagging the muscles, the insertions can be exposed adequately by applying 4-0 black silk sutures through the sclera anteriorly and using them for traction on the globe. Trying to rotate the eye by holding the soft tissues with forceps leads to tearing of the tissues.

5. Rectus muscles are tagged by using the railroad method. A curved Steven scissors is used to dissect sharply under the rectus. Once the tips are seen on the other side, a muscle hook is pushed under the muscle using the scissors as guide. If a buckle is located under the muscle, it is easy to dissect under the muscle with the scissors. Blind hooking of the muscles as in primary surgery should never be done.

6. Sharp dissection should be done to separate the tissues and expose the surface of the sclera. Blunt separation with cotton-tipped applicators has no role.

7. While placing a new buckle under a muscle, the adhesion of the muscle to the sclera all along its length should be cut, before trying to push the buckle underneath the muscle.

8. Retreatment of break is needed if the revision surgery is being done beyond seven days of primary surgery or if the previous treatment was not adequate.

break should also be evaluated. Sometimes a shallow detachment at the posterior edge of the break can be missed and one may assume the original break to be flat. Attention should also be paid to the anterior edge of the retinal break, which may not be well-supported. Repeated examination of the fundus with scleral depression may be needed to detect missed or new breaks. One should also evaluate the status of vitreous traction. Significant medial haze or vitreous membranes can potentially hide a small break. Locations where one can miss a break are the posterior pole in high myopia. Breaks can be hidden in areas of chorioretinal atrophy and staphyloma. Tiny breaks at the edge of vitreous base can also be hidden if the vitreous is condensed and semiopaque. Proliferative vitreoretinopathy is usually obvious if it is the cause of recurrence.

The planning of the management would depend upon the identification of the cause of the redetachment. The following options exist:

1. *Gas injection*: Simple injection of gas/air followed by positioning (pneumatic retinopexy) can reattach the retina in cases of retinal breaks that are on the buckle. If the procedure is done within the seven days of the primary surgery, retreatment of the break for retinopexy is not needed. Inferior breaks that are in similar location cannot be closed with gas injection usually. Pneumatic retinopexy and prone positioning can sometimes be used to manage recurrent

detachments due to macular holes that were present in addition to the buckled peripheral break.

2. *Revision buckling:* Revising the buckle may be the best option in case of inadequate buckle. The revision may involve just shifting the buckle posteriorly, adding an extra element, such as Pruett's meridional buckle or replacing the buckle with a larger one. In case of a new break, an extra buckle may need to be placed.

3. *Parsplana vitrectomy:* Vitrectomy procedures have become the most important way of managing recurrent retinal detachment. A definitive management is possible in most cases. This approach enables clearance of medial opacities, precise identification of the tiny breaks that missed detection by ophthalmoscopy and removal of all vitreous traction on the breaks. Superior breaks that are not on the buckle can also be managed by vitrectomy with internal tamponade without revising the buckle. Inferior breaks that are posterior also do well with this approach. However, inferior and relatively anterior breaks may still need additional buckle to support the break. Eyes with proliferative vitreoretinopathy are managed by pars plana vitrectomy with gas or silicone oil tamponade.

RESULTS OF SCLERAL BUCKLING AND PNEUMATIC RETINOPEXY

Scleral Buckling

Anatomical Results

Sharma and associates reported a series of 601 eyes that underwent primary scleral buckling by one surgeon. The anatomical reattachment was achieved in 86% of the eyes after a single procedure, which improved to 90% with additional procedure. Predictors of poor anatomic outcome were preoperative presence of choroidal detachment, significant vitreous opacification, circumferential buckle of more than 2 quadrants, need for intravitreal injection of air or fluid, and occurrence of postoperative vitreal inflammation.

Visual Results

Tani and associates found the following factors to be predictive of better anatomical success—preoperative vision better than 20/50, partial retinal detachment, retinal tears located at or anterior to equator, absence of giant retinal tear, absence of preoperative hypotony (IOP < 5 mmHg), ocular hypertension (IOP > 20 mmHg), nondrainage procedure, a single operation with less than 50 cryo applications, and noncircumferential buckle.

Pneumatic Retinopexy

In a series by Tornambe and associates, 73% of cases of pneumatic retinopexy had retinal reattachment with one surgery vs 84% with scleral buckle group. However, with reoperations, the success was equal in both groups indicating the pneumatic retinopexy does not adversely affect the final outcome even if it fails necessitating a scleral buckle subsequently. The visual results were better with pneumatic retinopexy compared to scleral buckling possibly because of the increased trauma associated with the scleral buckling. In addition, pneumatic retinopexy is decidedly a less morbid procedure with early rehabilitation and absolute lack of any effect on the extraocular movements. In the scenario of recurrent retinal detachment, Sharma and associates had a success rate of 69.4% with pneumatic retinopexy in a series of 36 eyes. They found that pneumatic retinopexy failed to reattach the retina in case of break on the slope of the buckle or posterior to the buckle.

PROLIFERATIVE VITREORETINOPATHY

Definition

Proliferative vitreoretinopathy may be defined as a non-neoplastic growth and contraction of cellular membranes in the vitreous cavity and on both surfaces of the retina. It is the most common cause of failure of retinal reattachment surgery. Proliferative vitreoretinopathy can be considered as an attempted repair process that has gone away and is caused by a retinal break. The present term is the most accepted and was preceded by nomenclature, such as massive vitreous traction and periretinal proliferation. Some consider it not as a disease entity, but as an endpoint of several stimuli due to various diseases.

Classification

The 1983 classification developed by the Retina Society was the commonly used one, although there are several limitations to the same (Table 30.6).

Table 30.6: Classification of proliferative vitreoretinopathy (Retina Society)

Grade	Name	Clinical signs
A	Minimal	Vitreous haze, pigmentary clumps
B	Moderate	Wrinkling of inner retinal surface
		Rolled edges of tears, retinal stiffness Vessel tortuosity
C	Marked	Full-thickness fixed retinal folds
C1		One quadrant
C2		Two quadrants
C3		Three quadrants
D	Massive	Fixed retinal folds in four quadrants
D1		Wide funnel shape
D2		Narrow funnel shape
D3		Closed funnel shape

The silicone oil study group's classification is more elaborate and descriptive. The presence of anterior proliferative vitreoretinopathy and subretinal fibrosis have been given due cognizance in this classification (Table 30.7).

Table 30.7: Definitions of terms used in proliferative vitreoretinopathy classification

Type 1: Focal contraction—A star fold in the posterior retina

Type 2: Diffuse contraction—Confluent irregular folds in posterior retina. Remainder of retina drawn posteriorly and the disc may not be visible.

Type 3: Subretinal contraction—Napkin ring or clothesline type of subretinal bands in posterior retina

Type 4: Circumferential contraction—Irregular retinal folds in the anterior retina; peripheral retina within vitreous base stretched inward

Type 5: Perpendicular contraction—Involves anterior retina as a smooth circumferential fold of retina at insertion of posterior hyaloid.

Type 6: Anterior contraction—Circumferential fold of retina at insertion of posterior hyaloid pulled forward; trough of peripheral retina anteriorly; ciliary processes stretched with possible hypotony; iris retracted.

Certain terms were defined as follows:

Grades A and B are the same as Grades A and B of Retina Society Classification. Grade CP is subclassified into P1 to P4 depending upon the number of quadrants involved of posterior retina with focal and/or diffuse and/or subretinal contraction (types 1-3) and Grade CA is subclassified into A1 to A4 depending upon number of quadrants of anterior retina involved with circumferential and/or perpendicular and/or anterior traction of the retina (types 4-6). In addition, a detailed drawing is made with symbols depicting each one of the types. Since the location on the drawing is precise, the quantification of proliferative vitreoretinopathy is easier.

Pathogenesis

Despite the identification of several biochemical factors from the eyes with proliferative vitreoretinopathy and in experimental studies, the exact sequence of events and the relative importance of each of these factors and their effects on cellular behavior are not as yet clear. The following discussion is a distillate of the mass of information available on this subject.

Information from Clinical Studies

1. Preoperative proliferative vitreoretinopathy and preoperative choroidal detachment have been identified as important predictors of postoperative proliferative vitreoretinopathy in several studies.
2. Cryo has been found to increase risk of proliferative vitreoretinopathy, especially if the treatment is extensive and if done in the presence of curled posterior edges of horseshoe tears.
3. Other factors, such as extent of retinal detachment, presence of vitreous hemorrhage, signs of uveitis, use of air tamponade, etc. have also been suggested as risk factors, but have not been proved.

Information from Basic Studies

1. Cells participating in the proliferative vitreoretinopathy process: Retinal pigment epithelial cells, retinal glial cells and possibly macrophages.
2. Changes in retinal pigment epithelial cells: With the onset of rhegmatogenous retinal detachment, retinal pigment epithelial cells undergo dedifferentiation, migration and proliferation.
3. Glial cells of retina also dedifferentiate, migrate and proliferate on both sides of retina.
4. Stimulus for the retinal pigment epithelial changes consequent to the rhegmatogenous retinal detachment is the lack of contact with photoreceptors. Retinal and matrix derived signals are believed to allow normal differentiation of retinal pigment epithelial cells and downregulate the growth promoting autocrine loop.
5. Autocrine loops help self-sustain the proliferative response by retinal pigment epithelial cells. Retinal pigment epithelial cells have receptors to growth factors liberated by them and so respond by proliferation.
6. Autocrine loops also sustain the proliferative response of epiretinal membranes, wherein the factors liberated by the cells of the membranes act to perpetuate the proliferative response.
7. Factors possibly involved in the occurrence of proliferative vitreoretinopathy:
   a. Platelet-derived growth factor (PDGF) is a chemoattractant and mitogen for both retinal pigment epithelial and retinal glial cells related to wound repair response.
   b. Vascular endothelial growth factor (VEGF)—although more often associated with vasoproliferative disorders, the relative ischemia caused by the detached retina can stimulate liberation of VEGF, which can contribute to the membrane formation.
   c. Epidermal growth factor (EGF) and insulin-like growth factor-1 (IGF-1) are serum derived and can contribute to proliferation.
   d. Cytokines liberated by the retinal pigment epithelium may indirectly contribute by recruiting macrophages.
   e. Fibronectin derived from serum stimulates the RPE to migrate.
8. Breakdown of blood-retinal barrier is responsible for bringing in the serum-derived growth factors (endocrine), such as Fibronectin, EGF and IGF-1 into the vitreous cavity following the occurrence of retinal detachment.
9. Retinal pigment epithelial cells are more responsive to the growth factors in the presence of retinal detachment.

Pathology

The most important characteristic of proliferative vitreoretinopathy is the formation of membranes in the vitreous cavity and on both sides of the retina. The origin of the membranes is fairly well-established to be the retinal pigment epithelial and the retinal glial cells with contribution from the macrophages. The membranes of proliferative vitreoretinopathy have been classified as complex membranes (Foos and associates), in contrast to simple membranes with no contractile features (e.g. prepapillary membranes) and intermediate membranes (e.g. idiopathic epiretinal membrane in front of macula, etc.). Majority of the membranes have myoblastic features. Intracellular actin filaments have also been found in the membranes by immunofluorescent techniques. The classification (silicone oil study group) detailed above also gives an insight into the macroscopic pathology seen in the cases of proliferative vitreoretinopathy.

Management

Surgical Management of Rhegmatogenous Retinal Detachment with Proliferative Vitreoretinopathy

As has been alluded to, proliferative vitreoretinopathy is the most important cause of recurrent retinal detachment. The management has undergone a dramatic change with the advent of vitrectomy techniques by Machemer. Prior to vitrectomy era, high and broad buckles and injection of air were the only tools available for the management of these difficult problems.

Do All the Cases of Rhegmatogenous Retinal Detachment with Proliferative Vitreoretinopathy Need Vitrectomy?

Scleral buckle can be effective in the management of most cases of Grades A and B and some cases of Grade C1. If the fixed fold is not located in the vicinity of a reasonably anteriorly located break, a buckle should be able to result in anatomical reattachment of the retina. One has, of course, to contend with the fact that an eye with preoperative proliferative vitreoretinopathy is at a higher risk of developing postoperative proliferative vitreoretinopathy. In most other situations, one has to resort to vitreoretinal procedures.

When to Operate in an Eye with Proliferative Vitreoretinopathy?

It is well-known that mature membranes are easier to remove compared to immature ones. The incidence of recurrent proliferative vitreoretinopathy is also expected to be more if one operates in the active stage of the disease. Hence, in cases of early proliferative vitreoretinopathy, waiting for a few days can theoretically be helpful in the reduction of recurrent proliferative vitreoretinopathy. However, from the visual recovery perspective, it would be obviously important to operate early. Hence, it is difficult to define the ideal time frame for surgical intervention.

Role of Buckle along with Vitrectomy

A peripheral buckle is placed along with vitrectomy in cases of rhegmatogenous retinal detachment with proliferative retinopathy by most surgeons. One can argue that since a vitrectomy relieves all traction, there is no need for the buckle. However, one should realize that a total vitrectomy in that sense of the word is never possible. A peripheral buckle helps support the vitreous base. Very often, the buckle is not placed to support any break directly, especially in the presence of a superior break. However, a relatively anteriorly located inferior break may need to be buckled, especially if gas tamponade is used. In the case of a 360° retinal tear or retinotomy, it is obvious that a peripheral buckle has no role to play.

Role of Lens Sacrifice

In the presence of significant lens opacity, there is no controversy in the concept of removing the lens to enable the management of the retinal detachment properly. However, in the presence of a clear lens or only minimal lens opacity, an important decision has to be taken whether the lens needs to be sacrificed or not. It is best not to take rigid stance regarding the lens sacrifice.

Advantages of Lens Removal

The obvious advantage of removing the lens is the ability to see the periphery better and more importantly to reach the periphery better. A better debulking of the peripheral gel vitreous can be done. Fluid-air exchange is also easier since visualization in an aphakic eye with air does not need any special contact lens. Any treatment in the form of retinopexy with endolaser will be easy in an aphakic gas-filled eye. Peripheral retina can be easily treated by indenting the sclera. Postoperatively, it will be easier to visualize the fundus and to perform any additional treatment, such as fluid-air exchange.

Disadvantages of Lens Removal

The downside of lens removal is the fact that the patient is being made aphakic with need to wear contact lenses or to go through additional surgery for scleral fixated IOL. In addition, during the fluid-air exchange, there can be occurrence of Descemet's folds that can interfere with visualization. This problem is more likely to occur in cases where an ab externo removal of the lens was needed due to a relatively hard lens. The pupil is also likely to become smaller during the lens removal and can be a source of problem.

There are certain cases wherein lens removal is mandatory. These are cases with significant anterior proliferative vitreoretinopathy. In case of recurrent retinal detachment after previous vitreoretinal surgery and in most cases of traumatic retinal detachments with PVR, one would need to sacrifice the lens.

Procedure of Lens Removal

Most lenses can be removed using the cutter or the fragmatome through the sclerotomies. Very hard lenses need extracapsular cataract surgery. One can deliver the nucleus and close the wound. The capsule and the cortical matter can be removed using the cutter through the sclerotomies. Option of retaining the anterior or posterior capsule to enable a later introduction of IOL may not be ideal. The capsule can serve as a scaffold for the reproliferation to take place.

Role of Intraocular Lens Sacrifice

The concepts are different for the IOL. The need for removal of the IOL is far less than that for crystalline lens. Reaching the periphery does not damage the IOL even if instruments touch the lens. However, the problems posed by the presence of IOL are several.

- There could be visualization difficulties due to the presence of after-cataract, IOL deposits, and posterior synechiae between the IOL and the sphincter.
- The IOL could get displaced during fluid-air exchange as in the case of iris-supported lenses.
- Very often, eyes with rhegmatogenous retinal detachment and proliferative retinopathy occurring after-cataract surgery tends to have a relatively murky peri-intraocular lens environment. The IOL could be decentered, sometimes to an extreme degree. There could be vitreous in the wound or adherent to the capsular tears. Pigment on the IOL can be significant.

Hence, removal of IOL may be indicated in some cases mainly to improve visualization. It must be emphasized that one should not compromise on the adequacy of visualization and treatment in an attempt to save the IOL. One can salvage a few cases by controlled excision of the after-cataract to give adequate pupillary space and by removing the deposits on the IOL using gentle scraping under viscoelastic.

Extent of Vitrectomy

Vitrectomy involves base excision in most cases of proliferative vitreoretinopathy. If only posterior proliferative vitreoretinopathy exists and one is preserving the lens, only limited debulking is possible. In all cases of anterior proliferative vitreoretinopathy, careful base excision is needed. Base excision can be done using scleral indentation. High cutting rate and low suction is required. Bimanual surgery may be needed in difficult cases of severe proliferative vitreoretinopathy. Abnormal vitreoretinal adhesions can, on occasions, be very posterior and prevent adequate base excision.

Membrane Peeling Techniques

Various instruments have been devised to perform this step of the procedure, such as pics, spatulas, forceps, etc. Important points to remember are (Fig. 30.14):

- Traction should be tangential and not anteroposterior in order to avoid iatrogenic retinal breaks.
- Very fine membranes can be lifted by using membrane scratcher.
- Presence of fine membranes may not be obvious and one has to take the guidance from the contour of the retina and the blood vessels.
- In general, a total relief of traction is aimed at.

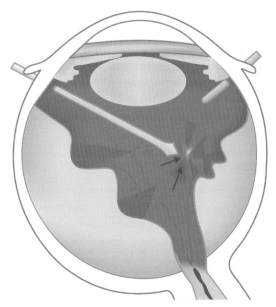

Fig. 30.14: Schematic diagram showing fixed folds. A microvitreoretinal blade is being used to initiate the dissection. (Modified with permission from Travis A Meredith, MD)

Subretinal Band Removal

Subretinal fibrosis can be extensive as a network of tissue or isolated bands. These bands can be located near the posterior pole or in the periphery. Isolated bands can be removed by retinotomy placed closed to or on top of the band in an accessible position. Extensive bands may need two or more retinotomies to access the entire circumference. Spatulas are used to mobilize the membranes before grasping them with forceps. Extensive tissues need large peripheral retinotomies and reflection of the retina to be able to remove all the membranes. Peripapillary napkin ring can be especially difficult to remove since the space available between the retina and the retinal pigment epithelium is less.

Role of Retinotomies and Retinectomies

- *Drainage retinotomy*: Mostly a superior and relatively anterior location is chosen so that it can be well-tamponaded by the air/gas. Too anterior a location may make it difficult to drain properly. The retinotomy is made using a cautery.
- Retinotomy for removing subretinal traction.
- *Relaxing retinotomy*: This is performed to relieve traction and enable the settlement of the retina when maximum membrane peeling could not relieve the traction. In most cases, a peripheral retinotomy is needed. The extent of retinotomy is dependent upon the amount of traction. In severe cases of proliferative vitreoretinopathy, a 360° retinotomy may be needed. It is better to err on the side of too much rather than too little. Radial retinotomy is almost never done since it can extend posteriorly into the functional retina. Only very rarely is this required. A relaxing retinotomy is never done before maximum membrane peeling has been performed.

- *Relaxing retinectomy*: Very often, the anterior retina beyond the retinotomy is excised since it can be a scaffold for reproliferation. Focal areas of contracted retina are also excised totally to create a large break and a relaxed retina. The retina around the sites of incarceration (posterior and anterior perforation sites) also needs to be cut so that there is a clear area between the edge of the retinotomy and the incarceration site.

Retinal Reattachment

Retina is reattached using either fluid-air exchange or direct fluid-oil exchange or with the use of perfluorocarbon liquids. Fluid-air exchange is done by insufflating the eye with air and simultaneously evacuating the vitreous and subretinal space with flute or other similar needle. Subretinal fluid removal is done through a preexisting retinal break or drainage retinotomy. In most cases, drainage retinotomy is not needed. Even through a relatively anterior retinal break, adequate drainage can be accomplished. If the break is on the buckle and does not permit flattening of the posterior retina, one can use a small bubble of perfluorocarbon liquid to flatten the posterior retina and then perform the fluid-air exchange, thus effectively flattening the whole retina. Fluid-oil exchange uses similar principles except that it is a slower procedure with risk of hypotony during the procedure, and risk of subretinal migration of oil if the traction is not adequately relieved. If a similar situation occurs with fluid-air exchange, reinfusing fluid can easily bring the subretinal air out. This permits addressing the problem area of unrelieved traction, and re-performing fluid-air exchange. However, with oil, it can be a messy affair to bring the subretinal oil into the main bubble in the vitreous cavity and performing the additional membrane surgery to address the unrelieved traction.

Uses of Perfluorocarbon Liquids

Perfluorocarbon liquids are heavier than water and very useful in the management of proliferative vitreoretinopathy. A small bubble placed in the posterior pole enables the dissection of anterior proliferative vitreoretinopathy by holding the posterior retina down (Fig. 30.15). It enables the detection of fine membranes. The extent of relaxing retinotomy can be fine-tuned with the help of perfluorocarbon liquid. Perfluorocarbon liquid enables the performance of 360° retinotomy with ease without the risk of the retina folding back.

Retinopexy

Retinopexy is preferably done with endolaser, which has the least risk of inducing retinal pigment epithelial cell liberation. In most cases of proliferative vitreoretinopathy, 360° treatment may be needed in addition to the treatment of the obvious retinal breaks. The performance of vitreous base excision also leads to occurrence of tiny breaks near the vitreous base and the ora serrata—hence the need for 360° treatment.

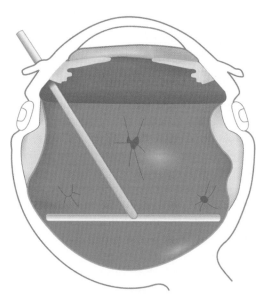

Fig. 30.15: Schematic diagram showing injection of perfluorocarbon liquids. Being heavier than water, the liquid reattaches the retina posteriorly facilitating the dissection of membranes anteriorly. (Modified with permission from Travis A Meredith, MD)

Choice of Tamponade

The choice is between long-acting gas and silicone oil (Figs. 30.16 and 30.17). The long-acting gas that is especially recommended for cases of proliferative vitreoretinopathy is perfluoropropane (C_3F_8). Short-acting gases like SF_6 may not be ideal. The choice of oil vs gas is not clear and mostly is dependent on the individual surgeon's choice and experience (Table 30.8). In general cases, with recurrence following use of gas, and cases needing large retinotomies, need silicone oil tamponade. Inability of the patient to maintain posture could be another important reason for use of oil. Where oil is used, it can be directly exchanged with perfluorocarbon liquid or fluid or alternately one can do fluid-air exchange first and then perform air-silicone oil exchange. The results from the silicone oil study group showed equal success with gas or oil in primary surgery in eyes with proliferative vitreoretinopathy.

Table 30.8: Gas versus oil

1. Rigid maintenance of postoperative posture may not be as important with silicone oil as with gas.
2. Inferior breaks do better with silicone oil compared to gas; although compared to superior breaks, inferior breaks lead to recurrence more often with both gas and oil.
3. Postoperative visualization of the fundus is easier with silicone oil and this permits laser photocoagulation comparatively easily.
4. There is no restriction on air travel with silicone oil.
5. The patient can have useful vision through oil while there is little useful vision possible through a gas-filled eye.
6. There is need for additional surgery in all cases filled with silicone oil for the removal of the same.
7. Recurrence of retinal detachments in a gas-filled eye spread fast and tend to be total, while oil tends to have some stabilization effect and restricts the spread of retinal detachment.

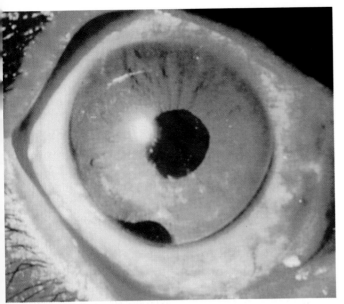

Fig. 30.16: External photograph showing the Ando 6 o'clock iridectomy. The iridectomy helps keep the oil away from the cornea by allowing entry of aqueous into the anterior chamber (Reprinted with permission from the Indian Journal of Ophthalmology)

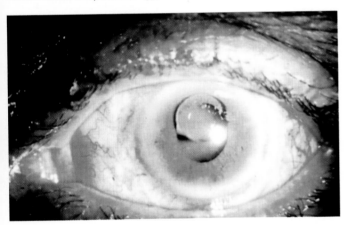

Fig. 30.17: Silicone oil bubble in the anterior chamber. This indicates significant zonular dehiscence (Reprinted with permission from the Indian Journal of Ophthalmology)

Silicone Oil Removal

Silicone oil removal should be attempted in most cases unless the condition is not satisfactory. Usually, one waits for three to four months before contemplating the same. However, in cases of traumatic proliferative vitreoretinopathy and recurrent proliferative vitreoretinopathy, it may be wise to keep the oil in the eye for a longer time. However, it is not a good practice to wait for the removal of the oil till complications arise, since the complications are not always reversible. At the time of removal of oil, one has to make sure that the retina is totally attached and there are no open retinal breaks. During the oil removal, very often additional membrane peeling is needed since some amount of reproliferation is very common. Peripheral unrelieved traction and fibrosis may also need attention even if the same is anterior to retinopexy scars. Recurrence of retinal detachment after oil removal is a real possibility and

the incidence is minimized by meticulous pre-oil removal examination of the eye and combining the oil removal with additional surgery.

Results

The results from most studies may not be comparable since the variability of the disease is great. However, with the advent of the classification by the retina society, some degree of comparability has emerged in the various series reported. In general, eyes with anterior proliferative vitreoretinopathy do much worse than those with only posterior proliferative vitreoretinopathy. In the pre-vitrectomy era, it was found that the success with simple buckling was less than 20%. Anatomical success in the range of 60 to 70% is reported in several series with the modern vitreoretinal techniques. Functional results are expected to be poor considering the severity of the problem. Ambulatory vision is most often achieved, with occasional cases recovering good reading vision. The results of the silicone oil study group are summarized in Table 30.9.

Table 30.9: Summary of the results from the multicentric trial conducted by silicone oil study group

1. Rates of anatomical reattachment of the retina are higher with per fluoropropane gas (C_3F_8) compared with sulfur hexafluoride (SF_6).

2. Rates of anatomical reattachment of the retina are equal with silicone oil (1000 centistokes) and C_3F_8.

3. Relaxing retinotomies were more often needed in eyes undergoing repeat vitreous surgery.

4. In eyes needing relaxing retinotomy also, C_3F_8 and silicone oil had equal retinal reattachment rates.

5. Macular pucker after surgery for proliferative vitreoretinopathy:
   a. 15% cases had macular pucker at 6 months postoperative period.
   b. Macular pucker more common with aphakic and pseudophakic eyes compared to phakic eyes (3 times more).
   c. Macular pucker more with large retinal breaks.
   d. No difference between eyes filled with gas or oil.
   e. Visual acuity worse in eyes with macular pucker.

6. Oil removal
   a. Oil removed eyes had more incidence of complete retinal reattachment than oil retained eyes.
   b. Oil removed eyes had better visual acuity than oil retained eyes.
   c. Oil removed eyes had better visual acuity and less incidence of hypotony than gas-filled eyes.

7. Intraocular pressure
   a. Greater chance of chronic raised pressure (more than 25 mmHg) in the silicone oil-filled eyes.
   b. Greater chances of chronic hypotony in eyes filled with gas.
   c. Chronic hypotony associated with recurrent retinal detachment, poor visual 'acuity and corneal opacity.
   d. Diffuse retinal contraction anterior to the equator predicts the occurrence of chronic postoperative hypotony.

8. Decreasing trends of visual recovery with increasing severity of proliferative vitreoretinopathy seen.

9. If successful anatomical result is achieved and retained up to 3 years, long-term stability chances are very high.

RECENT INNOVATIONS IN THE MANAGEMENT OF PROLIFERATIVE VITREORETINOPATHY

Considering the unsatisfactory and unpredictable nature of the results, various innovations have been tried—some surgical and some pharmacological.

Endoscopic Surgery

This method of approach involves use of an endoscope to visualize relatively inaccessible areas, such as the anterior proliferative vitreoretinopathy. However, the applicability of this technique as of today is limited and does not enhance the surgical result in most cases compared to routine techniques using binocular visualization. The possible indications for the use of the endoscope are:

- To visualize behind the iris and remove membranes.
- To be able to complete the surgery if the visualization becomes bad during the surgery, especially when laser retinopexy has to be performed (e.g. small pupil and corneal Descemet's folds).
- To perform vitreoretinal surgery and plan penetrating keratoplasty as a second-stage procedure in cases with significant corneal opacity. In some cases of corneal blood staining, the opacity may ultimately clear and may not need a keratoplasty at all. In such cases, the endoscopic performance of vitrectomy precludes the need for a combined keratoplasty and vitrectomy.

Erbium:YAG Laser Vitrectomy

Noncontact vitrectomy using Erbium:YAG laser was tried with apparently some advantages. However, the technology still has limitations and more wide application is possible only with further developments.

Pharmacological Modulation

Perhaps the most important area that is likely to be beneficial in improving the results of the management of proliferative vitreoretinopathy is drug therapy. Having considered the pathogenesis, one realizes how difficult it is to know when the disease is active and which of the multitude of the factors are responsible for the initiation and perpetuation of the disease at a given point of time. Hence, it has not been possible to target any one of the given factors. Most approaches involved use of antimetabolites or anti-inflammatory agents.

a. *Steroids*: Steroids have been tried as intravitreal injections since inflammation has been shown to release factors that modulate occurrence of PVR. Machemer's experiments have shown the tolerance of the retina to intravitreal triamcinolone acetonide. However, the efficacy was not found in vivo possibly due to the lack of prolonged action on the disease process.

b. *5-Fluorouracil (5-FU)*: This antiproliferative agent has been tried in animal experiments and in humans, but has not been shown to be very effective.

c. *Combination drugs*: Triamcinolone and 5-FU have been tried in experimental animals as co-drugs and have been shown to reduce the incidence of proliferative vitreoretinopathy when administered in slow release devices.

d. *Combination of dexamethasone and heparin*: It was tried with BSS during vitrectomy. In this study, the authors did not find any statistically significant difference between the two groups in terms of retinal reattachment rate although the study group had slightly better results.

e. *Daunorubicin*: It has been tried in a randomized trial conducted in Europe. The results show no statistical significant difference between the success after one surgery as well after multiple surgeries between the study and control groups. However, the number and frequency of reoperations needed was significantly less in the daunorubicin group. Hui and associates have shown in experimental animals that if triamcinolone is given during the inflammatory phase and daunorubicin is given in the proliferative phase, the success rate of preventing occurrence of proliferative vitreoretinopathy is high. Retinoic acid was tried in experimental animals and was found to be effective in reducing the incidence of proliferative vitreoretinopathy and this drug could be administered in silicone oil. However, no human studies are available.

f. *Others drugs*: Other drugs tried in experimental conditions are calcium antagonists (nifedipine), Taxol (a potent inhibitor of contraction of fibroblasts), monoclonal antibodies linked to toxin against transferring receptors in fibroblasts, interferon-α, trapidil (a PDGF inhibitor), suramin (a trypanocidal drug that can also block the binding of growth factors), integrins, etc.

GIANT RETINAL TEAR

Introduction

Giant retinal tears are defined as retinal tears with circumferential extent of more than 90°. The success rate of reattachment with scleral buckling procedures was about 30%. The introduction of vitrectomy has made significant improvement in their management. The other important developments that improved the success of their management are the introduction of perfluorocarbon liquids, gases and silicone oil. The use of perfluorocarbon liquids has enabled the surgery to be performed in supine position and has almost eliminated the problems of slippage of the retina posteriorly, thus improving the success rate of reattachment of fresh giant retinal tears to nearly 90 to 95%.

Etiology

Myopia is perhaps the most common risk factor for giant retinal tear. Nearly 40% of patients with giant retinal tear have myopia of more than 8 diopters. Trauma is a cause of giant retinal disinsertion rather than a tear and involves the upper nasal or lower temporal quadrants. A large area of chorioretinal atrophy or lattice degeneration can develop giant retinal tear along its posterior edge. Giant retinal tears are common in diseases, such as Marfan's syndrome, Ehler-Danlos syndrome and Wagner-Stickler syndrome. Nasal giant retinal tear is known to be associated with nasal coloboma of the lens. Both penetrating and blunt injury can be associated with giant retinal tear. Pars plana vitrectomy can be rarely complicated by postoperative occurrence of giant retinal tear. Attempted removal of dislocated lens fragments by the limbal approach during cataract surgery is also associated with the high-risk of giant retinal tear, especially inferiorly. Bilateral occurrence of giant retinal tear, following laser assisted *in-situ* keratomileusis (LASIK) has been reported. Retinitis pigmentosa associated with hearing loss (Usher's syndrome) has also been associated with giant retinal tear, although the causal relationship has not been established. Giant retinal tear could also result from relaxing retinotomies and retinectomies performed during surgery for cases of retinal detachment with severe proliferative vitreoretinopathy. The idiopathic and traumatic varieties are seen more commonly in males. Bilaterality is reported in 13% of cases. There is one report of idiopathic giant retinal tear occurring in identical twins bringing in the possible influence of genetics in the causation of giant retinal tear.

Clinical Presentation

One has to differentiate between giant retinal tear and dialysis. The pathogenesis, pathology and management are totally different. A giant retinal break is caused by vitreous traction occurring on the anterior edge of the flap. Hence, the posterior edge of torn retina does not have any vitreous adhesion. In contrast, a dialysis occurs within the vitreous base and the vitreous remains adherent to the posterior edge of the tear. Posterior vitreous detachment is absent in most cases. Avulsed vitreous base is often made out along with the dialysis. In echographic studies, Genovesi and associates showed the presence of vitreous synersis in primary giant retinal tear; while in cases of disinsertion, the vitreous was adherent to the posterior retinal flap. Significantly, there was no evidence of synersis in eyes with giant retinal tear secondary to IOL implantation although posterior vitreous detachment was present.

Variables

The giant retinal tear may extend to any degree circumferentially beyond 90°. They may also possess posterior extensions (horns) at the limits of the circumferential tear. The extent of these horns is variable. The flap of giant retinal tear is almost always inverted if the tear is more than 180°. The vitreous gel may enter the tear. This may be an important feature to identify since simple buckling surgery will not suffice if the vitreous is under the retina. There can be other retinal tears involving other quadrants associated with a giant retinal tear. Proliferative vitreoretinopathy of variable severity can occur. In view of the fact that a large area of retinal pigment epithelium is exposed, the risk of proliferative vitreoretinopathy is substantial. The proliferative vitreoretinopathy also tends to progress rapidly. The risk of proliferative vitreoretinopathy was found to be higher in cases with preoperative proliferative vitreoretinopathy and when cryo was used in comparison to use of photocoagulation. Profuse hypotony and choroidal detachment are also very common. Pars plana epithelium can be detached in the area of giant retinal tear and indicates vitreous traction.

Management

Broadly, the management revolves around the use of scleral buckling or vitreoretinal surgical techniques. Most cases of dialysis can be managed by scleral buckling, since the retinal tear is not inverted and is supported by the vitreous gel. Most other cases need vitreoretinal techniques. Occasional cases of dialysis of more than 3 clock hours have been managed by pneumatic retinopexy.

Technique of Scleral Buckling

Scleral buckling involves use of a relatively broad buckle. Broad buckle is needed to compensate for the relatively posterior point where the central edge of the retinal tear usually settles. In general, any tear with more than 30° circumferential extent will tend to gape significantly. This tendency is even more exaggerated in case of giant retinal tears. To counter the problem of gape in the center, one has to use a shallow buckle and use additional internal tamponade with a bubble of air or expansile gas. In view of the large size of the tear, drainage away from the site of the tear is not possible. Hence, one can expect liquid vitreous to drain in case of giant retinal tear. Where the tear is filled with gel vitreous, drainage can lead to incarceration of vitreous in the drainage site. Cryopexy tends to be extensive in view of the extent of the tear and hence is not the ideal choice for retinopexy. Laser photocoagulation using the indirect laser delivery system on the buckle after the drainage of fluid may be a better option and reduces the risk of proliferative vitreoretinopathy. Although the principles of surgery are the same, in case of a giant retinal dialysis, the surgery of scleral buckling is relatively simpler due to the presence of vitreous gel support to the break as was explained earlier.

Vitreoretinal Surgery

Most cases need vitreoretinal surgical techniques to attach the retina. The surgical technique has evolved over a period of time due to the several contributions listed before. The primary problem the surgeon faced is one of difficulties to keep the inverted flap of retina everted during and after the surgery. There is tendency for the flap to slip and result in circumferential folds that can sometimes involve the macula, especially in case of a temporal giant retinal tear.

Management of Inverted Flap

Historically, several maneuvers have been tried, including retinal incarceration, retinal suturing, retinal screws, retinal tacks, etc. The basic aim of all these techniques was to divide the free margin of the retinal tear into the three or four segments of 20 to 30 degrees each, which enables the settlement of the retina with fluid-air exchange without the retinal slippage. Prone fluid-air exchange was a good technique to flatten the retina, wherein air was injected in front of the disc after vitrectomy. This technique was technically difficult, especially for the anesthetist. Direct silicone oil-fluid exchange was tried by some surgeons with the belief that since the oil flows in much more slowly than the air, there is time for positioning the retinal flap using the intraocular instruments. This again does not work always and there is tendency for the fluid to get trapped posteriorly. Leaver and associates tried posterior retinotomies to drain the trapped posterior fluid. Zivojnovic popularized the use of the silicone brush needle, which is less traumatic to the retina and hence permitted the smoothening of the folds under the silicone oil to a certain extent. Despite all these improvisations, the trauma to the retina was rather significant. The retinal pigment epithelium was also often disturbed under the edge of the tear due to the manipulations. Most of these techniques have become redundant with the advent of perfluorocarbon liquids.

Present Technique

Choice of visualization system

Some type of wide field visualization system is useful in the surgery for GRT. This enables a panoramic view of the fundus, including the peripheral edge of the tear, which is very essential during certain steps. The BIOM (binocular indirect ophthalmomicroscope), the AVI system or their equivalents serve the purpose admirably. Even the Landers' wide field lens or prism lens in combination with an air bubble in the anterior chamber (in aphakic eyes) gives a good panoramic view. In phakic highly myopic eyes, the visualization is extremely difficult during fluid-air exchange even with −80 diopter lens. In the absence of AVI or BIOM, one can utilize auto indirect ophthalmoscopy by taking the microscope away from the eye and having no precorneal lens. The image is inverted, but the visualization is very good.

Surgical Technique

Routine pars plana vitrectomy is performed. Care is taken while introducing the infusion cannula since there could be choroidal detachment. The vitrectomy is relatively simple since there is total vitreous detachment posteriorly. The periphery has to be debulked. This can sometimes pose problems since the free edge of the tear may keep coming in the way of the cutter. The detached pars plana epithelium can also keep prolapsing through the sclerotomies. It is best to place a bubble of perfluorocarbon liquid to stabilize the posterior pole while cleaning the periphery.

Lens Management

Clear lens need not always be sacrificed. With scleral indentation, enough vitreous base debulking can be done without touching the lens. In very high myopes, it may be best to sacrifice the lens since this may help them incidentally with regards to the spectacle correction needed postoperatively (akin to clear lens extraction for optical purpose).

Intraocular Lens Management

In most cases, the IOL need not be removed. If the posterior capsule is opaque, a large enough opening made in the center can enable good visualization with the help of scleral indentation. However, if the capsular opacification is very dense or the IOL is decentered grossly, it may be best to remove the same.

Management of Edge of Tear

In all but the most recent giant retinal tears, the edge may show some contraction. In most cases, this may not pose a problem and can be smoothened with a spatula under the perfluorocarbon liquid or silicone oil. If the edge is too much contracted due to intraretinal fibrosis, it is best to cauterize and excise the edge. This is again best done with a bubble of perfluorocarbon liquid on the posterior pole. If the giant retinal tear is more than 300°, it is best to convert it into a 360° giant retinal tear so that peripheral traction can be totally eliminated.

Management of the Anterior Flap

The anterior flap of the retina is functionless and is a source of problem during and after the surgery. The flap keeps coming in the way of introducing instruments. It can fibrose postoperatively leading to potential recurrent retinal detachment. For these reasons, it is best to excise the anterior flap.

Management of Proliferative Vitreoretinopathy

In the presence of proliferative vitreoretinopathy, the technique has to be suitably altered. The presence of giant retinal tear does not permit the retina to offer resistance for easy peeling. Hence, membrane peeling can become difficult. It is best to remove the membranes on the posterior pole to start with. A bubble of perfluorocarbon liquid stabilizes the posterior pole while membranes anteriorly can be peeled. In giant retinal tears more than 180°, peeling can be difficult even with perfluorocarbon liquid. Bimanual surgery with forceps and spatula is very useful. One can use the coaxial illumination of the microscope since this part of the surgery is done relatively anteriorly. Alternatively, a fourth port can be made for the illumination or the light pipe can be placed on the contact lens to permit bimanual surgery. Once the preretinal membranes are removed, the subretinal space is explored directly. The giant retinal tear permits direct inspection of the undersurface of the retina. The removal of the membranes is as from the preretinal surface. One should specifically look for napkin ring membranes around the disc. Removal of these membranes must be done carefully since the membranes are very close to the retinal pigment epithelium on one side and to the peripapillary retina on the other. There is a risk of retinal pigment epithelium/choroidal damage as well as damage to the peripapillary retina, which can lead to large field defects. In case of tough napkin rings, one may have to segment them at one or two places before attempting to remove them off the subretinal surface. Fine preretinal membranes are more easily identified under the perfluorocarbon liquid. Diligent attempt must be made to remove all the membranes. In most cases of giant retinal tear with significant proliferative vitreoretinopathy, one ends up converting it into a 360° giant retinal tear.

Role of Perfluorocarbon Liquids

Perfluorocarbon liquids are heavier than water liquids. They form a separate meniscus with water and silicone oil. They can be injected and extracted through a small-bore needle. Being heavier than water, they displace the subretinal fluid anteriorly and flatten the retina from behind forwards. They are clear and hence permit visualization and treatment of the retina with endophotocoagulation. This permits the surgery to be done in the supine position. They are used as instruments during the surgery and removed at the end of the surgery by being replaced with either gas or silicone oil (Figs 30.18 and 30.19).

Retinal Reattachment

Perfluorocarbon liquids are injected over the optic disc. Slow injection is made into the bubble. Rapid injection from a height leads to multiple small bubble formation. Although they tend to coalesce, some of the small bubbles can migrate under the retina. As the bubble is enlarging, the retina gets reattached by

displacing the subretinal fluid forwards. Space has to be created for the expanding bubble of perfluorocarbon liquid. Usually, with a good vitrectomy, the intravitreal fluid is able to find its way back up through the infusion cannula to normalize the IOP. If the residual vitreous gel in the vicinity of the infusion cannula blocks this reverse flow of fluid, the IOP can go up. By withdrawing one of the instruments, one can allow leak of fluid quickly and normalize the IOP. Alternately, one can use a combined instrument that allows injection of perfluorocarbon liquid and egress of the intravitreal fluid. One can inject enough perfluorocarbon liquid to evert the flap. Total coverage of the edge of tear with perfluorocarbon liquid is not needed. Following the perfluorocarbon liquid injection, one can do either fluid-silicone oil exchange or fluid-air exchange as the case may be.

Technique of Air Fluid/Air Perfluorocarbon Liquid and Silicone Oil Fluid/Silicone Oil Perfluorocarbon Liquid Exchange

Perfluorocarbon liquid forms a convex meniscus anteriorly. This point has to be borne in mind during these exchanges. The most important step is to totally flatten the retina anterior to the perfluorocarbon liquid before evacuating the perfluorocarbon liquid. To facilitate the same, the flute or extrusion needle or back flush needle is placed near the edge of the retinal tear while injecting air or silicone oil with the eye relatively straight. If the eye is tilted too much towards the tear, the perfluorocarbon liquid bubble shifts in that direction, leading to a large pocket of subretinal fluid 180° away. This remains trapped since the perfluorocarbon liquid bubble seals the edge of the retinal tear. By keeping the eye relatively straight during this step, one can evacuate all of the subretinal fluid. Wide-angle visualization is very useful during this step since it permits the visualization of the periphery without tilting the eye too much. Once the retina anterior to the perfluorocarbon liquid is totally dry,

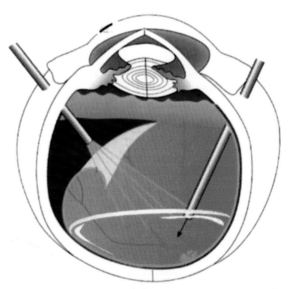

Fig. 30.18: Perfluorocarbon liquids are heavier than water and are used to flatten the retina in a giant retinal tear with retinal detachment (Modified with permission from Travis A Meredith, MD)

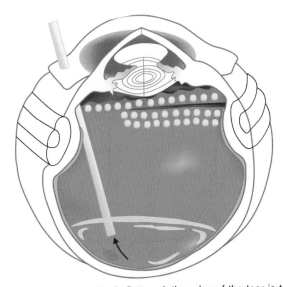

Fig. 30.19: Once the retina is flattened, the edge of the tear is treated with laser photocoagulation and the perfluorocarbon liquid is replaced with either gas or silicone oil. (Modified with permission from Travis A Meredith, MD)

the removal of the perfluorocarbon liquid posteriorly is very easy. Despite these precautions, air exchange tends to produce some slippage in the case of large giant retinal tears (more than 180°). Silicone oil and perfluorocarbon liquid exchange leads to less or no chance of slippage of the retina posteriorly. Hence, in most cases of giant retinal tears, more than 180°, silicone oil is recommended. For the above reasons, where silicone oil tamponade is decided upon it is advisable to do a direct fluid-silicone oil exchange and not to perform air-fluid exchange first and then do an air-silicone oil exchange. The choice of gas vs silicone oil is difficult and often is dependent on the surgeon's choice. In a study by Batman and associates, gas was found to be as good as oil in a series of 22 eyes with giant retinal tear. Perfluorophenanthrene has been used as an intraoperative tool and short-term postoperative tamponade in a series by the Vitreon Collaborative Study Group.

Retinopexy

The choice of retinopexy is photocoagulation. Photocoagulation can be done either with the endophotocoagulator or with the indirect delivery system. In view of the extensive treatment needed and the area of retinal pigment epithelium exposed, cryo will be a poor choice. The risk of proliferative vitreoretinopathy occurring postoperatively is rather high with cryo. The edge of the retinal tear is treated with 3 to 4 rows of moderate intensity laser photocoagulation. The untorn ora serrata is also treated to make it a 360° retinopexy. This improves the long-term success of the surgery by reducing the recurrences from leak occurring from untreated areas due to traction. In eyes with no retinal detachment in areas other than the area of giant retinal tear, the treatment can be restricted to the tear and the ora in the immediate vicinity. Care must be taken to cover the posterior horns properly.

Role of Peripheral Buckle

The role of a peripheral buckle is debated. There are reports of equally good success without a peripheral buckle. Krieger and associates reported a technique of good vitreous base shaving to eliminate the need for a peripheral buckle. Most surgeons prefer the protection offered by a buckle, especially when the lens is not sacrificed. In a series by Verstraeten and associates the reoperation rate was 14% in eyes that had scleral buckling, while 45% of eyes without primary scleral buckling had recurrent retinal detachment. In case of a 360° giant retinal tear or where one is converted into 360° giant retinal tear, peripheral buckle has no role.

Iridectomy

Six o'clock iridectomy is mandatory in all silicone oil-filled aphakic eyes. It makes sense to perform the iridectomy before the silicone oil injection. Performing iridectomy under oil is relatively difficult and any bleeding that is likely to take place from the edge of the iridectomy may be difficult to remove from the surface of the oil.

Postoperative Positioning

Tears less than 180° will need positioning on one side or prone positioning. More than 180° tears require a predominantly prone position. In general, silicone oil-filled eyes require less rigid positioning than gas-filled eyes. Although silicone oil also floats like gas over the fluid, the oil does not shrink in size with time, hence fluid currents are absent under the oil. In the absence of traction, the retina is not lifted up due to the lack of fluid currents. This is one reason why inferior unbuckled tears tend to do better with oil compared to gas.

Recurrent Retinal Detachment

Recurrences are mostly due to proliferative vitreoretinopathy. The recurrences are more dramatic and rapid in gas-filled eyes compared to oil-filled eyes. The management of recurrent detachment under oil differs from that without oil. In general, the approach should be more aggressive in the second surgery, i.e. lens may have to be removed if it was left behind first time. The IOL may also need to be removed to facilitate better management of the vitreous base area. The principles of membrane surgery are the same as discussed under primary surgery with PVR. However, in oil-filled eye with limited proliferative vitreoretinopathy, one can perform additional surgery under silicone oil, by connecting the infusion cannula to a syringe containing silicone oil. If the proliferative vitreoretinopathy is extensive, it is better to remove the silicone oil and re-do the surgery totally.

Silicone Oil Removal

In general, in fresh giant retinal tears without proliferative vitreoretinopathy, silicone oil can be safely removed 6 to 8 weeks after the surgery. In case of proliferative vitreoretinopathy at first or recurrent surgery, oil is best left behind for 3 to 4 months. The eye should be evaluated carefully before planning oil removal. Problems in the periphery can go unnoticed only to lead to recurrent detachment after the oil removal. Presence of skip areas of treatment, traction in the periphery, shallow detachment in the periphery, posterior epiretinal membranes, etc. should be consciously looked for. Peripheral detachment of retina anterior to the barrage of laser may be less dangerous than one spreading beyond the laser barrage. In the first instance, one can get away with excising the peripheral retina with the tractional membranes anterior to the laser barrage. There is no need for additional tamponade. Failure to relieve this traction can lead to spread of the tractional forces beyond the laser and leads to recurrences. In case of even shallow detachment of retina being present beyond the laser barrage, one has to modify the surgical procedure. In addition to relieving the traction by peeling and retinectomy anteriorly, one may have to use additional tamponade in the form of gas or in the worst-case scenario, reinjection of oil. Additional laser is also done to the previously detached areas. Preretinal membranes present posteriorly without fluid are of no concern. Even if extensive, they can be removed without need for additional treatment.

Fellow Eyes with Giant Retinal Tear

Freeman and associates reported 51% incidence of retinal breaks in the fellow eye of nontraumatic giant retinal tear. Sixteen percent of fellow eyes developed retinal detachment. Retinal breaks without detachment consisted of giant retinal tear in 13% eyes, retinal tears in 12%, holes in 10% and dialysis in 0.4%. In general, fellow eye involvement with giant retinal tear was seen within 3½ years of first eye treatment for giant retinal tear. Freeman identified high myopia (>10 D) and increasing white without pressure as risk factors for giant retinal tear in fellow eye. Fellow eyes are recommended prophylactic treatment of all retinal holes and tears. However, the role of prophylactic scleral buckling in eyes with progressive white without pressure is controversial.

MANAGEMENT OF DISLOCATED LENS AND INTRAOCULAR LENS

Introduction

This spectrum of diseases encompasses dislocation of whole crystalline lens, lens nucleus, lens fragments and IOL. The problems facing each one of these are unique and need to be discussed separately although there are some common features. The role of the anterior segment surgeon is also important while managing a complication during cataract surgery. Improper management at that stage cannot only create unnecessary retinal problems, but can also make the subsequent management by the vitreoretinal surgeon difficult. In many situations more than one option is available and the exact course of action ultimately depends upon what the surgeon is most comfortable with.

Clinical Scenario

1. Dislocated Crystalline Lens
   a. Spontaneous
   b. Post-traumatic
2. Dislocated lens fragments/nucleus/cortex
   a. Secondary mostly to intraoperative complications of cataract surgery
   b. Occasional cases of spontaneous absorption of lens matter and dislocated nucleus secondary to hypermaturity
3. Dislocated intraocular lens
   a. Dislocated IOL with vitreous disturbance
   b. Capsular fibrosis leading to zonular dehiscence and dislocation of IOL along with capsule
   c. Trauma-related dislocation
   d. Presence of additional IOL

Dislocated Crystalline Lens

Clinical Evaluation

The clinical evaluation includes the identification of the cause of the dislocation, and the associated damage to the anterior and posterior segment. The dislocated lens can be related to conditions, such as Marfan's syndrome, Marchesani's syndrome, Homocystinuria, etc. Retinal detachment can coexist in some of these cases. Trauma-related dislocated lens might be associated with retinal dialysis, vitreous base avulsion, macular damage, vitreous hemorrhage, secondary glaucoma and retinal detachment. The dislocated lens can be clear, partly opaque or totally cataractous. The lens may be mobile or fixed to the retina by fibrosis due to the long-standing condition. The lens may be leaking proteins and causing uveitis or secondary glaucoma. The total scenario dictates the type of management of a given case.

Management Options

- Observation
- Lens removal with correction of aphakia using contact lens
- Lens removal with correction of aphakia using anterior chamber or scleral fixated IOL
- Lens removal with correction of posterior segment problem with or without IOL
- Lens removal with treatment of glaucoma with or without IOL.

Observation: A dislocated lens is not always an indication for surgical intervention. A clear lens not causing any reaction can be left alone provided the patient is willing for the correction of aphakia with contact lens or aphakic glasses. If, however, there is any other indication for surgery, such as retinal detachment or glaucoma, it is best to combine the same with removal of dislocated lens. In contrast, a subluxated lens can impose optical problems due to inability to correct properly either the aphakic or the phakic portions of the pupil and by itself be an indication for surgical intervention.

Lens removal: A subluxated lens can sometimes be managed by routine ab externo techniques if sufficient zonular support is present and there is no vitreous disturbance. Endocapsular ring is useful for these cases. In case of dislocated lens and those cases of subluxated lenses with little zonular support and vitreous disturbance, the lens removal needs vitreoretinal surgical techniques. A pars plana vitrectomy is the first step. The removal of the lens depends on the hardness of the nucleus. A soft lens can be removed using the vitreous cutter itself. A relatively hard nucleus would need the ultrasonic fragmentor (Table 30.10). One uses the fragmentor only after performing core vitrectomy. The nucleus is lifted away from the retina with suction and then is fragmented in the midvitreous cavity. A very hard nucleus is sometimes not amenable for fragmentation. Such lenses may have to be brought into the anterior chamber and extracted ab externo. Several techniques have been described to bring the lens into the anterior chamber.

1. *Spearing*: The lens can be speared using a sharp microvitreoretinal blade and brought up.
2. *Use of perfluorocarbon liquid*: Perfluorocarbon liquids can be used to float the lens up to pupillary area from where it can be delivered.

3. A technique has also been described wherein the eye can be filled with air and the lens can be reached with a straight cryoprobe from the limbal wound under direct visualization.

Once delivered to the pupillary area, the lens can be extracted via a limbal incision using a wire vectis.

Table 30.10: Tips in using ultrasonic fragmentation

1. The ultrasonic fragmentor should never be used close to the retinal surface.

2. Lens fragments can fly away from the fragmentor tip. Some surgeons use a small bubble of perfluorocarbon liquid on the surface of the retina to protect the macula from the flying hard fragments. Using minimum power required helps in reducing this problem to some extent.

3. If lens milk appears, one must realize that the suction is blocked and continued use of the ultrasound energy can lead to scleral burns around the sclerotomy.

4. Fragmentation should never be used in vitreous gel. The ultrasound energy does not emulsify the vitreous and the suction can lead to retinal breaks.

5. In the presence of retinal detachment, fragmentation of the lens becomes difficult with the risk of sucking and damaging the retina being real. A bubble of perfluorocarbon liquid can make the job relatively simple by keeping the retina down. The suction used to lift the lens from the surface of detached retina should be gentle to start with; and once the lens/fragment is lifted up, the suction is increased to the desired level.

Correction of coexisting retinal detachment: Once the lens is removed, the correction of retinal detachment is by the usual techniques depending upon the presence or absence of proliferative vitreoretinopathy, etc. It is important to note that in the presence of dislocated lens, correction of retinal detachment by simple scleral buckling techniques is unlikely to succeed.

Correction of aphakia

1. The correction of aphakia can be by using postoperative glasses or contact lenses.

2. One can place an anterior chamber lens. The Kelman four-point flexible open loop IOL is the desired lens. Adequate iris diaphragm is important to prevent possible dislocation of the IOL.

3. One can also place a scleral fixated IOL. This is the ideal choice in the case of iris damage and in cases needing combined antiglaucoma surgery with the removal of dislocated lens.

The IOL is not considered if there is coexisting retinal detachment.

Dislocated Nucleus/Lens Fragments/Cortex

This complication occurs commonly during cataract surgery although trauma can result in a similar complication. With the growing popularity of phacoemulsification and the relatively longer learning curve, this complication is fairly commonly seen, especially in a country wherein this procedure is just becoming standard of care. Depending on the stage of surgery at which the posterior capsular rent occurs, there could be dislocation of whole nucleus, fragments or only cortex material. Patients

with retained lens fragments can present with glaucoma, uveitis, corneal edema, etc. Margherio and associates described an incidence of 52.4% of raised IOP beyond 25 mmHg, 69.6% of uveitis, and 50.8% of corneal edema. Timely referral to vitreoretinal surgeon can result in good prognosis.

The management of this complication by the cataract surgeon during the initial surgery is as important as the subsequent management by the vitreoretinal surgeon. Certain guidelines for the cataract surgeons are shown in Table 30.11.

Table 30.11: Guidelines for the cataract surgeon

1. One should never try to blindly fish in the vitreous with vectis for the dislocated nucleus. This results in iatrogenic retinal breaks that complicate the issue.

2. Anterior vitrectomy should be done with the automated vitrector to clear the anterior chamber and pupillary area of all vitreous. Specifically, there should be no vitreous in the wound.

3. The choice of introducing an IOL at this stage would depend upon what the estimate of the surgeon is of the hardness of the nucleus and of course the available support for the lens. One should not be bent upon introducing an IOL. If conditions are good the vitreoretinal surgeon managing the dislocated lens can always introduce the IOL under more controlled conditions after having managed the vitreous well.

4. If, however, the vitreous has been well cleared and there is a good support for the IOL, one can introduce a PC IOL in front of the anterior capsule. In the presence of a hard nucleus, one avoids the IOL since on occasions, one may have to remove the hard nucleus through the ab externo approach.

5. The patient must be referred to a vitreoretinal surgeon at the earliest.

Subsequent Management

Observation: Cases of minimal cortex in the vitreous can be observed, since very often the cortex gets absorbed without any sequelae. However, if significant cortical material is left over, it can cause inflammation and glaucoma. Most cases of dislocated nucleus or nuclear fragments will cause problems given sufficient time. Studies have shown that the removal of these before one week resulted in better visual results.

Surgical Management

The technique of surgery is relatively simple. A routine three-port vitrectomy is done. Cortex and epinucleus can be removed with vitreous cutter while nucleus needs ultrasonic fragmentation using 20-gauge fragmentor. The principles of use of fragmatome have already been detailed. Perfluorocarbon liquids can be used to float the lens fragments making it easier to emulsify them with ultrasonic fragmentor. Theoretically, the presence of perfluorocarbon liquid on the macula is said to protect the same from flying particles of lens matter (Figs 30.20 and 30.21). Any vitreous adherent to the capsule remnants should be cleaned. The periphery of the retina is inspected with indirect ophthalmoscopy using scleral depression. Any retinal tears are managed with cryotherapy and fluid-air exchange. In cases where IOL has not been implanted during the first surgery, one decides on the possibility of the same at the stage after the

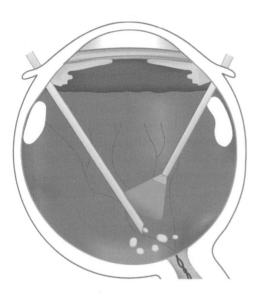

Fig. 30.20: Vitrectomy is done to access the dislocated lens fragments on retinal surface (Modified with permission from Travis A Meredith, MD)

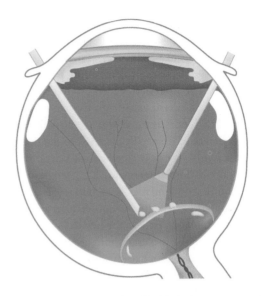

Fig. 30.21: Use of perfluorocarbon liquids helps to remove the lens fragments with ultrasonic fragmentor with relative safety (Modified with permission from Travis A Meredith, MD)

successful removal of the lens remnants. The capsular remnants are preserved to enable possible placement of the IOL in front of the anterior capsule. The exact extent and location of the tears in the anterior and posterior capsule have to be inspected. This is made easy with the help of the endoilluminator. The direction of placement of the IOL can be decided based on this information. If the capsular support is not enough, one can place an anterior chamber lens or a scleral fixated IOL.

Gonvers described a technique of one port vitrectomy in a series of cases with lens nucleus dislocation during phacoemulsification. He used a combined instrument of cutter with infusion sleeve with coaxial illumination of the microscope providing illumination. Schechter described a technique of using a glass slide on the cornea to flatten the same and facilitate viewing the posterior segment when there is no access to precorneal contact lens. He recommends the use of this device with the vitreous cutter and infusion sleeve to perform posterior vitrectomy and remove lens cortical droppings by anterior segment surgeon. For an unaccustomed anterior segment surgeon, such an adventurous approach can be disastrous and hence this approach is not to be recommended. Boscher and associates have attempted endoscopic management with moderate success for the management of dislocated lens nucleus as well as IOL. The authors have used the endoscopic approach to emulsify the fragments as well as to manage retinal breaks. The presumed advantage of this technique is the ability to localize the lens fragments in the vitreous base. The other manipulations have also been made easier despite the presence of corneal edema impairing visualization.

Dislocated Intraocular Lens

Dislocation of IOL can take place during the cataract surgery or subsequently. During the surgery, dislocation is due to inadequate identification of the extent of capsular damage and inability to identify the correct plane of introduction of the IOL.

In addition, if the vitreous has not been managed properly, the strands of vitreous can pull the IOL into the vitreous cavity if it is already precariously positioned. The IOL may be subluxated with one of the haptics still in the pupillary area or it may be totally dislocated. Depending upon the amount of optic in the pupillary area, the subluxation can be significant or insignificant. Insignificant subluxation is fairly common, but does not affect the vision. A dislocated IOL can be in the vitreous gel or may lie on the retinal surface if the vitreous is liquefied.

A decentered or subluxated IOL can be associated with problems, such as uveitis, glaucoma and CME. There can be associated retinal detachment especially since the vitreous has been disturbed and possibly not managed properly. On occasions, anterior segment surgeons have placed AC IOL with one dislocated IOL in the vitreous cavity. This situation if accompanied by retinal detachment is definitely an avoidable one.

Management

Presence of dislocated IOL is not always an indication for surgery. One can observe an IOL that is otherwise not causing any problems in the form of retinal damage if there is no other associated posterior segment problem needing surgical intervention and if the patient is willing for correction with aphakic glasses or the contact lenses. The moving IOL bothers some patients. Retinal detachment associated with dislocated IOL would definitely be an indication for the removal of the IOL and management of the retinal detachment internally.

Management of subluxated intraocular lens (decentration): Significant subluxation causes visual symptoms, such as diplopia and could also cause inflammation and glaucoma. Such cases can be approached in several ways. The deciding factors are the presence of adequate capsular support, amount of vitreous disturbance and how it was managed during the first surgery. If there is no vitreous in the anterior chamber and if one haptic of the IOL is visible in the pupillary area, one can adopt minimally invasive procedures. The visible haptic can be anchored to the sclera by a variety of maneuvers. One technique involves use of 27-gauge needle, with prolene suture pushed out of the needle as a loop. The loop is threaded around the haptic after the needle with the loop is pushed into the eye at the proposed site of anchorage. Once engaged, the needle is pulled out and the loop is tightened. The needle attached to the thread can be used to take a scleral bite in the bed of the scleral flap and the flap is next sutured. Similar technique has been described using the prolene suture with long needle used in reverse. The hub of the needle is pushed through a scleral track created in the bed of a scleral flap. The long end of the needle is used as a handle to guide the loop of the prolene suture around the haptic after the procedure is similar to what was described with the needle technique. If vitreous is in the anterior chamber, one would need to combine these techniques with pars plana approach to clean the pupillary area and the IOL of all the vitreous gel. On occasions, the IOL may be seen with broken haptics. Such IOLs would need to be explanted and replaced by another IOL. Management of dislocated intraocular lens: Dislocated IOL would need to be retrieved and then either explanted, exchanged or repositioned.

Retrieval of the intraocular lens: Dislocated IOL should be brought to the anterior segment before any further manipulation. This retrieval technique depends upon the location of the IOL and the state of the vitreous. Very often, one haptic may be still engaged in the capsule. In this situation, the IOL is first gripped with an intraocular forceps and the vitreous around the same is removed with the cutter before explantation of the IOL. If the IOL is in the anterior vitreous, similar technique is possible wherein the IOL is first gripped with forceps before the vitreous is removed around the same. However, the IOL in the posterior vitreous or on the retina needs a different technique for its retrieval. As a first step, the vitreous is removed in the center

and a peripheral debulking is done. To try and engage the IOL directly with a forceps can invite damage to the retina since the IOL is lying flat on the retina. One may be able to easily grasp the haptic, but this can break with disastrous results. It is important to lift one edge of the optic and present the same for the grasp by the forceps. This is achieved by two different maneuvers. One can place a bubble of perfluorocarbon liquid under the IOL and lift one edge. Alternately, one can use suction of the flute needle to gently lift the IOL and then grasp the edge of the optic with a forceps. A technique of using the vitreous pic to engage the dialing hole of the IOL has been described. One can, of course, use liberal quantity of perfluorocarbon liquid and float the IOL till the pupillary area and then deliver the IOL safely (Figs 30.22 and 30.23).

Explantation of the intraocular lens: Once the IOL is grasped with an intraocular forceps, the other intraocular instrument is removed and the sclerotomy is plugged. Through an ab externo incision, the IOL is shifted to the grip of an external forceps by handshake technique and the IOL is delivered. One can reopen the old cataract incision if the wound is not more than 1 week old. Some surgeons have even extracted the IOL through an enlarged sclerotomy. This technique is less than ideal since large sclerotomies can be associated with higher incidence of vitreous prolapse and retinal dialysis, hypotony and hemorrhage. It is also difficult to close the sclerotomies to water tightness, especially if one has to perform surgery for retinal detachment subsequently. Once a dislocated IOL has been explanted, one has to decide on the management of the aphakia. If, there was associated posterior segment problem in the form of retinal detachment, the eye is left aphakic. If, however, the posterior segment is otherwise normal, one has the option of implanting a new AC IOL or a scleral-fixated IOL.

Repositioning the intraocular lens: Repositioning the dislocated IOL is possible in some cases. The capsular support should be carefully assessed. The IOL can be brought in front

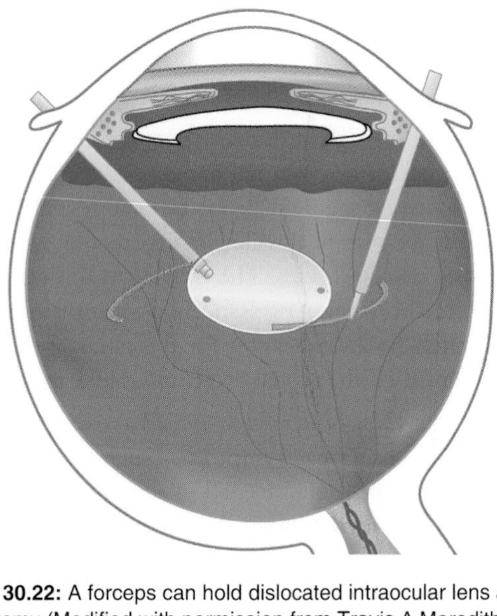

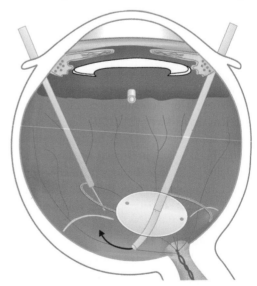

Fig. 30.22: A forceps can hold dislocated intraocular lens after vitrectomy (Modified with permission from Travis A Meredith, MD)

Fig. 30.23: Perfluorocarbon liquid injection can help float the intraocular lens making it easier to grip the same with forceps (Modified with permission from Travis A Meredith, MD)

of the remnants of the capsule and placed in the axis that gives the best support to the haptics. This, however, requires considerable manipulation using intraocular forceps and simultaneously an instrument via limbus, such as iris retractor or another forceps. If the capsular tear through which the IOL has dislocated, has contracted due to fibrosis, the opening needs to be enlarged deliberately to enable the bringing forward of the IOL. If there is no capsular support to place the IOL, one has to consider scleral fixation of the same IOL (Fig. 30.24).

Scleral fixation of the dislocated intraocular lens: There are several techniques of fixating the IOL to the sclera. A 10-0 prolene suture is used for the fixation. A scleral flap usually protects the extraocular part of the suture. Alternately, one can bury the suture in a scleral groove. The sutures are placed in the ciliary sulcus.

Several techniques have been described to fix the IOL at the ciliary sulcus without explanting the IOL. The lasso technique described by Lawrence and Hubbard uses slipknots of 10-0 prolene that are made outside and taken inside through the sclerotomies and placed around the haptics of the IOL in the vitreous cavity. The other end of the suture that is already passed through the ciliary sulcus is pulled to position the IOL. Koh and associates described the use of two corneal tunnels for passing the loop of suture to be placed around the haptic of the dislocated IOL that has been brought into the anterior chamber. Tsukasa and associates describe the use of cow hitch knot to engage the haptic of the IOL that has been brought into the anterior chamber and then anchoring the IOL to the scleral sulcus. Other techniques described the suturing to the sclerotomy lip as well as three- and four-point fixations.

Using perfluorocarbon liquids in liberal quantities and bringing the IOL into the pupillary area can be very useful in these techniques, since the IOL will remain there for the manipulations. Alternately, one can explant the IOL and reimplant it after tying the sutures to the haptic outside the eye.

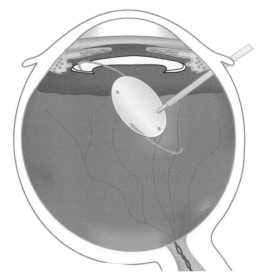

Fig. 30.24: The intraocular lens can be repositioned in the sulcus provided the capsular support is adequate (Modified with permission from Travis A Meredith, MD)

Implanting a new intraocular lens: This may be the option in case of damage to the dislocated IOL—either preexisting or during attempts at retrieval or when the implanted IOL is known to be of wrong power. One can implant an anterior chamber or scleral-fixated IOL. If one is implanting a new scleral fixated IOL, there is the option of using an intraocular with eyelets. This permits the passage of the suture through two points in the scleral bed and the eyelet of the IOL. The knot tied outside can be rotated into the eye. This technique significantly reduces the risk of erosion and exposure of the knot in the future.

Presence of a second intraocular lens in the pupillary area: The presence of a second IOL in the pupillary area can be a difficult problem to solve. One may have to remove both the IOLs and reimplant one of them. Some authors have removed the dislocated IOL via an enlarged sclerotomy without disturbing the IOL in the pupillary area. The problems associated with this technique have already been described.

Associated retinal detachment: As was mentioned, simple scleral buckling procedures should not be adopted in the presence of dislocated IOL with retinal detachment. It is best to remove the IOL and manage the retinal detachment internally. The use of perfluorocarbon liquid has already been alluded to in similar circumstances with crystalline lens dislocation.

ENDOPHTHALMITIS

Introduction

Endophthalmitis is a devastating condition of the eye with serious implications for the vision and the structure of the eye. By definition, endophthalmitis is the inflammation of the coats of the eye except the sclera and the term panophthalmitis defines the involvement of the sclera and the Tenon's capsule. Although technically endophthlamitis can define any severe inflammation of the eye, in most circumstances one understands the term to mean one of infective etiology. Endophthalmitis can be caused by exogenous infection secondary to trauma or surgical intervention. Endogenous infection is due to spread of infection from the bloodstream.

The virulence of the organism and the dose of the organismal contamination most often decide the course of the disease. However, in the circumstance of endogenous infection, the immunity of the individual can be an important factor. The subsequent course of the infection would depend upon the rapidity with which the treatment is initiated and the sensitivity of the organism to the drugs administered. Surgical treatment can only facilitate the cure, but cannot be the sole deciding factor for the outcome of the treatment.

Clinical Presentation

Postoperative Endophthalmitis

Infection is most often seen after cataract surgery since this is the most commonly done surgery in the eye. However, any surgery that invades the eyeball is at risk of intraocular infection. Vitreoretinal surgeries are at less risk possibly, because of the high volume of the fluid that passes through the eye that may wash off the contaminants. As a clinical spectrum, the infection may manifest as:

(1) acute presentation, and (2) chronic presentation.

Time of onset

The usual time of onset of the infection is between 48 and 72 hours. However, hyperacute infection, such as those with *Pseudomonas aeruginosa* and *Bacillus* species can manifest by 24 hours, while those caused by low-virulent organisms like *Propionibacterium acne* and fungi can manifest several days to weeks later. Delayed manifestation can also be due to secondary contamination as in cases occurring after suture removal and cases of bleb-related endophthalmitis. True delayed manifestation can also occur after Nd:YAG capsulotomy when the sequestered organisms get liberated into the vitreous cavity and cause clinical symptoms despite the fact that the cataract surgery might have been done several months before.

Symptomatology

Pain has been quoted as the commonest symptom. However, in the era of phacoemulsification with IOL implantation, the visual rehabilitation is fast enough for the vision reduction to be an important presenting symptom. Severe cases can present with significant mucopurulent discharge and lid swelling.

Signs

Depending on the severity, one may find evidence of external reaction in the form of lid edema, mucopurulent discharge, and conjunctival and circumciliary reaction. Corneal involvement is often seen in cases of *Pseudomonas, Bacillus* and fungal infections. A fast progressing corneal ring abscess can be seen in both *Pseudomonas* and *Bacillus* infections, while fungal infections tend to be very indolent. In cases of cataract surgery, abnormalities of the section can also be found. Anterior chamber may show variable amounts of flare and cells and frequently a hypopyon. The IOL or the pupillary area may be covered by fibrin. A fundal red glow will be absent in the case of vitreous reaction. On occasions, one may find the fibrin to be all round the IOL obscuring the visualization of the fundus. If vitreous visualization is possible, one may find exudates in the vitreous cavity and on the retinal surface.

Cataract surgery with IOL is associated with a specific type of chronic and recurrent infection wherein the organisms are sequestered in the capsular bag. P. acne and fungi are commonly associated with this type of presentation, although cases have been reported with Acinetobacter calcoaceticus. Common presentation in this type of situation is one of recurrent inflammations that is responsive to steroids, only to recur. The initial presentation can mimic mild postoperative sterile inflammation. Dilated slit-lamp evaluation can reveal plaques on the posterior capsule that are suggestive of the location of colonization of the organisms.

In fungal endophthalmitis, the presentation can be variable. The chronicity of the infection and the frequency of corneal involvement have already been alluded to. There can be granuloma formation in the pupillary area or near the section. The posterior segment may remain surprisingly clear for many days.

Endogenous Endophthalmitis

Endogenous endophthalmitis occurs usually in the clinical setting of an identifiable systemic problem. The patient may be immunocompromised or might have received prolonged intravenous infusions. A source of sepsis may be sometimes obvious. But it is not uncommon to find cases with no apparent source of infection despite a clinically classical presentation of endogenous endophthalmitis. The condition can be bilateral, but not invariably so. Even in bilateral cases, the involvement in the two eyes need not be symmetrical. In contrast to the exogenous infection, the presentation is predominantly in the posterior segment to start with. There can be occurrence of choroidal abscesses with vitreous exudates. Anterior segment involvement follows afterwards with hypopyon, etc.

Traumatic Endophthalmitis

Endophthalmitis can follow perforating injury with or without intraocular foreign body. The presence of intraocular foreign body definitely increases the risk of infection. Studies have shown that if the foreign body is removed within 24 hours, the risk of endophthalmitis is reduced significantly. The clinical diagnosis is usually straightforward in the circumstance of perforating injury that is obvious. However, instances of injury with thorns, contaminated needles and broomsticks being forgotten or ignored are not uncommon. In the context of a child, the injury may be undisclosed until the infection becomes clinically obvious. The site of injury is also small and can escape detection. Chronic granuloma occurring after such injuries is not uncommonly seen in this country, wherein the definitive treatment is delayed unduly. In cases with lens trauma, the diagnosis may sometimes be confused with lens-induced inflammation.

However rare, one must be alert to the presence of gas in the eye that can indicate infection with clostridial organisms. Foamy discharge has also been identified as an indicator of clostridial infection.

Bleb-Related Endophthalmitis

Conjunctival blebs secondary to glaucoma surgery or accidental blebs after routine cataract surgery can get infected long after the surgery. The clinical picture is like any other exogenous endophthalmitis with the additional picture of blebitis being evident. Sometimes blebitis without intraocular inflammation may be present for several days before the infection is evident inside the eye. In case of severe bleb infection, scleral necrosis around the site of bleb can lead to fistula at this site.

Corneal Involvement with Endophthalmitis

Corneal involvement is common with endophthalmitis caused by Pseudomonas and Bacillus species and fungi. The cornea may be involved as a ring infiltrate or a localized area of infection next to the cataract section. Severe corneal involvement can preclude any view of the posterior segment and prevent routine vitrectomy.

Panophthalmitis

If endophthalmitis is not adequately treated or if the infecting organism is virulent, the eye can go into panophthalmitis. This condition is indicated by the restriction of extraocular movements, proptosis and usually loss of perception of light.

Ultrasonographic Features of Endophthalmitis

Very often, the view of posterior segment is not possible and one has to rely on the ultrasonography to evaluate the same. The commonest feature is the presence of variable echoes in the vitreous cavity. The choroid is usually thickened due to the inflammation. Retinal detachment is a poor prognosticating factor and indicates severe necrosis of the retina secondary to severe infection. Such cases are usually not salvageable unless the retinal detachment is unrelated to the infection as in the case of infection secondary to retinal detachment surgery.

Management

Diagnosis

The clinical diagnosis is fairly obvious in most cases. Mild cases of postoperative inflammation can be mistaken for sterile inflammation. In such cases, involvement of the vitreous cavity and presence of pain are strong indicators of infection.

Microbiological Investigations

The importance of obtaining cultures of intraocular specimens cannot be overemphasized. Cultures are required for the confirmation of the diagnosis, identification of the organism and selection of the appropriate antibiotic.

Specimens for Processing

Conjunctival swab perhaps is of no value in the management of endophthalmitis. Anterior chamber tap and vitreous tap are the commonest specimens obtained. In addition, corneal scrapings can be used in the case of corneal infiltration. Postsurgically, the explanted IOL can be also cultured.

Collection of Specimens

The anterior chamber tap can be obtained with the help of a 27-gauge needle and a 2 cc syringe under topical anesthesia. A 30-gauge needle is likely to get blocked with the fibrin. The vitreous specimen can be obtained with a needle, or the vitrectomy cutter. In the outpatient setting, a needle is commonly used to get the vitreous specimen via the pars plana. However, there is risk of inducing traction on the retina that is already likely to be edematous. In the operating room setting, it is easy to obtain the specimen using the vitreous cutter with the suction port connected to syringe. New devices are available that enable the collection of vitreous specimen in the outpatient setting without traction on the vitreous. These 23-gauge cutters (Visitec, Sarasota, FL, USA) have the tip shaped like a microvitreoretinal blade and permit the penetration of the globe and collection of the specimen with the same instrument. The sclerotomy does not need suturing. In general, the vitreous tap yields greater positive results on cultures than anterior chamber tap. In addition to the vitreous acting as a good culture medium, the aqueous has been identified to contain a factor that inhibits the growth of the bacteria in vitro.

Processing of the Specimens

The specimens must be transported to the microbiology laboratory immediately. All air in the syringe is expelled and a needle is attached to the syringe and the needle is stuck in a rubber cork. The whole assembly is placed in a sterile test tube and transported. At the microbiology laboratory, the specimen is processed immediately. Smears are made for Gram's staining, KOH preparation and calcofluor staining. Culturing is done in blood agar, chocolate agar, pre-reduced blood agar, brain-heart infusion broth, Robertson's cooked meat broth and thioglycolate broth. Sabouraud's dextrose agar is used for fungal isolation. In case in-house microbiological facilities are not available, and delay in processing the specimen is anticipated, one should inoculate the specimen in liquid media and transport the same to the laboratory.

Interpretation

Cultures are considered positive if significant growth of the same organism is seen in two or more media or if confluent growth is seen on one or more solid media at the site of inoculation. It is considered equivocal if there is growth only in one liquid medium or there is scanty growth in solid media.

Repeat cultures are needed in cases where clinical response is not good despite apparently correct antibiotic administration. Contaminants misleading the clinician are not uncommon. Fungus is especially likely to be missed initially and be wrongly treated as bacterial infection.

Medical Therapy

Medical therapy revolves around the use of antibiotics and steroids. The choice of antibiotic is ideally decided, based on the identification of the organism. However, from the practical perspective, it is not possible to wait for culture report for the drug administration. From the clinical diagnosis, one chooses a mixture of broad-spectrum antibiotics to cover both Gram-positive and Gram-negative bacteria. If fungus is strongly suspected, antifungal drugs are administered.

Route of Administration

Topical: Frequent topical administration of antibiotics and steroids can penetrate the cornea and have useful affect on the anterior segment. Topical atropine is used to keep the pupil dilated and to reduce ciliary spasm.

Subconjunctival injections: This mode of administration of antibiotics and steroids does not have any advantage over frequent topical instillation and in addition is painful for the patient. Neither topical instillation nor subconjunctival injection can achieve significant levels in the vitreous cavity.

Intracameral injection: Injection of the drugs into the anterior chamber is not indicated, since frequent topical instillations reach significant levels in the anterior chamber. However, injection of vancomycin in the capsular bag may be useful in cases of suspected P. acne infection with little or no posterior segment involvement.

Intravitreal injection: This is the most accepted mode of delivery of the drugs to the posterior segment in cases of endophthalmitis. The drugs are administered via pars plana. In aphakic eyes, one may be able to inject the drugs through the limbus into the vitreous cavity. The dosages of most of the commonly used antibiotics and steroids have been well-worked out.

Choice of Antibiotics

The commonest antibiotics administered for bacterial endophthalmitis are a combination of vancomycin (1 mg) and amikacin (125 micrograms). This will cover most of the Gram-positive and Gram-negative organisms. Ceftazidime can be used in the place of amikacin in order to reduce the risk of macular toxicity. Other antibiotics can be administered based on the culture and sensitivity report. For bleb-related endophthalmitis, vancomycin is strongly recommended due to the common occurrence with Streptococcus and the fact that many of these strains are resistant to cephalosporins.

Systemic administration: Role of systemic antibiotics has been severely questioned by the endophthalmitis vitrectomy study at least for the cases of post-cataract surgery endophthalmitis. The same rules, however, do not apply for the other types of endophthalmitis. In cases of endogenous endophthalmitis, it is of great importance to administer intravenous antibiotics. Systemic antibiotics are also recommended for traumatic endophthalmitis.

Role of steroids: Steroids are needed to control the inflammation-mediated damage to the sensitive structures like retina, while the antibiotics are controlling the infection. In most cases, intravitreal steroid can be administered along with the antibiotics if fungus is not suspected. Alternately, one can wait for 24 hours for the antibiotics to act and then administer the intravitreal dexamethasone or put the patient on systemic steroids. Usually, 360 to 400 micrograms of dexamethasone is injected.

Other medications: Topical cycloplegic is usually administered. The IOP needs to be closely monitored and acetazolamide tablets or topical beta-blockers may have to be administered if it is raised. Raised pressure can be commonly seen in fungal endophthalmitis.

Vitrectomy

Vitrectomy enables the removal of bulk of the infected material, removes the toxins that are liberated by the bacteria, helps procure specimen for microbiological processing and allows better penetration of the antibiotics into the eye. However, it must be understood that the appropriate antibiotic in adequate dosage is needed for the control of infection. Vitrectomy can only hasten and facilitate the process. If the organism is resistant to the antibiotic administered, the infection recurs despite a vitrectomy (Table 30.12).

Table 30.12: Tips to perform vitrectomy

1. Six mm cannula is used to clear the edematous ciliary body so that accidental suprachoroidal infusion can be avoided.

2. High cutting rate and low suction are used.

3. The peripheral vitreous is avoided for fear of inducing peripheral retinal dialysis.

4. Surface retinal exudates are left alone. Attempts to remove them with flute needle suction can lead to retinal breaks.

5. Corneal edema can affect visualization. Most often, the visualization improves once the exudates in the anterior chamber are removed. Corneal epithelium is removed if need be. Use of viscoelastics in the anterior chamber can reduce the Descemet's folds significantly. Descemet's folds are especially common after IOL explantation.

6. Wound dehiscence: If the surgical wound gives way, resuturing needs to be done with long bites of interrupted sutures to avoid cheese wiring. Areas of scleral necrosis are occasionally seen in the cases of bleb-induced endophthalmitis. Such cases may need patch scleral grafting to correct the tissue loss.

Indication for Vitrectomy

Endophthalmitis vitrectomy study has shown that immediate vitrectomy is not needed in all cases of post-cataract surgery endophthalmitis. In cases presenting with better than hand motions vision, vitreous tap and intravitreal injection has resulted in as much success as immediate vitrectomy in control of the infection. However, the vitreous cavity clearance was faster in eyes undergoing vitrectomy. In eyes presenting with only perception of light vision, immediate vitrectomy resulted in better success (three-fold increase in the frequency of achieving 20/40 or better vision). However, these recommendations hold good only for post-cataract surgery endophthalmitis.

Immediate vitrectomy is recommended in cases of suspected fungal endophthalmitis since debulking allows the relatively weak antifungal antibiotics to act better. In cases of injury with retained intraocular foreign body presenting with infection, immediate surgery is indicated. Chronic infection due to sequestered organisms in the capsular bag after cataract surgery with IOL implantation can only be managed by surgery, which often involves removal of the intraocular lens.

Surgical Procedure

Three-port pars plana vitrectomy is performed. An attempt is made to perform only core vitrectomy for the fear of creating iatrogenic breaks since the retina is edematous. The undiluted initial vitreous aspirate is collected for microbiological purposes. In case of severe infections, one may add antibiotic in the infusate. However, this gives no control over the amount of antibiotic that is administered into the eye. The initial steps of the surgery are done with infusion provided by the 30° bent long cannula since very often the 4 mm cannula tip is not visible and there is a possibility of choroidal detachment being present. Following the initial vitrectomy, the infusion cannula tip can be visualized and then one can switch to the three-port vitrectomy.

Management of the Intraocular Lens

Since postoperative endophthalmitis is commonest after cataract surgery, one would expect to be confronted fairly commonly with the problems of IOL while managing the endophthalmitis. Where the IOL and the capsular bag are clear, there is no need to touch the IOL. In cases with exudates on the IOL, visibility of the fundus can be severely impaired. Very often, the fibrin can be removed using a needle or a forceps under viscoelastic. Sometimes exudates can be trapped between the posterior capsule and the IOL. On occasions, one can create a posterior capsulectomy with the vitreous cutter and remove the trapped exudates. In severe cases, one should not hesitate to remove the IOL. Most cases of fungal endophthalmitis and eyes with sequestered organisms in the capsular bag, such as Propionibacterium endophthalmitis would need IOL removal along with the capsular bag.

Procedure for the Removal of Intraocular Lens

In most cases of recent post-cataract surgery endophthalmitis, the old incision can be reopened. The anterior chamber is filled with viscoelastic. The IOL is lifted with a dialing hook and delivered with a forceps. Silicone lenses can be slippery and may need toothed forceps to get a grasp for explantation. The wound should be closed with 10-0 interrupted sutures. Long bites should be taken since the tissue is likely to be edematous. Possible problems associated with IOL removal are Descemet's folds, hyphema, etc.

Management in the Presence of Corneal Involvement

Mild corneal edema does not interfere with the vitreoretinal procedures. Removal of corneal epithelium can improve the visualization sufficiently to perform a simple core vitrectomy. However, if the cornea is badly infiltrated, one can perform corneal grafting along with vitrectomy. A large graft is needed in these circumstances. Hence, once vitrectomy is completed with the largest of the available temporary keratoprosthesis (8.2 mm), the corneal opening is enlarged to the required size of the graft. In most cases of endophthalmitis with severe corneal infection requiring combined corneal grafting with vitreous surgery, the posterior segment is also likely to be badly affected.

Cases with Retinal Detachment on Ultrasonography

The problem of retinal detachment with endophthalmitis has already been alluded to. If the infection was virulent and led to the occurrence of the retinal detachment, it is unlikely that any treatment will lead to recovery of vision. Such eyes have no or questionable light perception and usually end up getting eviscerated. Eyes operated for retinal detachment and getting infected postoperatively can have retina that is healthy looking. Under these circumstances, one has the option of controlling the infection and later on managing the retinal detachment. There are reports of primary correction of retinal detachment being done with the surgery for the endophthalmitis. In these cases, silicone oil tamponade is recommended since the risk of proliferative vitreoretinopathy is very high.

Second Intervention

1. *Repeat intravitreal injections:* In case of inadequate response, one may have to repeat the intravitreal injection of antibiotics. If the organism grown is found to be resistant to the initial antibiotic administered, injection of new antibiotic depending upon the antibiogram is warranted. Fungal endophthalmitis usually requires more than one injection for the control of the infection.

2. *Revitrectomy:* If there are recurrent vitreal exudates that do not clear despite the appropriate antibiotic therapy, one may be forced to reintervene surgically. If the IOL was not removed during the first surgery, it is usually removed during the second surgery. A simple vitreous wash out or outpatient fluid-air exchange will not work in these cases due to the presence of fibrin.

3. *Evisceration:* Evisceration as an end-stage procedure may be needed in the cases of uncontrolled infection and loss of light perception and in cases of panophthalmitis.

4. *Vitreoretinal procedures for retinal detachment:* Retinal dialysis and retinal detachment are not uncommon after vitrectomy for endophthalmitis if one considers the fact that the surgery is done in an eye with retinal edema. Once the infection is under control, one can perform vitreoretinal procedures to correct the retinal detachment. The incidence of proliferative vitreoretinopathy is very high and hence the resurgery should be done as soon as possible. Resurgery usually involves revision vitrectomy to clear the residual peripheral vitreous and internal tamponade with gas or silicone oil. In view of the propensity for severe proliferative vitreoretinopathy, silicone oil tamponade may be needed more often.

Complications

1. *Complications of infection:* Eyes with panophthalmitis would need evisceration. Uncontrolled infection despite maximum treatment would also need evisceration. Severely

inflamed eyes can go into phthisis bulbi despite control of infection.

2. *Complications of drug therapy:* Intraocular injection of aminoglycosides is associated with the occurrence of macular infarction. The current recommendation is to use amikacin instead of gentamicin, although macular infarction has been reported even with amikacin.

3. *Complications of surgery:* Vitrectomy can be associated with the occurrence of retinal tears and retinal detachment in view of the presence of retinal edema. The management of the same has already been discussed above.

Prognosis

The prognosis is better for bacterial infections compared to fungal infections. If the patient presents with better than perception of light vision, the prognosis is better. Infections with less virulent organisms, such as *Staphylococcus epidermidis* have better prognosis compared to organisms, such as *Streptococcus, Pseudomonas* and *Bacillus.* The prognosis is better if treatment is initiated immediately in the form of intravitreal injection of appropriate antibiotic. This perhaps is the most important message a cataract surgeon should note, especially in this country where immediate access to vitreoretinal surgeon may not always be available.

Routine Antiseptic Measures that can Reduce the Occurrence of Postoperative Infections

1. Improving the hygiene of the patients before and after the surgery. This especially applies to the rural patients and patients from the poor socioeconomic status.
2. Use of povidone-iodine (5%) in the conjunctival cul-de-sac preoperatively.
3. Strict adherence to sterilization precautions. Specifically, the phacoemulsification probe needs to be dismantled and autoclaved between two cases.
4. Precaution in inspecting the irrigating fluid just before its use.
5. Similar precaution should be exercised with viscoelastic solution.

Intravitreal Drug Dosage and Formulation

Intravitreal injection involves very minute dosages and hence it is important to be meticulous about the calculations. The possibility of the fluid in the needle contributing to the miscalculations should be kept in mind. This problem can be overcome by using stock solutions prepared by the pharmacist, wherein such facilities are available in a hospital. This involves use of separate empty sterile vials into which measured quantities are transferred. Such facilities are not, however, always available. Hence, methods of preparing intravitreal injections are described below:

1. *Vancomycin*
   a. To a vial containing 500 mg of the drug (powder), 10 cc of saline or BSS is added. 2 cc of the solution containing 100 mg of the drug is injected into a separate sterile empty vial. 8 cc of saline or BSS is injected into this vial. Each 0.1 cc of this solution will contain 1 mg of the drug.
   b. To a vial containing 500 mg of the drug (powder), 5 cc of saline or BSS is added. 0.1 cc of the solution containing 10 mg of the drug is aspirated into a 1 cc syringe and 0.9 cc of the saline or BSS is also aspirated into the same syringe. The mixture is mixed well with the help of an air bubble. 0.1 cc of this mixture contains 1 mg of the drug.

2. *Amikacin*
   a. From a vial of 2 cc containing 250 mg, 0.1 cc of the solution containing 12.5 mg of the drug is injected into a separate sterile vial. 9.9 cc of saline is injected into the vial. 0.1 cc of this solution contains 125 micrograms of the drug.
   b. From a vial of 2 cc containing 250 mg of the drug, 0.1 cc of the solution is aspirated into the tuberculin syringe and 0.9 cc of saline is aspirated. 0.9 cc of the mixture is expelled and a second dilution is done with saline or dexamethasone as the case may be. 0.1 cc of this mixture contains 125 micrograms of the drug.

3. *Ceftazidime*
   a. 10 cc of saline is injected into a vial containing 500 mg of the drug. One cc of the solution is injected into an empty vial and 1.2 cc of saline is added to the same. The solution contains 2.25 mg per 0.1 ml.
   b. 2.5 cc of saline is injected into the vial with 500 mg. 0.1 cc of the solution containing 20 mg of the drug is aspirated into a tuberculin syringe along with 0.9 cc of saline. 0.1 cc of this mixture contains 2 mg of the drug.

4. *Amphotericin-B*
   a. 10 cc of sterile water for injection is added to the vial containing 50 mg of the drug as powder. 0.1 cc of this solution is injected into an empty vial and to this 9.9 cc of sterile water is added. This solution contains 5 micrograms of the drug per 0.1 cc.
   b. 10 cc of the sterile water is added to the vial containing 50 mg of the drug. 0.1 cc of this solution containing 500 micrograms is aspirated into a tuberculin syringe along with 0.9 cc of sterile water 0.9 cc of this mixture is expelled and a second dilution of the residual 0.1 cc is done with 0.9 cc of sterile water. 0.1 cc of this mixture contains 5 micrograms of the drug.

Important Messages from the Endophthalmitis Vitrectomy Study

1. *Clinical Features*
   a. Commonest presentation was within 6 weeks.

b. Pain absent as symptom in 25% cases.

2. *Antibiotics*

a. Systemic antibiotics do not influence the outcome of treatment.

b. Most cases of Gram-positive coagulase negative micrococci were sensitive to vancomycin.

c. Most Gram-negative organisms were sensitive to both amikacin and ceftazidime.

3. *Role of Vitrectomy*

a. For eyes presenting with hand motion or better vision, tap/biopsy or vitrectomy yielded equal results.

b. For eyes presenting with perception of light only vision, early vitrectomy had better results.

4. *Cultures*

a. Culture positivity is higher with vitreous compared to aqueous.

b. Positive Gram's stain correlates with higher culture positivity, but negative Gram's stain does not indicate culture pattern.

c. Culture positivity equal with both tap and vitrectomy.

d. Source of coagulase-positive micrococci was mostly the patient's own flora.

e. Primary PC IOL associated more often with infection by Gram-positive coagulase negative micrococci, while AC IOL and secondary IOL are more often associated with infection by other Gram-positive and Gram-negative organisms.

5. *Needle Tap Biopsy vs Mechanized Cutter Biopsy*

a. No difference in yield of positivity on Gram's stain or cultures.

b. No difference in incidence of postoperative retinal detachment.

6. *Cultures vs Clinical Presentation*

a. Compared to coagulase-negative micrococci, other Gram-positive and Gram-negative organisms have higher incidence of onset before two days from surgery, corneal infiltration, section abnormalities, relative afferent pupillary defect, loss of red reflex and presenting vision of perception of light vision only.

b. Eyes with retinal vessel visibility unlikely to have Gram-negative infection and more likely to have culture negativity.

c. Pain does not predict infection with any particular group of organisms.

d. Coagulase negative micrococci is more often seen in diabetics.

7. *Cultures vs Visual Recovery*

a. Better than 20/100 visual recovery seen in 84% of eyes with coagulase negative micrococci, 50% of eyes with *staphylococcus aureus,* 30% of eyes with *streptococci,* 14% of eyes with enterococci and 56% of eyes with Gram-negative organisms.

b. Positive Gram's stain result and infection with other than coagulase negative Gram-positive organisms and Gram-negative organisms were associated with poor visual results.

c. Poor visual results correlate better with presenting vision rather than the microbiology of the infection.

8. *Additional Procedures*

a. Additional procedures required for complications of initial treatment (14%) or worsening inflammation or infection (86%).

b. Eyes needing additional procedures (especially earlier than 7 days) associated with poor visual results.

c. Reoperation rate higher with more virulent organisms and poor presenting vision.

9. *Post-treatment Retinal Detachment*

a. Incidence same with tap/biopsy or vitrectomy group.

b. More common with virulent organisms, poor presenting vision, open posterior capsule, and in patients needing early additional procedure.

c. Seventy-eight percent of eyes with retinal detachment that were reoperated had successful result.

d. Visual results in general are poor in eyes developing retinal detachment.

RETINOPATHY OF PREMATURITY

Introduction

Retinopathy of prematurity (ROP) is the present accepted term for what was known as retrolental fibroplasias. Terry in 1942 first identified the disease as a cause of blindness in premature infants. Oxygen was identified as an important causative factor leading to its curtailment and the consequent increase in infant mortality rate. The improved survival of very low birth weight infants has lead to increased incidence of this disease at the present time. The advent of indirect ophthalmoscope has enabled the identification of the early stages of the disease while the International Classification of ROP has enabled some uniformity of approach to the management of this disease.

Etiopathogenesis

Normal retina gets vascularity from the hyaloid vessel that is the only intraocular vessel in the embryology of the retina. At 8th month of gestation, the temporal retina beyond the equator is still totally avascular. Several factors in a premature infants eye make it susceptible to damage. The developing retinal vasculature is immature. It has more endothelial cells; and pericytes are just forming. The basement membrane of the newborn capillaries stain poorly with periodic acid-Schiff (PAS) staining and the level of vitamin E is very low in the periphery of the retina. In view of these factors, the premature retina is susceptible to noxious influences. Various factors are said to influence extensive gap junction formation in the spindle cells of the vanguard retina. This interferes with the maturation and migration of the capillaries. The activated spindle cells lead to abnormal vasculogenesis.

It is accepted that ROP is multifactorial in origin, the most important of the factors being the prematurity itself. The incidence and severity of the disease have been found to be inversely related to the birth weight. Shohat and associates found the incidence to be 52% in infants between 501 and 1,250 grams. Association with oxygen was found to be significant only for infants above 1,500 grams birth weight. Other risk factors are repeated blood transfusions, hypoxemia, respiratory distress syndrome, prolonged parenteral nutrition, intraventricular hemorrhage and septicemia. Factors, such as xanthine administration, phototherapy, etc. have also been blamed.

International Classification of Retinopathy of Prematurity

The adoption of international classification of ROP has brought in some uniformity in reporting of data on various management techniques. The ROP is classified according to the extent, location and severity. The location of the disease is depicted by the location from the optic disc. Zone 1 is the area within a circle drawn with the disc as the center and the perimeter lying 2 disc diameters temporal to the macula. Zone 2 is concentric to the zone 1 and abuts on the nasal ora serrata. The residual temporal crescent forms the zone 3. The number of clock hours affected describes the circumferential extent. The severity of the disease is graded into five stages.

Stages

Stage 1: Demarcation Line

This stage is characterized by the presence of a sharp demarcation line separating the vascularized posterior retina from the avascular anterior retina. Most premature babies have avascular retina without ROP, especially in the temporal periphery. However, this can be differentiated from the stage 1 by the fact that the vessels merge imperceptibly with the avascular portion.

Stage 2: Ridge Formation

In this stage, the line of separation acquires three dimensionality.

Stage 3: Extra Retinal Proliferation

In stage 3, the internal limiting membrane is broken through by the new vessel proliferation. The severity of this proliferation may be variable and can be sub-classified into mild, moderate and severe.

Stage 4: Partial Retinal Detachment

Retina can be detached due to traction, exudation or both. When the detachment is extramacular, it is called stage 4A; and once it involves macula, it becomes stage 4B.

Stage 5: Total Retinal Detachment

The detachment is almost always in the form of a funnel. This stage is sub-classified based on the configuration of the detachment into:

a. *Open-open*: Wherein the funnel-shaped detachment is open both posteriorly and anteriorly.
b. *Narrow-narrow*: Wherein the detachment has a narrow configuration both anteriorly and posteriorly.
c. *Open-narrow*: The funnel is open anteriorly, but narrow posteriorly.
d. *Narrow-open*: Wherein the funnel is narrow anteriorly and open posteriorly.

Most detachments have narrow-narrow or open-open configuration. Narrow-open configuration is extremely rare.

Plus disease: This defines the presence of dilated vessels. If it affects the iris, it is called anterior segment plus disease; and when it affects the retina, it is called the posterior segment plus disease. For the purpose of defining treatment indications, posterior segment plus disease is important.

Rush disease: This defines the presence of plus disease with zone 1 disease. It can be extremely severe and fast progressing.

Threshold disease: This is defined by the CRYO-ROP study group as stage 3 disease involving more than 5 continuous clock hours or 8 discontinuous clock hours with plus disease.

Prethreshold disease: When there is stage 2 plus disease involving 5 continuous or 8 discontinuous clock hours or there is stage 3 plus disease of less than 5 continuous or 8 discontinuous clock hours or there is zone 1 disease of any stage, it is called prethreshold disease.

Examination Protocol

A joint statement by the American Academy of Pediatrics, the American Association of Pediatric Ophthalmology and the American Academy of Ophthalmology has given some guidelines to monitor infants at risk of developing ROP.

1. Whom to Examine: Infants with birth weight of < 1,500 grams; infants with a gestational age of < 28 weeks; and infants over 1,500 grams if there has been unstable clinical course.
2. Who Should Examine: Ophthalmologist experienced in examining premature infants.
3. When Should One Examine: Examination should be done at 4–6 weeks of chronological age or between 31 and 33 weeks of postconceptual age. (Postconceptual age is defined as the gestational age + chronological age).
4. Follow-Up Examinations: The follow-up depends upon the results of the initial examination. If there is no ROP, but immature vasculature is present in the zone 2, follow-up examination is needed at 2-week intervals until the temporal periphery is vascularized normally. Infants with ROP or immature vessels in zone 1 need closer follow-up at weekly intervals until either the normal vascularization proceeds to temporal periphery or threshold disease develops.

Examination Procedure

The pupils are dilated with 2.5% phenylephrine and 1% tropicamide instilled twice at intervals of 15 minutes. Punctal occlusion is recommended to reduce risk of systemic absorption. The examination is preferably done at least 1 hour after a feed to avoid inducing vomiting and aspiration of milk. Binocular indirect ophthalmoscopy with scleral depression is done while the infant is restrained. Eyelids are usually separated by using Alfonso speculum (Figs 30.25 and 30.26). Scleral depression is done using a wire vectis or custom-made infant scleral depressor. Temporal periphery around the horizontal meridian is examined first. No anesthesia is required for the examination except topical anesthetics to facilitate transconjunctival depression. The findings are recorded as per the zonal, circumferential distribution and the recognized staging (Fig. 30.27).

Treatment

Treatment of Threshold Disease

Treatment is indicated within 72 hours of identification of threshold disease. The preferred mode of treatment is laser photocoagulation although cryo therapy was the modality used in the large multicentric trial conducted in the USA. Laser has several advantages. There is virtually no morbidity since no general anesthesia is needed. No conjunctival incision is required even in zone 1 or posterior zone 2 disease (unlike with cryo). The treatment can be spaced in 2 sessions if needed, unlike with cryotherapy, where in one would avoid repeated general anesthesia that is required for the treatment. There is no post-treatment reaction. Several studies have shown that the laser

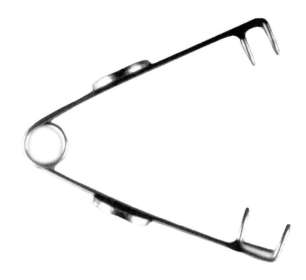

Fig. 30.26: Alfonso speculum is best suited for the examination of infants. Note the width of the two jaws of the speculum with one fitting into the other thus permitting easy introduction on the small palpebral fissure of premature infants

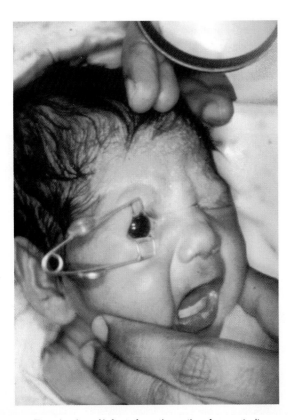

Fig. 30.25: Examination of infants for retinopathy of prematurity screening is done with binocular indirect ophthalmoscope. There is no need for general anesthesia

SANKARA NETHRALAYA
18, COLLEGE ROAD, CHENNAI – 600 006

R.O.P. EVALUATION FORM

Patient Name _____   MRD No._____

Gestational Age _____   Birth Date_____

Weight _____   Exam Date_____

ANTERIOR SEGMENT   OD   OS

iris rubeosis   yes no   yes no

corneal abnormality   yes no   yes no

suspect glaucoma   yes no   yes no

FUNDUS

	OD	OS
vitreous hemorrhage	yes no	yes no
plus disease	yes no	yes no
pre-threshold	yes no	yes no

(zone 1 and stage, zone 2 with stage 2+, zone 3 or zone 2 stage 3+but not reaching threshold clock hours. Need to examine in one week)

threshold   yes no   yes no
(zone 1 or zone 2 with stage 3+, 5 contiguous sectors or 8 composite sectors. Cryotherapy within 72 hours.)

OD Immature, no R.O.P._____   Mature _____

R.O.P Higher stage_____   Lowest zone_____   Total number clock hours _____

OS Immature, no R.O.P._____   Mature _____

R.O.P Higher stage_____   Lowest zone _____   Total number clock hours _____

Physician's Signature _____

Fig. 30.27: Standard chart is used to record the details of each visit of infants for retinopathy of prematurity screening

treatment is as effective as cryotherapy in inducing regression of the disease. Both diode and the argon green laser have been used. Diode laser is preferred in the case of presence of persistent pupillary membranes.

Technique of Laser Therapy

Alfonso speculum is used to keep the lids apart. Scleral depression is done with wire vectis. The avascular retina is treated from the ridge to the ora serrata. Burns are placed one burn width apart. If extensive treatment is needed as in the case of zone 1 disease, one may space the treatment in two sessions. In such a situation, first session should cover the area immediately anterior to the ridge. The anesthetist does cardiac monitoring throughout the treatment since oculocardiac reflex can occur during scleral depression.

Complications of laser treatment: The only significant complication is the possibility of cataract formation if treatment is done with green lasers for an eye with persistent pupillary membrane. Laser treatment needs lot more of patience to place the burns properly. Accidental foveal burn is extremely rare and should not occur in the hands of an experienced surgeon. Corneal burns have also been rarely reported.

Technique of Cryotherapy

Cryotherapy has been done under general anesthesia; subconjunctival anesthesia, as well as topical anesthesia with sedation. The principles of treatment remain the same, i.e. the avascular retina is treated avoiding the ridge itself. Contiguous spots are placed. Postoperatively treatment is done with steroid and atropine drops.

Complications of cryotherapy: Cryotherapy has lot more potential for complications than laser. Significant conjunctival reaction and lid edema are common. In extensive treatments, one may not be able to open the eyelids for the first few days. Conjunctival tears can occur while attempting to reach posteriorly. Intraocular hemorrhage has been reported in 22.3% of infants in the CRYO-ROP study. Inadvertent freezing of the optic nerve and macula, muscle laceration, globe perforation and late onset retinal detachment is the other complications reported. The scars caused by cryo are large. Anesthesia-related complications in the case of general anesthesia are many and perhaps are the most important reason why laser is becoming the desired modality of treatment.

Effect of the Treatment

The efficacy of treatment is indicated by the disappearance of the plus disease followed by the regression in the ridge. Next the vascularization proceeds beyond the ridge towards the ora serrata. On occasions, elevated blood vessels in the vitreous may remain for a longer time despite the regression of the ridge. These naked vessels regress usually with time. Some fibrosis can occur on the retina without inducing any traction on the retina and may be of no consequence. For total regression and normalization of the vascularization to take place, several

weeks may be needed. It is important to perform follow-up examinations at 1 to 2 weekly intervals. Additional treatment to skip areas may be done if the regression is not adequate.

Sequelae of Regressed Retinopathy of Prematurity

In most cases, ROP regresses without sequelae. In a few cases, there can be residual scarring. Depending on the location and extent of this scarring, the vision can be affected. Usually, there is some fibrosis in the temporal periphery. This can lead to variable extent of macular ectopia (Fig. 30.28). The temporal arcade is straightened. More severe scarring leads to occurrence of retinal fold formation. The size of the fold can be variable and usually involves the macula. Depending on the size of the fold, the rest of the retina is stretched. The stretched area of retina can have variable pigmentation and resemble areas of spontaneous retinal reattachment. Myopia is a frequent occurrence in children who were born premature even when ROP has not occurred. The degree of myopia can be quite high. Late onset rhegmatogenous retinal detachment is also a problem encountered on occasions. Strabismus is a known association of prematurity and could be sensory like in any other child or secondary to the macular ectopia. Those cases secondary to macular ectopia cannot be corrected by the squint surgery.

Treatment of Retinal Detachment

Stage 4 and beyond require surgical treatment. Surgical treatment is in the form of either scleral buckling or vitreoretinal surgical procedures.

Scleral Buckling

Scleral buckling is indicated in the cases of stage 4A and 4B and some cases of stage 5. Scleral buckling is done in the acute stage of the disease. The most common time of performance

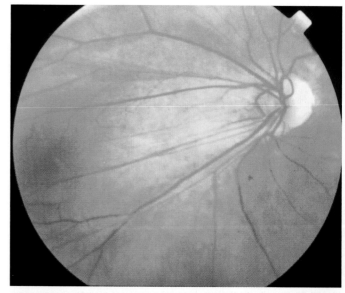

Fig. 30.28: Macular ectopia is not uncommon sequelae of regressed retinopathy of prematurity. The visual acuity depends upon the extent of the ectopia. The fibrous tissue in the temporal periphery causes the ectopia

of this procedure has been found to be around the term of a premature infant. The procedure is under general anesthesia. Cryo is done to the avascular retina if the treatment is not already done. A no. 240 or 40 band is used 360°. Scleral tunnels or mattress sutures are used to anchor the band in each quadrant. Indentation is aimed at the site of ridge. Subretinal fluid is not usually drained. Indentation is made possible by anterior chamber paracentesis. On occasions, the fluid may be significant enough to permit drainage of subretinal fluid.

Removal of the buckle: The buckle needs to be cut or removed a few months after its placement to prevent the intrusion of the band in a growing eyeball. Cutting the band without removing it may theoretically speaking allow some indentation effect to remain since the capsule around the band is left undisturbed. If one makes scleral tunnels at the first surgery, the band can be removed without disturbing the capsule.

Results of scleral buckling: Trese reported a 70% success in reattaching the retina in cases with stage 4A; 67% in cases with stage 4B; and 40% in eyes with stage 5, wherein scleral buckling could be done. Although anatomical attachment can be achieved in many cases, there can be distortion of the retina in the form of tractional folds and ectopia of the macula. It is the macular ectopia that usually dictates the amount of visual recovery.

Vitreoretinal Surgery

Stage 5 ROP that is not amenable to scleral buckling can only be managed by vitreoretinal surgery. Two approaches have been used for this purpose—the open-sky approach and the closed approach.

Pathoanatomy: The fibrovascular proliferation starts at the junction of the vascular and avascular retina. The proliferation into vitreous cavity is followed by traction anteriorly. This traction is able to pull the vascularized retina forwards, but the avascular retina remains adherent. In the process, the anatomy is grossly distorted with the double-layered retinal fold coming up as for anteriorly as behind the lens. Fibrosis proceeds along the posterior vascularized retina up to the disc. Anteriorly, the fibrosis bridges across the trough that is caused by the pulling forward of the retinal fold. Depending on the location of the original ridge and extent of the traction anteriorly by bridging tissue, the trough can be broad or narrow and deep or shallow. The fibrosis involves the anterior and posterior hyaloid as well as the vitreous cavity. Pars plana is not developed and ciliary processes are often drawn inwards by the transvitreal traction. The subretinal space may contain hemorrhage of variable extent and alteration. The detached retina undergoes contracture leading to closing of the funnel (Fig. 30.29).

Open-sky vitrectomy: Open-sky vitrectomy involves the removal of corneal button followed by dissection of the fibrous tissue from periphery to center. En bloc removal of the tissue is very often possible. However, visualization of the posterior pole is difficult. In addition, the duration of surgery is prolonged due to additional need for corneal surgery. The eye is also left

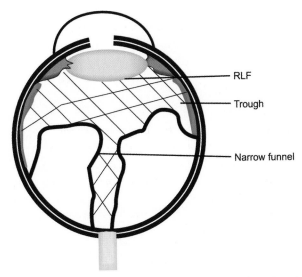

Fig. 30.29: Shows the pathoanatomy of stage 5 retinopathy of prematurity

hypotonous during the period of surgery with attendant risk of choroidal detachment. Hirose has reported a success rate of 38% in the cases of stage 5 ROP that were treated with open-sky vitrectomy.

Closed vitrectomy By virtue of its familiarity, the closed approach has been more popular. Triester and Machemer first tried surgery on ROP stage 5 in 1977. With better understanding of the pathoanatomy, the surgical technique has evolved. Two broad approaches are followed in the dissection of the tissue—the periphery to center and center to periphery. Periphery to center approach allows better tissue dissection, but the dissection is more difficult to initiate due to the difficult access of the periphery from inside. By using temporary iris retractors or by sacrificing the superior iris, one can access the periphery well and perform adequate dissection (Figs 30.30 and 30.31). The important principles are listed in Table 30.13.

Lens-sparing vitrectomy: Lens-sparing vitrectomy is occasionally possible in eyes with post pole tractional retinal detachment alone. This situation is encountered in zone I disease with good

Table 30.13: Principles of vitrectomy for stage 5 retinopathy of prematurity

1.	Most cases need lens removal
2.	Entry through iris root
3.	Bimanual surgery is often required under viscoelastic
4.	Tissue adherent to ciliary processes should be dissected all-round in order to open the trough
5.	Dissection into the funnel needs extreme caution to avoid retinal breaks
6.	Bleeding can be stopped by the sparing use of underwater diathermy
7.	During surgery, reattachment of retina is not possible. Hence, no attempt is done to do fluid-gas exchange
8.	Occurrence of retinal breaks spells disaster

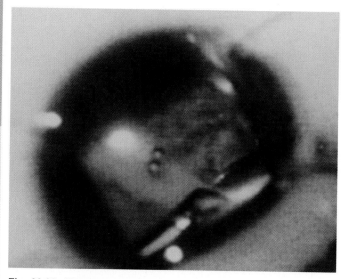

Fig. 30.30: Bimanual dissection in progress for stage 5 retinopathy of prematurity under viscoelastic fill (Reprinted with permission from the Indian Journal of Ophthalmology)

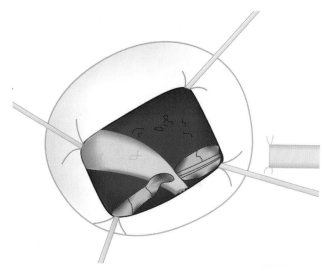

Fig. 30.31: Line diagram of Figure 30.30 (Reprinted with permission from the Indian Journal of Ophthalmology)

retinal ablation, since most of the peripheral retina is attached and lacered and since surgery is needed only around the posterior pole.

Results

The results are variable and unsatisfactory to say the least (Figs 30.32 and 30.33). Anatomical results depend on:
1. Funnel configuration,
2. Completeness of dissection, and
3. Nonoccurrence of retinal breaks.

Wide funnel configuration has the best prognosis (81% in open funnel vs 23% in closed funnel configuration). The visual results in eyes with attached retina are disappointing. Recordable visual acuity on Snellen's chart is seen only in occasional cases.

SURGERY FOR THE COMPLICATIONS OF DIABETIC RETINOPATHY

Introduction

The most common indication for vitreoretinal surgery happens to be the complications of diabetic retinopathy. The spectrum of pathoanatomy that one faces is so diverse that it may be important to discuss at length the anatomical factors that govern the disease pathology. Routine screening programs for diabetics have facilitated the recognition of diabetic retinopathy in early stages and their treatment with laser photocoagulation in many cases. Despite the same, progression to a stage requiring vitreoretinal surgery is not uncommon. In addition, in economically backward countries, such a routine screening

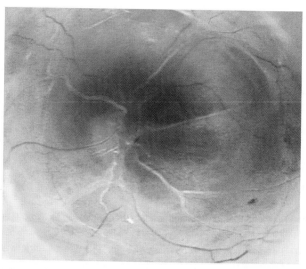

Fig. 30.32: Surgery for retinopathy of prematurity. Postoperative stage 5 retinopathy of prematurity that underwent lensectomy and vitrectomy. Retina is thin and atrophic with sclerosed blood vessels and is detached in the periphery

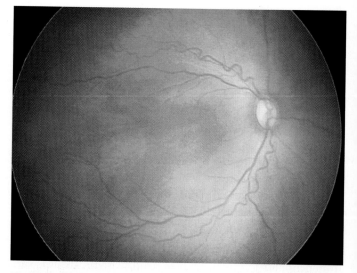

Fig. 30.33: Retinopathy of prematurity after treatment. Temporal drag has resulted in straightening of the arcade

program may not be in place and many patients seek the opinion of the ophthalmologist only at the first sign of visual loss.

Pathology

It is outside the scope of this chapter to discuss in detail the pathogenesis of diabetic retinopathy. The intent is more to concentrate on the anatomical changes that take place in the retina and vitreous that have a bearing on the surgical approach and outcome of treatment. Diabetic retinopathy basically is seen to be a duration-dependent response, although the degree of control of diabetes has a definite impact on the occurrence and progression of the disease as was evidenced by Diabetes Complication and Control Trial (DCCT) and the United Kingdom Prospective Diabetes Study (UKPDS). Through a combination of biochemical changes, hyperglycemia leads to endothelial degeneration and pericyte loss in addition to the thickening of basement membrane in the retinal blood vessels. Retinal ischemia secondary to closure of parts of retinal capillary bed leads to the liberation of angiogenic factors, notably the vascular endothelial growth factor. This, in turn, leads to the proliferative response that characterizes diabetic retinopathy. Initial changes, such as microaneurysms and intraretinal microvascular anomalies are of no surgical interest. Vascular incompetence can lead to exudation of fluid and lipids, especially in the macular area. Neovascular response initially starts as vascular outgrowths from the retinal blood vessels and this is followed by a variable fibrotic response. Although intraretinal hemorrhages occur in the initial stages of the disease, vision is affected only with preretinal and vitreous hemorrhage.

The occurrence of posterior vitreous detachment influences the progress of disease significantly. Both the timing and the extent of the same are important in defining the pathoanatomy and the occurrence or otherwise of tractional retinal detachment. The occurrence of retinal break during the course of the disease also influences the anatomy. Occurrence of full-thickness retinal break can lead to combined rhegmatogenous-tractional retinal detachment that can spread rapidly to involve the macula. The fibrosis can occur anywhere, but is more common in the posterior pole, especially along the arcades. The ongoing ischemia also leads to the thinning of the retina. The combination of these factors defines the surgical anatomy. The other factor that can influence the surgical anatomy is the presence and extent of photocoagulation scars.

Configurations

The common configurations one comes across are described below:

1. *Complete posterior vitreous detachment:* In this situation, the vitreous that is probably hemorrhagic is totally detached. This is relatively rare to come across in diabetic retinopathy. More commonly, there is at least one point of attachment at the site of fibrovascular proliferation.

2. *Posterior vitreous detachment with focal attachments:* These areas of focal attachments can be single or multiple. The disc is usually a site of such an attachment.

3. *Partial posterior vitreous detachment with broad attachments:* Vitreous may be separate from the peripheral retina, but adherent to broad areas of fibrous proliferation—usually along the arcades. The macular area can be bridged by tissue called trampoline membrane with the underlying retina being attached.

4. *Focal tractional retinal detachment:* In the presence of posterior vitreous detachment, traction at the point of attachment to fibrovascular tissue can lead to focal tractional retinal detachment. The extent of the detachment can vary. The focus of traction also can be a point focus or a slightly broader area.

5. *Broad-based tractional retinal detachment:* Partial posterior vitreous detachment in the presence of broad areas of adherence to the retina at sites of fibrovascular proliferation leads to the occurrence of broad-based tractional retinal detachment.

The Concept of Vitreoschisis and Second Membrane

Barring the simplest of the situations, one finds a second fibrocellular membrane extending anteriorly on the surface of the retina from the point of attachment of the apparently detached posterior vitreous. This membrane can vary in its thickness and anterior extent. Vitreoschisis with condensation of the residual vitreous into a membrane can partly explain this anatomy. It is important to identify and initiate dissection from the limit of this membrane in order to be at the correct plane of cleavage.

Tractional Retinoschisis

Traction-induced retinoschisis is not an infrequent finding in cases of diabetic retinopathy. The schisis may be associated with breaks in inner layer that can be mistaken for full-thickness retinal breaks. The tractional configuration of the detachment and the presence of retinal tissue visible through the retinal break can be assurance enough as to the partial-thickness nature of the break.

Other Factors

As has been alluded to, the retina can be variably thin and this can dictate the ease with which it can withstand the force required in the dissection of the overlying fibrovascular tissue. The vascularity of the fibrovascular tissue also is important since persistent and significant ooze in the presence of extensive tractional retinal detachment can sometimes be a nightmare situation.

Surgical Management

Pars plana vitreoretinal surgery has revolutionized the management of complications of diabetic retinopathy. The indications for the surgery have also been changing and expanding with increasing experience.

Indications for Vitrectomy

1. *Vitreous hemorrhage*: Traditionally, vitreous hemorrhage had been the commonest indication for vitrectomy in the cases of diabetic retinopathy. Tractional retinal detachment has replaced vitreous hemorrhage as the commonest indication. Traditionally again, one used to wait for 6 months to await possible natural clearance of the hemorrhage. Early surgery is needed in the case of bilateral condition or single-eyed patient with vitreous hemorrhage. If a wait and watch policy is adopted, intermittent ultrasonographic evaluation is needed to exclude possibility of underlying traction retinal detachment involving the macula.

2. *Tractional retinal detachment involving the macula*: Tractional detachment of the retina involving the macula, as has been alluded to, is the most common indication for vitrectomy in the present day. Extramacular tractional retinal detachment has been shown to progress very slowly and may not be an indication for vitrectomy. However, in the case of tractional retinal detachment threatening the macula and with the patient having good visual acuity, deciding to operate could be difficult. The risk-benefit ratio should be kept in mind while considering the surgical option. Extensive tractional retinal detachment all along the arcades with attached macula could also be a difficult situation to decide regarding surgery. Although these patients may have good visual acuity (depending upon the health of the macula), the gross tractional retinal detachment all around would limit the amount of field of vision.

3. *Combined rhegmatogenous-tractional retinal detachment*: Occurrence of full-thickness retinal break can lead to rhegmatogenous type detachment. Unlike the tractional retinal detachment, the combined detachment spreads fast and hence needs to be treated whether or not the macula is involved.

4. *Macular distortion:* Fibrosis in the vicinity of macula can lead to the distortion of macula leading to reduced vision although there may not be actual tractional retinal detachment of the macula.

5. *Rubeosis iridis with vitreous hemorrhage*: In the presence of rubeosis iridis, one would aim to clear the vitreous hemorrhage and perform endolaser on urgent basis without waiting for spontaneous clearance.

6. *Post-vitrectomy fibrin response with retinal detachment*: In this circumstance, there is rapid onset of rubeosis iridis with grave risk to loss of the eye. Early resurgery is indicated to correct the retinal detachment.

7. *Dense-premacular hemorrhage*: Dense hemorrhage trapped under a membrane in front of macula can sometimes have deleterious effect on the visual improvement if left behind for long time. Such hemorrhages are best removed early.

8. *Anterior hyaloid proliferation*: This response is typically seen following a vitrectomy. The proliferation usually starts at one of the sclerotomy sites and spreads along with the vitreous base. Depending on the severity of the problem, the proliferation can extend to 360°. This condition can only be corrected by aggressive vitrectomy with sacrifice of lens; and on many occasions, a 360° retinectomy with excision of the fibrovascular tissue.

9. *Macular edema resistant to photocoagulation*: This is an emerging indication for vitrectomy in diabetics. There is controversy as to the need to demonstrate premacular traction before subjecting the case for vitrectomy. Eyes with extensive subretinal lipids have been subjected to surgery with the removal of the lipids through retinotomy by some surgeons.

10. *Recurrent vitreous hemorrhage with retinal detachment*: In the presence of recurrent vitreous hemorrhage following vitrectomy, if the ultrasonography reveals retinal detachment, one has to intervene immediately and correct the same. Persistent retinal detachment in this situation can lead to the high-risk of rubeosis iridis. The detachment will be one of rhegmatogenous variety. One should be able to differentiate, on the ultrasonography between persistent tractional retinal detachment that may be taking time to settle and a fresh onset rhegmatogenous retinal detachment. The intraoperative notes of the first operation and the location of the ultrasonographically detected retinal detachment can guide the surgeon to the appropriate decision.

Contraindications

a. *Absence of light perception.*

b. *Inoperable retinal detachment*: This is easier said than defined. The type of cases that may be labeled inoperable would vary from surgeon to surgeon based on their experience. Most cases would fall under relative contraindications. Factors that push a case towards inoperability are presence of florid disease coupled with the absence of posterior vitreous detachment and presence of extensive retinal detachment in an eye with thin atrophic retina.

c. *Risk-benefit ratio issue*: Cases of chronic retinal detachments involving the posterior pole of several year's duration and with thin and atrophic retina have very little scope for visual recovery and probably are best left alone.

Anesthesia: Most cases can be done under local anesthesia with sedation. A good control of blood pressure during surgery is important to control the amount of bleeding intraoperatively. In cases needing prolonged surgery, the patients can become uncomfortable with gradual rise in blood pressure. Intermittent sedation can be very important in such cases. One must be cognizant of the fact that many of these patients can be suffering from multisystem diseases, such as associated ischemic heart disease, nephropathy, etc. Hence, a thorough evaluation by the physician preoperatively is a must.

Aspirin—to stop or not to stop: Since most of these patients have multisystem diseases, the likelihood of them being on aspirin is very high. The present-day recommendation is not to stop the aspirin before or after ocular surgery considering the benefit systemically of continuing aspirin. If it is possible to stop aspirin, it should be stopped at least 10 to15 days in advance since the life of the platelets is 10 to 15 days.

Surgical Procedure

Number of ports: Most cases can be managed by 3-port pars plana vitrectomy (Figs 30.34 and 30.35). However, combined retinal detachments with severe fibrovascular proliferation, may need bimanual surgery in which case, 4-port surgery may be resorted to. The fourth port in such situations is usually placed inferotemporally close to the 6 o' clock meridian. This port is used to introduce a light pipe that is handheld by an assistant.

Choice of observation system: This is the individual surgeon's option. However, in extensive detachments, a wide angle system scores over the routine Landers' type lens system.

High cut rate vs normal cut rate: Using the new high-speed cutters (> 800 cuts per min.) is sometimes advantageous in diabetic retinopathy. Most fibrous tissue can be removed with safety from the surface of the retina. The need for membrane dissection using the scissors can also be reduced.

Management of lens: Most cases can be managed by retaining the crystalline lens. Unplanned removal of lens may be necessitated in the case of accidental lens touch. Planned lens removal may be needed in case of significant lens opacity that hinders the successful completion of the vitreoretinal surgery. Dense posterior subcapsular cataract interferes with intraoperative visualization more than nuclear sclerosis or peripheral spokes of cortical cataract. Where cataract removal is needed, one can perform phacoemulsification with IOL along with the vitreoretinal surgery. Following phacoemulsification, IOL insertion can be either done before vitrectomy or at the end of vitrectomy. There are advantages and disadvantages for both the approaches. Inserting IOL initially will keep the posterior capsule stretched, but will introduce additional interfaces for visualization. Without IOL if vitrectomy is done, there is a risk of posterior capsule being accidentally removed since it is lax. A compromise approach is to fill the anterior chamber with viscoelastic till the completion of the vitrectomy and then introduce the IOL.

Management of preexisting intraocular lens: The IOL can pose a problem for intraoperative visualization when there are significant deposits on the IOL, or posterior synechiae have formed. In most cases, one can get reasonable visualization by removing the deposits with a needle under viscoelastic. In small pupils with posterior synechiae, one may have to use temporary iris retractors to keep the pupil dilated. It is only seldom that one is forced to remove the IOL.

Vitrectomy: The steps of vitrectomy will vary depending on the surgical anatomy.

1. Eyes with total posterior vitreous detachment are the easiest from the surgical perspective. A core vitrectomy with debulking of the vitreous is done. Subhyaloid blood is aspirated with a flute needle or other aspiration device (Figs 30.36 and 30.37).

2. Eyes with near total posterior vitreous detachment with attachments to one or two focal areas of fibrovascular proliferation are also easy to handle. The adhesion can be to the disc or elsewhere. The focal areas of proliferation can be trimmed and cauterized. Near the disc, very often there can be a membrane extending on to the peripapillary retina. Unless this membrane is identified and peeled towards the disc, traction on the peripapillary retina could be left behind.

3. *Focal tractional retinal detachment:* The focus of tractional retinal detachment in diabetic eyes is usually in the posterior pole especially along the arcades. Posterior vitreous detachment can be variable in circumferential extent. After removal of the anterior and midvitreous, an attempt is made to locate

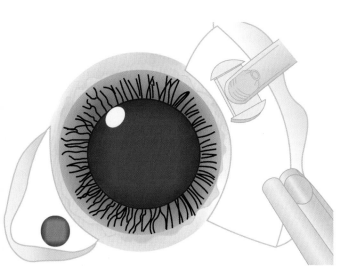

Fig. 30.34: Routine set up for 3-port pars plana vitrectomy (Modified with permission from Travis A Meredith, MD)

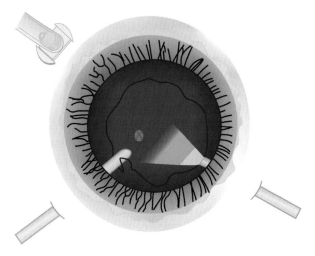

Fig. 30.35: Vitrectomy in progress using endoilluminator and vitrector (Modified with permission from Travis A Meredith, MD)

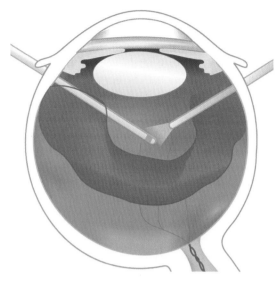

Fig. 30.36: Opaque vitreous being cleared by vitreous cutter (Modified with permission from Travis A Meredith, MD)

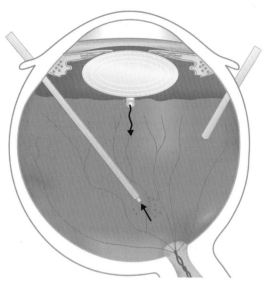

Fig. 30.37: Subhyaloid blood being evacuated by aspiration (Modified with permission from Travis A Meredith, MD)

the area beyond the traction retinal detachment, wherein posterior vitreous detachment is present. From this area, it may be easier to remove all the anteroposterior traction by going 360°. Areas with no posterior vitreous detachment also tend to develop posterior vitreous detachment as the dissection progresses all round. After the relief of anteroposterior traction, the preretinal tissue is removed.

4. *Extensive tractional retinal detachment*: These cases form the most difficult from the surgical perspective. The ease or otherwise of the dissection would depend on the extent of attachments, and the ability of the retina to withstand some amount of traction. Absence of posterior vitreous detachment adds to the problems.

5. *Membrane surgery*: Approaches to remove the preretinal tissue can vary with the individual surgeon's experience.

   a. *Segmentation*: In this technique, either the vitreous cutter or vertical scissors is used to cut the tissue into islands with single point attachment. The islands are trimmed and if need be cauterized. No attempt is made to remove all the tissue. This technique may be used by itself or as a prelude to delamination (Figs 30.38 A to D).

   b. *Delamination:* In this technique, an attempt is made to remove all the preretinal tissues. Usually, scissors with horizontally oriented blades are used. The curved scissors is an excellent instrument for this procedure. As was indicated in the pathoanatomy, it is important to identify the second membrane that extends anteriorly from the site of the attachment of the fibrovascular tissue and initiate the dissection from the same. This enables easier dissection. Loose attachments can be separated by blunt dissection, but firm attachments are cut with the scissors (Figs 30.39 to 30.41).

   c. *Peeling:* In general, peeling is avoided in diabetic vitrectomies since the risk of retinal break formation is

significant. However, there are situations when peeling can be done carefully and facilitates the removal of large areas of tissue.

   d. *Viscodissection:* Some surgeons have used injection of viscoelastic substances under the fibrovascular tissue to try and separate most of the loose attachments.

   e. *Bimanual dissection:* When the retina is relatively mobile and the fibrovascular tissue is firmly adherent, unimanual dissection can become very difficult. Using two active instruments can facilitate rapid dissection. Several techniques are available to facilitate this step:

   i. Use of fourth port: By using a fourth port, a handheld light pipe can be placed and kept in position by the assistant while the surgeon uses the two active instruments, such as scissors and forceps.

   ii. Use of combined instruments: Multifunction instruments, such as illuminated light pic, illuminated forceps and illuminated scissors can also help in this step (Fig. 30.42).

   iii. Use of coaxial illumination of the microscope: Some microscopes come with slit-illumination. Use of this facilitates the visualization of the fundus with the microscope illumination thus freeing the two hands of the surgeon for the active instruments.

   f. *En bloc dissection:* In this technique, the posterior vitreous is not cut off all round to start with. The persistence of anteroposterior traction acts to keep the membrane pulled anteriorly. This tractional force can be used to advantage. Through an opening made in the posterior hyaloid, delamination is done to cut off the vitreoretinal adhesions while they are kept taut. This technique, however, is possible only in a few cases (Figs 30.43A to 44).

   g. *Endpoint of membrane surgery:* If there is no retinal break formation, residual traction away from macula may not

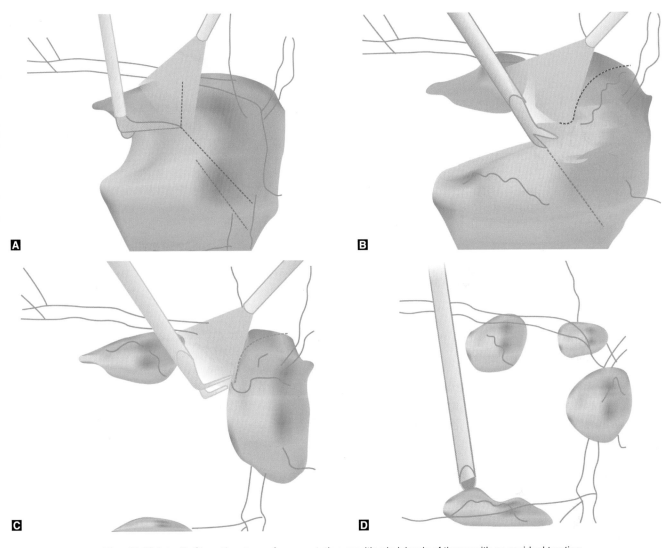

Figs 30.38 A to D: Show the steps of segmentation resulting in islands of tissue with no residual traction
(Modified with permission from Travis A Meredith, MD)

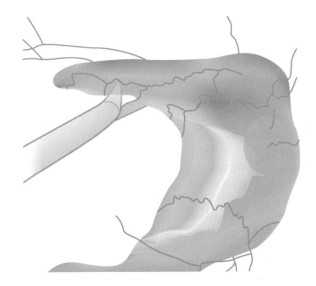

Fig. 30.39: Delamination procedure in progress. Horizontal bladed scissors is used to cut the nails of attachment of fibrovascular tissue (Modified with permission from Travis A Meredith, MD)

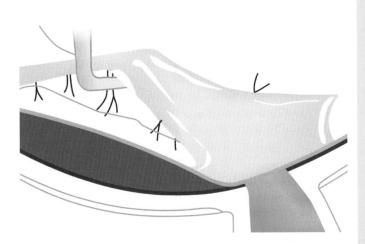

Fig. 30.40: A sharp pic is used to lift the fibrovascular tissue. Loose attachments can be peeled off using a pic-like device (Modified with permission from Travis A Meredith, MD)

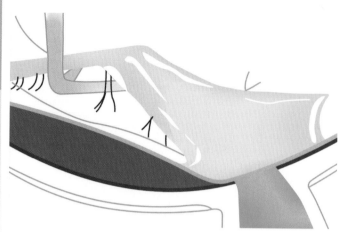

Fig. 30.41: Spreading blades of scissors can sometimes to be used to separate a relatively loose adhesion of fibrovascular tissue (Modified with permission from Travis A Meredith, MD)

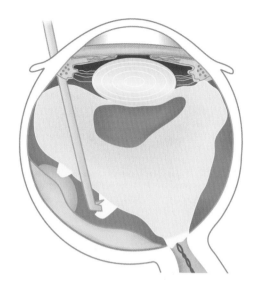

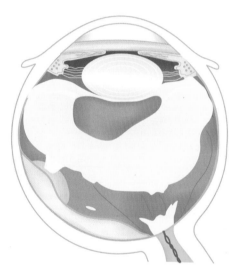

A

B

Figs 30.43A and B: En bloc dissection

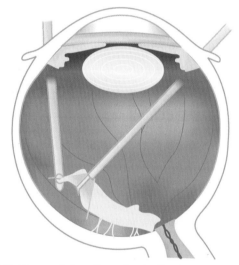

Fig. 30.42: Bimanual dissection using the illuminated pic and cutter (Modified with permission from Travis A Meredith, MD)

be a major issue. If, however, breaks form, total relief of traction should be aimed at for proper reattachment of the retina.

h. *Pulling the plug:* Removal of the fibrovascular tissue adherent to the disc may not be always necessary. In some cases, removal of this tissue leads to considerable relief of peripapillary traction. Cases with firmly adherent tissue can be left alone after trimming and cauterizing. Care must be taken to remove all the peripapillary extensions of the tissue.

6. *Hemostasis:* This could be an important issue in surgery on diabetic eyes. The vascularity as well as the altered blood rheology can be responsible for the intraoperative hemorrhage. Several maneuvers have been described to achieve hemostasis:

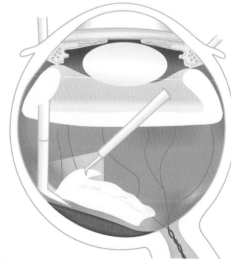

Fig. 30.44: Bimanual dissection using the illuminated pic and scissors to complete the en bloc dissection

a. *Raising the infusion pressure:* Hydrostatic pressure of the infusion fluid can be increased, by raising the infusion bottle height. Recent vitrectomy instruments come with pneumatic pressurization and enable rapid increase in the IOP. Care must be taken not to keep the pressure raised for too long a time to avoid ischemic damage to the retina.

b. *Use of cautery:* Endocautery can be used to cauterize elevated bleeders. 23-gauge instrument is ideally suited for this purpose. However, caution must be exercised in applying aggressive cautery on proliferative tissue adherent to disc since this can cause thermal papillitis. Cautery to surface retinal bleeders is fraught with the danger of retinal break formation in addition to the full-thickness retinal damage that occurs at site of the cautery. On occasions, surface retinal bleeders may need to be treated by cautery to facilitate the surgery.

c. *Use of pressure:* Mechanical pressure with a blunt instrument, such as tip of the cutter or heme stopper can control the bleeding in some cases. This involves delicate balance between the amount of pressure needed for hemostasis versus potential to damage the underlying RPE and choroid. Usually, a continuous pressure of at least one minute is needed to achieve hemostasis.

d. *Fluid air exchange:* Can sometimes produce hemostatis and permit the continuation of the surgery. The fluid is reinfused before proceeding with the surgery.

e. *Thrombin infusion:* This is a relatively rarely used technique. Bovine thrombin in infusion is expected to reduce the severity of bleeding. However, it is effective before the bleeding occurs and hence used in anticipation of bleeding.

f. *Perflurocarbon liquids and silicone oil:* These have been suggested to produce hemostasis.

7. *Retinal ablation:* Most cases would have had some amount of retinal photocoagulation before requiring vitreoretinal surgery. Intraoperatively, more treatment is usually added. Areas that could not be treated preoperatively are covered. In case of resurgery for recurrent vitreous hemorrhage, peripheral retinal ablation with cryo can be done. Photocoagulation is also done around the retinal holes if any (after fluid-air exchange). Peripheral cryotherapy is useful to treat peripheral retinal breaks, especially dialysis which can occur near sclerotomy sites.

8. *Fluid-air exchange and internal tamponade:* Fluid-air exchange is needed if there is preexisting or iatrogenic retinal break. Depending on the need, internal tamponade can be with air, long-acting gases, such as sulfur hexafluoride and perfluoropropane or silicone oil. Usually single break with well-relieved traction can be managed by air. Multiple breaks may need perfluoropropane gas or silicone oil. Before subjecting to fluid-air exchange one must make sure that all traction is relieved on the retina. Residual traction in an eye with retinal break will not permit reattachment of the same.

9. *Retinotomy:* In most cases of diabetic vitrectomy, a deliberate retinotomy is not needed and is avoided. Residual tractional retinal detachment usually settles postoperatively once the traction is relieved. There is no need to attempt to settle the same on the table. Subretinal bands that are present on occasion are usually left alone. Small pockets of subretinal altered blood can be present in the areas of tractional retinal detachment, even without retinal break. If peripheral, they are left alone; but if present in the macular area, drainage through a retinotomy may be needed. Likewise, surgery for subretinal exudates secondary to severe diabetic maculopathy also needs retinotomy to access the same.

10. *Retinectomy:* On occasions, the retina with the area of unrelieved traction may have to be excised before reattaching the same. In cases of anterior hyaloid proliferation, 360° retinectomy may be needed. Relaxing retinectomy is done after cauterizing the area to be excised to reduce the risk of bleeding.

Role of encircling band and scleral buckling: In most cases, encircling band is not necessary. In cases with residual peripheral traction, encircling band may be advantageous. Likewise, in eyes with extensive tractional detachment of retina extending up to ora serrata, encircling band may be useful. In eyes with peripheral retinal breaks and unrelieved traction, a broader buckle may be needed.

Intraoperative Complications

In addition to the complications common to all pars plana surgery, there are complications specific to surgeries on diabetic eyes:

1. *Corneal epithelial problems:* Corneal epithelium is likely to be loose and can give rise to edema and haziness very early on in the surgery and hence may need to be removed more often than in nondiabetics. However, knowing that epithelial healing can be delayed in diabetics, removal of epithelium should be avoided unless really needed.

2. *Intraoperative hemorrhage:* This is such an integral part of surgery for diabetic retinal complications that hemostasis has been discussed in the surgical procedure section.

3. *Retinal breaks:* The incidence of iatrogenic retinal breaks is depended on several factors:
   a. *Adhesion of the fibrovascular tissue:* This dictates the ease with which it can be dissected free.
   b. *Thickness of retina:* This reflects on the ability for the retina to withstand traction while dissecting the membranes.
   c. *Technique of dissection:* Peeling is more likely to give rise to breaks than delamination and segmentation.
   d. *Surgical expertise:* The experience of the surgeon would be important in keeping the retinal breaks to the minimum.
   e. Dialysis can occur near the sclerotomy sites due to the frequent introduction and withdrawal of instruments. Odd-shaped instruments, such as the vertical scissors are

also associated with greater incidence of retinal break formation.

Postoperative Complications

1. *Corneal epithelial defects*: For the reasons enunciated above, corneal epithelial defects can occur with increased frequency in diabetics. They are managed by the patching and instillation of hypertonic saline and lubricants.

2. *Recurrent vitreous hemorrhage*: This is the most common complication after vitreous surgery for diabetic retinal complications. Early postoperative vitreous hemorrhage is fairly common, but tends to resolve with time. However, recurrent hemorrhage can occur and be of variable severity. The cause of such a hemorrhage may not be obvious. Fibrovascular proliferation from the sclerotomy sites is an important cause. Identification of such a proliferation is possible using ultrasound biomicroscopy. Anterior hyaloid proliferation is a more severe proliferative response and is discussed elsewhere. Recurrent hemorrhage may need reintervention.

   a. *Outpatient fluid-air exchange*: In this technique, fluid in the vitreous cavity is exchanged with air. In phakic and pseudophakic eyes, the procedure is done via pars plana. Air is injected via one needle while the fluid is removed through another. Total replacement of fluid with air is not possible. Visualization of the fundus is not possible with any degree of clarity immediately after and hence additional treatment in the form of photocoagulation may not be possible immediately.

   b. *Needle fluid-fluid exchange*: The technique is done in supine position. One needle connected to infusion line and other connected to 5 cc syringe can be used. By sucking the syringe, fluid passively flows into the eye. Since 27-gauge needles are used, the height of the infusion bottle needs to be increased and the suction exerted should also be slow, to avoid collapse of the eye. The wash out of blood takes time. Clots and film of blood adherent to retinal surface cannot be removed by this technique. Agitation of the adherent blood is not possible since the jet of infusion is slow. However, this technique when effective, enables the treatment of retina with laser same time since the visualization is good. Wu and associates describe a device that enables homeostatic volume exchange of fluid. They have also recommended use of tissue plasminogen activator along with the above procedure to remove any clotted blood.

   c. *Vitreous lavage*: Vitreous lavage as a surgical procedure may need to be done in some cases especially if there is need to do additional procedure at the same time. This can sometimes be anticipated based on ultrasonography or intraoperative findings at time of first surgery. Where sufficient laser photocoagulation could not be done in the initial instance, it is better to do surgical vitreous lavage and perform additional treatment at the same time. Any eye with evidence of fibrovascular proliferation should be subjected to vitreous lavage and evaluation of the proliferation. Vitreous lavage can be a two- and three-port procedures based on the need. Additional membrane surgery may be needed in some cases due to reproliferation. Fibrovascular proliferation from sclerotomy sites may need to be trimmed and cauterized. This step is possible in case of pseudophakic and aphakic eyes with ease.

3. *Anterior hyaloid proliferation*: This is one of the more serious complications. There is a variable amount of fibrovascular proliferation circumferentially along the vitreous base. The process is usually initiated at the sclerotomy sites and goes all round. In the late stages, anterior hyaloid proliferation can lead to traction on the peripheral retina and ciliary body. Anterior hyaloid proliferation can be dealt with only by aggressive surgery. Phakic eyes may need lens removal. The vitreous base is carefully excised and the anterior hyaloid proliferation is dissected, if need be by bimanual dissection facilitated by scleral indentation. If peripheral retina is incarcerated in the anterior hyaloid proliferation, retinectomy is needed. Very often, silicone oil tamponade will be needed.

4. *Rubeosis iridis*: Rubeosis iridis is first detected along the pupillary margin and hence it is mandatory to look for the same under the higher magnification of slit lamp before dilatation. The common associations of this development are retinal detachment and anterior hyaloid proliferation. In the absence of these, aggressive retinal ablation is needed. Presence of retinal detachment or anterior hyaloid proliferation needs further vitreoretinal surgical procedures.

5. *Neovascular glaucoma*: The end stage of rubeosis iridis is the development of neovascular glaucoma. Treatment will be in the form of cyclophotocoagulation in addition to retinal ablation.

Results

The Diabetic Retinopathy Vitrectomy Study (DRVS) has demonstrated that early vitrectomy (surgery 1–6 months after the onset of hemorrhage) is beneficial in the case of severe vitreous hemorrhage (vision of 5/200) and resulted in 20/40 (6/12) or better vision in 36% patients compared to only 12% in the deferred group. This difference is more apparent in type 1 diabetics compared to type 2. The risk of losing light perception is similar in both groups for type 1 diabetics; while for type 2 diabetics, there was a trend towards less frequent incidence of no light perception in the deferral group. The results of the surgery in the present day could be better than what is seen in the DRVS since endolaser photocoagulation has become the norm now and not so during the study period. In surgery done for recent onset of macular detachments, macular attachment has been achieved in 66 to 88% in various reports. Visual acuity of 5/200 or better was achieved in 59 to 71%. About 10 to 20% of diabetic vitrectomies result in loss of light perception due to neovascular glaucoma. Eyes with combined retinal detachments have much less success rate (Figs 30.45 and 30.46).

SURGICAL TREATMENT OF VEIN OCCLUSIONS

Introduction

Retinal vein occlusions could be broadly classified as central and branch occlusions. The degree of visual disturbance and the ultimate prognosis is variable even among the two groups due to other variables. In this chapter, the stress will be on the surgical management (although controversial) of these two entities.

Central Retinal Vein Occlusion

Central retinal vein occlusion is caused by the occlusion of the central retinal vein at the lamina cribrosa. The event of thrombotic occlusion is presumably precipitated by compression by a thickened central retinal artery. The effect it has on the retinal circulation results in variable amount of ischemia. Fundus typically shows dilated, tortuous blood vessels, retinal hemorrhages and disc edema. The severity of each of these features can be variable. The nonischemic variety of central retinal vein occlusion has minimal hemorrhages and the visual acuity is usually better preserved. Presence of macular edema can lead to visual loss even in nonischemic variety. The typical blood and thunder appearance is seen usually in the ischemic variety wherein the disc edema is also prominent and visual loss can be severe. However, it has been difficult to define the level of ischemia with the clinical picture. Factors that have been used to identify the degree of ischemia include relative afferent pupillary defect, reduced b/a ratio on electroretinography, extent of capillary drop out on fluorescein angiography, visual acuity and the clinical picture. Of these, the clinical picture has been found to be the least reliable in judging the amount of ischemia. In addition, one has to also contend with the problem of progressive

ischemia due to worsening occlusion. The treatment of this condition was and has been unsatisfactory. Various medical treatments have been tried without success, including the use of anticoagulants. The central vein occlusion study group tried to test the efficacy of photocoagulation in preventing and treating iris neovascularization and concluded that photocoagulation in scatter format has no preventive role, but is useful once neovascularization of iris is noted. It has also been noted that laser for the macula edema has no beneficial role on the visual recovery although the macular edema may reduce.

Medical treatment has been found to be ineffective. Many drugs have been tried, including anticoagulants. McAllister and associates have described the technique of creating chorioretinal shunt using laser photocoagulation, thus creating an alternative path for the blood to flow out. In the experience of the authors, successful shunt could be created only in 33% of the cases. The authors used green laser to rupture the Bruch's membrane and green or YAG laser to rupture a venule, thus setting up a situation amenable for shunt formation. Several complications have subsequently been described with this technique by others, including the occurrence of choroidal neovascular membrane, progressive fibrovascular proliferation and retinal detachments.

Although traditionally surgery was never thought possible for central retinal vein occlusion, several surgical procedures have been tried. The most common technique described is one of radial optic neurotomy.

Radial Optic Neurotomy

Rationale behind this technique is to decompress the vein near the lamina cribrosa. A special neurotomy knife has been devised to incise the scleral ring nasally. After a routine 3-port pars plana vitrectomy, the knife is inserted radial to the ring and the scleral fibers were cut. Thus, the injury to the nerve fibers is minimized and the papillomacular bundle is avoided. Reports of successful results varied. Improvement is indicated by the disappearance of hemorrhages and edema rapidly.

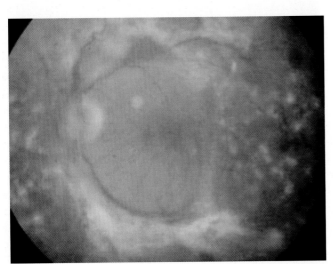

Fig. 30.45: Preoperative fundus picture of a case of diabetic retinopathy

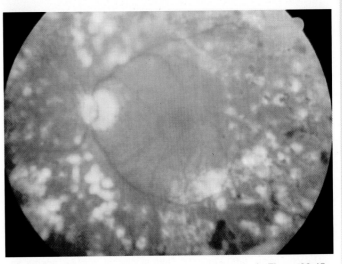

Fig. 30.46: Post-vitrectomy fundus picture of the eye in Figure 30.45

Spaide and associates suggested that the mechanism for relief of the edema may be not just release of pressure, but also occurrence of retinochoroidal collaterals at the site of incision. Potential complications with this technique include significant hemorrhage from the incision site, which in majority of cases could be controlled. Choroidal neovascularization at the site of incision has also been described. Not all ophthalmologists agree regarding the value and rationale of this surgical procedure.

Other treatment modalities tried include intravitreal injection of tissue plasminogen activator in an attempt to clear the thrombus in the vein and intravitreal triamcinolone for the macular edema.

Branch Retinal Vein Occlusion

Branch retinal vein occlusion (BRVO) typically affects the upper temporal vein. Pathogenetically, it is well-accepted that the hardened artery presses on the vein resulting in the occlusion. Visual loss in the acute phase is due to the presence of macular edema and hemorrhages in the macular area. Subsequent complications are due to the ischemia leading to neovascularization, occurrence of vitreous hemorrhage, retinal hole formation and retinal detachment; and on occasions, neovascularization of the anterior segment. Traditionally, treatment was directed towards the macular edema and the neovascularization. Branch retinal vein occlusion study has shown benefit of photocoagulation to the ischemic macular area in a modified grid fashion resulting in improved vision. However, eyes with macular ischemia are not likely to benefit by this treatment. Surgical treatment of BRVO was envisaged to relieve the pressure on the vein by the hardened artery. This is based on the observation that they both share a common adventitious sheath.

Sheathotomy

Three-port pars plana vitrectomy is done, including the induction of posterior vitreous detachment if need be. Sheathotomy knife is used to incise the common adventitious sheath between the artery and the vein at the crossing involved in the occlusive process. The site of occlusion is identified from the clinical picture and the fluorescein angiography. Peeling of the internal limiting membrane and intravitreal triamcinolone are optional steps in the surgical procedure. José García and associates describe a modification in the technique. They perform internal limiting membrane peeling over the site of AV crossing and then use a specially designed forceps to encircle the arteriole and lift it atraumatically. Using a bimanual technique facilitated by illuminated infusion, a microscissors is used along with the forceps to cut the adventitious sheath under the artery. Massaging of the vein is done to displace the thrombus and 25 micrograms of t-PA is placed over the site. Fluid-air exchange is done (Figs 30.47 to 30.50). Most authors have shown significant and rapid improvement both functionally in terms of visual acuity and reduction in macular edema evidenced on optical coherence tomography. Yamaji and associates have shown definite improvement in the venous perfusion following surgery using videoangiography.

SURGICAL TREATMENT OF INTRAOCULAR FOREIGN BODY

Introduction

Ocular injuries can be broadly classified into open and closed globe variety. Open globe variety is characterized by the dehiscence of ocular coats. This could result from blunt or penetrating trauma. While a blunt trauma results in dehiscence by inside out mechanism leading to rupture of the sclera at the weak points, a penetrating trauma is caused by a sharp instrument resulting in a clean sliced wound. Agents, such as knife, needle, etc. cause the trauma, but are not lodged in the eye. Small foreign bodies like metallic chips and bullets, flying at high speed tend to be lodged in the eye or may double perforate the eye and be lodged beyond the eyeball.

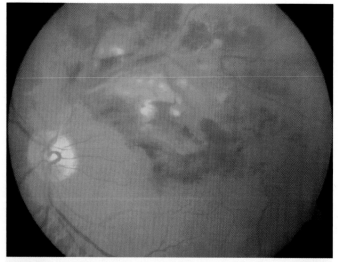

Fig. 30.47: Preoperative fundus picture of a case of branch retinal vein occlusion [vision- 6/60 (20/200)]. Note significant macular edema and hemorrhages

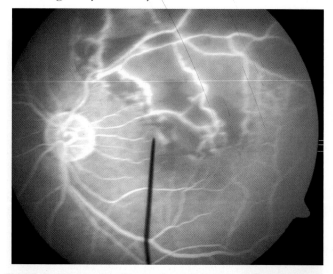

Fig. 30.48: Preoperative fluorescein angiographic picture of the eye in Figure 30.47. Note staining of the blood vessels and capillary drop out

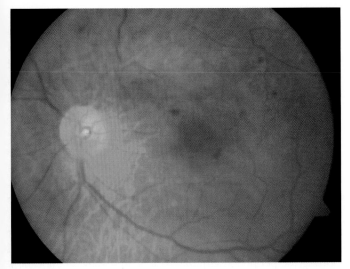

Fig. 30.49: Postoperative fundus picture of the eye in Figure 30.51 after sheathotomy, internal limiting membrane peeling and sectorial scatter photocoagulation [vision 6/12 (20/40)]. Note almost resolved macular edema

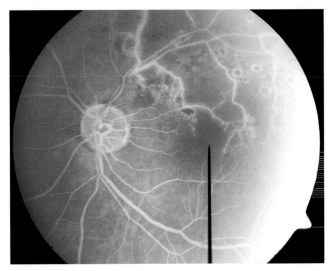

Fig. 30.50: Postoperative fluorescein angiographic picture of eye in Figure 30.47. Note grossly reduced leakage of dye from the blood vessels

Clinical Picture

It is outside the scope of this chapter to dwell in detail about the clinical presentation. Certain important features that have bearing on the management will be discussed.

1. *Type of injury:* Injuries while chiseling or working on lathe machines are usually associated with iron foreign bodies. Usually, the entry wound in these cases may be clean-cut wound and if small enough could be self-sealing. Injuries with shotgun are associated with multiple foreign bodies on the body, but the eye itself is affected by only one of these. Being a blunt, but high velocity missile, the damage to the internal structures is very severe. Likewise, double perforation is not uncommon. Injuries due to blast are associated with multiple small foreign bodies.

2. *Associated corneal/scleral/corneoscleral damage:* This is mandatory for the occurrence of intraocular foreign body. However, on occasions, the entry wound can be self-sealing or may not be evident.

3. *Associated infection:* Infection can be virulent as in *Bacillus* infection associated with contamination with soil. Injuries with vegetable matter are associated with fungal infection that presents as chronic infection with granuloma formation.

4. *Associated medial opacity:* Vitreous hemorrhage and lens opacification are common accompaniments of perforating injury. These can interfere with the assessment of the retinal damage. Corneal damage can also interfere with the assessment of the interior of the eye depending on the extent and location.

5. *Location of the intraocular foreign body:* Broadly speaking, the foreign body can be located in the anterior or posterior segment. In the anterior segment, it can be seen in the anterior chamber, angle, iris and the lens. In the posterior segment,

it may be lying in the vitreous cavity, on the surface of the retina or within the coats of the eye.

6. *Size and multiplicity of intraocular foreign body:* The size of intraocular foreign body can vary. Usually, metallic chips from chiseling tend to be smaller in size, while glass pieces from broken wind screen or spectacles tend to be larger in size. Blast injury and broken glass injury are also associated with more than one foreign body.

7. *Associated retinal damage:* Damage to the retina can be at the site of initial impact and the ricochet wound. The foreign body may lie in a different place after the impact. Retinal detachment is uncommon as presenting feature with intraocular foreign body unless the duration is long.

8. *Encapsulation:* Some amount of encapsulation is common even one day after injury.

9. *Siderotic changes:* Siderotic changes can occur depending on the iron content in the foreign body, location and duration since injury.

Evaluation

In addition to the clinical evaluation, keeping in mind the points discussed above, one may have to perform investigations before planning surgical management.

Ultrasonography

Performed as an office investigation, it can provide valuable information to guide in the management of a case of intraocular foreign body. The presence of the intraocular foreign body can be confirmed in the case of opaque media. The location can also be made out in a majority of cases. The presence of retinal detachment and on occasions, the posterior perforation site can be made out. Ultrasonography has been found to be more sensitive in picking up intraocular foreign body compared to CT scan in a series of siderotic eyes.

Radiology

CT scan has replaced plain X-ray in most instances. CT scan enables not only identification of all the foreign bodies, but makes it possible to identify its location in relation to the eye wall with precision. Associated trauma to the bones is also identified.

Management

Decision Regarding the Removal of the Intraocular Foreign Body

Although in most instances, the intraocular foreign body needs to be removed, in some cases, it can be left alone. An inert foreign body not causing mechanical damage to the structures of the eye in an eye otherwise not needing surgical intervention can be watched. Most glass foreign bodies are inert. If present in the vitreous gel, they can be observed. However, if the vitreous is liquefied and the foreign body is freely lying on the retinal surface, there is risk of retinal damage and the foreign body would need to be removed. A reactive foreign body on occasions may need to be left alone if the removal is likely to be more traumatic as in the case of foreign body impacted within the optic nerve or in macular area, which may not necessarily be a foreign body and may be associated with the risk of siderosis. An intraocular foreign body in a blind and otherwise inoperable eye can be left alone. If at all, such an eye is advised enucleation.

Decision Regarding the Timing of Surgery

Fresh cases of injury with intraocular foreign body should be handled immediately and intraocular foreign body should preferably be removed at the same time as the primary repair. This considerably reduces the risk of endophthalmitis. On occasions, the corneal wound may not permit proper vitreous surgery at the primary sitting. One may be forced to postpone the foreign body removal by a few days to permit improvement in the corneal condition. Knox and associates have shown that even in eyes with intraocular foreign body and endophthalmitis, immediate intravitreal injection of antibiotics followed by slightly delayed vitrectomy can still have desirable results. If the patient presents more than 4 to 5 days after the injury and has no evidence of infection, removal of the intraocular foreign body can be on a more planned basis. In the presence of established siderosis, the decision to remove the iron foreign body could be difficult. Risk of complications has to be weighed against the questionable benefit in retarding or halting the progression of siderotic changes. The removal of foreign body in such instances has not necessarily been shown to be complicated.

Decision Regarding the Approach to Remove the Intraocular Foreign Body

Foreign body in the anterior segment is removed from the limbal route. Foreign body in the vitreous cavity with no damage to the retina can be removed via pars plana without vitrectomy using a magnet. However, most foreign bodies in posterior segment are managed with pars plana vitrectomy. Direct posterior approach by scratch down sclerotomy over site of foreign body impaction is not usually performed. However, on occasions, such an approach may be useful.

Surgical Procedure

Initial Steps

Corneal/scleral/corneoscleral wounds may need to be sutured before proceeding with the vitreoretinal surgery in the case of significantly large wounds. Sometimes, previously sutured wounds may need to be resutured to perfection if leaks are seen during the surgery. The role of encircling band in supporting the peripheral vitreous base is unproven. The location of the sclerotomies may have to be in unconventional position because of the location of the injury site.

Management of the Lens

Clear lens is only very rarely sacrificed as in very large intraocular foreign bodies that cannot be removed from extended sclerotomy in the pars plana. Traumatized lens is usually removed during vitreoretinal surgery.

Vitrectomy

Three-port pars plana vitrectomy is done as a routine. The subsequent steps would depend upon the location of the foreign body and the status of the retina.

a. *Foreign body in the vitreous:* In this situation initially only core vitrectomy done. No attempt is made to induce posterior vitreous detachment. The residual vitreous acts like a cushion for the foreign body and may protect the retina from damage during the manipulations. Magnetic foreign bodies are picked up by intraocular magnet and once freed from the vitreous, are transferred to the better grip of the diamond-dusted foreign body forceps of Machemer. The foreign body is aligned with its long axis along the shaft of the forceps. The sclerotomy is enlarged to the required extent by approximate estimation and the foreign body is extracted. Subsequently, the sclerotomy is sutured to reduce its dimension to a 20-gauge sclerotomy. Posterior vitreous detachment is induced at this stage and the vitrectomy is completed. Peripheral retina is inspected for dialysis. This is especially common near the sclerotomy through which the foreign body has been extracted. Hidden trauma to the retina is also looked for and treated with laser if need be. Dialysis is treated with cryo and supported by gas tamponade with or without peripheral encircling band.

b. *Foreign body on retinal surface with encapsulation:* In this situation, posterior vitreous detachment is induced even before the removal of foreign body. The retina around the site of impaction is treated with laser photocoagulation. The treatment is done before attempting to remove the foreign body since these attempts can lead to localized retinal elevation or edema preventing adequate treatment later on. The capsule covering the foreign body is incised with a sharp microvitreoretinal blade. The foreign body is well exposed and lifted with magnet if magnetic. Nonmagnetic foreign bodies are directly held with forceps and removed. The steps of surgery are otherwise similar to what has been elucidated above.

c. *Foreign body in the peripheral vitreous/retina with clear lens*: Foreign body localized in the periphery may not be easily accessible/visible during vitrectomy. Once its location is confirmed with indirect ophthalmoscopy, scleral depression can facilitate the access to the foreign body.

d. *Foreign body in the ciliary body area:* These foreign bodies can be removed by scleral route via scratch down sclerotomy without vitrectomy.

e. *Foreign body deeply embedded in the posterior globe wall:* It may not be possible to be sure as to the extent of the foreign body that is within the eye and the extent beyond the eye. An attempt is made to remove the foreign body from inside by carefully cutting the capsule and if need be some retina around. Significant bleeding from choroid usually does not occur. If a large component of the foreign body is protruding outside the eye, it is best to remove from outside. The sclerotomies are plugged and the muscle disinserted if need be to gain better exposure of the posterior sclera. Since the area of foreign body may be camouflaged by blood and fibrosis, one may have to dissect carefully before identifying the same. Once the foreign body is identified, careful dissection of the sclera around the site is important. A suture is preplaced around the site before extracting the foreign body to facilitate quick closure of the posterior scleral opening. Further surgery is to repair the retinal damage internally.

f. *Removal of glass intraocular foreign body:* Glass foreign bodies pose a special problem in removal. They are usually multiple especially when caused by blast injury. The size can be fairly large, sometimes making it difficult even to grasp with the widest separation of the blades of the foreign body forceps. The surface can also be slippery and attempts to grasp the same can lead to retinal cuts caused by the sharp edges. Very thin slivers can get crushed if not handled properly. All varieties of glass are heavier than perfluorocarbon liquids and hence perfluorocarbon liquids cannot be used to float the glass pieces. Perfluorocarbon liquid can be used, however, to gently nudge the glass piece into a more vertical position, permitting better grip for the forceps. Since the retinal cuts caused by the sharp edge of glass piece tend to be linear, there is need to identify the same with cautery as soon as they occur.

g. *Extraction of the foreign body:* Once the forceps picks it up, generally the foreign body is removed via an enlarged sclerotomy as was described above. However, if the foreign body is large, it is brought out through the anterior route. A clear corneal or limbal groove is made. With the foreign body held with the forceps with one hand, the other hand is freed and one sclerotomy is plugged. The eye is entered with a blade and the incision is extended. The foreign body is maneuvered through the opening. External forceps can be used to transfer the foreign body from the intraocular forceps. The wound is closed with 10-0 nylon suture.

h. *Further surgery:* Before proceeding further with the surgery, one needs to reduce the enlarged sclerotomies to 20-gauge size. Further surgery would depend on the extent and type of posterior segment pathology. Retina in the meridian of sclerotomies needs to be examined carefully for the evidence of any dialysis. In view of the irregular surface of the foreign bodies, peripheral vitreous can be dragged while withdrawing the foreign body and can easily induce dialysis. The enlarged sclerotomy also facilitates the prolapse of the vitreous gel. All retinal breaks need to be treated with laser or cryo and appropriate tamponade with gas or silicone oil is used.

Role of Encircling Band

Encircling band is useful to support the peripheral vitreous base and to support peripheral breaks in association with internal tamponade.

Difficulties

1. *Difficulty in access:* Foreign body enmeshed in the peripheral vitreous may not be visible easily during vitrectomy. One needs to perform indirect ophthalmoscopy with scleral indentation to visualize the same. To access such a foreign body internally without damaging the lens could be difficult. High indentation facilitated by some induced hypotony may enable one to overcome the problem.

2. *Too small a foreign body:* A very small foreign body may be difficult to hold with foreign body forceps. Such foreign bodies are best grasped with regular intraocular forceps and extracted. On occasions even the flute needle can be used to suction hold a foreign body that is very small.

3. *Too large a foreign body:* Glass pieces can sometimes be very large and may be of odd shapes. Pyramidal shape can make it very difficult to grip it, since it keeps slipping off. The diamond-dusted Machemer's forceps is a must to remove these foreign bodies. It is best to hold these foreign bodies such that the narrower end is facing down so that the tendency is to slip anteriorly and not posteriorly. Once brought into the pupillary area, a quick ab externo delivery is needed using a strong toothed external forceps, such as Bishop-Harmon forceps.

4. *Foreign body stuck in the sclerotomy site:* If attempts are made to extract the foreign body using magnet itself without transferring to a forceps, the foreign body can get stuck in the peripheral vitreous near the sclerotomy site. Even a forceps held foreign body could get stuck if the sclerotomy has not been enlarged to the desired extent. This can be anticipated during the attempted extraction. Once it is felt that the foreign body will not come out, enlargement of sclerotomy can be done even with the forceps in the sclerotomy.

5. *The dropped foreign body:* Foreign body can drop on the retina under several situations:

   a. Foreign body can drop from its moorings, while vitrectomy is being performed. On occasions, one can grasp the foreign body after partial vitrectomy, free it from the vitreous around and deliver it before it drops. In the absence of vitreous detachment, foreign body dropping from the periphery onto the posterior pole may not be a cause for concern in view of the cushion of vitreous. In the presence of posterior vitreous detachment, there is a theoretical risk of the foreign body causing further mechanical damage to the retina, although this is expected only with large and heavy foreign bodies.

   b. Foreign body slipping from the forceps is not uncommon. Unless the foreign body is large, usually mechanical damage does not occur due to this impact on the retina. The presence of vitreous cushion helps prevent damage to some extent.

6. *The crumbling foreign body:* Iron foreign body in case of long-standing siderosis could be dissolved partially leaving behind a rusty crumpling foreign body. This can be difficult to bring out in one piece. The problem of thin slivers of glass pieces has already been alluded to.

7. *Multiple foreign bodies:* It is important to be aware that multiple foreign bodies can be present in an eye especially when the injury is caused by blasts.

Results

In general, prognosis for eyes with intraocular foreign bodies is better than perforating injuries due to other mechanisms. In a series by Greven and associates, 71% of the patients recovered 20/40 or better vision and nearly 85% recovered ambulatory vision. Prognosticating factors for better visual outcome included better presenting vision and hammering metal-on-metal type of injury. Poor prognosticating factors included poor presenting visual acuity, presence of relative afferent pupillary defect and vitreous hemorrhage. In case of glass intraocular foreign body, Gopal and associates have reported a 66.7% recovery of better than 20/200 (6/60) vision in a series of 51 eyes of 43 patients. Univariate analysis revealed that scleral entry wound, posterior segment intraocular foreign body, large size of intraocular foreign body and coexisting retinal damage were associated with poor anatomical outcome. Lower presenting visual acuity, hyphema, retinal damage, subretinal hemorrhage, detached retina and large intraocular foreign body were associated with a poor functional outcome. Multivariate analysis, however, identified retinal damage as the only significant factor associated with poor anatomical and functional outcome.

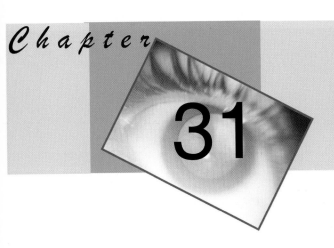
Macular Surgeries

Sandeep Saxena

Modern vitreous surgery through the pars plana is now one of the most effective tools for treating posterior segment diseases. Macular pucker, vitreomacular traction syndrome, macular hole, subfoveal choroidal neovascular membrane, submacular hematoma and diabetic macular edema comprise the spectrum of macular disease. Innovative and exciting developments in the field of macular surgery offer promise to patients with these conditions.

EPIRETINAL MEMBRANE

Epiretinal membranes are fine, nonvascular fibrotic membranes on the surface of the retina. They can cause a wrinkling or a puckering effect on the retinal surface, interfering with its function. These membranes can occur as a primary idiopathic disorder (Fig. 31.1), as a limited form of proliferative

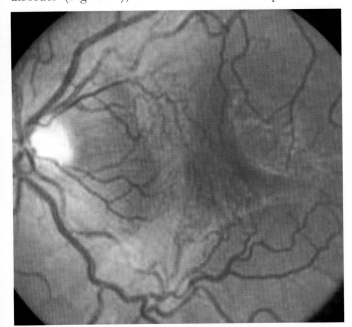

Fig. 31.1: Epiretinal membrane. Fine, nonvascular fibrotic membrane is visible on the surface of the retina

vitreoretinopathy after successful retinal reattachment surgery (Figs 31.2A and B), or as an associated finding in numerous other ocular disorders.

Etiopathogenesis

In idiopathic epiretinal membranes, glial cells of retinal origin proliferate through defects in the internal limiting membrane. Glial cells from the neurosensory retina migrating through breaks in the inner lamina are responsible for producing epiretinal membranes. These breaks were usually associated with posterior vitreous separation. Vitreous detachment might contribute to the development of these membranes through several mechanisms. Vitreous detachment can lead to retinal breaks, liberating retinal pigment epithelial cells into the vitreous cavity, which can subsequently attach to the posterior retina and proliferate. Disruption of the internal limiting membrane at the time of posterior vitreous detachment could allow fibrous astrocytes access to the retinal surface to proliferate and create an extracellular matrix. Vitreous hemorrhage, inflammation, or both at the time of vitreous detachment might stimulate cellular proliferation. In cases of epiretinal membrane formation before the vitreous detaches, glial cells may grow into the vitreous cavity. As the epiretinal membrane extends over the retina, a layer of vitreous is trapped against the inner limiting lamina. This relationship between the membrane and vitreous explains one mechanism by which spontaneous separation of epiretinal membranes could occur with subsequent vitreous separation. Other cell types that contribute to epiretinal membrane formation include fibrocytes, myofibroblasts, macrophages, inflammatory cells, hyalocytes, retinal pigment epithelial cells and vascular endothelial cells. Once formed, both idiopathic and secondary epiretinal membranes behave similarly. After an initial period of growth and contraction, epiretinal membranes are morphologically and visually stable in approximately 90% of patients.

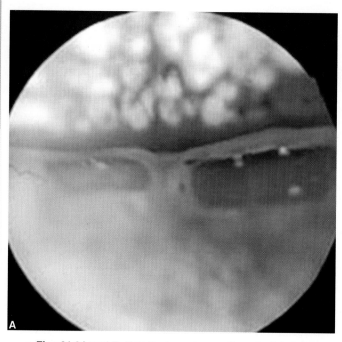
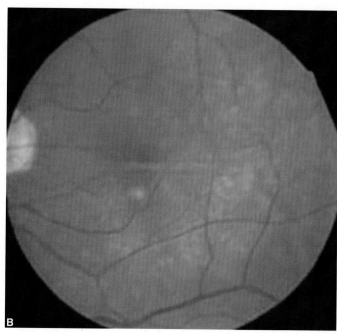

Figs 31.2A and B: Epiretinal membrane after retinal detachment surgery. (A) Open break on inferior buckle following successful retinal reattachment surgery, (B) Macular pucker as a limited form of proliferative vitreoretinopathy

Clinical Features

The majority of patients with symptomatic idiopathic epiretinal membranes are older than 50 years. Bilateral involvement occurs in 10 to 20% of cases. Visual symptoms from epiretinal membranes manifest as a continuum from no symptoms to severe visual dysfunction and are usually related to the severity of the membrane. In fact the majority of patients with idiopathic epiretinal membranes are asymptomatic. When minimally symptomatic, patients usually complain of mild metamorphopsia, and visual acuity remains 20/40 or better indicating that only the inner retinal surface is involved. In eyes with marked distortion of the retina patients may have severe metamorphopsia and visual acuity of less than 20/200. Less commonly, central photopsia, macropsia, or diplopia is noted. The level of vision may also be related to preexisting retinal detachment. In fact, vision is usually reduced further in eyes with epiretinal membranes that occur after retinal detachment. Mechanisms for these symptoms include tissue covering or distorting macula, vascular leakage with cystoid macular edema, low-lying traction macular detachment and obstructed axoplasmic flow.

The clinical characteristics vary according to the degree of the membrane. Gass has proposed a classification scheme for epiretinal membranes. Translucent membranes unassociated with retinal distortion are grade 0 (cellophane maculopathy). Membranes that cause irregular wrinkling of the inner retina are grade 1 (crinkled cellophane maculopathy). Opaque membranes that cause obscuration of the underlying vessels and marked full-thickness retinal distortion are grade 2 (macular pucker).

An asymptomatic patient may have a glinting, irregular light reflex caused by a subtle epiretinal membrane. These "cellophane membranes" usually do not have a distinct edge.

If the translucent membrane is more apparent, it can appear to cover the entire macula and even extend anteriorly beyond the vascular arcades. The full extent of an epiretinal membrane is best appreciated at the time of surgery, and sometimes idiopathic membranes can be stripped out past the equator. When internal membrane "contraction" or "shrinkage" is observed, there is an associated tractional effect on the entire inner retina, which produces fine retinal striae radiating from the center of the membrane, and tortuosity of retinal vessels (Fig. 31.3). However, the membrane can extend beyond the area of retinal striae. In more severe and visually debilitating epiretinal membranes, vascular tortuosity with tethering and straightening of vessels occurs distal to the center of membrane contraction (Fig. 31.4). If the membrane is centered distal to the macula, foveal ectopia can occur that causes complaints of diplopia. Occasionally, the epiretinal membrane lifts the sensory fovea off the retinal pigment epithelium in a subtle, shallow and tabletop manner. Cystoid macular edema may be present (Figs 31.5A and B). Pigmentation may also be present in the membrane. A high incidence of posterior vitreous detachment is noticed in eyes with idiopathic epiretinal membranes. Occasionally, spontaneous separation of epiretinal membrane from the retinal surface can result in improvement in visual acuity.

Surgical Case Selection

No absolute criteria exist for recommending vitrectomy for epiretinal membrane. Indications depend mainly on the visual

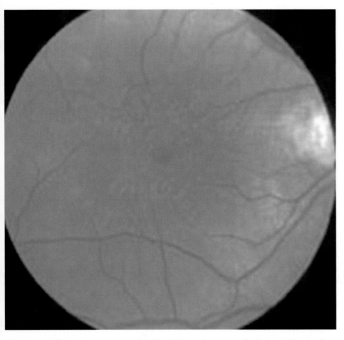

Fig. 31.3: Epiretinal membrane. Red-free photograph demonstrates fine retinal striae radiating from the center of membrane

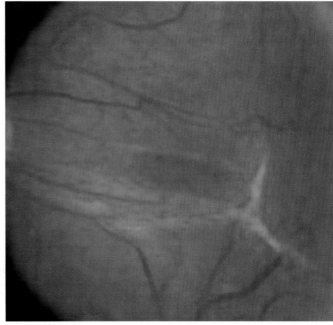

Fig. 31.4: Epiretinal membrane. Tethering and straightening of retinal vessels occurs distal to the center of membrane contraction

needs of each patient. The optimal time for the removal of epiretinal tissue is probably 6 to 8 weeks after the eye becomes symptomatic. The epiretinal membrane is mature after 6 to 8 weeks and usually can be removed completely. In idiopathic cases, membrane growth is generally slow and surgery is recommended when the patient has substantial impairment of vision or severe metamorphopsia. The postoperative visual acuity may improve if the membrane has been present for a few months; however, the potential for improvement is reduced if the membrane has been present for an especially prolonged time. Other

preoperative prognostic factors regarding final visual acuity include preoperative vision and the presence of cystoid macular edema. Eyes with preoperative visual acuity of 20/70 or better have an improved postoperative visual acuity after vitrectomy for macular pucker. However, such eyes have been found to improve significantly fewer lines overall compared with those eyes with visual acuity of 20/80 or worse. Therefore, unless the patient is seriously hampered by symptoms of metamorphopsia, vitrectomy for macular pucker is often not advocated unless the visual acuity is in the range of 20/70 or worse. The presence

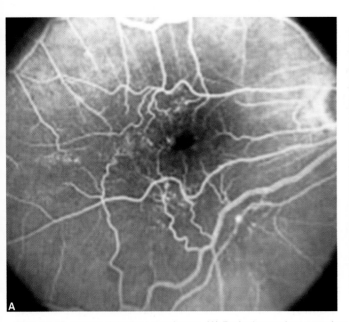

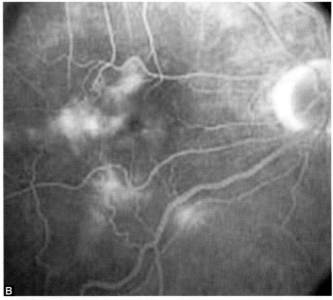

Figs 31.5A and B: Epiretinal membrane. (A) Retinal vascular tortuosity and capillary incompetence are seen in the early arteriovenous phase of fluorescein angiography, (B) Late frames of the angiogram demonstrate cystoid macular edema

of preoperative retinal vascular leakage and cystoid macular edema has been found to correlate with less visual improvement postoperatively.

Surgical Technique

A conventional vitrectomy technique is used in the management of macular pucker. A complete posterior vitreous detachment is nearly always present. Sometimes the vitreous is not separated from the retina in young patients and in eyes with membranes associated with inflammatory conditions. The entire central vitreous gel is removed in aphakic and pseudophakic eyes. The anterior portion of central vitreous gel is spared in phakic eyes to decrease the possibility of trauma to the lens. The most accessible edge of the epiretinal membrane is engaged with a vitreoretinal pic. This is followed by a slight to-and-fro motion with gentle elevation (Fig. 31.6). If there is no preexisting elevation of the edge, the pic is used to apply centripetal traction on the membrane near its margin, until the edge becomes elevated. Often radiating striae, present in the inner retina central to the margin of the membrane, aid in the identification of the edge. A barbed microvitreoretinal blade is often used to create a plane between the epiretinal membrane and internal limiting membrane. After the edge is identified and dissection started, a vitreoretinal pic is used to avoid fragmentation of the membrane. After a portion of the membrane has been separated from the retina, it is grasped with an intraocular forceps (Fig. 31.7). The membrane is usually removed as a single piece, although it may be necessary to engage it sequentially to tease it from the retinal surface. If an abnormally firm area of attachment to the retina is encountered, the membrane is amputated with an intraocular scissors or a vitrectomy probe. Once the epiretinal membrane is removed, the underlying retina may have an abnormal sheen and the inner retinal surface may appear wrinkled. Prominent whitening probably represents obstruction of retrograde axoplasmic flow in the inner retinal surface and disappears in 48 to 72 hours after surgery. This change is important to recognize to avoid misinterpreting it intraoperatively as an additional layer of membrane. Petechial hemorrhages commonly occur along the inner retinal surface as the membrane is removed and denote that separation occurs at the level of the internal limiting membrane. Such minimal bleeding is usually self-limited, but may require temporarily increased intraocular pressure by elevation of the infusion bottle. Finally, at the close of each vitrectomy the retina must be carefully inspected by indirect ophthalmoscopy with peripheral scleral depression to rule out iatrogenic peripheral retinal breaks at the time of surgery.

Dye-Assisted Epiretinal Membrane Removal Surgery

Trypan blue-assisted epiretinal membrane removal: Trypan blue concentration of 0.06% is obtained by further dilution of a commercially available 0.15% trypan blue solution with balanced salt solution. Then, 0.5 ml of a 0.06% trypan blue solution is dropped over the macula after fluid-air exchange or under continuous infusion over the posterior pole under direct visualization. After one minute the dye is removed. Visible epiretinal membrane is removed using an end-gripping forceps. If the retinal surface still has a glistening aspect without slight whitening as a sign of removed internal limiting membrane, the internal limiting membrane is incised and then peeled off using the end-gripping forceps.

Indocyanine green-assisted epiretinal membrane removal: Twenty-five milligrams of indocyanine green dye is reconstituted with 1.0 ml of sterile water. After the indocyanine green was completely dissolved, 4.0 ml of balanced salt solution is added to the solution to attain a final indocyanine green concentration of 0.5%. Then 0.6 to 0.8 ml of indocyanine green solution is instilled directly over the posterior pole using a 27-gauge blunt needle. The indocyanine green was left in the vitreous cavity for three minutes with scleral plugs in place. After removal of the indocyanine green with active suction, the internal limiting membrane is stained except in those areas where the epiretinal membrane is adherent to the internal limiting membrane. The staining is more intense in the posterior pole. The indocyanine

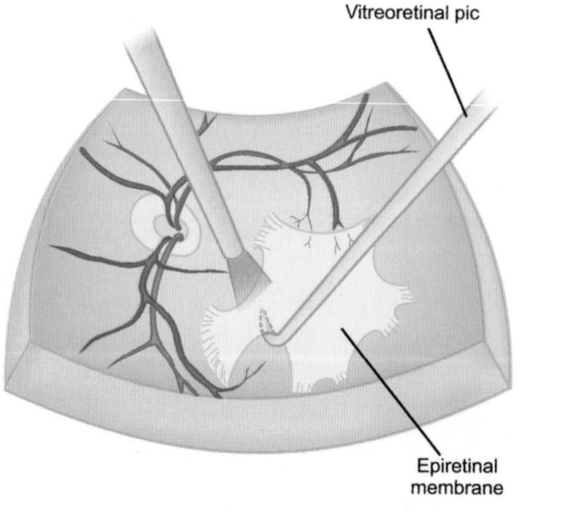

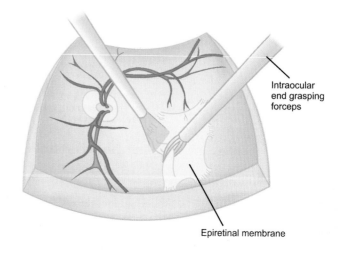

Fig. 31.6: The most accessible edge of the epiretinal membrane is engaged with a vitreoretinal pic

Fig. 31.7: Epiretinal membrane is grasped with an intraocular forceps

green-stained internal limiting membrane is cut and peeled off in a circular fashion. As a result, the internal limiting membrane is removed together with the epiretinal membrane.

Complications

Complications include peripheral retinal breaks, retinal detachment, retinal pigmentary epitheliopathy, postoperative nuclear sclerosis of the crystalline lens and peripheral visual field defects.

Role of Optical Coherence Tomography

Epiretinal membrane may be clearly separated from the retina with focal points of attachment or globally adherent (no observed separation). Secondary epiretinal membranes are more likely to be characterized by focal retinal adhesion than are primary epiretinal membranes. Primary epiretinal membranes tend to be globally adherent.

Optical coherence tomography is able to provide a structural assessment of the macula that is useful in the preoperative and postoperative evaluation of epiretinal membrane surgery. A significant correlation has been found between visual acuity and macular thickness before surgery and at the end of the postoperative follow-up. Macular thickness decreases after epiretinal membrane surgery, but the macular profile rarely returns to normal.

VITREOMACULAR TRACTION SYNDROME

Vitreomacular traction syndrome has been described as a distinct clinical entity. This syndrome comprises a broad spectrum of easily missed clinical findings, ranging from total peripheral vitreous separation with residual foveal attachment to multiple areas of subtle traction retinal detachment caused by persistent, focal, posterior and peripheral vitreous attachment. The hallmark of vitreomacular traction syndrome is persistent anterior to posterior traction on the macula via a directly observable, persistent vitreoretinal attachment. The vitreous attachment margin can be observed because it is separated peripherally. This allows sharp contrast between the linear profiles formed by the vitreous and optically clear postvitreous fluid. The attachment most commonly includes a one-to six-disc area zone centered on the fovea. It is usually contiguous with the optic nerve head, yielding a horizontally oriented oval or hourglass configuration of the margins. The zone of vitreous attachment also includes premacular tissue that mimics a macular pucker. The cystic macular changes stain with fluorescein and the extent of premacular tissue approximates the zone of persistent vitreous attachment.

Etiopathogenesis

The pathogenesis of vitreomacular traction syndrome is unknown. Two possible sequences may occur. Firstly, completion of subsequent vitreous separation may be prevented by epiretinal cellular proliferation. Secondly, an incomplete vitreous separation may lead to epiretinal membrane proliferation. The latter sequence seems more likely, because the visual loss tends to be progressive and the macular tissue has been observed in some cases to increase in size and extent with further follow-up. During posterior vitreous detachment the cortical vitreous can remain attached to the posterior pole and cause traction on the macula.

Clinical Features

The age, symptoms and clinical appearance of patients with vitreomacular traction syndrome are similar to those with idiopathic macular pucker. The symptoms include decreased vision, metamorphopsia and monocular diplopia. The visual symptoms may worsen gradually because persistent traction causes retinal vascular incompetence, leakage and cystic degeneration. Alternatively, spontaneous release of the traction can occur, resulting in visual improvement. Examination of the posterior pole may show subtle areas of traction retinal detachment, cystic macular changes, retinal striae, a thickened posterior hyaloid face, an epiretinal membrane and tractional changes on the optic nerve head. Persistent posterior vitreous attachment is best seen at the posterior margin of the vitreous attachment (Fig. 31.8). The characteristic area of residual posterior vitreous attachment and remacular tissue often involves a horizontally oriented, dumbbell-shaped area that encircles the macula and optic nerve head. Peripapillary vitreous traction appears as a ring of fibrous adherence lying on the optic nerve surface, the "fleshy doughnut" sign. Eyes may be categorized anatomically as having either "classic" vitreomacular syndrome (eyes with 360° midperipheral vitreous detachment) or "variable" vitreomacular traction syndrome (eyes with a variety of midperipheral areas of vitreous separation). There is a variable amount of fibrous proliferation ranging from a diffuse cellophane-like macular appearance in mild cases to more discrete, heavy fibrous bands in more

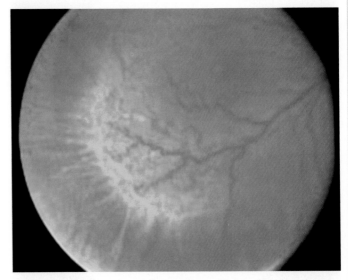

Fig. 31.8: Vitreomacular traction syndrome. The margin of persistent vitreous attachment in the inferotemporal macula is easily seen

severe cases. Although rare, persistent vitreomacular traction can lead to low-traction retinal detachment. Fluorescein leakage has been observed more frequently than for idiopathic macular pucker. However, many cases may not show leakage.

Surgical Case Selection

Correctly diagnosing the vitreomacular traction syndrome allows the surgeon to inform the patient of prognosis and therapy. Idiopathic macular pucker can mimic vitreomacular traction syndrome. The relation of the vitreous to the retina, even in cases with epimacular proliferation, is the predominant feature that separates idiopathic macular pucker from vitreomacular traction syndrome. In true epiretinal membranes, posterior vitreous separation is almost always present. Another diagnostic difficulty lies in differentiating vitreomacular traction syndrome from impending macular hole. The main distinguishing feature is the observation of direct vitreomacular traction. Visual acuity is typically better in stage I macular hole than it is in vitreomacular traction syndrome, although patients with mild cases of vitreomacular traction syndrome may have good vision. Central serous chorioretinopathy and cystoid macular edema can also mimic vitreomacular traction syndrome. The distinguishing features between these clinical entities can usually be best observed with slit-lamp biomicroscopy and optical coherence tomography.

Surgical Technique

A standard three-port vitrectomy is performed to remove anterior to posterior vitreous traction. In cases with formed vitreous membranes, the posterior hyaloid is identified and elevated in an "en bloc" fashion using a vitreoretinal pic or a bent needle. Subsequently, the posterior hyaloid is removed along with any contiguous preretinal tissue. Special care is taken to avoid direct macular trauma. Frequently, it is impossible to

determine the vitreoretinal relationship preoperatively. The vitreoretinal relationship can be determined intraoperatively using oblique intraocular illumination, noting the effect of gentle tractional forces on the macula.

Complications

Complications of vitreous surgery for vitreomacular traction syndrome include accelerated nuclear sclerosis, epiretinal membrane formation, retinal breaks, retinal detachment and macular holes.

Role of Optical Coherence Tomography

Optical coherence tomography is able to provide a structural assessment of the vitreomacular traction and is useful in the preoperative and postoperative evaluation of vitreomacular traction syndrome.

IDIOPATHIC MACULAR HOLE

Advances in the pathogenesis, classification and surgical intervention of idiopathic macular holes have generated a renewed interest in this entity. Better indicators of visual outcome as well as refinements in the surgical technique have led to improvements in the success of macular hole surgery.

Etiopathogenesis

Clinical characterization and theories on the pathogenesis of macular hole have continued to evolve. Gass proposed a theory whereby shrinkage of adherent cortical vitreous and subsequent tangential vitreous traction first cause a circumscribed foveolar detachment (stage I) followed by early retinal dehiscence (stage II), then enlargement of the macular hole with vitreofoveal separation (stage III) (Figs 31.9A and B) and finally complete posterior vitreous detachment (stage IV) (Fig. 31.10).

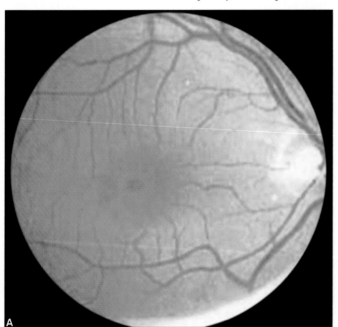
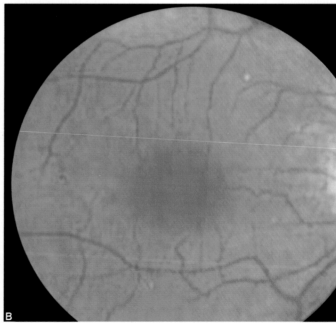

Figs 31.9A and B: Idiopathic macular hole. (A) Preoperative stage III macular hole. Visual acuity is 20/200, (B) Postoperative stage III macular hole. Visual acuity is 20/40

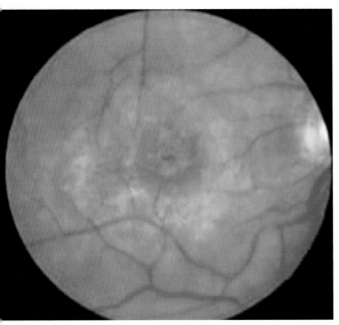

Fig. 31.10: Idiopathic macular hole. Retinal pigment epitheliopathy following vitrectomy and gas-fluid exchange for stage IV macular hole. Although the hole is closed, the patient sees a ring scotoma and visual acuity is 20/150

Clinical Features

Idiopathic macular holes occur most frequently in the sixth decade of life. Table 31.1 summarizes the biomicroscopic findings of various stages of macular hole. According to Gass, stage IA and IB lesions represent focal foveal detachments secondary to vitreous traction. A 100- to 200-μm diameter yellow spot is the earliest change observed. With progression, a 200- to 350-μm yellowish ring develops. Fine radiating striae are often seen surrounding the yellow ring. The vision is in the range of 20/25 to 20/70. Within several weeks to months, a

full-thickness dehiscence develops. This dehiscence often starts eccentrically, and then opens in a "can-opener" fashion to form a crescentic retinal defect, then a horseshoe-shaped hole, and finally a round hole with an operculum. In some cases, the dehiscence starts centrally, with gradual enlargement of the hole, and no operculum develops. A ring of retinal detachment usually surrounds the hole. As the hole enlarges, the vision generally decreases and within several months it progresses to a fully developed hole that measures approximately 500 μm in diameter. When present, the operculum is suspended over the hole by the detached vitreous cortex. With time, round yellow deposits on the central retinal pigment epithelium, epiretinal membranes that cause contracture of the internal limiting membrane, depigmentation of the pigment epithelium under the cuff of retinal elevation, and a pigmentary demarcation ring defining the outer margin of the retinal detachment may be observed. Vision is usually in the range of 20/70 to 20/400. Posterior vitreous separation from the macula and disc develops in a small percentage of cases. Eyes with idiopathic macular hole lose vision secondary to tissue dehiscence, cystic changes, and retinal cuff elevation with photoreceptor degeneration. Clinical observations have led to the impression that the macular hole and cuff enlarge secondary to persistent tangential traction from the vitreous, tangential traction from epiretinal membranes, and the development of large cystic spaces within the surrounding cuff. The incidence of apparent disappearance of idiopathic full-thickness macular holes was low. Improvement in visual acuity was greater in those cases in which macular holes disappeared in a relatively short period of time. Long-term follow-up of unoperated macular holes demonstrates progression in hole size and stage, vision loss which generally stabilizes at the 20/200 to 20/400 level, a redistribution and reduced number of yellow nodular opacities at the level of the retinal pigment epithelium, and the development of retinal pigment epithelial

Table 31.1: Biomicroscopic classification of idiopathic macular hole

Stage	Biomicroscopic findings	Anatomic interpretation
IA (impending hole)	Central yellow spot Loss of foveolar depression No vitreofoveolar separation	Early serous detachment of foveolar retina
IB (impending or occult hole)	Yellow ring with bridging interface Loss of foveolar depression No vitreofoveolar separation	For small ring, serous foveolar detachment with lateral displacement of xanthophyll; for larger ring, central occult foveolar hole with centrifugal displacement of foveolar retina and xanthophyll, with bridging contracted prefoveolar vitreous cortex
II	Eccentric oval, crescent, or horseshoe retinal defect inside edge of yellow ring Central round retinal defect Rim of elevated retina — with prefoveolar opacity — without prefoveolar opacity	Hole (tear) in contracted prefoveolar vitreous bridging round retinal hole, no loss of foveolar retina Hole with pseudo-operculum[a], rim of retinal detachment Hole, no posterior vitreous detachment from optic disc and macula
III	Central round ≥ 400 μm diameter No retinal defect Weiss' ring, rim of elevated retina — with prefoveolar opacity — without prefoveolar opacity	 Hole with pseudo-operculum, no posterior vitreous detachment Hole with no posterior vitreous detachment from optic disc and macula
IV	Central round retinal defect rim of elevated retina, Weiss' ring — with prefoveolar opacity[b] — without prefoveolar opacity	 Hole with pseudo-operculum and posterior vitreous detachment from optic disc and macula Hole and posterior vitreous detachment from optic disc and macula

[a] Pseudo-operculum contains no retinal receptors
[b] Prefoveolar opacity usually found near temporal border of Weiss' ring

atrophy surrounding the macular hole, resulting in a "bull's-eye" macular appearance. Macular hole may reopen after surgery. The cause of reopening might have been any anatomic stress such as epiretinal membrane formation or macular edema. However, in most of the reopened cases, no definite cause is evident.

Surgical Case Selection

A full-thickness macular hole is most accurately diagnosed clinically using a fundus contact lens and slit-lamp biomicroscopy and by optical coherence tomography. Amsler grid testing is sensitive in detecting any form of macular abnormality, but is not specific enough to be useful in establishing a diagnosis of macular hole, and preoperative testing has not been standardized. The Watzke-Allen test and to a greater degree the laser-aiming beam test further improve the accuracy of the diagnosis of full thickness macular holes (Figs 31.11A and B). The major advantage of these tests is that they are simple to perform, can be done in the office and are easily accessible. Watzke-Allen sign testing in all patients with clinically defined macular holes shows a break or thinning of the slit beam. Thinning of the beam is seen in both macular hole and pseudomacular hole cases. Therefore, thinning is not as specific as a total break in the slit beam in full-thickness macular hole. The laser-aiming beam test may yield similar diagnostic information, allowing the clinician to test focal areas of the retina for a scotoma. A 50 μm spot laser-aiming beam can be hidden in the macular lesion in all patients with clinically defined full-thickness macular hole. This contrasts with the finding in pseudohole eyes, which could detect the 50 μm spot. In addition, the inability to detect a 200- or 500 μm spot size is noted only by patients with macular holes. Thus, the absolute scotoma detected by the laser beam test is sensitive and specific for full-thickness macular holes. Other ancillary tests, such as focal electroretinography, scanning laser ophthalmoscopy, confocal laser tomographic analysis systems, monochromatic photography and laser biomicroscopy have been applied to the study of macular holes with some success. These modalities are not available or feasible for many clinical practices, however. Echographic features of idiopathic macular hole correlate reasonably accurately with clinical features. A pseudo-operculum is a focal condensation of the vitreous cortex suspended on detached invisible posterior hyaloid membrane, in front of either intact foveolar retina or full-thickness macular hole. It is demonstrable ultrasonographically. Its presence in the front of intact foveolar retina indicates evidence of vitreofoveal separation and low risk of developing a macular hole. Optical coherence tomography has been found effective in distinguishing full-thickness macular holes from partial thickness holes, macular holes and cysts. It has been successful in staging macular holes and providing a quantitative measure of hole diameter and the amount of surrounding macular edema. It can also detect small separations of the posterior hyaloid from the retina. Careful patient selection is critical to a successful outcome. The ideal candidate would be a patient with bilateral holes of relatively recent onset, with vision in the better eye less than or equal to 20/100. Patients with unilateral symptomatic holes with recently reduced vision to 20/70 or worse are also good candidates.

Surgical Technique

The surgical objectives for the repair of macular holes include relief of all tangential traction and retinal tamponade. Identification and removal of the cortical vitreous or posterior hyaloid and removal of fine epiretinal membranes around the hole relieve tangential traction. Tamponade is provided by total gas-fluid exchange with SF_6 or C_3F_8 and strict face-down positioning for at least one week. Most eyes with macular

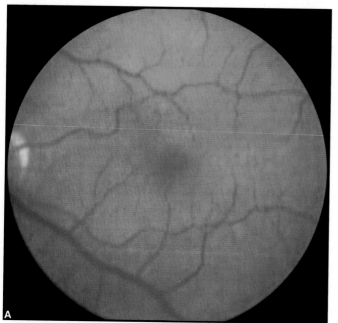 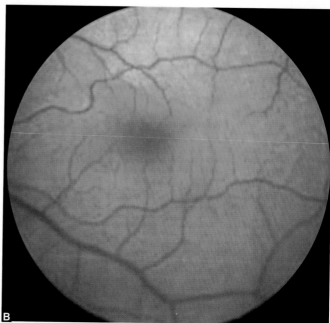

Figs 31.11A and B: Idiopathic macular hole. (A) Preoperative stage II macular hole. Watzke-Allen sign is present (B) Postoperative fundus photograph shows closed macular hole. Visual acuity is 20/25-1. Watzke-Allen sign is absent

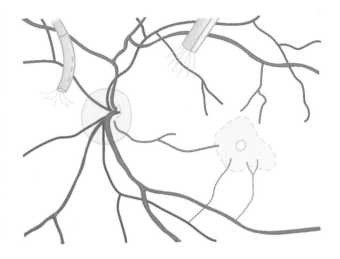

Fig. 31.12: A silicone-tipped cannula flexes once the cortical vitreous is engaged

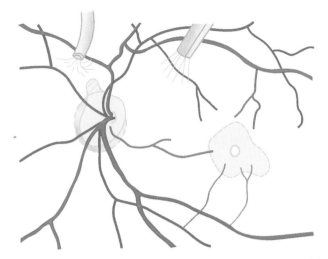

Fig. 31.13: With continuous suction and anterior-posterior-tangential traction, a posterior vitreous detachment can be created

hole have uniform intraoperative vitreous findings. A zone of collapsed vitreous fibers usually lies anterior to a posteriorly optically clear cavity. In most instances, the vitreous cortex or posterior hyaloid is invisible and remains attached to the underlying internal limiting membrane of the retina. In some cases, the presence of a focally detached vitreous is suggested by an operculum floating above the macular hole.

After surgical removal of the central vitreous, it is necessary to develop and/or complete a posterior vitreous detachment. Using active aspiration (150–250 mm Hg), a silicone-tipped suction cannula is gently swept over the retinal surface near the major arcades or the optic nerve. The area immediately around the hole is avoided. The silicone tip is noted to flex once the cortical vitreous is engaged (Fig. 31.12). This has been termed the "fish-strike sign" or "divining rod sign". Once engaged, a posterior vitreous detachment can be created by continuous suction with anteroposterior-tangential traction while the tip is moved over the retinal surface (Fig. 31.13). The dissection is carried from the area of initial detachment to adjacent attached areas in an attempt to complete the detachment from the posterior retina to the equatorial zone. Vitrectomy probe with "cutter off" is currently used to create posterior vitreous detachment. The cutter's large port engages the vitreous more firmly and is more efficient in peeling the cortex from the optic nerve. Once the posterior cortical vitreous is engaged near the optic nerve, it can be peeled from the nerve with continued suction and traction. It is common to create small disc and retinal hemorrhages during this process. Once the vitreous separates from the optic nerve it will usually separate easily to the posterior vitreous base with further gentle traction. Once the posterior hyaloidal dissection has been initiated, the vitreous cortex becomes visible as a thickened transluscent sheet, especially the oblique illumination. Occasionally, the disc attachments are so firm that tissue forceps or pic manipulation is required to complete the posterior vitreous detachment in these areas. A 36-gauge subretinal pic can be useful in engaging the posterior hyaloid near the optic nerve and then pulling off

Weiss' ring (Fig. 31.14). Frequently, an operculum is detected as a glial fragment attached to the vitreous cortex. Frequently, an operculum or pseudo-operculum can be detected as a luteal-colored fragment attached to the vitreous cortex. A ring of condensed vitreous (Weiss' ring) is observed over the disc corresponding to previous vitreopapillary attachment. If the vitreous cortex is not removed it will become apparent during the completion of the air-fluid exchange as a gelatinous substance on the retinal surface.

Fifty percent of operated eyes have some degree of epiretinal membrane proliferation. These epiretinal membranes, unlike typical epiretinal membranes, tend to be finer and more friable, and at times are densely adherent to the retina. The epiretinal membranes may be present surrounding the hole or can involve only a few clock hours. A microbarbed myringotomy blade is used to create an edge in the epiretinal membrane, which is grasped with tissue forceps and stripped. One disc area around the macular hole is checked and liberated from epiretinal membranes to ensure the relief of traction. During this maneuver, it is common to create small hemorrhages around the hole. Damage to the inner retina is avoided, an early sign of which may be the development of fluffy whitish areas.

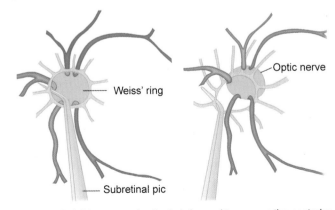

Fig. 31.14: A 36-gauge subretinal pic is used to engage the posterior hyaloid near the optic nerve and pull off the Weiss' ring

Internal Limiting Membrane Peeling

Rationale for internal limiting membrane peeling is as follows:

- Relaxation of tangential traction of internal limiting membrane itself
- Removal of possible cause of persistent fine retinal fold
- Removal of epiretinal proliferation
- Removal of diffusion barrier
- Differences between internal limiting membrane and retina

Surgical Technique

Internal Limiting Membrane Peeling

The first step is puncturing the internal limiting membrane with a sharp-tipped and barbed microvitreoretinal blade in the superior macula about half disc diameter away from the macular hole. Once the internal limiting membrane is punctured, the microvitreoretinal blade is drawn gently across the surface of the retina for a short distance until a small opening is created. There is typically a white "fluffy" appearance to this opening and occasionally a fleck of hemorrhage. A pic is advanced and wiggled slightly from side to side in an effort to engage only the internal limiting membrane and not the nerve fiber layer. Once a proper dissection plane is established, effort is made to tunnel beneath the internal limiting membrane in a counter-clockwise direction, creating a pocket to work in. An intermittent slight lifting motion is used to peel the internal limiting membrane off the nerve fiber layer ahead of the instrument tip. The internal limiting membrane is often not visible over the instrument tip, but a slight movement of the retina in the direction of the pic indicates that it has been engaged. Once the internal limiting membrane is elevated to this extent, it can be grasped with an internal limiting membrane or end-gripping forceps and peeled around the macular hole.

Indocyanine Green-Assisted Internal Limiting Membrane Peeling

Indocyanine green dye is prepared as follows:

(a) 25 mg of indocyanine green dye is diluted with 0.5 ml of distilled water. Then 4.5 ml of balanced salt solution (BSS) is added to make 0.5% solution.
(b) 25 mg of dry indocyanine green substance is first dissolved with 5 ml sterile distilled water. One milliliter of this solution was then diluted with 9 ml of BSS Plus. Indocyanine green with a concentration of 0.05% is then applied to stain the internal limiting membrane. 0.2 to 0.5 ml of diluted indocyanine green is placed/sprayed over the retina under normal infusion. The dye is washed out immediately. After removal of the indocyanine green, internal limiting membrane peeling is performed.

Internal limiting membrane peeling can be done as follows:

(1) Directly grasping the internal limiting membrane by forceps.
(2) Creating a tear/rent in internal limiting membrane by:
   i. Barbed microvitreoretinal blade or bent 28-gauge needle

ii. Tano's diamond-dusted membrane scraper: It is a useful tool for membrane separation during vitreous surgery. A diamond-dusted silicone cannula is fashioned from flexible silicone tubing with a beveled tip and coated with diamond fragments. It has been found to be particularly useful for removing residual vitreous cortex and epiretinal membranes from around the hole. It is also effective in removing "immature membranes" in proliferative vitreoretinopathy. The diamond-dusted silicone cannula is a useful tool for removing thin epiretinal membranes and vitreous cortex that may be difficult or nearly impossible to remove safely using other techniques.

iii. Silicone brush
iv. Suction with a back-flush needle

(3) Completion of internal limiting membrane peeling: The unstained, underlying retina is readily apparent in contrast to the green-stained internal limiting membrane. Subsequently, the flap of internal limiting membrane is easily grasped and peeled with a diamond-dusted intraocular forceps. Continuous curvilinear maculorrhexis is performed. The contrast enables the surgeon to monitor precisely the extent and the completeness of the internal limiting membrane peeling. Subtle frills of internal limiting membrane are not left at the edge of macular hole. The bare area free of internal limiting membrane is intended to be one disc diameter surrounding the macular hole. Persisting autofluorescence of the macular area or the optic nerve is observed up to three months after surgery.

Infracyanine Green-Assisted Internal Limiting Membrane Peeling

To prepare the infracyanine green solution (Laboratories SERB, Paris, France), a 25 mg vial of infracyanine green is dissolved in 5 ml of glucose 5% solution to obtain final infracyanine green concentration of 0.5% with an osmolarity of 309 mOsm/kg. After closure of the infusion line, 0.2 ml of this solution is instilled directly into the posterior vitreous cavity over the macula using a blunt cannula. After 2 minutes, the infusion line is reopened and the excess of dye was removed from the vitreous cavity using a backflush cannula. The internal limiting membrane that had been in contact with the dye is stained green diffusely.

Trypan Blue-Assisted Internal Limiting Membrane Peeling

0.5 to 1 ml of trypan blue 0.06% (VisionBlue, DORC International, the Netherlands) is injected under continuous infusion over the posterior pole under direct visualization, staining the internal limiting membrane. Alternatively, after fluid-air exchange, the dye is placed over the macula under air sufflation. Air fluid-exchange is done to aspirate the dye. A 20-gauge bent microvitreoretinal blade is then used to incise the membrane and diamond-dusted intraocular forceps are used to remove it in a circumferential manner 360° around the macular hole.

Currently, Brilliant Blue dye is being used for staining.

Triamcinolone-Assisted Vitrectomy

The preservative of triamcinolone acetonide is removed with a filter and rinsed with balanced salt solution. The triamcinolone acetonide particles (40 mg) are then resuspended in 2 ml of balanced salt solution. Following core vitrectomy, triamcinolone acetonide suspension is injected over the posterior pole. The posterior hyaloid is clearly observed. Separation of the hyaloid from the optic nerve head and posterior retina is then performed. Next, a subtotal vitrectomy was performed. The triamcinolone acetonide suspension is injected again over the posterior pole and excess triamcinolone acetonide is aspirated with a backflush needle. Numerous particles of triamcinolone acetonide are observed as white specks on the posterior retina. The internal limiting membrane is then grasped with an intraocular forceps and peeled in a circumferential manner around the macular hole. The peeled area was clearly observed as an area lacking the white specks left by the triamcinolone acetonide. Several particles of triamcinolone acetonide are observed on the peeled internal limiting membrane. Triamcinolone acetonide tends to stick to the residual vitreous cortex on the internal limiting membrane or to the internal limiting membrane itself. The peeled area of the membrane is clearly confirmed by the lack of white specks left elsewhere by the triamcinolone acetonide. The internal limiting membrane can be easily peeled in a circumferential manner as using indocyanine green. A small amount of triamcinolone acetonide often deposits in the macular hole, however. Local toxicity of triamcinolone acetonide to the neural retina and retinal pigment epithelium is unknown.

Prolonged intense illumination from the light pipe near the macula is avoided to prevent phototoxicity. A total air-fluid exchange is performed and effort is made to dehydrate the vitreous cavity. The shallow fluid in the base of the optic disc cup is aspirated repeatedly, with a soft-tipped cannula, until fluid no longer collects. A nonexpansive concentration of long-acting gas is exchanged for air. Postoperatively, strict prone positioning is prescribed. At the 1-week visit if the edges of the macular hole are flattened and imperceptible with flattening of the cuff of retinal detachment, anatomic success is assured. However, if the edges are still visible and the cuff elevated, anatomic failure is probable.

Tamponade

Gas: A nonexpansive concentration of long-acting gas (C_3F_8) is exchanged for air. Postoperatively, 24 hour-a-day strict prone positioning for 5–7 days is prescribed. Face-down positioning increases the buoyancy effect of gas bubble, which may augment the surface tension effects of intraocular gas tamponade, which in turn may enhance the anatomic closure of macular holes.

Silicone oil: Silicone oil eliminates the need for face-down positioning, allows immediate return of normal functioning and unrestricted air travel and possibly eliminates visual

field defects. It requires a second procedure to remove it after 2–3 months, and is possibly not as effective as gas tamponade. The rate of hole closure is significantly lower than for C_3F_8 gas. Silicone oil may be considered if: the patient is either unable or unwilling to maintain face-down position postoperatively, early return to normal activity is necessary, patient is monocular and postoperative air travel is required.

Successful macular hole closure is possible without face-down positioning. This technique may be an alternative for patients with macular holes in pseudophakic eyes that are unable to assume face-down posturing. Combining cataract surgery with this technique for macular hole repair is reasonable for phakic patients who cannot maintain prone positioning. Major disadvantages of combined surgery include the morbidity of the second procedure and removal of a visually insignificant cataract. This approach should be considered for those patients unable to tolerate face-down positioning.

After macular hole surgery, anatomically unsuccessful closure of the hole correlates with small enlargements in the diameter of the macular hole and its surrounding subretinal fluid cuff, and with a slight decrease in visual acuity. Macular hole closure after repeat surgery improves visual acuity outcome in the majority of retreated eyes.

Complications

Complications include nuclear sclerosis, peripheral retinal breaks, rhegmatogenous retinal detachment from a peripheral retinal break, enlargement of the hole, late reopening of the hole, retinal pigment epithelium loss under the hole, photic toxicity, endophthalmitis and ulnar neuropathy. Peripheral retinal tears may develop during stripping of cortical vitreous. A significant temporal field defect may occur in patients after otherwise uncomplicated surgery for macular holes. The most common visual field defect is dense and wedge-shaped and involves the temporal visual field. Two categories of scotomas have been observed: peripheral and relative arcuate. Some eyes develop increased intraocular pressure after vitreous surgery for macular hole and the increase occurs most frequently between two days and two weeks postoperatively.

Intravitreal indocyanine green-assisted internal limiting membrane peeling improves anatomic success in macular hole surgery, but it may potentially lead to unfavorable visual acuity outcome and peripheral visual field loss. Fundus fluorescence is observed after indocyanine green.

Miscellaneous

Combining cataract surgery with vitrectomy surgery may prevent a later second operation for postvitrectomy cataract formation. Biometry after macular hole surgery should be corrected by subtracting the depth of the foveolar crater (0.5 mm, the estimated depth of the foveolar crater) from the measured axial length. C_3F_8 gas has proved to be a more effective tamponade than silicone oil with respect to achieving initial closure of macular holes. Eyes receiving an oil tamponade required significantly more reoperations to achieve a similar rate of hole closure compared with eyes undergoing a gas tamponade. Final visual acuity was better for gas-operated eyes than for silicone-operated eyes.

A small macular hole appears to be closed by three days after vitrectomy with gas tamponade.

Role of Optical Coherence Tomography

Optical coherence tomography plays an important role in the diagnosis and management of macular hole. Macular holes have been assessed with optical coherence tomography before pars plana vitrectomy. Macular hole diameters were determined at the level of the retinal pigment epithelium (base diameter) and at the minimal extent of the hole (minimum diameter). Calculated hole form factor (HFF) was correlated with the postoperative anatomical success rate and best corrected visual acuity. The duration of symptoms was correlated with base and minimum diameter of the macular hole. In eyes without anatomical closure of the macular hole after one surgical approach, the base diameter and the minimum diameter were significantly larger than in cases with immediate postsurgical closure. There was a significant negative correlation between both the base and the minimum diameter of the hole and the postoperative visual function. In all patients with HFF >0.9 the macular hole was closed following one surgical procedure, whereas in eyes with HFF <0.5 anatomical success rate was less. Better postoperative visual outcome correlated with higher HFF. Preoperative measurement of macular hole size with optical coherence tomography can provide a prognostic factor for postoperative visual outcome and anatomical success rate of macular hole surgery.

The postoperative closure of idiopathic macular holes following vitreous surgery has been related to the preoperative macular hole diameter determined by optical coherence tomography, with lesions smaller than 400 μm demonstrating higher success rates. A trend toward greater visual acuity improvement was demonstrated for idiopathic macular holes smaller than 400 μm. Late reopening was only seen in macular holes that were 400 μm or larger measured by optical coherence tomography.

Vitrectomy surgery for impending macular hole based on optical coherence tomography has also been suggested. It is possible to repair macular holes by using optical coherence tomography to guide the dissection of the vitreous from the macular hole followed by limited vitrectomy. By using a less invasive approach, it may be possible to repair macular holes in less operative time and with fewer complications. A microspatula knife is used to dissect the connection between the vitreous and the retina previously delineated by optical coherence tomography. The posterior vitreous was not stripped from the retinal surface. Limited vitrectomy over the hole was performed to create a space for a gas bubble.

SUBMACULAR SURGERY

In the last several years, a surge of interest has been seen in submacular surgery. Candidates for this surgery consist primarily of individuals with subfoveal choroidal neovascularization and those with submacular hemorrhage.

Subfoveal Choroidal Neovascularization

Choroidal neovascularization is a principal cause of the loss of central visual function in adults. Choroidal neovascular membranes disrupt normal macular anatomy (including the critical photoreceptor-retinal pigment epithelial interface); leak serum or formed blood elements or both; and lead to irreversible loss of overlying photoreceptors.

When fibrovascular membranes grow beneath the center of the foveal avascular zone, the visual prognosis is generally poor. Choroidal neovascular membranes are most frequently caused by age-related macular degeneration and presumed ocular histoplasmosis syndrome, although neovascularization may be observed as a complication of other ocular conditions.

Management

With the advent of anti-VEGF therapy, surgical removal of choroidal neovascular membranes is currently not advocated in the cases of age-related macular degeneration.

Case Selection

The following clinical findings may suggest that the neovascular complex lies anterior to the retinal pigment epithelium:

- A well-defined edge with an abrupt transition to underlying retinal pigment epithelium,
- An anterior location apparent on stereoscopic viewing,
- A thin layer of subretinal blood outlining the edges of a neovascular complex and the subjacent retinal pigment epithelium, and
- A pigmented border (which corresponds to the rim of hypofluorescence occasionally seen angiographically) outlining the location of the membrane (Figs 31.15A and B). Some lesions that are indeed anterior to retinal pigment epithelium may lack a sharp border perhaps because of their recent onset. Additionally, fibrin may obscure the border with underlying retinal pigment epithelium.

Angiographic findings suggestive of an anterior location of the membrane include the following:

- A distinct boundary between the hyperfluorescence of the membrane and background
- Choroidal fluorescence
- A rim of blocked fluorescence between the two
- Compact angiographic appearance
- Homogenous hyperfluorescence
- Clearly visible lacy vascular pattern
- Anterior location apparent on stereoangiogram viewing

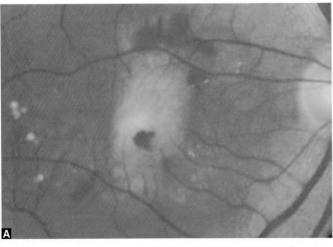

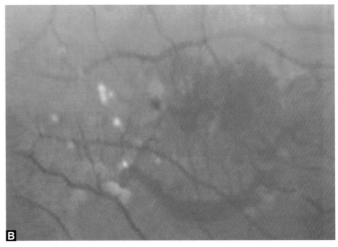

Figs 31.15A and B: Submacular surgery. (A) This compact subfoveal neovascular membrane appears to lie anterior to the retinal pigment epithelium, has a slightly pigmented border and is partially outlined by a thin layer of subretinal blood (B) A one-day postoperative photograph confirms that the membrane was anterior to retinal pigment epithelium and could be safely removed without damaging underlying structures

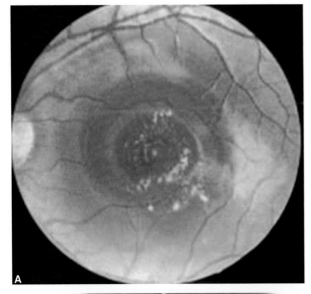

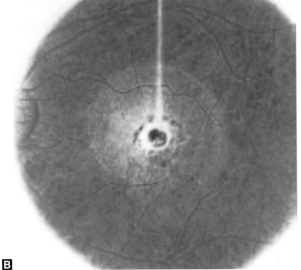

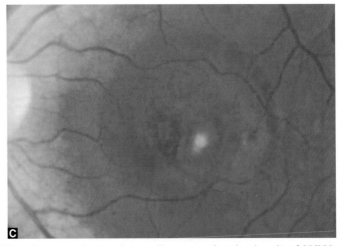

• Absence of late staining surrounding tissues (indicative of occult or subretinal pigment epithelium neovascularization) (Figs 31.16A to C). Membranes posterior to the retinal pigment epithelium tend to have clinical and angiographic findings that are the opposite of those for anterior membranes.

Surgical Technique

Current surgical technique is most effective in those cases in which the membrane lies predominantly anterior to the retinal pigment epithelium and thus can be removed without extracting large areas of retinal pigment epithelium.

Sclerotomy Site: A standard three-port pars plana vitrectomy is performed. The placement of sclerotomies is critical. The surgeon should study the angiogram and decide preoperatively where the retinotomy is to be placed to avoid damaging major vessels and to provide adequate access to the subretinal membrane. These factors usually dictate that the retinotomy be created in a straight

Figs 31.16A to C: Submacular surgery. (A) Compact, hyperpigmented subfoveal neovascular membrane with preoperative visual acuity of 20/200, (B) The angiographic appearance is favorable for surgical removal (C) The membrane is completely removed without disturbing underlying retinal pigment epithelium except for the focus of hypopigmentation at the ingrowth site. Visual acuity is 20/20-1

temporal location and thus the superotemporal sclerotomy should be made near the horizontal meridian.

Removal of posterior hyaloid: Although there are no data to support the importance of removing the posterior hyaloid, its removal is attempted in every case, as described earlier.

Retinotomy: The placement of retinotomy takes into account:

- The exact location and extent of the membrane under the fovea.
- The presence of presumed adhesions between the neurosensory retina and underlying tissue (previous photocoagulation scars and/or evidence of pigment migration into neurosensory retina or retinochoroidal vascular anastomoses).
- The dimensions of the subretinal instruments (specifically, the length of the angled instrument tips that determines how far away from the fovea the retinotomy can be made and still allow the tips to reach the membrane).
- The topographic anatomy of the neurosensory retina and nerve fiber layer.

In most cases, these factors dictate a straight temporal or slightly superotemporal location for the retinotomy (Fig. 31.17). However, a retinotomy can be created superonasal to the fovea (Fig. 31.18). With 33- and 36-gauge instruments, the retinotomies are small enough that no significant damage to the papillomacular bundle occurs. Besides being in the most advantageous location, the retinotomy should be as small as possible. Initially, the retinal surface was lightly diathermized and then the microvitreoretinal blade was used to tease open a small hole. A 120°-angled, sharply pointed 36-gauge subretinal pic is used to pierce undiathermized neurosensory retina. While intraocular pressure is raised, the tip can be pushed through neurosensory retina to achieve a very tiny retinotomy. As the pic is obliquely advanced through the neurosensory retina, transient blanching of the choriocapillaris may be seen. Rarely, the local retinal pigment epithelium underlying the retinotomy site may be scraped as the pic enters the subretinal space, but this can be avoided by gently lifting the pic as the retina is

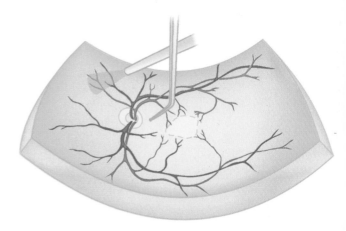

Fig. 31.18: For a right-handed surgeon in a left eye a retinotomy can be created superonasal to the fovea without significant damage to the papillomacular bundle

perforated. A small hemorrhage can occur as retinal capillaries are cut, but this always responds to the increased intraocular pressure and is limited.

Creation or enhancement of neurosensory detachment: After retinotomy, an angled 33-gauge infusion cannula is introduced beneath the retina and the balanced salt solution is infused to elevate the neurosensory retina (Fig. 31.19). This is accomplished by gently pushing on the plunger of a syringe that is connected to the hub of the needle by a short piece of tubing. To avoid trapping air bubbles within the tip, balanced salt solution is gently infused as the instrument is entered into the eye and before the subretinal space is entered. Slow infusion is very important, as this step can lead to the development of a retinal break, especially in the areas of strong chorioretinal adhesions. Excessive infusion pressure can tear the retina. A neurosensory detachment can also be created or enhanced by injecting balanced salt solution using a controlled infusion pump. As the fluid enters the subretinal space, attention is directed to the edges of the laser scars or adhesions to the underlying membrane, or both.

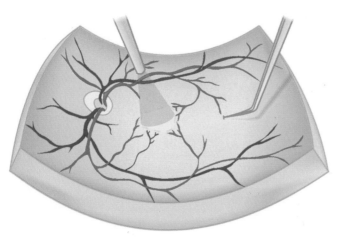

Fig. 31.17: For a right-handed surgeon in a right eye, a straight temporal retinotomy is often best

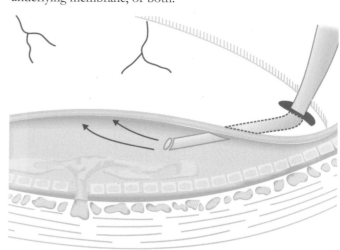

Fig. 31.19: A gentle infusion of balanced salt solution through a 33-gauge cannula creates a small neurosensory retinal detachment

Removal of neovascular membrane: The subretinal membrane is dislodged from the underlying retinal pigment epithelium and the overlying neurosensory retina with the aid of a pointed, 36-gauge subretinal pic (Fig. 31.20). The sharp end of the pic is very helpful in engaging the edges of the neovascular complex and facilitating its separation from the underlying retinal pigment epithelium. The pic is moved in a pivoting or rotating manner to avoid stretching or enlarging the retinotomy. In most cases, the neovascular complex dislodges easily from the underlying subfoveal retinal pigment epithelium, but remains attached to the edge of a laser scar or to the stalk of choroidal vascular ingrowth. Occasionally, horizontal subretinal scissors are necessary to cut firm adhesions. If the retina is not mobilized over the entire photocoagulation scar, separation is achieved at least far enough into the scar to allow manipulation and extraction of the membrane without tearing adjacent retina. Trauma to foveal photoreceptors from either the pic or scissors is avoided. A positive-action horizontal forceps is introduced (closed) through the retinotomy, which has usually enlarged during the subretinal manipulation. The opened blades are placed around the stalk or the adhesion, with the membrane in front of the blades. Gentle traction with the blades held closed breaks the connection (Fig. 31.21)). If traction on the retina is seen, the membrane is released and further separation of the complex from neurosensory retina is accomplished. If excessive tugging and displacement of retinal pigment epithelium are seen, consideration is given to using the subretinal scissors to cut the stalk rather than breaking it with the forceps. When the vascular connection from the choroid is about to be severed, the intraocular pressure is raised to approximately 80 mm Hg. Minimal hemorrhage is often encountered when the membrane is removed. The intraocular pressure is elevated for at least one minute and any evidence of rebleeding is observed while the pressure is slowly lowered. When these measures fail, hemostasis can be achieved by subretinal endophotocoagulation. Most membranes are easily grasped with horizontal subretinal forceps. Vertical action forceps may be needed to extract the relatively thin discs of neovascularization that have been disconnected from the choroid. Once hemostasis is achieved, the membrane is removed from the eye through the sclerotomy. Dividing a large membrane with intraocular forceps or a vitrector is preferable to enlarging the sclerotomy. Scleral plugs are placed and the retina is inspected with indirect ophthalmoscopy and scleral depression to verify that no peripheral tears have occurred.

A complete air-fluid exchange is performed. Standard extrusion needles or silicone-tipped needles are used to aspirate over the optic nerve. The angled 33-gauge cannula can be used to aspirate subretinal fluid at the retinotomy. This generally everts the edges of the retinotomy, allowing for better closure. If the retinotomy is small and the surgeon desires a small gas tamponade, balanced salt solution is gently reinfused over the optic nerve after the vitreous cavity has been dry for a few minutes. The eye is almost completely filled with fluid and the patient is asked to be face down postoperatively. In early cases, endolaser photocoagulation of the retinotomy was done. Smaller gauged instrumentation allows for the creation and preservation of a small retinotomy that does not require laser photocoagulation. This prevents thermal damage to neurosensory retina, retinal pigment epithelium and choriocapillaris, thus preserving extrafoveal retinal function and decreasing the size of a postoperative scotoma.

Complications

Two changes in the milieu that occur in the setting of choroidal neovascular membrane have a practical impact on surgical technique and visual prognosis: cystoid macular edema and fibrin- or photocoagulation-related retinal adhesion to choroidal neovascular membrane (Figs 31.22A and B and 31.23A and B). Cystoid changes render the fovea vulnerable to iatrogenic macular hole during fluid-assisted separation of the retina from the subjacent neovascular complex. Incomplete separation of the overlying retina from underlying choroidal

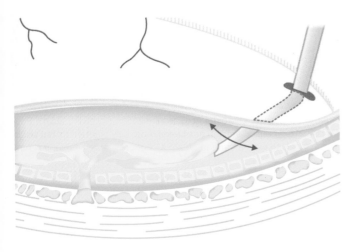

Fig. 31.20: The neovascular tissue is dislodged from underlying retinal pigment epithelium with the aid of a pointed, 36-gauge subretinal pic

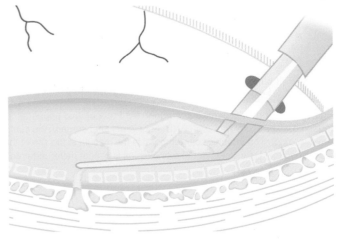

Fig. 31.21: Horizontal subretinal forceps are used to firmly grasp the neovascular tissue and slowly remove it from the subretinal space

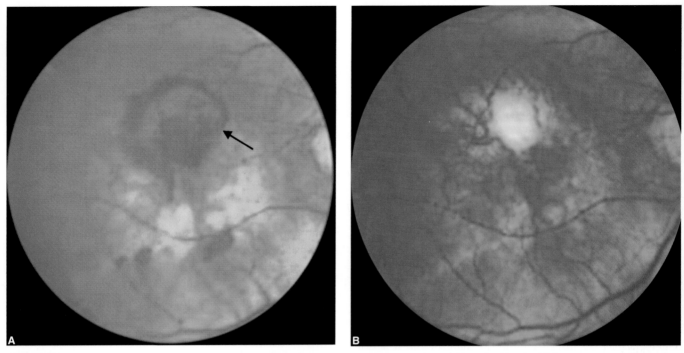

Figs 31.22A and B: Submacular surgery. (A) Fundus appearance of a neovascular membrane. Note the blood, which appears to outline a clear border between the neovascular complex and underlying tissue, (B) Postoperative clinical appearance. The atrophic white spot is the site of laser scar removal. The retinal pigment epithelium appears thinned where the membrane previously lay, but the tissue appears intact

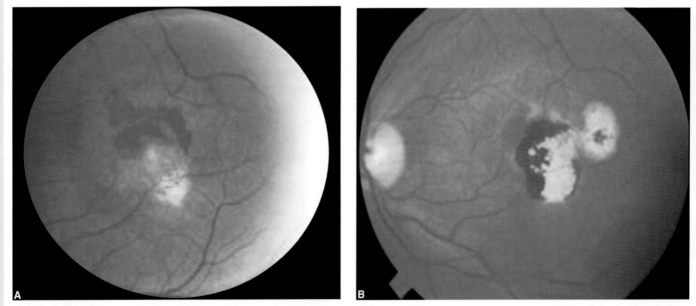

Figs 31.23A and B: Submacular surgery. (A) Preoperative appearance of recurrent subfoveal choroidal neovascularization (following laser). Best corrected visual acuity was 20/400, (B) Four years after surgery, the subfoveolar retinal pigment epithelium has become densely pigmented, but vision remains 20/20. The atrophic scar temporal in the macula is the site of the retinotomy, which was lasered to create a chorioretinal adhesion. It is now understood that laser treatment of retinotomies is almost never required

neovascular membrane or prior photocoagulation scar places the fovea at the risk of avulsion during membrane removal. Other intraoperative complications are subretinal hemorrhage, retinal tear and retinal detachment.

SUBMACULAR HEMORRHAGE

Blood beneath the neurosensory retina almost always originates from the choroidal circulation. Trauma to choroidal vessels can produce hemorrhage: from blunt or penetrating trauma, from inadvertent surgical trauma with a deep suture during scleral buckling or from drainage of subretinal fluid either internally or externally. In the absence of trauma, hemorrhage can occur secondary to choroidal neovascularization. Small hemorrhages frequently accompany the ingrowth of vessels from the choroid through Bruch's membrane. Extensive hemorrhages are believed to occur as a result of the rupture of large choroidal vessels that extend into fibrovascular complexes. Vessels in fibrovascular scars have been observed to have arterial and venous characteristics and are continuous with choroidal arteries and veins, respectively. Leakage of blood or serous fluid from the neovascular tissue leads to the detachment of the retinal pigment epithelium and produces pressure on the artery and vein as they enter the fibrovascular scar. This pressure reportedly leads to necrosis of the artery and, when it ruptures, massive hemorrhage occurs with the accumulation of blood under the retinal pigment epithelium, under neurosensory retina and in some cases in the vitreous cavity.

Mechanism of Retinal Injury

Subretinal blood is toxic to the outer retina and has been documented to cause irreversible photoreceptor damage. Laboratory animal studies have shown that the degree of retinal destruction is correlated with the duration of contact of the retina with hemorrhage. These animal studies show that damage can occur as early as one hour, with moderate to severe outer retinal destruction at 3 to 7 days and full-thickness retinal degeneration by day. Subretinal blood clots form a mechanical barrier between the retina and the retinal pigment epithelium. This can inhibit metabolic exchange between retina and retinal pigment epithelium. Retinal toxicity can result from iron liberated from hemoglobin that is released from degenerating erythrocytes. Subretinal blood clot adherence and retraction caused tractional forces on the photoreceptors, which led to outer retinal damage. The role of fibrin in causing retinal damage associated with subretinal hemorrhage has been defined. A fibrinolytic agent can be used to dissolve the fibrin meshwork, thereby preventing the shearing effect on the photoreceptors.

Hemorrhage is a frequent concomitant finding in age-related macular degeneration-associated maculopathy because of the intrinsic fragility of the vessels present in choroidal neovascularization. Subretinal blood either beneath the neurosensory retina or beneath the retinal pigment epithelium can have profound impact on the visual prognosis.

Blood presents a significant impediment to visualization of the pathologic process. Thus one objective in the management of hemorrhagic age-related macular degeneration is improving visualization to allow therapy. Subretinal blood (particularly thick blood) has long been considered toxic to photoreceptors and thus harmful to vision.

Thick subretinal hemorrhage causes necrosis of the overlying retina. Fragments of the erythrocytes infiltrate the retina and cross an intact internal limiting membrane to cloud the vitreous. Rapid necrosis of the retina occurs over thick subretinal hemorrhage and indicates the need for early displacement of the hemorrhage from the macula if function is to be preserved and breakthrough prevented.

Management

Early surgical intervention is required to avoid toxicity from subretinal hemorrhage.

Case Selection

Multiple preoperative, intraoperative and postoperative factors have an impact on the visual result following surgery for submacular hemorrhage. Preoperative factors, including the baseline health of the neurosensory retina and submacular retinal pigment epithelium, the presence of choroidal neovascularization, disciform scarring or previous foveal photocoagulation will determine the postoperative visual potential. The health status of the retinal pigment epithelium and neurosensory retina can also influence the tolerance of these tissues to the noxious effects of subretinal blood. Eyes with age-related macular degeneration may have more extensive and diffuse photoreceptor/retinal pigment epithelium dysfunction and less metabolic reserve than eyes without age-related macular degeneration (i.e. eyes with choroidal neovascular membranes due to presumed ocular histoplasmosis syndrome, macroaneurysm or idiopathic causes). This may partially explain why eyes without age-related macular degeneration are more likely to have visual improvement following surgery than are eyes with age-related macular degeneration. The duration of submacular hemorrhage may also be an important factor. Progressive photoreceptor destruction has been observed to occur for up to 14 days following the introduction of experimental subretinal hemorrhage. Postoperative visual function may also be affected by photoreceptor and/or retinal pigment epithelium trauma induced by surgical manipulations in the subretinal space as well as intraoperative and postoperative complications. In the absence of results from clinical trials, case selection remains unclear. The randomized, prospective Submacular Surgery Trial is comparing surgical removal of large submacular hemorrhage secondary to age-related macular degeneration. No randomization trials have been proposed for hematomas of other etiologies. Hence, at the present time only impressions regarding case selection can be offered. Relatively thin hemorrhages unassociated with choroidal neovascularization often do well with observation. Thick hemorrhage without known choroidal neovascularization may be appropriate for removal. Thick hemorrhages with probable choroidal neovascularization remain controversial. Recent-onset hemorrhages probably have a better surgical result than do older hemorrhages and may be appropriate for tPA use (Figs 31.24A and B).

Observation

Given the poor natural history of hemorrhagic age-related macular degeneration, observation is of limited appeal in cases

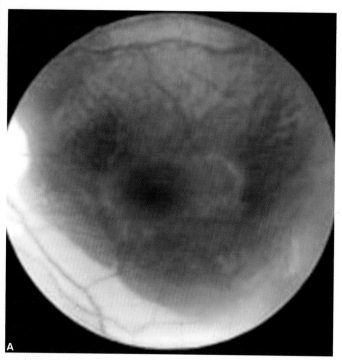
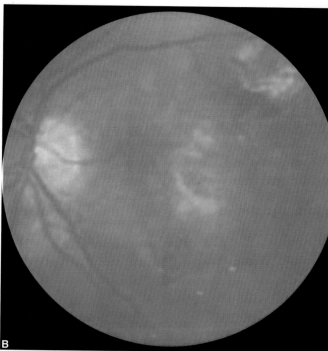

Figs 31.24A and B: Submacular hemorrhage. (A) The thickness of submacular hemorrhage is better appreciated on higher magnification, (B) Three months postoperatively, the macula is free of subretinal hemorrhage. The causative neovascular membrane was superotemporal. Visual acuity returned to 20/70

with thick subretinal hemorrhage. In cases with thin blood, watchful waiting may be reasonable. As a thin hemorrhage clears, indocyanine green imaging may become feasible and reveal treatable pathology.

Vitrectomy With Mechanical Clot Extraction, Without Tissue Plasminogen Activator (tPA)

Given the poor prognosis of hemorrhagic age-related macular degeneration with thick blood, many investigators have explored vitrectomy to remove the clot and associated choroidal neovascularization. Visual acuity has been almost universally poor (20/200) or worse, and a high rate of complications including retinal detachment with proliferative vitreoretinopathy have been common. Mechanical extraction of blood clot is also being evaluated in submacular surgery trials. Mechanical removal of the choroidal neovascular membrane/clot may be appropriate in select cases.

Vitrectomy With Clot Removal Following Subretinal Tissue Plasminogen Activator Injection

Tissue plasminogen activator (tPA) is an endogenous serine protease with a molecular weight of 70,000. Tissue plasminogen activator forms a complex with fibrin to activate plasminogen to plasmin, which in turn lyses fibrin into soluble degradation products, thus achieving clot lysis. Tissue plasminogen activator has a theoretical appeal in managing subretinal hemorrhage: facilitation of liquefaction of thick clots to allow extrafoveal displacement and modulation of the fibrin-neurosensory retinal interaction that may cause shearing of photoreceptors.

It is hypothesized that dealing with liquefied blood may be less traumatic to neurosensory retina than mechanical clot removal.

Surgical technique: Pars plana vitrectomy with posterior hyaloid removal is followed by subretinal injection of tPA (10–12 μgm per 0.1 ml). Twenty to forty minutes pass with tPA bathing the clot before active irrigation is done through the same or adjacent retinotomy to flush out the dissolved blood. Some blood always remains; the goal is to remove most of the thick, large clots. Some surgeons advocate grasping and removing the causative neovascular complex, if visible, whereas others intentionally leave it in place.

Pneumatic Displacement With or Without Tissue Plasminogen Activator

Subretinal hemorrhage can be managed with intravitreal tPA and gas injection without vitrectomy.

Surgical technique: The injection procedure was performed with the patient under retrobulbar anesthesia. Fifty micrograms of commercial recombinant tissue plasminogen activator (rtPA) solution in a volume of 50 microliters, is drawn in a tuberculin syringe and injected slowly into the midvitreous cavity through a 30-gauge needle. After an aqueous tap to reduce intraocular pressure, 0.5 ml of 100% sulfur hexafluoride gas is injected into the vitreous cavity. Both injections are administered via the pars plana in the superotemporal quadrant, 3 mm posterior to the limbus in pseudophakic patients and 3.5 mm posterior to the limbus in phakic patients. Patients were then instructed to maintain prone positioning for 72 hours. Whenever blood displacement from under the fovea is not complete, prone positioning is continued for an additional 24 to 48 hours.

Vitrectomy, Subretinal Injection of tPA and Fluid-Gas Exchange

A hybrid approach with the goals of maximizing clot lysis while minimizing the risk of trauma to the retina and retinal pigment epithelium can be taken.

Surgical technique: Following pars plana vitrectomy and posterior hyaloid removal, a bent 36-gauge needle is used to inject 25 or 50 micrograms of tPA per 0.1 ml directly into the clot. Complete fluid-air exchange is performed and the eye is left with a full fill of either 20% SF6 gas or air. Postoperatively, face down positioning is advised.

Special Considerations

Patients with neovascular age-related macular degeneration who are chronically anticoagulated (on warfarin) have a higher risk of this devastating complication.

Complications

Substantial postoperative complications have been seen following the surgical removal of subretinal hemorrhage. Postoperative retinal detachment, proliferative vitreoretinopathy, recurrent subretinal hemorrhage, subretinal fibrosis, cataract and optic atrophy have been reported.

VITRECTOMY FOR DIABETIC MACULAR EDEMA

Macular edema is a major cause of visual loss in a number of ocular disorders, including diabetes, retinal vein occlusion, postoperative edema (Irvine–Gass), uveitis, vitreomacular traction syndrome and retinitis pigmentosa. Breakdown of the blood–retinal barrier and vitreoretinal traction are probably the most relevant factors. Treatment of persistent macular edema remains a major challenge.

Clinical Characteristics

Diffuse diabetic macular edema is macular thickening due to diffuse leakage from a generally dilated macular retinal capillary bed in eyes with diabetic retinopathy. Sometimes it is further classified based on the presence of macular cysts. It is often bilateral. Hard exudates may be variable, from none to extensive. Attached posterior hyaloid often may be present and appears as thickened and taut. Fluorescein angiography reveals diffuse leakage from retinal capillaries and possibly from the choriocapillaris across the retinal pigment epithelium. There may be associated shallow (10 μm or greater) macular detachment detectable by optical coherence tomography. Associated systemic factors may include cardiovascular or renal fluid retention and systemic hypertension.

Rationale

In recent years it has become evident that the vitreous must play a role in various aspects of diabetic retinopathy. The exact role of the vitreous is however in many aspects still ill defined. There are structural changes of the vitreous, as for instance vitreous liquefaction and posterior vitreous detachment, which are associated with the occurrence and earlier onset of diabetic retinopathy. Further there are angiogenic and angioinhibitory factors in the vitreous, which influence neovascularization by the means of endothelial cell proliferation. Photocoagulation of the retina can cause structural changes (posterior vitreal detachment) and histological changes (increased hyalocytes activity), which can protect against the progression of proliferative diabetic retinopathy. The role of vitrectomy in protecting against proliferative diabetic retinopathy is generally related to the removal of the vitreal scaffold. But vitrectomy can also induce changes in the oxygenation of the eye. If complete detachment of the posterior vitreous can be achieved, it might be possible to further slow the progression of diabetic retinopathy. It is possible that in the future, manipulation of the vitreous by the means of enzymes and lasers can play a role in the treatment and prevention of diabetic retinopathy.

The physiologic mechanism of photocoagulation can be seen in the following steps. The physical light energy is absorbed in the melanin of the retinal pigment epithelium. The adjacent photoreceptors are destroyed and are replaced by a glial scar and the oxygen consumption of the outer retina is reduced. Oxygen that normally diffuses from the choriocapillaris into the retina can now diffuse through the laser scars in the photoreceptor layer without being consumed in the mitochondria of the photoreceptors. This oxygen flux reaches the inner retina to relieve inner retinal hypoxia and raise the oxygen tension. As a result, the retinal arteries constrict and the blood flow decreases. Hypoxia relief reduces the production of growth factors, such as vascular endothelial growth factor and neovascularization is reduced or stopped. Vasoconstriction increases arteriolar resistance, decreases hydrostatic pressure in capillaries and venules, and reduces edema formation according to Starling's law. Vitrectomy also improves retinal oxygenation by allowing oxygen and other nutrients to be transported in water currents in the vitreous cavity from well oxygenated to ischemic areas of the retina. Vitrectomy and retinal photocoagulation both improve retinal oxygenation and both reduce diabetic macular edema and retinal neovascularization.

Vitreous surgery may improve perifoveal microcirculation in the eyes of diabetic patients with cystoid macular edema and resolve the macular edema. Improvement of perifoveal microcirculation may be an important factor affecting visual outcome. In addition, the removal of the vitreous might have a beneficial effect due to a potential accumulation of growth factors and inflammatory cytokines in the vitreous gel. Leukocyte-mediated endothelial cell damage and apoptosis in experimental diabetes have been demonstrated to increase the vascular permeability. Also, vitreous levels of Angiotensin II and vascular endothelial growth factor have been reported to be elevated in diabetic macular edema patients irrespective of the status of posterior vitreous detachment. Angiotensin II and vascular endothelial growth factor may be induced in the eyes and be related to the pathogenesis. In another study, altered vitreous levels of interleukin-6 and vascular endothelial growth factor have been related to diabetic macular edema. Retinal traction by the posterior hyaloid membrane is involved in the pathogenesis of honeycombed cystoid changes in diabetic patients. In order to further improve fluid diffusion from the retinal tissue, a removal of the remaining barrier between the vitreous cavity and the retina might be a promising approach. The internal limiting membrane is thought to be formed by the footplates of the Müller cells. Peeling of the internal limiting membrane has been performed previously to reduce vitreoretinal traction and in combination with the removal of macular epiretinal membranes. How internal limiting membrane peeling reduces diabetic macular edema is unclear; however, it is likely that the peeling can only increase diffusion of fluid from the retinal tissue by eliminating the barrier function of the internal limiting membrane, a pseudomembrane formed by the endplates of Müller-cells, which is thought to act as a diffusion barrier between the retina and the vitreous. The blood-retinal barrier as evidenced by fluorescein angiography, in contrast, seems to be unaffected. Blood-retinal barrier breakdown as seen in persistent macular edema is the result of several pathophysiological alterations, which have been investigated clinically and experimentally, including increased passive permeability, structural defects of junction molecules and increased expression of permeability factors. It is much more likely that internal limiting membrane peeling merely reduces the diffusion barrier towards the vitreous and thus is more efficient in patients with preexisting interface alterations. With respect to the inflammation-mediated fluid accumulation, intravitreal application of triamcinolone in combination with internal limiting membrane peeling could be a promising approach. A reduction in the inflammatory response most likely plays a role.

Surgical Technique

The surgical technique includes pars plana vitrectomy that utilizes the standard three-port incisions. After core vitrectomy, the remaining cortical vitreous is aspirated with a flexible tipped cannula or a vitreous cutter to create posterior hyaloid detachment. After confirming the presence of a sheet-like posterior hyaloid membrane, including Weiss' ring, the remaining vitreous, up to vitreous base is removed.

Intraocular injection of triamcinolone acetonide during a vitrectomy visualizes the transparent vitreous and that this method helps surgeons to obtain complete separation of the posterior vitreous from the retina. A triamcinolone acetate aqueous suspension is left standing for 30 minutes, and the vehicle of triamcinolone acetonide is discarded. The remaining triamcinolone (40 mg) suspension is mixed with 2.5 ml of balanced salt solution. Next, 0.5 to 1.0 ml of triamcinolone suspension is injected with a 27-gauge needle into the midvitreous cavity. The triamcinolone granules are trapped in the gel structure of the residual vitreous cortex. After this procedure, residual vitreous cortex is typically seen on the retina as either a diffuse membrane or small islands. Residual posterior vitreous cortex could not be visualized without using the triamcinolone acetonide suspension.

Posterior hyaloidal separation can also be achieved using triamcinolone acetonide. A core vitrectomy was performed and 0.5 to 1.0 ml of triamcinolone suspension was injected with a 23-gauge needle into the midvitreous cavity. The triamcinolone granules were trapped in the gel structure of the vitreous. Then, posterior cortical vitreous appears as a white gel and a break of posterior hyaloid cortex appears on the temporal retinal vein. Next, the edge of the hyaloid cortex break is held by the gentle aspiration of the vitrectomy probe. The separation of the posterior hyaloid from the retina can be easily started from this edge by gentle cutting and mild aspiration (less than 50 mm Hg). During this procedure, the posterior hyaloid is clearly seen as a white colored vitreous. Even after this procedure, the residual vitreous cortex was sometimes left on the retina as islands. The thin layer of vitreous cortex that is visualized with triamcinolone acetonide is removed, using Tano's diamond-dusted membrane eraser or brush back-flush needle.

The internal limiting membrane is stained with 0.125% of indocyanine green dye under balanced salt solution. The dye is removed immediately after injection to minimize possible complication. Internal limiting membrane is removed using an asymmetric forceps or other micro-forceps.

In order to visualize the peripheral vitreous, a triamcinolone suspension is sprayed onto the peripheral vitreous, so that the peripheral vitreous appears as a white gel. Peripheral vitreous is removed as much as possible. Removal of peripheral vitreous after internal limiting membrane peeling can decrease the postoperative concentration of indocyanine green dye in the vitreous cavity, reducing its possible toxicity. Thereafter, an attempt is made to wash out the residual triamcinolone granules from the eye. The vitreous with triamcinolone is removed with a vitrectomy probe. Although small amounts of triamcinolone granules (<1 mg) are usually left on the inferior retina, they disappear within two weeks after pars plana vitrectomy. Results of surgery are shown in Figs 31.25A to D.

Complications

The intraoperative and postoperative complications include peripheral retinal tear, postoperative rhegmatogenous retinal detachment, neovascular glaucoma, recurrent or persistent vitreous hemorrhage, hard exudates in the center of the macula, postoperative epiretinal membrane formation, lamellar macular hole, full-thickness macular hole, angle closure glaucoma, persistent vitreous hemorrhage, choroidal detachment and intravitreal fibrin formation.

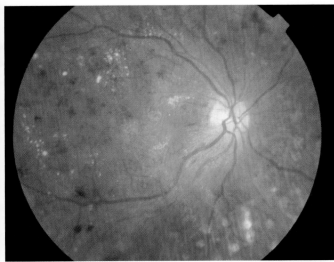

Figs 31.25A: A 69-year-old female with cystoid macular edema due to diabetic retinopathy. Fundus examination revealed taut posterior vitreous membrane. Visual acuity was 20/250 preoperatively (Prof Masahito Ohji)

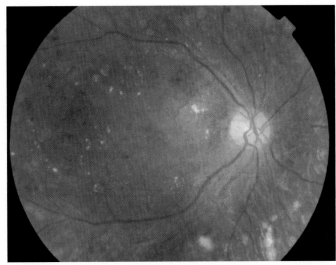

Fig. 31.25C: Macular edema was resolved following vitrectomy combined with internal limiting membrane removal (Prof Masahito Ohji)

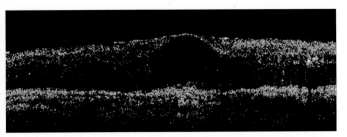

Fig. 31.25B: Optical coherent tomography disclosed marked cystoid macular edema (Prof Masahito Ohji)

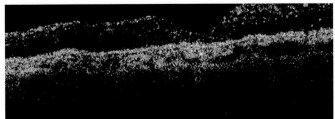

Fig. 31.25D: Optical coherent tomography showed the reduction of macular edema and recovery of foveal depression (Prof Masahito Ohji)

Role of Optical Coherence Tomography

Optical coherence tomography appears to be a useful tool in the diagnosis and management of diabetic macular edema and in the monitoring of the morphological changes after vitrectomy. Optical coherence tomography allowed the diagnosis of subtle vitreomacular traction and provided precise preoperative and postoperative assessments of macular thickness.

Diabetic macular edema vitrectomy study is a prospective, randomized clinical trial evaluating the role of vitrectomy with internal limiting membrane peeling versus standard therapy (grid laser photocoagulation) for diffuse diabetic macular edema.

MACULAR TRANSLOCATION

Macular translocation can be defined as any surgery that has a primary goal of relocating the central neurosensory retina or fovea intraoperatively or postoperatively specifically for the management of macular disease. Its role in the management of choroidal neovascularization in age-related macular degeneration has become less defined with the advent of anti-VEGF therapy.

Rationale

In the early, potentially reversible stages of neovascular age-related macular degeneration, visual deterioration may be secondary to such factors as subretinal fluid and hemorrhage in the fovea. In the later likely irreversible stages of the disease, fibrovascular proliferation causes the permanent damage of the photoreceptors. Therefore, by moving the neurosensory retina in an eye with recent-onset subfoveal lesion to a new location with presumably healthier retinal pigment epithelium and choriocapillaris away from the lesion, the fovea may be able to recover or maintain its visual function. In addition, moving the fovea away from such subfoveal lesions as choroidal neovascularization may permit the removal of the choroidal neovascularization or its destruction by laser photocoagulation.

Macular Translocation with 360-Degree Retinotomy

Crystalline lens removal is necessary to ensure visibility and maneuverability in the peripheral fundus in phakic eyes. Phacoemulsification and intraocular lens implantation are performed at the beginning of the surgery.

Core vitrectomy is performed via a standard three-port pars plana approach. The surgeon must either confirm or create a posterior vitreous detachment, since adherent vitreous may cause postoperative retinal detachment or proliferative vitreoretinopathy. However, it is often difficult to detect residual vitreous cortex intraoperatively by simple observation alone. Intravitreal injection of triamcinolone dramatically facilitates visibility of the vitreous cortex. After creation of the posterior vitreous detachment, peripheral vitrectomy is performed with scleral indentation. Removal of the peripheral vitreous is crucial for macular translocation with 360-degree retinotomy to facilitate the maneuvering of the retina during surgery and to prevent postoperative proliferative vitreoretinopathy.

The retinal detachment may be created with either transscleral or transretinal infusion of balanced saline solution into the subretinal space; the latter technique is often performed. A 39- or 41-gauge polyimide flexible needle may be used for the transretinal infusion. Balanced salt solution is infused into the subretinal space with the needle. A 20-gauge silicone-tipped needle might be used to complete the total retinal detachment. Intraocular pressure should be kept lower to facilitate enlargement of the retinal detachment. Fluid-air exchange might be necessary to complete the total retinal detachment at the posterior pole.

A circumferential 360-degree retinotomy is created using a vitreous cutter or scissors as peripherally as possible to preserve functioning retina, minimize exposed retinal pigment epithelium and prevent hemorrhage. The retina is then flipped, and the choroidal neovascular membrane and/or subretinal hemorrhage is removed under direct visualization using forceps.

The retina at the posterior pole is unfolded and flattened using liquid perfluorocarbon, followed by rotation of the retina. The retina is then gently rotated clockwise or counterclockwise around the axis of the optic nerve head using a soft-tipped cannula. After the retina is translocated to the appropriate position, additional perfluorocarbon liquid is injected to achieve complete retinal reattachment. Photocoagulation is applied to the peripheral retina and intentional retinal breaks made with a 39-gauge needle. Finally, perfluorocarbon is directly exchanged with silicone oil.

Silicone oil is usually removed 2–3 months late. Extraocular muscle surgery is performed if the patient complains of a tilted image or diplopia, but it could be performed simultaneously with translocation surgery.

Results of surgery are shown in Figs 31.26 to 31.28 B.

Limited Macular Translocation

Limited macular translocation is based on the concept of creating neurosensory retinal redundancy by shortening sclera/retinal pigment epithelium relative to neurosensory retina. This technique eliminates the need for large retinotomies and associated complications.

Pars plana vitrectomy is followed by the removal of posterior hyaloid. A 41-gauge cannula is used to create detachment of temporal retina by the means of self-sealing retinotomies. Scleral imbrication is created using in-pouching technique with scleral sutures or outpouching technique using clips. Fluid-air exchange is done and upright positioning is recommended for 24–36 hours. Postoperative laser photocoagulation to choroidal neovascular membrane is performed.

Results of surgery are shown in Figs 31.29 to 31.31.

Complications

Various postoperative complications can develop because macular translocation surgery involves many procedures. Retinal detachment and diplopia are the most important of the complications. Postoperative retinal detachment reportedly

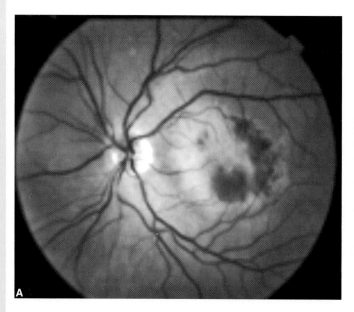
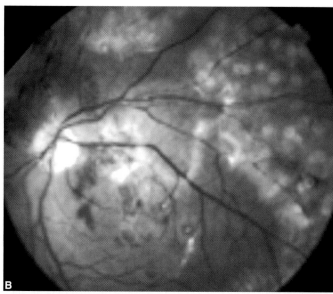

Figs 31.26A and B: Macular translocation with 360° retinotomy (A) Preoperative, (B) Postoperative (Dr Levent Akduman)

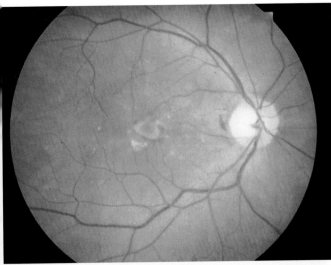

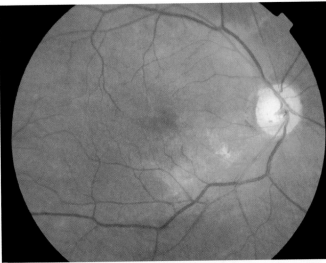

Fig. 31.27A: Macular translocation with 360° retinotomy: A 67-year-old male with subfoveal choroidal neovascular membrane due to age-related macular degeneration with visual acuity was 20/160 preoperatively (Dr Levent Akduman)

Fig. 31.27B: Macular translocation with 360° retinotomy: The retina was rotated upward by 25 degrees followed by counter-rotation of the eyeball. Visual acuity improved to 20/25 (Dr Levent Akduman)

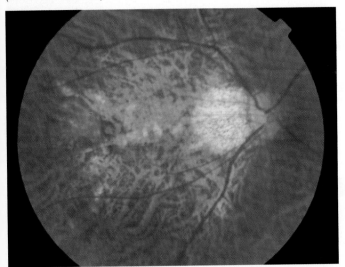

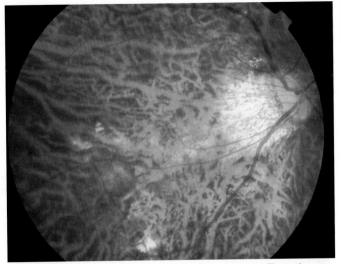

Fig. 31.28A: Macular translocation with 360° retinotomy: A 45-year-old male with subfoveal choroidal neovascular membrane due pathological myopia. Visual acuity was 20/200 preoperatively (Dr Levent Akduman)

Fig. 31.28B: Macular translocation with 360° retinotomy: The retina was rotated by 18 degrees followed by counter-rotation of the eyeball. Visual acuity improved to 20/15 and has been maintained until the last visit, three years postoperatively (Dr Levent Akduman)

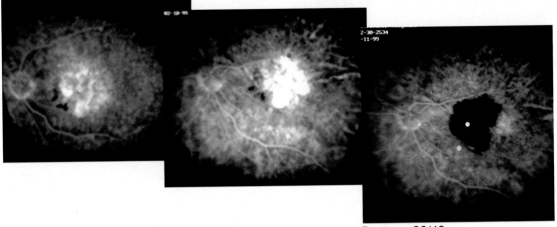

Pre-op=20/250

Post-op=20/40

Fig. 31.29: Limited macular translocation: Age-related macular degeneration with large subfoveal choroidal neovascular membrane. (Corresponding retinal landmarks are marked with color dots for comparison in preoperative and postoperative figures) (Dr Levent Akduman)

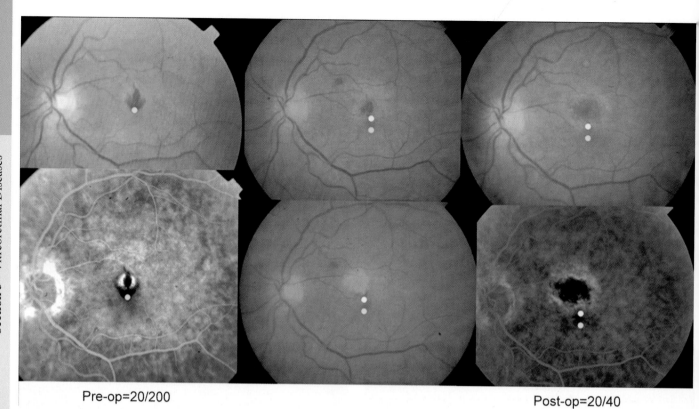

Pre-op=20/200

Post-op=20/40

Fig. 31.30: Limited macular translocation: Age-related macular degeneration with large juxtafoveal choroidal neovascular membrane with hemorrhagic edge extending subfoveally (Corresponding retinal landmarks are marked with color dots for comparison in preoperative and postoperative figures) (Dr Levent Akduman)

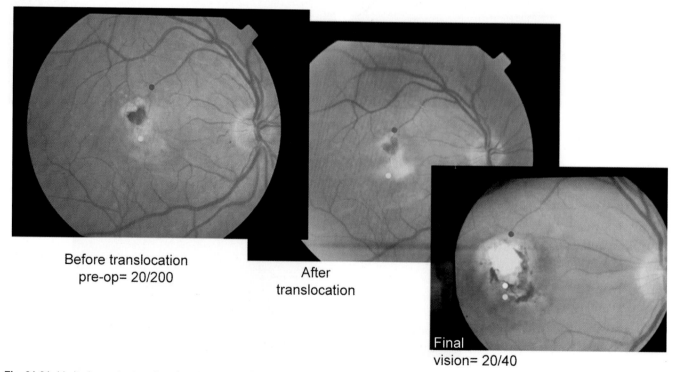

Before translocation
pre-op= 20/200

After
translocation

Final
vision= 20/40

Fig. 31.31: Limited macular translocation: A 21-year old punctate inner choroidopathy patient who initially had argon laser for juxtafoveal membrane, then subfoveal recurrence for which photodynamic therapy was performed and limited macular translocation and removal of choroidal neovascular membrane was done for persistent subfoveal choroidal neovascular membrane (Corresponding retinal landmarks are marked with color dots for comparison in preoperative and postoperative figures) (Dr Levent Akduman)

develops in 20 to 40% of cases. Although improvements in surgical techniques and surgical instruments reduced the incidence of retinal detachment, postoperative retinal detachment, including proliferative vitreoretinopathy is still the most serious complication.

MYOPIC FOVEOSCHISIS

Myopic foveoschisis is common in high myopia. Vitrectomy with vitreous cortex removal, internal limiting membrane peeling and gas tamponade could be useful to treat myopic foveoschisis in highly myopic eyes.

Tractional force of the epiretinal membrane may cause myopic foveoschisis. Optical coherence tomography has provided more information and indicated that different subtypes of myopic foveoschisis may have processes specific to their development. For instance, local posterior vitreous detachment at the posterior retina as well as a preretinal strand between the edge of the macular hole and the posterior vitreous surface often is observed in myopic foveoschisis in which a macular hole develops. This indicates that a macular hole associated with myopic foveoschisis may develop as the result of posterior vitreous detachment, which generates anteroposterior traction and consequent retinal tearing at the fovea. Another possible mechanism is retinal vascular traction on the retina.

Collagen fiber and cellular component are suggested to play an important role in developing myopic foveoschisis. Internal limiting membrane peeling may be essential for vitrectomy for myopic foveoschisis.

Surgical Technique

Surgery is performed under local anesthesia in most cases. Phacoemulsification is performed at the beginning of the surgery, followed by intraocular lens implantation. Core vitrectomy is performed with a standard three-port vitrectomy system. Vitreous cortex is visualized with the injection of triamcinolone acetonide. Visualization of vitreous cortex allows surgeons to confirm residual vitreous cortex. Although so-called posterior vitreous detachment is found in many cases, thin layer of vitreous cortex remains attached to the posterior retina in most cases. The thin layer of vitreous cortex that is visualized with triamcinolone acetonide is removed, using Tano's diamond-dusted membrane eraser or brush back-flush needle. Internal limiting membrane is stained with 0.125% of indocyanine green dye under balanced salt solution. The dye is removed immediately after injection to minimize possible complication. Internal limiting membrane is removed using an asymmetric forceps or other micro-forceps. Peripheral vitreous

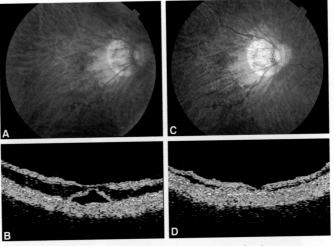

Figs 31.32A to D: Myopic foveoschisis. Preoperative fundus appearance of patients who underwent vitrectomy for myopic foveoschisis (A) Color fundus photograph shows almost normal fundus, except for myopic atrophy (B) However, OCT shows apparent foveal detachment and retinoschisis. Fundus appearance, 6 months after surgery (C) The color fundus image has not changed from preoperatively (D) However, the OCT image shows complete resolution of the foveal detachment and consequent visual improvement (Late Prof Yasuo Tano)

is removed as much as possible. Removal of peripheral vitreous after internal limiting membrane peeling can decrease the postoperative concentration of indocyanine green dye in the vitreous cavity, reducing its possible toxicity. Fluid-air exchange followed by injection of 20% sulfur hexafluoride is performed. Reoperation including complete vitreous cortex removal and internal limiting membrane peeling could be beneficial for patients with persistent myopic foveoschisis after primary surgery, indicating that vitreous cortex removal and internal limiting membrane peeling are critical in treating myopic foveoschisis. Vitrectomy for macular holes associated with myopic foveoschisis may be performed. Although significant visual improvement occurs in less than 50% of cases, vitrectomy can be beneficial for some cases. Results of surgery are shown in Figs 31.32A to D.

Role of Optical Coherence Tomography

After surgery; OCT typically shows that foveal detachment gradually resolves over time. Foveal detachment completely resolves soon after surgery in some cases; however, other cases can take longer than six months to resolve, probably depending on the viscosity of the subretinal or intraretinal fluid. Although there is a risk of macular hole formation even after surgery, 80 to 90% of patients have improved visual acuity. The surgery usually results in the stabilization of the fixation point in scanning laser ophthalmoscope microperimetry, indicating that retinal function has improved.

Step-by-Step Macular Surgery

EPIRETINAL MEMBRANE REMOVAL

Step-by-step epiretinal membrane removal is shown from Figs 31.33A to O:

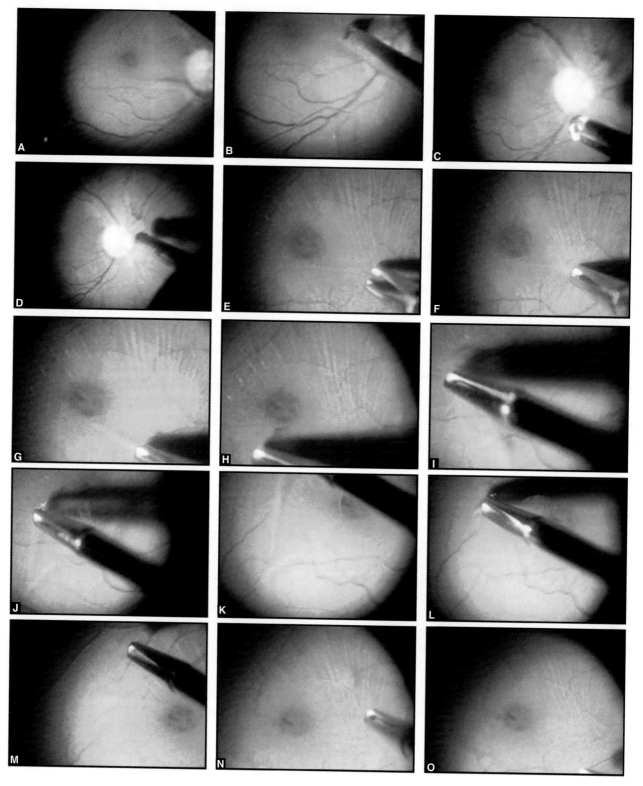

Figs 31.33A to O: Step-by-step epiretinal membrane removal (Dr Manish Nagpal)

TRIAMCINOLONE-ASSISTED EPIRETINAL MEMBRANE REMOVAL

Step-by-step triamcinolone-assisted epiretinal membrane removal is shown in Figures 31.34 A to L:

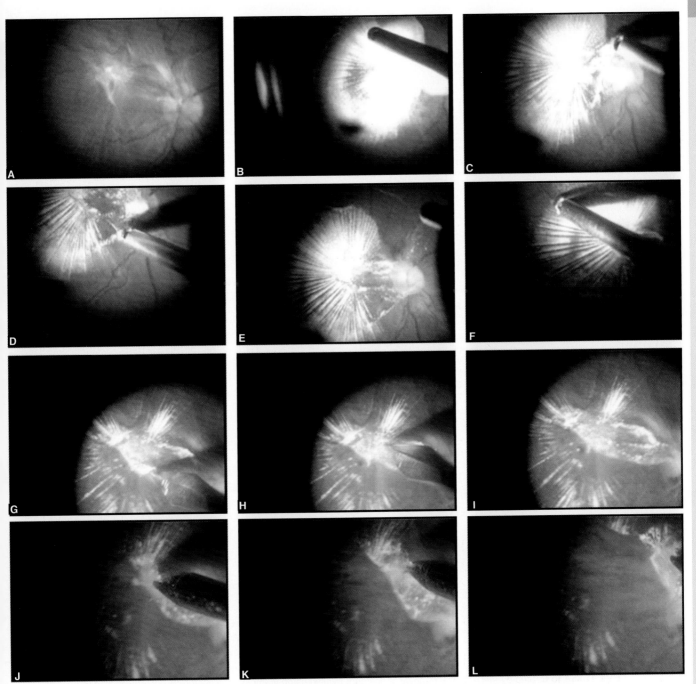

Figs 31.34A to L: Step-by-step triamcinolone-assisted epiretinal membrane removal (Dr Manish Nagpal)

POSTERIOR HYALOID REMOVAL USING TRIAMCINOLONE ACETONIDE

Step-by-step surgery for removal of posterior hyaloid using triamcinolone acetonide is shown in Figs 31.35A to L:

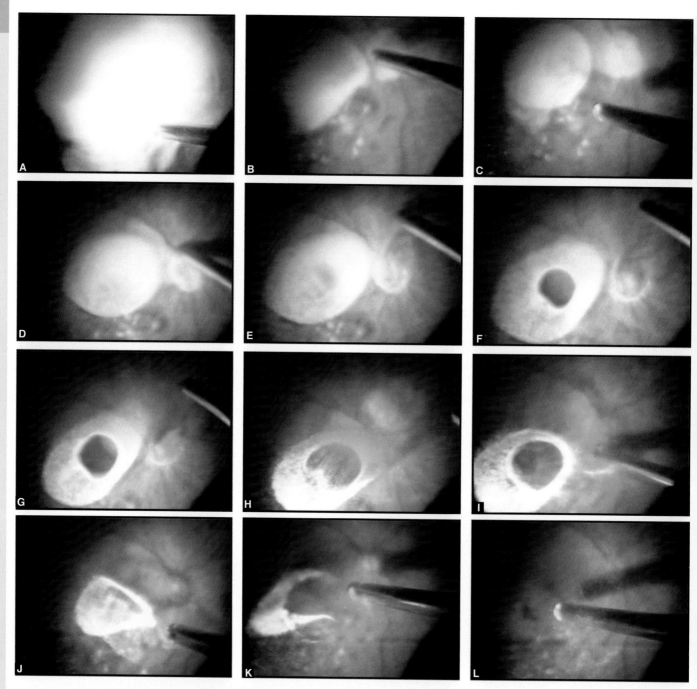

Figs 31.35A to L: Step-by-step surgical removal of posterior hyaloid using triamcinolone acetonide (Dr Manish Nagpal)

MACULAR HOLE SURGERY

Step-by-step macular hole surgery using trypan blue dye for epiretinal membrane staining and indocyanine green dye for internal limiting membrane staining is shown in Figs 31.36A to L:

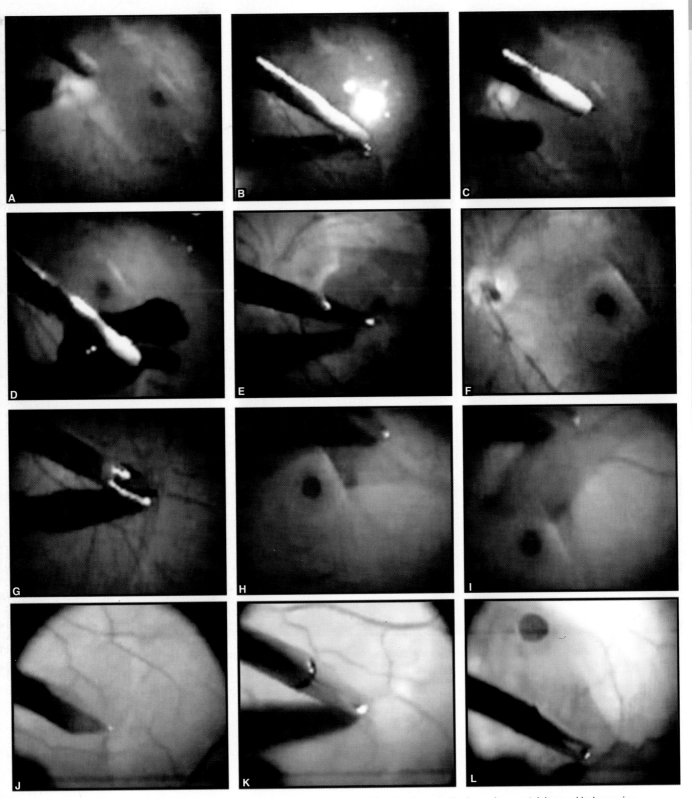

Figs 31.36A to L: Step-by-step macular hole surgery using trypan blue dye for epiretinal membrane staining and indocyanine green dye for internal limiting membrane staining (Dr Nazimul Hussain)

Step-by-step macular hole surgery using triamcinolone acetonide is shown in Figures 31.37A to L:

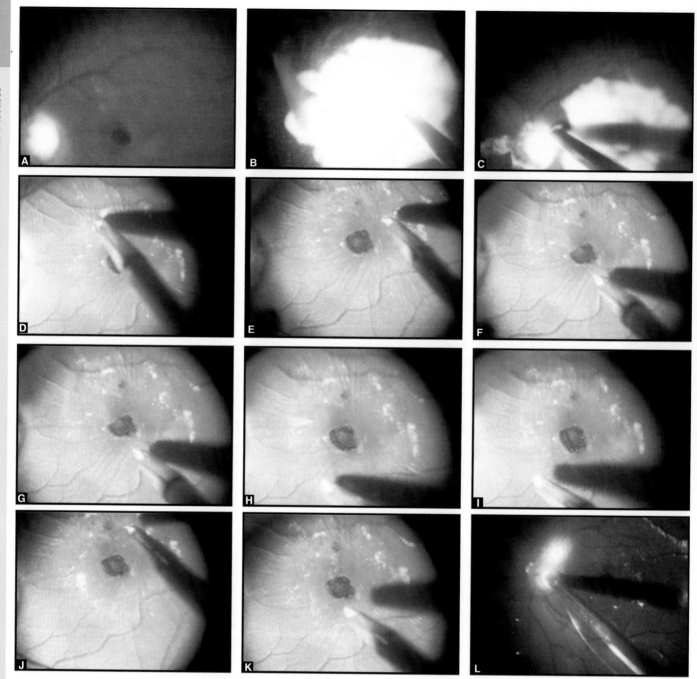

Figs 31.37A to L: Step-by-step macular hole surgery using triamcinolone acetonide (Dr Manish Nagpal)

Chapter 32

Hereditary Vitreoretinal Diseases

Parveen Sen, R Priya, J Manju

INTRODUCTION

Hereditary retinal degenerations are familial, bilaterally symmetrical disorders of the retina. The varied morphological picture in all these disorders is governed by the specific underlying genetic defect. Though the genetic defect is present at birth, the typical clinical picture is manifested at various stages of life in different disorders. These are diagnosed with the help of relevant history and clinical examination coupled with various investigations, including electrodiagnostic tests, fundus fluorescein angiogram, optical coherence tomography (OCT) and color vision with field evaluation.

A morphological classification of these hereditary disorders is usually done depending upon the histological layer of the retina primarily involved.

1. *Nerve fiber layer:* X-linked juvenile retinoschisis
2. *Photoreceptor layer:*
   a. Retinitis pigmentosa: It primarily affects the rods and cones and may present with typical or atypical clinical manifestation. Atypical forms of retinitis pigmentosa may be central (inverse retinitis pigmentosa), sine pigmento retinitis pigmentosa (retinitis punctata albescence) or sector retinitis pigmentosa. Retinitis pigmentosa may also be present with associated syndromes like Laurence-Moon and Bardet-Biedl syndromes.
   b. Leber's congenital amaurosis
   c. Cone dystrophy
   d. Cone-rod dystrophy
3. *Retinal pigment epithelium*
   a. Stargardt's disease
   b. Fundus flavimaculatus
   c. Vitelliform dystrophy
   d. Pattern dystrophy
   e. Dominant cystoid macular dystrophy
   f. Dominant drusen
4. *Bruch's membrane*
   a. Pseudoinflammatory dystrophy
   b. Angioid streaks
   c. Age-related macular degeneration
   d. Myopic macular degeneration
5. *Choroid:* Central areolar choroidal dystrophy
6. Vitreotapetoretinal Degenerations
   a. Goldmann-Favre syndrome
   b. Stickler's syndrome
   c. Wagner's syndrome

NERVE FIBER LAYER

X-Linked Retinoschisis

Introduction

X-linked retinoschisis is a hereditary, vitreoretinal degeneration that is one of the most common causes of juvenile macular degeneration in males. The disease was first described in 1898 by Haas. Microcystic changes seen at the fovea have been postulated to be secondary to splitting of the inner retina especially within the nerve fiber layer.

Molecular genetic studies have detected the gene causing X–linked retinoschisis. This gene codes for a polypeptide, RS1, called retinoschisin. This protein is thought to play an important role in cell to cell adhesion and maintains the integrity of the retinal neurons. Retinoschisin is mainly produced by the photoreceptors and the bipolar cells. Retinoschisin 1-deficiency is known to cause disorganization of all the retinal cell layers with splitting of the inner nuclear layer.

Clinical Presentation

Subjects usually present with symptoms of gradual decrease in vision in the second decade of life. Poor vision is due to foveal schisis. Some times the presentation may be in the form of a sudden decrease in vision due to vitreous hemorrhage/retinal detachment. In some cases, an infant is brought into the clinic by the parents with history of poor vision/fixation or strabismus. In the severe forms of the disease foveal schisis happens in the first year of life. Poor fixation at an early stage could

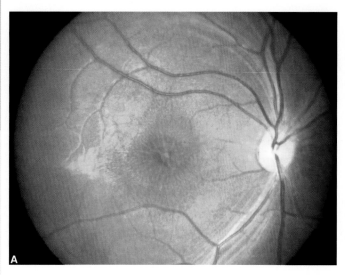
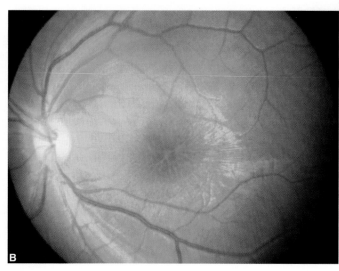

Figs 32.1A and B: X-linked retinoschisis. (A) Color fundus photograph of the right eye shows spoke wheel pattern
(B) Color fundus photograph of the left eye shows spoke wheel pattern

be secondary to foveal schisis or because of a large peripheral schitic cavity overhanging the macula. Surgical drainage of such a cavity may be indicated to promote macular maturation and prevent amblyopia.

Fundus picture is characterized by the presence of bilateral symmetrical picture of cystoid spaces at the fovea also described as the "bicycle-wheel" pattern (Figs 32.1A and B). Peripheral schisis is seen in nearly 50% of the subjects. Since the inner wall of the retina is very thin, formation of large inner layer breaks is seen. Vitreous degeneration is also seen giving "vitreous veils".

Investigations

Electroretinogram: Full-field ERG (ffERG) typically reveals a negative waveform in the response to a bright flash under scotopic conditions (Fig. 32.2). Multifocal ERG shows amplitude loss in multiple retinal areas (Fig. 32.3). Decreased amplitudes on mfERG are not restricted to the area of schisis suggesting a global pathology.

Optical coherence tomography: Optical coherence tomography is useful to document foveal schisis, even when it is not obvious clinically (Fig. 32.4).

Fluorescein angiography: Typically the cystoid spaces in X-linked retinoschisis do not show any leakage even in the late stages of the disease (Figs 32.5A and B).

Visual fields: A relative central scotoma is seen. Peripheral defects may be seen in patients corresponding to the areas of peripheral retinoschisis.

Treatment

Indications of surgery in a typical case of X-linked retinoschisis may include retinal detachment, vitreous haemorrhage because of bleeding of the fragile unsupported blood vessels in the inner layer of the schisis and drainage of an overhanging schitic cavity in infantile severe forms of X-linked retinoschisis.

PHOTORECEPTOR LAYER

Retinitis Pigmentosa

Introduction

Retinitis pigmentosa is a hereditary disorder, which may present as an autosomal recessive/autosomal dominant/sporadic inheritance pattern. X-Linked inheritance is the least common. The severity and the presenting features of the disease vary depending upon the inheritance pattern.

Clinical Presentation

Night blindness or nyctalopia is usually the first symptom. It is followed by progressive decrease in the visual field leading to tunnel vision in the late stages in typical cases. On fundus examination it is characterized by a triad of disc pallor, arteriolar attenuation and bony spicule pigmentation. The pigment alterations typically begin at the mid periphery (Fig. 32.6). Granular or mottled appearance of retinal pigment epithelium may be seen throughout the fundus even in the early stages of the disease. Visual acuity in retinitis pigmentosa may be preserved even in the very advanced cases. Causes of early decrease in visual acuity include atrophic macula, cystoid macular edema or central retinitis pigmentosa. Color vision defects depend upon the degree of central or cone involvement.

Investigations

Electroretinogram: Electroretinogram shows poor scotopic responses in early stages. In fully manifest disease photopic responses are also affected leading to a nonrecordable waveform (Fig. 32.7). Central response may be measurable using mfERG (Figs 32.8 and 32.9) in the early stages of the disease even in presence of an extinguished ffERG.

Visual fields: Typically, a progressive constriction of the fields with only a small island of vision remaining in the late stages is

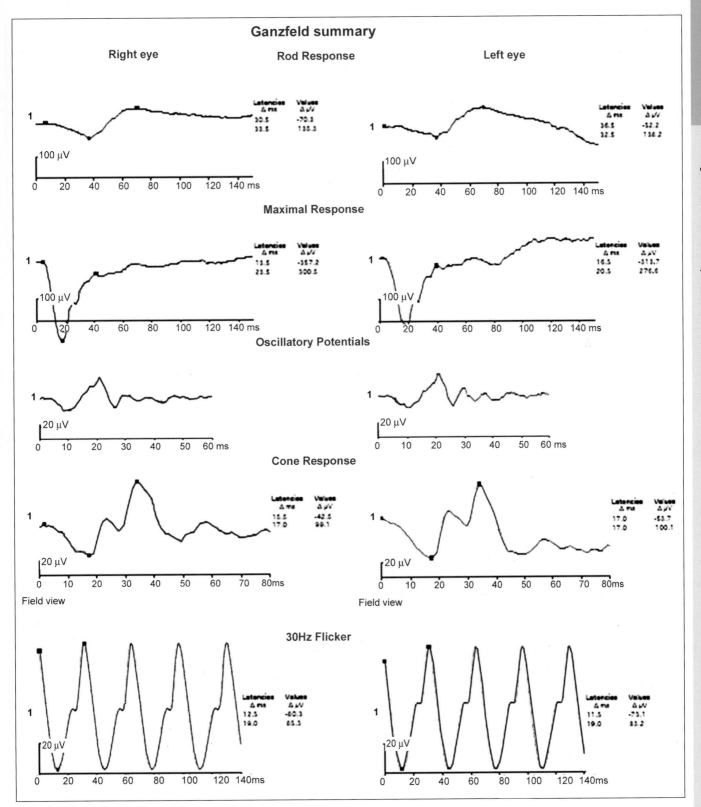

Fig. 32.2: Full-field ERG (ffERG) shows selective b-wave reduction in X-linked retinoschisis resulting in a negative-type ERG waveform in the scotopic combined response

Patient

Field view

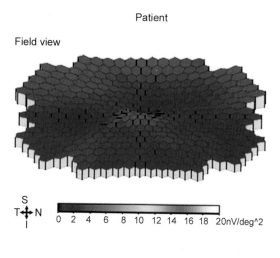

Fig. 32.3: Multifocal ERG of the left eye reveals multiarea decrease in amplitudes

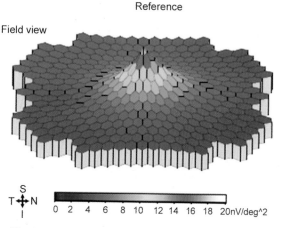

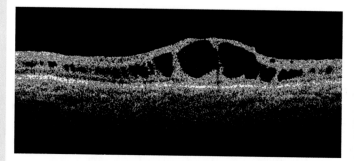

Fig. 32.4: Optical coherence tomography of the same patient shows hyporeflective spaces with vertical palisades

seen. Field defect usually begins as an annular mid-peripheral scotoma.

Optical coherence tomography: Optical coherence tomography helps to document cystoid/atrophic retina, which is the cause of poor vision in early stages (Figs 32.10A and B). Resolved cystoid macular edema after topical dorzolamide administration, which is the treatment of cystoid macular edema in retinitis pigmentosa, can also be documented on OCT (Figs 32.11A and B).

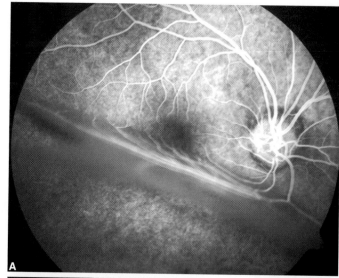

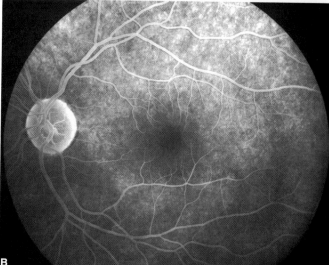

Figs 32.5A and B: Fluorescein angiograms of the right and the left eye. No leakage is seen in the cystoid spaces even in the late phase of the angiogram

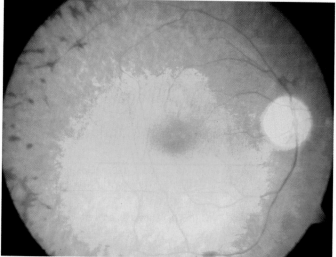

Fig. 32.6: Retinitis pigmentosa. Color fundus photograph of right eye shows waxy disc with arteriolar attenuation and retinal pigment epithelium. Pigment mottling typically seen in the midperiphery. The macular area still shows healthy retinal pigment epithelium

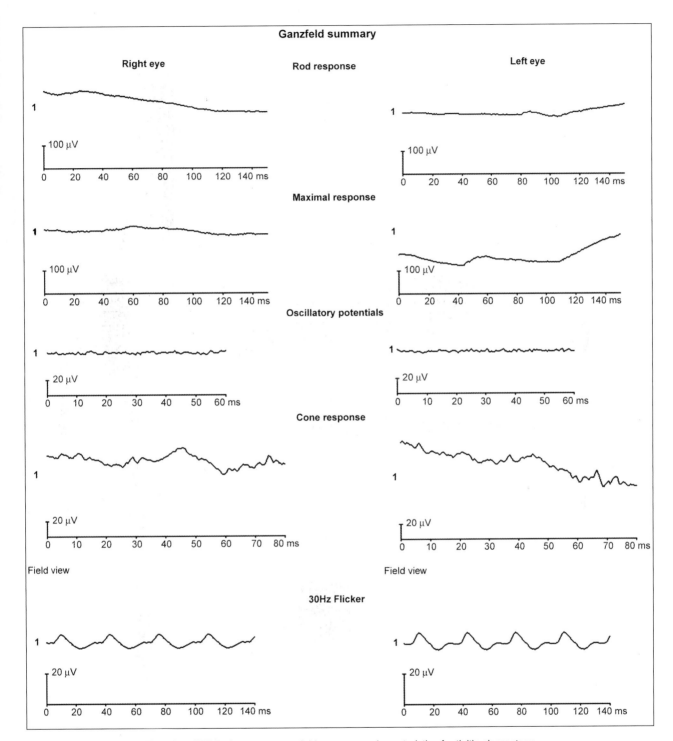

Fig. 32.7: ffERG shows nonrecordable response characteristic of retinitis pigmentosa

Fluorescein angiography: Fluorescein angiography reveals area of granular dysfunctional retinal pigment epithelium, which may be more widespread than seen clinically.

Treatment

Daily vitamin supplements, including vitamin A and E with or without antioxidants have been proposed by studies worldwide

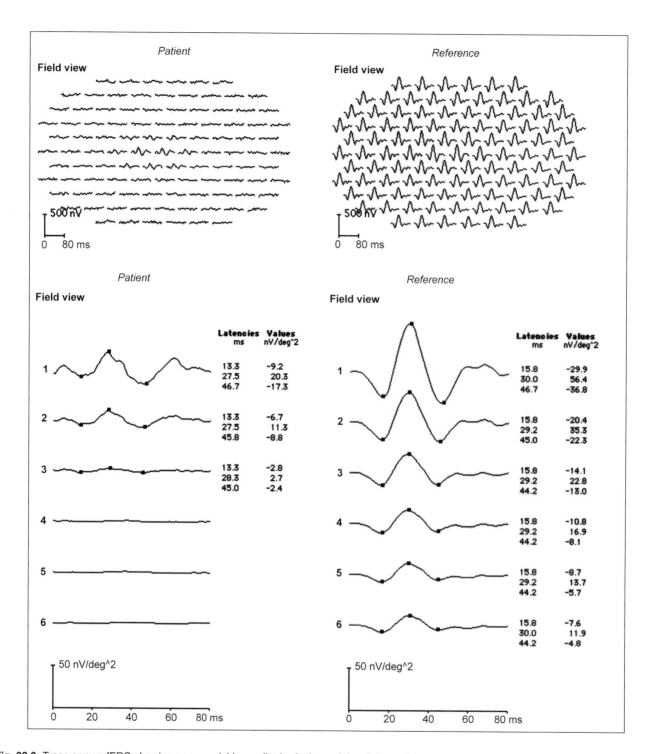

Fig. 32.8: Trace array mfERG showing nonrecordable amplitudes in the peripheral rings whereas some response can be picked up in the central two rings. Implicit times of the central areas are nearly normal

with limited success. Various studies have postulated the effectiveness electrical stimulation of the retina or the optic nerve using retinal or optic nerve prostheses in retinitis pigmentosa. However usefulness of these treatment modalities remains to be proved in a clinical setting. Visual function improvement has also been recorded in patients with artificial silicon retina microchip implanted in the subretinal space in these patients.

Atypical Forms of Retinitis Pigmentosa

Central Retinitis Pigmentosa

It is an atypical form of retinitis pigmentosa affecting the central retina in the beginning of the disease process (Figs 32.12A and B). These patients have poor vision in the day as well as the night.

Full-field ERG as well as mfERG may be nonrecordable.

Patient   Reference

Field view   Field view

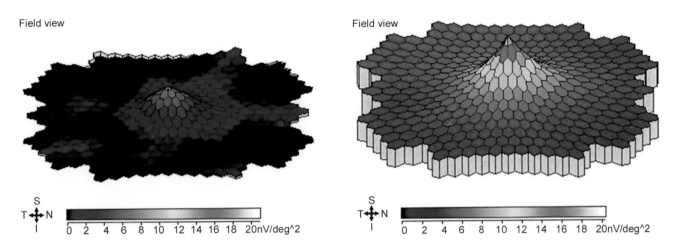

Fig. 32.9: Topographical mfERG plot shows preserved foveal peak corresponding to the normal macular retinal pigment epithelium on fundus photograph

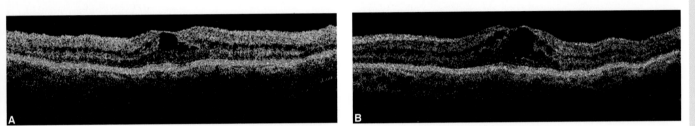

Figs 32.10A and B: Optical coherence tomography of the right and the left eye shows cystoid spaces involving the fovea and increased central macular thickness. The leakage is usually from the parafoveal and perifoveal capillaries

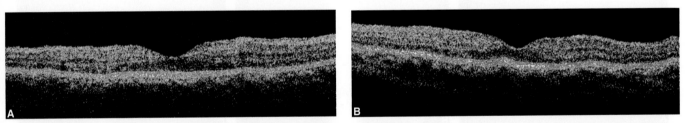

Figs 32.11A and B: Optical coherence tomography of both eyes shows resolved CME after systemic acetazolamide therapy

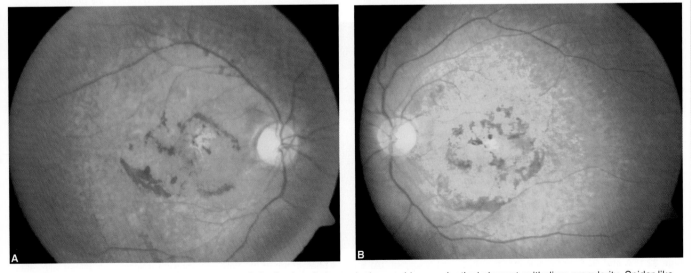

Figs 32.12A and B: Central retinitis pigmentosa. Color fundus photograph shows widespread retinal pigment epithelium granularity. Spider-like clumps form an "island around the macula". Optic atrophy and arteriolar attenuation are seen

Retinitis Punctata Albescence

Retinitis punctata albescens is an infrequently occurring form of autosomal recessive retinal dystrophy with early-onset severe night blindness and tiny, dotlike, white deposits in the fundus. Presence of disc pallor and vessel attenuation distinguishes this form of retinitis pigmentosa from other "white dot syndromes" of the retina (Figs 32.13A to 32.14C). Retinitis

punctata albescens is associated mostly with mutations in RLBP1 (retinaldehyde-binding protein gene).

Retinitis Pigmentosa with Coats' Response

Coats'-like changes that is, retinal telangiectasia and/or exudative detachment have been reported in as many as 1.2% to 3.6% of patients with retinitis pigmentosa (Figs 32.15 A to 32.16 C).

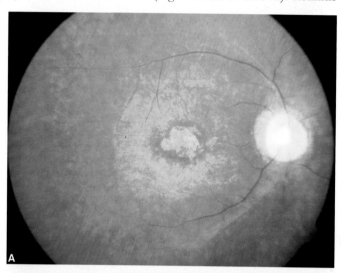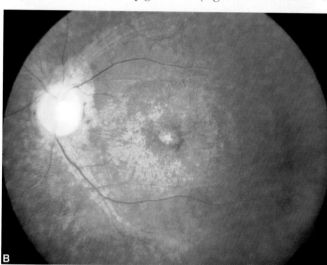

Figs 32.13A and B: Retinitis punctata albescence. Color fundus photograph of the right and the left eye shows disc pallor with marked arteriolar attenuation and bilateral atrophic macula. Presence of yellowish dots throughout the fundus is seen. Electroretinogram showed nonrecordable responses

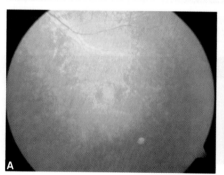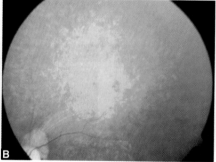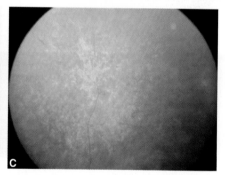

Figs 32.14A to C: Color fundus photograph of the same patient reveals absence of bony spicule pigmentation even in the periphery

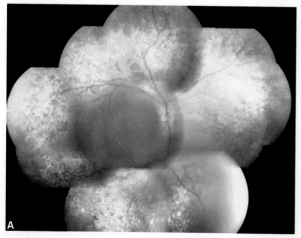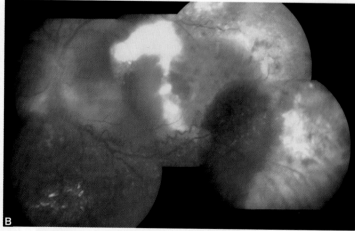

Figs 32.15A and B: Retinitis pigmentosa with Coats' response. (A) Fundus photograph of the right eye showing retinitis pigmentosa with retinal pigment epithelium granularity typically involving the equatorial and peripheral region. Arteriolar attenuation and bony spicule pigmentation is seen. (B) Fundus photograph of the left eye with retinitis pigmentosa and extensive subretinal extravascular lipid deposits

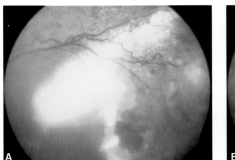
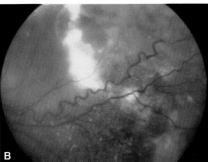
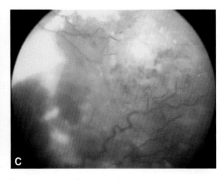

Figs 32.16A to C: Color fundus photograph showing dilated and tortuous telangiectatic vessels. These are usually formed secondary to chronic microvascular leakage associated with retinitis pigmentosa

Pigmented Para Venous Chorioretinal Atrophy

Pigmentary changes are seen in close distribution to the retinal veins. This is opposite to preserved para-arteriole retinal pigment epithelial atrophy seen in some patients with retinitis pigmentosa. Pigmented paravenous chorioretinal atrophy is a rare disorder, which is diagnosed primarily because of the typical fundoscopic appearance of retinal pigment epithelial atrophy and clumping in a paravenous distribution (Figs 32.17 A to 32.20 C).The scotopic ERG responses are markedly abnormal (Fig. 32.21). Pigmented paravenous retinochoroidal atrophy may occur in association with systemic infections or inflammation.

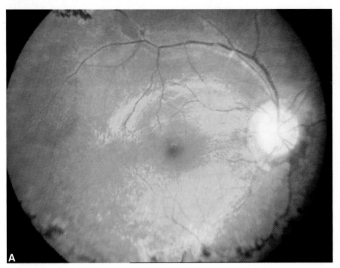
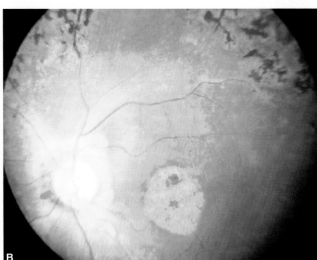

Figs 32.17A and B: Pigmented paravenous chorioretinal atrophy. Color fundus photograph of the right and the left eye shows retinal pigment epithelium granularity with associated pigment mottling along the major retinal vessels. Left eye shows an atrophic patch at the macula

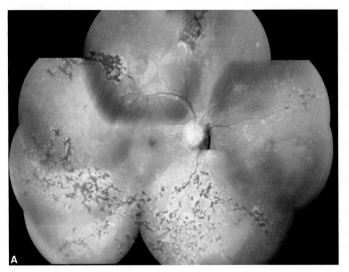
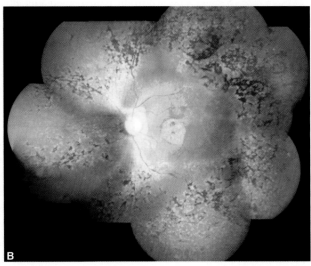

Figs 32.18A and B: Color montage photograph of the right and the left eye shows pigment migration along the vessels

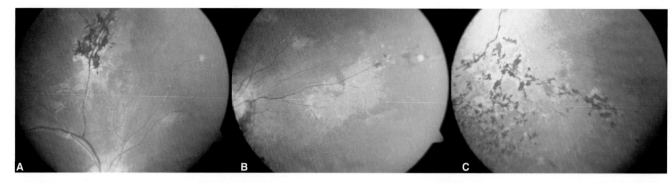

Figs 32.19A to C: Superonasal, nasal and inferonasal quadrants of the right eye showing paravenous distribution of the chorioretinal atrophy

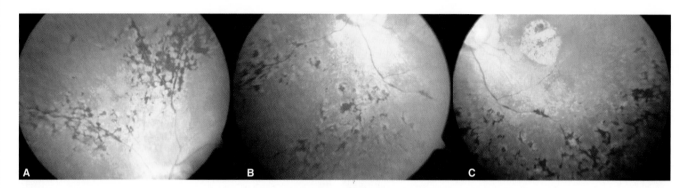

Figs 32.20A to C: Similar areas of pigment clumping seen along the veins in the nasal, superonasal, inferonasal and temporal quadrants of the left eye as well

Ocular Associations of Retinitis Pigmentosa

Include posterior subcapsular cataract, open-angle glaucoma, myopia, keratoconus and vitreous degeneration. Coats' like response may also be seen as described above. Regular follow-up of these patients is required to document the progression of the disease as well as for the management of these disorders.

Systemic Associations of Retinitis Pigmentosa

Retinitis pigmentosa may be part of a syndrome resulting from specific genetic defects.

Bassen-Kornzweig syndrome: This syndrome is also called abetalipoproteinemia. Deficiency in beta-lipoprotein results in intestinal malabsorption. Inheritance is autosomal recessive. Presenting signs include ptosis, progressive external ophthalmoplegia, retinitis pigmentosa and spinocerebellar ataxia. Presence of acanthocytosis in peripheral blood smear is diagnostic. Treatment with vitamin E may be useful for the improvement of the neurological signs.

Refsum's syndrome: Inheritance is autosomal recessive. It is caused by the deficiency of phytanic acid 2-hydroxylase resulting in excessive accumulation of phytanic acid. Systemic features include polyneuropathy, cerebellar ataxia, ichthyosis and cardiomyopathy and deafness. Ocular features include retinitis pigmentosa, cataract and prominent corneal nerves. Diagnosis is made by phytanic acid assay in the blood or tissues. Phytanic acid-free diet is required in the treatment.

Kearns-Sayre syndrome: It is caused by mitochondrial DNA mutations. Presenting features include ptosis with progressive external ophthalmoplegia. Systemic features include ataxia, myopathies with cardiac conduction defects, deafness and diabetes.

Usher syndrome: Inheritance is autosomal recessive. Congenital deafness associated with retinitis pigmentosa is used to refer to Usher's syndrome. It is classically subdivided into Type 1, the more severe variety and Type 2, the milder form of the disease. Type 1 has profound deafness with early onset retinitis pigmentosa with vestibular symptoms while type 2 has milder form of deafness and retinitis pigmentosa and no vestibular symptoms. Types 3 and 4 have also been recognized by many. Type 3 is used to define a syndrome of progressive deafness retinitis pigmentosa and vestibular ataxia. Type 4 is associated with mental retardation.

Friedreich's ataxia: Inheritance is autosomal recessive. Presenting features include spinocerebellar ataxia, cardiomyopathy, deafness and diabetes.

Bardet-Biedl syndrome: Bardet-Biedl syndrome is an autosomal recessive disorder. It is a genetically heterogenous disease. Up to 12 genes have been implicated in the pathogenesis of the disease. The Bardet-Biedl syndrome is characterized by five cardinal features: obesity, postaxial polydactyly, pigmentary retinopathy (Figs 32.22), mental retardation and central obesity. Non cardinal features include hepatic fibrosis, diabetes mellitus, reproductive organ abnormalities, endocrinological disturbances, short stature, hearing difficulties, developmental

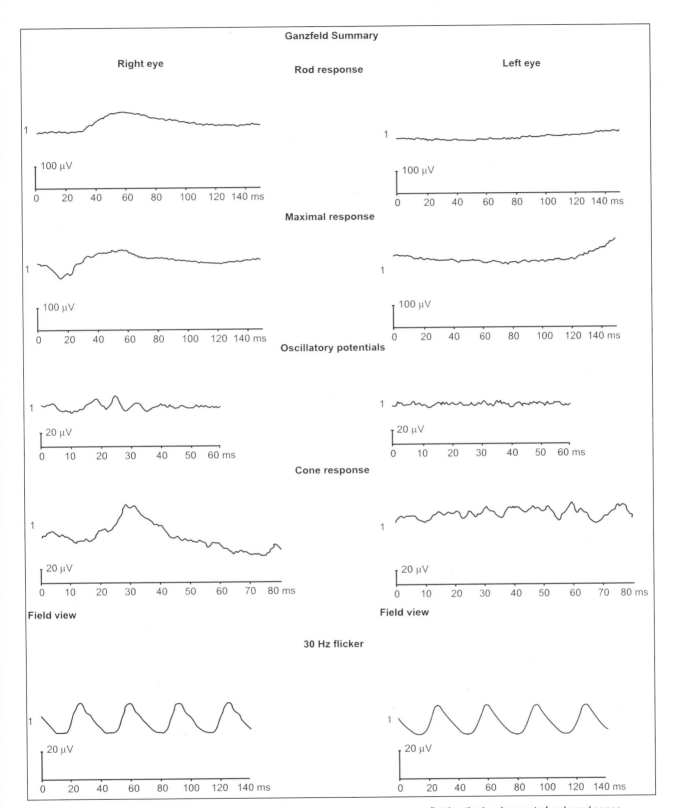

Fig. 32.21: Full-field ERG shows reduced photopic and scotopic responses reflecting the involvement of rods and cones

milestone delay and speech deficit. Other ocular abnormalities seen include astigmatism, strabismus, cataracts, color blindness, optic atrophy, and macular edema and degeneration. The progression of pigmentary retinopathy is rapid in these cases as against the people with typical retinitis pigmentosa. Full-Field ERG is usually nonrecordable by 10 years of age (Fig. 32.23).

Polydactyly seen is usually postaxial. In addition these patients may have short, broad hands and stubby fingers. Other features like clinodactyly or brachycephaly may also be seen. More than 2/3 rd of the subjects with this disease are known to be obese (Body mass index >25 kg/m^2) with a truncal distribution of fat. Renal disease is a major cause of morbidity in these patients.

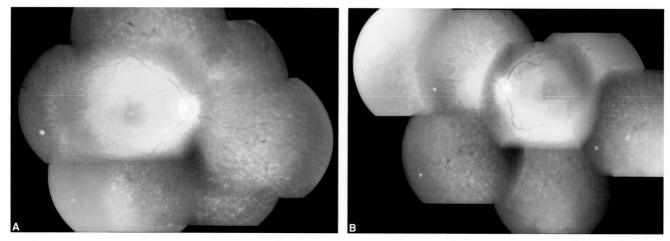

Figs 32.22A and B: Bardet-Biedl syndrome. Color montage of the right and the left eye shows widespread area of granular retinal pigment. Blood vessels are markedly attenuated with waxy pallor of the disc. Physical examination revealed spina bifida of the lumbosacral spine, polydactyly, obesity and mental retardation

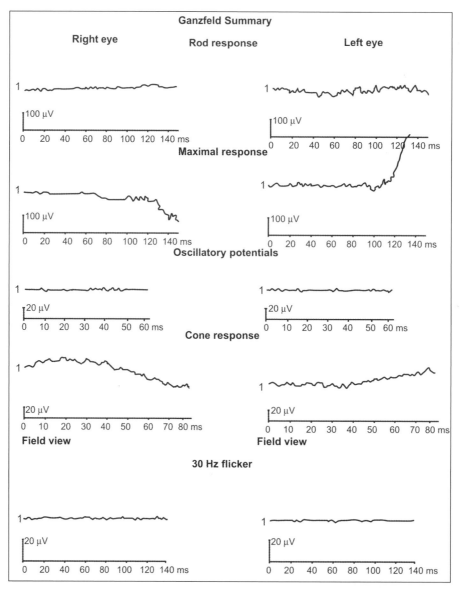

Fig. 32.23: Full-field ERG of the patient shows nonrecordable ERG confirming the diagnosis of retinitis pigmentosa

The common structural abnormalities include renal parenchymal cysts, calyceal clubbing, fetal lobulation, unilateral agenesis and dysplastic kidney. Learning disability, emotional disturbances and poor reasoning with obsessive compulsive trait may also be seen. Hypogonadism in males and delayed menarche in females is almost universal. Bardet-Biedl syndrome has been differentiated from the much rarer Laurence-Moon syndrome in which features like retinal pigmentary degeneration, mental retardation and hypogenitalism occur with a progressive spastic paraparesis. Polydactyly is usually not seen.

Leber's Congenital Amaurosis

Severe visual impairment, nystagmus with normal looking fundus in children less than one year of age without any other obvious cause is used as the diagnostic criterion for Leber's congenital amaurosis. Inheritance is autosomal recessive. Keratoconus, hyperopia and oculodigital sign are frequently seen in these patients. Fundus picture is near normal or in some cases tapetal reflex, retinal pigment epithelium granularity mild attenuation of retinal vessels, a bull's maculopathy or macular coloboma may be seen.

Other Genetic Disorders Associated With Night Blindness

Congenital Stationary Night Blindness

This group of disorders is classified into
1. Congenital stationary night blindness with normal fundi
2. Congenital stationary night blindness with abnormal fundi
   a. Oguchi's disease
   b. Fundus albipunctatus

Congenital stationary night blindness with normal fundi: It is a non-progressive disorder. Patient presents with difficulty of vision in the night with near normal visual acuity in daytime. Fundus examination is within normal limits. Inheritance may be autosomal recessive, autosomal dominant and X-linked recessive.

Investigations: Full-field ERG may be of two types:

Type 1 (Riggs type): Absent Scotopic ERG with reduced photopic response.

Type 2 (Schubert-Bornschein type): Negative wave on bright flash scotopic ERG due to absence of b-wave responsiveness (Fig. 32.24).

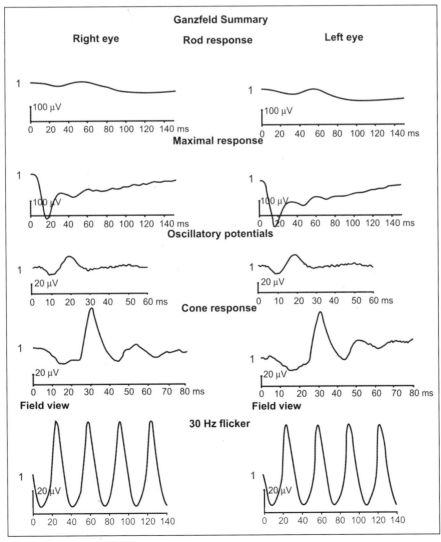

Fig. 32.24: Congenital stationary night blindness with normal fundi. Full-field ERG shows negative wave in the scotopic maximum combined response

Congenital stationary night blindness with abnormal fundi:

a. *Oguchi's disease:* Inheritance is autosomal recessive. Gene defects in the arrestin gene are associated with Oguchi's disease. Patient presents with the history of night blindness. Visual acuity remains unaffected. Fundus picture is characterized by a peculiar gray white discoloration of the retina giving it a metallic sheen (Figs 32.25A and B). This metallic sheen disappears after prolonged dark adaptation to reappear again on exposure to light (Mizuo's phenomenon). Full-field ERG responses show grossly reduced and delayed rod response and negative waveform in the combined response (Fig. 32.26).

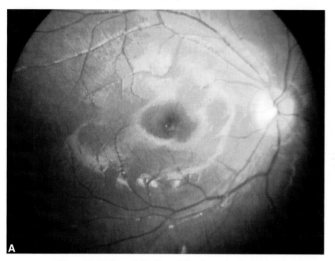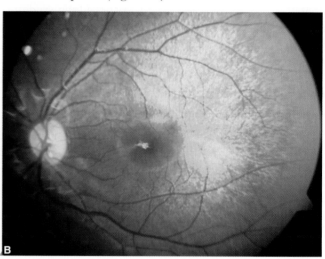

Figs 32.25A and B: Oguchi's disease. Color fundus photograph of the right and the left eye shows a peculiar gray white discoloration of the retina giving a metallic sheen

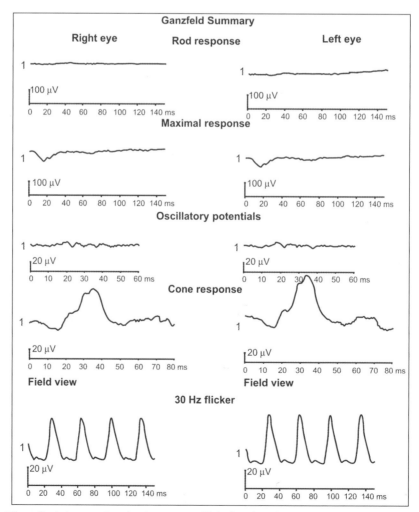

Fig. 32.26: Full-field ERG of the patient shows reduced rod response with both reduced amplitude and markedly increased implicit time. Negative waveform in the scotopic combined response is seen

b. *Fundus albipunctatus:* This also is a nonprogressive disorder. Nyctalopia is the only presenting feature. Visual acuity is usually preserved. Fundus picture reveals innumerable tiny white dots all over the fundus from the periphery to the center (Figs 32.27A to 32.29 B). Retinal vessels that are of normal caliber distinguish it from retinitis punctata albescence. Optic disc is unaffected; bony spicules are not seen. Delay in the regeneration of rhodopsin is the underlying pathology. Extensive dysfunction in the cone and rod system may be seen. On full-field ERG, a prolonged time for dark adaptation is required to produce normal amplitude electroretinograms in patients with fundus albipunctatus (Fig. 32.30).

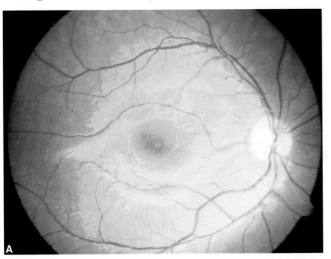
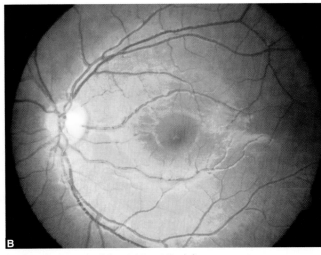

Figs 32.27A and B: Fundus albipunctatus. Color fundus photograph of the right and the left eye. Optic disc, macula and the retinal blood vessels are normal

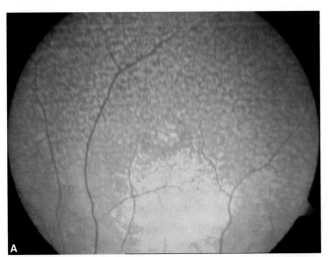
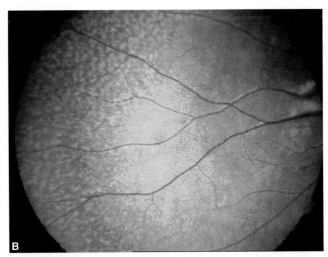

Figs 32.28A and B: Superior and nasal quadrants with innumerable tiny white dots extending from posterior pole to the periphery

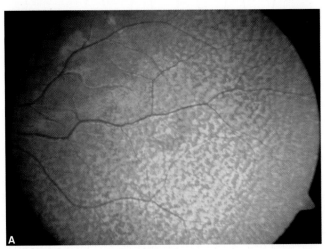
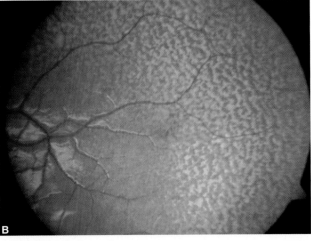

Figs 32.29A and B: Inferotemporal and superotemporal quadrants with yellowish dots

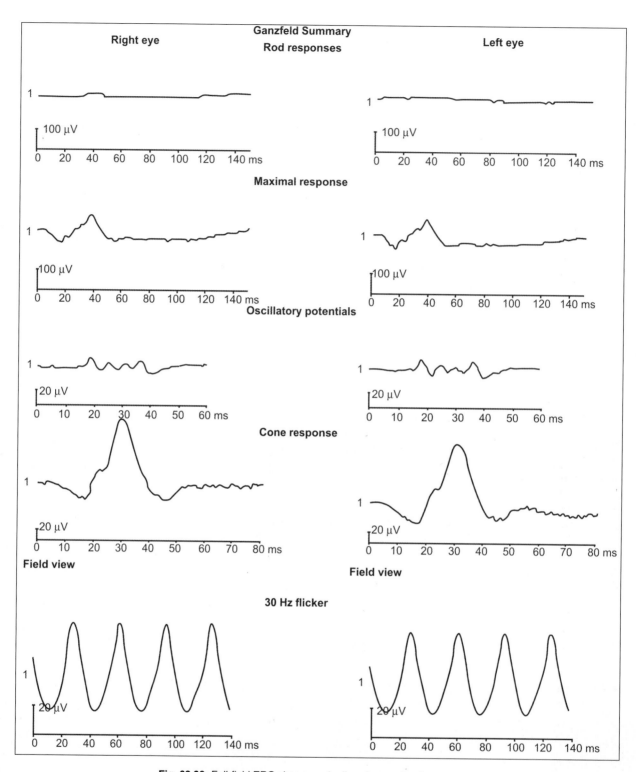

Fig. 32.30: Full-field ERG shows markedly subnormal rod responses

Progressive Cone Dystrophy

Introduction

Mode of inheritance is usually autosomal dominant with the onset of symptoms in early childhood.

Clinical Presentation

Presenting symptoms include diminution of vision, photo aversion, nystagmus and color vision defects. Photophobia and nystagmus though can be early signs of the disease; they are seen to diminish with increasing age.

Fundus examination can vary from near normal fundus to a classic bull's eye lesion in the macular region (Figs 32.31A to 32.32 B). Mild temporal pallor as well as mild arteriolar attenuation may be seen as the disease becomes more manifest.

Investigations

Fluorescein angiography: Presence of window defects corresponding to the area of RPE atrophy is seen at the posterior pole. In cases with bull's eye lesion, it may take the form of alternating rings of hyper fluorescence and hypofluorescence at the macular area (Figs 32.33 A to C).

Electroretinogram: In early stages may show mildly reduced photopic response. As the disease progresses the photopic response are markedly attenuated in ffERG and mfERG (Figs 32.34A and B and 32.35).

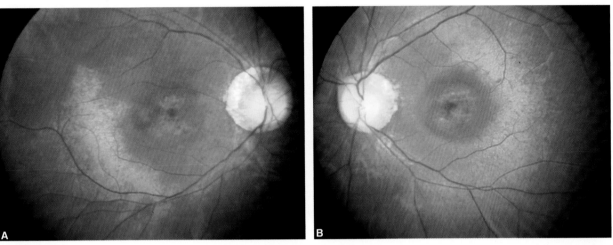

Figs 32.31A and B: Progressive cone dystrophy. Color fundus photograph of a patient presenting with blurring of vision and photophobia. A bull's eye like lesion is seen at the macula with a Mizuo-like metallic sheen. Mild temporal disc pallor and attenuation of the arterioles is evident

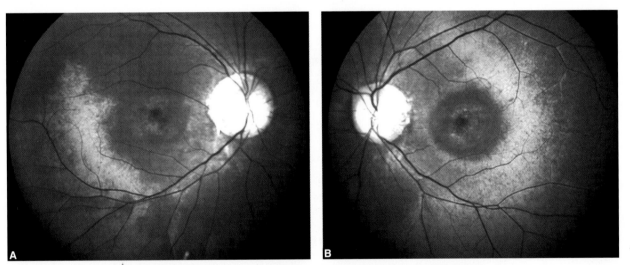

Figs 32.32A and B: Red free photograph highlights the macular lesion and tapetal reflex

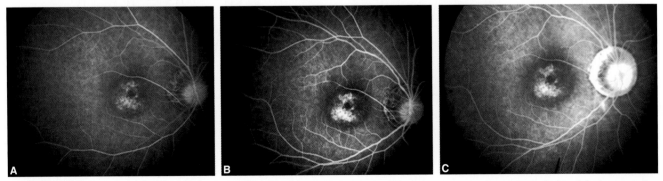

Figs 32.33A to C: Fluorescein angiography shows hypofluorescent center with a ring of hyperfluorescence due to transmission defects suggestive of bull's eye maculopathy. No changes are seen at the site of the tapetal reflex. Fluorescein angiography may sometimes pick up subtle retinal pigment epithelium alteration at the macula, which are not otherwise be visible on fundus examination

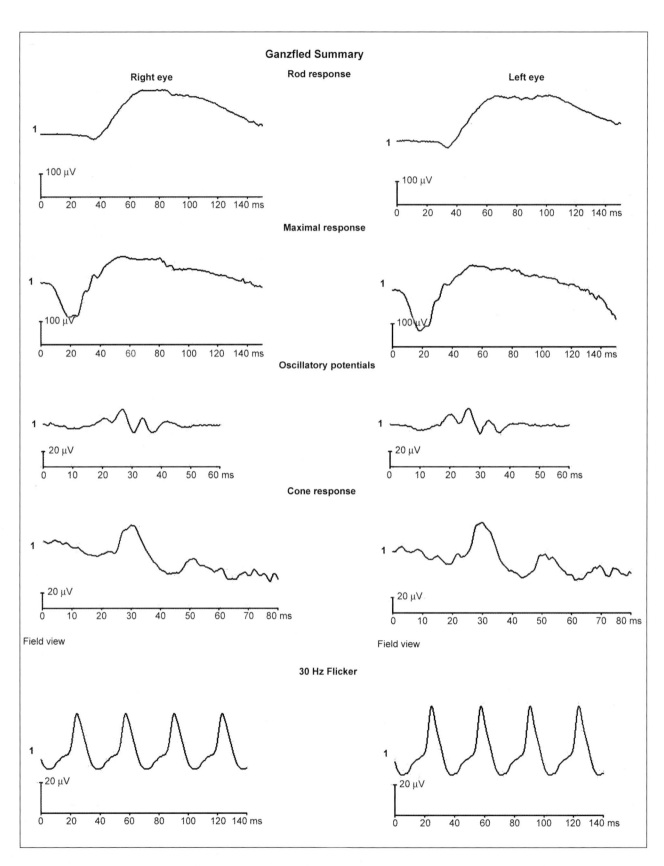

Fig. 32.34A

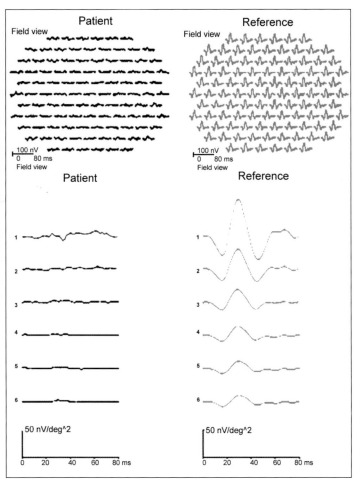

Fig. 32.34B

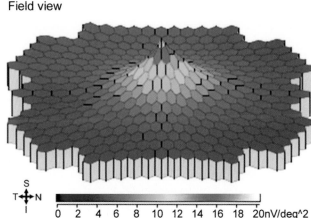

Fig. 32.35: 3-D topographical plot reveals markedly reduced responses

Figs 32.34A and B: (A) Full-field ERG showing subnormal cones. Rod responses are normal (B) Reduced multifocal responses in all the rings differentiate it from other macular dystrophies

Optical coherence tomography: Foveal thinning is seen corresponding to the bull's eye maculopathy.

Visual fields: Central scotoma is seen with the peripheral fields unaffected in the early stages of the disease.

Cone Rod Dystrophy

Introduction

Cone rod dystrophy is characterized by primary cone involvement, or, sometimes, by concomitant loss of both cones and rods.

Clinical Presentation

The predominant symptoms of cone rod dystrophy include decreased visual acuity, color vision defects, photoaversion and decreased sensitivity in the central visual field, later followed by progressive loss in peripheral vision and night blindness. The clinical course of cone rod dystrophy is generally more severe and rapid than that of rod cone dystrophy, leading to earlier legal blindness and disability. Fundus picture is similar to that of cone dystrophy in the early stages of the disease with the presence of temporal optic disc pallor, attenuation of the arterioles and macular atrophy (Figs 32.36A to 32.37 B). Late stages of the disease may show mild pigment alteration in the periphery similar to that seen in patients with retinitis pigmentosa.

Investigations

Fluorescein angiography: Widespread retinal pigment epithelium granularity is revealed (Figs 32.38A and B).

Electroretinogram: Involvement of the rod and the cone system is seen in ffERG and mfERG once the disease is fully blown (Figs 32.39A and B and 32.40).

Optical coherence tomography: Foveal thinning can be appreciated.

Visual fields: Central scotoma with ring and paracentral scotoma seen in the late stages of the disease.

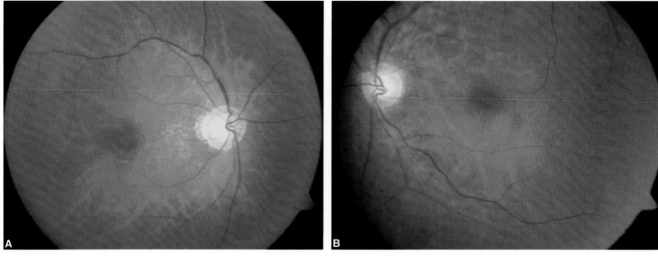

Figs 32.36A and B: Cone rod dystrophy. Fundus photograph of the right and the left eye shows temporal pallor of the disc with mild arteriolar attenuation and retinal pigment epithelium granularity in the periphery

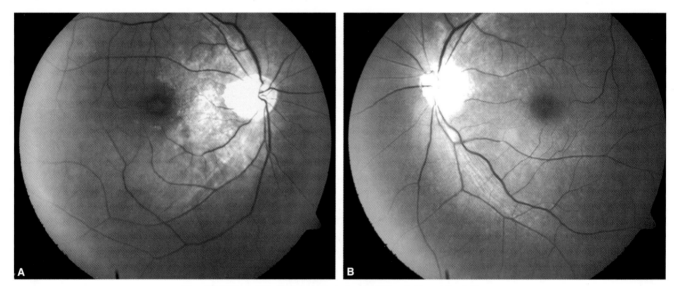

Figs 32.37A and B: Red free photograph of the right and the left eye

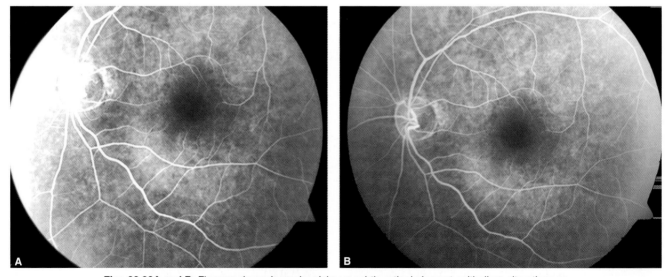

Figs 32.38A and B: Fluorescein angiography picks up subtle retinal pigment epithelium alterations as hyperfluorescence in the mid arteriovenous phase

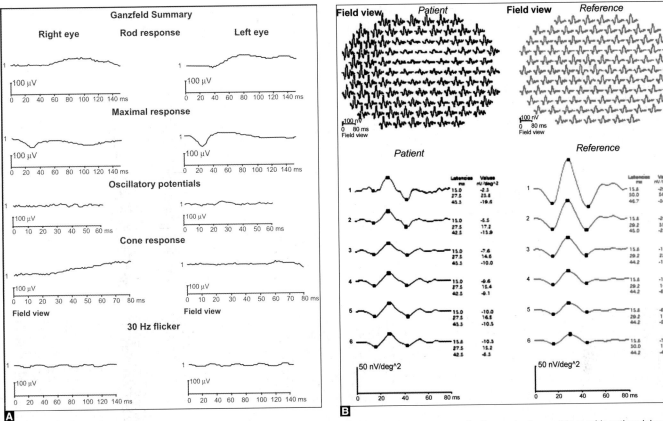

Figs 32.39A and B: (A) Full-field ERG revealed grossly reduced rod and combined responses under the scotopic conditions with extinguished photopic responses (B) Trace array reveals markedly reduced responses both in the central as well as peripheral rings

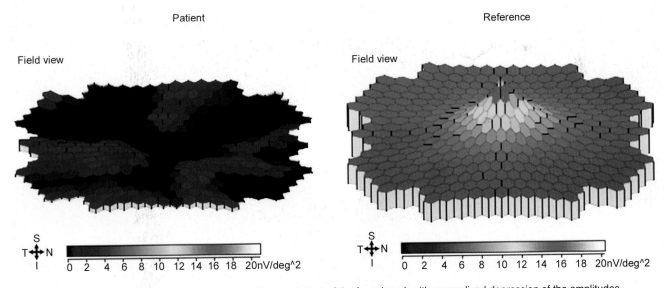

Fig. 32.40: 3D-topographical map on mfERG reveals loss of the foveal peak with generalized depression of the amplitudes

RETINAL PIGMENT EPITHELIUM

Stargardt's Dystrophy

Introduction

Inheritance is usually autosomal recessive. The most commonly identified gene for Stargardt's macular dystrophy is the ATP-binding transporter gene (ABCA4 gene), which is mapped to the short arm of the chromosome 1.

Clinical Presentation

Patients usually present in the first or the second decade of life with complain of gradual decrease in vision. There is no history of night blindness. The visual acuity may range from 6/60–6/9 depending upon the stage of the disease. Fundus picture is that of a well defined horizontally ovoid atrophic area (beaten bronze appearance) seen at the macula with or without few surrounding yellowish flecks (Figs 32.41A to 32.42 B). Optic disc and the retinal vessels are healthy. This is an important differentiating feature from the cone dystrophy, which in early stages of the disease may appear similar. Stargardt's disease and fundus flavimaculatus have been considered by many, as different morphological or phenotypic expression of the same disease.

Investigations

Fluorescein angiography: Central ovoid area of dystrophy is seen as hyperfluorescent because of the transmission defects. "Silent choroids" is due to the presence of abnormal lipofuscin like material, which gets deposited in the retinal pigment epithelium layer in these patients (Figs 32.43 A to 32.44 C). Though it is considered a pathognomic sign it may not be seen in all the cases of Stargardt's disease. The flecks may show hyperfluorescence in the late stages of the disease because of the overlying retinal pigment epithelium atrophy.

Electroretinogram: In patients with lesions confined to the posterior pole, the electroretinogram and electrooculogram are usually normal (Fig. 32.45) though color vision is affected in the early stages of the disease. MfERG is useful to detect central retinal dysfunction in Stargardt's macular dystrophy especially in patients with minimal fundus changes in which diagnosis of Stargardt's macular dystrophy may be difficult (Figs 32.46 and 32.47).

Optical coherence tomography: Increased reflectivity of the retinal pigment epithelium in the macular area due to lipofuscin deposits is observed (Fig. 32.48).

Visual fields: Central relative or absolute scotoma may be seen depending upon the severity of the disease. Peripheral fields remain unaffected.

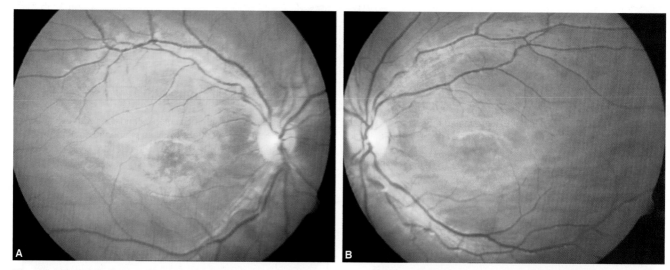

Figs 32.41A and B: Stargardt's dystrophy. Color fundus photograph of the right and the left eye shows atrophic macula with a tapetal reflex or bronze metal beaten appearance. Discs, vessels and periphery are normal

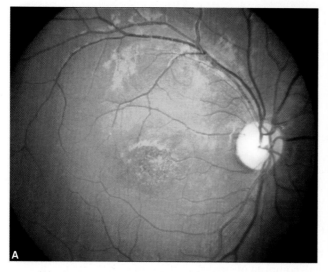
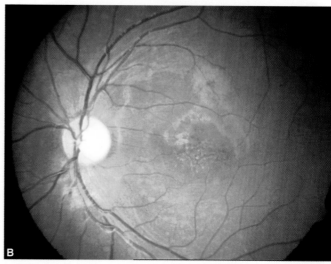

Figs 32.42A and B: Stargardt's dystrophy. (A) Color fundus photograph of the right eye with an atrophic macula and tapetal reflex (B) Color fundus photograph of the left eye of the patient with similar features .Very few flecks are seen

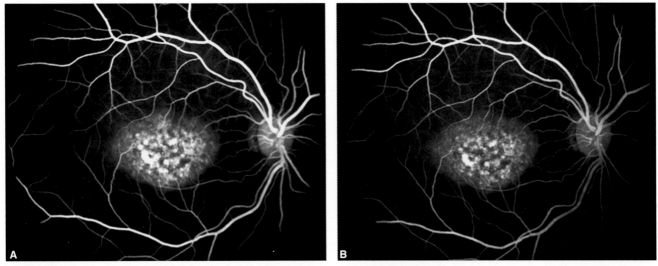

Figs 32.43A and B: Fluorescein angiography is characterized by the presence of silent choroids or the absence of the normal choroidal flush. Few irregular hyperfluorescent flecks are seen within the lesion

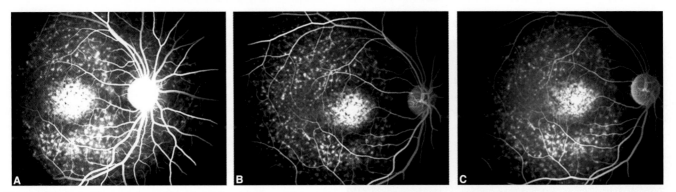

Figs 32.44A to C: Fluorescein angiography of the right eye of the same patient. Numerous flecks with early hyperfluorescence, which fades in the late phases are seen

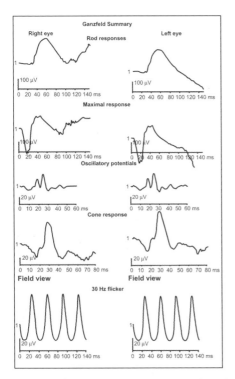

Fig. 32.45: ffERG is normal under both scotopic and photopic conditions

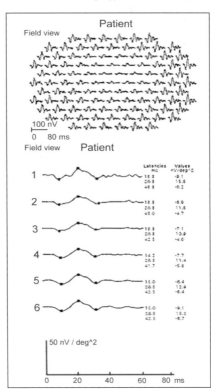

Fig. 32.46: Trace mfERG of the right eye reveals reduced amplitudes especially in the central rings

Patient

Reference

Field view

Field view

S
T✛N
I
0 2 4 6 8 10 12 14 16 18 20nV/deg^2

S
T✛N
I
0 2 4 6 8 10 12 14 16 18 20nV/deg^2

Fig. 32.47: 3-D mfERG showing inverted crater like appearance typical of Stargardt's disease

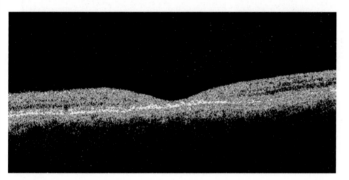

Fig. 32.48: Optical coherence tomography of the right eye showing increased reflectivity of the retinal pigment epithelium in the macular area due to lipofuscin deposits seen in Stargardt's disease

Fundus Flavimaculatus

Introduction

The term was first coined by Franceschetti in 1953 who first described the disorder. Inheritance of fundus flavimaculatus is autosomal recessive. ABCA4 gene mutation has been commonly associated in these patients as well.

Clinical Presentation

Patients usually present in the first or the second decade of life. Fundus picture is that of bilaterally symmetrical yellowish crescent shaped flecks (Figs 32.49A and B). These flecks may be present up to the equator. The degree of visual acuity loss and

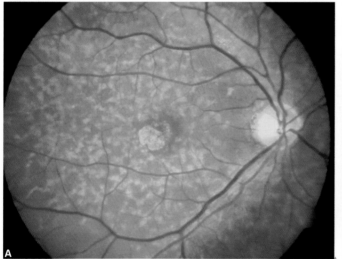

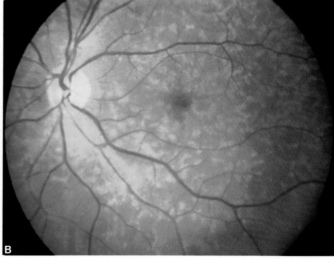

Figs 32.49A and B: Fundus flavimaculatus. (A) Color fundus photograph of the right eye shows atrophic macula with multiple irregular surrounding flecks at the posterior pole as well as beyond the arcades (B) Color fundus photograph of the left eye. Retinal pigment epithelium alterations at the macula is seen with surrounding flecks

color vision will depend upon the extent of macular involvement. Optic disc and the retinal vessels remain normal throughout the course of the disease. Morphologic changes and retinal function deterioration are more severe in patients with fundus flavimaculatus than in patients with Stargardt's macular dystrophy. The duration of the disease has a greater effect on patients with fundus flavimaculatus than on patients with Stargardt's macular dystrophy.

Investigations

Fluorescein angiography: Hyperfluorescence corresponding to the area of the flecks is seen. Usually the number of flecks seen on fluorescein is more than those seen on fundus picture (Figs

32.50A to C). Autofluorescence is usually high in patients with fundus flavimaculatus. Autofluorescence patterns in many studies have been shown to relate to functional abnormalities seen in these patients.

Electroretinogram and electrooculogram: They remain unaffected in the majority of the cases. Some cases may reveal subnormal photopic and scotopic responses in ffERG (Fig. 32.51). Multifocal ERG reveals mild to moderate generalized reduction of amplitude (Figs 32.52A and B).

Visual fields: Visual fields are usually unaffected.

Optical coherence tomography: Thickened retinal pigment epithelium may be revealed.

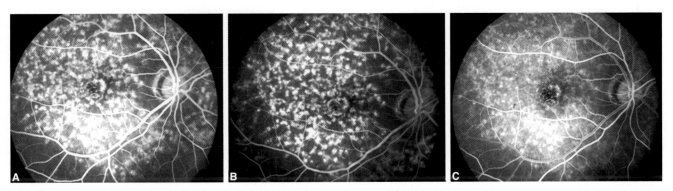

Figs 32.50A to C: Fluorescein angiography of the right eye shows transmitted fluorescence in the region of the flecks, which fades away in the late phase. Silent choroid is seen in the peripapillary region, in between the flecks and in the periphery

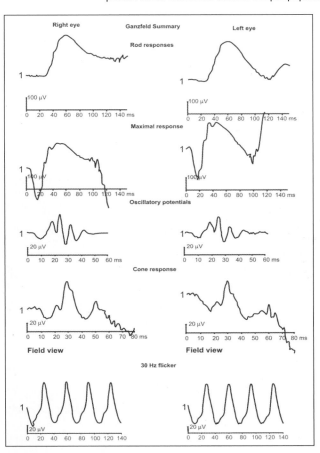

Fig. 32.51: Normal full field ERG

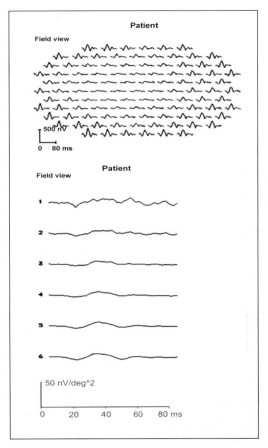

Fig. 32.52A: Trace arrays of the right eye with ring averages showing reduced amplitudes in all eccentricities

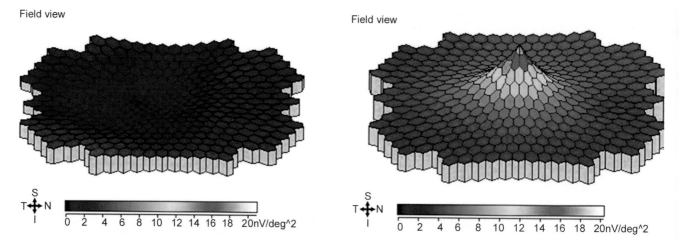

Fig. 32.52 B: Topographical display of the multifocal amplitudes showing generalized decrease in amplitudes at the posterior pole

Differential diagnosis of the fleck retina:
- Fundus albipunctatus
- Dominant drusen
- Multiple vitelliform disease
- Benign fleck retina syndrome.

Benign Fleck Retina Syndrome

Affected patients are asymptomatic with normal visual acuity (Fig. 32.53A to I).

Electrophysiological tests and visual fields are relatively unaffected.

Best's Disease or Vitelliform Dystrophy

Introduction

Inheritance is autosomal dominant with variable penetrance. Best's disease is caused by the VMD2 gene, which has been mapped to the chromosome 11q13. This gene codes for the protein bestrophin. Defective bestrophin disrupts the normal fluid transport across the retinal pigment epithelium resulting in a generalized retinal pigment epithelial abnormality that results in an abnormal accumulation of lipofuscin granules within the retinal pigment epithelium, macrophages in the subretinal space and within the choroid.

Clinical Presentation

Patient may be symptomless in early stages with diagnosis made on routine examination. Gradual decrease in vision is seen as the disease advances. Visual acuity and color vision may be normal in early stages of the disease. Fundus examination reveals a bilaterally similar picture. The macular features may differ depending upon the stage of the disease. The various stages described in the evolution of the disease include

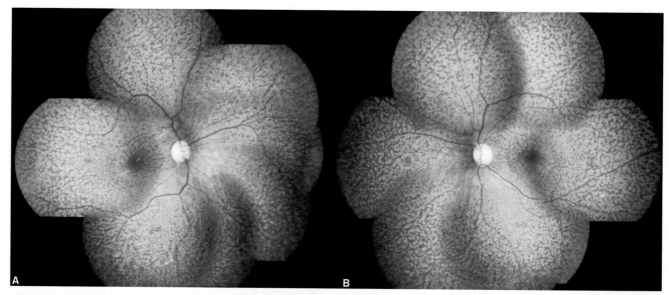

Figs 32.53A and B: Benign fleck retina syndrome. Color montage of the right and the left eye showing innumerable flecks scattered throughout the fundus

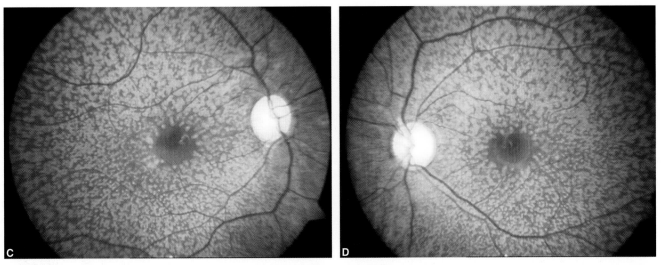

Figs 32.53C and D: Fundus photograph of the right and left eye shows yellowish white flecks; fovea is spared

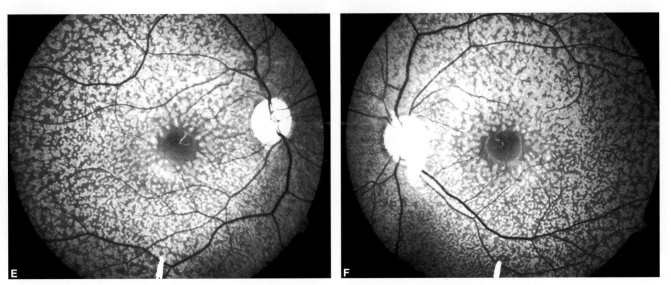

Figs 32.53E and F: Red free photograph of the same patient shows numerous flecks

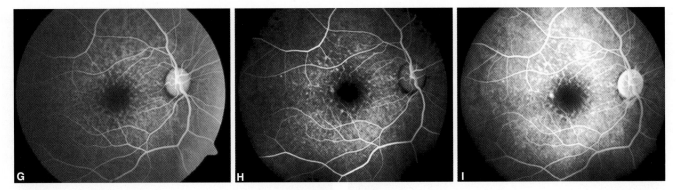

Figs 32.53G to I: FFA of the same patient shows irregular hyperfluorescence at the level of the flecks due to transmission defects

Stage 0: Normal fovea is seen in the early stages of the disease. EOG may be subnormal.

Stage 1: Previtelliform stage: A few yellowish spots may be seen at the fovea.

Stage 2: Vitelliform stage: It is a classically round and elevated lesion like an egg yellow (sunny side up) due to collection of lipofuscin in the retinal pigment epithelium (Fig. 32.54 A).

Stage 3: Scrambled-egg stage: It is formed by the disintergration of the vitelliform stage. This is usually associated with a decrease in vision (Fig. 32.54 B).

Stage 4: Cyst stage: It is observed when a fluid level appears with in the lesion due to the disintergration of its contents. This formation of a fluid level mimics a hypopyon and hence is called the pseudohypopyon stage (Fig. 32.54 C).

Stage 5: Atrophic stage: It is seen as the end stage in the older age groups. It is associated with a well defined area of chorioretinal atrophy (Figs 32.54D to 32.55 D).

Usually a single lesion is seen in these patients. However, multiple vitelliform lesions may also be seen in some individuals called as the "multiple vitelliform disease". Some subjects may have a late presentation or the "adult onset vitelliform disease".

Investigations

Fluorescein angiography: In the early stages of the disease, blocked choroidal fluorescence because of the presence of the lipofuscin pigment is observed. However, in the late stages of the disease hyperfluorescence may become evident due to the atrophy of the overlying retinal pigment epithelium (Figs 32.55 C to E). Angiogram is vital for the recognition and treatment of choroidal neovascularization, which may also be seen in this disease.

Electrooculogram: The Arden's ratio may be markedly reduced even in the presence of a normal electroretinogram (Fig. 32.55 F).

Electroretinogram: Full-field ERG remains unaffected (Fig. 32.55 G). Multifocal ERG amplitude decrease of the central response is usually correlated with visual acuity loss (Fig. 32.55 H and I). Multifocal ERG may serve as an indicator of the extent of retinal dysfunction. ERG and EOG helps to differentiate Best's disease especially the atrophic stage, from other forms of maculopathies like the cone-rod dystrophy and Stargardt's dystrophy.

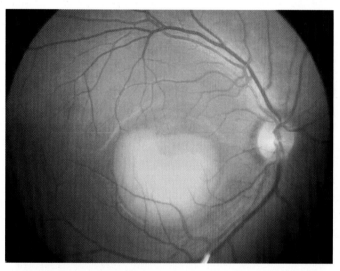

Fig 32.54A: Best's disease. Vitelliform stage shows egg yolk appearance on fundus examination

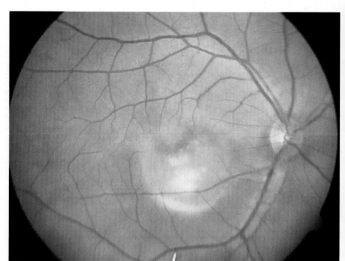

Fig. 32.54B: Vitelliruptive stage

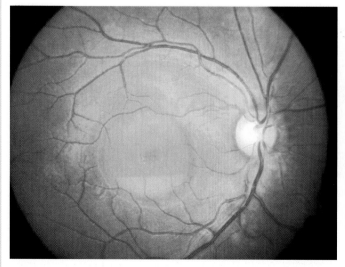

Fig. 32.54C: Pseudohypopyon stage: As the yellowish material disrupts the vitelliruptive stage and pseudohypopyon stage sets in

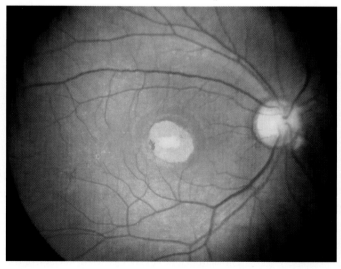

Fig. 32.54D: Atrophic stage is marked by the prominence of the large choroidal vessels

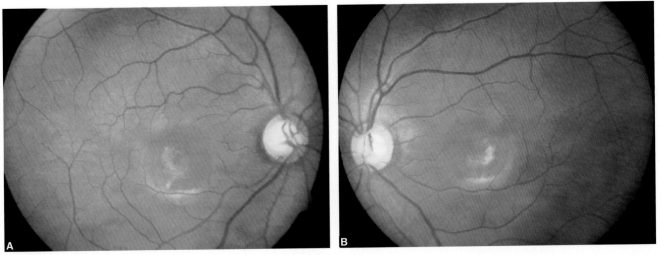

Figs 32.55A and B: Best's disease. Fundus photograph of the right and the left eye showing bilaterally symmetrical, well demarcated, round lesion at the posterior pole with few yellowish subretinal deposits suggestive of the vitelliruptive stage. Arden's ratio on electrooculogram was markedly reduced

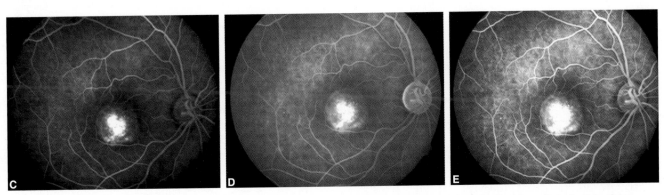

Figs 32.55C to E: Fluorescein angiography shows early hyperfluorescence with staining of the subretinal deposits in the late phase

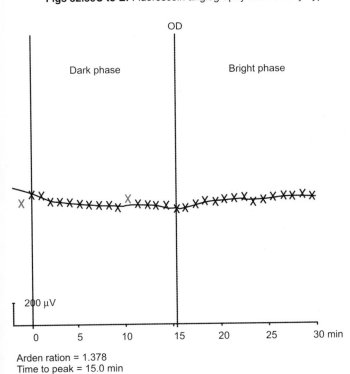

Arden ration = 1.378
Time to peak = 15.0 min

Fig. 32.55F: Electrooculogram of the same patient with an Arden's ratio of 1.378

Subretinal choroidal neovascular membrane is seen as a complication in some individuals (Figs 32.56A to F). Hence, these patients should be on regular follow-up to look for this complication.

Pattern Dystrophy

Introduction

Inheritance of pattern dystrophy is autosomal dominant inheritance with variable penetrance. Mutations in peripherin/RDS have been postulated by many to be associated with pattern dystrophy.

Clinical Presentation

Patients present with a moderate loss of vision in fourth to fifth decades of life. Metamorphopsia may be the presenting feature in some patients. It is characterized by the presence of bilaterally symmetrical picture of subretinal deposits at the fovea (Figs 32.57 A to D). These deposits form variable shapes giving rise to the typical pattern. In some cases the deposits may be

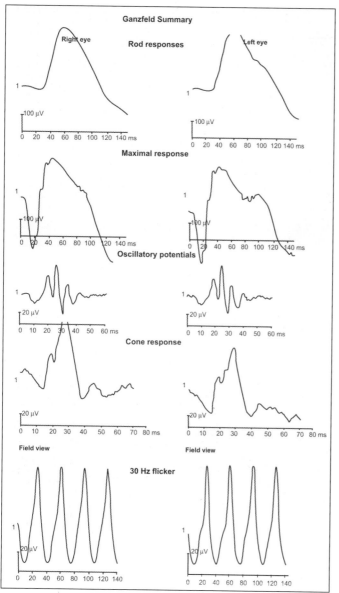

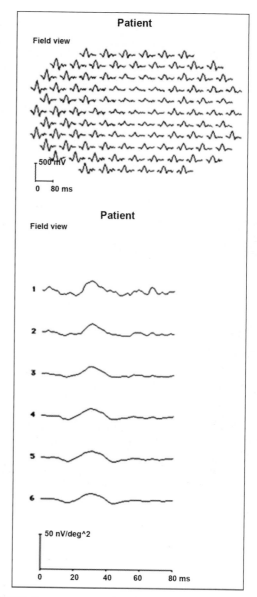

Fig. 32.55G: Normal full field ERG of the same patient

Fig. 32.55H: Trace array reveals reduced P1 amplitudes especially in central 5-10 degrees. Implicit times are normal

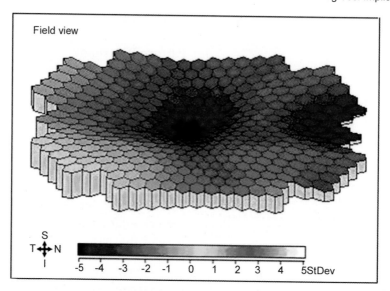

Fig. 32.55 I: 3-D topographical map shows central reduced responses

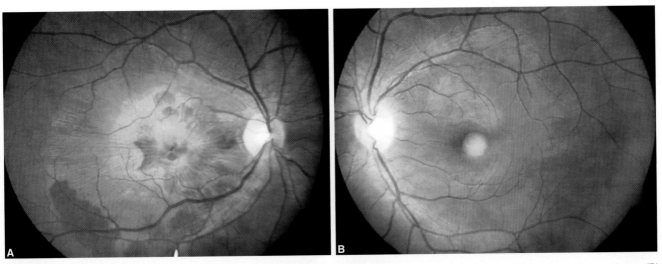

Figs 32.56A and B: (A) Best's disease. Color fundus photograph of the right eye shows classic subfoveal choroidal neovascular membrane (B) Color fundus photograph of the left eye shows well-defined vitelliform lesion

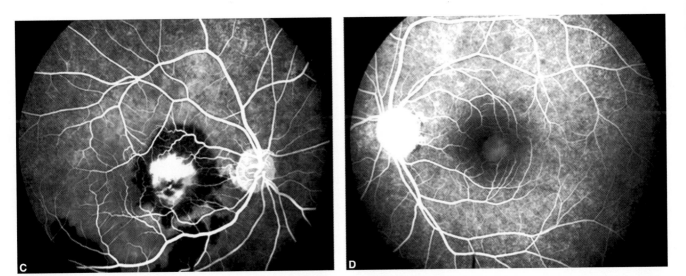

Figs 32.56C and D: (C) Fluorescein angiography of the right eye with intense hyperfluorescence of the lesion with fuzzy margins. Blocked fluorescence is seen due to subretinal blood (D) Fluorescein angiography of the left eye reveals mild hyperfluorescence of the vitelliform lesion

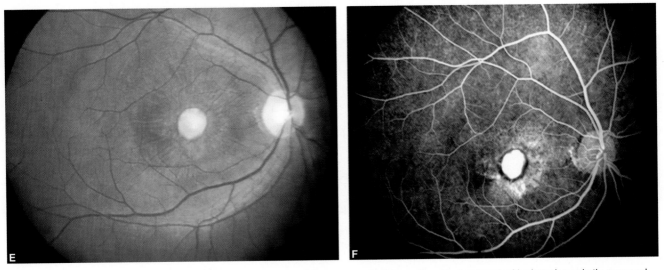

Figs 32.56E and F: (E) Color fundus photograph of the right of the same patient 6 months after treatment with photodynamic therapy and bevacizumab (F) Fluorescein angiography of the right eye post treatment showing marked decrease in leakage. Staining is seen in the late phase

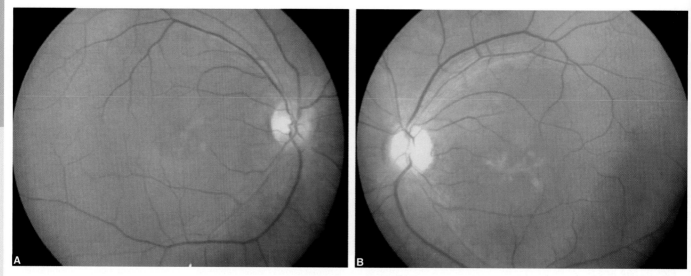

Figs 32.57A and B: Pattern dystrophy. Fundus photograph of the right eye shows subtle irregular subretinal deposits at the macula (B) Fundus photograph of the left eye shows similar subretinal deposits

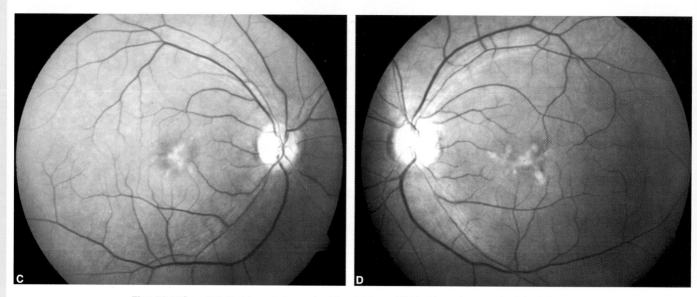

Figs 32.57C and D: Red free photograph of the right eye (D) Red free photograph of the left eye

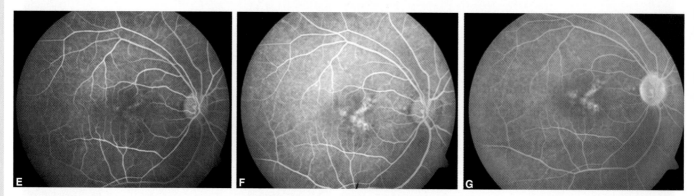

Figs 32.57E to G: Fluorescein angiography of the right eye. Central area of hypofluorescence is seen with radiating spokes like picture. A particular pattern is seen in the arteriovenous phase

present in the form of radiating lines. Macular atrophy is the cause of moderate visual loss in these patients.

Investigations

Fluorescein angiography: Deposition of the yellowish material in the subretinal space blocks choroidal fluorescence giving rise to the pattern on angiogram. The pattern thus formed is usually bilaterally symmetrical (Figs 32.57E to G).

Subfoveal choroidal neovascularization can be associated with eyes affected by the pattern dystrophy of the retinal pigment epithelium. Fluorescein angiography and OCT is vital for the follow-up of these patients.

Electroretinogram and electrooculogram: They are normal in these patients.

Visual fields: Visual fields are not affected other than an increase in the sensitivity of the central responses.

Dominant Cystoid Macular Dystrophy

Introduction

Dominant cystoid macular dystrophy is inherited as an autosomal dominant disorder.

Clinical Presentation

Clinical picture is that of bilaterally symmetrical picture of cystoid macular edema in a young patient without an underlying pathology. There is a moderate decrease in vision to begin with which may worsen with age.

Investigations

Fluorescein angiography: It may reveal leakage and hyperfluorescence from the perimacular capillaries.

Electroretinogram: Electroretinogram is normal though EOG may be slightly subnormal.

Optical coherence tomography: The presence of the cystic spaces at the macula may be revealed.

Dominant Drusen

Introduction

Dominant drusen is called Doyne honeycomb retinal dystrophy (DHRD), and malattia leventinese. Inheritance of this disorder is autosomal dominant with variable penetrance. The causative gene EFEMP1 has been mapped to the chromosome 2p16-21.

Clinical Presentation

Extreme variability is seen in the clinical expression of this dominant form of drusen and macular degeneration. Most subjects have fine macular drusen and good vision. It may be discovered on routine fundus examination. Frequent presenting symptoms include blurring of vision with or without metamorphopsia. Progression of the disease in late adulthood with

moderate visual loss may be seen in few affected individuals. Subjects may present in the second to third decades of life or later with symptoms of metamorphopsia with the development of choroidal neovascular membrane. Fundus picture is characterized by the presence of a large number of discreet, well defined hard drusen scattered all over the posterior pole. Usually these drusen are also seen nasal to the disc (Figs 32.58A and B). Visual acuity and color vision remain unaffected in most of the cases.

Investigations

Fluorescein angiography: Fluorescein angiography shows hyperfluorescent window defects due to RPE atrophy (Figs 32.59 A to N).

Electroretinogram and electrooculogram: They are normal (Figs 32.58 C to E).

Optical coherence tomography: Bumpy retinal pigment epithelium is revealed suggestive of macular drusen (Figs 32.59 O and P).

Visual fields: Visual fields remain unaffected.

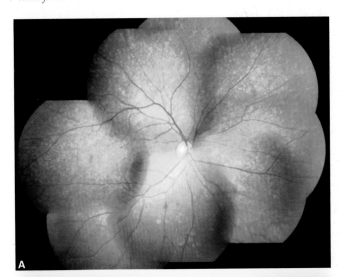

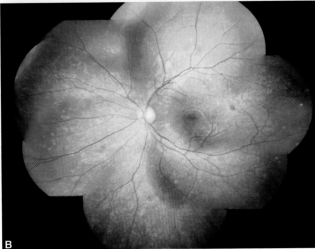

Figs 32.58A and B: Dominant drusen. Color montage of the right and the left eye show bilaterally symmetrical numerous white flecks or spots in the deep retinal layers spread all over the posterior pole suggestive of drusen

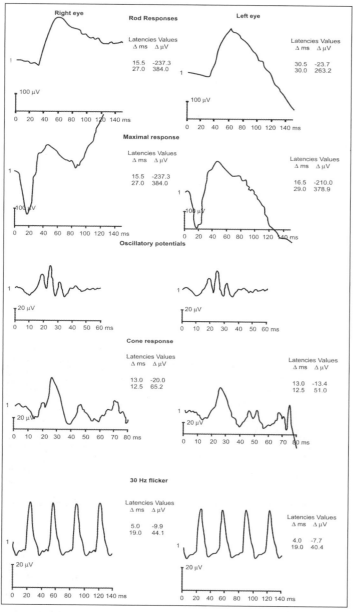

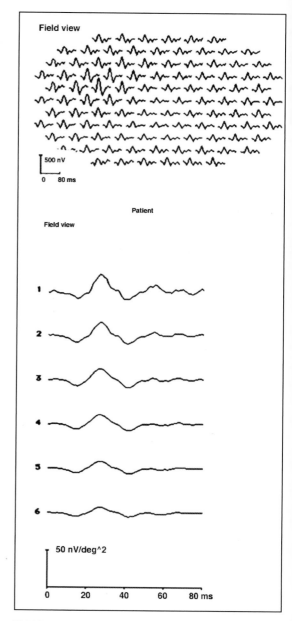

Fig. 32.58C: Full field ERG of the patient is normal

Fig. 32.58D: Trace array of the same patient shows reduced responses in all eccentricities

Fig. 32.58E: 3-D topographical map of the left eye of the patient shows foveal peak shifted (eccentric fixation)

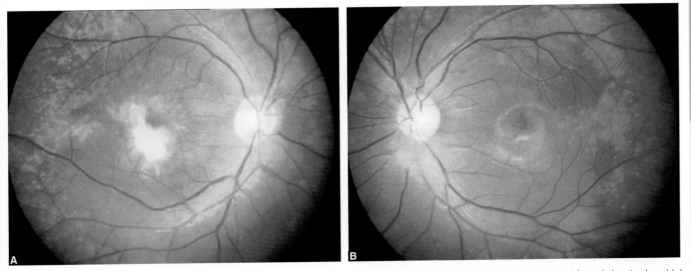

Figs 32.59A and B: (A) Dominant drusen. Color fundus photograph of the right eye shows peripheral drusen with scarred subfoveal classic choroidal neovascular membrane (B) Color fundus photograph of the left eye of the same patient with peripheral drusen and small active subfoveal classic choroidal neovascular membrane

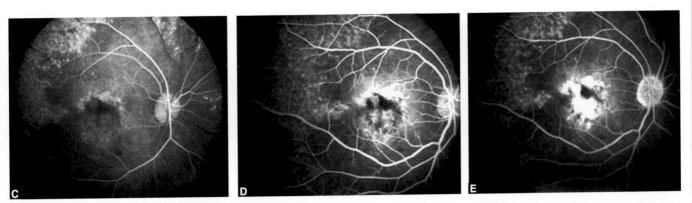

Figs 32.59C to E: Fluorescein angiography of the right eye shows scarred choroidal neovascular membrane with staining in the late phase

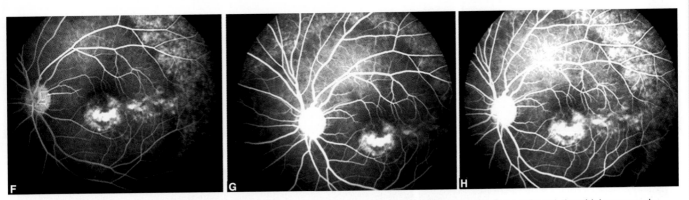

Figs 32.59F to H: Fluorescein angiography of the left eye of the same patient showing well defined active subfoveal choroidal neovascular membrane with early hyperfluorescence and leakage in the late phase

BRUCH'S MEMBRANE

Sorsby Pseudoinflammatory Dystrophy

Introduction

It is a rare disorder. Inheritance is autosomal dominant with complete penetrance. The causative gene has been recognized to be TIMP3 (Tissue inhibitor of metalloproteinase 3) mapped on the chromosome 22q12.13. The underlying pathology of the disease is believed to be the sclerosis and atrophy of the choroidal vessels with multiple ruptures in the Bruch's membrane which predisposes to the formation of the subretinal neovascularization.

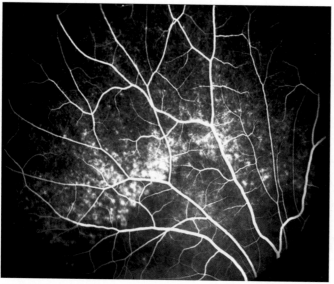

Fig. 32.59 I: Dot like hyperfluorescence in the superonasal quadrant is observed because of drusen

Clinical Presentation

The disease presentation is acute at about 40 years of age. Fundus picture is characterized by the presence of hemorrhages and exudates in the central retina to begin with. Retinal pigment epithelial atrophy is seen. The exudative stage is followed by the cicatricial stage. Peripheral involvement is seen late in the course of the disease.

Investigations

Fluorescein angiography: In early stages of the disease hyperfluorescence is seen due to leakage and the late stages of the disease window defects due to the loss of RPE and choriocapillaries appear as hyperfluorescence. Large choroidal vessels are seen.

Visual fields: Visual fields show presence of a large central scotoma which enlarges as the disease progresses.

Electroretinogram: Electroretinogram is normal initially; late stages however show subnormal photopic as well as scotopic responses.

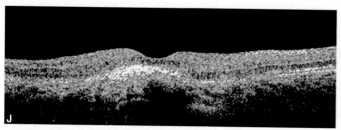
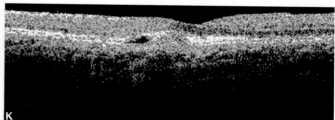

Figs 32.59J and K: (J) Optical coherence tomography of the right eye shows a subfoveal scarred choroidal neovascular membrane (K) Optical coherence tomography of the left eye showing a small subfoveal choroidal neovascular membrane with subretinal fluid

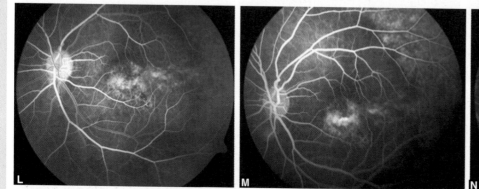
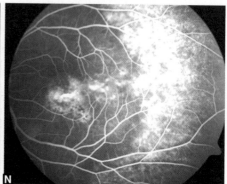

Figs 32.59L to N: Fluorescein angiography of the left eye posttreatment shows decrease in the leakage

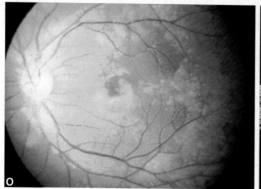
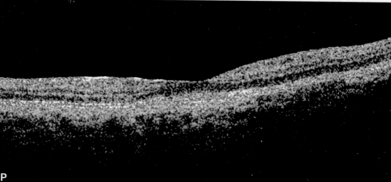

Figs 32.59 O and P: (O) Color fundus photograph of the patient posttreatment with photodynamic therapy and intravitreal bevacizumab (P) Optical coherence tomography of the left eye of the same patient 3 months after PDT with bevacizumab shows decrease in subretinal fluid

Angioid Streaks

Introduction

These are found associated with several conditions like pseudoxanthoma elasticum, osteitis deformans, sickle cell anemia and Ehlers-Danlos syndrome. Mode of inheritance depends upon the associated disease process.

Clinical Presentation

Angioid streaks usually develop in the second or third decade of life. Patient is usually symptomless unless there is development of choroidal neovascular membrane or subretinal hemorrhage. Presenting symptom then includes drop in vision and metamorphopsia. Growth of choroidal neovascular membrane occurs through the breaks in the Bruch's membrane. Choroidal neovascular membranes seen in patients with angioid streaks are recurrent and typically classic (Figs 32.60 A to D). Visual acuity is normal in the absence of a choroidal neovascular membrane unless the angioid streaks is seen to pass through the macula.

Investigations

Fluorescein angiography: Hyperfluorescence along the angioid streaks is seen in the arterial phase of the FFA due to window defects produced by the atrophic retinal pigment epithelium (Figs 32.60 E to G). Staining of the scleral margin is seen in the late phases. Once a choroidal neovascular membrane is seen, the features are typical of those of a choroidal neovascular membrane (Figs 32.60 H to J).

Visual fields: Visual fields are normal unless the condition is complicated by the presence of a choroidal neovascular membrane.

Electroretinogram: Electroretinogram remains unaffected throughout the course of the disease.

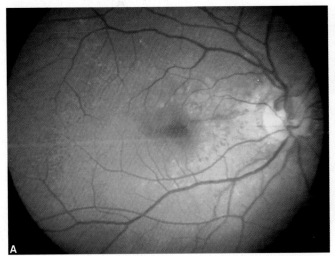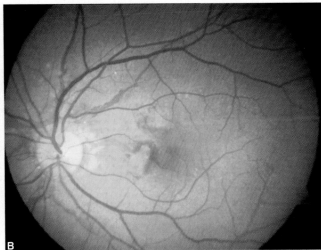

Figs 32.60A and B: (A) Angioid streaks. Color fundus photograph of the right eye reveals the presence of grayish crack like lines radiating from the disc (B) Color fundus photograph of the left eye with similar radiating lines

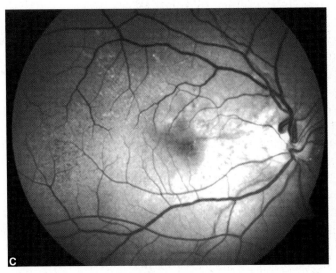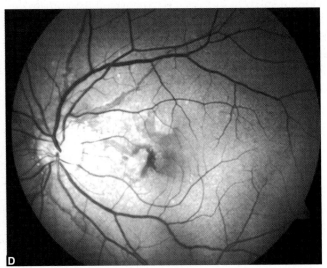

Figs 32.60C and D: (C) Red free photograph of the right eye (D) Red free photograph of the left eye

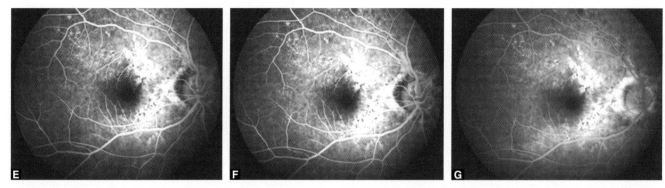

Figs 32.60E to G: Fluorescein angiography of the right eye of the patient with hyperfluorescent lines are seen radiating from the disc

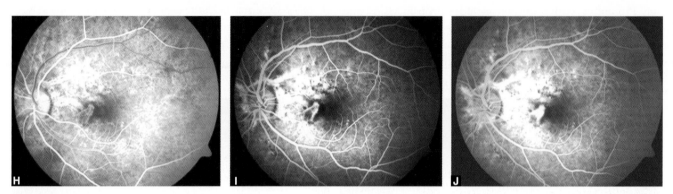

Figs 32.60H to J: Fluorescein angiography of the left eye with angioid streaks with a well defined classic choroidal neovascular membrane

CHOROID

Central Areolar Choroidal Dystrophy

Introduction

Central areolar choroidal dystrophy is inherited as autosomal dominant /autosomal recessive.

Clinical Presentation

Patients present with decrease in central vision in the fourth to sixth decades of life. Fundus examination reveals bilaterally symmetrical well-defined area of atrophy, which grows centrifugally with age. Atrophy of the neurosensory retina, retinal pigment epithelium and choroids is seen in these areas (Figs 32.61A and B). Central areolar choroidal dystrophy has been further classified into:
- Central choriocapillaris dystrophy with atrophy primarily involving the smaller choriocapillaries.
- Central total choroidal vascular dystrophy involving all the layers of the choroids, including the larger choroidal vessels.
  The area of macular atrophy may assume a horseshoe shape sparing the fovea till the end stage of the disease, which may explain the relatively unaffected visual acuity even in advanced cases. Low visual aids may help to improve near vision.

Investigations

Electroretinogram: It may be normal in early stages, but late stages invariably show reduced photopic as well as scotopic responses.

Reduced P1 amplitudes are seen in the central macula compared with normals in mfERG. These reduced responses may extend beyond the area of atrophy visible ophthalmoscopically.

Fluorescein angiography: Early phase of the FFA reveals the presence of large choroidal vessels in a well demarcated of choriocapillaris atrophy. The edges may leak from the intact choriocapillaris (Figs 32.61 C to E).

Visual fields: Central or paracentral scotomas are seen.

Bietti's Crystalline Retinopathy

Introduction

This disease was first decribed by Bietti in 1937. Inheritance is autosomal recessive. It is a slowly progressive disorder.

Clinical Presentation

Fundus examination characterized by the presence of crystalline deposits in all layers of the retina associated with well-defined focal areas of choriocapillaris and retinal pigment epithelium loss particularly at the posterior pole.

In some cases, cholesterol crystals are also seen on slit-lamp biomicroscopy in the superficial corneal limbus. The disease has been divided into three stages by Yuzawa and associates:
- *Stage 1:* Retinal pigment epithelial atrophy with uniform fine white crystalline deposits seen at the macular area (Figs 32.62 A to D).

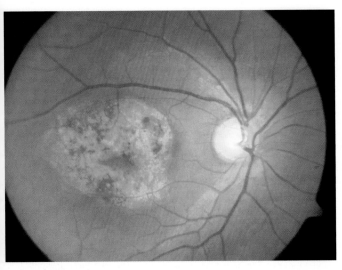

Fig. 32.61A: Central areolar choroidal dystrophy. Color fundus photograph of the right showing choroidal, retinal pigment epithelium and choriocapillaris atrophy with pigment stippling at the posterior pole. Optic nerve, blood vessels and peripheral retinas are normal

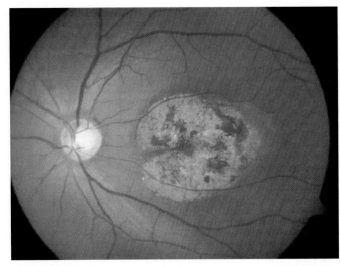

Fig. 32.61B: Color fundus photograph of the left showing bilaterally symmetrical area of choroidal, retinal pigment epithelium and choriocapillaris atrophy at the posterior pole

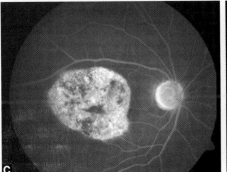 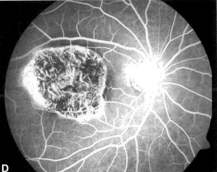 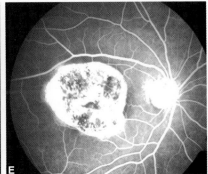

Figs 32.61C to E: Fluorescein angiography shows well-defined area of early hypofluorescence due to loss of choroidal capillaries. Leakage is seen at the edge from the intact choriocapillaris

- *Stage 2:* Retinal pigment epithelial atrophy extends beyond the posterior pole. Choriocapillaris atrophy in addition to the RPE atrophy appears markedly at the posterior pole.
- Stage 3: Retinal pigment epithelium-choriocapillaris complex atrophy is observed throughout the fundus.

Investigations

Fluorescein angiography: It reveals well-defined areas of hypofluorescence due to the loss of the choriocapillaris. The large choroidal vessels are unaffected. Late stages of the FFA may reveal the presence of staining at the margins of the atrophy (Figs 32.62 E to I).

Electroretinogram: Full-field ERG reveals reduced cone as well as rod responses (Figs 32.62 J to L).

Visual fields: Visual fields reveal the presence of bizarre scotoma corresponding to the areas of chorioretinal atrophy (Figs 32.62 M and N).

Choroideremia

Introduction

It has X-linked recessive inheritance with history of night blindness and field loss seen in patients since early childhood. It was first described by Mauthner in 1871. The gene causing choroideremia has been mapped to Xq13-q22.

Clinical Presentation

Hemizygous males usually develop night blindness in the first or second decade of life, followed by progressive peripheral visual field constriction and visual disability in late age. Heterozygous female carriers are mostly asymptomatic, but their fundi may show characteristic pigment changes in the midperiphery. Posterior subcapsular cataracts are seen in one third of these patients. Well-defined areas of chorioretinal atrophy (Fig. 32.63 A) may be seen in the periphery as in gyrate atrophy. It differs from gyrate atrophy by presence of normal ornithine levels.

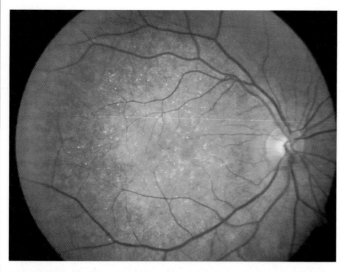

Fig. 32.62A: Bietti's crystalline retinopathy. Color fundus photograph of the right eye shows crystalline deposits in the retina predominantly at the posterior pole. Crystal deposits were not seen at the limbal or the paralimbal area on slit-lamp examination

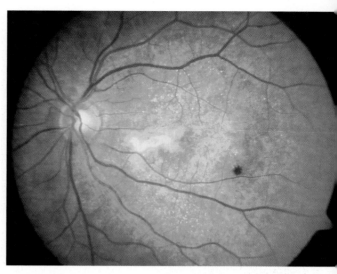

Fig. 32.62B: Color fundus photograph of the left eye shows crystalline deposits. A fibrous scar is seen in the parafoveal region

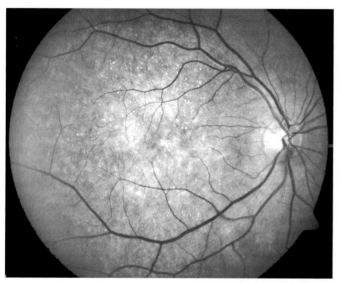

Fig. 32.62C: Red free photograph of the right eye

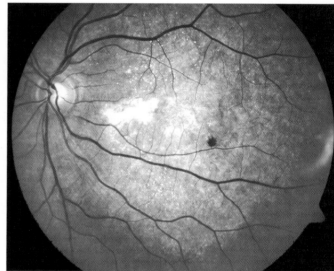

Fig. 32.62D: Red free photograph of the left eye

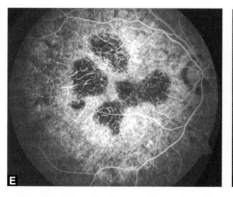
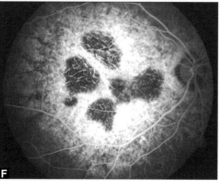
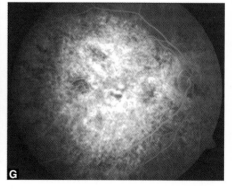

Figs 32.62E to G: Fluorescein angiography of the same patient highlights the well defined hypofluorescent focal areas of choriocapillaris and retinal pigment epithelium atrophy. The large choroidal vessels are prominent in the area of the atrophy

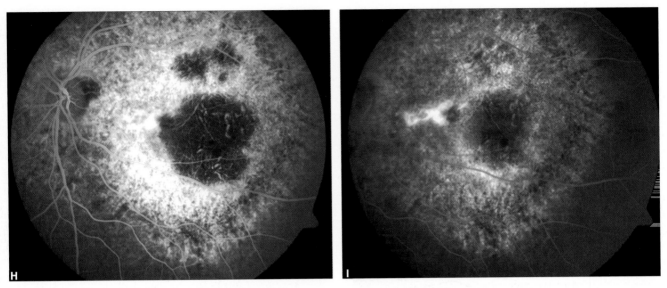

Figs 32.62H and I: Fluorescein angiography of the left eye

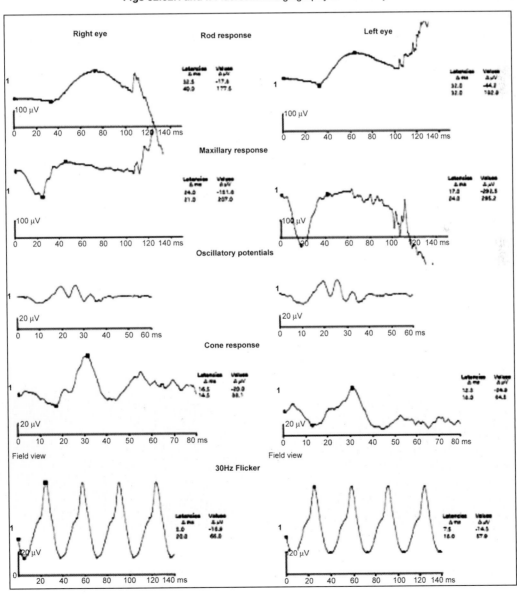

Fig. 32.62J: Full field ERG shows mildly reduced cone as well as rod responses

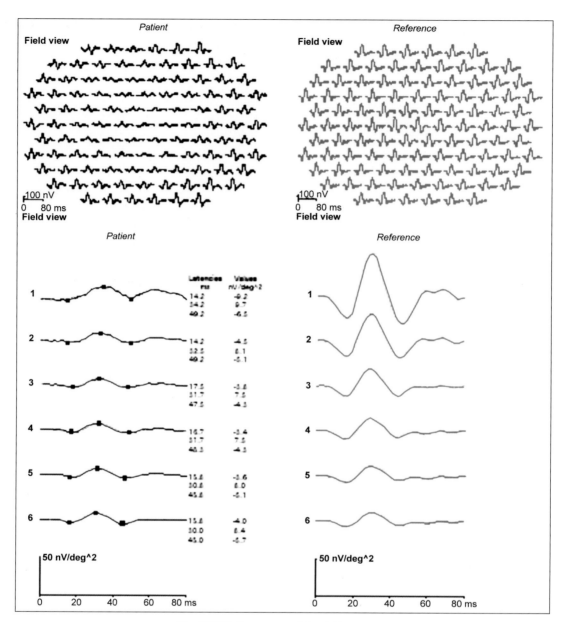

Fig. 32.62K: Trace array of the right eye

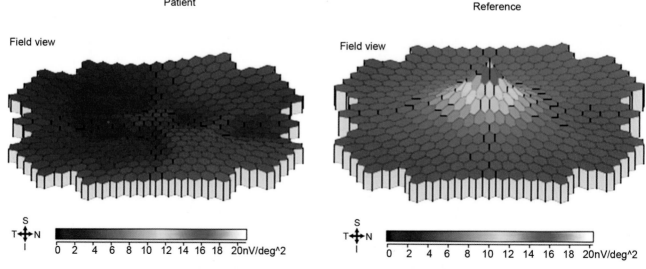

Fig. 32.62L: Topographical map of the right eye on mfERG picks up the particularly subnormal ERG in the areas of the chorioretinal atrophy

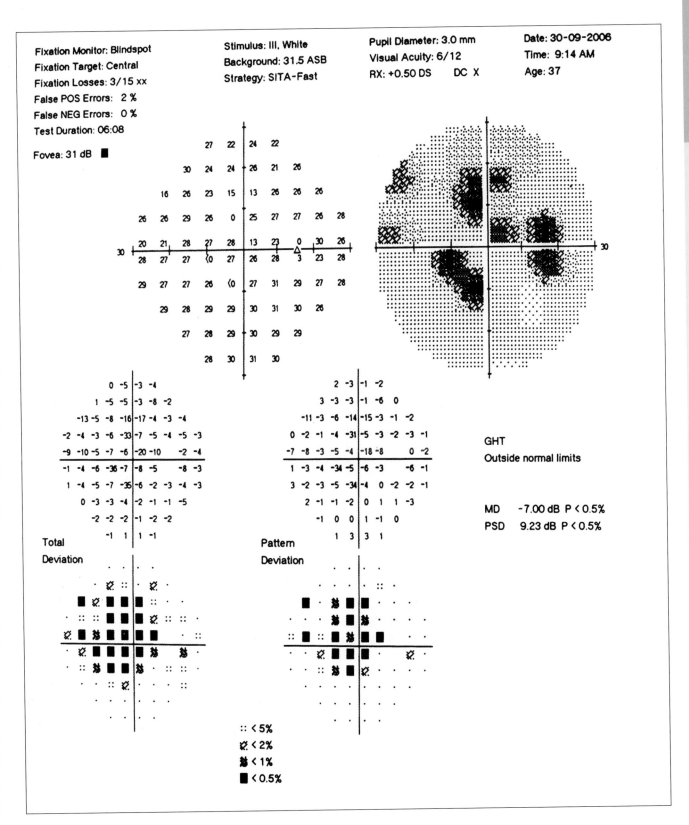

Fig. 32.62M: Visual field HVF 30-2 of the right eye shows paracentral scotomas

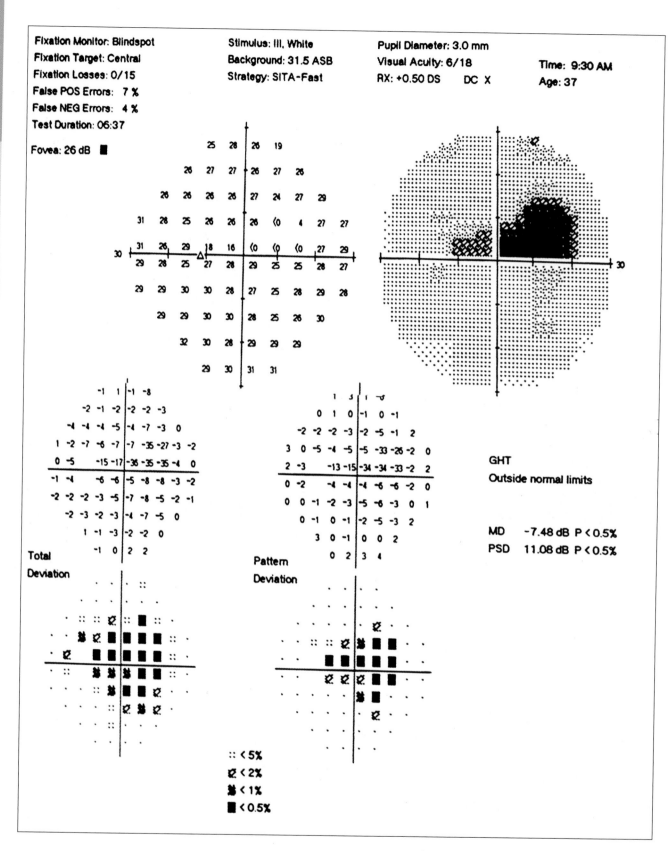

Fig. 32.62N: Visual field of the left eye

Investigations

Fluorescein angiography: Fluorescein angiography reveals areas of hypofluoresence with large choroidal vessels imaged well (Figs 32.63 B to D).

Visual fields: Visual fields reveal peripheral constriction of the fields early in the course of the disease.

Electroretinogram: Both rod and cone responses are reduced.

Gyrate Atrophy

Introduction

Inheritance of gyrate atrophy is autosomal recessive.

Clinical Presentation

Patients present with symptoms of night blindness and loss of peripheral vision in first decade of life. High myopia and/or astigmatism are seen in 90% of the cases. Posterior subcapsular cataract is seen in second or third decade of life. Several circular discrete areas of chorioretinal atrophy with scalloped margins

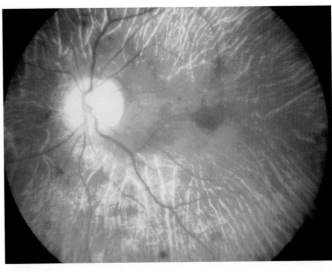

Fig. 32.63A: Choroideremia. Fundus photograph of the left eye showing extensive loss of the retinal pigment epithelium and choriocapillaris. Larger choroidal vessels are preserved. An island of preserved retinal pigment epithelium is seen at the fovea. Optic atrophy and arteriolar attenuation are not seen. Pigment clumps are seen

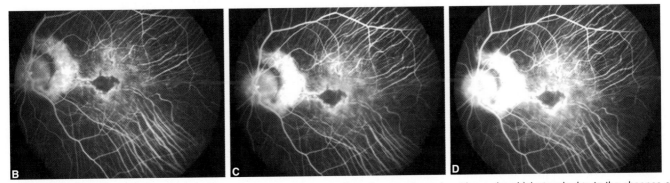

Figs 32.63B to D: Fluorescein angiography of the same patient shows scalloped areas of prominent large choroidal vessels due to the absence of the overlying retinal pigment epithelium and choriocapillaris. Small Island of intact retinal pigment epithelium is seen at the macula with leakage in the late phase from the intact choriocapillaris

are seen beginning in the midperiphery proceeding towards the periphery and center. These areas of atrophy finally involve the macula causing a drop in vision.

Investigations

Fluorescein angiography: Fluorescein angiography reveals presence of leakage at the edge of the scalloped lesions from the intact choriocapillaris. Larger choroidal vessels are seen within these circular lesions (Figs 32.64A and B) .

Visual fields: Peripheral constriction of fields is seen first followed by less of central vision.

Electroretinogram: In these cases, ERG may be nonrecordable early in the course of the disease (Figs 32.64 C and D). Increase in the serum ornithine levels is seen. Serum ornithine levels are raised due to reduced activity of ornithine aminotransferase. If started at an early age, long-term reduction of plasma ornithine levels by way of an arginine-restricted diet may slow the progression of the chorioretinal lesions in patients with gyrate atrophy.

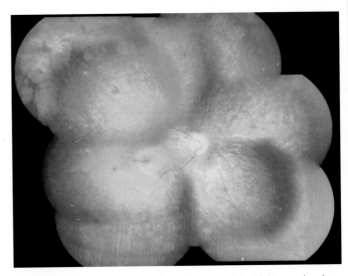

Fig. 32.64 A: Gyrate atrophy. Color montage of the right eye showing widespread chorioretinal atrophy. Atrophic patch is seen at the macula

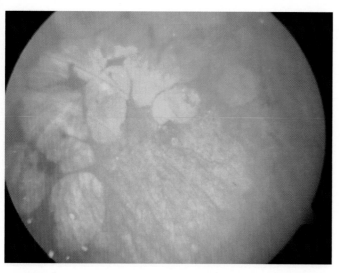

Fig. 32.64B: Color fundus photograph of the right eye showing the presence of discrete scalloped areas of chorioretinal atrophy

These patients may or may not be pyridoxine responsive. In a small subset of patients who are biochemically found to be pyridoxine responsive, long-term treatment with pyridoxine can reduce the levels of ornithine.

Ocular Albinism

Introduction

Albinism is associated with an inborn error of amino acid metabolism affecting the production of melanin in the body. It is characterized by changes secondary to a deficit melanin restricted to ocular structures only. When associated with a hypopigmentation of the skin and hair as well, it is called oculocutaneous albinism. Oculocutaneous albinism may be Tyrosinase-positive (incomplete) or Tyrosinase-negative (complete). Oculocutaneous albinism is autosomal recessive while

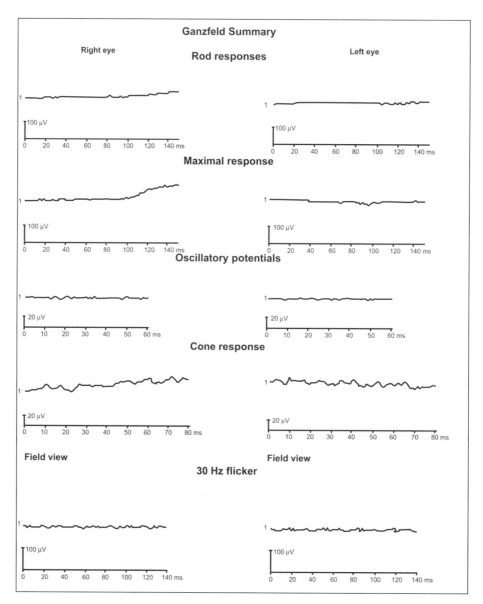

Fig. 32.64C: Full-field ERG of a case of gyrate atrophy. Nonrecordable waveforms are seen. Serum ornithine levels were 3.3 mg/dl (Normal 1mg/dl). Ornithine aminotransferase levels were reduced

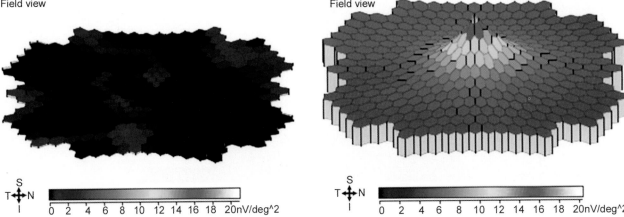

Patient   Reference

Field view   Field view

Fig. 32.64D: Three dimensional plot of mfERG showing markedly reduced responses both centrally as well as in the periphery as compared to normal

the ocular albinism is usually X-linked; though autosomal recessive inheritance is also known.

Clinical Presentation

Visual acuity is poor due to the presence of foveal hypoplasia. Pendular nystagmus is seen, which reduces with increasing age. Changes seen on fundus examination include depigmented fundus, foveal hypoplasia and optic disc hypoplasia (Figs 32.65 A to D).

HEREDITARY VITREORETINOPATHIES

This group of disorders includes conditions like the X-linked retinoschisis, Stickler's syndrome, Wagner's syndrome and Goldmann-Favre's syndrome.

Goldmann-Favre's Vitreoretinal Degeneration

Peripheral and foveal schisis are also seen in Goldmann-Favre's vitreoretinal degeneration. Inheritance is autosomal recessive inheritance.

Clinical Presentation

Features differentiating Goldmann-Favre's from XLRS include, night blindness since early childhood. Fundus picture shows foveal and peripheral schisis with predominant pigment clumping, arteriolar attenuation and waxy pale disc. Cataract formation is seen early in life. Visual acuity and color vision abnormalities are seen early in the course of the disease.

Investigations

Fluorescein angiography: Fluorescein angiography reveals the presence of widespread retinal pigment epithelium granularity. Foveal schisis when seen clinically does not reveal any

leakage on fluorescein angiography even in the late stages of the angiogram.

Optical coherence tomography: Presence of schisis cavities is confirmed on optical coherence tomography.

Electroretinogram: Electroretinogram is nonrecordable early in the course of the disease.

Stickler's Syndrome

Stickler's syndrome is also called hereditary arthro-ophthalmopathy. It is a collagen connective tissue disorder that is expressed in the vitreous as well as the cartilage. Inheritance of this disease is autosomal dominant.

Clinical Presentation

The presentation is typically in the form of a young child with high myopia and typical orofacial abnormalities. Fundus picture is that of pathological myopia with optically empty vitreous because of early liquefaction and degeneration. Peripheral multiple lattice degeneration patches are seen with unhealthy adherent vitreous. Retinal detachment is commonly seen. Hence there is need for regular follow-up and prophylactic laser photocoagulation of the peripheral retinal lesions. Other ocular associations include cataract, ectopia lentis and glaucoma.

Investigations

Electroretinogram: Electroretinogram is usually normal

Wagner Syndrome

Inheritance of Wagner syndrome is autosomal dominant with the gene linked to chromosome 5q14. Systemic abnormalities are not seen in this group of patients as seen in the Stickler's syndrome.

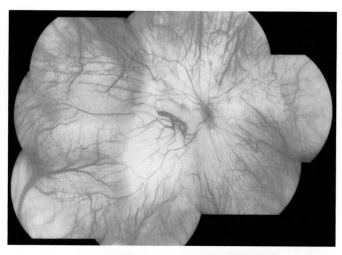

Fig. 32.65A: Ocular albinism. Color montage of the right eye showing prominence of the large choroidal vessels

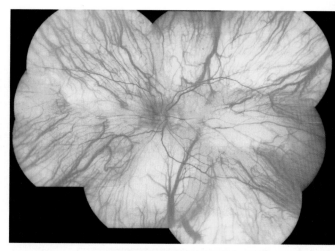

Fig. 32.65B: Color montage of the left eye showing prominence of the large choroidal vessels

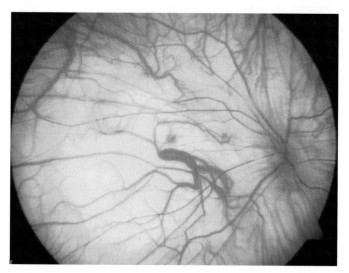

Fig. 32.65C: Color fundus photograph of the right eye with foveal hypoplasia as evident by lack of the foveal avascular zone

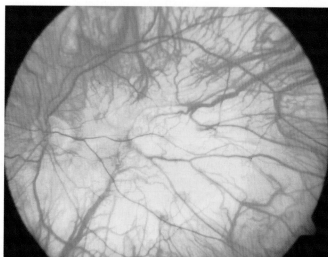

Fig. 32.65D: Color fundus photograph of the left eye. Choroidal blood vessels are seen crossing the normal site of the fovea

Clinical Presentation

Presentation is similar to Stickler's syndrome with myopia, early cataract, vitreous degeneration, chorioretinal atrophy, and perivascular pigmentation and sheathing. Retinal detachment is seen in up to 50% of cases. As apposed to that seen in Stickler's syndrome in these cases retinal detachment seen is usually tractional.

Investigations

Electroretinogram: Electroretinogram may be normal early in the course of the disease. However, the rods become subnormal as nytalopia sets in the later stages of the disease, the ERG may be nonrecordable.

Fluorescein angiography: Areas of progressive chorioretinal dystrophy may be revealed.

Visual fields: Visual fields primarily reveal peripheral constriction.

Prophylactic treatment of the peripheral lattice degeneration in these cases may reduce the risk of associated retinal detachment.

Familial Exudative Vitreoretinopathy

Familial exudative vitreoretinopathy is characterized by incomplete peripheral retinal vascularization. Inheritance is autosomal dominant; X-linked recessive cases may also be seen.

Clinical Presentation

Patient commonly presents with poor visual acuity and strabismus. Fundus picture is characterized by temporal straightening of the retinal vessels, which do not reach up to the periphery. Peripheral ridge formation with neovascularization and fibrovascular proliferation is also seen. Temporal macular and disc drag may also be seen in severe cases. These features may make differentiation for retinopathy of prematurity difficult. Absence of any history of prematurity in a normal birth weight child points towards the diagnosis of familial exudative vitreoretinopathy.

Treatment may be required in the form of laser photocoagulation of the telangiectatic vessels and to the avascular retina to prevent vascular response. Recent reports of the use of anti-VEGF injection have also been seen in familial exudative vitreoretinopathy.

DRUG TOXICITIES

Various drugs are known to be retinotoxic. Early damage may be restricted to the macula. Widespread damage may be seen in late stages.

Chloroquine Toxicity

Introduction

Antimalarials are used for a prolonged period in patients with arthritis. Hydroxychloroquine is less toxic as compared to chloroquine and other disease-modifying drugs. Because of its retinotoxicity, chloroquine is no longer the drug of choice.

Clinical Presentation

In early stages, the toxicity is limited to the macula (Figs 32.66 A to E).

Hydroxychloroquine Toxicity

Introduction

Hydroxychloroquine is safer than chloroquine, though, long term hydroxychloroquine use may also be associated with retinal toxicity.

Sight-threatening retinopathy in these patients is less at the recommended dose of 400 mg daily.

Clinical Presentation

Presentation may vary from a near normal looking macula to a bull's eye maculopathy (Fig. 32.67A and B). Damage caused by it is reversible in the early stages of the disease. Retinal toxicity due to hydroxychloroquine is monitored using investigations like visual acuity, Amsler charting, color vision, automated perimetry, ffERG (Fig. 32.67 C) and EOG.

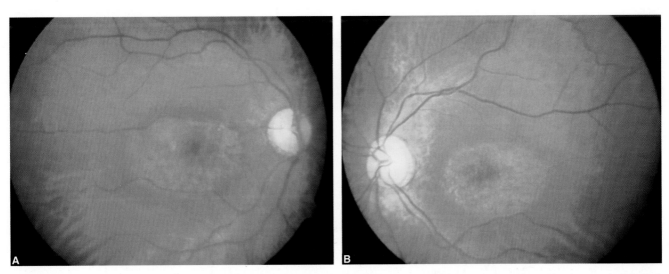

Figs 32.66A and B: Chloroquine toxicity. Fundus photograph of the right and the left eye showing hypopigmented patch at the macula in both the eyes who had been on chloroquine for the treatment of rheumatoid arthritis for several years

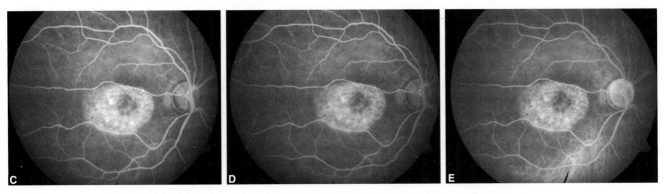

Figs 32.66C to E: Fluorescein angiography of the right eye showing a typical bull's eye maculopathy

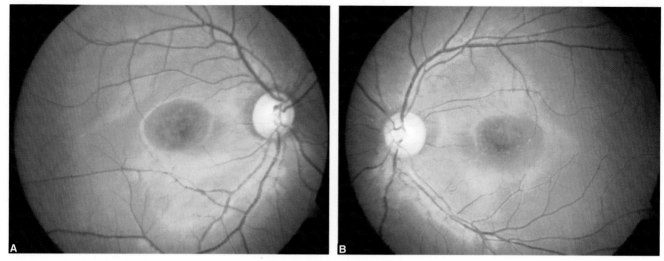

Figs 32.67A and B: Hydroxychloroquine toxicity. Fundus photograph shows symmetrical retinal pigment epithelium defects at the posterior pole with normal disc and the vessels

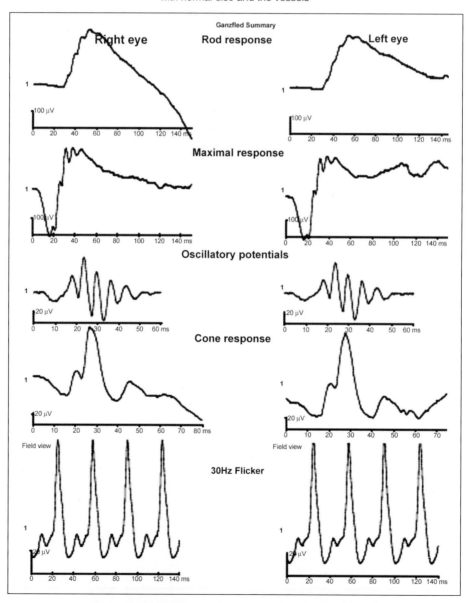

Fig. 32.67C: Photopic and scotopic responses are normal on ffERG

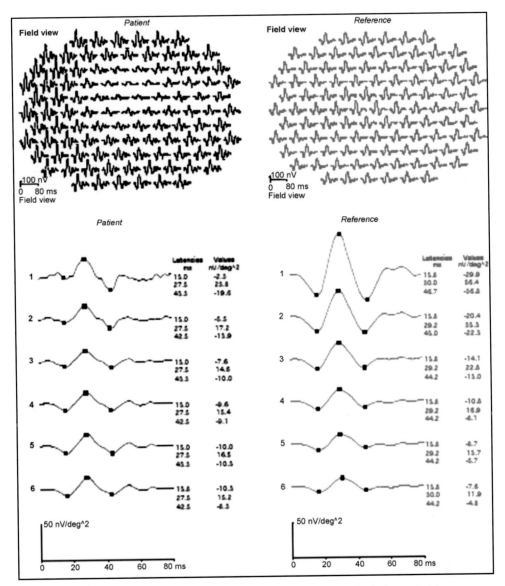

Fig. 32.67D: Trace array of the right eye shows reduced amplitudes in the central rings

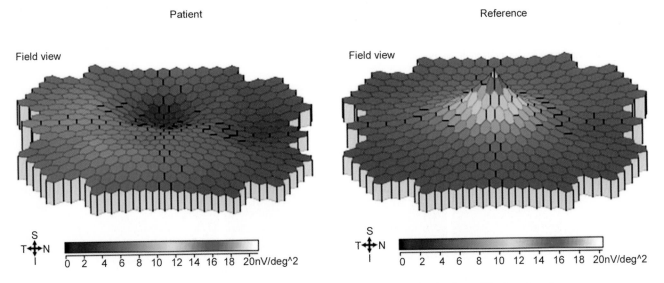

Fig. 32.67E: Three dimensional plot of the right eye amplitudes showing loss of the foveal peak

Investigations

Multifocal electroretinogram: Multifocal ERG can point towards macular toxicity due to hydroxychloroquine even when these investigations are normal (Figs 32.67D and E).

Fluorescein angiography: Fluorescein angiography reveals the presence of retinal pigment epithelium alteration with hyperfluorescence due to window defects (Figs 32.67F to H).

Desferrioxamine Toxicity

Desferrioxamine is used for the treatment of chronic iron overload and acute iron poisoning. Ocular toxicity secondary to prolonged treatment with desferrioxamine is known to cause night blindness, visual field defects, cataract, pigmentary retinopathy, maculopathy (Figs 32.68 A to H) and optic neuropathy. To avoid such complications, a routine ophthalmic screening is recommended for patients taking desferrioxamine.

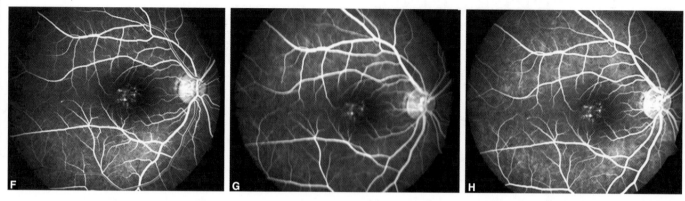

Figs 32.67F to H: FFA of the right eye shows hyperfluorescence due to window defects at the macula

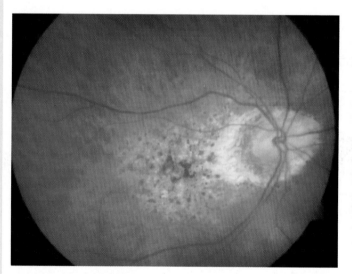

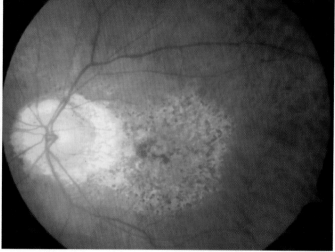

Fig. 32.68A: Desferrioxamine toxicity. Fundus photograph of the right eye showing pigment mottling of the macula

Fig. 32.68B: Fundus photograph of the left eye with similar findings

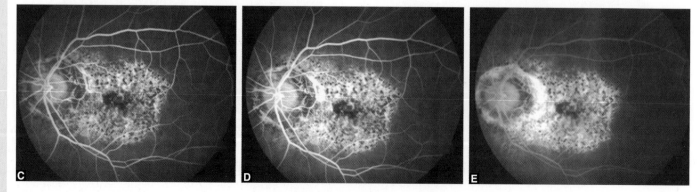

Figs 32.68C to E: Fluorescein angiography of the left eye shows hyperfluorescence at the macula due to underlying retinal pigment epithelium atrophy

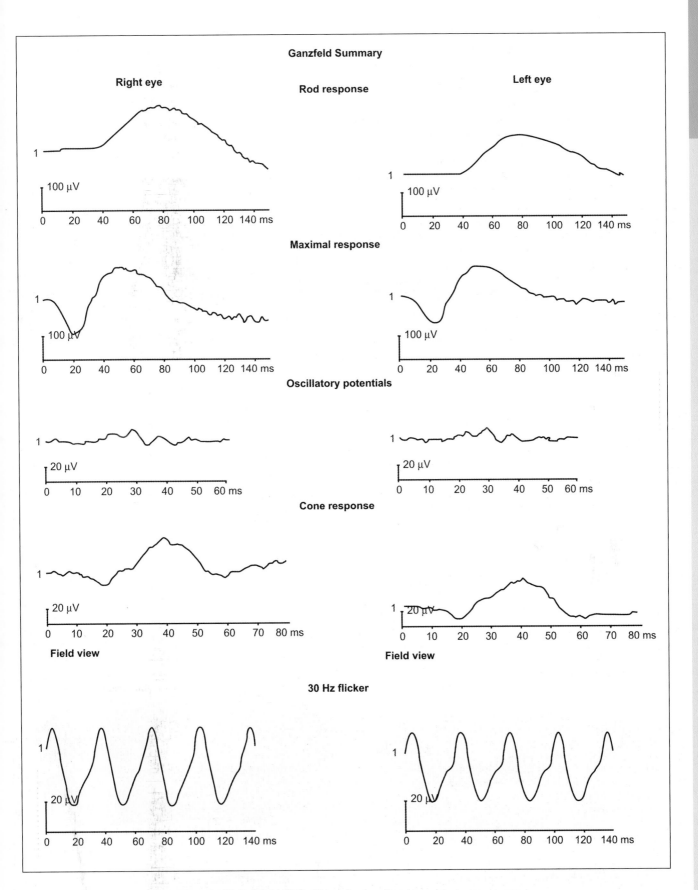

Fig. 32.68F: Full-field ERG with predominantly subnormal cone responses

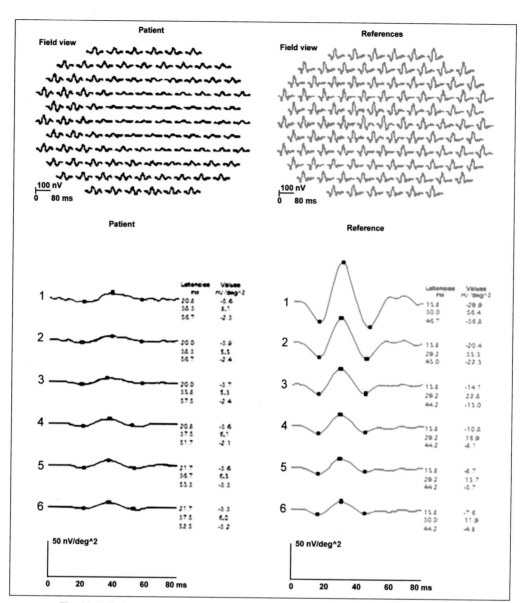

Fig. 32.68G: Trace array of the right eye shows reduced amplitudes in all eccentricities

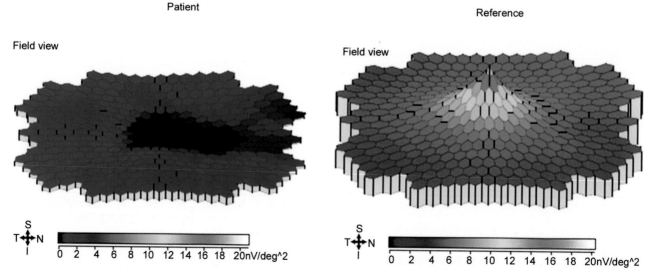

Fig. 32.68H: Three-dimensional topographical map of the right eye with foveal blunting as well as generalized reduction of macular responses

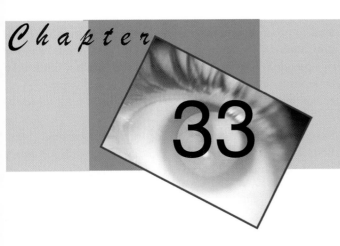

Chapter 33

Ocular Oncology

Mahesh P Shanmugam, Praveen R Murthy,
Krishna R Murthy

INTRODUCTION

Ocular oncology has become recognized as a separate subspeciality in ophthalmology. In the present chapter an overview of common intraocular tumors is given. Retinoblastoma and uveal melanoma being the most important intraocular malignancies, are dealt with in detail in the beginning of the chapter. This is followed by an account of intraocular vascular tumors, intraocular lymphoma, leukemia and other intraocular tumors.

RETINOBLASTOMA

Introduction

Retinoblastoma is the most common pediatric intraocular malignancy and the second most common primary intraocular malignancy in any age group. Petrus Pawius made first description of the tumor. Till 1809, the mortality due to this tumor was 100%. James Wardrop described the pathology of this tumor and advised enucleation as the primary modality of the treatment. Enucleation is still used all over the world, in the management of many cases of retinoblastoma.

Incidence

Retinoblastoma occurs in approximately 1 in 14,000–34,000 live births. Incidence in Indian patients is not available, but is not thought to be much different from that of other countries. No predisposition to the race, sex or laterality of the eye is noted. The majority of the cases of retinoblastoma are sporadic (no family history and no affected family members on ophthalmic examination).

Genetics

Although the hereditary form of retinoblastoma obeys Mendelian-dominant predictions, the retinoblastoma gene itself is recessive. In 1971, Knudson proposed the "two hit hypothesis" to explain the genetic events that are necessary for both heritable and nonheritable retinoblastomas.

Hereditary Cases

In hereditary cases, "first hit" (mutation) occurs at the germinal level in either the affected individual or in an asymptomatic parent. Therefore, all cells in the person posses the mutation effect. "Second hit" (mutation) is thought to occur at the somatic cell and occurs sometime during the development of the fetus. If it affects the retinal cells, retinoblastoma develops. The presence of germinal mutation in all the cells predisposes these patients to bilateral retinoblastomas and multifocal as well as other nonocular tumors, e.g. osteosarcoma which develops at a later age. 10 to 15% of unilateral patients may also harbor a genetic defect, thereby transmitting the defective gene to their offspring. These patients are also at an increased risk of nonocular tumors.

Nonhereditary Cases

In nonhereditary cases, both mutational events occur at the somatic cells during the development of the retina and in the same retinal cell. As both hits are somatic, the rest of the body carries no higher risk of developing other tumors. The probability of two independent hits occurring in the same retinal cells in both eyes or at several locations in the same eye is significantly less. Therefore, these patients are older and have unilateral, unifocal tumors.

Chromosome 13q14 Deletions and Esterase D

The specific area corresponding to retinoblastoma gene was identified on 14 band, on the long arm of chromosome 13 (13q14). This particular area of chromosome is fragile and alterations are easily induced. Approximately 5% of the retinoblastoma patients have a deletion of one homologue of chromosome 13q14 region. The esterase gene has also been localized to the region of 13q14 and demonstrates close linkage with the hereditary form of the retinoblastoma. Esterase-D was found to be half the normal level in persons with heterozygous deletion of 13q14. Patients with large deletions present with several abnormalities like mental retardation, microcephaly, broad prominent nasal bridge, hypertelorism, etc. in addition to retinoblastoma. This gene has been cloned and sequenced. Discovery of such a gene makes the prenatal diagnosis possible in high-risk groups.

Age at Diagnosis

The average age at diagnosis is 18 months. Bilateral cases are diagnosed earlier (12 months) than unilateral cases (24 months). Ninety percent of the cases are diagnosed before 3 years of age.

Clinical Features

The most common presentation of retinoblastoma is leukocoria (61%) and strabismus (22%). Other presentations in order of frequency are visual impairment (5%), asymptomatic (detected on routine fundoscopy) (4%), orbital inflammation and proptosis (2%), secondary glaucoma with red eyes (2%), unilateral pupillary dilatation (1%), and hyphema and heterochromia iridis (<1%).

On fundus examination, early retinoblastoma lesions are seen as slightly white, flat, translucent lesion in the sensory retina, which may be asymptomatic and are usually detected on routine fundus examination. If the lesion is at the macula, it causes strabismus.

Moderately advanced lesions may present as unilateral or bilateral "Leukocoria" - better known as "Cat's eye reflex". Light is reflected from the mass in the retina and causes a white reflex. The lens remains clear in most patients with retinoblastoma. Based on the growth pattern, the tumor can be classified into:

- Endophytic
- Exophytic
- Mixed (both endophytic and exophytic).

Endophytic Tumors

Endophytic lesions grow from the retina into the vitreous cavity (Fig. 33.1). They appear as ill-defined, yellowish mass with no retinal vessels overlying them. They are very friable and hence tend to produce vitreous seeding and can also simulate endophthalmitis. This tumor may present in the anterior chamber as a pseudohypopyon or as nodules at the pupillary border. An endophytic retinoblastoma can be diffusely infiltrative.

Exophytic Tumors

Exophytic lesions grow outwards into the subretinal space. Retinal vessels are seen over the tumor along with secondary retinal detachment. These tumors may simulate Coats' disease, especially when associated with a bullous retinal detachment (Fig. 33.2).

Mixed Tumors

These tumors have both endophytic and exophytic components.

Diffuse infiltrating retinoblastoma is characterized by a flat infiltration of the retina with no obvious visible mass lesion. This can lead to a delay in diagnosis and may simulate intraocular inflammation due to the presence of tumor cells in the vitreous and anterior chamber.

In advanced retinoblastoma, the tumor may spread into the optic nerve or may be associated with distant metastasis. Lamina cribrosa offers resistance to tumor spread and retrolaminar involvement indicates poor prognosis. Once the tumor reaches the subarachnoid space, it rapidly spreads intracranially.

Proptosis may be a sign of orbital involvement of retinoblastoma in which event local lymph nodes may also be involved. Distant metastasis to brain, spinal cord, skull bones, distant bones, viscera and lymph nodes may occur. They usually occur at a late stage and are rarely detected on systemic evaluation at the time of initial presentation.

Spontaneous regression of retinoblastoma can occur in about 1% of patients. It is often seen in eyes with phthisis bulbi and following an episode of severe inflammation. These lesions are usually flat and sometimes associated with calcific specks. The genetic implications in patients with spontaneously regressed retinoblastoma are the same as in the case of active tumor.

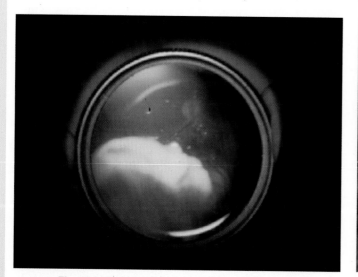

Fig. 33.1: Retinoblastoma. Endophytic retinoblastoma

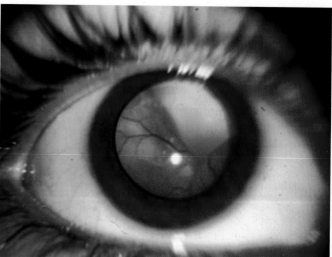

Fig. 33.2: Coats' disease. Bullous retinal detachment in Coat's disease

Extraocular spread of the retinoblastoma can occur by contiguous extension into the optic nerve and brain, while orbital extension occurs probably through scleral emissaries or through the ciliary body when there is epibulbar mass.

Distant metastasis occurs by hematogenous route via the choroid or through the anterior chamber angle to the lungs, bones and the brain. Lymphatic spread to the preauricular and cervical lymph nodes occurs when there is a massive extraocular extension.

Differential Diagnosis

Differential diagnosis of retinoblastoma includes:
- *Differential diagnosis of leukocoria*
  Congenital cataract, persistent hyperplastic primary vitreous, retinopathy of prematurity, toxocariasis, coloboma of the choroids and optic nerve, Coats' disease (Fig. 33.3), nematode endophthalmitis.
- *Differential diagnosis of vitreous seeds*
  Pars planitis, microbial endophthalmitis.
- *Other retinal tumors and simulating lesions*
  Retinal astrocytoma, myelinated nerve fibers

Evaluation of a Case of Retinoblastoma

- Relevant history
- Complete ophthalmic examination in the outpatient department
- Examination under general anesthesia.

As majority of the patients are under five years of age, a detailed ocular examination with indirect ophthalmoscope and scleral depression is often not possible without general anesthesia. Examination under anesthesia provides an opportunity to detect early lesion(s) in the opposite eye or other tumor foci in the same eye. During examination under anesthesia, the following steps are recommended:
1. *External examination:* This is performed using the magnification of operating microscope.

2. *Measurement of corneal diameter:* This is done to exclude microphthalmos or secondary buphthalmos.
3. Measurement of intraocular pressure.
4. Binocular indirect ophthalmoscopy with scleral depression of both eyes and fundus drawing denoting the site and extent of the tumor.
5. Gross systemic examination.

Ancillary Tests

Although retinoblastoma is most often a clinical diagnosis, certain ancillary tests are needed for confirmation. A list of ancillary tests required in the work-up of a case of suspected retinoblastoma is given in Table 33.1.

Table 33.1: Ancillary tests in a suspected case of retinoblastoma

1.	Ultrasonography of the eyeball and orbit.
2.	Computerized tomography of the orbit.
3.	Magnetic resonance imaging of the orbit.
4.	Cytology by fine needle aspiration biopsy (Figs 33.4A and B).*

(*Very rarely in an atypical situation, when clinical and ancillary evaluations fails to establish the diagnoses).

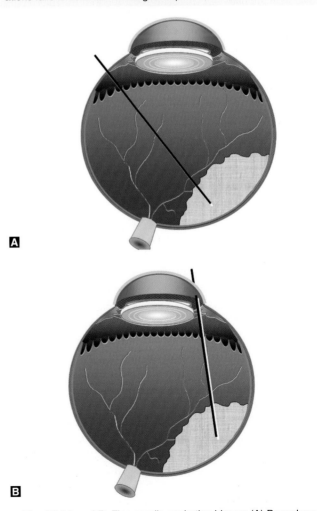

A

B

Figs 33.4A and B: Fine needle aspiration biopsy: (A) Pars plana approach, (B) Clear cornea approach

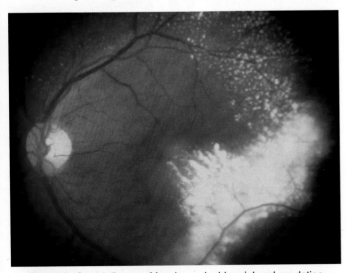

Fig. 33.3: Coats' disease. Macular and mid peripheral exudation

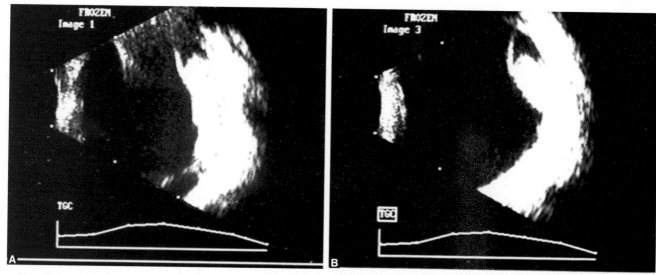

Figs 33.5A and B: B-scan ultrasonography in retinoblastoma. Ultrasonographic appearance of retinoblastoma is visualized. High internal reflectivity due to calcium and secondary retinal detachment is observed

Ultrasonography

Ultrasonography can pick up lesions as small as 2 mm. A-scan shows high intensity internal echoes throughout the mass lesion and orbital shadowing due to calcification (Figs 33.5A and B). B-scan may reveal following features:

1. A mass lesion with well-defined margins and numerous high internal reflective echoes.
2. *Foci of calcification:* This is one of the important diagnostic features on ultrasound and is seen in the majority of cases. One can reduce the amplification and can demonstrate the calcification selectively.
3. Attenuation or absence of normal soft tissue echoes in the orbit (orbital shadowing).
4. High reflectivity of calcium makes evaluation of the optic nerve and detection of extraocular disease with ultrasound difficult.

Computed Tomography (CT scan)

In a CT scan, retinoblastoma is seen as an intraocular mass with the foci of calcification (Fig. 33.6). Although CT scan and ultrasound can both detect retinoblastoma, CT scan has the advantage of detecting an extraocular extension, the presence of pinealoblastoma or intracranial metastasis. In a thin, 1.5 mm section, high resolution CT scan can detect 2 mm thick tumors. It is important to note that an extraocular extension is usually noncalcified. Therefore, a subtle extraocular extension may still remain undetected in CT scan. One may order a routine CT scan in the initial work-up of a retinoblastoma to rule out such extraocular spread of intracranial metastasis. An optic nerve spread is usually infiltrative and does not visibly enlarge the nerve in all cases; hence it may not be picked up on CT scan.

Magnetic Resonance Imaging (MRI)

A CT scan is more sensitive in detecting intraocular calcification than MRI, but extraocular extension of retinoblastoma is

better seen with MRI. It is useful when the CT scan is equivocal in case of an anticipated extrascleral spread. Retinoblastoma is moderately hyperdense to vitreous in T_1-weighted image and hypodense in T_2-weighted image. It can be used to differentiate between hemorrhage, exudates and active tumor. It is of use to demonstrate infiltrative spread along intracanalicular and cisternal portions of the optic nerve, subarachnoid seeding and involvement of the brain.

Metastatic Work-up

Systemic evaluation may be necessary in high-risk cases such as:

a. Suspected extrascleral spread
b. Optic nerve invasion on imaging studies
c. Presentation with glaucoma/orbital cellulitis

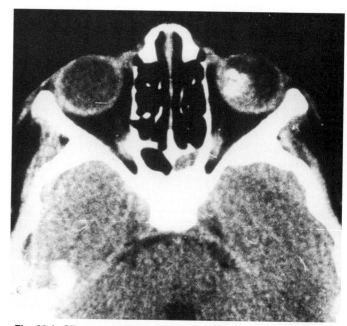

Fig. 33.6: CT scan in retinoblastoma. CT scan of the orbit showing an intraocular mass lesion with calcification suggestive of retinoblastoma

d. Anterior chamber seeding

e. Gross choroidal invasion

f. Suspected metastasis

Lumbar puncture, CT scan, bone marrow biopsy and routine blood investigations are adequate.

Examination of Parents and Siblings

It is important to examine the siblings of bilateral or genetically transmitted retinoblastoma patients so that the disease can be detected at an early stage and treated. Parents may harbor regressed retinoblastoma lesions, which may indicate the familial nature of the disease.

Pathogenesis

Retinoblastoma is a primitive neuroectodermal tumor of the retina. The exact histogenesis of this tumor is still not clear. Immunohistochemical and electron microscopic studies done on this tumor indicate that it arises from primitive multipotential neuroepithelial cells of early embryogenesis.

Histopathology

All eyes enucleated, as retinoblastoma must be examined histopathologically. Under low power, a basophilic mass with lightly eosinophilic areas due to the necrosis of tumor and/or multiple dense basophilic foci (due to calcification) within the areas of necrosis may be seen. The tumor may be well-differentiated or poorly differentiated. Poorly differentiated retinoblastoma consists of small- to medium-sized round cells with hyperchromatic nuclei and scanty cytoplasm. Huge mitotic figures are often observed.

A well-differentiated tumor may show: (i) rosettes, or (ii) fleurettes. Seventy percent of retinoblastomas are known to contain rosettes.

Rosettes are of two types:
- Flexner-Wintersteiner rosette
- Homer-Wright rosette

Flexner-Wintersteiner rosette is highly specific for retinoblastoma, but can be seen in other tumors, such as medulloepithelioma. Here columnar cells are arranged around a clear central lumen. The nuclei of the cells are arranged near the base of the tumor. The lumen contains hyaluronidase-resistant glycosaminoglycans, which are found between photoreceptor and retinal pigment epithelium.

In a Homer-Wright rosette, the cells are arranged radially around a central tangle of neural fibers. They are not specific for retinoblastoma and can be seen in neuroblastoma and medulloepithelioma.

Fleurettes represent further differentiation and are highly specific for retinoblastoma. They present as flower bouquet-like aggregates of tumor cells with bulbous eosinophilic processes projecting through the fenestrated membrane. They are seen in 6 to 10% of the retinoblastoma cases.

Sometimes one may see tumor cells clustered around blood vessels in some necrotic retinoblastomas. These have been termed as pseudorosettes, which are very nonspecific and are seen in many tumors in the necrotic state.

Management

Enucleation

When there is no chance of preserving useful vision in an eye with retinoblastoma it should be enucleated. Conservative management is contemplated if an eye has useful vision or some vision can be restored.

Enucleation is indicated in unilateral and bilateral retinoblastomas involving more than half the globe. Unilateral cases are usually diagnosed at an advanced stage, necessitating enucleation. Presence of glaucoma and anterior chamber involvement are also indications for enucleation.

Eyes with visual potential (unilateral/bilateral cases) are managed conservatively. Conservative management includes cryotherapy, laser photocoagulation, external beam radiotherapy, brachytherapy or plaque radiotherapy, chemoreduction, transpupillary thermotherapy and thermochemotherapy.

Cryotherapy

Triple freeze-thaw technique is utilized to treat primary or recurrent tumors that are anterior to equator and up to 4 mm in diameter and less than 3 mm thickness, without vitreous seeds. The treatment effect is noted within 3-4 weeks and it may be repeated if needed. Advantage of the cryotherapy is that it preserves the internal limiting membrane and Bruch's membrane, which act as natural barriers to tumor growth. Complications of the cyrotherapy are: vitreous hemorrhage, retinal holes, serous and rhegmatogenous retinal detachment. Posterior tumors are usually treated by the photocoagulation. However, if laser photocoagulation is not possible, a posterior tumor can also be treated with cryo, after incising the conjunctiva provided the tumor is away from the macula and optic disc. Recently cryotherapy is employed as a means of breaking down the blood retinal barrier thereby facilitating penetration of chemotherapeutic agents into the eye.

Photocoagulation

It can be used to treat primary or recurrent tumors, which are 3-4 mm in diameter, 2 mm thick, without vitreous seeding and not involving the disc or macula. Two rows of deep burns surrounding the tumor are indicated. The tumor is treated in multiple sessions until it is replaced by chorioretinal scar. Treatment effect is noted within 4 weeks. Photocoagulation delivered through an indirect ophthalmoscope is the preferred mode of delivery at present. Complications of laser photocoagulation are the same as cryotherapy.

External Beam Radiotherapy

Bilateral tumors of less than 15 mm in width, but larger than those treatable with laser or cryo, tumors adjacent to the disc and macula, multiple tumors with minimal vitreous seeding, are treated by external beam radiotherapy (EBRT). EBRT is recommended in orbital recurrence and also the anophthalmic orbit if the tumor has extended to the line of transection of the optic nerve. A two-field approach, using lens shielded anterior and temporal portals delivering 3500–4000 cGy in 200 cGy fractions, delivered over a 4-5 week period is recommended.

Complications of EBRT include cataract, rare radiation retinopathy, hypoplasia of bone and soft tissue of the face, failure of eruption of molars, eyelid damage, impairment of tear production and corneal toxicity. The incidence of second malignant neoplasms is high within the treatment field in genetically predisposed patients. The incidence of second malignant neoplasms within the irradiated field has been found to be as high as 29% while it is 8% outside the field, which is not significantly different from patients with bilateral retinoblastoma who did not receive radiation. Recent reports indicate increased risk of second malignant neoplasms in children less than 1 year of age.

Various patterns of regression are noted after radiation for retinoblastoma:

Type I : Calcific residue resembling cottage cheese
Type II : Avascular fleshy, translucent mass resembling fish flesh.
Type III : Combination of I and II.
Type IV : Flat chorioretinal scar as seen after laser, cryo
Type O   : Complete disappearance of tumor

Brachytherapy

Brachytherapy or plaque radiotherapy is a method of treating the intraocular tumor by localized radiation with episcleral plaque applicators (iodine-125 or ruthenium-106) (Fig. 33.7). The advantage of brachytherapy is that is limits normal tissue being irradiated and can be used in the case of reactivation

of tumor following EBRT, laser or cryo. It is commonly indicated for tumors less than 15 mm in diameter and 6 to 8 mm in height, at least 2 mm from optic disc and fovea with or without localized vitreous seeding. Regression patterns are as seen with EBRT.

Chemoreduction

Chemoreduction is currently the preferred treatment modality. 6–9 cycles of vincristine 1 to 5 mg/m², etoposide 150 mg/m² and carboplatin 560 mg/m² at three week intervals is advised for unilateral or bilateral disease in eyes with visual potential. Tumors that are larger than those amenable to photocoagulation or cryotherapy and those that were traditionally treated with radiotherapy can be treated with chemoreduction. The goal of the treatment is to chemoreduce the tumor to such an extent that the residue is destroyed with "sequential aggressive local therapy" comprising of laser photocoagulation, cryotherapy and transpupillary thermotherapy (Fig. 33.8). Role of subconjunctival chemotherapy is under investigation.

Transpupillary Thermotherapy

Transpupillary thermotherapy alone can be used to treat tumors less than 3 mm thick and 3 mm in diameter, in the absence of vitreous seeds. Multiple treatment sessions may be necessary (Figs 33.9A and B).

Posterior tumors are treated with a microscope adapter while peripheral tumors are treated with the indirect laser ophthalmoscope. Both the transpupillary thermotherapy and thermochemotherapy are performed with the 810 nm diode laser.

Thermochemotherapy

Combination of the focal transpupillary hyperthermia and systemic carboplatin for small posterior pole retinoblastomas was

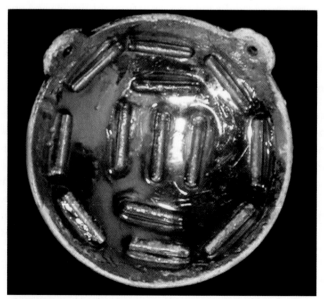

Fig. 33.7: Brachytherapy. Standard round, 15 mm, gold plaque with active iodine-125 seeds

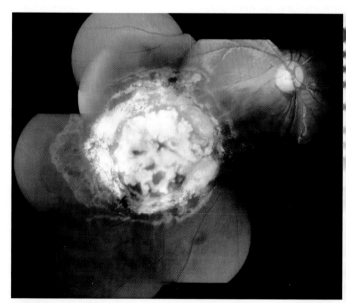

Fig. 33.8: Chemoreduction in retinoblastoma. Appearance of a regressed retinoblastoma following chemotherapy and laser photocoion for the residual tumor

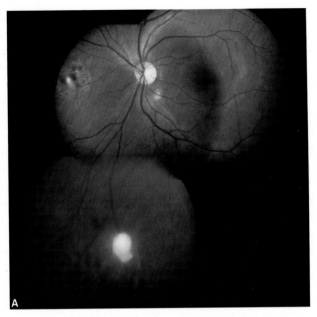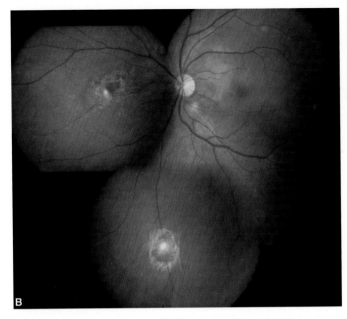

Figs 33.9A and B: Transpupillary thermotherapy in retinoblastoma: (A) Pretreatment appearance, (B) Posttreatment appearance.

first described by Murphree and associates. This utilizes the concept that hyperthermia 6-10°C above the baseline is synergistic with the platinum group of drugs. The heat facilitates cellular uptake of the drug, thereby increasing its effectiveness significantly. Thermochemotherapy is useful in primary or recurrent lesions smaller than 8 mm in diameter and 5 mm high. The technique involves continuous heating of the tumor over 20–30 minutes with diode laser within 2 to 3 hours after intravenous carboplatin. The treatment is repeated in cycles.

Prognosis

The survival rate of the retinoblastoma has increased considerably in recent years due to earlier diagnosis and improved treatment. Overall 5-year survival is around 90%. Patients with germinal mutations are more likely to die due to second nonocular tumors, which develop at a later age. Out of several histopathologic criteria that were correlated with the metastatic risk, only two factors, i.e. invasiveness of the tumor into the optic nerve and to ocular coats were found to be significant. Degree of choroidal invasion is thought to have a bearing on the prognosis. However, no significant worsening of the prognosis was found in an analysis of a large series of retinoblastoma cases. The degree of the optic nerve involvement is generally considered the most reliable single prognostic indicator. However, anterior chamber seeding and choroidal infiltration are also considered high risk factors for metastatic disease and adjuvant treatment in the form of multidrug chemotherapy is advised. As the mortality rates correlate with optic nerve involvement, the surgeon should ensure removal of the globe with at least 10 mm of the optic nerve. Involvement of the cut end of the optic nerve indicates poor prognosis and possible intracranial metastatic disease if adequate (at least 10 mm) length of the optic nerve was obtained during enucleation.

Clinical Staging Systems in Retinoblastoma

Reese-Ellsworth classification system (Table 33.2), for visual prognosis, is the most widely accepted classification system. Abramson's staging system takes extraocular disease also into consideration (Table 33.3).

Second Tumors in Retinoblastoma

Over 30 years, there is a 35% cumulative risk of developing nonocular second primary tumor, following irradiation, as against 6% without radiation. The risk of developing a second tumor increases with the age of the patient. Osteogenic sarcoma is

Table 33.2: Reese-Ellsworth classification system
(for visual prognosis)

Group I	**Very Favorable**
A.	Solitary tumor less than 4 disc diameter (DD) in size at or behind equator
B.	Multiple tumors none over 4 DD in size, all at or behind equator
Group II	**Favorable**
A.	Solitary tumor 4 to 10 DD in size, at or behind equator
B.	Multiple tumors, 4 to 10 DD in size behind equator
Group III	**Doubtful**
A.	Any tumor anterior to equator
B.	Solitary tumor, larger than 10 DD, behind equator
Group IV	**Unfavorable**
A.	Multiple tumors some larger than 10 DD in size
B.	Any lesion extending anteriorly to ora serrata
Group V	**Very Unfavorable**
A.	Massive tumor involving over half of retina
B.	Vitreous seeding

Table 33.3: Abramson's staging system

1. Intraocular disease
   a. Retinal tumors
   b. Extension into choroid
   c. Extension up to lamina cribrosa
   d. Extension into sclera
2. Orbital disease
   a. Orbital tumor
      • Suspicious (pathology of scattered episcleral cells)
      • Proven (biopsy-proven orbital tumor)
   b. Local nodal involvement
3. Optic nerve disease
   a. Tumor beyond the lamina cribrosa but not up to cut section
   b. Tumor at cut section of optic nerve
4. Intracranial metastasis
   a. Positive cerebrospinal fluid only
   b. Mass CNS section
5. Hematogenous metastasis
   a. Positive marrow/bone lesion
   b. Other organ involvement

the commonest such tumor, while fibrosarcoma, malignant melanoma, chondrosarcoma, leukemia, renal cell carcinoma, Ewing's sarcoma, thyroid carcinoma, rhabdomyosarcoma may also develop. The risk appears to be higher if a child younger than 1 year of age is treated with radiation. Hence, it is preferable to substitute chemoreduction, if possible in children less than 1 year of age.

Trilateral Retinoblastoma

The association of midline intracranial pineal tumor of suprasellar and parasellar neuroblastic tumors with bilateral retinoblastoma is called trilateral retinoblastoma and have been reported in 2.3% of the bilateral retinoblastomas. Pinealoblastomas occur during the first 4 years of life and are invariably fatal. There are early indications that chemoreduction may have a favorable role in managing pinealomas.

Follow-up

All retinoblastoma patients are to be followed up for tumor recurrence in the orbit following enucleation and occurrence of new tumors in the same or fellow eye. The RetCam, a digital contact wide field camera is useful in the follow-up of retinoblastoma patients (Table 33.4). The images obtained during

Table 33.4: The follow-up schedule for retinoblastoma patients

• Six weeks after initial therapy
• Every three months for first year
• Every four months for second year
• Every six months till fifth year
• Once a year, life long (especially heritable tumors)

different visits can be compared to assess tumor progression. The digital image can also be electronically mailed for seeking opinion or for conducting multicentric studies.

RETINOCYTOMA OR RETINOMA

Introduction

Gallie and associates first described retinocytoma in 1982 as retinoma and Margo and associates as "retinocytoma". It is considered a benign variant of retinoblastoma. It usually appears as a homogenous, translucent, gray, slightly elevated placoid tumor with the blood vessels of normal caliber. Histopathologically, it consists of smaller and less hyperchromatic nuclei, absence of necrosis and presence of fleurettes, calcification in non-necrotic areas. Gallie and associates hypothesized that it could be due to the inactivation of both suppressor genes occurring late in the development of the retina. They found 27 (1.9%) cases of retinocytoma in a series of 1,400 retinoblastomas examined microscopically. There are reports of retinoblastomas occurring in retinomas in later life.

UVEAL MELANOMA

Introduction

Uveal melanomas are malignant neoplasms that arise from neuroectodermal melanocytes within the choroid, ciliary body or iris. Uveal melanomas are the most common primary intraocular tumors. The average age of the detection of melanoma of the choroid and ciliary body is in the fifth and sixth decade. Iris melanomas are detected at a younger age owing to their visibility.

Uveal melanomas are rare in Indian population and appear at a relatively younger age (mean age 45.89 years, range 15–82 years). Some of the predisposing factors for the development of uveal melanoma include:
• Oculodermal melanocytosis
• Dysplastic nevus syndrome
• Uveal nevus
• Xeroderma pigmentosum
• Family history of melanoma
• Neurofibromatosis (various phakomatoses syndromes are described in Table 33.5)
• Intense recurrent sunlight exposure

Melanoma of Iris

Iris melanomas form 3% to 13% of all uveal melanomas and are rare in the Asian population. Most iris melanomas are believed to arise from active growth in preexisting nevi. Epidemiological studies suggest that sunlight exposure plays a role in the pathogenesis of iris melanomas.

Patients present with an iris mass, secondary glaucoma and pain or heterochromia. It commonly presents in the inferior iris

Table 33.5: Phakomatoses syndromes

Name	Other Names	Inheritance	Ocular Features	Extraophthalmic Features
Neurofibromatosis 1	von Recklinghausen's disease	AD on 17q11	Subcutaneous NF and plexiform NF of eyelid, Lisch nodules on iris, optic nerve glioma, absence of greater wing of sphenoid. congenital and infantile glaucoma, multifocal bilateral choroidal nevi, retinal astrocytic hamartoma.	Cafe au lait spots, axillary and inguinal freckles, cutaneous neurofibroma Neurofibromas and solid tumors of the CNS, skeletal deformities.
Neurofibromatosis 2	Central neurofibromatosis	AD 22q12	Combined hamartoma of the retina Juvenile posterior subcapsular or cortical lens opacities.	Bilateral vestibular schwannomas Acoustic neuroma with or without sensory neural deafness. widely scattered NFs, meningioma, glioma and schwannomas
Tuberous sclerosis	Bournevilles Disease	2/3 sporadic 1/3 familial chromosome 9q32,34 locus in familial cases AD	Retinal astrocytoma	Low grade CNS astrocytoma, mental deficiency, seizures adenoma sebaceum, ash leaf spots, Shagreen patch, subungual fibroma. Angiomyolipoma of kidney. Cardiac rhabdomyoma. Pulmonary lymphangioleiomyomatosis Benign cysts in various viscera like kidney liver or lung.
Sturge-Weber syndrome		No typical inheritance pattern	Diffuse choroidal hemangioma. Ipsilateral congenital or infantile glaucoma. Telangiectasia over conjunctiva and episclera.	Facial nevus flammeus. Ipsilateral leptomeningeal hemangiomatosis. Cortical atrophy and seizures.
von Hippel-Lindau syndrome		Ch 3p25-26	Retinal capillary hemangioma	Hemangioblastoma of brain and spinal cord. Renal cell carcinomas, pheochromocytoma, solid and cystic neoplasms of various visceral organs.
Wyburn-Mason syndrome		Nonfamilial	Arterio-venous malformation of retina Orbital AVMs	AVMs of the ipsilateral CNS
Ataxia Telangiectasia	Louis-Bar syndrome		Telangiectasia of bulbar conjunctiva and skin in butterfly area of face and neck, ocular motility disturbances	Progressive cerebellar ataxia. Humoral and cellular immunodeficiencies. Chronic sinopulmonary infections. High incidence of malignancy Radiosensitivity

AD — Autosomal dominant
AVM — Arteriovenous malformations

as a localized dark brown tumor. Iris melanoma may diffusely involve the iris presenting as an ill-defined mass or as a ring melanoma. Angle involvement by the tumor, pigment-laden macrophage blocking the angle, angle closure or neovascularization may cause secondary glaucoma. The patient may present with heterochromia iridum and iridis. Loss of iris crypts and architecture, replaced by a diffuse pigmented thickening of the iris indicates the diagnosis.

The malignant potential of the tumor can be assessed by:
- Size of the lesion
- Apparent cohesiveness
- Intense vascularity
- Effect on adjacent ocular tissue—involvement of ciliary body indicates a malignancy

Diagnosis

Iris melanomas should be differentiated from leiomyoma, metastatic disease and nevi of the iris and also from iris cysts, iridocorneal endothelial syndrome, Koeppe and Busacca nodules, Lisch nodules and primary iris pigment epithelial tumors. Pigmented tumor > 3 mm in diameter and 1 mm in thickness that replaces the stroma of the iris having three of the following five features indicate an iris melanoma. Photographic documentation of growth, secondary glaucoma, secondary cataract, prominent vascularity and/or ectropion irides is considered to be an iris melanoma.
- Serial photography of the lesion may be done to document growth especially when differentiation from a nevus is difficult.

- Gonioscopy and transillumination can be used to estimate the extent of the tumor and detect extension of the tumor into ciliary body.
- Indirect ophthalmoscopy to rule out ciliochoroidal involvement.
- Ultrasound biomicroscopy helps us to assess the shape, internal architecture and extent of the tumor. It can also be repeated serially to monitor the growth of the tumor.
- Anterior segment fluorescein angiogram may demonstrate tumor vasculature.
- Fine needle aspiration biopsy can be done in cases where diagnosis is in doubt.
- Incisional biopsy

Since iris melanomas are usually detected early there is no justification for an extensive metastatic work-up. However, in advanced lesions a work-up similar to choroidal melanoma is necessary.

Iris melanomas have to be differentiated from a primary ciliary body melanoma extending through the root of the iris and presenting in the anterior chamber. In such a case, transillumination, gonioscopy and ultrasound biomicroscopy will reveal the tumor to arise from the ciliary body. An iris nevus is flatter and less vascular than a melanoma, though it alters the normal anatomy of the iris (in contrast to a freckle, which does not alter the anatomy of the iris). The documented evidence of growth indicates a melanoma than a nevus though a nevus may also increase in size.

Management

Iris melanomas are generally less aggressive than ciliary body or choroidal melanoma. Mortality rate from iris melanomas varies from 0% to 11% depending on the presence or the absence of metastases (2% to 10%) and ciliary body involvement.

Small iris melanomas can be observed with serial photography and ultrasound biomicroscopy. Larger lesions can be excised by iridectomy or iridocyclectomy. Large, diffuse lesions may require enucleation. Selective, diffuse or large focal iris melanoma in a single-eyed patient may be treated by customized plaque therapy.

Patients should be monitored for the development of secondary glaucoma and extension.

Ciliary Body and Choroidal Melanomas

Melanomas may involve only the ciliary body or the choroid or may extend in to the adjacent tissue when they are called ciliochoroidal melanomas. Ciliary body melanoma is less common than choroidal melanoma, with a ratio of occurrence of 1 in 10.

Ciliary Body Melanoma

Patients with ciliary body melanoma may be asymptomatic or present with blurred or decreased vision due to the growth of the melanoma into the lens causing subluxation, lenticular astigmatism or cataract. Ciliary body tumors may also cause field loss due to associated retinal detachment. Erosion of the tumor into blood vessels in adjacent tissues or necrosis of the tumor can lead to hyphema or vitreous hemorrhage causing decreased vision or floaters. Ciliary body melanomas can push the iris diaphragm anteriorly or they can infiltrate the trabecular meshwork, producing acute angle closure prompting the patients to present with pain.

Clinical Features

An early sign of an occult ciliary body melanoma is a sentinel vessel, which is one or more dilated episcleral blood vessels feeding the metabolically active tumor and is visible through the conjunctiva overlying it. Difference of intraocular pressure of >5 mm Hg between the two eyes with hypotony of the involved eye may also be present, due to separation and disruption of the overlying ciliary epithelium decreasing aqueous production. Extrascleral extension of the tumor may lead to a subconjunctival nodule. The tumor may be seen in the anterior chamber growing through the root of the iris. Most ciliary body melanomas can be observed as a darkly pigmented mass posterior to the pupil. However, the degree of pigmentation may vary from a totally amelanotic tumor to highly pigmented one. In addition to the commonly seen dome-shaped tumor, the tumor may diffusely involve the ciliary body as a ring melanoma having a greater tendency to metastasize and grow extrasclerally. Tumor-induced glaucoma can occur due to the obstruction of outflow pathways by pigment cells, melanin-laden macrophages or tumor cells. Direct invasion of the angle by the tumor, neovascularization and angle closure may also cause secondary glaucoma.

Differential Diagnosis of Ciliary Body Melanomas

Acute and chronic angle closure, neovascular glaucoma, other tumors of the iris and ciliary body, such as leiomyoma, iris melanoma, melanocytoma, metastasis, adenoma, adenocarcinoma, medulloepithelioma, anterior extension of choroidal melanoma and intraocular extension of conjunctival melanoma should be considered in differential diagnosis. Iridociliary cysts and inflammatory, foreign body granulomas can also mimic ciliary body melanoma.

Choroidal Melanoma

Choroidal melanomas may be asymptomatic or present with blurred vision due to a subfoveal tumor, cystoid macular edema, retinal detachment, vitreous hemorrhage, cataract and blockage of the visual axis directly by the tumor. They may also present with floaters due to vitreous hemorrhage, pain and field loss. A necrotic tumor may also induce an inflammatory reaction. Few patients may present with a blind painful eye without prior diagnosis of uveal melanoma. Hence, it is better to do an ultrasound examination to rule out a melanoma in all blind eyes without an explanatory cause.

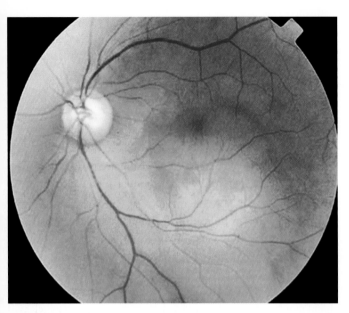

Fig. 33.10: Choroidal melanoma. Choroidal melanoma with overlying subretinal fluid

The typical choroidal melanoma appears as a dark brown, dome-shaped, solid tumor (Fig. 33.10). It can break through the overlying Bruch's membrane and form a dumbbell or collar button-shaped nodular mass under the retina. Diffuse melanoma (5%) may present as an ill-defined thickening of the choroid. The tumor pigment may vary from amelanotic to dense pigmentation and rarely the tumor may be multicentric or bilateral. Overlying retinal pigment epithelium and photoreceptor atrophy, drusen formation and retinal pigment epithelium detachment, cystoid degeneration of the retina, cystoid macular edema and choroidal neovascularization may occur as secondary effects. Secondary retinal detachment usually occurs. Severe ocular pain may occur when the tumor impinges on the posterior ciliary nerves. Melanomas may exhibit orange-colored lipofuscin pigment over their surface. Diffuse pigment indicates an active tumor while a localized pigment and drusen indicate a slow growing or a dormant tumor.

The tumor may grow anteriorly to involve the ciliary body, lens causing cataract, trabecular meshwork causing glaucoma, erode the blood vessels leading on to vitreous or anterior chamber hemorrhage. The tumor may also cause neovascular glaucoma secondary to rubeosis iridis and uveitis when undergoing necrosis. Patient may also present with subretinal hemorrhage and a posterior extrascleral extension that may cause proptosis.

Differential Diagnosis

Subretinal hemorrhage due to age-related macular degeneration might present as a dark red mass lesion, mimicking a melanoma. Choroidal hemangioma; choroidal detachment; choroidal nevus; melanocytoma; choroidal metastasis; choroidal osteoma; congenital hypertrophy of retinal pigment epithelium; retinal pigment epithelium tumors, such as adenoma and adenocarcinoma; combined hamartoma of the retina and retinal pigment epithelium; posterior scleritis and inflammatory granulomas due to sarcoidosis and tuberculosis may be mistaken for a melanoma.

Pathophysiology and Prognosis of Uveal Melanoma

Uveal melanoma arises from melanocytes in the uveal tract. Although uveal melanomas may grow de novo, most developed from a preexisting melanocytic nevus. Three distinct cell types, spindle A, spindle B and epithelioid are found. Presence of the latter type of cell is associated with more aggressive behavior and carries a poorer prognosis for the patient's survival. Callender's classification divides uveal melanocytic tumors into spindle cell nevi, spindle cell melanomas, necrotic melanomas, epithelioid cell melanomas and mixed cell melanomas. The latter two carry the poorest survival prognosis. Evaluation of vascular supply of the tumor, age at presentation, presence of extrascleral extension, mitotic rate, nucleolar area, quantification of nucleolar organizer regions, and tumor size and cell type have been used to evaluate the prognosis. Tumor features, such as larger size, anterior location, transcleral extension, growth through Bruch's membrane, optic nerve extension, lack of pigmentation and histologic characteristics, such as mitotic activity and cell type have been found to correlate with increased mortality.

Uveal melanomas tend to metastasize to the liver, lung, CNS, bone and skin. Less frequently, the tumor can grow transclerally, through emissary channels and spread locally into the orbit and conjunctiva. An overall mortality rate of approximately 30% to 50% occurs from uveal melanoma within 10 years from diagnosis and treatment. Most often, it is related to the development of distant metastasis. Peak incidence of metastasis occurs during the first year after diagnosis. Ciliary body tumors are detected late due to the location and that they are asymptomatic in the early stages. This increases the risk of hematogenous metastasis in these patients.

Diagnosis

The premanagement evaluation of uveal melanoma should include a thorough physical examination, with particular attention to the hepatic abdominal region, the skin and subcutaneous tissues, which are frequent sites of metastatic spread. Hepatic function tests (serum levels of gamma-glutamyl transpeptidase, lactic dehydrogenase, glutamic-oxaloacetic transaminase), ultrasound/CT scan examination of the abdomen are essential to rule out hepatic metastasis. However, the imaging studies will not exclude micrometastasis (smaller than 1–2 cm in diameter). X-ray of chest is also indicated to rule out lung metastasis, though it is often negative. These investigations are to be repeated six monthly after treatment, for early diagnosis of metastatic disease. However, most patients do not have any evidence of metastasis at the time of presentation.

Ultrasonography

B-scan usually shows a solid mass with a biconvex or mushroom shape. The tumor shows a relative brightness on the vitreal side and a relative darkness on the choroidal or basal aspect. Acoustic hollowing and choroidal excavation are also seen (Fig. 33.11).

Standardized A-scan reveals high surface spike with low amplitude internal reflectivity, with a decremental reduction of spike height from the surface to the depth of the mass. This is termed as positive angle kappa. A scan echoes may also show fluctuation of echo height indicating the vascularity of the tumor, this is however difficult to elicit. Ultrasound biomicroscopy has high resolution for ciliary body abnormalities, including melanomas. It can differentiate tumors of the ciliary body from those of choroidal origin and help define the anterior border.

Fundus fluorescein angiography picture depends on the shape of the tumor, its intrinsic and overlying pigmentation and presence or absence of healthy retinal pigment epithelium over the tumor. Choroidal melanomas typically are hypofluorescent in early frames and may show prominent intratumor blood vessels (double circulation). In the later frames, there is leakage from the tumor and in late frames, there is staining of the entire tumor and some leakage into the subretinal fluid. Pinpoint spots of hyperfluorescence appear in the choroidal phase of the fluorescein angiography corresponding to the areas of retinal pigment epithelium loss.

Malignant melanomas are hypofluorescent throughout indocyanine green angiography.

CT scan can image most choroidal and ciliary body melanomas and a majority of them show enhancement on contrast CT.

In MRI, malignant melanomas of the choroid and ciliary body appear bright (hyperintense) with respect to vitreous on T_1-weighted images and dark (hypointense) with respect to vitreous in T_2-weighted images.

In rare situations, when the diagnosis could not be made with reasonable certainty with above methods, fine needle aspiration biopsy may be necessary to obtain tissue specimen. It is usually advised when it is difficult to differentiate a melanoma from a metastatic disease or if the patient insists on a histopathological diagnosis prior to the therapy.

Management

The choice of treatment modality for a particular patient depends on multiple factors:

Visual acuity: Eyes with salvageable vision are treated conservatively, while those with no visual potential are enucleated.

Intraocular pressure: Choroidal melanomas with increased intraocular pressure are an indication for enucleation as they seldom respond to conservative treatment.

Size of the tumor: Small melanomas (2–3 mm thick) are usually observed periodically for the evidence of growth and other signs of malignancy. Medium (3–5 mm) and large (5–10 mm thick) may be observed, irradiated, locally resected or enucleated depending upon other factors. Extra large (>10 mm thick, 15 mm in diameter) are usually enucleated.

Location of the melanoma: Eyes with tumors close to and involving the optic nerve are enucleated, while tumor located at the equator can be irradiated and an anterior tumor can be resected depending on the size of the tumor and other factors.

Growth pattern of the tumor: Eyes with diffuse tumors and those associated with large extrascleral extensions may need to be enucleated or exenterated.

Activity of the tumor: Documented growth on follow-up, presence of subretinal fluid and an abrupt elevation from the Bruch's membrane suggest an active tumor, needing treatment. Drusen on the tumor surface indicates chronicity. Hazy and ill-defined orange pigment over the tumor indicates activity while well-defined pigment indicates dormancy.

Status of the opposite eye: In a one-eyed patient, all attempts are made to conservatively manage the tumor.

Age of the patient: Enucleation may not improve the systemic prognosis in patients over 65 years of age and hence older patients are managed conservatively.

General health of the patient: Sick patients who obviously cannot tolerate surgery or those with metastatic disease are managed conservatively.

Treatment Modalities

Melanomas may be periodically observed, enucleated, resected or irradiated depending on the factors detailed above.

Periodic Observation

Dormant, small- and medium-sized tumors, slow growing small- and medium-sized tumors in sick and one-eyed patients may generally be observed periodically after proper documentation with color fundus photograph and ultrasonography.

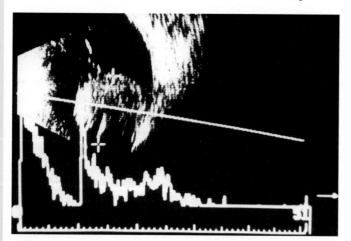

Fig. 33.11: B-scan ultrasonography in choroidal melanoma. B-scan shows characteristic appearance of malignant melanoma of the choroid

Enucleation

In the recent years, there has been a shift away from enucleation in the management of uveal melanomas. This shift is not attributed only to the increased risk of mortality after enucleation. The recognition that spindle cell tumors are less malignant and small melanocytic tumors behave biologically dormant with little tendency to grow and metastasize has prompted physicians to conservatively manage these tumors.

Large tumors producing visual loss and of a size that cannot be managed by conservative methods, small- or medium-sized tumors with optic nerve invasion, posterior uveal melanomas with total retinal detachment or severe glaucoma however are managed by enucleation. A "no touch technique" has been advocated to prevent hematogenous dissemination of the tumor.

Local Resection

Indications

Ciliary body tumors, not extending more than 4 clock hours of pars plicata, choroidal melanoma not greater than 15 mm in diameter, centered at the equator can be considered for iridocyclectomy or partial lamellar sclerouvectomy respectively if the retina is spared and penetrating sclerochorioretinovitrectomy if the retina and sclera are involved.

The technique involves localization of the tumor on the sclera, dissection of partial thickness scleral bed, resection of a thin layer of the sclera with the tumor leaving the overlying retina intact, if there is no retinal involvement. The presence of secondary retinal detachment overlying the tumor aids resection of the tumor without damaging the retina. Preoperative barrage laser photocoagulation or cryotherapy 2–3 mm surrounding the tumor is done, if retinal involvement is noted, in an attempt to keep the retina attached postoperatively. In such a situation, the infiltrated retina with the tumor is removed with open-sky vitrectomy through the scleral window. The sclera if involved is also removed and replaced with donor scleral graft.

Complications of this procedure include retinal detachment, cataract formation, vitreous hemorrhage, expulsive hemorrhage, chronic cystoid macular edema, anterior segment ischemia, tumor recurrence, hypotony and wound leak and preretinal fibrosis. Resection is generally preferred for anterior tumors with a small base and greater height in younger patients.

Internal Resection

This involves preoperative photocoagulation around the tumor, followed by vitrectomy and internal removal of the tumor piece-meal in posteriorly located tumors that are not amenable to lamellar sclerouvectomy. Short-term results of both techniques do not report increased metastatic risk. Combining brachytherapy with resection and pre-enucleation radiation is said to reduce the risk of tumor recurrence and metastasis.

Photocoagulation

Photocoagulation has been tried for malignant melanoma of the choroids, but not with the same success as for retinoblastoma. (1) Small nasal melanoma; (2) temporal peripheral small melanoma located away from macula and outside the arcade can be treated with laser photocoagulation. The tumors should be less than 3 mm in height and 9 to 10 mm in basal diameter without secondary retinal detachment. They should not be closer than 1 disc diameter from the disc. Less than 5% of melanomas meet the criteria laid down for use of photocoagulation. Multiple treatment sessions may be necessary before satisfactory regression of the tumor.

Retinal break formation, choroidoretinovitreal neovascularization near the edge of treatment, branch retinal vein occlusion, secondary macular edema and corneal and iris burns are known complications of photocoagulation treatment.

Photodynamic Therapy

The combination of tunable dye laser and a suitable photo-activated dye has been attempted in the management of malignant melanomas. Hematoporphyrin dye derivative is the most commonly used dye. The efficacy of this treatment is still under trial.

Radiotherapy

External Beam Radiotherapy

Pre-enucleation radiotherapy has been advocated to decrease the mortality rate following enucleation, but its value is currently debatable. Post-enucleation irradiation to the orbit has been found to decrease the mortality. The COMS study failed to show any benefit of pre-enucleation radiation in decreasing mortality. Regular external beam radiotherapy is not used in the management of choroidal melanoma due to the large dose involved that will invariably cause radiation-related complications leading to blindness. Post-enucleation irradiation may be useful in cases where extrascleral extension is noted intraoperatively.

External Beam Particle Radiotherapy

The charged particle radiation consists of the usage of helium ions and protons and the benefit lies in the fact that relatively large doses can be delivered to the tumor specifically. The high-energy charged particles have minimal scatter and a well-defined, finite, energy dependent range. The entire tumor can be treated uniformly and due to the inherent Bragg peak effect; unnecessary radiation to the normal tissue is avoided.

Uveal melanomas up to 24 mm in diameter and 14 mm in height have been treated with charged particle irradiation. Tumors involving the fovea, optic nerve head, those with small extrascleral extension can also be managed by this technique. The technique involves localization of the tumor with transillumination and indirect ophthalmoscopy and suturing four,

2.5 mm tantalum rings as localization markers. The treatment is then planned using a computer, thereby choosing the correct direction of the beam, which entails minimum radiation to normal structures, but also complete treatment of the tumor and 1.5 mm of surrounding normal tissue. Approximately 70 gray equivalents of cobalt-60 are delivered in five sittings over 7 to 10 days.

The five-year survival rate following proton beam radiation has been to be comparable with of plaque therapy. Complications include those of the surgery, such as transient diplopia, intratumor hemorrhage and those related to radiation, such as madarosis, epiphora due to punctual occlusion, dry eye, cataract formation, rubeosis iridis, neovascular glaucoma, radiation vasculopathy, papillopathy, maculopathy, macular edema, neovascularization of the retina and vitreous hemorrhage.

The disadvantage of the current charged particle radiation systems is that they are expensive to install and maintain.

Brachytherapy

The current relative indications of plaque therapy are:
1. Selected small melanomas that are documented to be growing or that show clear-cut signs of activity on the first visit.
2. Most medium-sized and some large choroidal and ciliary body melanomas in an eye with potential salvageable vision.
3. Almost all actively growing melanomas that occur in the patients' only useful eye.

If a melanoma exceeds 15 mm in diameter and 10 mm in thickness, one should anticipate visual morbidity from radiation therapy and enucleation should be strongly advised. Local recurrence, usually requiring enucleation, occurs at a rate of about 12% to 16%. Complications include cataract, rubeosis, scleral necrosis, keratopathy, radiation retinopathy and optic neuropathy, but at a reduced rate compared with external beam irradiation.

There is no statistically significant difference in the survival between patients treated with plaque radiotherapy (cobalt-60, iodine-125) and those treated with enucleation. The COMS study group is currently evaluating this issue in relation to the management of medium-sized melanomas.

Combined plaque radiotherapy and laser photocoagulation or thermotherapy has been used recently to increase the likelihood of complete local tumor destruction particularly in patients with tumor adjacent to the optic disc. Currently, binuclid plaques (combination of iodine-125 and ruthenium-106) are also being evaluated in managing uveal melanoma (Fig. 33.12).

Transpupillary Thermotherapy

In transpupillary thermotherapy (TTT), infrared laser is used to elevate the temperature of the tumor to 45–60°C, which is below photocoagulating temperatures. This causes vascular occlusion and death of the tumor cells up to a depth of 3–9 mm. Transpupillary thermotherapy has found wide use in treating small melanomas (<3 mm in thickness) that are away

from the disc and macula. With proper selection of tumors 94% of treated small choroidal melanomas showed regression. Vitreous and subretinal hemorrhage, epiretinal membrane formation with traction on the retina, retinal vascular occlusion and retinal break formation are the known complications.

VASCULAR TUMORS OF CHOROID

Introduction

Most vascular tumors of the retina and choroid indicate the presence of a phakomatosis, though they may occur without evidence of systemic disease. Work-up of a patient with suspected phakomatosis should include family history and also examination of the family members if necessary.

Choroidal Hemangioma

Choroidal hemangioma is a benign vascular tumor that is composed of large, dilated choroidal blood vessels. These vascular hamartomas can occur in two distinct forms—the circumscribed choroidal hemangioma and diffuse choroidal hemangioma (Figs 33.13 and 33.14A and B). The circumscribed tumor has no extraocular associations while the diffuse type can be associated with facial nevus flammeus or variations of Sturge-Weber syndrome. Cavernous hemangioma of the choroid is the most common vascular tumor of the uveal tract.

Circumscribed Choroidal Hemangioma

Circumscribed choroidal hemangiomas are relatively rare hamartomatous vascular tumors that appear in the posterior pole and are not associated with systemic disease. The tumor is generally diagnosed in patients between 20 and 40 years of age. The tumor is almost always unifocal and unilateral with bilateral

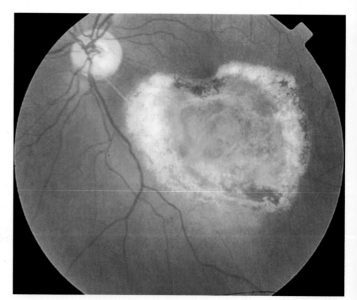

Fig. 33.12: Choroidal melanoma. Regression of choroidal melanoma following transpupillary thermotherapy

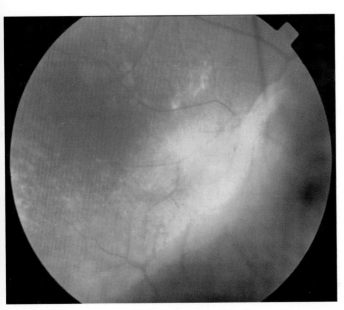

Fig. 33.13: Diffuse choroidal hemangioma showing typical 'tomato catsup' appearance

cases being extremely rare. Circumscribed choroidal hemangiomas can clinically simulate amelanotic melanomas and other choroidal masses.

Clinical Features

Circumscribed choroidal hemangioma appears as a discrete, smooth, round or oval, orange-red mass located in the posterior pole. The tumor may be homogenous in appearance or may show retinal pigment epithelial proliferation or fibrous metaplasia on its surface. The tumor may range from 3 to 18 mm (mean 7 mm) in diameter and 1 to 7 mm in height (mean 3 mm). The tumor is usually located posterior to the equator with most often in the macular or peripapillary region.

Subfoveal tumors tend to produce visual impairment early in life as a result of unilateral, ipsilateral hyperopia secondary to the anterior displacement of the retina by the underlying choroidal tumor. Patients with parafoveal tumors may remain asymptomatic up to adulthood, until they develop a secondary exudative retinal detachment that may extend into the central macular area. The tumor is usually not recognized until it causes a gradual or sudden onset of blurred vision or when the patient develops metamorphopsia in the third or fifth decade of life. The retina over a circumscribed choroidal hemangioma often develops severe secondary cystoid retinal degeneration. Occasionally, a total retinal detachment can occur and lead to neovascular glaucoma. The tumor may blanch on depression indicating the vascularity of the tumor.

Diagnosis

Ancillary tests can help in differentiating a choroidal hemangioma from other nonpigmented intraocular tumors.

Fluorescein angiography: Circumscribed choroidal hemangiomas show some characteristic features on fluorescein angiography, but they are not pathognomic. Fluorescein angiography shows irregular linear hyperfluorescence of the large choroidal vessels within the tumor, which is seen in the prearterial or early arterial phases. In the arterial and venous phase, there is progressive staining of the tumor with the pinpoint foci of hyperfluorescence. In the late phases, intraretinal hyperfluorescence is seen due to the diffuse leakage of dye in to the cystic spaces in the retina overlying the tumor. A similar pattern of fluorescence can be observed with some choroidal melanomas.

Indocyanine green angiography: Indocyanine green angiography reveals characteristic findings in circumscribed choroidal hemangiomas. The maximum fluorescence is typically hyperintense and is seen at an average of 1.2 minutes after injection.

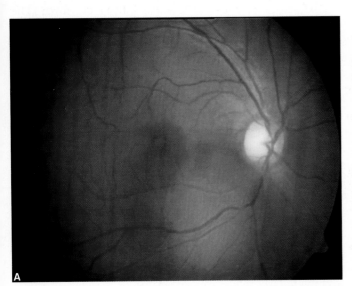
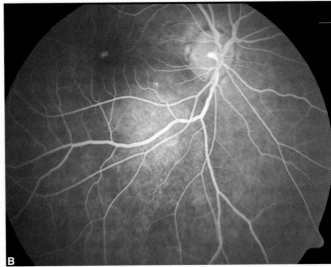

Figs 33.14A and B: Circumscribed choroidal hemangioma. Discrete, smooth, round, orange-red mass located in the posterior pole (A). Fluorescein angiography shows linear irregular hyperfluorescence (B)

A lacy diffuse fluorescent pattern is seen. In the late phases, a washout of the dye, which appears as hypofluorescence of the tumor is seen. A rim of hyperfluorescence is seen surrounding the tumor in the late frames.

Ultrasonography: On A-scan ultrasonography, circumscribed choroidal hemangiomas demonstrate an initial high spike on the anterior surface of the hemangioma and high internal reflectivity with no significant shadowing. With B-scan, the tumor shows a rounded or placoid, choroidal tumor pattern with a distinct anterior border and acoustic solidity. The characteristic findings of acoustic hollowness and choroidal excavation seen in choroidal melanomas are almost never seen with a circumscribed choroidal hemangioma. Occasionally, high reflective echoes can be noticed over tumor surface due to dense fibrous or osseous metaplasia of the overlying retinal pigment epithelium.

Computed tomography: Computed tomography can help substantiate the diagnosis of circumscribed choroidal hemangiomas and in the evaluation of size and shape of the tumor. Circumscribed choroidal hemangiomas show moderate enhancement with contrast material.

Magnetic resonance imaging: On Magnetic resonance imaging, circumscribed choroidal hemangioma is relatively hyperintense with respect to the vitreous in T_1-weighted images and isointense to the vitreous in T_2-weighted images. The tumor shows a marked enhancement on gadolinium administration. On the other hand, a choroidal melanoma is hyperintense to the vitreous in T_1-weighted images and hypointense to the vitreous on T_2-weighted images.

Radioactive phosphorus uptake test: Radioactive phosphorus uptake test (the P-32 test) is an invasive diagnostic method and is utilized only if ancillary tests fail to help in the differential diagnosis. Circumscribed choroidal hemangiomas produce a negative result with the P-32 uptake test in the majority of cases. In the occasional borderline positive case, the uptake is lower than for a comparable sized melanoma.

Pathology

On histology, they can be classified into predominantly capillary, predominantly cavernous or mixed types depending on the prevailing type of blood vessels. The capillary type is rare and is composed of small blood vessels with inconspicuous endothelial cells separated by loose connective tissue. The cavernous type is more common and consists of large, thin-walled, blood-filled vascular channels lined by a flat endothelium and separated by thin intervascular septa. A mixture of both types can be seen in many tumors. Extensive cystic changes are generally present in the outer retinal layers overlying the tumor and may coalesce to form retinoschisis. The retinal pigment epithelium overlying the tumor may show fibrous or osseous metaplasia. The pigmented rim seen clinically is caused by irregularly compressed choroidal melanocytes at the margin of the hemangioma.

Differential Diagnosis

Amelanotic choroidal melanoma: A typical circumscribed choroidal hemangioma has a red-orange color, which is never seen with a choroidal melanoma. Sometimes, when the choroidal melanoma breaks through the Bruch's membrane, large congested vessels may appear on the surface of the tumor and may produce a hemangioma-like picture. In reality, such vessels are not seen with a choroidal hemangioma. The characteristic findings of acoustic hollowness and choroidal excavation seen in choroidal melanomas on ultrasonography are almost never seen with a circumscribed choroidal hemangioma.

Choroidal metastasis: Choroidal metastasis usually has a dull or creamy yellow appearance in comparison to the red-orange color of a choroidal hemangioma. Circumscribed choroidal hemangioma are always unilateral and unifocal whereas choroidal metastasis are often multifocal and bilateral.

Central serous retinopathy: Both central serous retinopathy and circumscribed choroidal hemangioma can be clinically similar in the sense that both conditions can produce metamorphopsia due to recurrent subretinal fluid in the foveal area. Indirect ophthalmoscopy demonstrates the absence of a tumor and fluorescein angiography shows central serous chorioretinpathy type leaks.

Posterior scleritis: Posterior scleritis can sometimes resemble a circumscribed choroidal hemangioma, but is usually associated with inflammatory signs and choroidal folds.

Management

The management of choroidal hemangioma varies with the severity of symptoms and the presence or absence of exudative retinal detachment. In asymptomatic cases no treatment is necessary as circumscribed choroidal hemangioma rarely increases in size and remains quiescent for months or years and the patient should be observed every six months.

Treatment is usually considered in cases with visual loss due to serous retinal detachment involving the fovea. The various treatment options are photocoagulation, microwave thermotherapy, external beam irradiation, proton beam therapy, brachytherapy (EBRT) and cobalt-60 radiotherapy and recently, transpupillary thermotherapy and photodynamic therapy.

Photocoagulation: Photocoagulation is the most widely accepted mode of treating a choroidal hemangioma. Argon laser has been commonly used for treatment. The main aim of treatment is to create a chorioretinal adhesion so as to facilitate the reattachment of the retina and resolution of subretinal fluid. In cases of extensive retinal detachment, surgical drainage of subretinal fluid can be carried out to allow photocoagulation and saline or gas may be injected in the vitreous to flatten the retina.

Diffuse Choroidal Hemangioma

Diffuse choroidal hemangioma is a benign vascular tumor that has poorly defined borders and extends over a broad area of the posterior choroid. It is characteristically associated with cutaneous, ocular or central nervous system findings. It is generally associated with an ipsilateral facial hemangioma, sometimes as part of the Sturge-Weber syndrome. The Sturge-Weber syndrome (encephalotrigeminal angiomatosis) is characterized by the presence of a leptomeningeal hemangioma variably associated with a facial nevus flammeus and abnormalities of the underlying cerebral cortex with intracranial calcification. Precise incidence of diffuse choroidal hemangioma in patients with Sturge-Weber syndrome is not known. A series of 35 patients with this syndrome found an incidence of 31% of diffuse choroidal hemangioma and a 100% incidence of facial nevus flammeus. The diffuse choroidal hemangioma is generally unilateral and ipsilateral to the facial hemangioma, but may be bilateral if facial nevus flammeus is bilateral or of it is associated in variants of Klippel-Trenaunay-Weber syndrome.

Clinical Features

It is extremely rare for the diffuse choroidal hemangioma to occur as an isolated finding without facial nevus flammeus or some of the other manifestations of the Sturge-Weber syndrome. Diffuse choroidal hemangioma is usually diagnosed at a young age, either because the associated facial hemangioma prompts a fundus examination or due to visual impairment caused by hyperopic amblyopia or from a secondary retinal detachment. The pupil shows a brilliant red reflex (tomato-catsup fundus) in the involved eye in contrast to the normal reflex in the opposite pupil. Lens and vitreous cavity are usually clear.

Diffuse choroidal hemangioma on ophthalmoscopy reveals a diffuse red-orange thickening of the posterior choroid, which is mainly seen in the macular area. Cystoid degeneration in the overlying retina over the tumor surface with retinal pigment epithelial disruption commonly occurs. The overlying retinal vessels may appear tortuous. In comparison to circumscribed choroidal hemangioma, the diffuse choroidal hemangioma is frequently large and often extends anterior to the equator. The diffuse choroidal hemangioma can produce a total secondary retinal detachment, cataract and leukocoria. Ipsilateral congenital glaucoma can develop, particularly when the upper lid is involved by the nevus flammeus. Asymmetry of the optic disc can be documented with the enlargement of the optic cup. Vascular, mechanical and developmental causes offer the most plausible mechanisms to explain the pathogenesis of glaucoma in encephalotrigeminal angiomatosis.

Diagnosis

A diagnosis of diffuse choroidal hemangioma should be considered in a child with facial nevus flammeus and ipsilateral visual loss. Ultrasonography demonstrates a markedly thickened choroid with medium to high internal reflectivity with an overlying retinal detachment. Fundus fluorescein angiography reveals diffuse leakage similar to circumscribed choroidal hemangioma, but with more widespread involvement. Magnetic resonance imaging features are similar to circumscribed choroidal hemangioma.

Pathology

Diffuse choroidal hemangioma is characterized by an intermixed proliferation of small and large blood vessels and is usually classified as a mixed hemangioma. Fibrous transformation of the proliferated retinal pigment epithelium is observed in over 50% of diffuse choroidal hemangiomas in Sturge-Weber syndrome.

Management

Diffuse choroidal hemangioma is a difficult condition to manage. Treatment in the form of refraction, corrective lenses and amblyopia therapy is indicated if unilateral, subfoveal tumor causes hyperopia. With extensive secondary retinal detachment, drainage of subretinal fluid through a posterior sclerotomy and injection of saline and or scleral buckling with pars plana vitrectomy and injection of gas and endolaser may be recommended.

Glaucoma filtering surgery may be performed to lower the intraocular pressure, but serous or hemorrhagic choroidal detachments may occur during surgery. EBRT in the dose of 1250 to 2000 cGy in divided fractions has been utilized for treatment of diffuse choroidal hemangiomas. Radiation leads to resolution of the retinal detachment in most cases and control of glaucoma in some cases.

VASCULAR TUMORS OF RETINA

Introduction

Vascular tumors of the retina include the following:

- Capillary hemangioma of the retina
- Cavernous hemangioma of the retina
- Racemose hemangioma
- Vasoproliferative tumor of the retina

Capillary Hemangioma of the Retina

Capillary hemangioma of the retina may occur as a phakomatosis with central nervous system and systemic tumors when it is called von Hippel-Lindau syndrome. It may occur without systemic disease as well. It is genetically transmitted in an autosomal-dominant mode with incomplete penetrance and variable expressivity. von Hippel-Lindau syndrome is linked to a defect in the short arm of chromosome 3 (3p 25-26).

Ocular Features

The ocular lesions are usually diagnosed between 10–30 years of age. The early angioma appears as a yellow spot between a feeding arteriole and a draining venule (Figs 33.15A and B). As the angioma increases in size, the supplying vessels increase in diameter and become tortuous. Visual acuity decreases due to exudation or secondary retinal detachment involving the macula. An appearance of dilated pair of vessels in the posterior pole with macular exudates should prompt one to examine the periphery for a capillary angioma. Multiple or bilateral

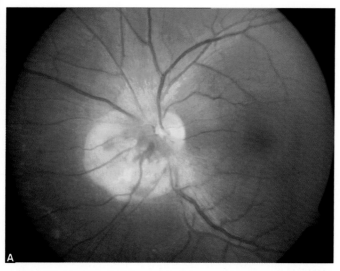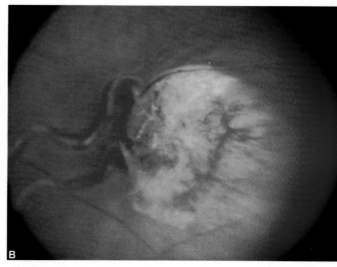

Figs 33.15A and B: Capillary hemangioma. (A) Capillary hemangioma at the optic nerve head. (B) Capillary hemangioma with a feeding arteriole and a draining venule

angiomas indicate the presence of von Hippel-Lindau tumor and screening for central nervous system or systemic disease should be done. The exudation in the macular region may be due to a steal phenomenon or a subretinal migration.

Some authors believe that two forms of disease exist—the exudative form and the vitreoretinal form. In the vitreoretinal form, epimacular membranes are formed, which cause macular traction detachment and decreased vision. Traction on the angiomas can lead to "free floating" angiomas in the vitreous, vitreous hemorrhage and a combined traction rhegmatogenous retinal detachment can also occur.

Angioma of the optic nerve head may occur. This differs from the retinal angioma in that no feeder arteriole or a draining venule is seen. The orange-red lesion is ill-defined, involves an eccentric part of the optic disc with exudation involving the peripapillary region and simulates papilledema.

Without treatment, most eyes progress to total retinal detachment, neovascular glaucoma and a painful blind eye.

Differential Diagnosis

The retinal angioma may be mistaken for Coat's disease (no paired dilated vessels in coat's disease), racemose angioma (no tumor between the arteriole and venule in racemose angioma), intraretinal macroaneurysm (occurs along an arteriole without a draining venule), retinal cavernous hemangioma (multiple sac like aneurysmal dilatations), familial exudative vitreoretinopathy and nematode endophthalmitis.

The disc angioma may simulate papilledema, optic neuritis, peripapillary choroidal neovascular membrane and optic disc granuloma.

Pathology

The lesions are made of a proliferation of capillaries that usually replace full thickness retina with benign proliferation of endothelial cells and pericytes.

Diagnosis

The diagnosis can be made most often on indirect ophthalmoscopy with the classic picture of an orange tumor with a feeding arteriole, draining venule associated with macular exudates. A fundus fluorescein angiogram may however be necessary to delineate early lesions that are not visible on clinical examination. These lesions fill early phases of the angiogram and leak profusely later. The paired vessels are well delineated as well.

Management

Early treatment of retinal capillary angiomas leads to better visual results. Early stages of the angiomas without retinal detachment are treated with laser photocoagulation. It is preferable to use green, yellow or blue-green wavelength to treat these lesions, as red or infrared lasers may not be absorbed well. Lesions <2 mm are treated with direct photocoagulation. For lesions 3 to 5 mm, it is preferable to try occlusion of the feeder vessels—the arteriole in the first session and the venule later. The angioma as such can be treated in subsequent sessions. Hemorrhage from the tumor and increase in secondary retinal detachment may occur as complications.

For tumors larger than 5 mm, it is preferable to use triple freeze-thaw cryotherapy. A conjunctival incision is usually necessary to treat posteriorly placed tumors, while anterior tumors can be treated without the same. Postoperative increase in the exudative detachment is commonly seen, which settles with time. Hemorrhage from the tumor may also occur.

If the tumors that are associated with a bullous retinal detachment, drainage of the fluid, cryotherapy and scleral buckling may be necessary. Advanced vitreoretinal form of the disease may need vitrectomy to relieve tractional or rhegmatogenous retinal detachment. Some authors have tried internal (vitreoretinal route) or external (transscleral route) resection of single large tumors. Eyes with advanced disease that needs surgical intervention usually have a poor visual prognosis.

Transpupillary thermotherapy, plaque brachytherapy, proton beam irradiation and external beam radiation therapy have been employed in the management of retinal and disc angiomas.

Systemic Features

In contrast to most phakomatosis, von Hippel-Lindau syndrome does not have major cutaneous features. Angiomas, nevi or café-au-lait spots may occasionally be seen.

Cerebellar hemangioblastoma is the classic central nervous system lesion of von Hippel-Lindau syndrome. It usually causes cerebellar symptoms in the fourth decade of life and can be imaged on a CT scan. Treatment is in the form of surgical resection if possible.

Unilateral or bilateral pheochromocytomas, renal cell carcinomas, and cysts of the kidney, pancreas and epididymis may occur in these patients. It is thus important to follow-up patients of von Hippel-Lindau syndrome with periodic neurological and systemic evaluation.

Cavernous Hemangioma of the Retina

Cavernous hemangioma of the retina is also recognized as a phakomatosis with the involvement of the retina, skin and the central nervous system. It appears to have an autosomal-dominant mode of inheritance (Fig. 33.16).

Ocular Features

The ocular involvement is usually asymptomatic if situated in the periphery or may cause loss of vision if involving the macula. One patient with a superonasal cavernous angioma has been noted to have associated cone dysfunction. The lesion appears as a cluster of dark red saccules with associated fibroglial proliferation. No feeder arteriole or draining venule is usually seen though some authors have noted twin vessels to be associated with this tumor. The lesion is nonprogressive or may enlarge minimally over time. The tumor may rarely cause vitreous hemorrhage, but does not cause exudation. The differential diagnosis of this lesion includes those listed for capillary hemangioma of the retina.

The lesion consists of endothelial-lined venous aneurysms interconnected by narrow channels. Associated cystic degeneration of the retina may occur.

The diagnosis is evident on fundus examination, but the fundus fluorescein angiogram is quite characteristic. These lesions have a slow blood flow, which leads to the separation of the plasma from the blood cells, which settle down within the saccule. Fluorescein enters the saccule slowly and fills the supernatant plasma, enhancing the fluid level, creating a "fluorescein cap".

No treatment is required for this lesion. If vitreous hemorrhage occurs, cryotherapy, photocoagulation and low-energy plaque may be used to treat these tumors.

Similar lesions involving the central nervous system may lead to seizures and other neurological symptoms. Hepatic cavernous angiomas may also occur. Cutaneous angiomas may involve the back or the neck.

Racemose Hemangioma

Racemose hemangioma is more of a vascular malformation than a tumor and if associated with systemic disease, is called the Wyburn-Mason syndrome. No definite hereditary pattern has been noted (Fig. 33.17).

Arteriovenous communications in Wyburn-Mason syndrome have been classified in to three types. In the first type, an abnormal capillary plexus is interposed between the arteriole and the venule. These lesions do not cause symptoms

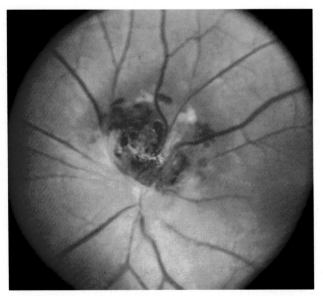

Fig. 33.16: Cavernous hemangioma of the retina

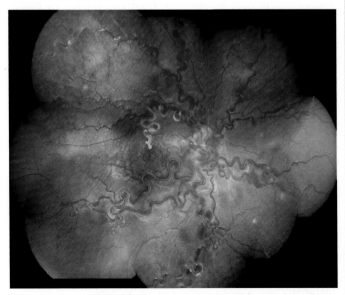

Fig. 33.17: Racemose hemangioma

and are not usually associated with cerebral involvement. In second type, no capillary bed is found and direct arteriovenous communication exists and the patients experience few visual symptoms. Associated cerebral vascular malformation may be found. In third type, patients have more complex and extensive arteriovenous malformation with visual loss and increased risk of cerebral disease. One or more dilated arterioles emanate from the disc, travel for a variable distance in the retina, form arteriovenous communication and return to the disc. No associated exudation or retinal detachment is found.

The clinical appearance is characteristic and a fluorescein angiogram may show rapid filling of the arteriovenous communication without dye leakage.

Most lesions are stationary and do not need treatment. However, visual prognosis is poor. Spontaneous intracranial hemorrhages may lead to neurologic symptoms. Bones of the skull, maxilla and mandible may be involved; causing massive bleeding during dental extraction. Orbital vascular malformations may cause proptosis.

Vasoproliferative Tumor of the Retina

These solitary tumors commonly involve the inferotemporal or inferior quadrants of the retina. They may occur without any antecedent cause, but are associated with prior uveitis, retinitis pigmentosa, Coat's disease and familial exudative vitreoretinopathy and toxoplasma scars. They appear as solitary mass lesions with minimally dilated feeder vessels, associated with intraretinal and subretinal exudation and hemorrhage, secondary retinal detachment, premacular fibrosis, tractional retinal detachment, retinal pigment epithelium hyperplasia, macular edema and vitreous hemorrhage. Some patients may have multiple or diffuse tumors. The pathogenesis of these lesions is unclear.

Fluorescein angiography shows early filling and late leakage and dilated feeder vessels. If progressive exudation causes loss of vision then cryotherapy, photocoagulation or plaque brachytherapy may be necessary. Epiretinal proliferation may need vitreous surgery.

OCULAR METASTASIS

Introduction

Carcinoma can metastasize to involve the eye. Ocular metastasis is most commonly seen in the uveal tract. The choroid is the commonest site of metastasis due to its vascularity. The commonest malignancy to metastasize to the eye is from the breast, followed by lungs and gastrointestinal tract in women; and lungs, kidney and the gastrointestinal tract in men. Metastasis can also involve the optic nerve, neural retina and rarely the vitreous. Ocular metastasis are unilateral and unifocal in 80% of cases on presentation. Most patients with ocular metastasis have a mean survival of six months.

Patients are commonly present with blurred or distorted vision. Usually, pain is absent, but can occur in cases with extensive metastasis or secondary glaucoma.

Fundus examination shows unifocal or multifocal creamy white or yellowish placoid, minimally elevated subretinal mass lesions. Rarely the lesion may be dome shaped and elevated into the vitreous cavity. It is often associated with serous retinal detachment, which can be extensive. Some metastatic tumors exhibit characteristic color, e.g. renal cell carcinoma— reddish-brown, malignant melanoma—skin-black, etc.

Metastatic carcinoma to the optic disc may appear as a swollen disc or as an infiltrative mass over the optic disc. It is usually associated with profound visual impairment. The retina is rarely involved. Vitreous involvement may appear as vitreous opacities. Metastasis to the iris may be seen as a mass lesion over the iris. They can be a source of spontaneous hyphema and pseudohypopyon.

Investigations

Evaluation by an oncologist is essential in patients without an obvious primary tumor.

Fluorescein Angiography

Metastatic choroidal tumors appear hypofluorescent in the early frames and show diffuse hyperfluorescence in the late frames. There may be pooling of dye under the serous retinal detachment.

Ultrasonography

Flat and irregular, medium reflective, multiple hyperechoeic lesions, with associated disproportionate serous retinal detachment can be imaged. A scan shows high amplitude internal echoes.

Fine Needle Aspiration Biopsy

This is done only when the primary site of malignancy is not found or if the tumor mimics an amelanotic melanoma from which it cannot be differentiated with certainty. It should be done in conjunction with an experienced cytologist. Cytologic interpretation helps in confirming the diagnosis of metastasis and may sometimes identify the primary tumor.

Differential Diagnosis

Amelanotic malignant melanoma, bullous central serous retinopathy, posterior scleritis, inflammatory granuloma (tuberculosis, sarcoid granuloma), and other choroidal tumors, such as hemangioma, Vogt-Koyanagi-Harada's syndrome may all mimic choroidal metastasis.

Management

Ocular metastasis usually responds to the same treatment as the primary.
• Chemotherapy and hormonal therapy

- Radiotherapy-external beam radiation or plaque radiation
- Enucleation of painful blind eyes

Rarely excision of a solitary metastasis or enucleation of the eye can be done if only a solitary metastasis is expected (carcinoid tumor).

PRIMARY INTRAOCULAR LYMPHOMA

Introduction

Primary intraocular lymphoma is a subtype of lymphoma, formerly called as reticulum cell sarcoma. It is a non-Hodgkin's large cell lymphoma (Fig. 33.18).

Patients usually belong to the age group of 60–70 years and commonly are present with diminished vision and floaters. Retinovitreal involvement is associated with CNS lymphoma, while choroidal involvement is common with systemic lymphoma.

Ocular examination reveals a uveitis like clinical picture. There may be signs of anterior uveitis with cells and keratic precipitates with diffuse cellular infiltration of the vitreous. These cell clumps differ from vitreous cells associated with vitritis in that they are larger and are clumped together. There may be accumulation of lymphoma cells in the subretinal pigment epithelial space. These appear yellow-white, geographic, with pigmentation due to clumping of retinal pigment epithelium at the borders (leopard skin appearance). Small satellite lesions can occur at the vicinity of larger lesions. An associated exudative retinal detachment may also occur.

Differential Diagnosis

- Chronic idiopathic vitritis
- CMV retinitis
- Metastatic carcinoma
- Pars planitis

Fundus fluorescein angiogram and ultrasound are not diagnostic. The diagnosis requires a strong index of suspicion,

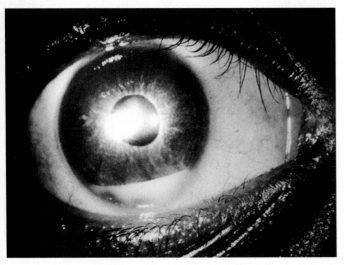

Fig. 33.18: Primary intraocular lymphoma

particularly in elderly patients presenting with signs of chronic uveitis not responding to steroids. Diagnostic vitreous biopsy may demonstrate malignant lymphoid cells with cytological features of large lymphoid cells. Rarely a fine needle aspiration biopsy may be necessary to prove the diagnosis.

Patients with primary intraocular lymphoma frequently develop independent primary foci of lymphoma in the central nervous system. All cases diagnosed as intraocular lymphoma should undergo an MRI scan of the brain to rule out CNS lymphoma and these patients should be followedup for the subsequent development of CNS lymphoma.

Management

Primary intraocular lymphoma responds to low dose ocular radiation. Chemotherapy and whole brain irradiation can be combined for patients with CNS lymphoma. Prognosis for life in patients with CNS lymphoma is poor.

INTRAOCULAR LEUKEMIA

Introduction

The leukemias are malignant transformations of the blood forming cells of the body. They include lymphocytic and myelogenous groups. Intraocular deposits of leukemic cells have been noted in 31% of patients postmortem. Clinical signs of ocular leukemia are seen less commonly. Eye changes indicate advanced disease and suggest an unfavorable prognosis. Intraocular leukemia can occur even if the peripheral blood smear and the bone marrow biopsy suggest disease remission.

The ocular manifestations of leukemia include leukemic infiltrates of the cornea, sclera, iris, vitreous, retina, choroid and optic nerve. Pseudohypopyon, iris nodules, secondary glaucoma and rubeosis are other anterior segment manifestations. The retina may show cotton wool spots, Roths' spots (white-centered retinal hemorrhages), microaneurysms, periphlebitis, optic disc swelling and venous occlusive disease. Overlying retinal pigment epithelial disturbance with resultant degeneration and clumping (leopard spot pattern) may be seen. Retinal changes may be due to associated hematologic abnormalities, such as anemia, hyperviscosity, thrombocytopenia and not always due to leukemic infiltration.

A history of treated leukemia is important in suspecting the diagnosis. In patients with pseudohypopyon or vitritis, cytological analysis of the aqueous tap or vitreous aspirate/biopsy may be necessary. Treatment is as that of the primary disease, which includes chemotherapy and radiation.

CHOROIDAL OSTEOMA

Introduction

It is an uncommon, benign, acquired, bony tumor of the choroid, which presents in young healthy females in the second

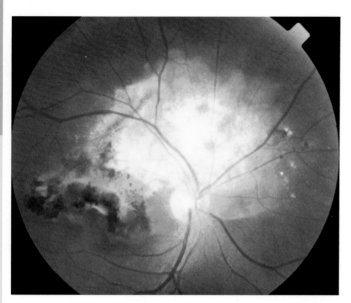

Fig. 33.19: Choroidal osteoma

or third decades of life. It is unilateral in 70 to 80% of cases (Fig. 33.19).

Patients usually present with painless progressive loss of vision over several months or years or abrupt reduction of central vision with metamorphopsia. Sometimes the lesions are noticed on routine eye examination.

The tumor appears as a yellow-orange, well-defined, juxtapapillary or circumpapillary choroidal mass.

Surface of the tumor may be relatively flat or visibly uneven with depressions and elevations. Margins are irregular and tufts of short branching vessels, which originate deep within the tumor, may be seen. These vascular tufts are believed to emerge from the marrow spaces onto the surface of the tumor. Hence, they are not neovascular tissue.

Degeneration of overlying retinal pigment epithelium and neurosensory retina can cause loss of vision. Development of a choroidal neovascular membrane may also decrease vision.

Diagnosis

Ultrasonography and computed tomography are useful for confirming a presumptive diagnosis. Choroidal osteoma appears as highly reflective plate like lesion that shows orbital shadowing. Fluorescein angiography shows patchy, early hyperfluorescence and late diffuse hyperfluorescence. An associated choroidal neovascular membrane will show early lacy hyperfluorescence with late leakage. On indocyanine green angiography, early hypofluorescence of the mass with superimposed hyperfluorescent intralesional blood vessels and late diffuse hyperfluorescence is seen.

Differential Diagnosis

* Amelanotic choroidal melanoma
* Choroidal nevus

* Metastatic carcinoma of the choroid
* Choroidal hemangioma
* Metastatic calcification

Management

Choroidal osteomas have no malignant potential and can be observed. The tumor may enlarge and rarely may partly regress as well. If a choroidal neovascular membrane was to develop, it can be treated with laser photocoagulation.

MEDULLOEPITHELIOMA

Introduction

Medulloepithelioma is a rare primary intraocular neoplasm that arises from non-pigmented epithelium of the ciliary body usually in the first decade of life. The tumor may rarely arise from the iris. It is derived from neuroectoderm (Fig. 33.20).

Medulloepithelioma may vary from a benign proliferation to a frankly malignant lesion, with invasive capability but low metastatic potential.

The child may present with a red eye, elevated intraocular pressure, change in the color of the iris, a visible mass on the iris or visual impairment.

Medulloepithelioma of the ciliary body typically appears as a tan to white lesion involving the ciliary body, causing a notch in the lens, cataract and subluxation. It may be associated with the formation of cysts, some of which may be free floating in the anterior chamber.

Medulloepithelioma of the iris appears as a tan to pink mass that replaces the peripheral iris and fills the angle. Such tumors often show intrinsic blood vessels.

Common complication of medulloepithelioma is neovascular glaucoma. In young patients with unexplained neovas-

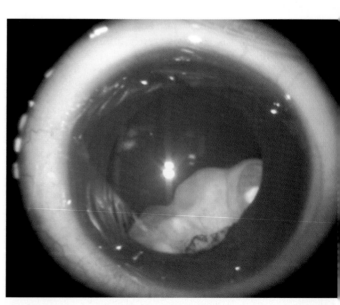

Fig. 33.20: Medulloepithelioma

cular glaucoma or acute-angle closure glaucoma and a normal fundus, medulloepithelioma should be ruled out.

Investigations

- B-scan ultrasonography/B-scan with stand off and ultrasound biomicroscopy may show the ciliary body tumor.
- CT, MRI scan: Bigger tumors can be imaged on the scans, provided the tumor is big enough and the scan slices are thin enough.

Differential Diagnosis

- Retinoblastoma
- Amelanotic malignant melanoma of ciliary body
- Leiomyoma of ciliary body
- Nematode granuloma
- Juvenile xanthogranuloma

Management

- Iridocyclectomy or cyclectomy for small-circumscribed lesions.
- Enucleation for large lesions, recurrent lesions after excision and blind eye.

RETINAL ASTROCYTOMA

Introduction

Retinal astrocytomas are glial tumors arising from the optic nerve head or the retina (Fig. 33.21). Though these tumors have a predilection to the posterior pole they may occur anywhere on the retina. The tumor may manifest in two clinical forms:

- As a glistening, white-yellow calcified tumor, which has well-defined borders and multiple small excrescences, so called mulberry or fish egg lesions.
- As a flat, gray-white tumor that is round or oval and has a smooth surface.

The visual acuity may be decreased if optic disc or macular involvement is present. Rarely vitreous hemorrhage may occur.

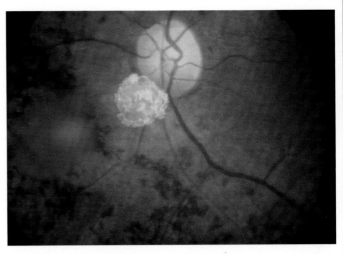

Fig. 33.21: Retinal astrocytomas

Systemic Associations

Astrocytomas are commonly associated with patients with tuberous sclerosis. They may also occur less commonly in patients with neurofibromatosis and retinitis pigmentosa.

Ancillary Tests

Ultrasonography

Astrocytomas appear as well-demarcated, oval mass with a sharp anterior border, acoustic solidity and lack of choroidal excavation. Orbital shadowing due to the presence of calcification may be seen.

Fluorescein Angiography

The calcified astrocytoma may demonstrate autofluorescence in preinjection photographs. There is diffuse hyperfluorescence in the late phases due to leakage from the tumor vessels.

Management

Treatment is usually not necessary as they are relatively stable and do not affect the visual acuity. Laser photocoagulation may be tried for those tumors with serous exudates threatening the fovea.

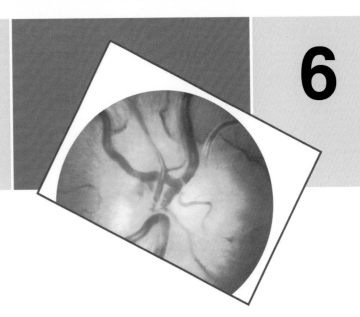

Diseases of Optic Nerve

34. Optic Nerve Disorders

34

Optic Nerve Disorders

Radhika Tandon, Lalit Verma

INTRODUCTION

Optic nerve transmits visual information from the retina to the lateral geniculate body. Afferent fibers for the pupillary light reflex also leave the eye via the optic nerve. The optic nerve consists of axons arising from the retinal ganglion cells, which are second order neurons of the afferent visual pathway. Therefore, the optic nerve is actually a portion of the central nervous system and is a tract, not a peripheral sensory nerve. Only the anterior portion of this tract is termed the optic nerve, the optic chiasma is the X-shaped partial decussation and the optic tract is the posterior or retrochiasmatic continuation of the same fiber tract to its termination at the lateral geniculate body.

The optic nerve is about 5 cm long and is broadly described as consisting of four portions. The intraocular portion or optic disc or optic nerve head is 1 mm long, the intraorbital part is 25 mm long, the intracanalicular portion is about 9 mm long and the intracranial part is approximately 16 mm long.

Optic nerve receives its blood supply mainly from 3 major sources:

(a) Choroidal vessels (optic nerve head and retrolaminar portion)
(b) Short posterior ciliary arteries (optic nerve head and prelaminar segment)
(c) Pial arterial network derived from the ophthalmic portion artery in the optic canal and orbit before the ophthalmic artery passes through the nerve sheath 8 to 12 mm behind the globe and travels inside the nerve as the central retinal artery.

Optic nerve carries approximately 1.2 million axons from the eye. These axons originate from the retinal ganglion cells. Ninety percent of the retinal ganglion cells are concentrated in the macula and overall 80% of the optic nerve fibers originate from the macular region. Hence, diseases of the macula can mimic optic nerve diseases and vice versa.

DIAGNOSIS OF OPTIC NERVE DISORDERS

Optic nerve diseases may present with acute, severe visual loss manifesting as a drop in visual acuity along with a disturbance of color vision, contrast sensitivity and visual field. On the other hand, mild neuropathies may cause only minimal visual loss and hence are difficult to diagnose. Early diagnosis can in some instances, such as a pituitary adenoma causing chiasmal compression, prevent profound irreversible visual loss if timely intervention is successful. Moreover, the relative absence of dramatic clinical signs and appearance of a normal fundus in such situations can further hamper the physicians' clinical diagnostic abilities.

Some optic neuropathies and maculopathies may have similar symptomatology, such as acute painless monocular visual loss in a young adult could be the presenting feature of both central serous retinopathy and some cases of optic neuritis. Another example is sudden severe unilateral visual loss in an elderly diabetic individual could be due to anterior ischemic optic neuropathy, ischemic diabetic maculopathy or even age-related macular degeneration with an occult subretinal neovascular membrane.

Common symptoms of optic nerve disorders
- Dimness of vision
- Patchy black spots in the visual field
- Desaturation of colors
- Pain in or behind the eye, increasing with eye movements in some diseases

Common signs in optic nerve disorders
- Decreased vision (visual acuity, color vision, contrast sensitivity, stereo acuity, visual field defect)
- Relative afferent pupillary defect
- Abnormality of the optic nerve head on funduscopy

Differential diagnosis of optic nerve and macular diseases is shown in Table 34.1.

Table 34.1: Differential diagnosis of optic nerve and macular diseases

Clinical features	Optic nerve diseases	Macular diseases
Visual loss	Yes	Yes
Visual acuity	Variably reduced	Markedly reduced
Pain	Sometimes	Rarely
Color vision	Markedly reduced	Slightly reduced
Visual field	Variable	Normal or central scotoma
Refractive error	Unaffected	Sometimes hyperopic shift
Amsler grid	Central scotoma	Metamorphopsia
Visual evoked response	Marked delay in latency	Small delay in latency
Photo stress	Normal	Abnormal

OPTIC NEURITIS

Optic neuritis is a clinical entity with a complex spectrum that embraces idiopathic, immune-mediated and infective optic neuritides. Inflammatory diseases of the adjacent paranasal sinuses, brain and meninges, cranial base and orbit, contiguously involving the optic nerves are also included.

Fifteen to twenty percent cases of multiple sclerosis present to an ophthalmologist as optic neuritis and 35 to 40% of multiple sclerosis patients develop optic neuritis at some point in the course of the disease.

Optic neuritis commonly involves the younger age group (mean age at onset, 30 years). It is rare in children and is also rare in patients > 50 years. Ischemic optic neuropathy is a more common cause of acute loss of vision in the older age group. Females are more commonly affected than males.

Clinical Symptoms

The initial attack is unilateral in most adults and bilateral in 30%. Bilateral involvement is more common in children. It usually presents with a triad of loss of vision, ipsilateral pain and dyschromatopsia. Associated symptoms include impairment of depth perception (Pulfrich's phenomenon), apparent dimness of light intensities, movement phosphenes and visual obscurations in bright light and Uhthoffs' symptom of decreased vision following increase of body temperature, such as with exercise or hot bath. Asymptomatic cases may be detected by routine ophthalmic or neurologic examination by the presence of mild dyschromatopsia, temporal pallor of optic disc, nerve fiber layer defects and abnormal visual evoked potential (VEP) tests.

Loss of vision is usually acute, progressing rapidly within hours or days and may vary from complete failure of vision to asymptomatic patients with 6/6 vision. In majority of cases visual acuity begins to improve in second to third week and may be near normal by fourth week. In small percentage of cases vision does not improve at all.

A rare variant of optic neuritis—chronic progressive demyelinating optic neuropathy is characterized by slowly progressive visual loss without remission. It is due to protracted production of micro plaques involving the whole cross section of the affected optic nerve.

Pain is seen in 50 to 80% of unilateral optic neuritis cases. In typical cases, pain is experienced as a dull ache or sinus pain with or without tenderness of the globe. Eye movements may aggravate it. The cause of pain is not known. It may be due to tight fit of the swollen optic nerve in the optic canal. It may be due to inflammation and swelling, stretching the nerve sheath and since the sheath of the superior rectus muscle is closely related, eye movements, especially up gaze, often aggravate pain.

Uhthoff's symptom is episodic transient obscuration of vision with exertion. The other provocating factors for Uhthoff's symptom include—hot bath or showers, hot weather, stress, anxiety, anger, hot food or drink and is seen in isolated optic neuritis and in multiple sclerosis and may also be associated with toxic optic neuropathy due to chloramphenicol, Friedreich's ataxia and Leber's hereditary optic neuropathy.

Clinical Signs

Reduced visual acuity, dyschromatopsia, reduced contrast sensitivity, field defects, relative afferent pupillary defect and disc changes.

Visual acuity is reduced and may vary from mere perception or light to asymptomatic 20/20 vision. Color vision is abnormal in patients with acute and recovered optic neuritis. Both red/green and blue/yellow color vision defects are seen. Color vision defects are highly sensitive indicators of previous attack of optic neuritis. In mild or asymptomatic cases, this may be detected by comparing the brightness and the hue of a red-colored object with that of the normal eye.

Most patients with optic neuritis complain of imperfect vision even with a visual acuity of 20/20. These patients when examined for contrast sensitivity show reduced contrast sensitivity. The pattern of loss may be variable—high, medium or low spatial frequencies may be selectively affected or all spatial frequencies may be affected. The measurements of peak contrast sensitivity is an effective indicator of subclinical optic neuritis, but this is not useful to differentiate optic neuritis from maculopathies and also in distinguishing organic from nonorganic visual loss (as it is a subjective test).

Visual field defects during an attack and after recovery of optic neuritis may be variable. The cardinal defect is widespread depression of sensitivity, which may be pronounced centrally producing central scotoma. When vision is severely impaired, confrontation field-testing should be done.

In the presence of normal fellow eye relative afferent pupillary defect is present in symptomatic optic neuritis. This is best elicited by swinging flash light test. A relative afferent pupillary defect can be detected even in the presence of one unreactive pupil (due to mydriatics, synechiae, miotics, oculomotor palsy, trauma, etc.) by comparing the direct and consensual response of the single reactive pupil. Relative afferent pupillary defect can be roughly quantified by using graded neutral density filters in front of the normal eye and increasing the density of the filter till the reaction is realized.

On fundus examination the appearance of optic disc may be normal, swollen, blurred and/or hyperemic. There may be peripapillary hemorrhages around the disc. Recovered optic neuritis patients may show normal disc or disc pallor (temporal pallor or total disc pallor). Retinal hemorrhages associated with optic neuritis and multiple sclerosis and retinal venous sheathing, due to periphlebitis retina and nerve fiber layer defects are also seen. Retinal venous sheathing is characterized by deposits of small round or ill-defined confluent white exudate along peripheral veins and may be accompanied by overlying vitritis. Nerve fiber layer defects precede the development of optic atrophy and these are better appreciated in red free light examination (seen as slits in nerve fiber striations in arcuate fiber bundles).

Differential Diagnoses

Unilateral optic neuritis: Includes ischemic optic neuropathy, rhinogenous optic neuritis, Lyme borreliosis optic neuropathy, syphilis, HIV-related optic neuritis and nonorganic visual loss.

Simultaneous or sequential bilateral optic neuritis: Devic's disease, immune-mediated optic neuropathy, nutritional amblyopia, Leber's hereditary optic neuropathy and functional blindness.

Prognosis

Although irreversible optic nerve damage occurs in most of the patients, prognosis for recovery of Snellen acuity is good. But there is significant risk of recurrence. The incidence of recurrence is greater in patients with Uhthoff's symptom.

Conversion to Multiple Sclerosis

The risk of developing multiple sclerosis within two years after optic neuritis is about 20% and 40% within five years without regard to MRI findings. The presence of clinically silent brain lesions on MRI at the time of onset of optic neuritis has been shown to be associated with the increased risk of subsequent development of multiple sclerosis.

Treatment

Based on optic neuritis treatment trial recommendations, treatment with intravenous methylprednisolone 250 mg every 6 hours (or single dose of 1000 mg) for three consecutive days followed by two week course of single daily dose of oral prednisolone 1mg/kg/day should be considered, especially if MRI shows multiple signal abnormalities in periventricular white matter consistent with multiple sclerosis or if a patient has a need to recover vision faster. Oral prednisolone alone in standard dosages should be avoided because it leads to a greater risk of recurrences.

Optic Neuritis in Children

Optic neuritis in children differs from adults by being more often anterior, bilateral and usually occurs within one to two weeks after a viral infection or vaccination and is steroid sensitive. In contrast to optic neuritis in adults, it is less often associated with the development of multiple sclerosis.

Neuroretinitis

Neuroretinitis is characterized by optic disc swelling and stellate maculopathy in presence of acute visual loss in one eye (Fig. 34.1). They may be associated with some infectious disease or idiopathic—"Leber's idiopathic stellate neuroretinitis".

It affects all age groups, but is more common in third to fourth decades of life. Usually painless and vision may be 6/6 to light perception only with dyschromatopsia. It is usually a self-limiting disorder with good visual recovery. Typically the disc swelling resolves over 6–8 weeks and stellate maculopathy resolves slowly over 6 to 12 months.

Neuroretinitis can be infectious or parainfectious (immune mediated) and may be caused by cat scratch disease, syphilis, lyme disease and leptospirosis. Neuroretinitis is one condition, which is not associated with multiple sclerosis. Patient with neuroretinitis should have detailed history taking regarding possibility of severally transmitted diseases, cat scratches, skin rashes, tick bites, lymphadenopathy, fever and flu-like illness. Complete physical and ocular examination should be done to rule out any infectious process and serologic tests should be done to confirm the diagnosis. Treatment of neuroretinitis is by treating the underlying infectious or inflammatory conditions.

Infectious and Parainfectious Optic Neuritis

Optic neuritis can result either from direct viral or bacterial infection of optic nerve or from immunological response to systemic or central nervous system infection. Parainfectious optic neuritis usually follows the onset of viral or bacterial infection by one to three weeks. It is commonly seen in children

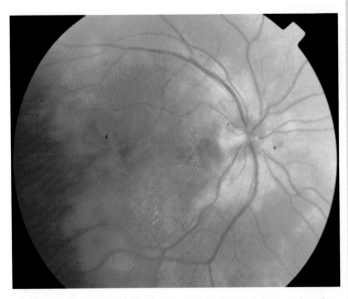

Fig. 34.1: Neuroretinitis. Optic disc swelling and stellate maculopathy are the characteristic features

and is usually bilateral. These patients usually have excellent visual recovery even without treatment. But corticosteroids may hasten recovery.

Optic neuritis may occur in association with both DNA and RNA viruses like adenovirus, coxsackievirus, cytomegalovirus, hepatitis A virus, HIV type I, measles, mumps, and rubella and varicella-zoster viruses. Bacterial infections producing optic neuritis include syphilis, lyme disease, cat scratch disease, anthrax, B-hemolytic streptococci, brucellosis, tuberculosis and typhoid.

Postvaccination Optic Neuritis

Optic neuritis can occur after vaccinations and in such case is usually bilateral. It commonly occurs after influenza vaccine. Others include BCG, hepatitis B virus, rabies virus, tetanus toxoid, combined measles, mumps and rubella virus. Usually optic neuritis is of anterior variety and onset is within one to three weeks after vaccination and visual recovery is common.

Inflammatory Optic Neuritis

Sarcoidosis may produce anterior or retrobulbar optic neuritis producing granulomatous inflammation of optic nerve. It may be characterized by the lumpy white appearance of optic disc associated with overlying vitritis and anterior chamber reaction. This characterized by dramatic response to steroids, but vision may decline with tapering of steroids.

A typical optic neuritis may also be seen in systemic lupus erythematosus, polyarteritis nodosa and other vasculitides. Optic neuritis in these cases is most likely due to ischemic demyelination of axonal necrosis or both. Diagnosis is confirmed by the presence of systemic signs and symptoms of disease and by serologic testing. Treatment is with steroids and may require usage of immunosuppressives.

NEUROMYELITIS OPTICA (DEVIC'S DISEASE)

Unilateral or bilateral optic neuropathy associated with transverse or ascending myelopathy. It usually occurs in children and young adults, but may be seen in all ages. Both sexes are equally affected. Devic's disease may develop in patients with systemic lupus erythematosus, pulmonary tuberculosis and sarcoidosis.

Scattered lesions of demyelination affect the brain, optic nerve and spinal cord. White matter is principally affected. Optic nerve and spinal cord are invariably damaged and cerebrum may be involved in some cases.

Devic's disease differs from multiple sclerosis by the following:
- Cerebellum is almost never affected neuromyelitis optica
- Gliosis is almost never seen in neuromyelitis optica
- Excavation of affected tissue with formation of cavities is common in neuromyelitis optica
- Cerebral subcortex is relatively unaffected in neuromyelitis optica

Clinical Features

Visual loss caused by damage to anterior visual pathway and paraplegia due to spinal cord damage. Systemic features may be mild febrile illness, sore throat, headache and fever. Visual loss is almost always bilateral, but one eye may be affected first, followed by second within hours to weeks. Pain in or around eyes may be seen in some cases. Visual field defects are variable as the foci of demyelination that affect optic nerves are irregular.

Fundus picture varies from normal disc appearance to mild disc swelling to substantial disc swelling and may be associated with dilated veins and peripapillary exudates. Ultimately, most patients develop disc pallor regardless of their initial appearance. Visual recovery usually occurs in patients with neuromyelitis optica and usually begins within one to two weeks.

Visual loss may precede or follow the onset of paraplegia. The interval between the manifestations may be days to months. The onset of paraplegia is usually sudden and severe and may be associated with fever. The paraplegia varies from paraplegia in flexion to paraplegia in extension to paraplegia with the loss of deep tendon reflexes. Most patients recover motor function to some extent, but have some residual paraparesis.

Diagnosis

During the acute phase of neuromyelitis optica, CSF shows evidence of inflammation as lymphocytosis pleocytosis or rise in protein concentration. The CSF glucose concentration is normal. MRI may show T_2-weighted signals. It may be differentiated from multiple sclerosis by the following:

- Neuromyelitis optica is not uncommon under the age of 10 years whereas multiple sclerosis is rarely seen in children under 10 years age.
- Bilateral optic neuritis and myelitis is rarely seen in multiple sclerosis.
- Bilateral simultaneous blindness is unusual in multiple sclerosis.

Treatment

There is no specific treatment for neuromyelitis optica. Only treatment includes supportive treatment in patients with severe myelitis. Administration of intravenous steroids may reduce the severity of the attack and hasten the recovery.

PAPILLEDEMA

Papilledema literally means edema of the optic nerve head or papilla (Fig. 34.2), however conventionally it has come to be used only for that category of optic disc edema, which is secondary to raised intracranial pressure. Optic disc edema due to other causes is not described as papilledema and this group may include various etiologies (Table 34.2).

Table 34.2: Causes of optic disc edema

Disease	Laterality	Visual acuity	Visual field	Color	Other
Nonarteritic AION	Usually unilateral	Normal or decreased	Nerve fiber bundle defect	Decreased	Small optic disc and small cup in fellow eye; diabetes/hypertension
Arteritic AION	May be bilateral	Usually markedly decreased	Nerve fiber bundle defect	Markedly decreased	Headache, claudication, polymyalgia rheumatica, scalp tenderness.
Papillitis (Optic Neuritis)	Unilateral	Usually decreased	Nerve fiber bundle defect (often altitudinal)	Decreased	Pain with eye movement, focal neurologic signs, demyelinating disease
CRVO	Unilateral usually	Usually decreased	Generally decreased	Decreased	Four-quadrant retinal hemorrhages, hypertension/glaucoma
Hypertensive optic neuropathy	Bilateral	Decreased	Enlarged blind spot, generalized constriction	Decreased	Elevated blood pressure, cotton wool spots, retinal hemorrhages
Diabetic papillopathy	Unilateral	Normal or mildly decreased	Normal or enlarged blind spot	Decreased, may be normal	Diabetes (often poorly controlled and insulin-dependent)
Uveitis/Scleritis	Unilateral	Often normal unless macular folds/fluid	Enlarged blind spot	Often normal	Ocular pain, injection, AC and vitreous reaction, collagen vascular disorder
Hypotony	Unilateral	Mildly decreased depending on macular status	Enlarged blind spot	Normal	Low IOP, abnormal gonioscopy, intraocular surgery/trauma
Neuroretinitis	Unilateral	Decreased depending on macular status	Enlarged blind spot, nerve fiber bundle defect	Normal	Viral prodrome, positive tests for Lyme disease, syphilis, toxoplasmosis
Optic nerve tumor/Infiltration	May be bilateral	Decreased	Nerve fiber bundle defects, generally decreased	Decreased	Progressive visual loss, disc pallor in fellow eye, leukemia, intracranial involvement, sarcoidosis

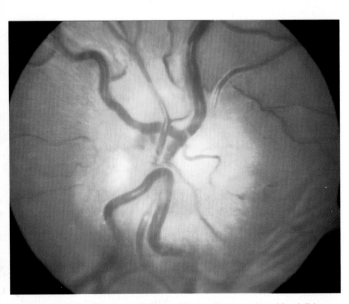

Fig. 34.2: Papilledema. Edema of the optic nerve head is visible

Pathogenesis

Various mechanisms have been proposed to explain the occurrence of papilledema and generally held belief is that there is an obstruction of both fast and slow components of axonal transport causing accumulation of axoplasm at the lamina cribrosa resulting in swelling of axons. It is unclear as to how obstruction of axonal transport is compatible with a normal conduction of nerve impulses or normal visual acuity. It is also not clear as to what causes the obstruction of axoplasmic flow. While some have postulated that it is due to mechanical reasons or due to transmission of intracranial pressure to retinal ganglion cells; other postulate that ischemia caused by disturbances of autoregulation contributes to axonal transport obstruction.

Optic nerve head swelling is an important clinical sign and warrants careful evaluation, as it may be an indicator of an underlying serious systemic or neurological disease. It is important to remember that the optic nerve is not really a nerve like the peripheral nervous system, but is actually a tract or a part of the central nervous system.

Accordingly, it is covered by the leptomeninges—the dura, arachnoid and pia mater. Therefore, any disease process affecting the meninges can easily and contiguously spread to the optic nerve as well and/or often the optic nerve may be affected in cases of meningitis. The dura surrounding the nerve fuses with the sclera anteriorly and at the orbital apex, it is continuous with the periorbita of the optic canal and then merges with the intracranial dura. The arachnoid and pia are also continuous with their intracranial portions. The subarachnoid space around the optic nerve is continuous with the intracranial space and CSF flows freely in this subarachnoid space along the optic nerve.

Symptoms and Signs

The diagnosis of papilledema is made on the basis of a careful ophthalmoscopy and general examination. Papilledema is optic disc edema due to raised intracranial tension and therefore, the clinical features are mainly dominated by symptoms and signs attributable to raised intracranial tension, for example, headache, seizures, and nausea and vomiting, etc. Papilledema may also be diagnosed in a setting where the patient is not acutely ill and the signs of raised intracranial tension may not be so apparent. The patients vision is generally not affected, which is an important differentiating feature from papillitis and ischemic optic neuropathy. However, visual acuity can also be decreased in some cases of papilledema due to macular folds or exudate and changes of secondary optic atrophy in chronic papilledema. Another visual symptom patients may report is that of transient visual obscurations. These are brief, abrupt episodes of decreased visualization, usually lasting only a few seconds where the decrease may vary from mild blurring to complete blindness and it may affect either one eye alone or alternate eyes or rarely both eyes simultaneously. The common feature in all cases is the brevity of the symptoms and the rapid and complete visual recovery. These observations are often precipitated by sudden changes in posture from reclining to more erect. The pathogenesis of these observations has not been clearly established. However, they are widely believed to be caused by the transient episodes of compression or ischemia of the optic nerve.

Similar transient visual obscurations also occur as a part of the symptom complex of migraine, as well as due to transient ischemic attacks or seen in carotid occlusive disease. These observations, however, last longer than those seen in papilledema, usually minutes to hours. Amaurosis fugax due to carotid occlusive disease lasts about 5–15 minutes and emboli in the central retinal artery or more peripheral arterioles may sometimes be seen on fundus examination. Transient monocular visual loss may also sometimes be seen as a feature of retinal migraine where it lasts for 15–20 minutes and is frequently accompanied or followed by headache.

Visual field defects manifesting as an enlarged blind spot is a common finding in patients with papilledema. Various mechanisms have been suggested for this, including lateral displacement of the peripapillary retina that has been observed in pathological specimens. Another mechanism which has been proposed is that the peripapillary retina is elevated by subretinal fluid causing an acquired hyperopia and a refractive scotoma, which can be reduced to near normal size by the use of progressively stronger plus lenses. Other early field defects have also been described with papilledema, such as arcuate scotoma and nasal steps that are commoner nasally than temporally as seen with most optic nerve affections.

Another field defect associated with papilledema is constriction of the visual field, which occurs during chronic papilledema that is developing optic atrophy and is thus a late sign.

Decrease in central visualization may occur in various different situations:

- There may be permanent loss of visualization as the optic disc goes into atrophy after the stage of chronic papilledema and is usually a gradual process.
- The macula may be involved by exudates or hemorrhages for example, a retinal star or half star, which may cause decrease visualization.
- It may occur due to effect of the underlying disease on the optic nerve, for example, meningitis.

Diplopia may be another symptom in such patients as raised intracranial tension can lead to VIth nerve paresis, which may be unilateral or bilateral and may cause diplopia. Other miscellaneous abnormalities of visual function, for example, abnormal contrast sensitivity may be seen in cases with full visual field, 6/6 vision and normal color vision.

Other signs of associated disease may be seen, i.e. specific localizing signs attributable to tumors of the central nervous system.

Ophthalmoscopic Appearance of Papilledema

Papilledema has been classified into 4 stages:
(1) Early
(2) Established
(3) Chronic
(4) Atrophic

The various features of papilledema evolve as follows:

Hyperemia of the optic disc is an early feature and occurs due to the dilation of capillaries on the surface of the disc. However, the color of the normal disc varies and this variation may be more marked with significant refractive errors; but if there is evidence that the optic discs have changed in color, then it is definitely significant.

Blurring of the peripapillary nerve fiber layer causes them to appear striated. Looking for opacification of the nerve fiber layer at the superior and inferior poles of the optic disc is useful in diagnosing early papilledema.

Swelling of the optic disc is the hallmark of papilledema and should be specifically looked for by slit-lamp biomicroscopy using a +90D or +78D lens.

Blurring of the disc margins because of the disc edema is most distinct at the inferior and superior margins in the early stages. Various congenital anomalies may be associated with indistinct disc margins hence this sign may be sometimes difficult to interpret if present in isolation. Of course this sign is of great importance if the appearance has been seen to change on follow-up.

Hemorrhages on the disc and in the nerve fiber layer seen as thin radial streaks on the disc or near its margin are often associated with capillary and venous dilatation and microaneurysms.

Absence of venous pulsations tends to occur when the intracranial tension exceeds about 200 cm of water, but intracranial tension fluctuates widely in patients especially when there is raised intracranial tension. Also 20% of the normal population may have absent spontaneous venous pulsations and this sign may not be very useful. The observation of spontaneous venous pulsations indicates that loss of spontaneous venous pulsations present earlier, indicates raised intracranial tension.

Enlargement of retinal veins and blurring of surface vessels due to opacification of overlying nerve fibers are signs that develop as edema progresses.

Cotton wool spots and exudates may form and in severe cases, circumferential retinal folds may be seen around the disc, called Paton's lines.

The physiological cup is obliterated only in very late stages unlike the cases of optic neuritis where the cup is lost early. In contrast the degree of disc elevation is marked in established papilledema as opposed to papillitis. In well-established papilledema the degree of disc elevation over the surface of the retina can be as high or higher than 4 diopters as determined by the lenses used in the direct ophthalmoscope to focus the surface of the disc compared to the retina. In papillitis, elevation is usually in the order of 1–2 diopters only.

With chronicity exudates form on the disc, resembling drusen the disc becomes atrophic and the retinal vessels become narrow and sheathed. Optociliary shunt vessels may also be seen.

The classical attributes of papilledema, which distinguish it from other causes of disc edema (example papillitis) are – normal visual acuity, normal pupillary reactions and the fact that it is almost always bilateral. However, in late stages visual acuity can be affected and an afferent pupillary defect also appears when atrophy sets in. Also, there are conditions when the raised intracranial tension may cause only unilateral disc edema, i.e. (a) cases of antecedent optic atrophy in one eye because if there aren't enough nerve fibers to swell, papilledema cannot occur, (b) foster Kennedy syndrome in patients having a frontal lobe or olfactory groove tumor develop optic atrophy on the ipsilateral side due to the compression of the nerve and as the tumor enlarges develop papilledema on the contralateral side due to raised intracranial pressure, and (c) congenital anomaly of the optic nerves wherein the perineural sheaths may be abnormal, thus closing off or blocking the perineural spaces, d) it may be bilateral asymmetric papilledema.

Diagnosis

The mainstay of diagnosing papilledema is a careful ophthalmoscopy and slit-lamp biomicroscopy. In doubtful cases, fluorescein angiography may be helpful, which shows disc capillary dilatation, leakage, aneurysm formation in early frames and leakage of dye beyond disc margins in late frames.

The other investigation that may be used is an ultrasonographic examination. It can determine whether the optic nerve diameter is increased and also whether this diameter is caused by increased volume of CSF surrounding the nerve. A thirty-degree test can also be performed during ultrasonographic examination. The diameter of the retrobulbar optic nerve between the inner aspects of the arachnoid sheaths is first measured in the primary gaze and then again when the patient changes his gaze to a position of 30 degrees eccentricity. In cases of papilledema, the diameter is more in the primary gaze and decreases on 30° side gaze implying the presence of a compressible substance, presumably CSF surrounding the optic nerve, which is pushed out when the nerve becomes relatively taut on lateral gaze.

Patients suspected to have papilledema should be advised urgent neuroimaging preferably contrast enhanced MRI to look for an intracranial space occupying lesion, hydrocephalus or enhancement of the meninges. If the brain scan is normal, a lumbar puncture to measure CSF pressure is performed to rule out pseudotumor cerebri. Cerebrospinal fluid should be examined for protein, glucose, cell count and cell morphology to look for any likelihood of infection or malignancy.

Treatment

In cases of papilledema due to either a mass less or block in the ventricular system or interference with the absorption of CSF, the obvious treatment is to tackle the primary pathology. However, there are other cases where either there is no specific treatment or the mass cannot be removed. There are also patients suffering from pseudotumor cerebri or benign intracranial hypertension, which require other forms of treatment. In cases of pseudotumor cerebri, osmotic agents, diuretics and corticosteroids may be used in the acute phase. The patient is kept on close follow-up monitoring symptoms (predominantly headache), visual acuity and fields.

The surgical treatment options are: (a) multiple lumbar punctures—in this, the needle used for lumbar puncture creates on opening in the dura through which CSF leaks out. With several punctures a "sieve" is created, which allows sufficient egress of CSF, (b) shunt procedure—for example, ventriculoperitoneal or lumboperitoneal shunt. Since, the former is difficult to perform. The latter is a simpler and more popular alternative and (c) another described procedure is that of optic nerve sheath fenestration.

ISCHEMIC OPTIC NEUROPATHY

Ischemic optic neuropathy (ION) is a frequent cause of loss of vision in the elderly population where there is infarction of some portion of the optic nerve due to ischemia. It may be anterior or posterior.

Anterior ischemic optic neuropathy (AION): In this condition, there are visible changes on ophthalmoscopy in the form of disc edema and associated features like peripapillary hemorrhages.

Posterior ischemic optic neuropathy (PION): In this condition, there are no visible changes on ophthalmoscopy as the ischemia process affects the retrobulbar portion of the optic nerve.

Ischemic optic neuropathy may also be classified according to etiology, as arteritic and non-arteritic.

Arteritic ischemic optic neuropathy: This condition occurs in patients with giant cell or temporal arteritis.

Non-arteritic ischemic optic neuropathy (NAION): This condition, sometimes called idiopathic, is usually associated with a variety of risk factors for atherosclerosis, i.e. diabetes mellitus, hypertension, smoking, etc. and the patients also show features of atherosclerosis of vessels elsewhere in the body.

Clinical Features

As already mentioned, ischemic optic neuropathy is mainly a disease of the elderly. The nonarteritic variety generally has a relatively lower age of presentation occurring most frequently in the fifth and sixth decades. The arteritic form occurs most commonly in patients in their sixth and seventh decades. The peak incidence of NAION is usually 60–65 years while that of AION is between 65–70 years. However, ION may also be found in much younger patients especially when associated with other diseases like diabetes and hypertension. The other clinical features are:

- *Sudden visual loss:* This is the commonest presenting complaint. The visual acuity level may be variable ranging from 6/6 (with only slight blurring of vision) to no light perception. The visual acuity is usually much worse in the arteritic form compared to the nonarteritic form. This visual loss may slowly deteriorate further over a period of few hours to a few days. Patients with ION may complain of transient visual obscuration as a premonitory symptom. The ischemic event and loss of vision often occurs during the early morning.

- *Visual field defect:* An altitudinal field defect especially affecting the lower field is considered to be the hallmark of an ischemic event causing segmental damage of the optic nerve. However other field defects may also be seen, i.e. central scotomas, arcuate defects and generalized constriction of the field.

- *Loss of color perception*: It is expected in any disorder affecting the optic nerve. The point to be remembered is that the color vision loss in ION is usually proportional to the level of visual acuity unlike in optic neuritis where the loss of color visualization is much more severe as compared to the level of visual acuity. Also loss of color visualization is a prominent and early feature of compressive optic neuropathies, but the loss is gradual unlike the sudden dramatic loss in ischemic optic neuropathy and optic neuritis.

- *Afferent pupillary defect:* A relative afferent pupillary defects is almost always found in cases of ischemic optic neuropathy. The only exception being cases with preexistent damage to the retina or optic nerve of the other eye or the rare cases of bilateral simultaneous and symmetric ION in which cases both pupils will have sluggish pupillary light reflexes.

Ophthalmoscopic appearance: As already mentioned, the ophthalmoscopic appearance is normal in the cases of posterior ischemic optic neuropathy. In anterior ischemic optic neuropathy, there is disc swelling, which could be generalized or sectoral. The swollen part of the disc, i.e. the ischemic part is pale, but in sectorally infarcted discs the rest of the disc may appear hyperemic (Fig. 34.3). The disc swelling in anterior optic neuropathy is characteristically described as "pallid disc edema". The disc edema in patients with giant cell arteritis can sometimes even be chalky white. Peripapillary nerve fiber layer hemorrhages, cotton wool spots and narrowing of retinal arteries may also be seen.

It has also been described that eyes suffering from non-arteritic ischemic optic neuropathy may structurally have "discs at risk" meaning that these eyes have small optic discs, with a small physiologic cup and elevation of the disc margin by a thick nerve fiber layer giving the appearance of a small disc with crowding of the axons as they pass through a small scleral canal. Since the cup-disc ratio of fellow eye is the same or differs by less than 0.1 in over 90.7% persons; looking at the disc of the fellow eye may be informative in the cases of ischemic optic neuropathy. It has been suggested that a small cup may be associated with either arteritic or non-arteritic ischemic optic neuropathy. While a normal or large cup should make one suspect an arteritic etiology. Fluorescein angiography shows delayed optic disc filling in the cases of anterior ischemic optic neuropathy and this is much more marked in the cases of arteritic AION where there also occurs a marked delay in choroidal filling consistent with posterior ciliary artery occlusion (Fig. 34.4). After an attack of ischemic optic neuropathy, the disc edema gradually resolves and optic atrophy ensues. Eventually, these cases will develop optic disc pallor after about 4–6 weeks. Hemorrhages and exudates resolve and there is further narrowing of retinal arterioles. In arteritic cases, the disc subsequently often develops cupping resembling that seen in glaucoma. Though earlier it was thought that ischemic optic

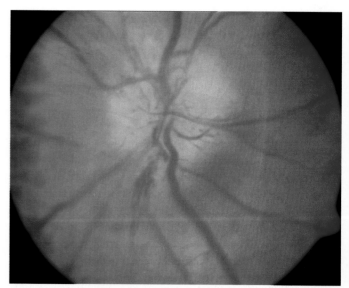

Fig. 34.3: Anterior ischemic optic neuropathy. The ischemic part is pale

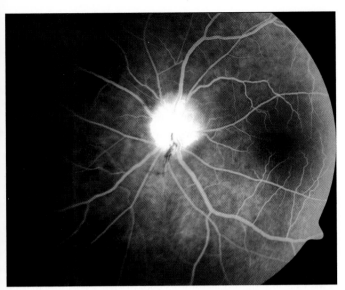

Fig. 34.4: Anterior ischemic optic neuropathy. Fluorescein angiogram shows delayed optic disc filling

neuropathy is caused by a completed infarct with no chance of visual improvement, many recent studies have shown that visual improvement does take place over prolonged periods. However, it is uncommon in arteritic cases to have significant visual improvement.

- *Other eye involvement*: This occurs much more frequently in cases of arteritic ischemic optic neuropathy where 25% to 30% of cases develop ION within days or weeks if prompt and appropriate therapy with corticosteroids is not given. However, other eye may get affected even in cases of nonarteritic ischemic optic neuropathy with incidence quoted from 15% to 33%. Also in these cases, the interval to second eye involvement is much longer ranging from few months to few years. In this respect, it is important to remember that the picture of optic atrophy in the previously affected eye and disc edema in the fresh eye gives a picture similar to Foster Kennedy syndrome, the correct diagnosis of pseudo Foster Kennedy syndrome can be made out by the fact that the eye with disc edema shows pale disc edema as well as a unilateral ipsilateral afferent pupillary defect or a relative afferent pupillary defect, which are not seen in true Foster Kennedy syndrome.
- *Associated clinical features:* Various associated clinical features include polymyalgia rheumatica, scalp tenderness and jaw claudication in giant cell arteritis as well as features of arteriosclerotic disease elsewhere in the body may also be seen.

Management

Any patient with suspected ischemic optic neuropathy must have the blood pressure recorded and a blood sample taken for estimation of blood glucose level, glycosylated hemoglobin level, serum lipid profile and the erythrocyte sedimentation rate (ESR). The latter is tested as an emergency and there are newer testing techniques designed to give quicker preliminary results.

A raised ESR favors an arteritic etiology and warrants a temporal artery biopsy for confirmation of the diagnosis. Early treatment with high dose systemic corticosteroids is crucial in preventing other eye involvement and temporal artery biopsy, if not possible immediately can be deferred by 24–48 hours. A positive biopsy report is helpful, but a negative result does not rule out giant cell arteritis as "skip" lesions are known to occur and one must rely on one's clinical judgement. The treatment of ischemic optic neuropathy is generally disappointing and the visual prognosis of the affected eye is quite poor.

Medical

Medical treatment has virtually no role in nonarteritic cases except in taking care of the associated disease. The use of levodopa-carbidopa combination therapy has been tried with some success. In case of giant cell arteritis, however, prompt steroid therapy should be started not only to take care of the systemic features, but also to prevent other eye involvement. A diagnosis of giant cell arteritis is supported by finding a high ESR in an elderly patient with other features suggestive of giant cell arteritis and is proved by a temporal artery biopsy, but this should not delay the initiation of treatment. Treatment is generally begun with intravenous methylprednisolone 1 gm/day along with 80 mg of oral prednisolone per day as a single daily dose in the morning. After three days, the intravenous steroids can be stopped and oral steroids are reduced to 60 mg/day, which can be further tapered gradually to reach a maintenance dose of about 10 mg/day. The duration of treatment is governed by the patient's symptoms and ESR values. The usual duration of maintenance therapy is about 1–2 years, but may be longer.

Surgical

Optic nerve sheath decompression has been tried in the cases of nonarteritic ischemic optic neuropathy. However, the results were not gratifying. The percentage of cases showing improvement was roughly the same as seen for spontaneous improvement. In addition, optic nerve sheath decompression had its own complications. A multicentric, randomized clinical trial, the ischemic optic neuropathy decompression trial for cases of nonarteritic ischemic optic neuropathy ceased recruitment for optic nerve sheath decompression midway as it became clear that patients assigned to surgery did not have a better outcome and did slightly worse than patients assigned to follow-up only.

OPTIC ATROPHY

Optic atrophy as the name suggests is an atrophy of the optic nerve head (Fig. 34.5). Any optic neuropathy can lead to optic atrophy. Once clinical optic atrophy is established the ophthalmoscopic appearance of the optic disc is often nonspecific and not helpful in determining the underlying cause. Nevertheless some clinical features are useful in certain cases, such as

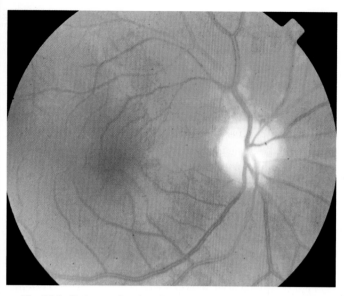

Fig. 34.5: Optic atrophy. Atrophy of the optic nerve head is visible

presence of gliosis and a dirty gray color and indistinct margins indicating a "secondary" optic atrophy, a term that is reserved for situations where the disc was previously swollen. A chalky white disc with clear distinct margins is labeled as "primary" optic atrophy though the underlying etiology could be anything, such as posttraumatic optic atrophy, compressive optic atrophy and drug-induced optic neuropathy to name a few. Acquired cupping of the optic disc is of course typical of glaucoma, but can also occur following ischemic optic neuropathies, such as giant cell arteritis and sometimes following compressive optic neuropathies, such as a pituitary adenoma compressing the chiasma. Finally, optic atrophy is also a possible consequence of lesions in the retina in which case, the disc may acquire a waxy yellow appearance as is seen in retinitis pigmentosa and is termed "consecutive" optic atrophy.

It is well to remember that optic atrophy can also occur as a consequence of diseases affecting the optic chiasma and optic tract, but does not occur in lesions that affect the visual pathway proximal to the lateral geniculate body that is lesions from the optic radiation to the occipital cortex.

The clinical features of optic atrophy include a triad of (a) visual loss, (b) an afferent pupillary defect and (c) the ophthalmoscopic appearances of a pale optic nerve head with or without attenuation of the vessels. Visual loss need not always manifest as a marked decrease in visual acuity. Other changes, such as visual field defect, color vision deficit or disturbance in contrast sensitivity may also occur in varying degrees and in different proportions. Another aspect of visual function is stereoacuity or accuracy of depth perception. There is normally a linear relationship between stereoacuity and Snellen visual acuity. However, this linearity is lost in certain disorders like optic neuritis or postneuritic optic atrophy and other conditions while produce optic nerve damage and may not return even if visual acuity returns to normal.

LEBER'S HEREDITARY OPTIC NEUROPATHY

This disorder primarily affects males in western or Caucasian populations. It is inherited by mitochrondrial transmission. Genetically at least six mutations in the mitochondrial DNA have been identified. Between 50% to 60% patients have a mitochondrial point mutation at the nucleotide position 11,778. 50% men and 20% women who have inherited the 11,778 defect have been shown to develop optic neuropathy in pedigree studies. It has been suggested that this specific mitochondrial DNA mutation can only be expressed when matched with a specific X-chromosome allele.

Leber's hereditary optic neuropathy manifests with the rapid loss of vision in both eyes either simultaneously or sequentially in young adults, mostly males. Visual field defects are initially central scotomas, which rapidly become centrocecal in location. Fundus examination should be performed to carefully look for specific findings namely (a) circumpapillary telangiectatic microangiopathy; (b) swelling of the nerve fiber layer around the disc and (c) the absence of leakage of dye from the disc or peripapillary region on fluorescein angiography.

Ultimately, optic atrophy develops late in the course of the disease. Eventually, about 15% of patients recover useful vision in one or both eyes. Visual recovery may take many years. Those with the 11,778 mutations have been found to have a uniformly poor visual prognosis.

There is no effective treatment available. A blood sample should be sent for testing for known Leber's mutations. Genetic counseling should be offered. Patients have been known to have a significantly high incidence of cardiac conduction defects so a cardiology consultation should be advised.

RADIATION OPTIC NEUROPATHY

This is a delayed effect, which may manifest 1 to 5 years after radiation therapy. It is more likely to occur following radiation therapy to the eyes orbit, paranasal sinuses, nasopharynx and occasionally the brain. Visual loss can be acute or gradual and is often severe. Disc swelling and retinopathy may or may not be evident or present (Fig. 34.6). There is no specific or effective treatment. Corticosteroids may be helpful in some cases.

TOXIC OPTIC NEUROPATHY

Also called metabolic optic neuropathy by some is characterized by bilateral painless acute or gradual progressive loss of vision. Clinical features include poor vision, abnormal color vision, bilateral centrocecal or central scotomas and either a normal optic disc or signs of temporal disc pallor or frank optic atrophy on ophthalmoscopy.

Common etiologic agents include tobacco/alcohol abuse, severe malnutrition with thiamine (vitamin B_1) deficiency, drug-induced (ethambutol, isoniazid, chloramphenicol, digitalis, chloroquine, streptomycin, chlorpropamide and lead) and

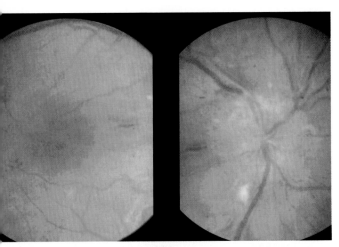

Fig. 34.6: Radiation optic neuropathy and retinopathy. Disc swelling and retinopathy is visible

pernicious anemia, which is usually due to a problem with vitamin B_{12} absorption.

Treatment includes (a) withdrawal of the offending agent after consulting the primary treating physician for substitute medication, (b) thiamine 100 mg orally twice a day, (c) folate 1 mg orally daily, (d) multivitamin tablet daily and (e) vitamin B_{12} 1000 mg intramuscularly once a month for pernicious anemia, which is treated in coordination with the patients physician.

COMPRESSIVE OPTIC NEUROPATHY

This includes intrinsic nerve diseases, such as optic nerve glioma or external compression due to a space-occupying lesion involving the nerve sheath, such as a meningioma or a mass in the orbit or intracranially compressing the optic nerve, chiasma or tract. Compressive optic neuropathy can also occur due to raised intraorbital pressure in conditions like severe dysthyroid eye disease and pseudotumor of the orbit. In these cases, the mechanism could be both, direct pressure or indirect damage due to posterior or anterior ischemic optic neuropathy from vascular compromise.

The patient presents with slowly progressive visual loss though occasionally the loss may be acute or sometimes suddenly noticed. Important signs include a visual field defect, which is central in lesions distal to the chiasma, bitemporal hemianopia if there is chiasmal involvement or incongruous homonymous hemianopia if involving the optic tract. Additional features may include proptosis and/or restriction of extraocular movements in the case of orbital lesions. Fundus appearance of the disc can be normal, pale or even occasionally swollen. Sometime optociliary shunt vessels are visible. These are small peripapillary vessels that shunt blood from the retinal vein to the choroidal venous circulation.

Investigation includes visual fields of both eyes and neuroimaging with coronal and axial views with CT or MRI of the orbit and brain.

Treatment depends on the etiology. Treatment essentially involves removing the compressive lesion as and when possible. If surgical removal is likely to cause more damage than the lesion itself, such as optic nerve glioma and meningiomas then it is recommended to adopt a wait and watch policy. These lesions are monitored with serial record of visual acuity and visual fields in consultation with a neurosurgeon. If there is any evidence of extension and intracranial involvement, surgical excision may be indicated.

In cases of acute inflammatory conditions threatening the optic nerve such as severe dysthyroid eye disease or orbital cellulitis with orbital abscess immediate measures to decompress the orbit will be required. In case of dysthroid eye disease, high dose steroids are given initially and orbital decompression performed if there is inadequate response in the first 48 hours.

DRUG-INDUCED TOXICITY

There are several drugs, which can lead to a toxic optic neuropathy. The usual presentation is a bilateral progressive visual loss, which is usually gradual but can be rapid occasionally. Clinical examination of the eye yields few positive clinical signs in early stages. Apart from decreased visual acuity, the patients will have defective color vision and bilateral central scotomas. Fundus appearance may be totally normal leading to the evidence of optic atrophy later on in the course of the disease.

Careful history taking, including detailed medical, social, diet, work and family history at the appropriate time is a key to diagnose these cases giving one the opportunity to initiate timely remedial measures.

Drugs, which can lead to this condition, include ethambutol, isoniazid, chloramphenicol, chlorpropamide and ethchlorvynol (placidyl). Other conditions that cause a similar clinical picture include nutritional optic neuropathy, i.e. "tobacco-alcohol amblyopia"; vitamin B_{12} and folate deficiency; heavy metal and methanol poisoning; hereditary optic atrophy and infiltrative disorders, such as carcinomas, lymphoreticular diseases; and granulomatous disorders, such as sarcoidosis, syphilis and tuberculosis.

Regarding drug toxicity from antitubercular drugs and with ethambutol in particular, the neuropathy can be both idiosyncratic and dose related. In general, ethambutol toxicity is less common in doses of 15 mg/kg/day and much higher in a dose of 20–25 mg/kg/day.

Once the suspected offending agent is determined, treatment begins with the cessation of the drug. Stop any associated alcohol and tobacco use and institute a well-balanced diet, including B complex vitamin supplements. Treatment with hydroxycobalamin 1000 mg intramuscularly once a month may be added. The treating physician must be consulted in case a different drug needs to be substituted for ethambutol. As most antitubercular regimes include both ethambutol and isoniazid (INH) and as toxicity with ethambutol is much more common than with INH, one should discontinue ethambutol first. Only if INH is specifically still believed to be responsible, should it be stopped too. Another consideration to be kept in mind is whether there is direct infiltrative involvement of the optic nerve due to the tuberculosis infection itself. Ultrasound examination of the optic nerve and nerve head can sometimes help to pick up infiltrative neuropathy.

Timely intervention can reverse the neuropathic process and vision improves gradually over several months and the patient often regains useful vision. However, if the diagnosis is missed and the insult to the nerve from the offending agent continues, the damage can be permanent and irreversible.

TRAUMATIC OPTIC NEUROPATHY

Damage to the optic nerve can occur in closed head injuries particularly when a rotational or shearing force is transmitted to the frontal areas. The blow is typically ipsilaterally to the frontal area and is usually severe enough to produce a loss of consciousness. The damage to the nerve is produced by shearing forces that may be induced in the relatively immobile canalicular portion of the nerve by the movement of the brain from the frontal impact. The damage could be by direct disruption of the nerve fibers or indirect damage by disruption of the blood supply. Edema or hemorrhage can also be factors, inducing nerve damage by compressing the nerve within the optic canal. In addition, a fracture of the wall of the optic canal may produce a bone fragment directly exerting pressure on the optic nerve. Rarely blunt trauma can lead to optic nerve damaged in the orbit producing an optic nerve head avulsion.

Optic nerve injuries are usually unilateral, but less commonly optic chiasmal damage can occur in blunt head injuries producing bilateral visual loss.

Apart from decreased vision, signs include a field defect (Fig. 34.7) and relative afferent pupillary defect. If the optic nerve head is avulsed, it is visible ophthalmoscopically as a defect in the papillary region and may be accompanied by hemorrhage. Sometimes damage to the intraorbital part of the nerve may lead to a picture resembling a central artery occlusion. However, in most cases, traumatic optic neuropathy affects the canalicular part of the nerve and the fundus appearance is usually normal with the disc pallor typical of optic atrophy developing after three to four weeks. Earlier, onset of pallor implies a significant disruption of the optic nerve head blood supply.

In most cases, the visual loss is maximum from the time of impact, but in some cases, the visual loss is delayed by few hours, and progresses over the next few days. Computed tomography should be performed to look for a fracture of the canal with a bone fragment pressing on the nerve and for the preserve of hemorrhage in the nerve sheath, both of which are indications for surgical intravenous. Mega dose intravenous corticosteroids: Dexamethasone 3–5 mg/kg/day or Methylprednisolone 20–30 mg/kg/day has been reported to be effective in some cases. Visual evolved potentials help in monitoring response to therapy particularly when the visual acuity is very poor. Treatment should be instituted within 24 to 48 hours and then

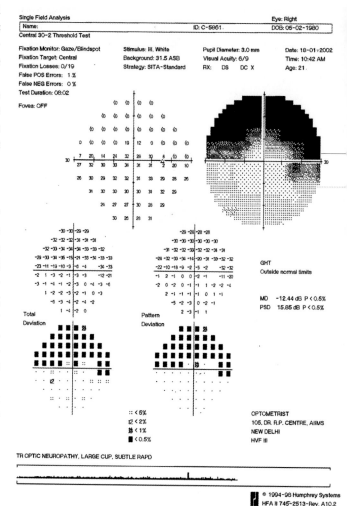

Fig. 34.7: Traumatic optic neuropathy. Visual field defect is visible

if improvement occurs one can switch to oral steroid therapy, which is tapered over the next two weeks. If there is no visual improvement within one or two days of mega dose steroids and particularly if there is documented worsen presumably from edema or hemorrhage within the nerve or canal, optic canal decompression through either a transethmoidal or transfrontal approach should be performed. Another indication for optic canal decompression in such cases is if vision worsens as steroids are tapered.

UNCOMMON AND MISCELLANEOUS OPTIC NEUROPATHIES

Papillophlebitis

This is an ill-defined disease usually seen in young adults. It is characterized by unilateral disc swelling and optic nerve function is variably affected. Disc swelling can be marked and scattered retinal hemorrhages are also occasionally seen. Diagnosis is usually clinical, but a CT to rule out a compressive lesion is advisable.

The cause of this condition is unknown. Inflammation of the central retinal vein has been postulated. The lesion has also been considered to be a part of the spectrum of Eales' disease. No specific role of corticosteroid therapy has been proven. Differential diagnosis includes other forms of vasculitis and infiltrative optic neuropathies.

Partial Central Vein Occlusion

This represents a syndrome similar to papillophlebitis, but usually occurs in older individuals. Again disc swelling is marked with relatively preserved optic nerve function. Scattered retinal hemorrhages and dilated retinal veins are present. Optociliary shunt vessels may form. Visual function generally remains good and neovascular glaucoma is rare.

Diabetic Papillopathy

This is an uncommon condition seen in young juvenile insulin-dependent diabetic patients in their teens or twenties. The cases present with unilateral or bilateral blurred vision with insidious onset and may even be asymptomatic and could be detected incidentally. Involved discs are swollen with telangiectatic vessels overlying the disc surface. Vision is not severely affected and visual field defects could be central scotomas or arcuate pattern defects. The presence of telangiectatic vessels overlying the swollen disc is characteristic and useful in diagnosis. When the condition is bilateral, neuroimaging is mandatory to rule out an intracranial space-occupying lesion. Pseudotumor cerebri is another important differential diagnosis and neurosurgical consultation and documentation of CSF pressure may be needed.

Disc edema generally resolves over several months. Visual field defects tend to be irreversible. No treatment is specifically recommended. The cause is not established. There does not appear to be any relationship with the degree of glycemic control or the presence of diabetic retinopathy. It is clinically different from ischemic optic neuropathy by two features namely (a) diabetic papillopathy is often simultaneously bilateral and (b) optic nerve function is often not impaired in diabetic papillopathy.

Parasitic Infestation of the Optic Nerve

Cysticercosis cellulose has rarely been found to be present within the optic nerve. The condition may mimic optic neuritis, papillitis, neuroretinitis or unilateral severe disc edema. Visual loss is profound. Diagnosis is often delayed or missed as the condition is often mistaken for an optic nerve tumor on neuroimaging. Ultrasonography is helpful in detecting the cyst with a highly reflective pinhead lesion within the cyst representing the scolex.

Careful examination of CT or MRI scans performed with 1mm sections is also helpful in detecting the scolex. Treatment includes use of high dose steroids to reduce inflammation, as the visual loss is believed to be due to toxins released by the dying parasite. Medical treatment with oral albendazole and surgical removal of the cyst have both been tried, but with poor results. This could be due to delayed presentation and late diagnosis in few cases reported so far.

Thyroid-Related Optic Neuropathy

Optic neuropathy of Graves' disease is caused by the compression of the nerve at the apex of the orbit by enlarged extraocular muscles. Visual loss is usually gradual, but a rapid deterioration has also been seen to occur. There is no direct relationship between the severity of optic neuropathy and the amount of proptosis in fact in some patients, optic neuropathy occurs in the absence of any apparent proptosis. In our experience, proptosis is often a natural mechanism to decompress the orbit and those patients with tight orbits and no proptosis are more likely to develop features of optic nerve dysfunction. Clinically, the optic nerve head may be normal, swollen or even pale at presentation.

Clinical work-up for evidence of neuropathy includes recording of visual acuity, color vision and visual fields. Additional tests include measuring amount of proptosis, amount of lagophthalmos, slit-lamp examination for exposure keratopathy, recording of intraocular pressure and testing of ocular motility.

Treatment is determined by the extent of nerve involvement and has to be planned on an individual basis. The treatment options include systemic steroids, orbital decompressive surgery or orbital radiation. If visual loss is mild with minimal field defect, oral steroids with careful follow-up is the norm. Additional measures, such as sleeping propped up, avoidance of smoking and eye protection are advised.

If visual loss is not controlled by these measures or is severe from the outset then high dose intravenous methylprednisolone 1 gm/day is administered. If vision does not improve within 24–48 hours then orbital decompression is required.

In patients who cannot be given systemic steroids for any reason, the surgical option remains. In those not considered fit for surgery or in whom other measures are only partially effective orbital radiation (2000 rad in 10 doses over a fortnight) is an alternative.

Sarcoid Optic Neuropathy

Granulomatous infiltration of the optic nerve can occur in patients with sarcoidosis. Fundus appearance may be typical with a white lumpy swelling of the optic nerve head. Visual involvement can vary from no loss to severe loss. Corticosteroids are usually effective. Optic nerve involvement could be isolated or combined with ocular or CNS involvement.

Shock Optic Neuropathy

Any patient, who becomes suddenly hypotensives due to systemic shock, is at risk for developing this condition. Elderly people with compromised circulation may be more prove. The presentation is with blurred vision and field defect usually

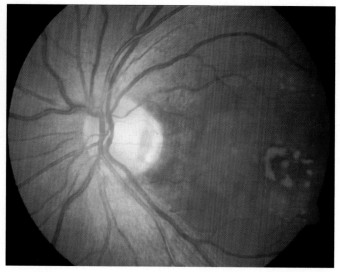

Fig. 34.8: Optic disc pit. A small crater-like depression in the optic nerve head can be discerned very well

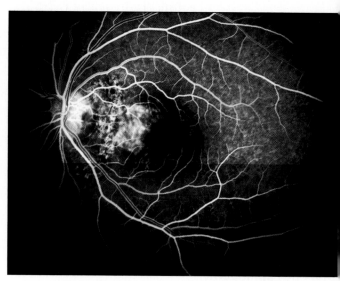

Fig. 34.9: Optic disc pit. Fluorescein angiogram

noticed when the patient is recovering from the systemic illness. Disc appearance may be edematous. The clinical appearance resembles ischemic optic neuropathy. Disc hemorrhage may also be seen. Visual field defects are generally nerve fiber bundle pattern defects or altitudinal loss. Visual loss is generally permanent. In later stages, disc pallor or even cupping may occur mimicking glaucoma.

CONGENITAL ANOMALIES OF THE OPTIC DISC

These include optic disc coloboma, morning glory syndrome, optic nerve hypoplasia, tilted disc, optic disc drusen, optic disc pit, etc. It is important to recognize these disorders and avoid unnecessary further investigations and at the same time in certain conditions, such as optic disc coloboma and morning glory disc there may be specific indicators of the possibility of an underlying intracranial or endocrine abnormality requiring further investigation, such as neuroimaging and treatment.

Optic Disc Pit

An optic disc is a congenital developmental abnormality where there is a small crater-like depression in the optic nerve head (Figs 34.8 and 34.9). It is worth noting that acquired pit-like lesions have been documented in patients with normal tension glaucoma. The pathogenesis is not established. Histologically, the lesion is an outward herniation of rudimentary neuroectodermal tissue into a depression within the nerve substance. The lesion appears oval or round in shape and the base may

be whitish, gray or yellowish in color. Pits most commonly are found in the temporal region of the disc, but can as well occur in any other part of the disc. They may be associated with adjacent peripapillary retinal pigment epithelial changes. It has been noticed that the affected disc may be slightly larger normal disc in unilateral cases.

Optic disc pits have variable visual field defects. The field defect may not show specific correlation with the morphology of the pit. The most common field defect is an arcuate pattern field defect, which is paracentral in location and may be connected to an enlarged blind spot.

Unlike optic nerve head coloboma, optic disc pits are not associated with intracranial malformations and hence detection of a pit does not warrant neuroimaging.

Optic disc pits are often associated with serous retinal detachments in the macular region. The subretinal fluid has been postulated to originate either from the vitreous cavity or the subarachnoid space surrounding the optic nerve. It has been shown that the fluid initially produces an inner retinal layer separation akin to a retinoschisis involving the posterior pole. An outer retinal layer hole develops subsequently, through which the intraretinal fluid escapes to enter the subretinal space producing a typical sensory macular detachment. If vision is profoundly affected the preferred method of therapy used to be photocoagulation at the disc margin to block the flow of subretinal fluid to the macular region. A newer approach to treatment is internal tamponade to displace the subretinal fluid from beneath the macula.

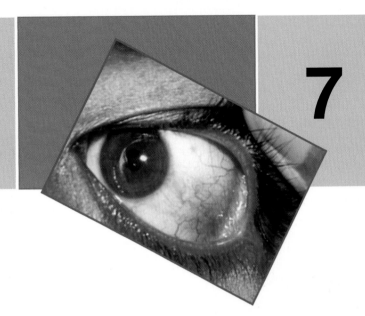
Diseases of Lid, Orbit and Lacrimal System

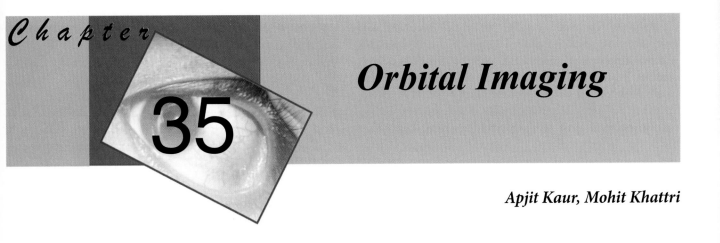

Chapter 35

Orbital Imaging

Apjit Kaur, Mohit Khattri

INTRODUCTION

Diagnosis of orbital diseases is made clinicoradiological and confirmed on histopathological and immunohistochemical studies.

The recent advances in orbital imaging allow the clinician to identify not only the location of the lesion and its relation to adjacent structures, but also its tissue characteristics computerized tomographic scanning (CT Scan), magnetic resonance imaging (MRI) and ultrasonography (USG) are the radiological tools. These tests are complementary to each other and are not mutually exclusive.

B-SCAN ULTRASONOGRAPHY

Standardized echography includes A-scan, B-scan and Doppler echography. Information obtained from ultrasonography of the orbit includes size and shape of the lesion, borders, and tissue composition (cystic or solid). Ultrasonography is used primarily as an adjunctive imaging modality. It is particularly useful in the evaluation of lesions that involve the globe and adjacent anterior orbit and to differentiate cystic from solid lesions. Doppler echography additionally provides information concerning vascularity. In most of the centers, however, CT scan and MRI are preferred over orbital ultrasonography in the evaluation of orbital lesion and its surgical planning.

CT SCAN

CT scan provides good visualization of all orbital tissue and surrounding bones. Intravenously administered contrast medium increases the visualization and suggests the vascularity of the lesion. Lacrimal gland and extraocular muscles are normal contrast enhancing structures. Inflammatory lesions and tumors with rich vascularity show contrast enhancement. Evaluation for foreign body, thyroid ophthalmopathy and bony lesions do not warrant IV contrast injection. 2 mm slices are

suited for orbital imaging in both axial and coronal sections. However, lesions within the eyeball, those in the region of optic canal and very small radiopaque foreign bodies require thinner slices of 1 mm.

Axial and coronal views both should be used for orbital and CNS lesions.

The axial sections are obtained parallel to the infraorbitomeatal line. The coronal sections are obtained roughly perpendicular to the infraorbitomeatal line.

The planes of axial sections can be obtained from the *"scanogram,"* which is the first frame of the CT scan film. Although axial sections give adequate information and reformatted coronal and sagittal images can be constructed from them, yet the quality of directly taken coronal images is superior to that of reformatted images. Coronal sections give additional information about the intracranial and paranasal sinus compartments. Bone window permits detail evaluation of the bony structure.

Thus, clinical suspicion of site, extent and nature of disease guide the radiologist in performing the CT scan.

"Hounsfield units" (HU) represent a scale of radiation attenuation values of tissues. The Hounsfield number can range from 1000 to +1000 HU or above. Higher the number, greater is the attenuation of X-rays, indicating higher tissue density. Hounsfield number hence can help in the differential diagnosis.

The only disadvantage of CT scan is exposure to radiation. The radiation dose is approximately 5 cGy per imaging plane, which is not cataractogenic.

MAGNETIC RESONANCE IMAGING (MRI)

Magnetic resonance imaging provides images of the orbital soft tissue in equal or slightly better detail than CT scan. Bony details and calcifications are not well visualized with this technique. It is contraindicated in patients with ferromagnetic foreign bodies, cardiac pacemakers and cochlear implants. Its greatest advantage lies in the fact that it is a radiation-free procedure.

Magnetic resonance imaging for orbit is recorded using head coil, short repetition time (TR) and short echo time (TE). A combination of postcontrast T_1 weighted image and a noncontrast T_2 weighted image is best to optimize MRI efficacy. Normal anatomy is better demonstrated by the T_1 weighted images, whereas T_2 weighted images demonstrate pathological changes well. Most of the orbital tumors are hypointense on T_1 and hyperintense on T_2 and show enhancement with Gadolinium complex of diethylenetriamine penta-acetic acid (Gd DTPA). T_1 weighted images provide more spatial resolution. Vitreous, muscles and large vessels appear hypointense while fat appears hyperintense in T_1 images. T_2 images provide more contrast resolution.

For optic nerve imaging, additional sagittal section is employed.

The contrast used for MRI, Gd DTPA is indicated for delineation of inflammation and vascularity of lesions. Magnetic resonance angiography remains the gold standard for imaging orbital and central nervous system vascular lesions.

Limitations of MRI include poor bony details due to its low hydrogen proton content and image distortion due to ferromagnetic objects. It is contraindicated in patients with metallic foreign bodies (ferrous), aneurysm clips, cochlear implants and cardiac pacemakers. MRI has certain advantages over CT; there is no radiation exposure or need for awkward head positioning.

Role of ultrasonography, CT scan and MRI scans for detecting orbital pathology are shown in Figures 35.1 to 35.20.

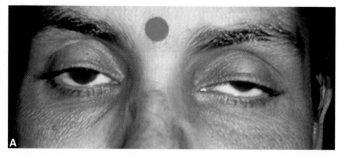
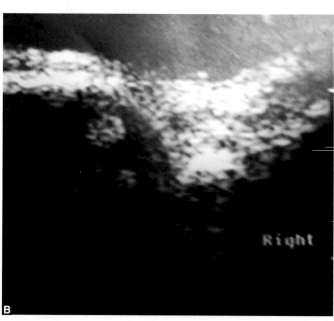

Figs 35.1A and B: Cysticercosis: (A) A middle-aged female presented with intermittent, progressive painful ptosis of left upper lid for past six months. (B) B-scan shows hypoechoic cystic lesion with a hyperechoic shadow of a scolex within it suggestive of cysticercosis

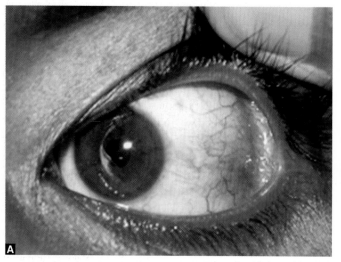
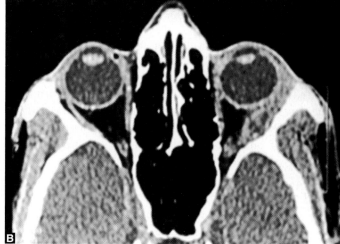

Figs 35.2A and B: Cysticercosis: (A) A middle-aged patient with an unexplained hyperemia associated with mild pain in lateral canthal area of the left eye. (B) Axial CT scan of the same patient revealed a localized, well-defined lesion in the temporal part of the left orbit. Excisional biopsy proved it to be cysticercosis

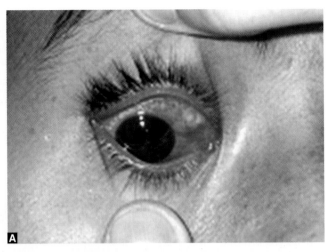

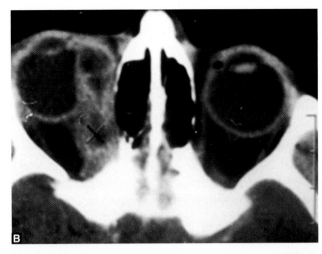

Figs 35.3A and B: Orbital pyogenic infection: (A) A young boy presented with chemosis and congestion in left eye. A localized episcleral abscess was seen in the superomedial quadrant of the right eye. (B) Axial CT scan of the same patient showing a lesion in the medial part of the right orbit. It had well-defined margins, with multiple loculi and variable density within the loculi. The findings are in concordance with the diagnosis of orbital abscess

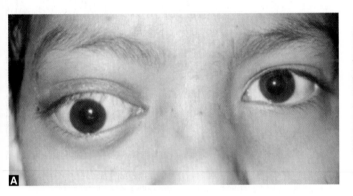

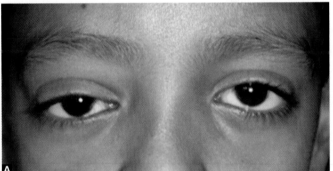

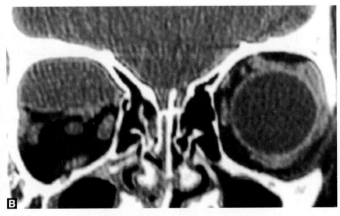

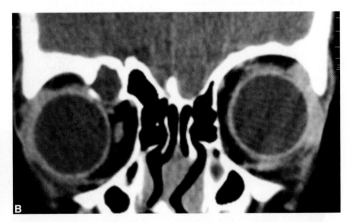

Figs 35.4A and B: Orbital trauma: (A) Subperiosteal hematoma. A young boy sustained blunt trauma on the right side of face one week prior to presentation. The eyeball was in down and out position. (B) Coronal CT scan of the same patient showing a well-defined lesion in the superior part of the right orbit. The lesion was isodense with the orbital soft tissue. Blood was aspirated from the lesion

Figs 35.5A and B: Orbital trauma: (A) Post-traumatic bone cyst. A young boy sustained head trauma following fall from moving vehicle. He presented with drooping of the right upper lid associated with swelling over the right upper lid below the eyebrow. A bony mass was palpable in the superomedial part of the right orbit. (B) CT scan of the same patient revealed fracture in the region of roof of orbit. Fractured bone fragment, enclosing a hypodense area, was seen abutting the right eyeball

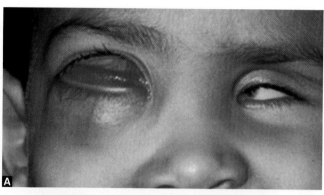

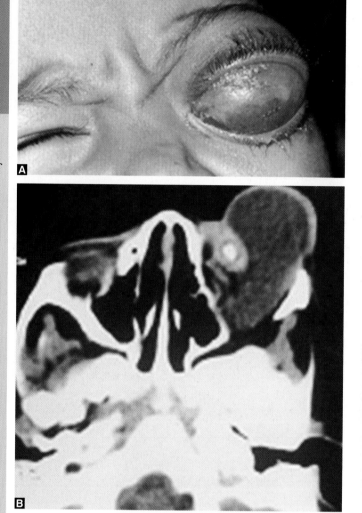

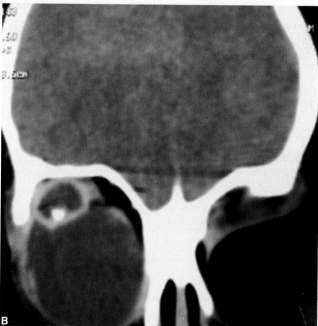

Figs 35.6A and B: Microphthalmia with cyst: (A) A small child presented with a large congenital swelling in the region of the left upper eyelid, causing the lower eyelid to be pushed inferiorly and resulting in exposure related tissue changes. A clinical diagnosis of congenital cystic eyeball was made due to the position of the cyst and absence of an identifiable eyeball. The right eyeball was normal (B) Axial CT Scan of the same patient showed a small rudimentary calcified eye in relation to the medial wall of a cyst that was filled with hypodense substance

Figs 35.7A and B: Microphthalmia with cyst: (A) A child presented with swelling in the region of right lower eyelid and a small nonfunctional eyeball since birth. On examination, the right side had a soft cystic swelling in the region of the right lower eyelid. The eyeball could be palpated below the right upper eyelid. The left eyeball was microphthalmic and esotropic (B) Coronal CT scan section of the above patient shows a large, hypodense cystic lesion, displacing the right eyeball superolaterally

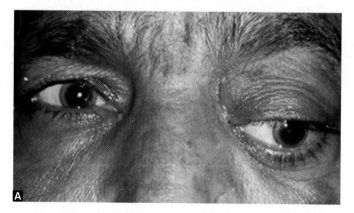

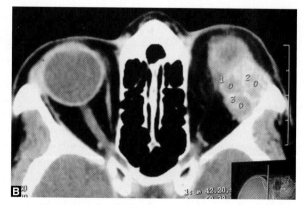

Figs 35.8A and B: Lacrimal gland tumor: (A) An elderly female presented with down and out proptosis of the left eyeball along with diminution of vision (B) Axial CT scan of the same patient revealed a large mass of variable density in the superolateral quadrant of the left orbit

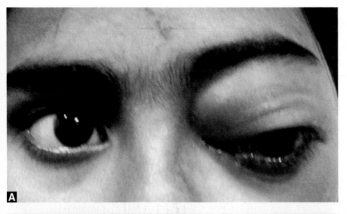

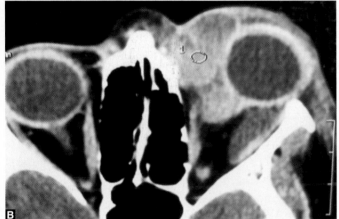

Figs 35.9A and B: Orbital hemangioma: (A) A young female presented with fullness over the left upper lid and abaxial down and out proptosis. (B) Axial CT scan of the same patient, showing well-defined multiloculated mass in the superomedial orbit, displacing the eyeball. Radiological diagnosis of cavernous hemangioma was made

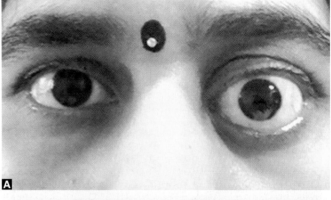

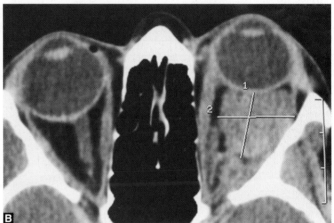

Figs 35.10A and B: Orbital hemangioma: (A) A middle-aged female presented with painless axial proptosis of left eye for a long duration. Examination revealed marginally raised orbital tonometry, full ocular movements and 20/20 vision. (B) Axial CT scan of the same patient, showing a well-defined retro-ocular intraconal mass of heterogeneous density, engulfing the optic nerve

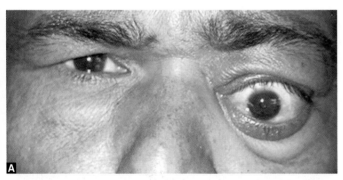

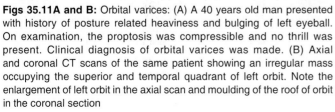

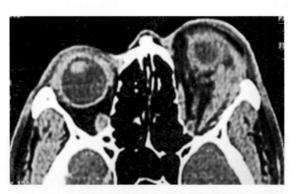

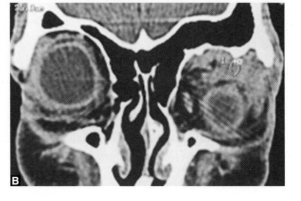

Figs 35.11A and B: Orbital varices: (A) A 40 years old man presented with history of posture related heaviness and bulging of left eyeball. On examination, the proptosis was compressible and no thrill was present. Clinical diagnosis of orbital varices was made. (B) Axial and coronal CT scans of the same patient showing an irregular mass occupying the superior and temporal quadrant of left orbit. Note the enlargement of left orbit in the axial scan and moulding of the roof of orbit in the coronal section

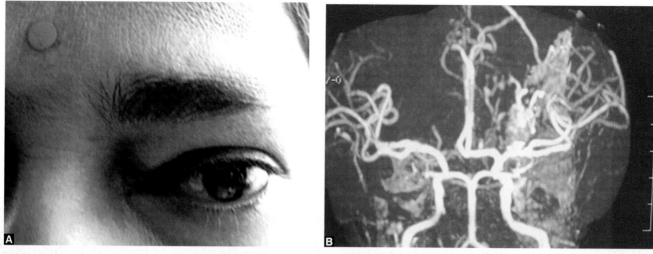

Figs 35.12A and B: Arteriovenous malformation: (A) A middle-aged female presented with heaviness and diffuse redness of left eye for a long duration. On examination, a knuckle like elevation was seen in the left superomedial quadrant. Thrill was palpable over the elevation. Clinical diagnosis of arteriovenous malformation was made. (B) Magnetic resonance angiography of the same patient revealed arteriovenous malformation

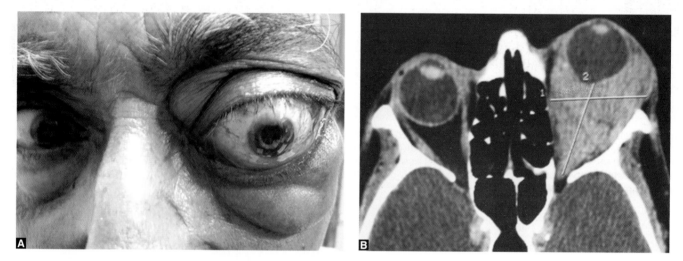

Figs 35.13A and B: Lymphoproliferative disorder: (A) An elderly male presented with a long standing, painless protrusion of the left eyeball with adequate of the left eyelids. A soft to firm mass was palpable below the upper and lower eyelids in all quadrants. Orbital tonometry was raised. (B) Axial CT scan of the same patient, revealed a diffuse hyperdense infiltrative mass, occupying the entire left orbit, destroying tissue planes. Orbital bones were intact. Biopsy was consistent with lymphoproliferative disorder

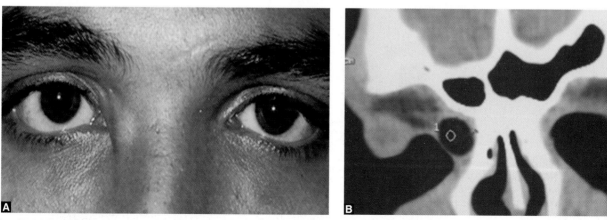

Figs 35.14A and B: Anterior orbital dermoid: (A) A young man presenting with a small cystic swelling in the lacrimal sac region on the right side. (B) Coronal CT scan of the same patient showing a small well-defined hypodense mass owing to the presence of fat inside the mass located anteromedially in the right orbit

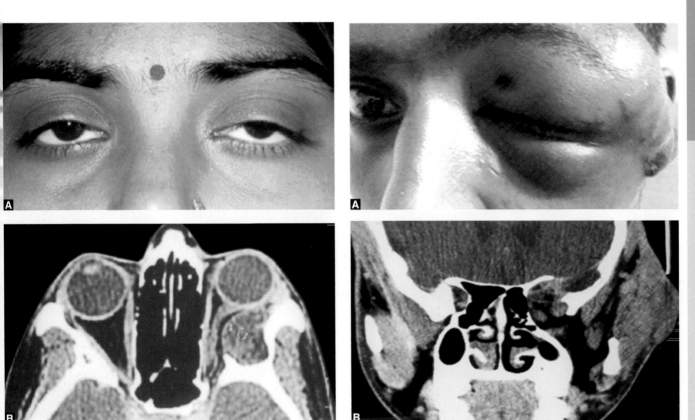

Figs 35.15A and B: Posterior orbital dermoid: (A) A middle-aged female presented with dull ache behind the left eyeball, associated with minimal ptosis of left upper lid. Orbital tonometry on the left side was raised. Best-corrected visual acuity was 20/20 in both the eyes. (B) Axial CT scan of the same patient showing a large, posterior, hypodense lesion causing scalloping of the left lateral orbital wall. Note the variable density and the displacement of the optic nerve

Figs 35.16A and B: Orbital neurofibroma: (A) A young male presented with large, boggy, irregular swelling, with surface discoloration extending from the left eyelids to the left temporal region. Clinical diagnosis was consistent with plexiform neurofibroma. (B) Coronal CT Scan of the same patient revealed a bony defect in the region of the sphenoid bone. Note the large soft tissue mass in the temporal region. Radiological diagnosis was consistent with plexiforn neurofibroma

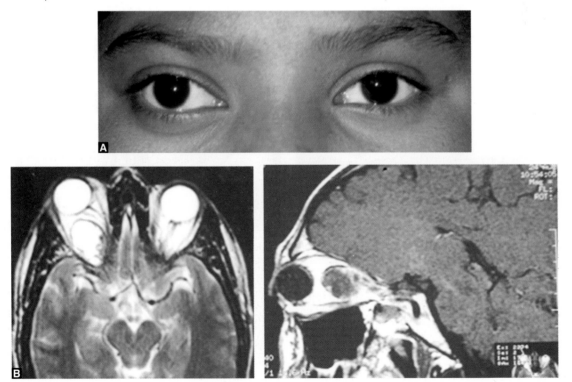

Figs 35.17A and B: Optic nerve glioma: (A) A young child presented with history of loss of vision in right eye along with painless proptosis. (B) T_2 and T_1 weighted MRI scans shows findings consistent with right optic nerve glioma

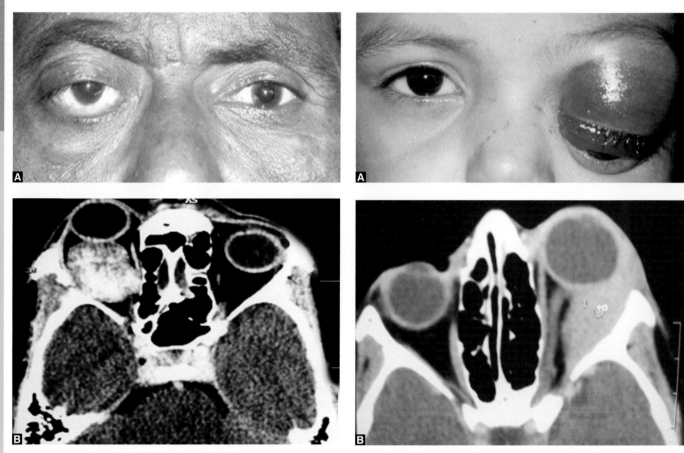

Figs 35.18A and B: Optic nerve sheath meningioma: (A) A middle-aged male presented with axial proptosis of long duration associated with diminution of vision. (B) Axial CT scan shows a mass in the right retrobulbar intraconal region with patchy intense enhancement

Figs 35.19A and B: Orbital rhabdomyosarcoma: (A) A 5 years old child presented with painful proptosis of left eye of one week duration. (B) Axial CT Scan of the same patient revealed a large infiltrative mass occupying the lateral part of the left orbit. Biopsy was consistent with rhabdomyosarcoma

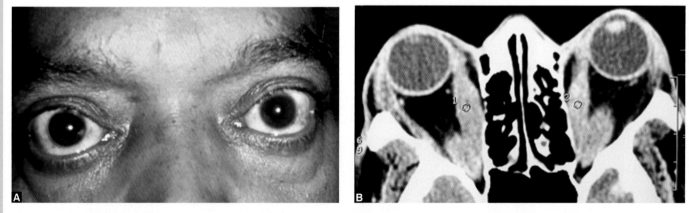

Figs 35.20A and B: Thyroid ophthalmopathy: (A) A middle-aged male presented with bilateral lid retraction of both eyelids. Clinical diagnosis of thyroid ophthalmopathy was made. (B) Axial CT scan shows enlarged rectus muscle bellies on both sides. Note the sparing of the tendons

Diseases of the Eyelid and Orbit

Santosh G Honavar, Milind N Naik,
Geeta K Vemuganti, G Chandra Sekhar

PTOSIS

Ptosis results from suboptimal functioning of the levator palpebrae superioris muscle, either because of developmental dystrophy or acquired deficit. Based on the possible etiopathology as determined by clinical evaluation and specific investigations, a practical classification of ptosis is suggested for routine use (Table 36.1).

Table 36.1: Classification of ptosis

Classification of Ptosis
I   Congenital Ptosis
   A. Congenital simple ptosis
   B. Congenital complicated ptosis
      1. With extraocular muscle deficit
         a. Strabismus
         b. Extraocular motility restriction
         c. Superior rectus underaction
         d. Double elevators' underaction
      2. With synkinesis
         a. Marcus-Gunn phenomenon
         b. Congenital III nerve palsy with aberrant regeneration
      3. With blepharophimosis syndrome
II Acquired Ptosis
   A. Mechanical
      1. Eyelid edema
      2. Eyelid tumors
      3. Blepharochalasis
      4. Dermatochalasis
   B. Neurogenic
      1. III nerve palsy
         a. Vascular
         b. Compressive
         c. Disruptive
      2. Horner's syndrome
      3. Ophthalmoplegic migraine
   C. Myogenic
      1. Myasthenia gravis
      2. Muscular dystrophies
      3. Chronic progressive external ophthalmoplegia
      4. Aponeurotic
         a. Levator dehiscence
         b. Levator disinsertion
   D. Traumatic
      1. Laceration
      2. Orbital fracture
      3. Ocular, periocular and orbital surgery
III Pseudoptosis
   A. Loss of support
      1. Microphthalmos, phthisis bulbi
      2. Enophthalmos
   B. Hypotropia

Evaluation of Ptosis

A thorough and objective preoperative evaluation is the vital initial step in the diagnosis of the type of ptosis and its appropriate management. Medical history should include the time (congenital, acquired) and mode of onset (sudden, gradual) of the ptosis, a history of its improvement or worsening since its onset, diurnal variation in the amount of ptosis, history of injury or surgery and other associated ocular and systemic symptoms. Review of patient photographs if available, may help better understand the temporal sequence of onset and progression of ptosis that may be helpful in cases where an accurate history may not be forthcoming.

Examination of a patient with ptosis would include the following components:

General examination: Examination of the face for facial asymmetry, head posture (chin elevation, head tilt), frontalis overaction, signs of periocular or eyelid inflammation or tumors, presence of enophthalmos and deep supratarsal sulcus (suggestive of aponeurotic ptosis) and evident signs of injury. Other features that may be important include telecanthus (defined as the intermedial canthal distance more than half of the interpupillary distance), epicanthus and blepharophimosis (Fig. 36.1). Assessment of orbicularis function and ocular signs of myasthenia gravis are important if myogenic ptosis is suspected.

Visual acuity: Best-corrected visual acuity assessment.

Eyelid inspection: Inspection of the eyelid skin for the signs of laxity and the presence, location, position and multiplicity of

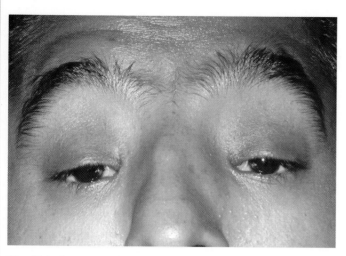

Fig. 36.1: A young patient with blepharophimosis syndrome showing reduced horizontal palpebral fissure, epicanthus inversus and ptosis. Also note the bilateral frontalis overaction

the lid crease. The upper lid crease is a helpful anatomic landmark. It is positioned generally 7–9 mm above the lash line. The eyelid margin-to-eyelid crease distance (margin-crease distance) should be measured with the patient looking down and compared with the contralateral eye. This is essential to plan the positioning of the lid crease during skin-approach levator resection surgery. A relatively higher lid crease in the presence of fair or good levator action indicates aponeurotic ptosis (Fig. 36.2). The prominence of the lid crease may also directly relate to the degree of levator function.

Amount of ptosis: There are several ways of assessing the amount of ptosis. In a patient with unilateral ptosis, the difference in the vertical palpebral aperture in primary position is a good method to measure ptosis provided the contralateral lower eyelid is symmetrically positioned and there is no compensatory retraction of the contralateral upper eyelid. Comparison of the margin reflex distance (MRD1, the linear distance between the corneal light reflex with the eye in primary position and the upper eyelid margin) is a reliable method, but allowance has to be made for the abnormal position of the contralateral upper

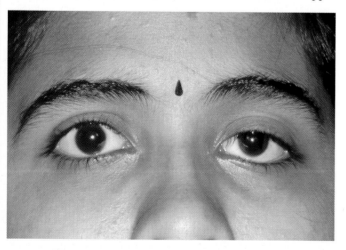

Fig. 36.2: Left acquired aponeurotic ptosis. Note the higher lid crease on left side

eyelid. It may be necessary to express MRD1 as a negative value if the ptosis is severe enough for the upper eyelid to cover the corneal light reflex. In such cases, a clear ruler is held in front of the cornea and the ptotic lid is lifted up to view the corneal light reflex. With the ruler is well aligned with the reflex, the ptotic eyelid is dropped and the amount of drop beyond the reflex is recorded as a negative MRD1 value. Measurement of the palpebral aperture and MRD1 are not applicable in a patient with bilateral ptosis. Beard described a simple method wherein the vertical corneal diameter is assumed as 11 mm, the pupil diameter as 3 mm and the amount of the normal upper lid coverage of the cornea as 2 mm. With these assumptions, if the upper eyelid is positioned at the upper edge of the pupil, the ptosis is measured as 2 mm. If it is at the corneal light reflex the ptosis is considered to be 3.5 mm and if it is at the lower edge of the pupil, then the ptosis is considered to be 5 mm. The amount of ptosis may be classified as mild (2 mm or less), moderate (3 mm) and severe (4 mm or more).

Levator function: Assessment of levator function is helpful in determining the appropriate surgical procedure to be used for ptosis correction. By the Berke's method, excursion of the upper eyelid from extreme down gaze to extreme up gaze is a measure of levator function. The frontalis muscle should be fixed with examiner's thumb with direct posterior pressure over the forehead just above the eyebrows to prevent any transmission of force from the frontalis muscle to the upper eyelid. Normal levator function ranges from 12–17 mm. The levator function is classified as poor (4 mm or less), fair (5 to 7 mm) and good (8 mm or more). It may be difficult to objectively assess levator function in younger children. Some clues to the poor levator function include head posture, frontalis overaction and the absence of lid crease. Eliciting Iliff's sign involves eversion of the upper eyelid as the child looks down. Spontaneous reversion of the eyelid indicates fair to good levator function.

Palpebral aperture in various positions of gaze: Relative difference in the height of the palpebral aperture is an indicator of the etiology of ptosis. The palpebral aperture in the ptotic eye in down gaze will be equal to or larger than the contralateral side in congenital ptosis (Figs 36.3A and B). This is because of failure of the dystrophic levator muscle to relax in downgaze on reciprocal innervation. In contrast, in aponeurotic ptosis, the palpebral aperture in downgaze on the involved side will be smaller than the normal side. In both congenital and acquired ptosis, the difference in the level of the eyelids is maximal on upgaze, except in the cases of aberrant regeneration of the third nerve where the ptotic lid may appear more elevated than the normal side.

Synkinetic movements: Marcus-Gunn jaw winking phenomenon is a common synkinesis associated with congenital ptosis (Fig. 36.4). It should be suspected in the presence of variable ptosis and levator action. Marcus-Gunn phenomenon is characterized by the movement of the ptotic eyelid corresponding with the action of muscles of mastication. Synkinesis could be with any of the masticatory muscles, including pterygoids, mylohyoid and digastric. In order not to miss synkinesis, it is preferable to

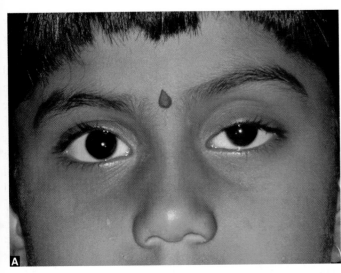 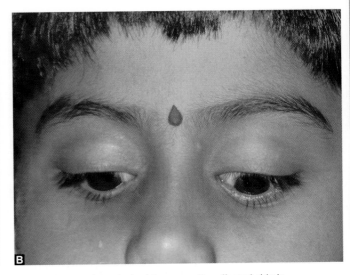

Figs 36.3A and B: A case of left congenital ptosis. Compared to the right eye, the palpebral fissure on the affected side is narrow in the primary gaze, (A) but wider in downgaze (B)

ask the patient to perform a range of maneuvers that includes sideward movements of the jaw, opening and closure of the mouth and protraction of the jaw. Synkinesis could be graded as follows: mild (maximum elevation of the ptotic lid to the nonptotic position), moderate (maximum elevation up to the superior limbus) and severe (maximum elevation beyond the superior limbus with scleral show). An objective grading involves measurement of the range of synkinesis: mild (2 mm or less), moderate (3 to 4 mm) and severe (5 mm or more).

Strabismus and extraocular movements: Presence of strabismus, more specifically hypotropia, hypertropia and dissociated vertical deviation need to be noted. Defective extraocular movement and the presence of diplopia should be objectively quantified.

Bell's phenomenon: The eye normally moves upwards and outwards on closure of the eyelid. This is a protective brainstem reflex, which may be deficient in patients with ptosis. Poor Bell's phenomenon may result in postoperative corneal complications.

Bell's phenomenon is elicited by lifting the upper eyelid to non-ptotic position while the patient gently attempts to close the eye. Bell's phenomenon is considered good if more than two-thirds of the cornea disappears behind the elevated upper eyelid. It is considered fair if one-thirds to two-thirds of the cornea moves up behind the upper eyelid. Poor Bell's phenomenon is characterized by little (<1/3) movement of the cornea. The movement of the eyeball could be inverse (upward and inward), reverse (downward) or perverse (movement in different directions).

Routine examination: Routine ocular examination with specific attention to refraction, tear film abnormality, corneal sensation and pupillary anomaly (miosis in Horner's syndrome and mydriasis in third-nerve palsy). Visual fields may be essential to establish functional deficit in a patient with aponeurotic ptosis.

Drug tests: Neostigmine or edrophonium test may be used to initially screen if myasthenia gravis is suspected. Phenylephrine is

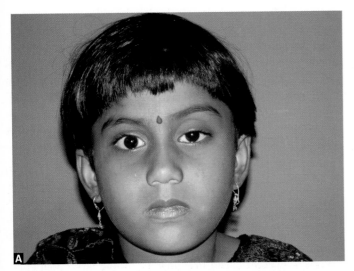 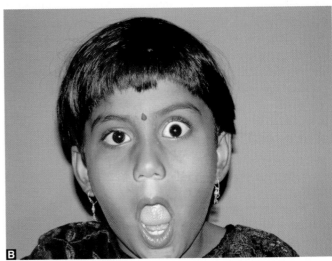

Figs 36.4A and B: Patient with left congenital ptosis with Marcus-Gunn phenomenon

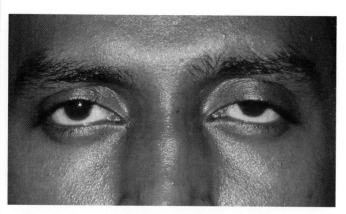

Fig. 36.5: A young patient with bilateral acquired myogenic ptosis. Edrophonium test confirmed ocular myasthenia gravis

used to diagnose ptosis in Horner's syndrome and to determine the feasibility of müllerectomy.

Systemic examination: Systemic evaluation to rule out associated diseases, such as myasthenia gravis and muscular dystrophies when myogenic ptosis is suspected (Fig. 36.5).

Management of Ptosis

The decision regarding the management of ptosis depends mainly on the etiology of ptosis, age of the patient and the magnitude of functional and cosmetic deficit. For congenital ptosis, surgery is ideally performed after about 4 years of age when ptosis can be better assessed and the child is cooperative for postoperative management. However, in cases where there is high risk of amblyopia or there is head posture, early surgery may be considered. This could be a temporizing procedure, such as a reversible tarso-frontal sling initially and a permanent procedure could be planned when the child is older.

The cause of mechanical ptosis is primarily managed, followed by a levator surgery where required. The management of acquired ptosis of neurogenic etiology may involve a period of observation ranging from 6 to 12 months for spontaneous recovery. Surgery may be performed for residual ptosis and following correction of strabismus. The management of myogenic ptosis is difficult. Medical management is the initial modality of choice in myasthenia gravis. Ptosis correction in patients with myasthenia gravis or chronic progressive external ophthalmoplegia may precipitate corneal complications or manifest diplopia. Crutch glasses are an option in very severe cases with the high risk of exposure keratitis. A reversible tarso-frontal sling with deliberate undercorrection may be considered where the risk of corneal complications is less likely.

TUMORS OF THE EYELID

The three most common malignant tumors of the eyelid include sebaceous carcinoma, squamous cell carcinoma and basal cell carcinoma, in order of frequency of occurrence. In the West, basal cell carcinoma is the commonest eyelid malignancy, followed by squamous cell carcinoma and sebaceous carcinoma.

Sebaceous Carcinoma

Sebaceous carcinoma is considered an aggressive tumor and the most lethal of all eyelid malignancies, with a 5-year mortality rate exceeding 20% reported in most series. It is essential to recognize these lesions early in the resectable stage. However, atypical clinical presentation or features that simulate other common benign conditions result in delayed diagnosis and inappropriate management. The incidence of clinical and histological misdiagnosis has been reported to be as high as 50%.

Incidence

The relative incidence of sebaceous carcinoma among all eyelid malignancies has been variably reported, although most series indicate an incidence between 1% to 6%. Sebaceous carcinoma is worldwide in distribution, but there appears to be a significant difference in the reported incidence between the eastern and western countries. In a collaborative study of eyelid malignancies from the USA and China, the relatively increased incidence of sebaceous carcinoma in the Orientals was established. In the Boston population, sebaceous carcinoma accounted for 1.5% of all eyelid malignancies, while in the Shanghai population, the incidence was 33%. A recent series from India confirmed the relatively high preponderance of sebaceous carcinoma among the Asian-Indian population.

Sebaceous carcinoma predominantly occurs in adults after 30 years of age, with the mean age being about 65 years. It is rarely found in younger individuals, specifically those who are immunocompromised or have received external beam radiotherapy for heritable retinoblastoma. There is a female preponderance.

Clinical Presentation

The tumor usually arises from the meibomian glands of the tarsus. It affects the upper eyelid two to three times more frequently than the lower eyelid, possibly because of relatively more numerous meibomian glands located there. Less commonly, it may arise from the Zeis glands of the cilia and sebaceous glands of the hair follicles of the skin, eyebrows and caruncle.

The clinical presentation of sebaceous carcinoma depends on the site of origin and shows great variability. The most common presentation is that of an enlarging mass that often clinically simulates a chalazion. In most cases, especially those of meibomian origin, the tarsus and the deeper structures of the eyelid are involved with no fixity, erosion, or ulceration of the skin. Apart from the common clinical presentation as a nodular mass (Fig. 36.6A), the other variants include a noduloulcerative or an ulcerative lesion. Ulceration is common on the tarsal and palpebral conjunctival aspect, but cutaneous ulceration may manifest rarely in advanced cases. When viewed through the conjunctiva, the yellow-white color and the lobular architecture of the tumor may be apparent (Fig. 36.6B). A complete everted eyelid examination of the tarsal, palpebral and fornicial conjunctiva is mandatory to determine the extent

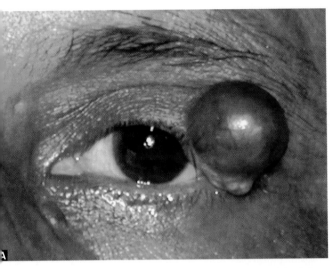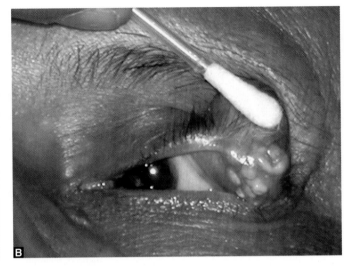

Figs 36.6A and B: Sebaceous gland carcinoma of the left upper lid seen as a nodular mass (A) Eyelid eversion demonstrates the extensive conjunctival component as well as loss of lashes (B)

of the tumor. Meibomian gland carcinoma generally causes loss of definition of meibomian orifices. When the tumor arises from the Zeis gland, it is located at the lid margin and madarosis typically occurs, sometimes with an ulceration of the eyelid margin. It is not uncommon to find a diffuse variant of sebaceous carcinoma that involves the meibomian as well as the Zeis glands or both the lids.

Intraepithelial involvement of sebaceous carcinoma may completely dominate the clinical picture and may masquerade as unilateral blepharoconjunctivitis (Fig. 36.7) or superior limbic keratoconjunctivitis. The subtle primary tumor in such situations is overlooked in several cases leading to misdiagnosis of chronic blepharitis or blepharoconjunctivitis. Rare cases of primary intraepithelial sebaceous carcinoma without a manifest eyelid tumor have been reported.

Orbital extension of sebaceous carcinoma occurs in about 6 to 16% of cases and may be the initial presentation in the Asian population. Orbital extension is seen in a high proportion of cases with recurrence and is associated with an increased mortality rate of up to 75%. Sebaceous carcinoma locally metastasizes in about 17 to 23% of cases to preauricular and cervical lymph nodes and the parotid gland and needs to be looked for at the initial visit and subsequent follow-up. Sites of distant metastasis include lung, liver and brain.

Management

Primary management of sebaceous carcinoma consists of complete surgical excision with full-thickness eyelid resection, including 3–5 mm of clinically tumor-free margins (Fig. 36.8). It is recommended that the surgical margins be monitored by frozen sections to ensure that there is no residual tumor. Some workers have advocated Moh's fresh-tissue technique for the intraoperative monitoring of resection margins. It is also recommended that multiple map biopsies from several sites in the bulbar, forniceal and palpebral conjunctiva be taken to identify areas of intraepithelial tumor invasion. Residual intraepithelial

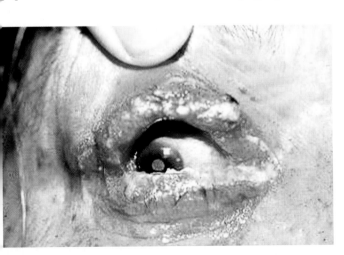

Fig. 36.7: Patient with right diffuse sebaceous gland carcinoma involving both the lids and the ocular surface presenting with a blepharoconjunctivitis like picture

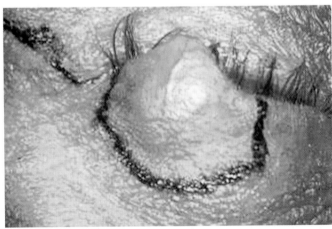

Fig. 36.8: Surgical resection margin for the excision of sebaceous gland carcinoma of the upper lid

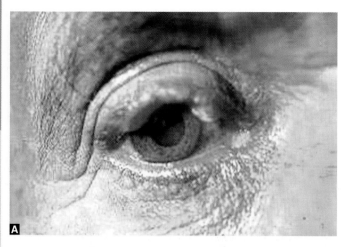
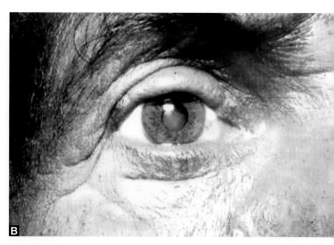

Figs 36.9A and B: Preoperative (A) and postoperative (B) photographs of a patient with right upper lid sebaceous gland carcinoma after Cutler-Beard surgery

tumor is treated with double freeze-thaw cryotherapy. The resulting surgical coloboma can be treated with appropriate lid reconstruction (Figs 36.9A and B). Orbital exenteration is indicated when orbital invasion or extensive intraepithelial neoplasia is present. Documented regional lymph node metastasis can be managed by radical neck dissection and external beam radiotherapy. Orbital external beam radiotherapy is reserved for patients who are not good candidates for surgery. This modality may, however, be palliative because sebaceous carcinoma is not known to be very radiosensitive.

Histopathology

Histopathologically, sebaceous carcinoma demonstrates lobules and cords of poorly differentiated infiltrative sebaceous cells (Fig. 36.10). The cells are large, polygonal with abundant vacuolated to slightly basophilic cytoplasm with large vesicular nucleus with prominent nucleoli. The cells show high mitotic activity. Special oil red O stain on frozen sections is used to demonstrate lipid. Histopathologic patterns may be lobular, comedoacinar, papillary or mixed. Morphological patterns, however, are not found to correlate with local and systemic prognosis. In contrast to the relative lack of importance of the histopathologic patterns, both the degree of differentiation and degree of invasiveness have a substantial effect on prognosis. Sebaceous carcinomas are also classified as well differentiated, moderately differentiated and poorly differentiated based on the differentiation towards sebaceous gland cells; and as minimally infiltrative, moderately infiltrative and highly infiltrative groups.

One of the distinct features of sebaceous carcinoma is its tendency for intraepithelial spread. It is reported to occur in 44 to 80% of cases. The origin of intraepithelial neoplasia is uncertain. It may result from an intraepithelial migration of tumor cells from a primary site of origin in the meibomian or the Zeis gland, or there may be an in-situ development within the conjunctival epithelium. The prognostic significance of intraepithelial neoplasia remains controversial, primarily because its biological potential is poorly understood. Despite the controversy concerning the prognostic significance of intraepithelial neoplasias, its diagnostic significance is unquestioned.

Prognosis

Between 9 and 36% of sebaceous carcinomas recur usually within the first five years after surgical excision. Local recurrence occurs in the eyelid and orbit in 6 to 17% of cases. In 1 to 28% cases, recurrence involves the regional lymph nodes. Regional lymph node involvement is the commonest form of metastasis of sebaceous carcinoma. Lymph nodes may show skip invasion. Cervical and supraclavicular lymph nodes may be involved without clinical involvement of preauricular and submandibular nodes. The tumor usually spreads by direct extension and through the lymphatics, but may hematogenously metastasize to distant sites, including the brain, skull, liver and lungs.

Sebaceous carcinoma is perhaps the most lethal of all eyelid malignancies. Overall mortality rates ranging from 23 to 41% have been reported. The rather high mortality rate of 41%

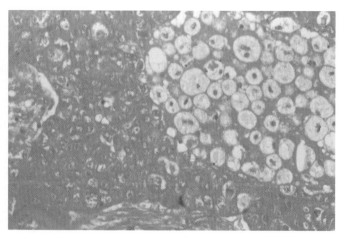

Fig. 36.10: Photomicrograph of sebaceous gland carcinoma of the lid showing large polygonal cells with vacuolated cytoplasm and hyperchromatic nuclei (hematoxylin and eosin, x 250)

reported in the Chinese series probably reflects a higher incidence of advanced cases in their series. Although clinical presentation of sebaceous carcinoma is similar to the Chinese series in Indian population, mortality rates are not high. Recognition of prognostic factors and appropriate treatment has improved the prognosis of sebaceous carcinoma. In a series covering six decades, there was 24% mortality prior to 1970s, but no tumor-related deaths in patients managed after 1970.

Various clinicopathologic features of sebaceous carcinoma that were associated with a bad prognosis have been identified. These include duration of symptoms greater than six months, tumor diameter exceeding 10 mm, involvement of both upper and lower eyelids, multicentric origin, highly infiltrative pattern, poor differentiation, and pagetoid, vascular, lymphatic and orbital invasion. In this series, mortality was 28% when sebaceous carcinoma involved the upper eyelid, 0% when it involved the lower eyelid and 83% when it was multicentric and involved both the eyelids. Sebaceous carcinoma arising from the glands of Zeis had an excellent prognosis. The mortality was 9% in patients with a histopathologically well-differentiated tumor in contrast to 30% in patients with moderately differentiated tumors and 60% in those with poorly differentiated tumors.

Conclusion

Sebaceous carcinoma is a rare, but aggressive malignant tumor usually arising from the tarsal meibomian glands and glands of Zeis. The tumor is found in greater frequency in the Orientals and Asian-Indians. It may commonly masquerade as less aggressive lesions, such as a chalazion or blepharoconjunctivitis, leading to delayed diagnosis and treatment. Factors associated with prognosis include clinical characteristics, such as tumor size, orbital invasion and metastasis and histologic characteristics, such as multicentricity, poor differentiation, infiltration and invasion of vascular and lymphatic channels. We recommend wide excision with frozen section controlled tumor-free margins for localized tumors, exenteration for orbital disease or for diffuse intraepithelial neoplasia and radical neck dissection with radiotherapy for documented lymph node metastasis. Map biopsy to determine the extent of intraepithelial neoplasia and cryotherapy for localized involvement may be acceptable, but needs periodic monitoring for recurrence. Topical mitomycin-C application is an encouraging new modality under trial for early or residual intraepithelial disease. Although considered the most malignant and fatal of all lid tumors, there has been a recent improvement in the prognosis of patients with sebaceous carcinoma. Improved prognosis is believed to be due to increased clinical suspicion, early diagnosis and aggressive treatment. All patients need to be followed up closely for local recurrence, regional lymph node involvement and metastasis.

Squamous Cell Carcinoma

Squamous cell carcinoma of the eyelid is a relatively rare neoplasm accounting for about 12% of all malignant tumors of the eyelid. It occurs in elderly individuals with fair skin and chronic sun exposure. There is a wide geographic variation in the relative frequency of occurrence of squamous cell carcinoma. It is more common in Caucasians living in North America, Europe and Australia, as compared to the ethnic Asian populations.

Squamous cell carcinoma could occur de novo or infrequently arise from several existing premalignant lesions, including Bowen's disease, actinic keratosis and reactive (chemical, irradiation) keratoses. There is a genetic predisposition to squamous cell carcinoma in individuals with xeroderma pigmentosum, an autosomal recessive inherited disorder of defective DNA repair.

Early lesions are commonly in the form of rough scaly patch with crusting, erosions and fissures, eventually developing into an ulcer. Ulcers are typically shallow with an erythematous base and sharply defined indurated and elevated borders. In addition to the common ulcerative form, squamous cell carcinoma may manifest as a papillomatous growth at the lid margin (Fig. 36.11), a nodular variant, a cyst or even a cutaneous horn. Rarely, it may clinically simulate verrucae and keratoacanthoma resulting in delayed diagnosis. Conversely, some malignant, precancerous or benign tumors may mimic squamous cell carcinoma. Basal cell carcinoma and squamous cell carcinoma may present with virtually identical features. The only point of difference may be the presence of keratin in squamous cell carcinoma accounting for the typical pearly white edges. Precancerous conditions, such as actinic keratosis and Bowen's disease may be clinically indistinguishable from squamous cell carcinoma. Benign conditions that may clinically simulate squamous cell carcinoma include inverted follicular keratosis, keratoacanthoma, tricholemmoma and pseudoepitheliomatous hyperplasia.

There has been a controversy whether squamous cell carcinoma is found more commonly in the upper or the lower eyelids. It has been shown that it is more common in the lower eyelid with a ratio of 1.4 to 1, although not as pronounced as in basal cell carcinoma. Squamous cell carcinoma arises frequently at the eyelid margin and in the medial canthal area as opposed to extramarginal locations.

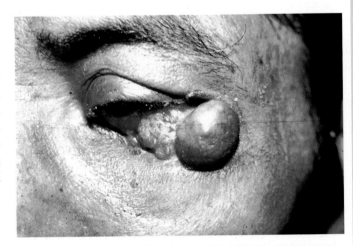

Fig. 36.11: Squamous cell carcinoma of the left lower lid showing a papillary growth along with a nodular component

Following local extension into dermis, deeper invasion into connective tissue and periosteum are the main routes of orbital spread and metastasis. Orbital invasion of squamous cell carcinoma of the eyelid may be associated with perineuritic spread resulting in ptosis and ophthalmoplegia before the development of proptosis. Involvement of the orbital nerves provides a route for intracranial extension of this neoplasm. In general, lymphatic spread occurs to the preauricular nodes if the tumor is in the upper eyelid or the lateral canthus and submandibular nodes if the tumor is in the lower eyelid or medial canthus. Reported incidence of regional lymph node metastasis varies from 1 to 21%.

The management of squamous cell carcinoma of the eyelid mainly consists of adequate excision with clinically clear margins under frozen section control. Squamous cell carcinoma is relatively radio-resistant. Therefore, radiotherapy is reserved only for patients in whom surgery cannot be performed. Smaller tumors may respond to cryotherapy while extensive lesions with orbital infiltration are managed with orbital exenteration.

Histopathologic stages of squamous neoplasia of the eyelids include intraepidermal squamous dysplasia, intraepidermal squamous cell carcinoma and invasive squamous cell carcinoma. Invasion of the dermis is the diagnostic hallmark of invasive squamous cell carcinoma. Broders developed a system of grading squamous cell carcinoma based on the proportion of differentiating cells. However, it is now generally recognized that, in addition to the number of differentiating cells, the degree of atypical tumor cells and the depth of invasion are important in grading the malignancy. In tumors of high grades of malignancy, increasing degree of cellular anaplasia is manifested by irregularly shaped and sized cells, enlarged nuclei, abnormal mitosis and the loss of intercellular bridges.

The prognosis of squamous cell carcinoma of the eyelid is correlated with several factors, including the presence of predisposing conditions, such as radiation therapy or xeroderma pigmentosum (Fig. 36.12), the histologic grade of malignancy and the site of the lesion. The mortality rates have been variably reported ranging from 0% to as high as 40%. It may be lowered considerably prompt diagnosis and treatment. Higher grades of malignancy are associated with increased rates of morbidity and mortality.

Basal Cell Carcinoma

Basal cell carcinoma is the most frequent malignant eyelid lesion in the West and represents more than 90% of all periocular malignant tumors. Most lesions occur in fair skinned individuals, e.g. the Irish or Scandinavians, compared to the pigmented races. Its prevalence in the Asian population is intermediate between the Whites and Blacks. It displays a considerable diversity of appearances, both clinically and microscopically. The distribution favors the lower lid to approximately 70%, whereas the medial canthus, the upper lid and the lateral canthus follow in frequency. It is usually present in the adult or the elderly.

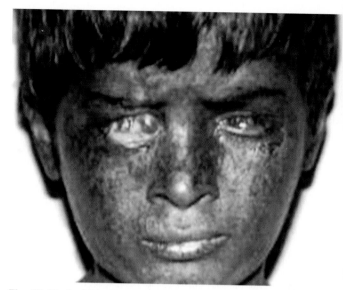

Fig. 36.12: A child with xeroderma pigmentosum with squamous cell carcinoma of the right lower lid and conjunctiva. Note the typical skin pigmentation

Exposure to actinic radiation appears to play an important role in the development of basal cell carcinoma and thus is seen more often in the "outdoor" types of individuals (e.g. cowboys, fishermen, golfers, sailors, etc.). The malignant cells arise from the so-called basal or germinal cells of the epidermis. This layer lies above the basement membrane and separates the dermis from the epidermis. Tumor enlargement occurs from the change in the basal cells that increase in size, proliferate and reach into the dermis and form, in most cases, a nodular tumor. The margin enhances in substance as its center suffers a diminution of blood supply that then breaks down to produce a crusted, umbilicated center. The central crust may loosen and give rise to episodes of bleeding. It is often this feature that initiates the patient's visit to his or her physician.

Clinical Appearance and Histopathology

Clinically, basal cell carcinoma may be divided into:

Localized form (nodular, ulcerative, cystic): The localized nodular and noduloulcerative subtype is the most common mode of presentation (75%). It begins as translucent papules with pearly appearance and telangiectatic vessels. With increasing growth, central umbilication, erosion or ulceration appears leading to the typical pearly, rolled margin (so-called rodent ulcer) (Fig. 36.13). Pigmentation in basal cell carcinoma is common in the Asians and may clinically mimic a malignant melanoma. Histologically, nodular and noduloulcerative basal cell carcinoma consists of large, well-defined basaloid lobules of varying shape and form. It consists of small, hyperchromatic cells with scanty cytoplasm. Characteristically, tumor cells show a parallel alignment at the periphery of the lobules, forming peripheral palisading (Fig. 36.14).

Diffuse form (morpheaform, sclerosing): It accounts for 15% of all basal cell carcinomas, consisting of a flat or slightly depressed

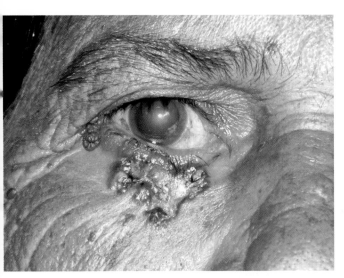

Fig. 36.13: Patient with right lower lid pigmented basal cell carcinoma showing an ulcerated growth with raised edges

indurated plaque, with a poorly demarked clinical margin. It lacks the obvious translucency as in the noduloulcerative form. Because of these features, morpheaform basal cell carcinomas are difficult to treat as they notoriously exceed the clinically visible tumor range. Additionally, morpheaform basal cell carcinoma is characterized by its deep invasion into the dermis and even the subcutis. Such morpheic eyelid tumors may invade the orbit and the paranasal sinuses. Histologically, there is intense stromal fibrous proliferation and peripheral palisading is usually nonexistent.

Superficial form (multifocal): Superficial basal cell carcinomas are seen almost exclusively on the trunk, presenting as multifocal slowly growing scaly red patches. The erythematous appearance may suggest a diagnosis of psoriasis, however, the peripheral translucent rolled border and the central epidermal atrophy provide the correct diagnosis.

Fibroepitheliomatous tumor of Pinkus: Fibroepitheliomatous basal cell carcinoma of Pinkus occurs mainly on the trunk as a

nodular, firm polypoid lesion. Translucency if present reveals the true nature of this lesion. Histopathology shows elongated strands of basaloid cells, which are connected to the epidermis and contain horn cysts.

Additionally, three clinical syndromes are associated with basal cell carcinoma:

Nevoid basal cell carcinoma syndrome (Gorlin-Goltz syndrome): It is an autosomal dominant form of basal cell carcinoma seen in adolescence or early childhood. The eyelids are involved in up to 25% of cases. Histologically, these tumors are usually superficial and indistinguishable from the noninherited form of basal cell carcinoma. Widespread systemic involvement, including hypertelorism, cataract, glaucoma, colobomas of the choroid and optic nerve, skeletal abnormalities, hypogonadism and central nervous system tumors are associated with this syndrome.

Linear unilateral basal cell nevus: It is a rare syndrome characterized by a unilateral linear eruption of nodular basal cell carcinoma, striae-like areas of atrophy and multiple comedones. It neither increases with age nor enlarges.

Bazex syndrome: It shows autosomal dominant inheritance and is characterized by multiple basal cell carcinomas on the face, developing between late childhood and adolescence. This syndrome also displays congenital hypotrichosis and "ice-pick marks" on the extremities caused by atrophic dermal follicular changes.

The mortality rate of basal cell carcinoma is reported from 2% to as high as 4.5%. Morphea or sclerosing lesions in the area of the canthi display a particular tendency towards invasion of the deeper structures of the orbit and the nasal sinuses. These tumors, as a rule, do not metastasize; however, in 0.02 to 0.1% such tumor spread is reported and may occur via hematogenous or lymphatic spread.

Basal cell carcinoma can be adequately managed by complete excision with edge control. All types of therapy for basal cell carcinoma have their advocates and every form of treatment has its advantages and disadvantages. In cases with orbital invasion by basal cell carcinoma, orbital exenteration is essential. The following are the presently applied principal forms of therapy of basal cell carcinoma.

Management

Micrographic (Mohs) Surgery

A combination of micrographic surgery for excision of basal cell carcinoma followed by direct reconstruction ensures predictable tumor removal and the most functional and cosmetically acceptable reconstructive result. The application of the fresh tissue micrographic surgical approach with its continuous histologic control of margins affords a very low recurrence rate. The reported recurrence rate with this management is as low as 1.9% for primary lesions. Mohs' surgery, however, is time consuming and requires a dermatologist trained in micrographic surgery.

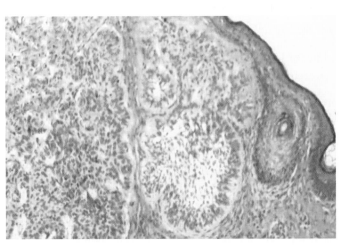

Fig. 36.14: Photomicrograph of a section of the skin showing nests of basaloid cells with palisading of the basal cells at the periphery (hematoxylin and eosin, x 250)

Excision with Frozen Section or Permanent Section Control

This involves the removal of the tumor with numerous marginal sections being subjected to either frozen section or permanent paraffin-embedded biopsies. Only after these biopsies are reported as being free of tumor is the second stage of reconstruction begun.

Radiotherapy and Electron Beam Therapy

Radiotherapy or electron beam therapy can be used to treat basal cell carcinoma. Well-standardized X-ray therapy of basal cell carcinoma in the periocular area usually involves doses in the total range of 35 Gy given in fractionated doses, with cure rates reaching 96%. Loss of lashes, ectropion and obstruction of the tear ducts, may occur as radiation side effect.

Chemotherapy

Systemic and local chemotherapy has been used in patients with basal cell carcinoma who refuse extensive surgery or are medically unfit to undergo surgery. Local application of cisplatin and doxorubicin was accomplished by iontophoresis. Such therapy potentially widens the scope of available methods for treatment of extensive basal cell carcinomas in selected cases.

Cryotherapy

The treatment involves two to three freeze-thaw cycles attaining a tissue temperature of -40°C with an advantage of low rate of complications and relative ease of application. The 5-year recurrence rate, however, can be up to 5%.

Photodynamic Therapy

The method consists of intravenous injection of hematoporphyrin derivative (HpD) given 48 hours prior to the application of laser light (630 nm) of an argon-pumped dye laser system and is effective in treating superficial tumors.

Carbon-dioxide Laser Treatment

It is a viable option for superficial tumors where the tissue temperature is raised to approximately 100°C, which vaporizes the cells under treatment and also coagulates small blood vessels. The affected region is permitted to granulate and scarring is minimal.

PROPTOSIS

Proptosis is the hallmark of orbital disease and can be defined as the displacement of the eyeball in the anterior direction.

Classification of Proptosis

Proptosis can be classified differently under the following categories. Each of these subcategories should be considered in the evaluation of an affected patient. Although this classification does not cover all the possible diagnoses, it can assist the clinician in the diagnostic thinking during patient evaluation:

A. Etiology
1. Dysthyroid orbitopathy
2. Inflammatory (excluding dysthyroid orbitopathy)
3. Tumors and cysts
B. Laterality
1. Unilateral
2. Bilateral
3. Direction
4. Axial
5. Non-axial
C. Time of onset
1. Childhood
   a. Congenital
   b. Acquired
2. Adulthood
   a. Duration
      i. Acute
      ii. Subacute
      iii. Chronic
   b. Clinical course
      i. Stationary
      ii. Progressive
      iii. Regressive
      iv. Pulsating
      v. Intermittent
      vi. Positional

Evaluation of a Case of Proptosis

The treatment of proptosis depends upon the underlying cause. In spite of availability of imaging techniques like CT scan, some basic steps in the clinical evaluation of a patient with orbital disease should be followed. Obtaining a basic history and performing a thorough clinical examination can often make the correct diagnosis made clinically. The differential diagnosis obtained by a clinical examination can be further refined by appropriate imaging studies. Imaging also helps decide the surgical plan. An incisional or excisional biopsy may be required to obtain a final histopathologic diagnosis.

Krohel, Stewart and Chavis described the six "Ps" of orbital history and physical examination, which is an easy way to remember the key steps in orbital history taking and physical examination. The six "P"s they described are:

Pain: It is caused by inflammation, infection, acute pressure changes and bone or nerve involvement.

Progression: It describes any change in symptoms (and the rate of change) occurring over a period of time since the onset. Some orbital disorders progress quickly, whereas others take months or years to develop.

Proptosis: Measurement of proptosis is done with an exophthalmometer that measures the anterior projection of the eye as the anteroposterior distance between the lateral orbital rim to the corneal apex. Proptosis implies an anterior displacement of the globe. Globe ptosis is the term used when the eye is pushed down by a mass. Axial proptosis is usually secondary to intraconal masses whereas extraconal lesions cause non-axial proptosis. The direction of globe displacement can give a clue to the possible underlying pathology (Table 36.2).

Table 36.2: Relationship of eyeball displacement to tumor etiology

Displacement	Etiology
Axial Displacement	
• Enlarged extraocular muscles	Thyroid orbitopathy
• Intraconal mass	Cavernous hemangioma
• Optic nerve tumor	Optic nerve meningioma
Non-axial Displacement	
Inferior Displacement	
• Lacrimal gland	Benign mixed tumor or lymphoid tumor
• Frontal sinus	Mucocoele
• Orbital roof	Sphenoid wing meningioma
Lateral Displacement	
• Ethmoid sinus	Abscess or mucocoele
Superior Displacement	
• Maxillary sinus	Carcinoma
• Orbital fat	Lymphoid tumor
Medial Displacement (rare)	
• Enophthalmos	Scirrhous carcinoma of the breast

Palpation: Palpation includes the exploration of the orbital rim and the superior as well as inferior fornices to look for any anterior mass. If present, its size, shape and position are noted. Other features like compressibility, tenderness and condition of the overlying skin give further clues.

Pulsation: Pulsations will be visible only in a classic pulsatile lesion. Presence of thrill or an audible bruit suggests an arteriovenous malformation.

Periocular changes: Abnormalities in skin, conjunctiva or the eye can give a clue to the diagnosis, i.e. lid lag in thyroid ophthalmopathy or a salmon patch of conjunctiva in a lymphoma.

Diagnosis

Several ancillary diagnostic techniques have been applied in the evaluation of patients with suspected orbital tumors. With the advent of newer imaging techniques, invasive procedures like phlebography and arteriography are rarely necessary.

Ultrasonography is an excellent method of characterizing intraocular tumors, but it is inferior to CT and MRI in the characterization of orbital tumors.

CT scan is the primary imaging technique for evaluation of any patient with proptosis. Orbital imaging serves two purposes: it provides diagnostic information and it helps to plan the orbitotomy. Magnetic resonance imaging has a role in vascular and demyelinating lesions as well as tumors with intracranial spread.

ORBITAL CELLULITIS

Infections of the orbit and periorbital tissues are an important subset of orbital inflammatory disease because they are potentially life threatening and demand prompt and specific management. Modes of presentation and treatment options differ according to the inciting factor, which can be bacteria, fungi or parasites.

Bacterial Infection

Orbital infections are most commonly caused by bacteria and are best categorized by patient's age, site of origin and anatomic location, because these factors serve to indicate the most likely organism, direct antibiotic selection and determine the prognosis.

Infection reaches the orbit by one of the three methods: implantation, local extension or hematogenous spread. Implantation occurs usually in association with a traumatic break in the skin. Local extension is exemplified by spread from a contiguous sinusitis and hematogenous spread may occur from a multiplicity of distant sites.

The most commonly encountered bacteria in children are *Staphylococcus aureus, Streptococcus* species and *Hemophilus influenzae.* The organisms most commonly isolated in adult bacterial infections include *Staphylococcus aureus* and *Streptococcus species.*

Most bacterial orbital infections present with periorbital pain, swelling, increased local temperature and redness. Fever is commonly present. Preseptal infections may simply present with eyelid edema, erythema and an abscess (Fig. 36.15). Postseptal infections are characterized by ophthalmoplegia, proptosis and chemosis (Fig. 36.16). Postseptal infections may present as a diffuse inflammation, localized inflammatory mass and finally, as a subperiosteal abscess. Orbital apex involvement, meningitis or cavernous sinus thrombosis are particularly severe manifestations of orbital infection.

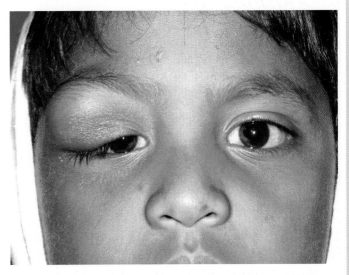

Fig. 36.15: A child with right preseptal abscess of the upper lid. Note that the conjunctiva is not inflamed

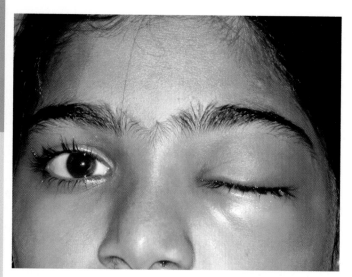

Fig. 36.16: Patient with left orbital cellulitis characterized by lid edema, conjunctival chemosis, proptosis and restricted motility

Diagnostic methods include physical examination (motility, vision, proptosis and fever), white blood cell count with differential, cultures (pus, blood and sinus drainage), orbital ultrasound and CT scan. The CT scan is the imaging modality of choice for patients with suspected orbital cellulitis (Fig. 36.17).

After appropriate work-up, all periorbital and orbital infections should be treated with broad-spectrum antimicrobial agents preferably by intravenous route. Selected cases of adult preseptal cellulitis can be managed on an outpatient basis with oral antibiotics with frequent monitoring. The appropriate antibiotic choice should be made in consultation with the internist or pediatrician. In the newborn period, staphylococcal species are the most common organisms and in children younger than the age of four, *H. influenzae, S. aureus* and *Streptococcus species*. Thus, treatment in the child younger than four years old should include coverage for *H. influenzae* and gram-positive cocci and

penicillin can be appropriate for gram-positive coverage. In penicillin-allergic patients, divided doses of vancomycin, 40 mg/kg/day every six hours, can be administered. Cefotaxime, a third-generation cephalosporin that covers all the most common sinus pathogens with the exception of Clostridium difficile, can be given in a dosage of 80 to 120 mg/kg/day in four divided doses. If anaerobic bacteria are suspected, metronidazole can be added in doses of 7.5 mg/kg given on a six hourly basis.

Once congestive and orbital inflammatory signs diminish, oral antibiotics can be substituted. Dicloxacillin, 25 to 40 mg/kg/day in four divided doses or augmentin (amoxicillin and clavulanate potassium), 40 mg/kg/day in divided doses given on an eight hourly basis, can be substituted.

Sinusitis should be treated with the appropriate antibiotics and possibly with the surgical drainage. Consultation with an otorhinolaryngologist is appropriate. The risk of *Haemophilus influenzae* and the threat of meningitis in children require a second or third-generation cephalosporin to be included as therapy. Most abscesses should be drained, however, several subperiosteal abscesses, can be successfully managed medically.

Fungal Infection

In contrast with bacterial infections, which tend to occur in otherwise healthy individuals, fungal infections have a predilection for the debilitated host. Most common fungal orbital infections are caused by the phycomycosis and ascomycetes classes of fungi. mucor and rhizopus are two genera implicated in human orbital phycomycosis infection, which may present as pulmonary, disseminated, gastrointestinal, cutaneous or rhino-orbital-cerebral forms. Rhino-orbital-cerebral progression begins in the nose, spreads to the maxillary sinus and then to the ethmoids and orbit. The organism causes the thrombosis and infarction of involved tissues and can spread to the central nervous system.

Diabetics and immunocompromised patients are predisposed and present with foul-smelling seropurulent discharge. Other present complaints include localized pain, fever, headache and lethargy. The involved tissues on intranasal examination are necrotic, with a dark discoloration that resembles clotted blood. Orbital apex involvement results in ophthalmoplegia, ptosis and periorbital numbness secondary to trigeminal nerve injury. Sedimentation rate and white blood cell counts are often elevated. Biopsied tissue reveals nonseptate branching hyphae. A CT scan is almost indispensable for defining the extent of fungal granuloma.

Management includes a combined surgical and medical approach, including early recognition, correction of acidosis, debridement of necrotic tissues, sinus/orbital drainage and intravenous antifungals. Mortality rates range from 15 to 35%.

In contrast to the fulminant infection associated with mucor or rhizopus, infections with aspergillus tend to be more indolent, with symptoms lasting from months to years.

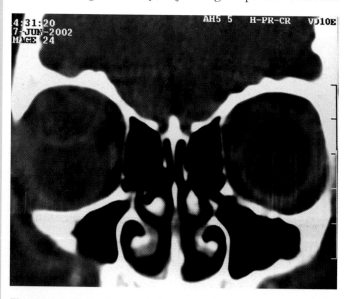

Fig. 36.17: Coronal computed tomography scan of the patient in Fig. 36.16 showing superior subperiosteal abscess with ring contrast enhancement

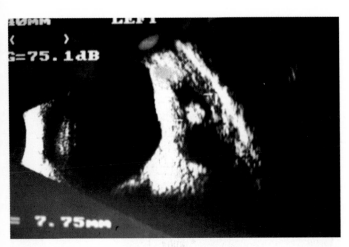

Fig. 36.18: B-scan ultrasonography of orbital myocysticercosis showing the cyst with central echodense scolex

Presenting symptoms include a gradually progressive exophthalmos associated with a chronic fibrosing granulomatous inflammation of the sinuses. Correct diagnosis depends on a high index of suspicion and a biopsy. The treatment for aspergillus is the same as for Phycomycetes: wide surgical debridement in conjunction with systemic antifungal therapy. Amphotericin-B, alone or in combination with 5-fluorocytosine or rifampicin is the option available to the clinician. Irrigation of the debrided tissues and reversal of immunosuppression should be accomplished if possible. The mortality associated with the diagnosis is high. Prompt, aggressive management is necessary for therapeutic success.

Parasitic Infection

Parasitic orbital infections are endemic in some parts of the world, including South America, Africa and the Middle East. Cysticercosis is the most common parasitic orbital infection found in our country.

Cysticercus cellulosae eggs from the intermediate host (pigs) are ingested by the human in the form of raw pork. The cysticerci are preferentially disseminated to the eye and brain, with orbital involvement affects the rectus muscles and can be well demonstrated on B-scan ultrasonography (Fig. 36.18). Rarely, rupture of the cyst mat lead to secondary orbital inflammation. Laboratory work-up, including ELISA for anticysticercal antibodies may be nondiagnostic. Medical therapy with albendazole (15 mg/kg body weight once daily for four weeks) along with steroids is the most appropriate primary therapy. Medical therapy generally results in resolution over 3–6 weeks with minimal residual functional deficit. Surgical excision is reserved for patients with suboptimal response to medical therapy.

CYSTS

A true orbital cyst is any closed cavity or sac within the bony orbital confines that is lined with epithelium and contains a liquid or semisolid material. Orbital cysts can be broadly classified into two groups:

Congenital or developmental: They are present at birth, but some may not be manifested for many years. These include dermoid and epidermoid cysts, cystic teratomas, encephaloceles, congenital cystic eyes and perioptic hygromas.

Acquired: They arise from neighboring sinuses or adjacent adnexal structures. These cysts include mucoceles, dacryoceles and epithelial inclusion cysts.

Parasitic encystment is more often an inflammatory granuloma than a cyst, although "cyst" is commonly used in reference to the manifestation of these infestations. Hematic "cysts" or "chocolate" cysts are not lined with epithelium, but are a fibrous encapsulation of blood or blood products. Only true orbital cysts are discussed in this chapter and although hematic cysts are not lined by epithelium, they are discussed here because of their importance in the differential diagnosis of true orbital cysts.

Dermoid and Epidermoid Cysts

Dermoid and epidermoid cysts are choristomas arising from subcutaneous epidermal rests or epidermal tissues trapped along bony suture lines during embryonic development. If the cyst wall contains skin appendages, such as hair follicles, sweat glands or sebaceous glands, the cyst is termed as a dermoid cyst. If skin appendages are absent, the cyst is termed as an epidermoid cyst.

On examination, there is a painless, smooth, ovoid, firm and rubbery mass protruding from beneath the superior orbital rim, most commonly in the superotemporal quadrant (Fig. 36.19). The mass is immobile and not attached to the overlying skin. Rarely it may pass through bony suture lines to extend intracranially or into the temporalis muscle fossa. CT scan shows a well-defined low-density mass with bony expansion of the corresponding orbital wall (Fig. 36.20).

Surgical removal is the treatment of choice and the approach is dictated by the location of the cyst. In the majority of cases, the cyst can be reached through a skin incision placed directly over it. A posteriorly located cyst requires an appropriate orbitotomy, whereas intracranial extension requires neurosurgical

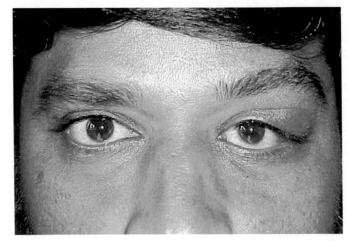

Fig. 36.19: Patient with angular dermoid in the left superolateral orbit

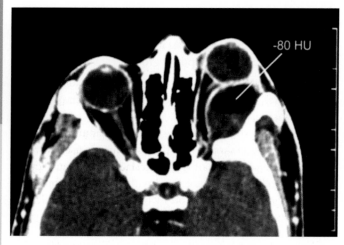

Fig. 36.20: Computed tomography scan of the same patient showing the cyst in the extraconal space with localized bone scalloping

consultation and possibly a craniotomy. Complete removal of the cyst wall is curative. Histopathologically, the dermoid cyst wall contains hair follicles, sweat glands or sebaceous glands (Fig. 36.21).

Teratomas

Teratomas are choristomas derived from all three germinal anlagen, ectoderm, mesoderm and endoderm. Majority of them present at or shortly after birth and imaging reveals the multicystic nature and intracranial extension if any. Most teratomas are benign, although some seen in newborns may be malignant. Tumor growth and unacceptable cosmetic appearance dictate the surgical removal of an orbital teratoma. Excision of the cyst and rarely exenteration may be necessary to affect a complete cure.

Meningoencephalocele

During embryonic development, failure of the fetal fissures to close leads to a congenital dehiscence in the bony cranium. This allows meningeal tissue to herniate into the orbit

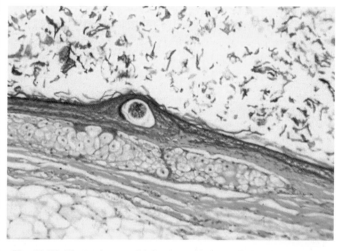

Fig. 36.21: Photomicrograph of a dermoid cyst wall showing skin with adnexa (hematoxylin and eosin x 50)

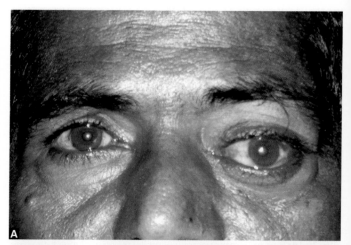

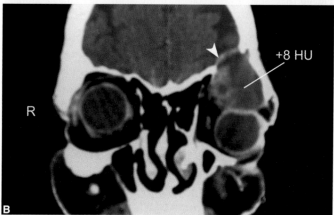

Figs 36.22A and B: A case of traumatic meningoencephalocele (A) Note the radiolucent nature of the temporal half of the mass on coronal scans, which showed a Hounsfield value consistent with fluid (B)

forming a cystic structure filled with cerebrospinal fluid—an orbital meningocele. If the brain protrudes inside the meningeal sac, it is called an encephalocele or meningoencephalocele. Posttraumatic meningoencephaloceles are more commonly seen after head injury with orbital roof fracture (Fig. 36.22).

Cephaloceles are rare and present in infancy as a slow growing, painless, anterior protrusion between the nose and eyebrow, which may show pulsations. There may be mild increase in size on crying. Orbital signs are limited to the mass effect and surgical treatment is indicated in all cases. Small encephaloceles require exposure, ligation and excision, whereas larger ones require craniotomy.

Microphthalmos with Cyst and Congenital Cystic Eye

Failure of the fetal fissure to close at the four weeks of development results in the proliferation of neuroectoderm through the opening, leading to the formation of an orbital cyst. The resulting eye is defective at birth and smaller. This condition is referred to as microphthalmos with cyst. In contrast, congenital cystic eye results from failure of the primary optic vessels to involute. The eye is filled with both solid and cystic forms of dysplastic neuroglial tissue (Fig. 36.23). Management of both involves excision of the cyst and/or globe along with orbital implant followed by prosthesis for cosmesis.

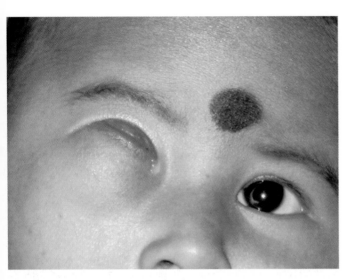

Fig. 36.23: An infant with right microphthalmos with orbital cyst. There was conjunctival prolapse and bony orbital expansion

Mucocele

Destruction of sinus ostia due to recurrent inflammation, trauma or intrinsic mucosal disease results in a mucus-filled sinus or mucocele, which can expand slowly to involve the orbital cavity. Mucocele usually presents in an adult with the history of recurring sinusitis, trauma or previous sinus surgery. Mucoceles of sphenoid or posterior ethmoid sinus usually produce axial proptosis (Fig. 36.24) and may cause ophthalmoplegia and ptosis. Radiographic analysis, including CT, serves to delineate the origin and extent of the mucocele. The treatment of mucoceles is surgical. Frontal and frontoethmoidal mucoceles are approached subperiosteally with the extirpation of diseased mucosa. Reestablishing sinus drainage avoids recurrence. Sphenoid sinus mucoceles are approached intranasally.

CYSTS OF THE OPTIC NERVE SHEATH

A cystic change in an optic nerve sheath filled with cerebrospinal fluid has been called perioptic hygroma or arachnoid cyst of the optic nerve sheath. Most patients are adults present with the

signs of optic nerve damage. Visual prognosis in these cases is guarded and the role of surgical treatment (optic nerve fenestration) is uncertain.

Dacryocele

Distended nasolacrimal sac with entrapped mucoid material is called a dacryocele. A congenital dacryocele manifests at birth as a firm bluish swelling in the medial canthal area, at or below the medial canthal tendon. Surgical intervention is indicated in the cases of dacryocystitis, cellulitis and recurrent dacryoceles.

Hematic Cysts

A hematic cyst is the accumulation of hematogenous debris within a cavity lined with fibrous tissue. Proptosis, globe displacement and motility disturbances are the usual presenting signs. They are thought to be due to trauma with an incompletely absorbed orbital hemorrhage that elicits a granulomatous inflammation and fibrous encapsulation. Treatment includes evacuation of cyst contents, removal of the fibrous wall lining and hemostasis to prevent recurrence.

Simple Cysts

Retention and implantation cysts are common in the eyelids and conjunctiva and orbital involvement is usually secondary. They are of little functional significance, although they may cause cosmetic embarrassment. Retention cysts originate in the glandular appendages of the conjunctiva and adnexal structures, whereas implantation cysts arise from the misplacement of surface epithelium into the orbit as a result of trauma or surgery. Treatment includes removal of the entire cyst or electrodesiccation of the epithelial lining.

VASCULAR LESIONS

Vascular lesions of the orbit display a wide range from the exceedingly benign to locally aggressive and highly malignant lesions. They comprise 10 to 15% of all orbital tumors. Here

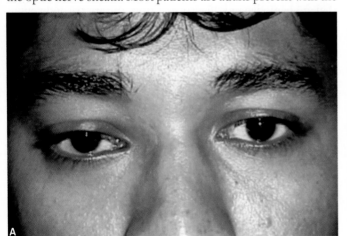

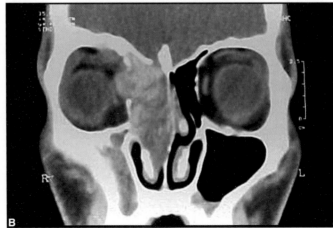

Figs 36.24A and B: Young male with downward and outward displacement of the right globe due to ethmoidal polyp with orbital extension (A). CT scan shows the deficient medial orbital wall with extension of the polyp into the orbit (B)

we shall discuss the most commonly encountered vascular orbital tumors.

Capillary Hemangioma

Capillary hemangioma is a benign orbital hamartoma composed of closely packed capillaries. It represents 18% of vascular lesions in all age groups, and has no specific racial or ethnic predisposition. It is more common in males than in females. It is usually apparent at birth or within the first eight weeks of life and is generally unilateral.

Involvement of the superficial dermis of the lids results in a raised, dimpled intensely red lesion called a strawberry mark (Fig. 36.25), whereas deep dermis or anterior orbital involvement creates a blue-appearing tumor with a spongy texture. The mass deepens in color and becomes more prominent when the child cries. If confined to the orbit, the child may present with slowly growing proptosis. There may be occasionally similar hemangiomas in the skin elsewhere and rarely in the viscera. Capillary hemangiomas of the eyelid and anterior orbit can usually be diagnosed on the basis of clinical examination. The differential diagnosis includes nevus flammeus (port-wine stain), congenital hydrops and rhabdomyosarcoma. Nevus flammeus is associated with the Sturge-Weber syndrome and is flat and noncompressible. Congenital hydrops is present at birth, is firm to palpation, and has associated signs and symptoms of naso-lacrimal duct obstruction. Deep capillary hemangiomas may be difficult to differentiate from rhabdomyosarcoma, thus necessitating biopsy.

B-scan ultrasonography demonstrates an irregular mass with high internal reflectivity and rapid blood flow. CT scan reveals an irregular, poorly circumscribed mass, which generally shows marked contrast enhancement. On gross examination, the capillary hemangioma is a circumscribed, soft red mass with a multinodular surface. Microscopically, the tumor is a proliferation of true capillary units consisting of endothelial cells surrounded by pericytes. It is composed of lobules of cells separated by fibrous tissue septa. High power microscopy demonstrates florid proliferation of well-differentiated capillary endothelial cells and numerous small capillaries. Mitotic activity may be present and calcification is rarely seen in longstanding cases.

Notable feature of capillary hemangioma is its remarkable ability to undergo spontaneous involution, usually by the age of 2 to 3 years. Cutaneous hemangiomas can be directly observed to regress, especially if there are no symptoms. Periodic examination to look for amblyopia and astigmatic refractive errors is all that is required. Management of large and symptomatic capillary hemangiomas can be done with the use of corticosteroids by either local or oral route.

Indications for treatment include:
- Occlusion of the visual axis secondary to tumor growth
- Induced strabismus
- The presence of anisometropia sufficient to cause amblyopia
- A rapidly growing tumor with the potential to occlude the pupillary axis

Corticosteroids shrink hemangiomas because of their vaso-constricting abilities and the recommended dose is 40 mg/ml of triamcinolone with 6 mg of betamethasone mixed in a single syringe and a total of 2 ml is injected directly into the lesion with a 30 G needle. Rapid involution is noted within three days and continues for two weeks. If regression is incomplete or clinically inadequate, a repeat injection is then recommended four to six weeks later. Radiotherapy is employed only for very extensive tumors in low superficial doses of 500 cGy in two to five sittings. Other treatment modalities include surgical excision diathermy; cryotherapy, yttrium aluminum garnet (YAG) laser photocoagulation and sclerosing agent are not commonly used today. Visual prognosis of the involved eye varies with the size of the tumor and the extent of associated amblyopia.

Lymphangioma

Lymphangiomas are congenital lymphovenous malformations that are hemodynamically isolated from the arterial and venous orbital circulation. Lymphangiomas are benign tumors that may involve the eyelids, conjunctiva or the orbit (Fig. 36.26). They most often are present during childhood. There is no preference for race, sex or laterality. Deep lymphangiomatous lesions are classically present with the acute onset of a fulminant proptosis resulting from spontaneous hemorrhage within the orbit. Proptosis may also occur in the presence of an upper respiratory tract infection, reflecting the proliferating lymphoid elements in the connective tissue trabeculae of the tumor.

The infiltrative tumor mass may compress the globe or optic nerve, causing refractive errors, secondary glaucoma, congestion of the optic nerve and visual field deficits. On computed tomography, an infiltrative, multi-lobulated cystic tumor with irregular outlines is apparent (Fig. 36.27). Phleboliths may be present.

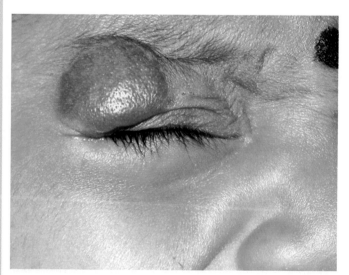

Fig. 36.25: A child with right upper lid capillary hemangioma showing a raised reddish compressible lesion

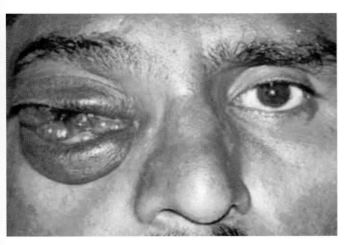

Fig. 36.26: Patient with extensive right lymphangioma involving the lids, conjunctiva and the orbit

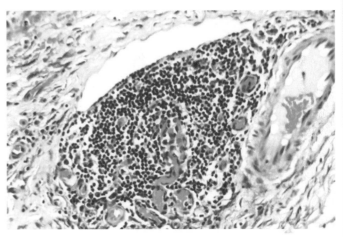

Fig. 36.28: Cystic spaces of lymphangioma showing prominent lymphoid follicles within the walls of the cystic spaces (hematoxylin and eosin, x 50)

The management of lymphangiomas is challenging. Systemic steroids have limited success and radiotherapy has no role in treating these lesions. Complete surgical excision is often difficult if not impossible; because of the infiltrative nature of the tumor. Limited success has been achieved with the carbon dioxide laser, which cauterizes while the tumor is being excised. Complications of surgery include optic nerve dysfunction secondary to hemorrhage, orbital fibrosis and recurrences.

On gross examination, lymphangiomas are non-capsulated tumors composed of cystic spaces filled with blood or clear fluid. On histologic examination, lymphangiomas consist of endothelial channels of variable sizes with lymphatic fluid and admixed erythrocytes. Connective tissue septa between the vascular channels may contain the foci of lymphoid cells (Fig. 36.28).

Cavernous Hemangioma

Cavernous hemangioma of the orbit is the most common benign orbital tumor of adults. It represents 3% of biopsies of all orbital masses and is cited as the most common vascular tumor of the orbit. It is a tumor composed of large dilated veins lined by thin endothelial cells.

Presentation is usually in the fourth to fifth decade of life as a unilateral, solitary tumor. There is no predilection for race or ethnicity. The typical history is of slowly developing axial proptosis over a 3 to 5-year period (Fig. 36.29) with mild degree of blurred vision. Pain, diplopia and other symptoms are characteristically absent. Cavernous hemangiomas are typically located within the intraconal space and motility is only slightly restricted. Horizontal choroidal folds in the macular area may be noted. B-scan ultrasonography shows rounded, regular, sharply defined lesion with high internal reflectivity. CT scan shows a well-circumscribed oval intraconal mass in the orbital tissues with mild to moderate contrast enhancement (Fig. 36.30). Venography and arteriography contribute little to the diagnosis of this tumor.

Surgical treatment is recommended for optic nerve compression as evidenced by visual field defects, optic nerve

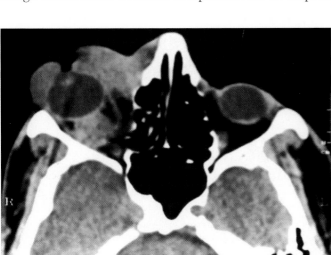

Fig. 36.27: CT scan of the same patient showing the extent of the lymphangioma. Note the irregular margins and the heterogenous consistency

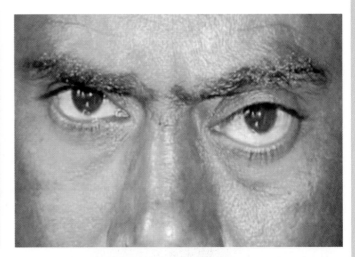

Fig. 36.29: Middle-aged patient with right proptosis and hypoglobus of longstanding duration

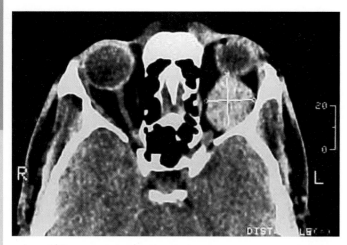

Fig. 36.30: Coronal CT scan of the same patient showing an intraconal, well-defined, homogeneous mass

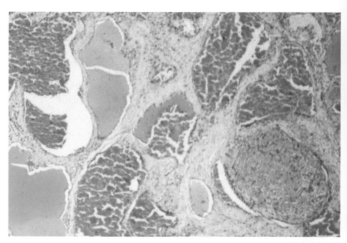

Fig. 36.32: Photomicrograph showing large blood-filled cystic spaces characteristic of cavernous hemangioma (hematoxylin and eosin, x 125)

swelling or pallor. Additional indications include diplopia and bothersome cosmesis. The surgical approach is most often a lateral orbitotomy with complete excision. On gross examination cavernous hemangiomas appears as a spongy, violaceous, well encapsulated mass (Fig. 36.31). Histologically it shows large, closely packed and congested vascular spaces separated by fibrous connective tissue septae (Fig. 36.32).

Carotid-Cavernous Fistula

Carotid-cavernous fistulas are direct communications between the internal carotid artery and the cavernous sinus. These shunts may arise spontaneously or may be the sequelae of severe head trauma. In either case, a rent is created in the intracavernous portion of the internal carotid artery, allowing blood to flow directly into the cavernous sinus leading to elevated pressure within its branch veins, including the ophthalmic vein. Clinical signs (Fig. 36.33) include chemosis, orbital swelling, episcleral venous congestion, elevated intraocular pressure, retinal hemorrhages and ischemia. Third and sixth-nerve palsies

may be associated. A thorough evaluation requires the use of contrast angiography with selective injection of the internal and external carotid arteries. Treatment is indicated when vision is threatened. The treatment options are embolization, electrothrombosis of the fistula, balloon obliteration and direct surgery.

Orbital Varix

Variable proptosis dependent on a change in head position is strongly suggestive of an orbital varix. These anomalies consist of either a single segmental dilatation of a vein or a tangle of ectatic vascular channels. Varices may be primary congenital lesions or secondary acquired lesions or the sequelae of intracranial or orbital arteriovenous malformations. They are present with the classical findings of proptosis and pain, which increase with Valsalva maneuver (Fig. 36.34). CT scan with contrast will demonstrate the enlarged vessels. The management of varices is conservative. Surgery should be performed only when vision is threatened or when the deformity is severe.

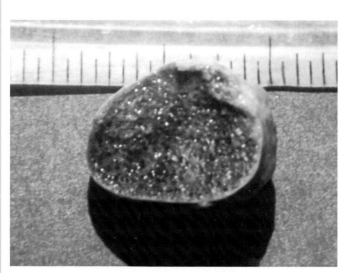

Fig. 36.31: Gross cut specimen of a cavernous hemangioma showing its spongy violaceous appearance

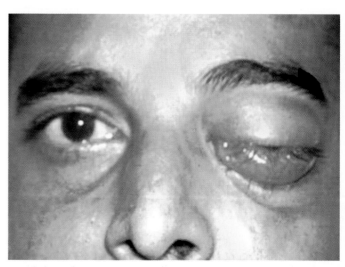

Fig. 36.33: Patient with left carotid cavernous fistula with proptosis, conjunctival congestion and chemosis

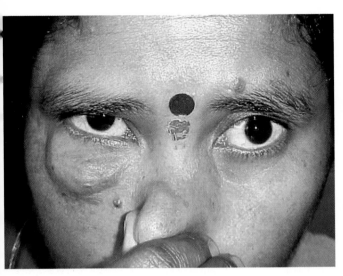

Fig. 36.34: A case of right inferior orbital varix, which becomes more prominent on Valsalva maneuver

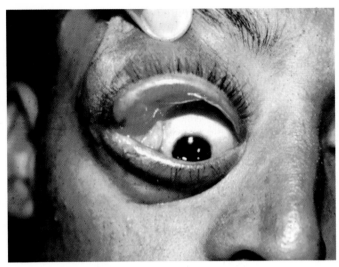

Fig. 36.35: Right plexifom neurofibroma of the upper lid showing the lid and conjunctival component of the tumor

NERVE SHEATH TUMORS

A number of peripheral nerves and related structures in the orbit can give rise to tumors. These include III, IV, V and VI cranial nerves and the ciliary ganglion and they are ensheathed by Schwann cells in contrast to the optic nerve, which is a tract of the central nervous system. Neurofibromas and neurilemmomas are the most common orbital peripheral nerve sheath tumors.

Neurofibroma

Neurofibroma is the most important peripheral nerve tumor of the orbit and is characterized histopathogically by combined proliferation of Schwann cells, endoneural fibroblasts and axons. Orbital neurofibromas can be of three types: plexiform, diffuse and localized. The plexiform type is considered pathognomonic of neurofibromatosis, whereas the other two types are rarely associated with it.

The exact incidence of neurofibromas is not known precisely because many cases are subtle and not histopathologically confirmed. It is reported to be 2% of all orbital cases in one series. The clinical features vary with the type of neurofibroma. The localized type usually occurs in a young or middle-aged adult with painless proptosis and downward displacement of the globe owing to its classic location in the superior orbit. The diffuse variety represents an intermediate lesion between the localized and plexiform types and presents with unilateral proptosis. In many cases, it involves both the eyelid and orbital structures. The plexiform type usually becomes apparent in the first decade of life and the patient has characteristic signs of neurofibromatosis (Fig. 36.35). There is facial asymmetry and palpable orbital mass. Concurrent swelling of the temporal fossa may be present. Buphthalmos may occur due to congenital or secondary glaucoma. Occasionally a pulsating proptosis may be seen due to the congenital absence of orbital roof.

They tend to cause an expansion of the orbital dimensions and sometimes cause bony fossa formation. The diffuse or plexiform type of neurofibroma should be examined for the signs of neurofibromatosis. CT scan shows circumscribed orbital mass in the superior orbit in the localized variety and cannot be differentiated from other soft tissue tumors. The diffuse type shows an irregular mass on imaging.

On gross pathology, localized tumor appears as a well-defined, firm, pinkish-white mass and the diffuse variety appears irregular and poorly defined. Microscopically they are composed of Schwann cells and fibroblasts within a mucoid matrix (Fig. 36.36). Special stains for acid mucopolysaccharides (alcian blue) and immunohistochemical studies can help in the diagnosis. Some neurofibromas are dominated by a mucoid matrix and are called myxoid neurofibromas.

Management of the localized tumor includes surgical excision if it shows increase in size or cosmetic blemish. Although not encapsulated, their removal is generally not problematic

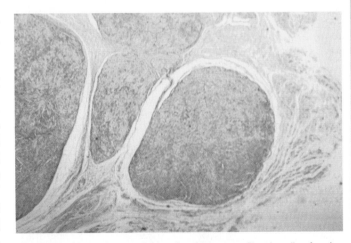

Fig. 36.36: Photomicrograph showing thick nerve fiber bundles forming nodules separated by thick collagenous stroma suggestive of neurofibroma (hematoxylin and eosin, x 50)

and superior orbitotomy with extraperiosteal approach is the most preferred method of excision. The management of plexiform and diffuse variety is much more complex and thus a conservative approach is preferred. Surgery is indicated in the case of threatened vision and bad cosmesis. Generally a partial excision or debulking surgery is performed.

Prognostically orbital neurofibromas are generally benign and have no tendency to metastasize. The localized and diffuse variety recur rarely even after an incomplete excision, whereas plexiform neurofibromas are more apt to recur. In patients with neurofibromatosis, malignant transformation of the cutaneous tumor occurs in up to 10% of the cases.

Schwannoma (Neurilemmoma)

Neurilemmoma is a peripheral nerve tumor of Schwann cells that are derived embryologically from the neural crest. It accounts for 1% of all biopsies of orbital tumors. It is usually present in individuals between the ages of 20–70, there is no predilection for sex or laterality. Most of the cases are unilateral and the patient presents with slowly progressive painless proptosis and downward globe displacement of insidious onset (Fig. 36.37). Occasionally they may arise from the sinuses and simulate a chronic sinusitis. Most orbital neurilemmomas are not associated with neurofibromatosis. On B-scan ultrasonography, the lesion shows round configuration with good sound transmission and CT scan shows a well-defined ovoid to fusiform lesion with its long axis in the anteroposterior direction.

On gross pathology, the tumor is firm to rubbery and may have tan to yellow discoloration (Fig. 36.38). Microscopically, two distinct cellular arrangements are seen within most neurilemmomas (Fig. 36.39). The Antoni A pattern is rather solid and consists of closely arranged spindle shaped cells and the nuclei have a palisading configuration. The Antoni B pattern consists of less orderly arranged stellate cells in a myxomatous or mucoid matrix. This pattern is similar to that seen in some

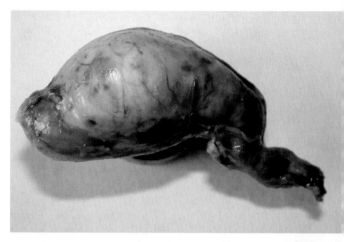

Fig. 36.38: Gross photograph of an orbital schwannoma showing a firm rubbery mass with yellow areas

neurofibroma. Special stains and immunohistochemical techniques may be useful in the diagnosis and its differentiation from neurofibroma and other neural tumors. Alcian blue is negative whereas S-100 protein and Bodian stain for axons are positive in neurilemmomas.

Most orbital neurilemmoma are progressively growing tumors that eventually require treatment. They are radio-resistant and require surgical treatment. Superior or lateral orbitotomy with extraperiosteal approach is the surgery of choice. Orbital exenteration may be necessary in advanced cases. Prognosis for vision is good following surgical excision, but incomplete excision may result in local recurrence many years later. Malignant transformation is extremely rare, but is reported.

LACRIMAL GLAND LESIONS

Mass lesions of the lacrimal gland fossa represent 13% of all orbital space occupying lesions. Almost 50% of all these lesions are of epithelial origin and 50% of non-epithelial origin. Of the

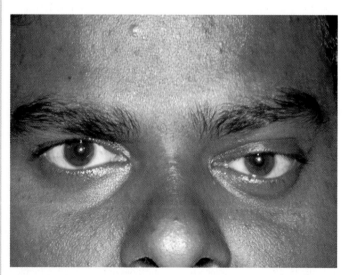

Fig. 36.37: An adult with insidious onset left proptosis with downward globe displacement

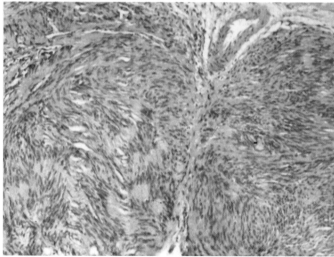

Fig. 36.39: Photomicrograph of a schwannoma showing the Antoni A and B pattern (hematoxylin and eosin, x 250)

epithelial tumors, pleomorphic adenoma accounts for 50% of the cases, adenoid cystic carcinoma for 25% and various other primary carcinomas account for 25%. Among the non-epithelial lesions, about 50% are lymphoid tumors and 50% comprise various inflammatory pseudotumors.

Epithelial Cyst (Dacryops)

It is a cyst of the palpebral lobe of the lacrimal gland resulting from the obstruction of one of the secretory ducts of the lacrimal gland. It characteristically occurs in young adults or middle-aged patients as unilateral or bilateral painless nontender fluctuant mass in the forniceal conjunctiva superotemporally. It may enlarge following crying or exposure to irritants. Following secondary inflammation, a fistula may develop (fistulizing dacryops). It is not attached to the bone and generally shows no osseous changes. The differential diagnosis includes a dermoid cyst, conjunctival epithelial cyst and eosinophilic granuloma. Histopathologically it is composed of one-to-two cell-layered epithelium containing clear fluid and normal lacrimal gland tissue is usually identified adjacent to the cyst. No treatment is required for small and asymptomatic cyst, whereas larger and symptomatic lesions can be excised transconjunctivally or via lateral orbitotomy.

Pleomorphic Adenoma

Pleomorphic adenoma is the most common benign epithelial tumor of the lacrimal gland. It is composed of both epithelial and mesenchymal elements and accounts for 3 to 5% of all orbital tumors, 25% of all lacrimal gland fossa masses and 50% of epithelial tumors of the lacrimal gland. It is characteristically a tumor of adults and slightly more common in males. The patient presents with a slowly progressive nontender mass in the anterior portion of the orbit superotemporally producing proptosis and downward as well as medial displacement of the globe (Fig. 36.40). There is absence of pain, diplopia or visual disturbance. CT scan shows a round to oval well-circumscribed mass in the lacrimal gland fossa and bony fossa formation is

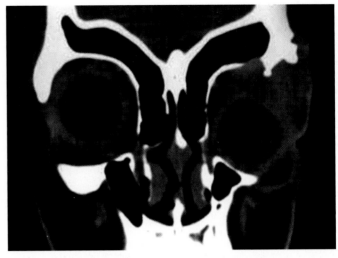

Fig. 36.41: Coronal CT scan of the same patient showing a well defined soft tissue mass in the left superotemporal orbit with bone fossa formation

common (Fig. 36.41). On gross pathology it is an encapsulated mass with nodular irregularities on the surface. But the capsule is rarely breached. Microscopically, it is composed of epithelial and mesenchymal elements. The former takes the form of ducts, cords or squamous pearls, whereas the latter include the myxoid and chondroid tissue (Fig. 36.42). Both these tissue components are necessary for the diagnosis of pleomorphic adenoma.

The management in these cases includes excision of the tumor completely with its capsule without prior biopsy (Fig. 36.43). Failure of complete excision or rupture of the capsule may lead to recurrence or malignant transformation.

Primary Carcinoma

Primary carcinomas constitute 49% of the epithelial tumors of the lacrimal gland comprising of adenoid cystic carcinoma (30%), pleomorphic adenocarcinoma (9%), de novo adenocarcinoma (7%), mucoepidermoid carcinoma (2%) and other miscellaneous carcinomas (1%).

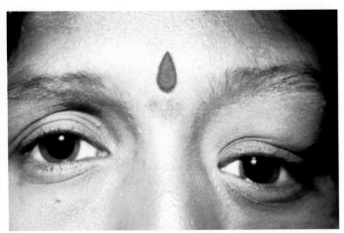

Fig. 36.40: A patient with an orbital mass in the superotemporal orbit, with downward and medial displacement of the globe

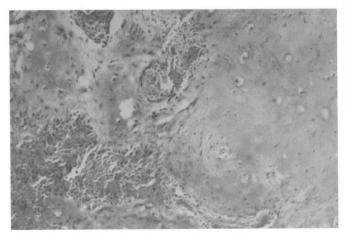

Fig. 36.42: Photomicrograph of pleomorphic adenoma showing variegated appearance with glandular elements, cartilaginous foci and myxoid stroma (hematoxylin and eosin, x 125)

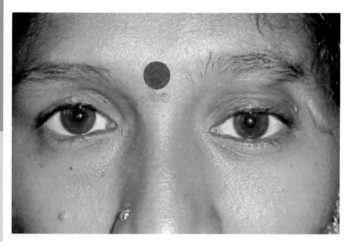

Fig. 36.43: Same patient after complete excision via lateral orbitotomy approach. Note the surgical scar of lateral orbitotomy

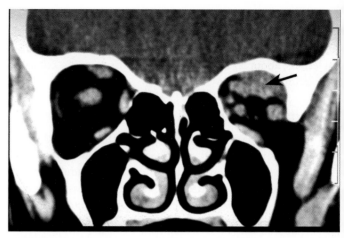

Fig. 36.45: Coronal CT scan of the same patient shows homogeneous irregular soft tissue mass occupying the entire superolateral orbit. The tumor has crossed the vertical midline of the right orbit

The patient is usually a young or middle-aged adult presenting with unilateral progressive proptosis and downward and medial displacement of the globe (Fig. 36.44). It is slightly more common in females. Malignant lacrimal gland tumors are more likely to cause pain, blepharoptosis and diplopia; the duration of symptoms is usually short. CT scan demonstrates a round ovoid or elongated soft tissue mass with irregular outline (Fig. 36.45). Erosion of bone occurs with more aggressive lesions. Foci of calcification are suggestive of but not absolutely diagnostic of malignant lacrimal gland tumors.

Adenoid cystic carcinoma is characterized by solid areas or cords of malignant epithelial cells clearly defined from the adjacent connective tissue (Fig. 36.46). The various histologic subtypes include Swiss cheese variant, sclerosing form, basaloid form, comedocarcinoma variant and tubular pattern.

Areas of malignant change in a pleomorphic adenoma characterize pleomorphic adenocarcinomas. The mass contains fewer glandular structures and more anaplastic features than those of pleomorphic adenomas.

Mucoepidermoid carcinoma shows diffuse proliferation of anaplastic squamous cells with abundant vacuolated cytoplasm. Special stains are positive for mucin within the cytoplasm. There is considerable controversy about the management of malignant lacrimal gland tumors. Extraperiosteal incisional biopsy should be done to confirm the presence of malignant nature. Orbital exenteration with the removal of adjacent bone is recommended. In case of advanced tumors, postexenteration supplementary external beam radiotherapy of 4000 to 5000 cGy to the entire orbit, including the orbital apex and the superior orbital fissure should be considered.

Prognosis of patients with lacrimal gland tumors is generally poor. Adenoid cystic carcinoma, especially the basaloid histopathologic pattern has a very poor prognosis. Generally pleomorphic adenocarcinomas have a better prognosis.

METASTASES

A metastatic cancer to the orbit is a malignant neoplasm that has spread by the way of hematogenous routes to the orbit

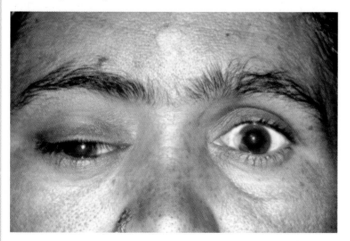

Fig. 36.44: A case of right lacrimal gland tumor, with infero-medial globe displacement

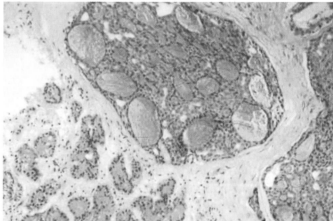

Fig. 36.46: Photomicrograph of a section of adenoid cystic carcinoma of the lacrimal gland showing the classical cribriform pattern (hematoxylin and eosin, x 250)

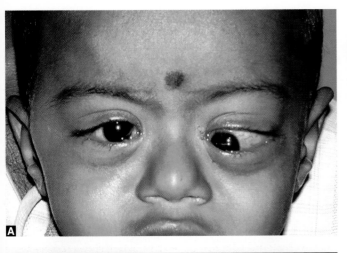

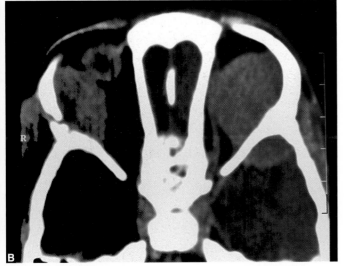

Figs 36.47A and B: A three-year-old child with bilateral orbital secondaries from Wilms' tumor (A) The CT scan shows classical crossroad sign with involvement of the orbit, temporal fossa and middle cranial fossa, with the tumor epicenter within the lateral orbital wall (B)

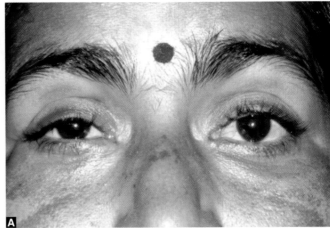

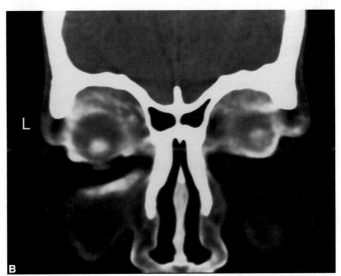

Figs 36.48A and B: Patient with bilateral orbital metastases from breast carcinoma. The patient had enophthalmos and restricted motility (A) Coronal CT scan of the same patient showing anterior orbital extraconal lesions. Incisional biopsy confirmed the diagnosis (B)

from distant primary site. They account for 1 to 13% of all orbital masses. Around 30 to 60% of patients develop ophthalmic signs and symptoms prior to the diagnosis of the primary tumor. Orbital metastatic tumors however are less common than uveal metastases. There are clear distinctions between adults and children with regard to the type and location of the primary tumor.

In adults, most tumors arise from epithelial structures of the breast, prostate, lung, gastrointestinal tract, kidney, thyroid and other organs. In children, they are more likely to arise from embryonal neural tumors and sarcomas. Thus, in children,

neuroblastoma, Ewing's sarcoma and Wilms' tumor (Figs 36.47A and B) are more important considerations. Breast cancer accounts for the greatest number of orbital metastases (Figs 36.48A and B), followed by lung, prostrate and gastrointestinal tract. The majority of them are unilateral. The patient usually presents with a short duration of diplopia, proptosis or ptosis. The metastatic tumors are often poorly differentiated and have little resemblance to the primary tumor. Immunohistochemistry and electron microscopy may be helpful in establishing the correct diagnosis. The patient requires a thorough search for the primary; and treatment depends on the stage of the systemic disease.

Arnab Biswas

INTRODUCTION

Diseases of the lacrimal system predominantly include various congenital anomalies, congenital and acquired dacryocystitis and lacrimal sac tumors. Newer treatment techniques have been developed for better results.

CONGENITAL ANOMALIES

The following congenital problems that can affect the nasolacrimal system:

Dacryostenosis: Dacryostenosis is a frequent condition in which the terminal end of the nasolacrimal duct under the inferior turbinate fails to canalize completely in the newborn period. Clinical symptoms may be produced in the newborns.

Anomalies of the sac: A diverticulum of the lacrimal sac may occur. A congenital fistula of the lacrimal sac is more common (Figs 37.1A and B).

Anomalies of the puncta: Congenital atresia, supernumerary or double puncta (Fig. 37.2), and congenital slits of the puncta

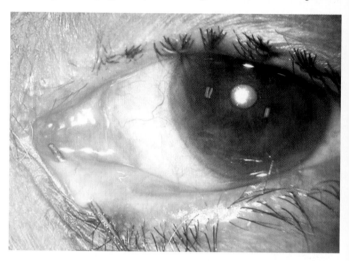

Fig. 37.2: Double punctum: Such an anomaly is likely to be present since birth. A probe has been passed through the double puncta

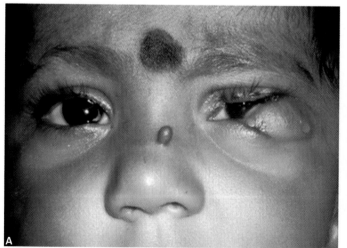

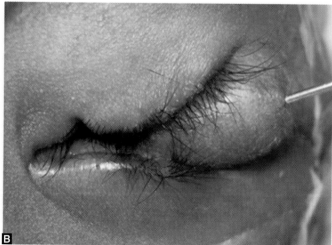

Figs 37.1A and B: Congenital fistulae: Complex developmental anomaly of the lid. There is coloboma of the upper lid, the lateral part of the lower lid has deviated downwards. An abnormal excess tissue bridges the lateral part of the upper and lower lid. Note a small tear drop within the abnormal bridging tissue. The point of tear drop is actually a congential fistulous tract from the sac opening into the skin. (A) The fistulous track has been traced and a probe has been inserted through it(B)

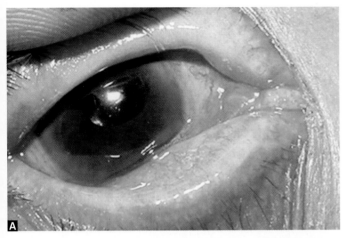

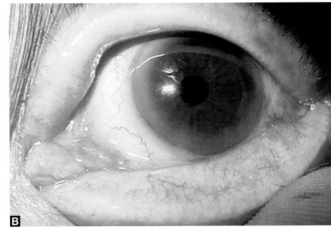

Figs 37.3A and B: Punctal stenosis: The upper and lower punctum cannot be made out even on high magnification. It is a case of punctual stenosis secondary to cicatrization in a case of Stevens-Johnson syndrome

may occur. Lateral displacement of the puncta may occur in some congenital syndromes, such as blepharophimosis.

Anomalies of the canaliculi: Absence or failure of the canalization of the lacrimal canaliculi may occur in association with punctal atresia.

Common causes of punctal stenosis include congenital causes, trauma, viral infections and autoimmune disorders (Figs 37.3A and B).

CONGENITAL DACRYOCYSTITIS

Congenital dacryocystitis results from nasolacrimal duct obstruction and can lead to various clinical manifestations, which include the following (Fig. 37.4).

Amniotocele: This condition occurs in neonates as a distention in the lacrimal sac. Amniotic fluid enters the sac during gestation age. It is retained by a nonpatent nasolacrimal duct, and is trapped in the sac by the valves. It results in the presence of a tense large swelling in the region of the sac area immediately after birth. Probing the nasolacrimal duct is usually curative.

Dacryocystitis (acute mucocele or pyocele): This condition occurs as an acute distention and inflammation in the lacrimal sac region

and can occur in the neonatal period (Fig. 37.5). Systemic antibiotic and even a surgical incision over the sac to drain the pus may be necessary in some cases.

Watering and matting: Newborns who have congenital dacryostenosis may not develop acute dacryocystitis with a mucocele or pyocele of the sac in the early neonatal period, but may have tearing with a chronic mucopurulent discharge, which usually manifests at two weeks. Topical antibiotics should be administered, and the parents must be instructed in the proper technique of lacrimal sac compression and massage. More than 90% of these cases clear and become asymptomatic with conservative management. Under normal circumstances, these children with mild-to-moderate symptoms of epiphora and lid crusting can be monitored for the first year of life. Probing may have to be done after the first year if symptoms do not improve.

Causes

In congenital dacryocystitis, the incomplete canalization of the nasolacrimal duct (specifically at the valve of Hasner) plays an important role in pathogenesis.

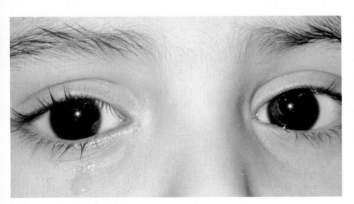

Fig. 37.4: Congenital nasolacrimal duct obstruction: Matting of the eye lashes with watery discharge in the right eye is seen

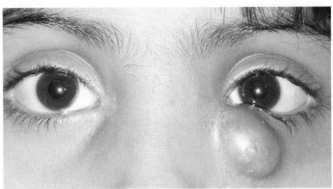

Fig. 37.5: Acute mucocele: Congenital nasolacrimal duct obstruction usually remains chronic, but in some cases where no intervention has been done, may present as a case of acute dacryocystitis with abscess formation

Management

The following management strategies may be employed:

- *Children <12 months:* Conservative management with topical antibiotic and lacrimal massage.
- *Children >12 months:* Diagnostic and therapeutic probing may be performed.
- *Failed primary probing:* Repeat probing is considered with silicone intubation or balloon dacryoplasty.
- *Failed secondary probing or child above three years:* Dacryocystorhinostomy is considered.

Medical

Congenital nasolacrimal duct obstructions spontaneously resolve in 90% of the cases in the first year of life.

Lacrimal massage with digital pressure over the sac area and milking it downwards helps in speeding up this natural resolution.

Topical antibiotics are useful for mucopurulent discharge, but the only treatment of efficacy for those patients who do not resolve spontaneously is surgery.

Surgical

- *Probing:* Probing cures more than 90% of congenital nasolacrimal obstructions. Prognosis for probing decreases exponentially with the increasing number of probing and the age of the patient. It is usually not successful after the third time or after three years. A soft stop indicates resistance at the common internal opening (valve of Rosenmüller). A hard stop indicates the probe has reached the medial wall of the lacrimal sac/bone. A grating, scratchy sensation indicates a false passage.
- *Nasolacrimal intubation:* It has been advocated as an alternate procedure to dacryocystorhinostomy (DCR) in children who have failed probing. Success rates of 80 to 95% have been reported, but most patients have only been probed twice or less and are younger than two years. Prognosis is poor for those patients with previous dacryocystitis and for

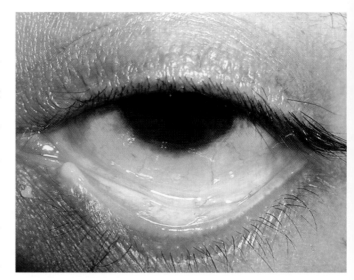

Fig. 37.6: Canaliculitis: The inferior punctum is pouting out. There is a localized purulent collection within the canaliculi

those patients in whom an obstruction is encountered during the procedure.

- *Balloon catheter dilatation of the nasolacrimal system with or without silicone tubing:* This procedure has slightly better results than intubation alone. Most probing failures occur as a result of upper sac or mid duct obstructions and are not amenable to cure by instrumentation. Repeat probing procedures and intubation can cause serious complications, including false passages, canalicular scarring and stenosis.
- *Dacryocystorhinostomy:* This is still the gold standard procedure when other measures fail.

CANALICULITIS

Introduction

Canaliculitis is caused by the infection of the canaliculi (Figs 37.6 to 37.7 B). Usually, it is chronic. It may also be iatrogenic

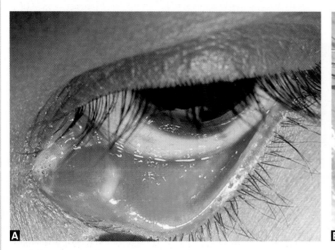

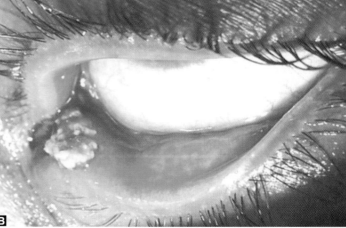

Figs 37.7A and B: Canaliculitis: Inflamed lower punctum with discharge spilling out is observed (A). Yellowish concretion-like granules are observed coming out through the punctum upon pressure over the inflamed canaliculi (B)

after the instrumentation or placement of silicone plugs in the treatment of dry eyes.

Clinical Features

Symptoms: Patient complains of watering, irritation or heaviness of the medial portion of the affected eyelid.

Signs: Edematous, "pouting" punctum and erythema of adjacent conjunctiva near the medial canthus may be present. On application of pressure mucid, sometimes hemorrhagic regurgitation presents from the punctum. Yellowish concretions may be expressed from the punctum. These are sulfur granules produced by *Actinomyces israelii.*

Causes

The most common pathogens of canaliculitis are *Actinomyces israelii* and *Nocardia* species. Recent case reviews have shown mixed flora associated with infection. Species isolated include *Staphylococcus* species, *Escherichia coli, Haemophilus* species, *Pseudomonas aeruginosa, Klebsiella oxytoca, Arcanobacterium haemolyticum* and *Mycobacterium chelonae.* Iatrogenic instrumentation especially during trauma to the canaliculi during syringing or plugging can also give rise to canaliculitis, but sulfur granules are usually absent.

Treatment

The concretions should be removed with gentle pressure and massage over the canaliculi using a cotton swab. Hot compression over the medial portion of the lid may give some relief. Irrigation with an antibiotic solution may help. Systemic antibiotics, usually amoxicillin or azithromycin for 1–2 weeks can help in refractory cases. Topical antibiotics—are usually used. This rarely achieves complete resolution due to the inability of antibiotics to penetrate concretions. Canaliculotomy (two or three snip procedure) with curettage is the definitive treatment.

INFLAMMATORY DISORDERS OF THE LACRIMAL SYSTEM

Acute Dacryocystitis

Acute dacryocystitis is manifested by the sudden onset of pain, erythema and edema overlying the lacrimal sac region (Fig. 37.8).

Clinical Features

The tenderness is characteristically localized in the medial canthal region, but may extend to the nose, cheek, teeth and face. Frequently, a purulent discharge is noted from the puncta. Conjunctival congestion and preseptal cellulitis often occur in association with acute dacryocystitis. Epiphora is invariably usually present, and a palpable mass over the sac area can be observed. Some may present with fever, prostration and an elevated leukocyte count.

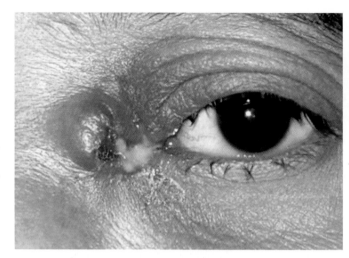

Fig. 37.8: Acute dacryocystitis: Features of acute inflammation in the region of the lacrimal fossa are observed. There is purulent material coming out from the puncta near the medial canthus. Syringing or probing should not be carried out in this acute situation, as it may worsen the condition

Causes

Both aerobic bacteria and anaerobic bacteria have been cultured from pediatric and adult patients with dacryocystitis.

Investigations

In most patients, a clinical diagnosis of acute dacryocystitis is made. Laboratory investigation includes a complete blood count to assess the degree of leukocytosis. Blood cultures and cultures of the ocular surface, nose and lacrimal sac discharge may prove useful in determining the appropriate antibiotic therapy in refractory cases.

Complications

Complications include mucocele (Fig. 37.9), fistulae formation and chronic conjunctivitis. More serious sequelae of acute

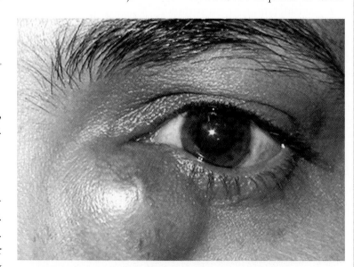

Fig. 37.9: Mucocele: In chronic dacryocystitis, the nasolacrimal duct is as such closed. In association if the upper canalicular passage becomes stenosed or closed, the collection within the lacrimal sac may get blocked resulting in such a situation

dacryocystitis include extension into the orbit with the formation of an abscess and development of orbital cellulitis.

Treatment

Acute dacryocystitis with orbital cellulitis necessitates hospitalization with intravenous antibiotics. Appropriate neuroimaging studies should be obtained and surgical exploration and drainage should be performed for the focal collections of the pus. Broad spectrum intravenous empirical antimicrobial therapy for both gram-positive and negative organisms should be initiated immediately. Blood cultures and cultures of the lacrimal secretions should be obtained prior to the start of antibiotic therapy. Hot compression may help in the resolution of the disease. Impending perforation should be treated with a stab incision of the skin. Purulent infection of the lacrimal sac and skin should be treated similarly. Hospitalization is not mandatory unless the patient's condition appears serious. Treatment with broad spectrum oral and systemic broad spectrum antibiotics is appropriate. Cultures of the lacrimal fluid should be obtained. Dacryocystorhinostomy is the treatment of choice. The surgery should be performed 4–6 weeks post-acute attack to prevent failure.

Chronic Dacryocystitis

Introduction

In chronic dacryocystitis the lacrimal sac is distended with minimal inflammation, there is usually suppurative or mucoid discharge from the punctum on pressure over the lacrimal fossa. In some cases lacrimal fistula may result (Figs 37.10 and 37.11).

Pathophysiology

The inferior part of the nasolacrimal duct becomes stenosed and obstructed following a chronic low-grade inflammation. Structural abnormalities of the midface should also be taken into consideration. Nasal pathology like: hypertrophied infe-

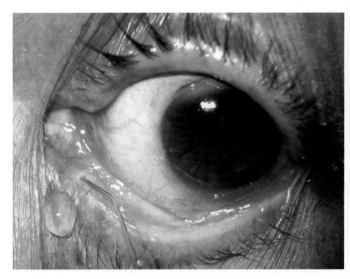

Fig. 37.11: Lacrimal fistulae: Small tear drop just inferior to the punctum is observed. This is the site of a fistulous track, through which fresh water comes out on performing syringing through the lower punctum

rior turbinate, deviated nasal septum, nasal polyp and allergic rhinitis can predispose to dacryocystitis.

Causes

The bacteriology of dacryocystitis mimics normal conjunctival flora in most instances. The most common aerobic organisms isolated from the lacrimal sac in adults with dacryocystitis include *S. epidermidis*, *S. aureus*, *Streptococcus*, *Pseudomonas* and *Pneumococcus* species. *S. epidermidis* is the most common isolate followed by *S. aureus*. The most common anaerobic organisms isolated from the lacrimal sac in adults with dacryocystitis include *Peptostreptococcus*, *Propionibacterium*, *Prevotella* and *Fusobacterium* species. Rarely, fungi have been isolated from infected lacrimal sacs (commonly associated with dacryolith formation).

Clinical Features

Watering or tearing is the most common presentation of chronic dacryocystitis. The lacrimal sac may become obstructed in the nasolacrimal duct from retained secretions forming a large secular retention (mucocele). Matting of lids is caused by the obstruction of drainage of the mucous layer of the tear film with the collection of debris and denuded epithelial cells from the surface of the eye. Chronic conjunctivitis may occur. Patient may also be present for the first time as a case of acute dacryocystitis

Imaging Studies

Simple syringing of the lacrimal system can clinch the diagnosis in most cases. It will manifest as the regurgitation of fluid through the opposite punctum.

CT scans may be done when one suspects malignancy or mass as a cause of dacryocystitis.

Dacryocystography and dacryoscintigraphy are useful adjunctive diagnostic modalities when the anatomical abnormalities of the nasolacrimal drainage system are suspected.

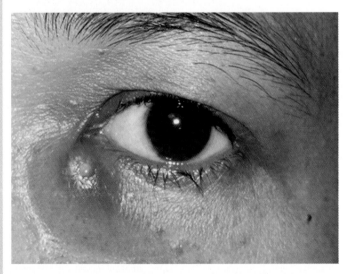

Fig. 37.10: Lacrimal fistulae: A small fistula has developed at the region where the lacrimal abscess had spontaneously ruptured

Subtraction dacryocystography with CT scan is also very sensitive to study the anatomy of the lacrimal sac and surrounding structures.

Other Tests

- *Schirmer basic secretor testing:* This test ensures that epiphora is not related to hypersecretion or abnormal lid function or position.
- *Baseline tear secretion measurement:* This can be measured with the Schirmer basic secretor test.
- *Nasal endoscopy:* This investigation is sometimes useful in assessing the etiology of dacryocystitis. Tumors, papillomas, hypertrophy of the inferior turbinate, nasal septal deviation and inferior meatal narrowing may be noted as the causes of dacryocystitis.
- *Jones dye test:* With the Jones I dye test, the functional and anatomical obstruction of the nasolacrimal system can be assessed. A positive result indicates no anatomical or functional blockage to tear flow. A negative result indicates a lacrimal drainage system problem (i.e. anatomical or functional blockage).

A Jones II dye test is used to determine the presence or absence of anatomical obstruction of the nasolacrimal outflow system. A positive Jones II dye test (colored fluid from the nose) indicates a patent system anatomically. In light of a negative Jones I dye test, a positive Jones II dye test indicates either partial obstruction of the nasolacrimal system or a false-negative Jones I test. A negative Jones II eye test (clear fluid from the nose) indicates functional blockage of the nasolacrimal system. This is common with the horizontal laxity of the lower eyelid or flaccidity of the canalicular system. If no fluid can be irrigated with the Jones II test, complete nasolacrimal obstruction is present.

Histologic Findings

Chronic inflammation and fibrosis of the lacrimal sac are present in varying degrees. Focal ulceration and loss of goblet cells are not uncommon. Focal abscesses and granuloma formation have also been noted in the lacrimal sac.

Management

Dacryocystorhinostomy (DCR): It is the standard treatment for nasolacrimal duct obstruction, with success rates consistently above 90%. It consists of creating a direct connection between the lacrimal sac into the nose, bypassing the blockage and allowing tears to drain normally again.

In cases of chronic dacryocystitis, the correction of the precipitating factor may be beneficial as in: occasionally, infracting of the inferior turbinate bone, submucous resection of the turbinate, and/or lacrimal outflow probing may be a successful treatment of dacryocystitis.

Acute cases are best treated surgically after the infection has subsided with adequate antibiotic therapy. For acute dacryocystitis, dacryocystorhinostomy is preferred after several days of

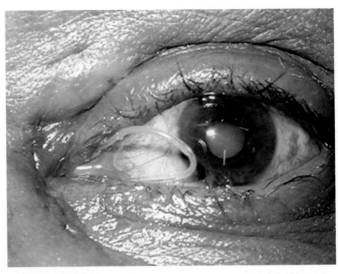

Fig. 37.12: Stent: A lacrimal intubation was done in a case of repeat dacryocystorhinostomy operation. The tube had slipped out and is prolapsing out following a finger nail injury

initiating antibiotic therapy. Stent is required in failed cases (Fig. 37.12).

External dacryocystorhinostomy: External dacryocystorhinostomy has been the gold standard, since Toti described the initial dacryocystorhinostomy operation in 1904. However with more understanding and refinement in instruments in nasal endoscopy, transnasal endoscopic dacryocystorhinostomy are giving at par results.

Endonasal approach of dacryocystorhinostomy: Surgeons are using the endonasal approach to dacryocystorhinostomy surgery with or without a laser. This may be the first line of management in patients with chronic dacryocystitis.

Lacrimal sac fistulization into the nose (dacryocystorhinostomy) can be performed successfully via a transcanalicular approach using a CO_2 or KTP laser. Instead of approaching the nasolacrimal duct system by exposing it externally, the transcanalicular approach involves introducing a special atraumatic cannula into the nasolacrimal duct from the lower punctum of the eye. A thin laser fiber is introduced into the cannula, and the whole procedure can be viewed using a nasal endoscope. With the laser fiber in contact with the bone, the laser energy is delivered to cause a vaporization of the bone, and entry of the laser fiber into the nose. This allows the stenosis of the nasolacrimal duct to be obviated.

Laser dacryocystorhinostomy has several advantages over conventional dacryocystorhinostomy. Some of these advantages include: Bloodless procedure, time efficiency, no external scar resulting in better cosmetic results, faster patient recovery, repeatability and preservation of ligaments and muscles of the internal canthus.

Balloon dacryoplasty: Balloon dacryoplasty has been popularized in the last several years. It appears to have a lower long-term success rate than the previous treatment modalities. It may be used in patients with circumscribed focal stenoses or occlusions of the nasolacrimal duct and is contraindicated in acute dacryo-cystitis, dacryocystolithiasis, and the post-traumatic obstruction of the nasolacrimal duct. In one study, the long-term success rate of balloon dacryoplasty was 60 to 70%.

LACRIMAL SAC TUMORS

Tumors involving the nasolacrimal drainage system are rare and more than 90% of these tumors are of the epithelial origin (Figs 37.13A and B).

Majority of lymphomas involving the lacrimal sac are secondary to systemic lymphoreticular malignancy. Primary non-Hodgkin's lymphoma of the lacrimal sac is a rare neo-plasm (Figs 37.14A and B).

Important suspicious and differentiating points from chronic dacryocystitis are as follows:

Lacrimal sac tumors are rare. Mass is present above medial canthal tendon. Lacrimal syringing reveals that fluid may pass to nose or blood may reflux from punctum. CT orbit may show extent of mass. Dacryocystography may show filling defect. There may be associated overlying skin ulceration, telangiectasia and lymph nodes. It may originate from skin or nasal mucosal tumors. Squamous cell carcinoma is the most common malignant tumor being more common than adenocarcinoma.

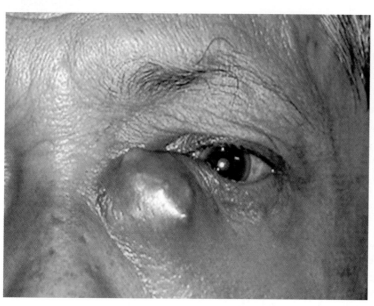

Fig. 37.13A: Lacrimal sac tumor: This middle-aged man presented with a hard soft tissue mass over the lacrimal fossa, with overlying skin excoriation and ulceration. Fine needle aspiration cytology from the mass confirmed presence of malignant cells

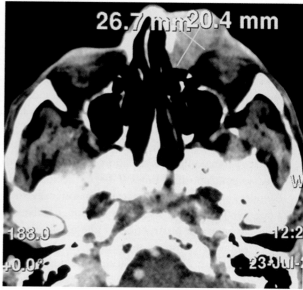

Fig. 37.13B: Lacrimal sac tumor: CT scan axial section shows a large mass occupying the whole of lacrimal fossa

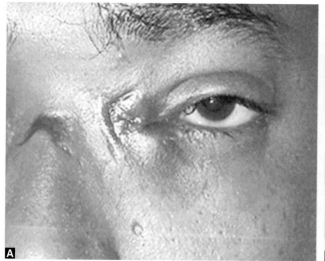

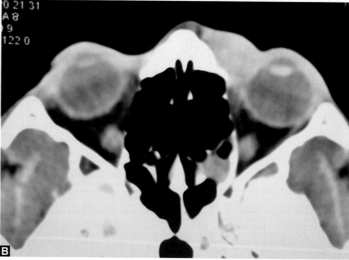

Figs 37.14A and B: Lacrimal sac lymphoma: This middle-aged gentleman had undergone a dacryocystectomy operation (left side) two months back on the basis of a clinical diagnosis of mucocele (Note the curvilinear scar of previous surgery). He is again presented with a very rapidly increasing swelling in the lacrimal fossa with resulting telecanthus formation. On examination the swelling was very hard. A repeat exploration and removal of the mass followed by histopathological evaluation confirmed it to be a lymphoma (A). CT scan axial section shows a globular mass occupying the whole of lacrimal fossa (B)

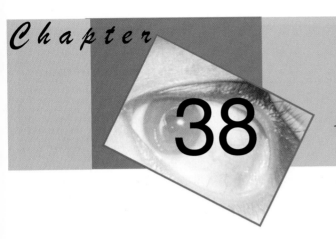

Eyelid and Lacrimal Surgeries

Milind N Naik, Santosh G Honavar

INTRODUCTION

Ophthalmic plastic and reconstructive surgery as a specialty is relatively new, but the art has been practiced from time immemorial. Its present and rapidly evolving form is a product of developments in the basic discipline, an understanding of periorbital anatomy and disease, and improvement in surgical equipments and techniques.

EYELID SURGERY

Ptosis Surgery

Timing of Ptosis Surgery

Congenital ptosis: The decision regarding the management of congenital ptosis depends mainly on the age of the patient and the magnitude of functional and cosmetic deficit (Figs 38.1A to D). Cosmetic correction of congenital ptosis is ideally performed after about four years of age when accurate ptosis measurements can be obtained and child is cooperative for postoperative management. However, in cases where there is a high risk of amblyopia or abnormal head posture, early surgery may be considered. This could be a temporizing procedure, such as a reversible tarso-frontal sling. A permanent procedure could be planned later when the child is older. Acquired ptosis can be of various types (Figs 38.2A to D), and the management plan therefore varies with the etiology.

Acquired aponeurotic ptosis: This can pose either a functional or cosmetic problem. The decision to operate is generally guided by the patient's needs.

Mechanical ptosis: It is primarily managed by addressing the cause, and levator surgery is performed only for residual ptosis if required.

Neurogenic ptosis: The management of neurogenic ptosis may involve a period of observation ranging from 6–12 months for spontaneous recovery. Surgery may be performed for residual

ptosis and following the correction of strabismus. *Traumatic ptosis* caused by direct injury to the levator muscle needs secondary ptosis repair after a period of 4–6 months.

Myogenic ptosis: The management of myogenic ptosis is difficult. Medical management is the initial modality of choice in myasthenia gravis. Ptosis correction in patients with myasthenia gravis or chronic progressive external ophthalmoplegia may precipitate corneal complications or manifest diplopia. Crutch glasses are an option in very severe cases with a high risk of exposure keratitis. A reversible tarso-frontal sling with deliberate undercorrection may be considered where the risk of corneal complications is less likely.

Choice of Surgery for Congenital Ptosis

Surgical approach to congenital ptosis is considered based on laterality, severity, levator function, Bell's phenomenon, associated elevator underaction and the presence of Marcus-Gunn phenomenon.

Bilateral mild congenital ptosis may be left untreated unless the patient is cosmetically conscious about the problem. It is usually associated with good levator action and hence the bilateral simultaneous Fasanella-Servat procedure may be optimal. Other options are levator plication or a small levator resection.

Bilateral moderate congenital ptosis is associated with good-to-fair levator action and is of cosmetic and functional consequence. It is best treated with bilateral simultaneous levator resection.

Bilateral severe congenital ptosis usually has associated poor levator action. Most patients have a head posture and may need to be treated early in childhood. A tarso-frontal sling is a good option in such cases. The amount of correction should depend on the adequacy of Bell's phenomenon.

The choice of surgery for mild to moderate unilateral congenital ptosis is no different from bilateral cases. In severe unilateral cases, options available include a unilateral tarso-frontal sling, supramaximal levator resection or the "Whitnall's sling". Unilateral sling is less preferred due to asymmetry in downgaze,

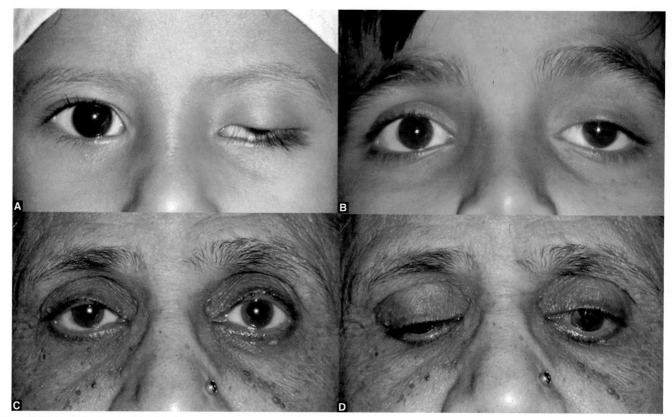

Figs 38.1A to D: One year old child with severe left congenital ptosis. Risk of amblyopia warrants early ptosis correction (A). 12-year-old male with mild 3 mm left congenital ptosis. Surgery is elective, and indicated for cosmetic reason (B). Acquired right aponeurotic ptosis (C), with eyelid drooping more in down gaze (D)

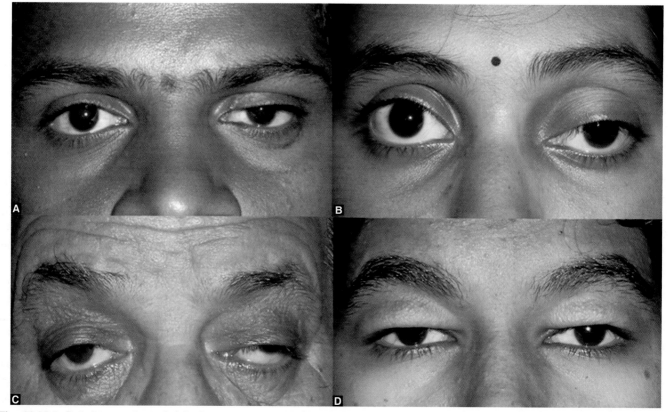

Figs 38.2A to D: Left traumatic ptosis following the repair of subtotal eyelid avulsion. Note the upper eyelid scar (A). Left traumatic third nerve palsy with ptosis and hypotropia (B). Bilateral severe myogenic ptosis and exotropia in a patient of chronic progressive external ophthalmoplegia (C). Bilateral blepharochalasis with acquired mechanical ptosis. A levator dehiscence is also likely in this case (D)

nd the lack of motivation on the part of the patient to use a nilateral sling.

Ptosis with associated Marcus-Gunn phenomenon calls or a discussion with the patient and the family regarding their erception of cosmesis and a mutual decision. Where Marcus-Gunn phenomenon is mild to moderate, ptosis alone could be orrected. For severe Marcus-Gunn phenomenon, the com-plete disinsertion of levator muscle along with a tarsofrontal ling would be necessary. Some surgeons advocate a bilateral arsofrontal sling to achieve symmetry in downgaze.

Choice of Surgery for Acquired Ptosis

Aponeurotic ptosis is the most common cause of acquired ptosis in clinical practice. It could be primary without any detectable precipitating factor or secondary to contact lens use, trauma, eyelid edema or inflammation, and following intraocu-lar surgery. Ptosis could result from either the dehiscence of the levator aponeurosis or its complete or partial disinsertion. Surgical approach would thus involve exploration for the defect in levator aponeurosis followed by reinsertion, plication or resection. Levator resection in such cases should be carefully judged because overcorrection is a common complication.

Surgical Techniques for Ptosis Correction

There are several surgical techniques described for ptosis cor-rection. An experienced surgeon modifies the original proce-dure to suit his convenience resulting in several versions of each surgical technique.

Fasanella-Servat Procedure

The Fasanella-Servat procedure classically involves tarsocon-junctivo-mullerectomy. Best results are achieved in up to 2 mm congenital ptosis with minimum 10 mm levator action. In such cases, 2 mm of tarsectomy is performed for every 1 mm of ptosis. The procedure could also be used for mild neurogenic or myogenic ptosis, and for residual ptosis following levator resection procedure. Laxity of the anterior lamina and tendency to entropion are relative contraindications for the Fasanella-Servat procedure. The surgical steps of the modified Fasanella-Servat procedure are as follows (Figs 38.3A to 38.6D):

Anesthesia: The surgery can be performed under local or general anesthesia.

Traction sutures: The upper eyelid is everted, and three 4-0 trac-tion sutures are placed at the upper border of the tarsal plate. Another set of three traction sutures is placed, starting from forniceal conjunctiva, and exiting at the eyelid margin.

Tarsal-conjunctival resection: The required amount of tarsal resec-tion is then marked over the everted tarsus staying parallel to the eyelid margin, and the tarsus is excised with radiofrequency monopolar cautery. The preplaced forniceal sutures allow easy approximation of the cut ends of the tarsus and conjunctiva.

Wound closure: A 6-0 catgut suture is placed over the eyelid skin at the medial end of the tarsal wound, and the needle is brought out on the conjunctival side. The cut edges are sutured with the 6-0 catgut in a continuous manner. The suture end is finally exteriorized at the lateral edge of the wound and sutured to the eyelid skin.

Levator Resection

Levator resection has several variations. The approach could be transconjunctival or transcutaneous. Transconjunctival approach is best used in cases with moderate ptosis and fair levator action. It could also be used for the correction of residual ptosis following the skin approach levator resection. The conjunctival approach is more difficult than the transcu-taneous approach because of altered anatomic orientation. Skin approach levator resection is more popularly practiced. The procedure of skin approach, levator resection surgery is described below (Figs 38.7A to 38.9D).

Anesthesia: Local anesthesia (frontal nerve block) is preferred for adults, while general anesthesia is necessary for children.

Incision: Eyelid crease incision is placed maintaining symmetry with the contralateral eye.

Exposure of orbital septum: The orbicularis is separated, and sub-orbicularis dissection is carried out to expose the orbital septum and upper half of the tarsal surface.

Exposure of levator aponeurosis: The orbital septum is now cut all through its extent, exposing the pad of fat. Whitnall's ligament will be visualized on retracting the overlying pad of fat as a whitish fascial condensation running across the junction of the muscular and aponeurotic part of the levator, about 14–18 mm from its insertion.

Levator disinsertion: The levator aponeurosis is disinserted at the upper edge of the tarsus and freed from the underlying con-junctiva by blunt dissection. The medial and the lateral horns are cut only if better exposure is required.

Levator resection: Three double-armed sutures (either 6-0 vicryl or 6-0 prolene) are passed about 2 mm from the upper border, one in the center and one each at the junction of the middle third of the tarsus with the medial third and the lateral third. The sutures are then passed through the levator aponeurosis between 18–24 mm from its tarsal insertion.

Assessment of lid height: The sutures are tightened with temporary knots to achieve a predetermined lid height and a natural con-tour. The placement of upper eyelid during surgery is based on the levator action (Table 38.1).

Formation of eyelid crease: The redundant stump of aponeurosis is excised, and lid crease is formed with three interrupted 6-0 vicryl sutures passed through the orbicularis muscle, including the levator stump.

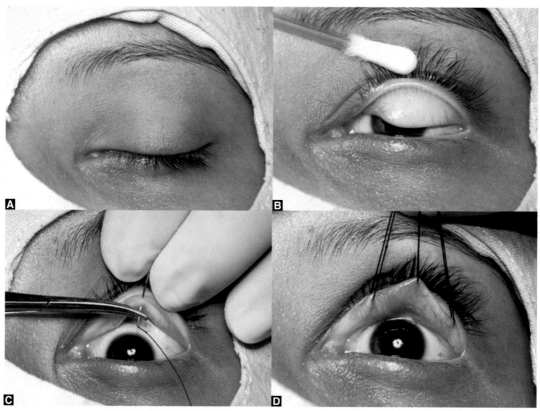

Figs 38.3A to D: Modified Fasanella-Servat procedure. Eyelid position under anesthesia (A) and adequate tarsal height (B). Traction sutures are placed at the upper border of tarsus with 4–0 silk sutures (C and D).

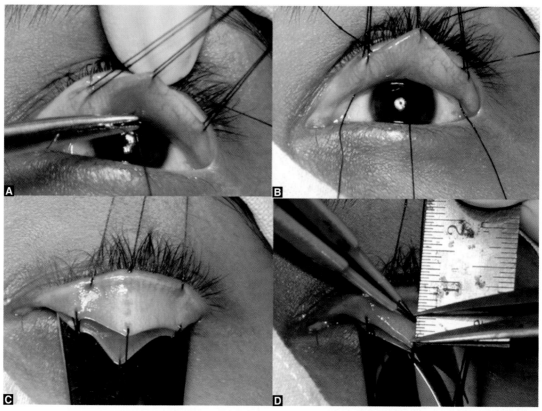

Figs 38.4A to D: Modified Fasanella-Servat procedure. A set of three forniceal stay sutures are placed, starting from conjunctival fornix, and exiting at the eyelid margin through the full thickness of the eyelid (A and B). The upper tarsus is stretched over an eyelid spatula (C), and the required amount of resection is marked (D)

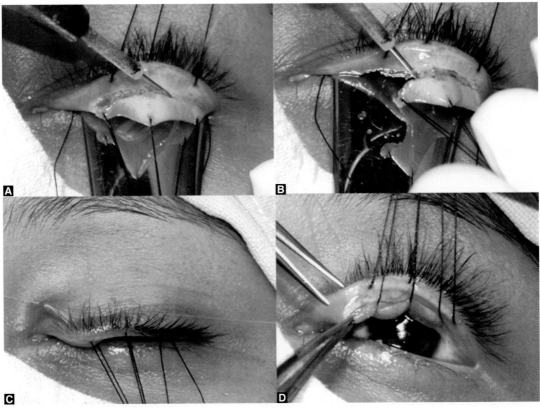

Figs 38.5A to D: Modified Fasanella-Servat procedure. The tarsus is marked along the line of excision with a monopolar cautery (A), and full thickness excision is performed along the entire extent (B). A skin suture is placed with 6-0 catgut at the medial end of tarsal excision, and the needle is brought out on the conjunctival side to close the tarsal wound (C and D). Note that the forniceal stay sutures help to keep the cut edges together

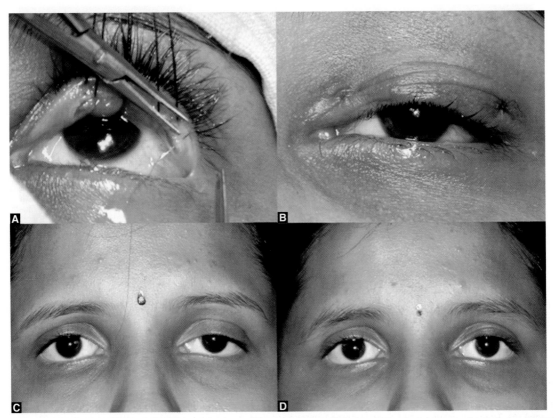

Figs 38.6A to D: Modified Fasanella-Servat procedure. Tarsal wound is closed with continuous 6-0 catgut suture and exteriorized onto the eyelid skin at the lateral end for the final knot (A and B). Preoperative and postoperative photograph of the patient with left mild congenital ptosis who underwent the Fasanella-Servat procedure (C and D)

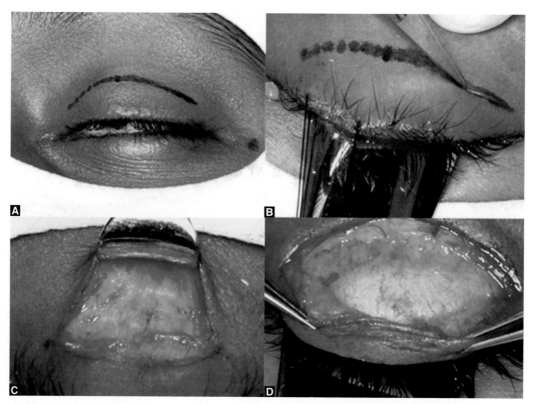

Figs 38.7A to D: Skin approach levator resection surgery. Upper eyelid crease incision is marked and skin incision is placed (A and B). Orbicularis is separated to expose the orbital septum (C), and the superior tarsal surface (D)

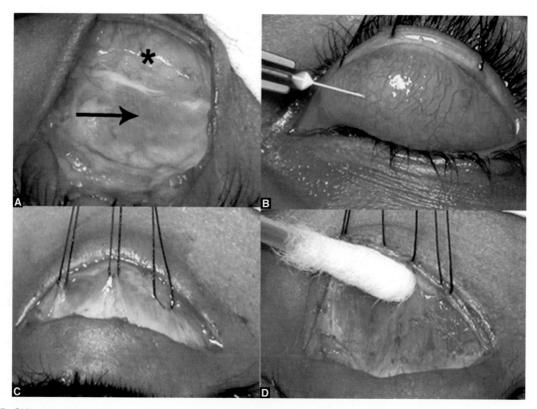

Figs 38.8A to D: Skin approach levator resection surgery. The orbital septum is incised to expose the preaponeurotic fat pad (asterix) and levator aponeurosis (arrow) (A). The conjunctiva is lifted away from the levator aponeurosis by subconjunctival injection of xylocaine (B), and 4-0 silk traction sutures are placed through the levator aponeurosis at its insertion (C). The levator is then disinserted, and separated from the underlying Muller's conjunctiva by blunt dissection (D)

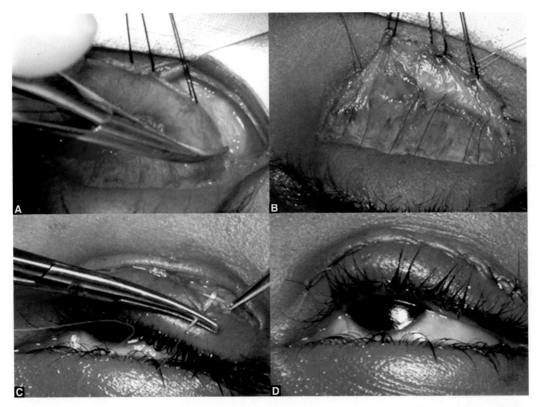

Figs 38.9A to D: Skin approach levator resection surgery. Medial and lateral horns are cut if necessary (A), and three cardinal sutures are passed from the tarsus through the levator muscle at the desired height (B). Orbicularis muscle is closed with interrupted 6-0 vicryl sutures (C), and skin is closed with 6-0 prolene continuous suture (D)

Table 38.1: Guidelines for the intraoperative placement of the eyelid position based on levator action, during congenital ptosis surgery via skin approach under general anesthesia

Levator action	Eyelid position
2–3 mm	At upper limbus
4–5 mm	1–2 mm below the limbus
6–7 mm	2–3 mm below the limbus
8–9 mm	3–4 mm below the limbus
10–11 mm	6 mm below the limbus

Wound closure: The skin is then closed with continuous 6-0 prolene and a Frost suture is applied.

Tarsofrontal Sling

Tarsofrontal sling is an ideal procedure for bilateral moderate to severe ptosis with poor levator action. It can be performed unilaterally in rare situations, such as following levator excision for Marcus-Gunn phenomenon, severe unilateral ptosis with poor levator action where levator resection will not benefit and cases needing a reversible procedure. Tarsofrontal sling can be performed with nonabsorbable synthetic materials, including 3-0 ethibond suture, 3-0 prolene suture, Silicone or Goretex. Autogenous fascia lata is, however, considered the best sling material. The sling can be performed with either the single triangle pattern or the pentagon pattern. Although the synthetic slings have a recurrence rate of 20 to 30%, they have the advantage of reversibility, minimal lagophthalmos, and the absence of donor site morbidity. The procedure of tarsofrontal sling surgery using the silicone rod sling is described below (Figs 38.10A to 38.12D).

Anesthesia: The surgery is performed under general anesthesia.

Marking the incisions: Eyelid incisions are marked over the upper eyelid one centimeter apart, 3–4 mm away from the lash line. The central brow incision lies 10–12 mm above the superior border of the eyebrow. The lateral and medial brow incision is marked above the eyebrow, in line with the lateral and medial canthus.

Skin incisions: Stab incisions are then made with Bard Parker knife. Eyelid incisions are placed in the skin and orbicularis, whereas brow incision is up to the frontalis muscle.

Passing the silicone rod: The needle attached to the silicone rod is then bent to maneuver it through stab incisions in the suborbicularis plane. It passes from the central brow incision to the lateral brow incision, lateral eyelid incision, medial eyelid incision, medial brow incision and back to central brow incision.

Adjustment of eyelid height: The silicone sleeve is then fed over the two ends of the silicone rod, and eyelid height adjusted to the desired level. The sleeve is transfixed with 6-0 prolene suture, and sutured to subcutaneous tissue within the brow incision. The silicone rods are cut short, and the ends buried within a subcutaneous pocket just above and adjoining the central brow incision.

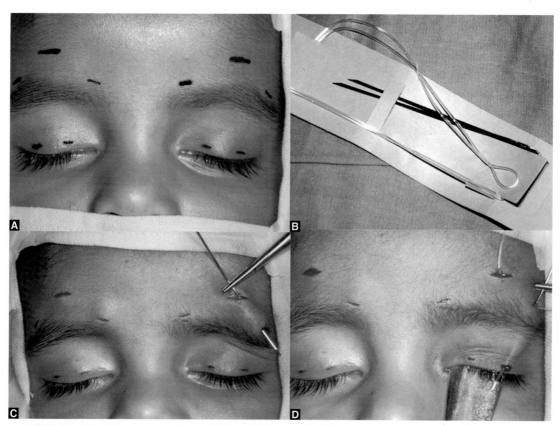

Figs 38.10A to D: Silicone rod sling procedure for bilateral severe ptosis. Eyelid markings made as described in the text (A). Silicone rod sling with a pre-swaged needle at either end, and a silicone sleeve (B). Stab incisions are placed over the eyelid and brow markings, and the needle is passed in the suborbicularis plane from central brow incision to lateral brow incision (C). The needle is then passed towards the lateral eyelid stab incision, while the eyeball is protected by a lid guard (D)

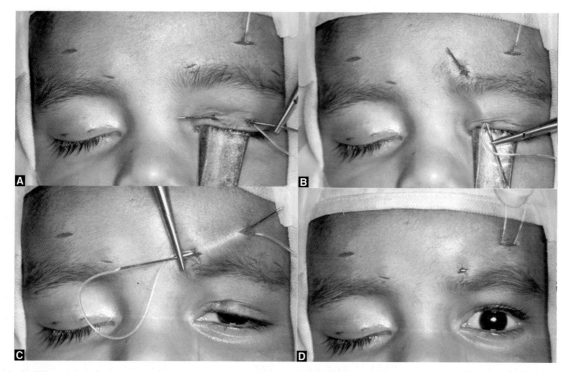

Figs 38.11A to D: Silicone rod sling procedure. Needle being passed through the suborbicularis plane toward medial eyelid incision (A), medial brow incision (B) and finally out through the central brow incision (C). The silicone rods are held under tension to look for eyelid lift and contour (D). Similar procedure is repeated for the right eye

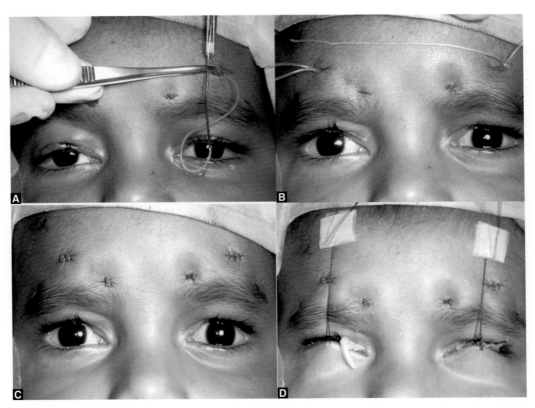

Figs 38.12A to D: Silicone sleeve is passed over the two ends of the silicone rod that are brought out through the central brow incision (A). The eyelid height is adjusted to the desired level by applying traction over each end of the silicone rod (B). The silicone sleeve can be transfixed to subcutaneous tissues with 6-0 prolene suture. Cut ends of silicone rods are tucked into superior subcutaneous pocket, and the wound is closed with interrupted 6-0 prolene sutures (C). Frost suture is placed before applying a patch (D)

Wound closure: The brow stab wounds are then closed with interrupted 6-0 prolene sutures. Frost suture is placed before patching the eye.

Complications

Undercorrection is the most frequent complication of congenital ptosis surgery (Figs 38.13A to D). Undercorrection may improve as the edema subsides, and persisting undercorrection may be treated with repeat surgery after 4–6 months. An obviously undercorrected eyelid immediately after surgery should be corrected within a week or two. Overcorrection is rare in congenital ptosis but could easily occur following surgery for acquired ptosis. Various methods to treat overcorrection include downward traction over lashes against forced upgaze, downward traction over the eyelid with forceps (requires local anesthesia), and surgical correction. Localized lid contour abnormalities are treated by loosening the cardinal suture for localized peaking, and further small levator resection for localized flattening. Lid crease abnormalities include absence of a crease, improper position and overhanging skin. Lid crease abnormalities may require the reformation of the eyelid crease at the desired level. Conjunctival prolapse occurs if the forniceal attachment of the levator is disturbed during posterior dissection. It usually improves without treatment, but may require fornix formation sutures or the excision of excess conjunctiva in some cases.

EYELID RECONSTRUCTION

Eyelid reconstruction is indicated for eyelid colobomas that are congenital, or acquired following trauma or tumor resection (Figs 38.14A to D). Any surgery that involves the repair or reconstruction of the eyelids must, if one is concerned to produce an optimal result, be carried out against the background of a thorough understanding-not simply a knowledge- of the detailed anatomy of the eyelids. As pointed out by Landolt in 1881, the eyelids can be thought of as two lamellae, an anterior lamella consisting of skin and orbicularis muscle, and a posterior consisting of tarsus with the closely applied conjunctival layer, and those structures that act as eyelid retractors. The combination of these two most important lamellae must be restored in any procedure involving eyelid reconstruction. Therefore, the repair and reconstruction of eyelids can be considered to fall into two basic categories. First, there are those procedures confined to the anterior lamella, i.e. the skin and orbicularis—the partial thickness of the eyelid; second, there are procedures involving both anterior and posterior lamellae-full thickness of the eyelid. Although in theory, lesions may

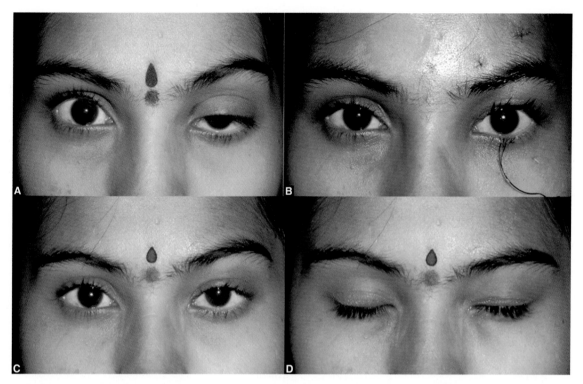

Figs 38.13A to D: A 22-year-old female with left severe congenital ptosis (A). Same patient one day postoperatively (B), and six weeks postoperatively following Silicone rod sling surgery (C). Note the absence of lagophthalmos on gentle eyelid closure due to the elasticity of the silicone rod (D)

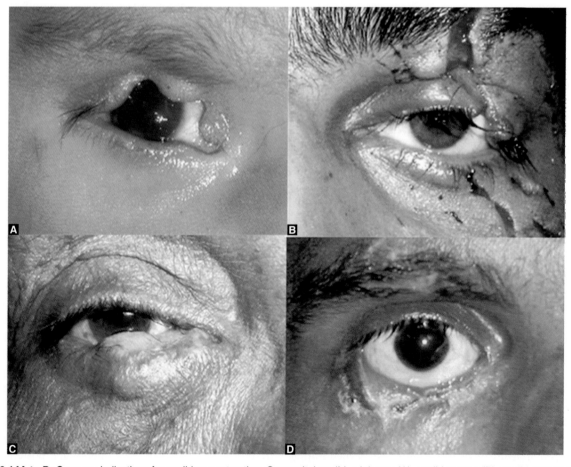

Figs 38.14A to D: Common indications for eyelid reconstruction. Congenital eyelid coloboma (A), eyelid trauma (B), eyelid tumors (C) and traumatic eyelid coloboma (D)

affect the posterior lamella alone, such as epidermoid inclusion cyst within the tarsus, such instances are extremely rare, and partial thickness lesions should, in this chapter, be taken to mean the involvement of the anterior lamina only.

Anterior Lamellar Defects

Anterior lamellar defects represent defects in the eyelid skin and orbicularis muscle. There are several options for the repair of skin and muscle defects in the periocular area (Table 38.2).

Healing by Granulation

Small lesions away from important anatomical landmarks would heal by granulation. This method is usually applied for lesions near the eyelid margin (Figs 38.15A to D), or near the canthi, especially if the equal amount of defect lies above and below

Table 38.2: Options for the reconstruction of anterior lamellar defects of the eyelid and periorbital region

- Healing by granulation
- Primary closure
- Primary closure with undermining
- Free skin graft
- Myocutaneous advancement flap

the canthus. The healing, however, may take weeks or months in a few patients.

Primary Closure

Primary closure with or without undermining is generally a better option than healing by granulation. It is performed in areas where redundant skin is available adjacent to the defect. Areas of the face that typically have redundant skin include glabella, upper eyelid skin, and temple. There is little redundant skin available in the lower eyelid or medial canthus area. In old patients with wrinkled and saggy skin, primary closure can be performed without difficulty. In young patients as well as in areas of scalp and forehead, however, undermining may be necessary. Knowledge of tissue planes, preservation of blood supply, and avoiding nerve injury is important for undermining. Within the orbital rims, tissue undermining should be done in the preseptal plane, whereas outside the orbital rims, it should be in the subcutaneous plane. Undermining in the area of forehead and scalp should be done deep to the frontalis muscle, in the loose areolar tissue superficial to the periosteum. Undermining should effect minimum tension on the skin closure. Deep anchoring sutures to the underlying periosteum should be placed whenever necessary to take the tension off the subcutaneous tissue.

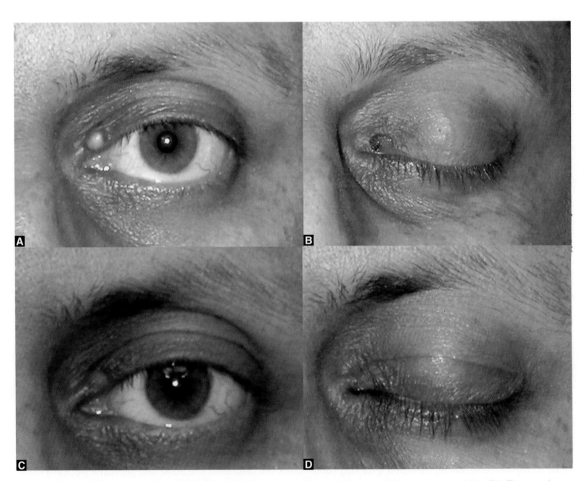

Figs 38.15A to D: Paramarginal upper eyelid epithelial inclusion cyst (A). Defect left to epithelialize after excision (B). Two weeks post-excision (C and D), showing near total healing with no evidence of eyelid malposition

Free Skin Graft

Free skin grafts are harvested from a donor site and transferred to fill an anterior lamellar defect. The recipient site provides the vascular supply for graft survival. Two types of skin grafts are used for eyelid reconstruction—full thickness skin grafts and split thickness skin grafts. In full thickness skin grafts, the epidermis as well as the dermis is transferred to the recipient bed. The donor site must be hairless, and requires surgical closure, thus limiting the size of the graft available. However, full thickness grafts heal with less contracture than split thickness grafts, thereby making the full thickness technique better suited for eyelid reconstruction (Figs 38.16A to D), where contracture can cause ectropion, lid retraction or lagophthalmos. Donor site of the same skin color, texture, and thickness is used for skin grafts. Donor sites for full thickness skin grafts include retroauricular skin, upper eyelid skin, preauricular skin, supraclavicular and skin from upper inner arm. Split thickness skin grafts are used rarely, and are generally harvested from the thigh skin. They can survive even on bare bone, but produce considerable shrinkage, and provide a poor color and texture match at the recipient site. Split thickness skin grafts are used only for defects too large for full thickness grafts, and where myocutaneous flap is not possible.

Myocutaneous Flaps

Myocutaneous flaps involve the rotation of adjacent skin and orbicularis into the eyelid defect, and provide the best means to repair anterior lamellar eyelid defects. When designed correctly, myocutaneous flaps provide the locally available tissue, derive their own blood supply and innervation, and provide a good color match and high success rate of healing with minimal contracture. Temporal transposition flap and cheek rotation flap are examples of myocutaneous flaps (Figs 38.17A to D).

Full Thickness Eyelid Defects

Although full thickness eyelid repair has been traditionally described by the size of the eyelid coloboma, all these techniques are a continuum of treatments (Table 38.3).

Small Defects (Pentagon Excision)

Small defects up to 25% of eyelid can be closed primarily. After a pentagon excision has been performed, the wound edges are approximated to assess the tension. A canthotomy and cantholysis may be required at this stage for apposition without tissue tension. The technique of primary repair of eyelid margin following pentagon excision is described in detail below for an eyelid papilloma involving the anterior lamella and the

Table 38.3: Commonly performed procedures for full thickness eyelid reconstruction

- Primary closure (with and without cantholysis)
- Tenzel's semicircular flap
- Sliding tarsal flap with skin/myocutaneous flap
- Cutler-Beard or Hughes procedure

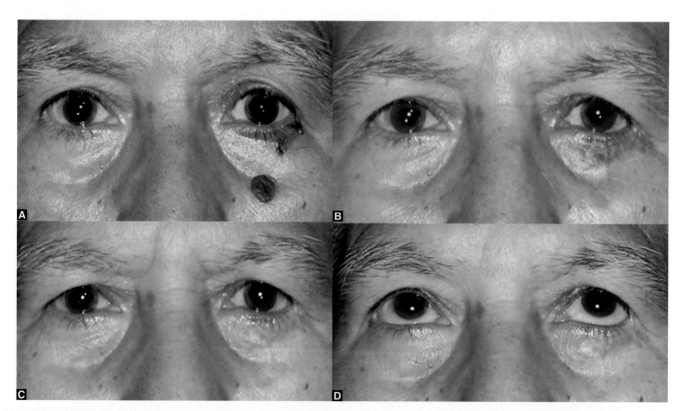

Figs 38.16A to D: A 60-year-old female with left lower eyelid pigmented basal cell carcinoma and malar skin papilloma (A). Early (B) and late (C and D) postoperative appearance. The basal cell carcinoma was excised, and defect replaced by a full thickness skin graft. The defect created by papilloma excision was undermined, and closed to obtain a vertically aligned wound

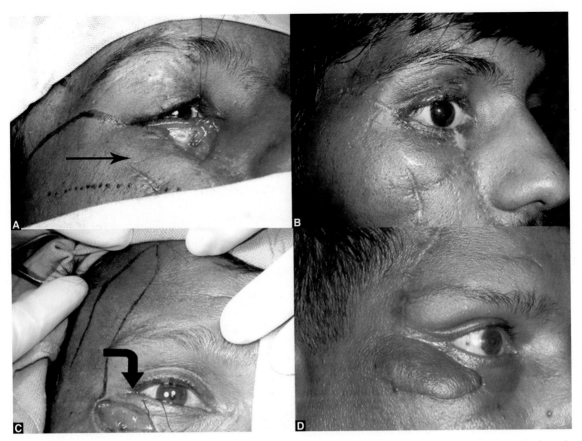

Figs 38.17A to D: Cheek rotation flap for traumatic right lower eyelid anterior lamellar defect. The incision extends above the lateral canthus, and curves down toward the tragus. Subcutaneous dissection is carried out up to a centimeter below the lower end of the defect, to move the flap medially (arrow) (A). Three months postoperative appearance (B). Extent of temporal transposition flap marked to cover the lower eyelid defect after the excision of basal cell carcinoma (C). The flap is rotated in the area of the defect, and primary closure of the temporal defect is performed. Six weeks postoperative appearance with residual flap edema (D)

lid margin (Figs 38.18A to 38.20D). The steps of eyelid margin repair are as follows:

Anesthesia: Local anesthetic with epinephrine is injected into the area of excision. Alternatively, infraorbital nerve block can be performed for the lower eyelid.

Marking the pentagon: The area to be excised is marked in a pentagon fashion with its vertical limbs maintaining a 3:2 proportion to the apical triangle.

Excision of the pentagon: The full thickness of the eyelid margin is incised along the marking with #11 Bard Parker blade, and skin incision is made along the entire extent of the pentagon. Full thickness pentagon is then excised along the skin incision with a straight scissors. The eyelid coloboma generally appears larger than the excised pentagon.

Assessment of wound tension: The wound edges are then approximated with fine forceps to assess wound tension for primary closure. If necessary, canthotomy and inferior cantholysis are performed at this stage to reduce wound tension. A lateral canthotomy is performed first in the usual manner. Within the skin anteriorly, and the conjunctiva posteriorly lies the inferior crus of the lateral canthal tendon. Cantholysis involves cutting the inferior crus, to allow the mobilization of the eyelid medially.

Alignment of eyelid margin: A vertical mattress suture is placed at the eyelid margin passing through the meibomian orifices with 6-0 silk suture. Slight eversion of the eyelid margin is desirable upon tightening the mattress suture. Additional simple sutures can be placed at the eyelid margin along the lash line and gray line if necessary.

Apposition of the tarsal plate: The tarsal plate is then aligned in a lamellar fashion with two or three interrupted, partial thickness 6-0 vicryl sutures.

Orbicularis closure: The orbicularis is then closed with interrupted 6-0 vicryl sutures.

Skin closure: The skin is finally closed with interrupted 6-0 silk sutures.

Moderate Defects (Tenzel's Semicircular Flap)

Medium defects up to 50% can, in some instances, be closed by primary closure with canthotomy and cantholysis. However, eyelid margin closure should be thought of as a series of steps that allow the surgeon to mobilize the cut ends of the margin until the wound can be closed without tension. To begin with, the wound edges should be apposed to consider the possibility of primary closure. If the wound is likely to be too tight,

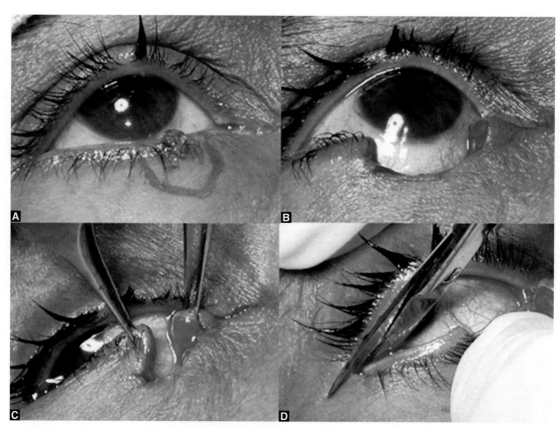

Figs 38.18A to D: Pentagon excision for right lower eyelid marginal papilloma. Pentagon is marked around the lesion (A). The full thickness of eyelid pentagon is excised (B). Note that the pentagon appears larger after excision, but its edges can be approximated to assess the feasibility of primary closure (C). A lateral canthotomy (D) and inferior cantholysis is performed if required, to allow the medial mobilization of the lateral eyelid tissue

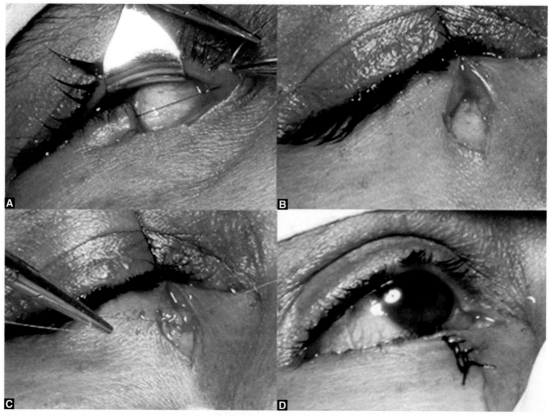

Figs 38.19A to D: Marginal vertical mattress suture is placed with 6-0 silk suture (A and B). The tarsus is approximated (C), followed by orbicularis, with 6-0 vicryl interrupted sutures. Skin is closed with interrupted 6-0 silk sutures (D)

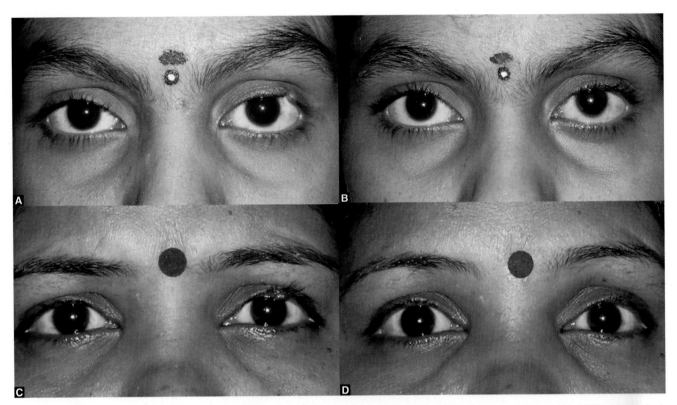

Figs 38.20A and D: Preoperative and postoperative photographs of the patient with upper eyelid traumatic coloboma (A and B) and marginal papilloma (C and D) treated with pentagon excision

a canthotomy and cantholysis should be added. If the wound is still unlikely to close, a Tenzel's semicircular flap should be raised. The technique of Tenzel's semicircular flap is described below (Figs 38.21A to 38.25D).

Marking the excision area: The pentagon is marked in the usual manner with a 3 mm margin from the clinical border of the tumor. The semicircular flap is then marked from the lateral canthus, curving away from the eyelid that requires excision. More commonly, performing Tenzel's flap would be an intraoperative decision, in cases where primary closure is not possible inspite of canthotomy and cantholysis. We therefore recommend curving the canthotomy incision superiorly during the reconstruction of lower eyelid, and vice versa for the upper eyelid.

Local anesthesia: Local infiltration or nerve block is sufficient for the eyelid excision. Subcutaneous local infiltration along the marked Tenzel's flap provides sufficient anesthesia. The procedure, however, is likely to be prolonged with the intraoperative frozen section control of resection margins, and therefore general anesthesia is preferable.

Excision of the pentagon: Pentagon excision is then performed in the usual manner as described earlier.

Mobilization of the Tenzel flap: A canthotomy and superior cantholysis is then performed. After assessing the wound apposition, Tenzel's myocutaneous flap is raised in the suborbicular plane. This will mobilize the skin and muscle medially.

Closure of pentagon: As you mobilize the Tenzel's flap, the eyelid margin would appose without tension. The vertical mattress suture is then placed at the eyelid margin, and pentagon excision is performed as described before.

Anchoring of the flap: The flap is then anchored to the periosteum of the lateral orbital rim with one or two 4-0 prolene sutures. This anchoring suture must be placed slightly superiorly, and on the inner aspect of the lateral orbital rim to pull the new lateral canthus inward toward its natural position of insertion.

Wound closure: The flap is then closed with interrupted 6-0 silk sutures.

Large Defects (Cutler-Beard Procedure)

Large full thickness defects of the eyelid require lid-sharing procedures. Cutler-Beard is the most commonly performed two-stage eyelid sharing procedure. Here, a width of the full thickness lower eyelid below the tarsal plate is used to reconstruct the upper eyelid defect. Reverse Cutler-Beard procedure can also be used for lower eyelid defects. The technique of Cutler-Beard procedure performed for an upper eyelid sebaceous gland carcinoma is described in below (Figs 38.26A to 38.30D):

Stage I

Anesthesia: The procedure is usually performed under general anesthesia.

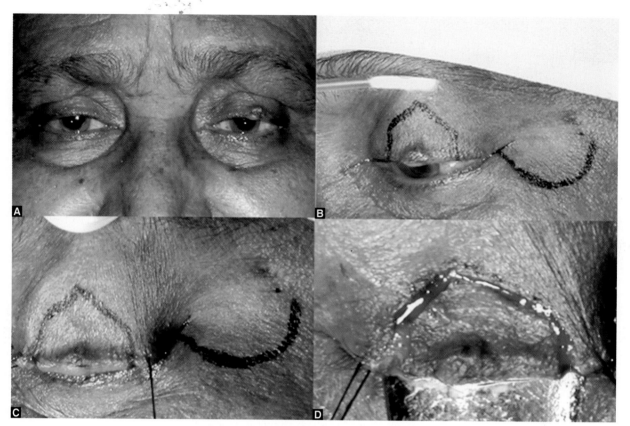

Figs 38.21A to D: Upper eyelid sebaceous gland carcinoma (A). Pentagon is marked around the lesion with wide margins. Tenzel's semicircular flap is marked to show its extent (B). Marginal full thickness incisions (C), and skin incision along the pentagon (D)

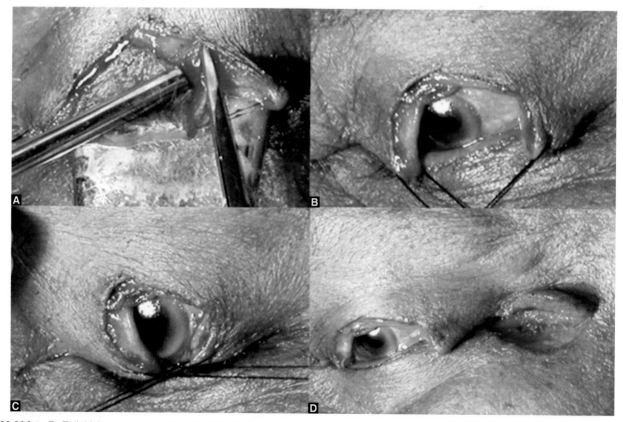

Figs 38.22A to D: Full thickness pentagon excision along the skin incision with straight cutting scissors (A and B). Cut margins are approximated to assess the possibility of primary closure without undue tension, which is possible in this case (C). Semicircular flap raised in the suborbicularis plane (D). Superior cantholysis allows the further mobilization of the eyelid tissue medially

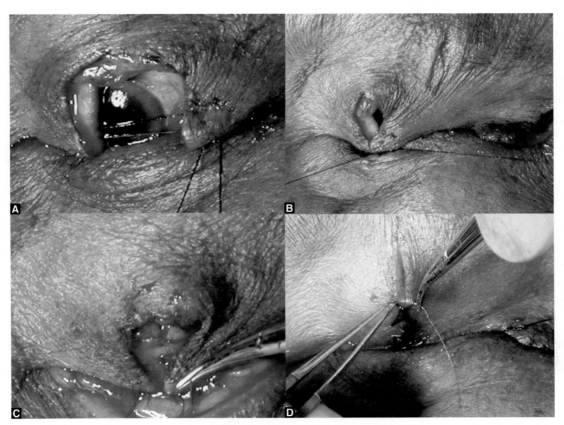

Figs 38.23A to D: Eyelid pentagon can now be closed in a standard manner. Marginal 6-0 silk vertical mattress suture is placed (A and B), and layered closure of the eyelid (C and D) is then performed

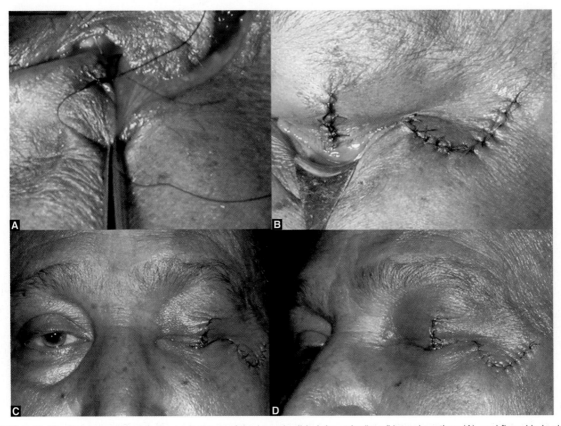

Figs 38.24A to D: The flap is anchored to the periosteum of the lateral oribital rim at its "new" lateral canthus (A), and flap skin is closed with interrupted 6-0 silk sutures (B). Appearance of the eyelid on the first postoperative day (C and D)

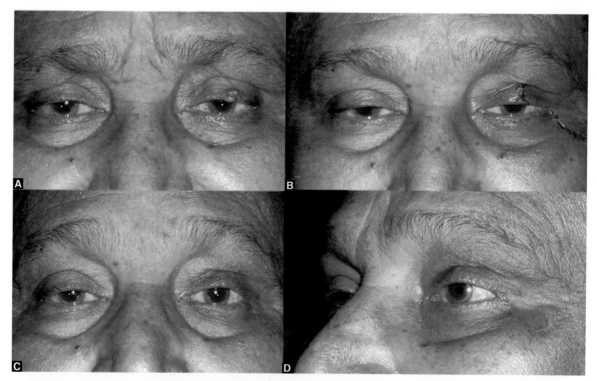

Figs 38.25A to D: Preoperative (A), and postoperative photographs of the patient at one week (B), and six weeks (C and D)

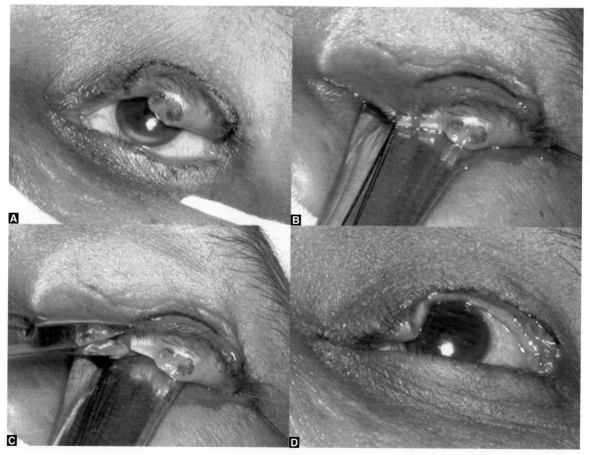

Figs 38.26A to D: Cutler-Beard Stage I procedure: Area of excision marked in a rectangular fashion (A). Full thickness marginal cuts, and skin incision performed along the marking (B). Full thickness excision completed with a straight scissors (C). Upper eyelid coloboma after the excision of tumor (D)

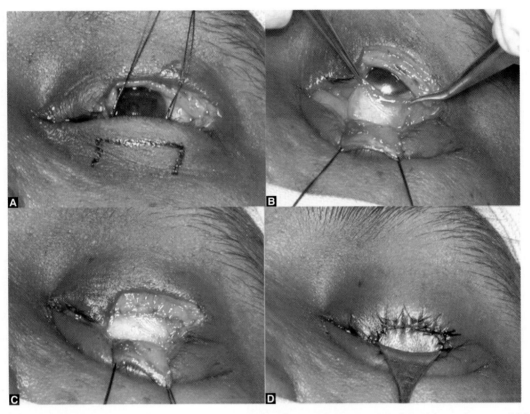

Figs 38.27A to D: Lower eyelid flap marked, starting 4–5 mm below the lower eyelid lash line (A). Full thickness lower eyelid flap created, and brought up under the lower eyelid margin (B). The anterior and posterior lamella of the flap is separated. Posterior lamella is sutures to the levator and conjunctiva of upper eyelid coloboma (C), and skin is sutured with interrupted 6-0 silk sutures (D)

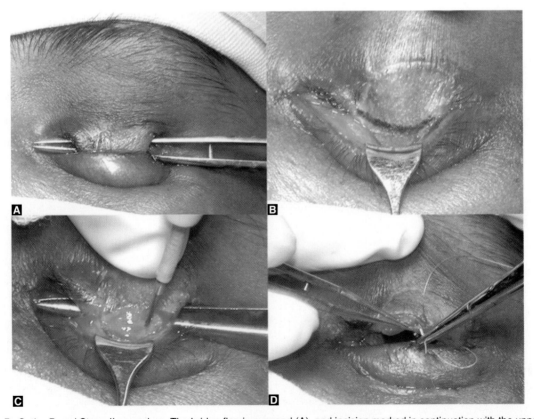

Figs 38.28A to D: Cutler-Beard Stage II procedure. The bridge flap is exposed (A), and incision marked in continuation with the upper eyelid margin on either side, with convexity downwards (B). Skin is incised with Bard Parker blade, and soft tissue incised differentially to obtain a longer length conjunctiva (C). The conjunctival edge is rolled outwards, and sutured to skin edge with continuous 6-0 vicryl sutures (D)

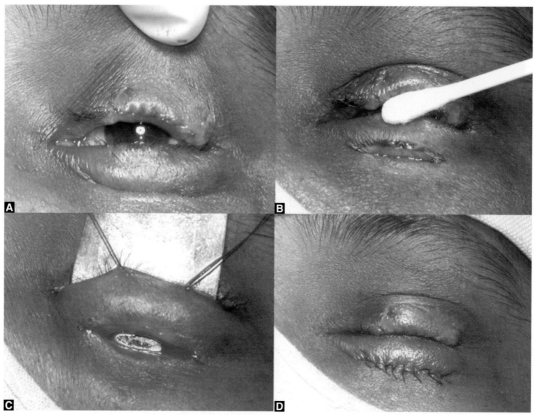

Figs 38.29A to D: Cutler-Beard Stage II procedure. Appearance of the upper eyelid margin after the two epithelial edges are sutured (A). Upper border of the lower eyelid wound is marked (B) and freshened with Bard Parker blade (C).The posterior lamella of the lower eyelid is sutured to the lower border of the tarsus with 6-0 vicryl sutures, and skin is closed with interrupted 6-0 silk sutures (D)

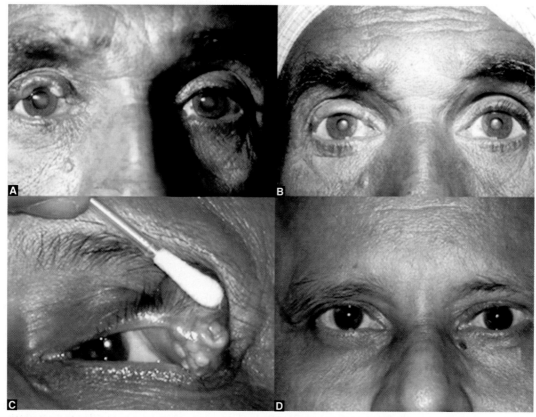

Figs 38.30A to D: Preoperative and postoperative photographs of the patient with upper eyelid sebaceous gland carcinoma treated with the Cutler-Beard procedure

Marking the excision: A rectangular area of excision is marked along the upper eyelid. Three mm wide margin is left from the clinical border of the tumor.

Excision of upper eyelid mass: The upper eyelid excision is done similar to a pentagon excision, except that the excised area is rectangular in shape.

Lower eyelid flap: The lower eyelid flap is marked, starting 3–4 mm below the lash line. Its horizontal extent is equal to the horizontal extent of the upper eyelid defect when its two ends are approximated with minimal tension. The lower eyelid skin incision is placed, and deepened to reach full thickness in one area, to complete full thickness incision with a straight scissors. The flap is then brought superiorly, below the lower eyelid margin. The two lamellae are separated, and differentially sutured to corresponding lamellae in the upper eyelid. Care is taken to correctly appose the posterior lamellar edge to the cut edge of levator muscle.

Stage II

The second stage is performed minimum six weeks after the first stage to allow the adequate vascularization of the bridge flap. The procedure is as follows:

Anesthesia: The procedure can be performed under general or local anesthesia.

Marking of incision: The lower eyelid margin is retracted, and incision is marked on the bridge flap, starting at either junction of the upper eyelid margin with the bridge flap with convexity downwards.

Incision and suturing: The bridge flap is then incised differentially along the marking, leaving the conjunctival end longer than the skin flap. The conjunctiva is then sutured to the skin with continuous 6-0 vicryl suture. The lower eyelid wound edges are freshened, and sutured in layers.

Complications

Common complications following eyelid reconstruction include localized eyelid defect, notching or malposition. Upper eyelid entropion is common following the Cutler-Beard procedure, and requires the electrolysis of offending skin hair. Lymphedema following reconstruction with periocular flaps usually settles with time, and does not require any treatment.

Eyelid reconstruction is a specialized and interesting arena at the crossroads of ophthalmic plastics and facial plastic surgery. A myriad of techniques are available for the reconstruction of anterior lamella and full thickness eyelid defects. A sound knowledge of the periorbital anatomy and surgical techniques of eyelid reconstruction will help the surgeon to achieve a gratifying functional and cosmetic outcome.

ECTROPION

Ectropion of the eyelid is defined as an eversion of the eyelid margin away from the eyeball (Figs 38.31A to D).

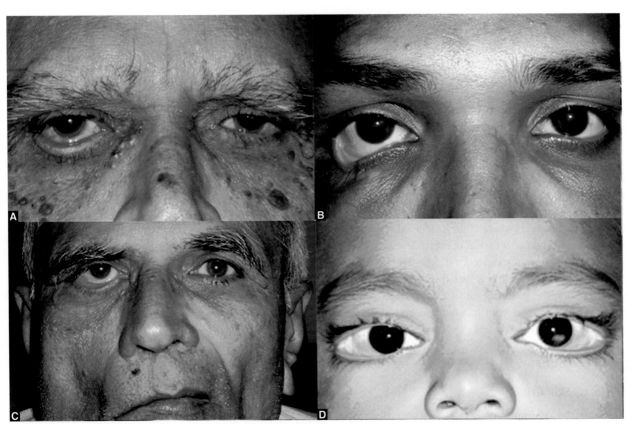

Figs 38.31A to D: Etiology of eyelid ectropion. Senile ectropion (A), cicatricial ectropion (B), paralytic ectropion following facial palsy (C), and congenital ectropion (D)

Congenital ectropion of the upper or lower eyelid is extremely rare.

Acquired ectropion, however, is more common in the lower eyelid and the following three etiologic types are recognized: cicatricial, paralytic and involutional.

Cicatricial ectropion is caused by the shortening of the anterior lamella, either due to trauma or cicatricial skin disease. Cicatricial ectropion can either affect the lower or upper eyelid.

Involutional ectropion is caused by horizontal eyelid laxity, and there is generally a progression from eyelid laxity to punctal ectropion, medial ectropion, and finally generalized ectropion of the entire lower lid.

Paralytic ectropion is caused by the loss of normal orbicularis muscle tone following facial nerve palsy. Involutional and paralytic ectropion almost always affect the lower eyelid, and there is no upper eyelid equivalent for the same.

Choice of Surgery

The type and cause of ectropion are usually obvious from history and examination.

After the etiology of ectropion is identified, the treatment plan can be made.

Cicatricial ectropion is treated by lengthening the shortened anterior lamella with a full thickness skin graft.

Involutional ectropion, as described earlier, is a spectrum extending from eyelid laxity to punctal ectropion, medial ectropion, and generalized ectropion. Medial ectropion may require surgical intervention, and the removal of a 5 mm spindle of conjunctiva and retractor directly beneath the punctum, and parallel to the eyelid margin may be necessary. Prominent medial ectropion can be treated with the Byron Smith "lazy T" procedure or the medial tarsal strip procedure. There is, however, a risk of damaging the patent canalicular system, and deep fixation of the medial canthal tendon is difficult. If ectropion is generalized, horizontal lid tightening procedures are advocated. Earlier this was achieved by performing pentagon excision or the Kuhnt-Szymanowski procedure. Anderson later suggested directing attention to the lateral canthal tendon, and introduced the lateral tarsal strip procedure. The ease in performing the tarsal strip procedure has made it the preferred technique of correcting lower eyelid ectropion in majority of cases. Paralytic ectropion is also commonly treated with the lateral tarsal strip procedure, but more tightening is usually necessary, along with spacer to lengthen the posterior lamella. It is often somewhat more complicated to treat than involutional ectropion due to associated lagophthalmos, corneal exposure, and brow ptosis.

Surgical Techniques

Full Thickness Skin Grafting

Shortening of the anterior lamella causes cicatricial ectropion. Lengthening of the anterior lamella usually with a full thickness

eyelid graft returns the scarred eyelid to its normal position (Figs 38.32A to D). Frequently, the lateral tarsal strip operation is used in conjunction with lower eyelid full thickness skin grafts. The steps of the surgery are as follows:

Anesthesia: General anesthesia is preferred for the skin grafting procedure.

Skin incision: Eyelid incision is marked 2–3 mm from the eyelid margin to extend beyond the cicatrix on either side. Ideally, it should extend beyond either canthus for good correction.

Scar excision: The anterior lamella is incised, and subcutaneous scar tissue is excised to allow the posterior lamella of the eyelid to return to its normal position. The anterior lamellar defect would thus become obvious, and is measured.

The lateral tarsal strip procedure is performed at this stage if surgery involves the lower eyelid.

Harvesting the graft: Graft size to be harvested is marked 10 to 20% more than recipient bed measurements. This is to allow for postoperative graft contracture. A full thickness graft is harvested from the donor site after the injection of xylocaine and adrenaline in the subcutaneous plane. Posterior surface of the excised skin graft is "defatted", and multiple holes or small stabs are made in the graft skin to allow the postoperative escape of serous collection.

Graft suturing: The graft is sutured into the defect with interrupted 6-0 prolene sutures. Quilting sutures can be passed through the full thickness of the graft to anchor it to the recipient bed.

Lateral Tarsal Strip Procedure

Involutional ectropion is the most common type of ectropion, and can be corrected by the lateral tarsal strip procedure. This procedure is one of the most useful procedures in eyelid surgery, and is used alone or as an adjunct in the management of senile and paralytic ectropion, as well as senile entropion.

The steps of lateral tarsal strip procedure are as follows:

Anesthesia: The procedure can be performed under local anesthesia. Infiltration is given along the inner aspect of lateral orbital rim, lateral third of lower eyelid, and conjunctiva.

Incision: A lateral canthotomy incision is placed, and the orbicularis is dissected to expose the periosteum of the lateral orbital rim. An inferior cantholysis is then performed.

Formation of tarsal strip: A tarsal strip is formed by splitting the anterior lamella off the posterior lamella for a distance of 5–7 mm from the lateral canthus. Skin, muscle and lashes are freed from the tarsus. The lower border of the tarsus is freed from the attached conjunctiva, and the conjunctiva over the posterior tarsal surface is scraped off. Shorten the tarsal strip if necessary.

Anchoring the tarsal strip: Reattach the tarsal strip to the inner aspect of lateral orbital rim periosteum with two interrupted 4-0 prolene or vicryl sutures, to achieve adequate horizontal

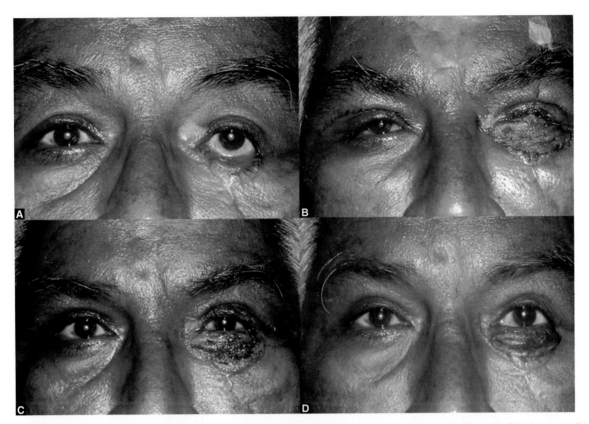

Figs 38.32A to D: Patient with left lower eyelid cicatricial ectropion following eyelid trauma (A). Full thickness skin graft of the lower eyelid extending beyond the canthi (B). Note the quilting sutures that anchor the graft to its bed, and the Frost suture to maintain the graft under stretch. The medial canthal tendon has been anchored to the periosteum of the anterior lacrimal crest. Two weeks (C) and six weeks (D) postoperative appearance showing the restored lower eyelid position. Pigmentation of grafted skin reduces with time

tension. The insertion could move higher on the orbital rim depending upon the desired height of the lower eyelid margin.

Wound closure: Trim the anterior lamellar lash line beyond the lateral canthus, and close the canthotomy and skin incision in layers with 6-0 vicryl and 6-0 silk or prolene respectively.

Kuhnt-Szymanowski Procedure

This procedure provides the differential shortening of the anterior and posterior lamella of the eyelid (Figs 38.33A to 38.34 D). It should, however, be preferred in patients with excessively lax anterior lamella, without lateral canthal tendon laxity.

Anesthesia: The procedure can be performed under local anesthesia.

Skin incision: The skin incision is marked 2 mm below the inferior punctum to the lateral canthus, and extended obliquely downwards below the lateral canthus. The skin flap is raised without orbicularis muscle to expose the posterior lamella.

Pentagon excision: An appropriate-sized pentagon is excised to shorten the remainder of the posterior lamella behind the skin flap.

Anterior lamellar shortening: Replace the skin flap, and draw it up and laterally to mark the excess skin. Excise the superior and lateral excess skin.

Wound closure: Close the pentagon by a standard technique, and subciliary incision with continuous 6-0 prolene suture.

Complications

Skin graft necrosis can result from the poor vascularization of the graft, or the collection of hematoma that interferes with its nutritional supply. Incomplete correction of cicatricial ectropion due to the contracture of full thickness graft requires repeat skin grafting. Recurrence of senile or paralytic ectropion is uncommon, and may require further horizontal eyelid tightening.

Senile and paralytic ectropion are the most commonly encountered types of entropions in ophthalmic practice. While senile ectropion can be corrected in majority of cases by the lateral tarsal strip procedure alone, paralytic ectropion has other eyelid abnormalities to attend in addition. Cicatricial ectropion commonly requires a full thickness skin graft.

ENTROPION

Entropion is the inward turning of the eyelid margin. It is most commonly seen as an aging phenomenon produced by the attenuation or detachment of the lower eyelid retractor and associated with horizontal eyelid laxity. Forceful eyelid closure causes the preseptal orbicularis muscle to override the tarsus,

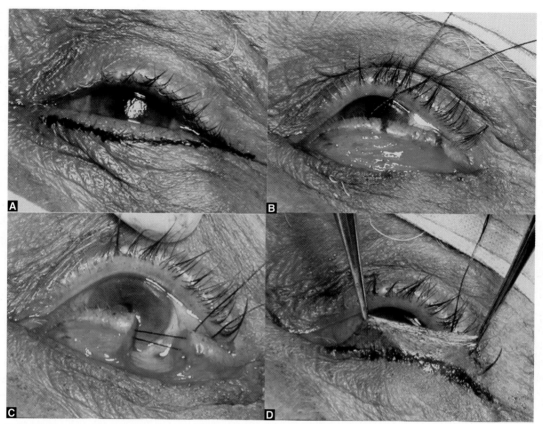

Figs 38.33A to D: Kuhnt-Szymanowski procedure. Skin incision placed 2 mm below the lash line from inferior punctum to lateral canthus and beyond (A). Skin flap raised without orbicularis, and pentagon is marked for excision assessing the eyelid laxity (B). Full thickness pentagon is excised, and closed in a standard manner (C). Excess anterior lamellar skin is marked for excision (D)

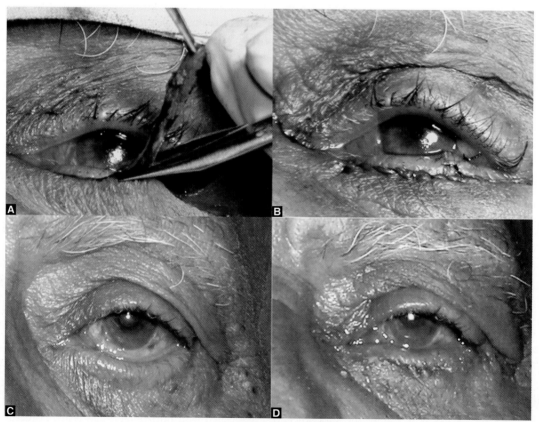

Figs 38.34A to D: Excess anterior lamella is excised (A), and subciliary incision closed with interrupted 6-0 prolene sutures (B). Preoperative and one week postoperative photograph of the patient who underwent the left lower eyelid Kuhnt-Szymanowski procedure (C and D)

resulting in the inward turning of the eyelid. Entropion may be classified as congenital, involutional (senile), spastic and cicatricial.

Congenital Entropion

Congenital lower eyelid entropion is caused by the hypertrophic fold of skin, subcutaneous tissue and orbicularis muscle that particularly affects the medial part of the lower eyelid (Figs 38.35A to D). It should be differentiated from epiblepharon in which there is a similar fold, but the eyelid margin itself remains in a normal position. In both these conditions, eyelashes may touch the cornea, but will not necessarily cause damage as the lashes are often very soft and child's cornea is remarkably tolerant to eyelash contact. Retractor aponeurosis disinsertion has been identified as the cause. Resection of skin and pretarsal orbicularis muscle has also been considered a successful method of managing these cases. Congenital upper eyelid entropion is extremely rare, and presents as congenital horizontal tarsal kink. It is associated with congenital corneal ulcers, and needs surgical correction.

Involutional Entropion

Involutional entropion is the most common type of entropion, and is caused by laxity or the disinsertion of lower eyelid retractors, horizontal eyelid laxity, and overriding of preseptal orbicularis over the pretarsal orbicularis. A multitude of surgical procedures have been advocated for the correction of entropion, reflecting various pathophysiologic features of the disorder. Eyelid everting suture repair is an excellent temporizing procedure. In eyelids with a minimal degree of horizontal lid laxity, such treatment may suffice indefinitely. It may also be useful in patients with spastic entropion, until the irritating focus has resolved. Surprisingly, till date, no single procedure has been proved to be the treatment of choice for the correction of lower eyelid senile entropion. A combined procedure to eliminate horizontal lid laxity and repair lower lid retractors is recommended for lower eyelid senile entropion. The preferred procedure for involutional entropion thus consists of a lateral tarsal strip procedure along with and repair of the lower eyelid retractors (Jones procedure). The lateral tarsal strip procedure has already been described with the management of ectropion. The Jones procedure is described below:

Anesthesia: The procedure is performed under local anesthesia.

Skin incision: A lateral canthal incision is created and continued medially as the subciliary incision.

Exposure of retractors: A skin muscle flap is elevated to expose the orbital septum. The orbital septum is penetrated and orbital fat identified and retracted inferiorly. The lower eyelid retractor is identified as a white fibrous structure beneath the fat pad. It is commonly found to be disinserted from its normal attachment to the lower border of the tarsus.

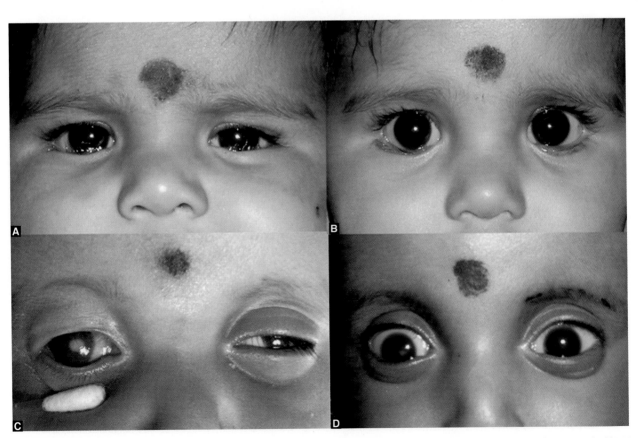

Figs 38.35A to D: Preoperative and postoperative photographs of an infant with bilateral lower eyelid congenital entropion treated with retractor reinsertion (A and B), and neonate with right upper eyelid congenital entropion (Tarsal kink syndrome) treated with tarsal fracture and rotation (C and D)

Plication of retractors: The superior edge of the lower eyelid retractor system is identified and carefully attached to the inferior tarsal border. If the attachment is intact, the retractors are plicated.

Horizontal lid tightening: A lateral tarsal strip procedure as described earlier is then performed to tighten the eyelid horizontally.

Wound closure: Redundant skin, if any, is draped over the lid margin and is excised as in a lower lid blepharoplasty. The orbicularis and skin is closed in layers with 6-0 vicryl and silk respectively.

Cicatricial Entropion

Cicatricial entropion is caused by the contraction of the posterior lamella of the eyelid drawing the eyelid margin toward the globe (Figs 38.36A to D). It may result from chemical or thermal injury, trachoma, chronic allergies, or ocular medications. In addition, conjunctival cicatricial changes may result from mucous membrane disorders, such as Stevens-Johnson syndrome and ocular cicatricial pemphigoid. Worldwide, upper eyelid entropion is most frequently encountered as sequelae of trachoma.

Mild degree of lower eyelid entropion can be treated with eyelid everting sutures. This, however, is likely to have a temporary effect. Mild to moderate degrees of cicatricial entropion are best treated with a Weis procedure (transverse tarsotomy), or tarsotomy with rotational sutures. This procedure, ideally described for lower eyelid, consists of fracturing the tarsus approximately 2 mm below the eyelid margin and passing double armed sutures so as to evert the eyelid margin. A modified Tenzel tarsal trough procedure is a variation of the Weis procedure in which full thickness tarsal incision is avoided. For upper eyelid, tarsal wedge resection would be the procedure of choice in cases that have an intact or thickened tarsus. A specially designed Radiofrequency monopolar tip facilitates the removal of tarsal wedge.

Severe posterior lamellar contracture requires lengthening of the posterior lamella by a suitable graft. An ideal graft should provide a mucous membrane and a rigid supporting structure; possible materials include autogenous tarsus and conjunctiva, nasochondral mucosa, hard palate mucosa, full thickness buccal mucous membrane and ear cartilage, or donor sclera from eye banks. The procedure of tarsal wedge resection is described below (Figs 38.37A to 38.39D).

Anesthesia: The procedure is performed under local anesthesia.

Skin incision: Lid crease incision is placed along the entire extent of the eyelid, and the anterior tarsal surface is exposed.

Tarsal wedge excision: A wedge-shaped partial thickness groove is made in the tarsus approximately 4 mm away from the lash line,

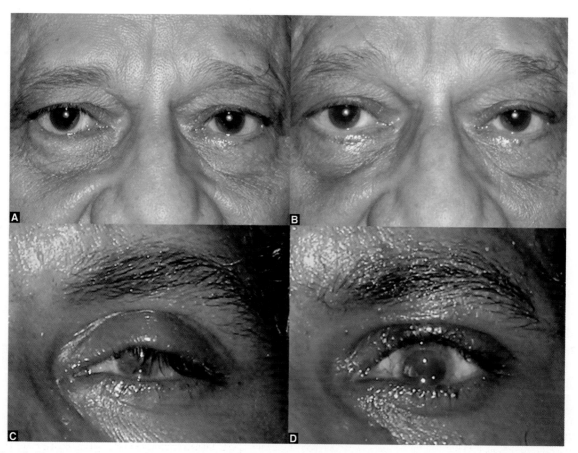

Figs 38.36A to D: Preoperative and postoperative photographs of right lower eyelid senile entropion treated with Jones procedure and lateral tarsal strip (A and B), and left upper eyelid cicatricial entropion following chemical injury treated with tarsal wedge resection (C and D)

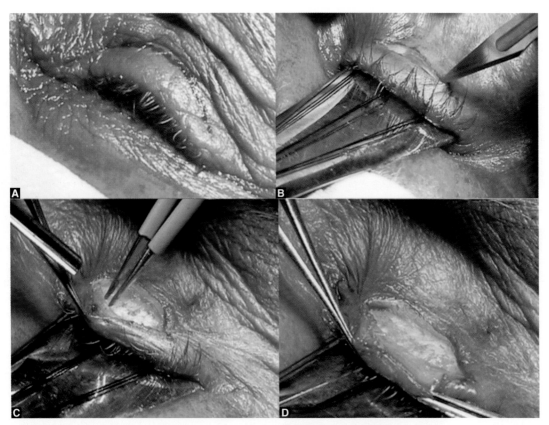

Figs 38.37A to D: Tarsal wedge resection. Eyelid traction sutures are placed, and upper eyelid crease incision is made (A and B). Orbicularis is separated to expose the anterior tarsal surface (C and D)

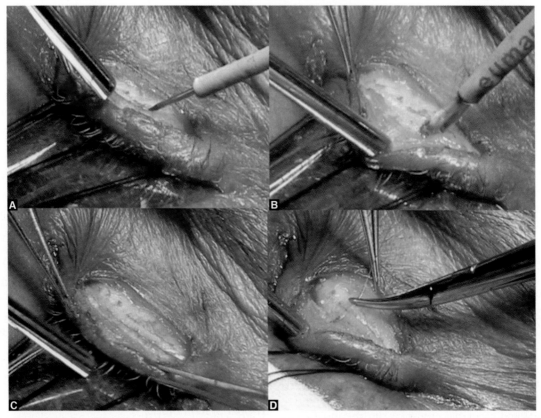

Figs 38.38A to D: Tarsal wedge resection. Marking is made along the entire extent of tarsus 4 mm away from the lash line with Radiofrequency monopolar cautery (A). Partial thickness tarsal wedge is resected along the marking with triangular tip Ellman monopolar cautery (B). Tarsal surface seen after the excision of tarsal wedge (C). Double-armed 6-0 vicryl sutures are passed across the wedge (D), and can be brought out through the skin 2 mm above the lash line

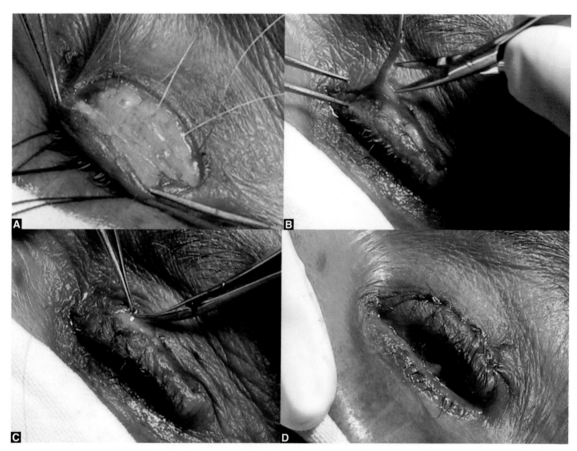

Figs 38.39A to D: Tarsal wedge resection. Three 6-0 vicryl sutures passed across the tarsal wedge (A) and tightened to evert the distal tarsus. Skin muscle strip excised from the upper edge of skin incision (B). Orbicularis and skin is closed in layers with 6-0 interrupted sutures (C and D)

along its entire horizontal extent reaching up to 80% of tarsal thickness. The wedge can be excised either with Bard Parker blade, or Radiofrequency monopolar cautery.

Suturing the tarsal wedge: Double-armed 6-0 vicryl sutures are then passed from the distal tarsus toward the proximal tarsus. Each end can be brought out through the skin near the lash line before tying. The sutures are tightened to evert the distal eyelid margin.

Wound closure: Skin muscle excision can be performed at the upper edge of skin incision to enhance eyelid margin eversion. Splitting of the two lamellae at the gray line can also enhance the everting effect of the wedge resection. The orbicularis and skin is then closed in layers.

Complications

Following the correction of congenital entropion, the scars may be unsightly in the first few weeks, but usually improve within a few weeks. Undercorrection or recurrence of cicatricial entropion may require a repeat procedure of the mucous membrane graft after 4–6 months. Following Jones procedure, overcorrection can be treated with the early release of sutures.

Involutional and cicatricial entropion are the most commonly encountered types of entropion. A Jones procedure combined with horizontal eyelid tightening is the procedure of choice for involutional entropion. Eyelid everting sutures and the Weis procedure are suited for lower eyelid cicatricial entropion, whereas tarsal wedge resection for upper eyelid cicatricial entropion. Posterior lamellar grafts are reserved for severe cicatricial entropion. Congenital lower eyelid entropion is rare, and must be differentiated from epiblepharon. Lower lid retractor reinsertion and skin muscle excision are the procedures to correct congenital entropion.

LACRIMAL SURGERY

The diagnosis of lacrimal system disorders requires a meticulous history taking, and a thorough clinical evaluation. Ancillary tests of lacrimal function, when properly and selectively applied, aid in the diagnosis. Tearing, the most frequent symptom is probably the most nonspecific. History and clinical examination should rule out the common causes of pseudoepiphora. The cause of true epiphora is then localized to the specific anatomic site, and the management is planned accordingly.

Congenital Lacrimal Disorders

Abnormalities of the Puncta and Canaliculi (Upper System Block)

Failure of the embryonic epithelial bud to open on the eyelid margin results in various grades of atresia of the punctum and canaliculus. In *simple punctual agenesis*, there is a visible

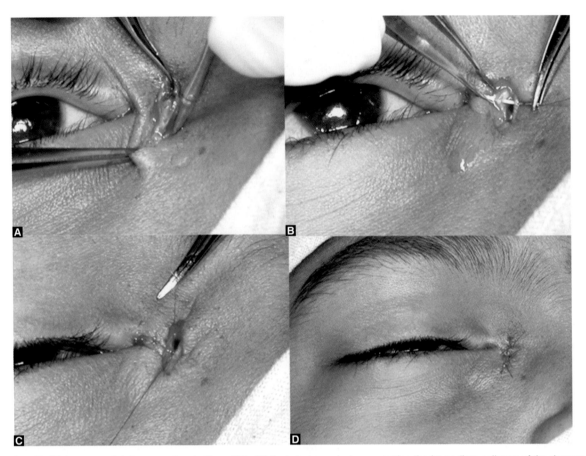

Figs 38.40A to D: Right congenital dacryocystocele (A and B). Clinical photograph demonstrating the immediate collapse of the dacryocystocele after probing (C) and appearance six months postprobing (D)

punctual papilla, and a membrane covering the punctual opening. Opening the membrane with a punctum dilator or fine needle cures the epiphora. The patency of nasolacrimal duct, however, should be confirmed. In *punctual agenesis with canalicular atresia*, the punctal papilla is absent. An avascular dimple at the medial aspect of meibomian gland orifices identifies the presumed location of the punctum. Treatment is difficult, and includes either a monocanalicular or bicanalicular intubation using the pigtail probe, retrograde canalicular intubation dacryocystorhinostomy, or a conjunctivo-dacryocystorhinostomy.

Abnormalities of the Lacrimal Sac

Congenital Lacrimal Fistulas

A congenital lacrimal fistula can originate from the lacrimal sac, or the canaliculus, and results from the canalization of a portion of epithelial cord that extends from the lacrimal sac to the surface of the skin. Simple excision of the fistula has been the most successful treatment. Repair of a congenital lacrimal fistula is described below (Figs 38.40A to 38.41D):

Anesthesia: This procedure is commonly performed in children, hence general anesthesia is required.

Lacrimal irrigation: The fistula opening is first identified, and lacrimal irrigation is performed to confirm the patency of the

nasolacrimal duct. If there is an associated nasolacrimal block, therapeutic probing, silastic intubation or dacryocystorhinostomy will be required in addition.

Incision: An appropriately sized probe is placed into the supernumerary duct, and an ellipse of skin is incised conservatively around the probe.

Fistulectomy: Fine subcutaneous dissection under the microscope is performed. The fistulous tract is dissected up to its junction with the lacrimal sac, where it is cut and excised.

Wound closure: The orbicularis and skin are then closed in layers with 7-0 or 6-0 vicryl sutures.

Congenital Dacryocystocele (Amniotocele)

Congenital dacryocystocele or amniotocele refers to a sterile accumulation of mucus or possibly amniotic fluid trapped in the nasolacrimal sac due to a one-way valve effect at the end of the nasolacrimal duct. Fluid can enter from below, but with poor exit of accumulated fluid, the dilated sac is seen as a bluish mass inferior to the medial canthal tendon. This swelling is frequently misdiagnosed as a hemangioma. For a congenital dacryocele without the signs of infection, one approach is to massage the lacrimal sac in an attempt to open the obstruction. Early probing, however, is the definitive treatment for congenital dacryocystocele (Fig. 38.42).

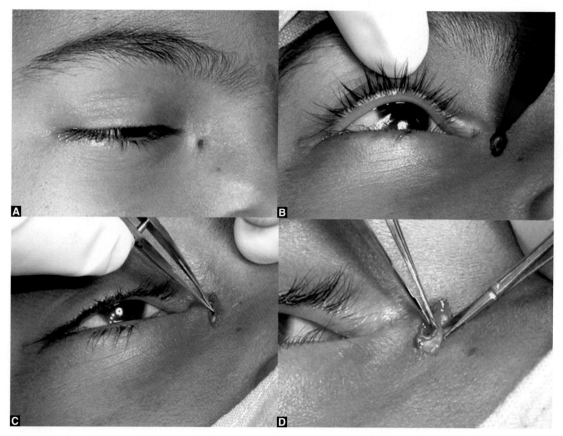

Figs 38.41A to D: Instrument set required for the therapeutic probing of the nasolacrimal duct includes Nettleships punctum dilator, a set of Bowman's lacrimal probes, and lacrimal irrigation cannula mounted on a syringe

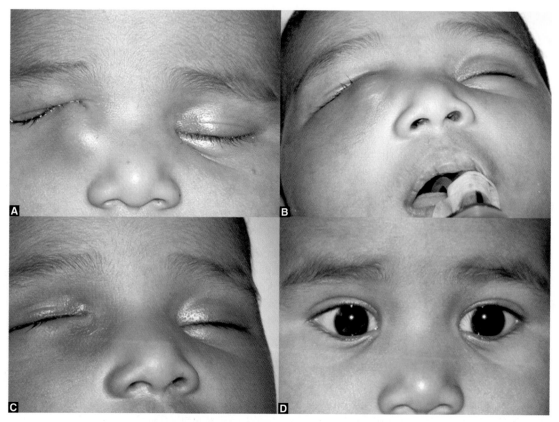

Figs 38.42A to D: Treatment process of congenital dacryocystocele

Neonatal Acute Dacryocystitis (Lacrimal Abscess)

Neonatal acute dacryocystitis is rare, and in addition to the history of preexisting epiphora, there are other signs of inflammation associated with fever. The treatment includes aspiration with a tuberculin needle to decompress the sac through a fine opening that will not fistulize, and the microbiological evaluation of the aspirate. A broad spectrum antibiotic is given intravenously until a more specific antibiotic can be identified by the cultures and sensitivity obtained from the aspirate. After several days, when the acute inflammation subsides, early probing is valuable in most cases to prevent the repeat episodes of acute dacryocystitis.

Congenital Lacrimal Disorders in Craniofacial Anomalies

Any of the lacrimal abnormalities described above can occur singly or in combination with craniofacial anomalies. Repair for each entity is identical to that described for routine lacrimal problems, but the timing of repair is different. Deformities, such as telecanthus, epicanthal folds, orbital volume problems, and many canthal deformities can be managed during the initial craniofacial reconstruction. Specific nasolacrimal problems, however, except for simple dacryostenosis or acute dacryocystitis, are best treated after major bone shifts or grafts. Unfortunately, good results are too easily undone by subsequent surgery, and repeat lacrimal procedures are particularly difficult and have significantly less potential for success.

Congenital Nasolacrimal Duct Obstruction

Congenital nasolacrimal duct obstruction is the most common cause of childhood epiphora. Its incidence is noted to be 30% in term babies, however, symptomatic block occurs in 2 to 6% cases. It is commonly caused by the failure of the canalization of the valve of Hasner, however, complete osseous obstruction may rarely occur. A relative narrowing causing decreased tear flow is a more common occurrence. Abnormalities within the nasal passages, such as deviation of the nasal septum or impaction of the inferior turbinate on the valve of Hasner, also may contribute to the obstruction of the duct. The symptoms begin commonly after three weeks of age with epiphora, matting of lashes and discharge. Evaluation includes office examination under good illumination to rule out associated lacrimal abnormalities and causes of pseudoepiphora. The management of congenital nasolacrimal duct obstruction can be either conservative or interventional. Conservative management should be done in most patients up to the age of 9–12 months. This involves presumptive topical antibiotics and lacrimal sac massage. Antibiotics should be used only in the presence of purulent discharge, and lacrimal sac massage should be demonstrated to the parents. The child can be followed up every two months till symptoms resolve, or probing is undertaken.

The correct timing for the initial probing of a child with nasolacrimal duct obstruction has been controversial. We recommend that initial probing be done when the child presents

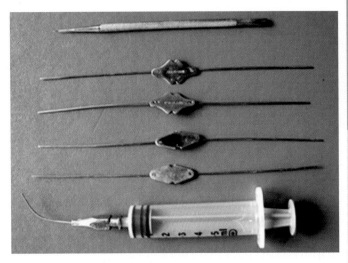

Fig. 38.43: Instruments required for congenital nasolacrimal duct obstruction

beyond the age of 9–12 months, or in case of failure of three months of conservative therapy.

We however prefer probing under general anesthesia with Laryngeal Mask Airway. Laryngeal mask is an excellent device that allows free access to the nose for the irrigation of fluids, and it maintains the airway, even if it becomes necessary to perform nasal endoscopy or Silastic intubation of the nasolacrimal system. The pediatric experience of the anesthetist and the hospital operating room staff is a critical factor in opting for a general anesthetic.

The minimum instruments required for probing the procedure are shown in Figure 38.43.

The procedure of probing is described below:

Anesthesia: General anesthesia with laryngeal mask airway is preferred.

Examination: Examine the eyelids and puncta, exclude fistula or mucocele by pressing over the lacrimal sac.

Lacrimal syringing: Dilate the upper punctum with Nettleship's punctum dilator. Perform lacrimal syringing to note the site and consistency of regurge. Establish patency of the lower canaliculus.

Probing: Select the appropriate-sized probe for the patient, and introduce the probe through the upper canaliculus- first vertically, and then horizontally, stretching the eyelid laterally. Feel or the "hard stop", and swing the probe gently vertically down the nasolacrimal duct. Correct position of the probe is indicated by its alignment with the trochlea, and the spring back test. The membrane can be perforated easily with a "pop" at the lower end of the nasolacrimal duct, and the probe is advanced further till the firm resistance of the nasal floor is reached. Visualizing the nasal end of the probe with a nasal endoscope confirms successful procedure.

Repeat syringing: After probing, repeat the syringing to confirm patency.

If one attempt of probing for congenital nasolacrimal duct obstruction is not successful, repeat probing can be performed if the initial finding was a membranous block. Bony obstruction encountered during probing can be relative or absolute. Absolute bony obstruction does not allow probing with the smallest available probe (#0000), and should be managed with dacryocystorhinostomy. For relative bony obstruction or a tight bony canal, either a graduated stepwise probing or reaming maneuver is required. If the obstruction is beyond the nasolacrimal duct, an infracture of the inferior turbinate is performed under general anesthesia. Failed probing can be managed either by repeat probing procedure, silicone intubation, balloon dacryoplasty or –dacryocystorhinostomy.

Acquired Lacrimal Disorders

Puncta and Canalicular Stenosis

Tissue atrophy due to age, cicatricial conjunctival disease or chronic use of topical medications can lead to acquired punctual stenosis. If dilatation of the punctum does not provide symptomatic relief, the one or two snip procedure can give good results. Viers three-snip procedure may be required in severe cases, and provides long lasting symptomatic relief.

Trauma, chronic infection, and repeated probing can lead to canalicular stenosis. Irrigation, diagnostic probing, and dacryocystography can document its degree and location. If partial, a monocanalicular or bicanalicular stent can be placed across the stenotic segment. If complete, a segmental microscopic resection and reconstruction can be performed. If both canaliculi are obliterated, a conjunctivo-dacryocystorhinostomy is indicated. Canalicular stenosis often co-exists with nasolacriml duct stenosis, and simultaneous repair with canalicular intubation and dacryocystorhinostomy may be indicated.

Nasolacrimal Duct Stenosis

Acquired nasolacrimal duct obstruction can present either as epiphora, mucoid discharge, or dacryocystitis. It can occur either as an involutional phenomenon (primary nasolacrimal duct obstruction), or secondary to sinus disease, nasal surgery or trauma (secondary nasolacrimal duct obstruction). If partial, i.e. symptomatic but allows forcible irrigation through the lacrimal system into the nasal cavity, silicone intubation can be helpful. The success rate of dacryocystorhinostomy, however, is higher in such cases.

Dacryocystorhinostomy is the current preferred technique for the treatment of complete acquired nasolacrimal duct obstruction. In the external dacryocystorhinostomy, the obstructed nasolacrimal duct is bypassed by forming an anastomosis of the lacrimal sac and nasal mucosa through a nasal ostium created by an external skin incision. The internal dacryocystorhinostomy, often facilitated by a nasal endoscope, creates the anastomosis from within the nasal cavity.

The technique of external dacryocystorhinostomy is described below.

Anesthesia: Local anesthesia in the form of infratrochlear nerve block along with local infiltration is adequate. The middle meatus should be packed with l/4-inch gauze tape impregnated with four percent xylocaine with or without adrenaline. Tilting the table to 30º head up and controlled sedation are useful adjuncts to minimize bleeding.

Skin incision: A curvilinear incision (8–15 mm in length) is placed through the skin along the anterior lacrimal crest, placed approximately 8 mm medial to the medial canthus, and starting from the level of the medial canthus. The orbicularis muscle is carefully separated with a sharp scissors down to the periosteum.

Exposure of lacrimal fossa: The periosteum is incised with a bipolar cautery or scalpel blade and reflected laterally to expose the lacrimal fossa. The anterior crus of the medial canthal tendon can be disinserted with the periosteum if wider exposure is needed.

Creating bony ostium: The frontolacrimal suture is then identified, and the bone is out-fractured. Serial bone punches are then used to enlarge the bony ostium to a minimum size of 15×15 mm diameter.

Raising mucosal flaps: The canaliculus is probed to tent up the lacrimal sac wall, and vertical incision is placed over the lacrimal sac extending from fundus to its junction with the nasolacrimal duct. Each end of the incision is then extended anteriorly to raise an anterior sac flap. The posterior sac flap is excised. Nasal mucosal flap is raised in a similar manner.

Suturing the flaps: The two flaps are assessed, and either flap can be trimmed if necessary to achieve taut approximation. If a lacrimal intubation is planned, it should be performed at this stage. The flaps are sutured with interrupted 6-0 vicryl or catgut sutures.

Wound closure: Orbicularis is closed with interrupted 6-0 vicryl, and skin with 6-0 silk sutures.

Lacrimal syringing is performed at this stage to confirm patency, and the nasal pack changed before patching the eye.

Lacrimal drainage system disorders are distinct in the pediatric and adult population. Therapeutic probing is the most common lacrimal procedure in children, whereas dacryocystorhinostomy in adults. Exact localization of obstruction by clinical evaluation and ancillary tests is important. Sound knowledge of anatomy and proper surgical technique provides relief of epiphora in majority of cases.

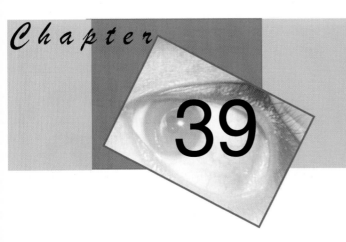

Chapter 39

Periorbital Rejuvenation

Milind N Naik, Rashmi Shetty

INTRODUCTION

Skin and subcutaneous changes are an important component of facial aging. Facial aging was traditionally attributed to gravitational descent, but is now recognized as a result of loss of facial volume. Moreover, with aging and sun damage, the skin loses its elasticity and tone, allowing wrinkles to form easily in response to underlying facial muscles. Botulinum toxin and soft tissue fillers have revolutionized the rejuvenation of the aging face. Botulinum toxin has evolved greatly over the past 30 years since its introduction in the 1970s for the management of strabismus. Today, apart from its varied therapeutic indications in ophthalmic plastic surgery, it is widely used for erasing dynamic facial rhytids, such as lateral canthal wrinkles (crow's feet), glabellar creases and horizontal forehead lines. Numerous soft tissue fillers ranging from bovine collagen to hyaluronic acid-derived products are currently available for static wrinkles and soft tissue augmentation.

The two primary hallmarks of facial aging include wrinkles and loss of subcutaneous volume. Wrinkles may develop as either hyperdynamic lines caused by the repetitive contraction of underlying facial musculature or as static wrinkles due to the additional thinning of dermis and loss of skin elasticity. Loss of subcutaneous fat, remodelling of underlying bony and cartilaginous structures, and gravitational changes from the loss of elasticity of the tissue also contribute to the facial changes that constitute aging.

Different aesthetic deficiencies warrant distinctive therapies. Although a given area of the face can present with different issues in diverse individuals, there are recurrent patterns for each facial area. Critical aging changes in the periorbital area include glabellar frown lines, horizontal forehead lines, crow's feet, and periorbital hollows. Descent of the forehead with age can lead to brow ptosis. An ophthalmologist can significantly contribute to the rejuvenation of the periorbital region and face.

Lasers and injectables are the two main treatment modalities for the nonsurgical rejuvenation of the aging face.

BOTULINUM TOXIN

Pharmacology

Botulinum toxin is an exotoxin produced by the naturally ubiquitous bacterium *Clostridium botulinum*, a gram-positive, spore-forming, anaerobic rod. The organism elaborates eight different exotoxins (A,B,C_1,C_2,D,E,F, and G), of which types A and B are most potent, and also represent the most commonly used commercial preparations. Intramuscular administration of Botulinum toxin acts at the neuromuscular junction to cause muscle paralysis by inhibiting the release of ACh from presynaptic motor neurons.

Three preparations of botulinum toxin are commercially available at present. Botox (Allergan, Inc, Irvine, CA, USA) and Dysport (Ipsen Pharmaceuticals, France) are the type A toxins. Myobloc (Elan Pharmaceuticals, San Diego, CA, USA) is the type B toxin. Type A toxin is easily producible in culture in a highly purified, stable and crystalline form. Type A toxin also has the longest duration of action, and a favorable ratio between biologically active and inactive neurotoxin.

Botox-purified neurotoxin complex is a sterile vacuum-dried purified extract of Botulinum toxin type A, produced from the fermentation of the Hall strain of *Clostridium botulinum* type A. Each vial of Botox contains 100 units (U) of *Clostridium botulinum* type A neurotoxin complex, 0.5 mg of human albumin, and 0.9 mg of sodium chloride in a sterile vacuum-dried solid without preservatives.

Toxin Reconstitution

Botulinum toxin type A (Botox: Allergan Inc, Irvine, CA, USA) is supplied in a vial containing 100 units (U) of vacuum-dried neurotoxin complex. Most clinicians reconstitute it with 2.5 to 3 ml of sterile, nonpreserved 0.9% saline prior to injection. However, a range of dilutions and injection volumes is acceptable. The reconstituted toxin is drawn into a tuberculin syringe via a fine gauge needle (30 G or 32 G) for final injection.

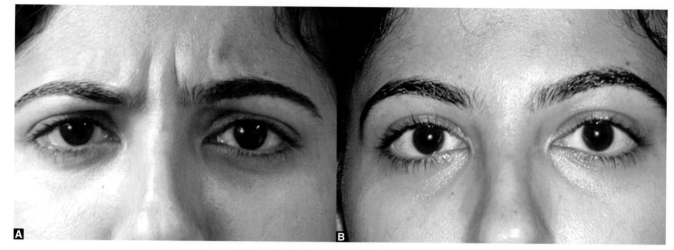

Figs 39.1A and B: Glabellar frown lines produced by the contraction of procerus, corrugator supercilii, and orbicularis oculi muscles (A). Note the elimination of frown lines upon attempted frowning two weeks after Botox injection (B)

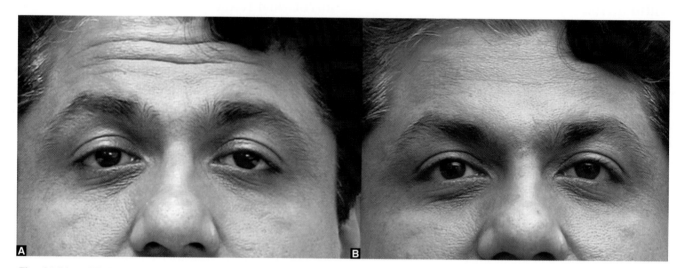

Figs 39.2A and B: External photograph demonstrating preinjection and postinjection photographs of horizontal forehead wrinkles treated with botulinum toxin chemodenervation of frontalis muscle. Each site is injected subcutaneously with 2.5 to 5 units of Botox

Treatment of Dynamic Facial Wrinkles

Dynamic facial wrinkles are the result of the activity of under-lying facial muscles, and are therefore amenable to treatment with Botulinum toxin. Repeated, prolonged effect of dynamic wrinkles can lead to the loss of subcutaneous fat, hyaluronic acid and collagen leading to static wrinkles. The dynamic wrinkles are most common over the upper third of the face (brow and periorbital region), and are amenable to management with chemodenervating agents.

Use of Botulinum toxin injection for dynamic wrinkles in the glabellar area was reported in 1992. Since then, its use has expanded to the midface, perioral and neck regions. In addition to its primary use, it has also been used to augment other procedures like chemical peels, laser resurfacing, brow lift, and fillers.

Glabellar Frown Lines

The glabellar wrinkles (Figs 39.1A and B) are caused by the actions of corrugator supercilii, depressor supercilii and procerus muscles. Injection into these muscles causes temporary paralysis that lasts up to six months, thereby eliminating these wrinkles. For treatment, 2.5 to 5 units of botulinum toxin type A (Botox) are injected at 5 to 7 sites into both corruga-tors and into the procerus muscle, with a median total dose of approximately 20 units.

Horizontal Forehead Wrinkles

The action of the frontalis muscle may, over years, lead to the development of horizontal forehead wrinkles. Injection of botulinum toxin type A (Botox) in 4 to 8 sites spaced evenly over the forehead may relax the muscle and soften these lines. The injections are typically given 2–3 cm above the orbital rim using 2.5 to 5 units per injection sites (Figs 39.2A and B).

Periocular Crow's Feet

The contraction of the lateral orbicularis fibers, zygomaticus and risorius muscles gives rise to dynamic wrinkles spreading out

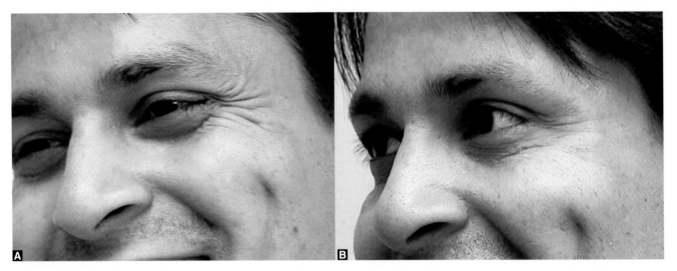

Figs 39.3A and B: Periocular dynamic crow's feet (A) can be significantly softened with botulinum toxin injection (B)

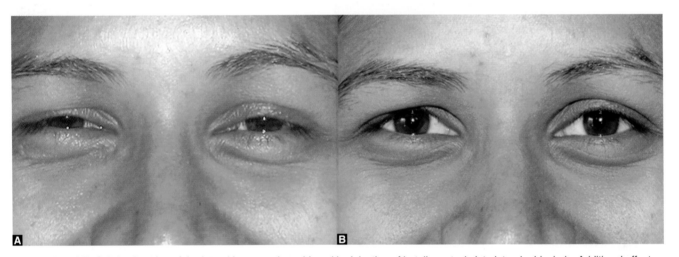

Figs 39.4A and B: Subtle elevation of the lateral brow can be achieved by injection of botulinum toxin into lateral orbicularis. Additional effect can be added by paralyzing the central frontalis in glabellar area

from the lateral canthus, known as the crow's feet (Figs 39.3A and B). Three to four injections of 2.5 to 5 units of Botox into lateral orbicularis oculi are required for the effective treatment of crow's feet. A study comparing 6, 12 and 18 units of botulinum toxin into the periocular area found no significant difference in the clinical response. Injection into the zygomaticus major can cause ipsilateral lip ptosis, and should thus be avoided.

Lower Eyelid Injection

Hypertrophic lower eyelid orbicularis oculi can be softened by a single lower eyelid injection of two units of Botox in the mid-pupillary plane. It widens the eye with reduction in infraorbital wrinkles (Fig. 39.4).

Chemical Brow Lift

Botulinum toxin can be used to create a chemical brow lift by selectively paralyzing the depressors of the eyebrow. Botulinum

toxin injections are given into the glabellar area (as described earlier) and lateral orbital orbicularis muscle (Fig. 39.5) below the eyebrow.

Botulinum toxin injection is very safe and effective, and has currently become the first cosmetic procedure a patient might receive owing to its excellent efficacy in reducing periocular dynamic wrinkles; the earliest sign of aging skin. Minimal downtime after injections and its ability to enhance the effect of fillers in certain areas makes it the most preferred noninvasive cosmetic procedure.

Soft Tissue Fillers

While botulinum toxin works well for dynamic wrinkles, soft tissue fillers are required for static wrinkles, preexisting facial defects, and for augmenting existing facial soft tissues.

Traditionally, loss of facial volume was thought to be due to descent of tissues as a result of gravity. However, it was demonstrated that the focal loss of volume can mimic descent

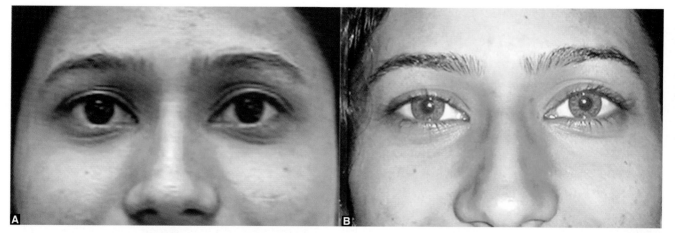

Figs 39.5A and B: Narrow palpebral fissure height, especially upon smiling can be widened by single Botox injection (two units) in the lower eyelid

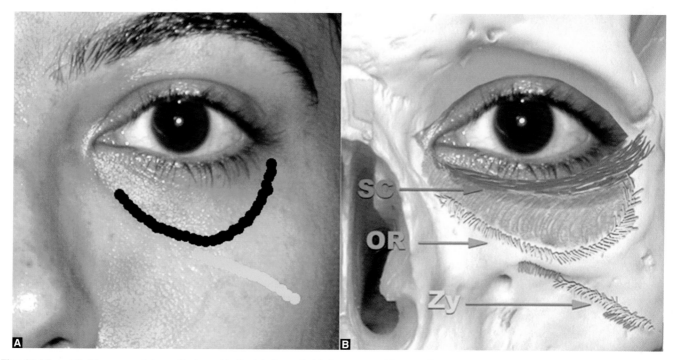

Figs 39.6A and B: The areas of deep attachment in the inferior periorbital area are orbital rim (OR) producing the orbital rim hollow, the confluence of retractors, tarsus and septum (SC) leading to the septal confluence hollow, and the zygomatico-malar (Zy) ligament producing the zygomatic hollow

of tissues in areas where skin is attached to deep structures. In the periorbital area, focal loss of volume along the orbital rim unveils the contours of orbital fat bound by arcus marginalis. So the significant change is not prolapse of the orbital fat or weakening of orbital septum, but unveiling of deeper contours caused by the focal loss of volume. There are three periorbital hollows of importance to the ophthalmologist while planning periorbital soft tissue augmentation: the orbital rim hollow, the zygomatic hollow and the septal confluence hollow (Fig. 39.6). Lifting the cheek surgically with a midface lift or permanent tear trough implant can fill the orbital rim and zygomatic hollows, but the same can be achieved by synthetic injectable fillers.

In the periorbital region, fillers are also used for static glabellar wrinkles, crow's feet and brow ptosis.

Since the introduction of bovine collagen (Zyderm and Zyplast; Inamed Aesthetics, Santa Barbara, CA, USA), several exogenous soft tissue fillers have been introduced in the last few years. These include human-derived collagen (CosmoDerm and CosmoPlast), hyaluronic acid-derived products (Restylane and Hylaform), and small particle-derived products (Radiesse and Sculptra).

The hyaluronic acids (Restylane) are the traditional volume filling products, in which the final result will be similar to the appearance at the time of injection, where "what you see is

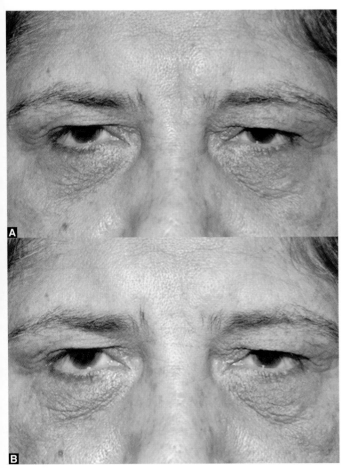

Figs 39.7A and B: Glabellar static furrows (A) treated with Restylane injection (B)

what you get". Alternative autogenous fillers are fat transplants, dermis and fascia.

Hyaluronic Acid Fillers (Restylane)

Hyaluronic acid is a glycosaminoglycan that consists of regularly repeating nonsulfated disaccharide units of glucuronic acid and N-acetylglucosamine. Four commercial preparations of hyaluronic acid formulation are available, of which Restylane (Medicis Aesthetics, Inc., Scottsdale, AZ, USA) is the most widely used product. It is available as a gel in the concentration of 20 mg/ml supplied in 1 ml and 0.4 ml disposable syringes along with a sterile 30 G needle.

Glabellar Furrows

Topical anesthetic in the form of lidocaine or prilocaine gel is most commonly used. Typically, 0.4 ml of Restylane is injected into the furrow (Figs 39.7A and B). A linear threading technique or the multiple puncture technique is used. Injection is performed during the withdrawal of the needle. The effect lasts up to six months when Restylane is used alone, but longer when it is used in combination with botulinum toxin.

Crow's Feet

Though botulinum toxin is effective in this area, treatment of crow's feet in the lower half could simultaneously paralyze the zygomaticus major muscle leading to unwanted facial distortions. A preferred practice in this region therefore is to immobilize the underlying muscle with botulinum toxin, and then treat the residual rhytides with not more than 0.2 to 0.3 ml of Restylane (Restylane *fine lines*) per side.

Brow Injection

The aging process leads to the drooping and receding of the brow, which can be raised with soft tissue fillers. Though surgical brow lift can produce dramatic results, sculpting of the brow with Restylane injection will project the brows to desirable arching contour. Taking into consideration the three-dimensional shape of the lateral brow fat pad, the technique of brow injection fills the brow rather than lifting it. Restylane (0.2–0.3 ml per side) injected just below the cilia in anterograde (push-ahead) technique fills and raises the superolateral margin, giving a youthful look.

Periorbital Hollows

The orbital rim hollow is located at or below the septal attachment along the orbital rim. Most patients have volume loss laterally in addition to the hollowing of medial tear trough. Best candidates for the soft tissue augmentation of periorbital

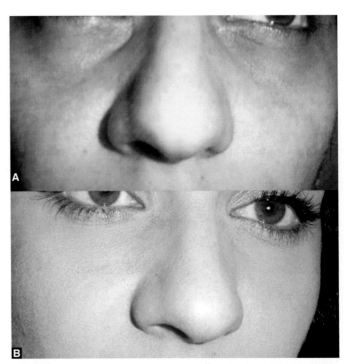

Figs 39.8A and B: Tear trough deformity (A) corrected by the deep injection of Restylane to achieve the soft tissue augmentation of the hollow. Note the young and rejuvenated look that is achieved (B)

hollows are younger patients with thicker skin and minimal to moderate volume loss.

The injection is placed deep subcutaneous, until the needle hits the bony orbital rim. The gel is placed at a level below the muscle, but above the periosteum. Approximately 0.2 ml Restylane per eye is required, and correction lasts for six months or more (Figs 39.8A and B). Gentle massage to distribute the hyaluronic acid filler within the tear troughs after injection is very useful.

Complications

Bruising, erythema and edema are usually transient. Tissue necrosis at the site of injection, and vascular embolism has been reported, but are extremely rare. Tissue necrosis is more common with glabellar injections; therefore novice injectors should be cautious in this area.

Botulinum toxin and soft tissue fillers have revolutionized the noninvasive management of facial wrinkles and soft tissue augmentation.

Orbital Surgeries

Santosh G Honavar, Milind N Naik

INTRODUCTION

Orbital surgery is one of the highly specialized branches at the crossroads of ophthalmology, neurosurgery and maxillofacial surgery. The orbit is a small space of 30 ml volume and is surrounded by bone, paranasal sinuses and cranial cavity. The complex of the eyeball and its neurosensory, motor and secretory appendages compacted within this small space, thereby posing a danger of functional impairment with slight mechanical insult. Surgery in this specialized area, therefore, lies in the domain of the experienced ophthalmic plastic surgeon that is familiar with the anatomy and physiology of the orbit and periorbital structures.

Over the last three decades, advances in investigative techniques, anesthesia and surgical techniques have vastly improved the operative potential for orbital diseases. Radiologic procedures, such as computed tomography (CT) and magnetic resonance imaging (MRI), allow the ophthalmic surgeon to accurately localize the lesion and plan the surgical approach. The use of hypotensive anesthesia, intraoperative magnification and special instrumentation allows meticulous dissection of orbital structures.

ORBITAL BIOPSY

The surgical approach to the orbit is influenced by the goal of the surgery. A well-encapsulated, cystic or solid, benign lesion located in an accessible surgical space (Fig. 40.1) is best excised completely. This is called an excisional biopsy. Incisional biopsy involves the removal of only a portion of the lesion for the purpose of establishing a histopathologic diagnosis. It is indicated for infiltrative lesions (Fig. 40.2) or those that need a complex surgical approach. The role of fine-needle aspiration biopsy is limited in the diagnosis of orbital lesions. It is used only for anterior orbital lesions that are potentially medically treatable, and is performed for suspected lymphoma, orbital inflammatory disease or metastases. Though fine-needle aspiration biopsy avoids the risks of general anesthesia and orbitotomy, an incisional biopsy should be preferred over a fine-needle aspiration biopsy in most accessible lesions.

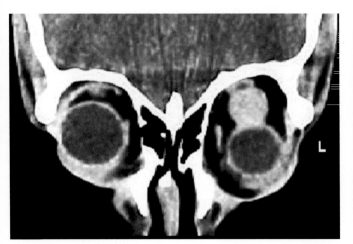

Fig. 40.1: Coronal scan showing left intraconal, well defined, homogeneous mass with smooth margins. Imaging characteristics suggest a benign well-encapsulated lesion that can be excised completely

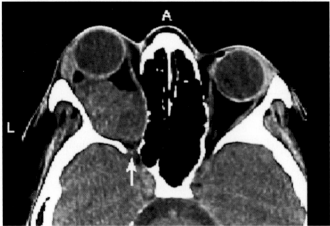

Fig. 40.2: Axial CT scan showing an irregular soft tissue mass filling entire left orbit, with possible intracranial extension through the widened superior ophthalmic fissure (arrow). Complete excision of this lesion would not be possible, thereby requiring an incisional biopsy for tissue diagnosis

OPERATIVE PRINCIPLES

Certain operative principles are especially necessary when operating within the orbit.

Bloodless Field

Differentiating normal and pathological tissue within the orbit is difficult. Moreover, the operative space is limited, thereby necessitating a bloodless field. Hypotensive anesthesia by an experienced anesthetist is recommended. A reverse Trendelenburg position not only reduces arterial flow, but also avoids venous backpressure within the orbit. Local hemostasis is obtained with monopolar and bipolar cautery, suction, direct and indirect packing, as well as bone wax.

Adequate Exposure and Visualization

Adequate lighting in the form of overhead lamps or fiber-optic headlights, magnification provided by surgical operating loupe, and careful retraction and use of hand-over-hand dissection technique ensures good visualization of orbital structures.

Proper Instrumentation

Malleable orbital retractors, periosteum elevators, fine tissue forceps and microdissectors are of utmost importance during orbital surgery. Modern mechanized bone cutting instruments and burrs are more convenient and less cumbersome than hand-operated saw or chisel.

Atraumatic Tissue Manipulation

Within the orbit, the surgeon has to remain close to the orbital mass and distract it from surrounding tissues rather than dissecting the orbital structures directly. Following appropriate orbital planes of dissection is extremely important.

Types of Orbitotomy

A myriad of clinical disorders can affect the orbit. The timing and approach of surgical intervention are based on the nature of the orbital disease process defined by clinical and imaging study. The basic indications for the surgery of the orbit are listed in Table 40.1.

The common surgical approaches to the orbit include anterior, lateral or superior orbitotomy. The orbit may be approached by any one route or by a combination of approaches. The position of the mass within the surgical space and its extent, its relation to the extraocular muscles and optic nerve, and the character of the lesion determine the specific choice.

Table 40.1: Basic indications for orbital surgery

1. Incisional biopsy
2. Excision of a cyst or mass
3. Repair and reconstruction
4. Abscess drainage
5. Decompression
6. Exenteration

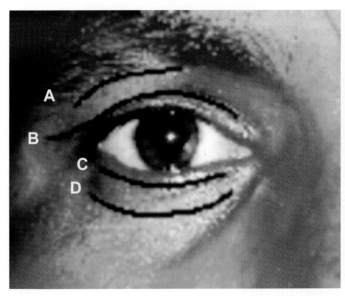

Fig. 40.3: Photograph showing anterior orbitotomy incision sites: (A) supraorbital incision, (B) upper eyelid crease incision, (C) subciliary incision and (D) lower eyelid crease incision

Anterior Orbitotomy

A majority of orbital procedures can be performed by an anterior orbitotomy through the skin or conjunctiva (Fig. 40.3). It can be used either for incisional biopsy of palpable orbital lesion anywhere within the orbit or for excising a well-defined anteriorly located tumors. When approached through the skin, the dissection may be either extraperiosteal or through the orbital septum (transseptal). Conjunctival approach could be transcaruncular for a medially located lesion or transforniceal for a lesion in the inferior orbit.

Lateral Orbitotomy

Lateral orbitotomy with or without removal of the lateral orbital wall provides good access to the extraconal and intraconal spaces of the orbit lateral to the optic nerve. It is commonly performed for intraconal tumors and lacrimal gland tumors. Access to the orbital apex, however, is limited in lateral orbitotomy.

Superior Orbitotomy

The superior approach to the orbit is either via transfrontal or temporofrontal (panoramic) incision. These approaches are in the domain of the combined ophthalmologic and neurosurgical team. It is commonly indicated for apical or combined apical and intracranial tumors, decompression of the optic canal, and compound trauma of the orbit and skull.

SURGICAL TECHNIQUE

While the knowledge of individual orbitotomy technique is essential, the practical application depends much upon the location of the tumor. One or a combination of these approaches can be used to obtain access to the desired surgical space of the orbit.

Table 40.2: Anterior orbitotomy approaches

Transcutaneous Transconjunctival
Upper eyelid skin crease incision
Lateral conjunctival incision
Supraorbital incision
Medial conjunctival incision (transcaruncular)
Medial (Lynch) incision
Lower eyelid incision
Subciliary incision

Approach to the Anterior Orbit (Anterior Orbitotomy Techniques)

Anterior orbitotomy techniques are used for the incisional biopsy of palpable orbital tumors or the excision of anteriorly located well-defined lesions. The various approaches to the orbit by anterior orbitotomy are given in Table 40.2.

Transseptal Approach

This route is an excellent approach for palpable superior orbital lesions in the extraconal space of the orbit. Common indications include lacrimal gland and orbital lymphomas. Transseptal incisions should be planned along the natural contours and folds of the eyelid, or can conveniently be placed over the most prominent part of the orbital mass. The upper eyelid skin crease incision and supraorbital incision are examples of transseptal orbitotomy (Fig. 40.3).

Steps of dermoid excision via transseptal anterior orbitotomy is described below (Figs 40.4A to 40.5D):

- The procedure can be performed under general or local anesthesia.
- A supraorbital skin incision is marked just below the eyebrow.
- Incision is placed along the marking, and orbicularis cut to expose the orbital septum.

- Septum is incised to expose the tumor, and blunt dissection is carried on all sides to separate the tumor from surrounding soft tissue.
- The tumor dissection is facilitated by gentle traction with a cryoprobe.
- Hemostasis is achieved. Orbicularis is closed with 6-0 vicryl and skin with 6-0 silk or prolene.

Extraperiosteal Approach

The anterior extraperiosteal approach is much suited for lesions occurring in the peripheral orbital space adjacent to the periosteum or arising from and involving the bone. Lesions commonly approached by this route include dermoid cysts, osteomas and subperiosteal abscess or hematoma. The skin incision is usually made at the orbital rim and carried up to the periosteum, which can be incised and elevated, thus exploring the extraperiosteal space. The supraorbital incision and lower lid incision are classic examples of this technique (Fig. 40.3). An alternative route of access in the lower eyelid is the subciliary incision through the skin and orbicularis to reach the orbital rim periosteum, and gives a cosmetically superior scar. The extraperiosteal approach, however, should be avoided for incisional biopsy of suspected intraorbital malignancy since periorbita provides a barrier against its spread.

Transconjunctival Approach

The medial transconjunctival anterior orbitotomy gives access to the medial rectus muscle, optic nerve as well as medial intraconal space for biopsy (Fig. 40.6A). The medial rectus muscle needs to be disinserted or retracted to enter the medial intraconal space. The medial transcaruncular incision gives excellent access to medial extraconal and subperiosteal space, and avoids a skin incision scar (Lynch), as well as avoids dissection around

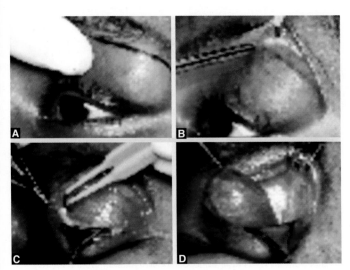

Figs 40.4A to D: Steps of transseptal anterior orbitotomy for a suspected dermoid cyst. Supraorbital skin incision (A). Skin incision and orbicularis separation (B). Tumor exposed after incising orbital septum (C). Cyst separated from surrounding soft tissue (D)

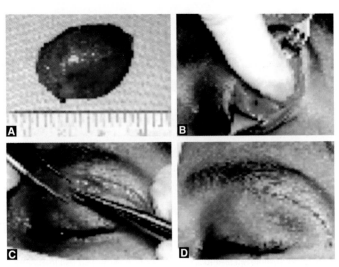

Figs 40.5A and D: Steps of transseptal anterior orbitotomy continued. Excised dermoid cyst (A). Palpation of lateral orbital rim to rule out bone defect (B). Orbicularis closure with 6-0 vicryl (C) and skin closure with 6-0 prolene (D)

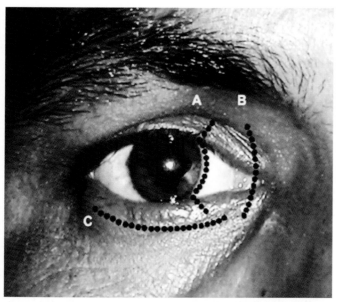

Fig. 40.6: (A) The medial transconjunctival anterior orbitotomy, (B) the medial transcaruncular incision and (C) lower eyelid transconjunctival approach are the most commonly performed transconjunctival orbitotomies

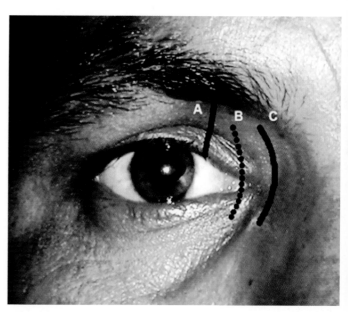

Fig. 40.8: Approach to the deep medial orbit. Vertical upper eyelid split anterior orbitotomy (A), Transcaruncular anterior orbitotomy (B), Transcutaneous frontoethmoidal anterior orbitotomy via Lynch incision (C)

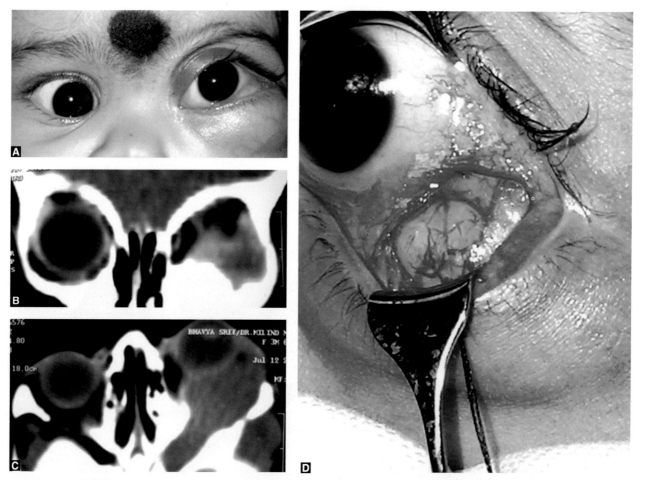

Figs 40.7A to D: Clinical and CT scan photographs of an infant with left inferior orbital soft tissue mass extending into pterygopalatine fossa through widened inferior orbital fissure (A, B and C). An incisional biopsy is performed via inferior transconjunctival anterior orbitotomy (D)

the lacrimal apparatus (Fig. 40.6B). The lower eyelid transconjunctival approach (Fig. 40.6C) gives you access to the inferior extraconal as well as extraperiosteal space; same areas as the transcutaneous route (Figs 40.7A to D). The transconjunctival incision can be combined with a lateral canthotomy and cantholysis to provide excellent exposure to the inferior and lateral orbit, yet avoiding a skin incision. Similarly, the lower eyelid transconjunctival incision can be extended medially into a transcaruncular incision to provide excellent access to inferior and medial subperiosteal spaces, orbital floor and medial wall.

Approach to the Deep Medial Orbit

It is difficult or impossible to reach the superior or medial orbit posterior to the equator, by the standard anterior orbitotomy approaches. Therefore, tumors within this orbital space require special surgical approach for excision (Fig. 40.8). These include vertical upper eyelid split anterior orbitotomy, transcaruncular anterior orbitotomy and transcutaneous frontoethmoidal anterior orbitotomy with a Lynch incision.

Vertical Upper Eyelid Split Anterior Orbitotomy

The postequatorial extraconal and intraconal space of the superior orbit cannot be reached by the standard eyelid crease incision. The vertical eyelid split approach allows access to these areas, as well as the medial orbit. The upper eyelid split anterior orbitotomy is described in detail below (Figs 40.9A to 40.12D):

The procedure is performed under general anesthesia. A vertical incision is marked on the upper eyelid at the junction of the medial third and lateral two-third. A scalpel blade is used to incise the eyelid margin. Full thickness eyelid incision is then extended along the marking with Stevens scissors, including the tarsus, levator aponeurosis, Müller's muscle and conjunctiva. The intraconal or extraconal space is then entered, using standard dissection techniques. The tumor is exposed, separated from surrounding soft tissue with blunt dissection, and extracted with the help of cyro probe. The forniceal conjunctiva is closed with wide spaced 6-0 vicryl sutures. Eyelid margin is sutures with 6-0 silk or prolene vertical mattress suture, and the full thickness eyelid defect is closed with standard full thickness eyelid closure technique. A frost suture can be placed for temporary protection of the cornea.

Transcaruncular Anterior Orbitotomy

The transcaruncular anterior orbitotomy provides access to the extraconal and subperiosteal space of the medial orbit. The main indications for this approach include medial wall fracture repair, drainage of subperiosteal hematoma, ethmoidectomy as a part of orbital decompression and medial extraconal or intraconal lesions. The procedure is described below (Figs 40.13A to D):

The procedure is performed under general anesthesia. Local anesthetic with epinephrine is injected within the medial bulbar conjunctiva and plica semilunaris. An incision is placed between the plica semilunaris and the caruncle for a variable length, and extending into the upper or lower conjunctival fornix as required. Stevens scissors is used bluntly to dissect a plane to the medial orbital wall, posterior to the posterior lacrimal crest. Additional retraction helps to reach the medial orbital wall. The indicated procedure is then performed in the required plane. Closure does not require periorbital sutures, and few absorbable conjunctival sutures are enough to close the wound.

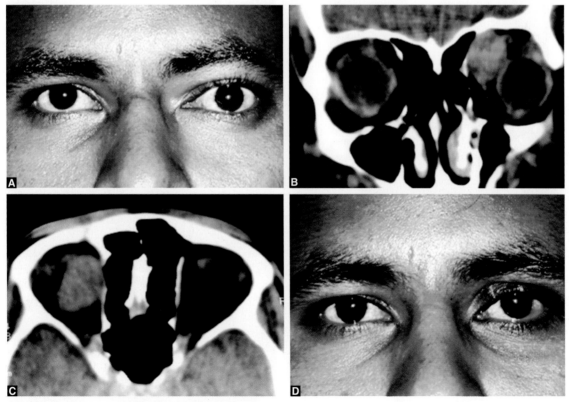

Figs 40.9A to D: Patient with left insidious proptosis (A), showing superomedial extraconal well-defined orbital soft tissue lesion on coronal (B) and axial (C) CT scan. Same patient six weeks after tumor excision via upper eyelid split anterior orbitotomy (D)

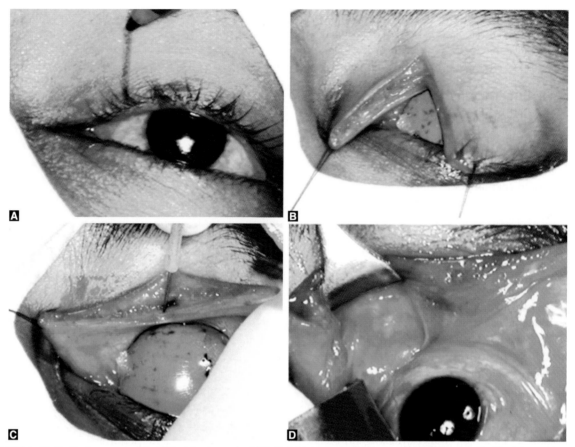

Figs 40.10A to D: Vertical upper eyelid split incision is marked (A). Full thickness division of eyelid (B). Conjunctival incision enters superior extraconal orbit (C). Exposure of tumor surface (D)

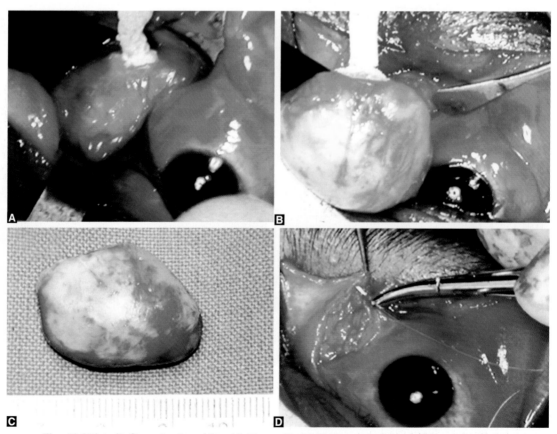

Figs 40.11A to D: Cryoextraction of the obital tumor (A and B). Gross photograph of the excised tumor (C) and closure of forniceal conjunctiva with vicryl 6-0 suture (D)

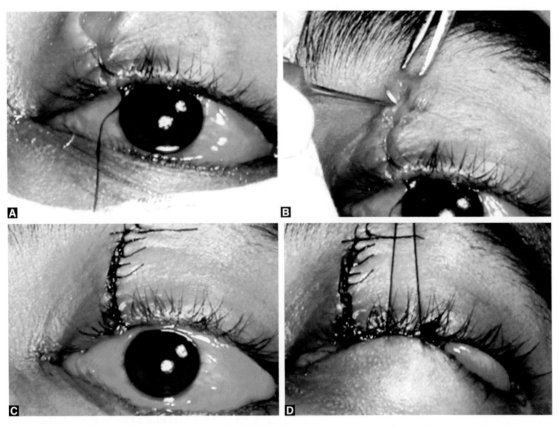

Figs 40.12A to D: Marginal vertical mattress suture placed with 6-0 silk (A). Tarsus and orbicularis closed in layers with 6-0 vicryl sutures (B). Skin closure with 6-0 silk sutures (C) and frost suture for corneal protection (D)

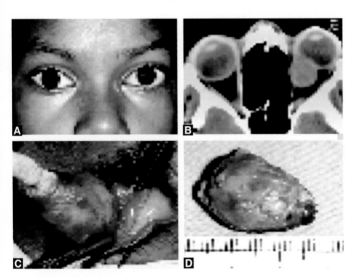

Figs 40.13A to D: Patient with left insidious proptosis (A) showing well-defined medial intraconal mass on axial CT scan (B). Cryoextraction of the mass via left medial transcaruncular incision (surgeon's view) being performed (C). Excised tumor mass (D)

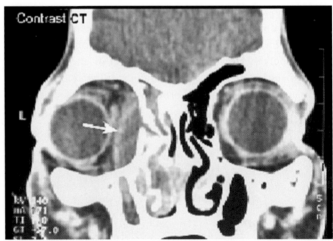

Fig. 40.14: Coronal CT scan with contrast showing left pansinusitis with medial subperiosteal abscess. Drainage can be performed via transcaruncular anterior orbitotomy or via Lynch incision

Transcutaneous Frontoethmoidal Anterior Orbitotomy (Lynch Incision)

The transcutaneous frontoethmoidal anterior orbitotomy or Lynch incision is used for access to the medial extraconal and subperiosteal spaces when a skin drain is required. The most common indication is medial subperiosteal abscess (Fig. 40.14).

An arched incision is placed from the medial canthal angle to the bridge of the nose in the concavity of the medial canthus. Retraction of the sac after elevation of the periosteum gives access to the medial orbital wall. The transcaruncular approach has now largely replaced the Lynch incision for drainage of medial subperiosteal abscesses.

Approach to the Deep Lateral Orbit (Lateral Orbitotomy)

Lateral orbitotomy with or without removal of lateral wall gives excellent approach to the intraconal and extraconal spaces of the orbit lateral to the optic nerve. Various incisions have been advocated to gain access to the lateral orbital wall. The two most popular approaches are the Berke-Reese incision and the Stallard-Wright incision (Fig. 40.15). The Berke-Reese incision involves a 3–5 mm horizontal incision after a complete lateral canthotomy. The Stallard-Wright incision is curvilinear, extending from lateral half of the eyebrow, toward the lateral bony orbital rim. Both incisions can provide good cosmesis with meticulous closure; however, the Stallard-Wright incision gives a better access to lacrimal gland fossa tumors, and does not require reconstruction of the lateral canthus. Eyelid crease approach is gaining popularity for being cosmetically advantageous with the scar hidden in the upper eyelid crease. The steps of lateral orbitotomy with bone removal are the following:

Lateral orbitotomy is performed under general anesthesia. Traction sutures are placed through the lateral rectus and superior rectus with 4-0 silk for future identification. A corneal shield is placed. Skin incision is marked along the lateral sub-brow region, curving down in S-shaped continuation in line with the lateral canthus. Skin is incised along the marking and orbicularis cut to expose the superolateral orbital rim. The periosteum is incised 2 mm posterior to the lateral orbital rim, and dissected off the orbital rim posteriorly, toward temporalis fascia. The temporalis fascia is opened, and temporalis muscle is separated and retracted laterally to expose the external aspect of the lateral orbital wall. The periorbita on the inner aspect of the orbit is elevated. The bony incisions are planned next. Generally, the superior incision is at or above the frontozygomatic suture and the inferior cut is at the junction of the zygomatic arch to the lateral orbital rim or lower, if demanded

by the size and location of the tumor. A mechanized saw is then used for bone cuts, while the assistant provides continuous saline irrigation and suction. Preplaced holes can be drilled into the bone for later repositioning the rim. The bone is then out-fractured with a ronguer, and additional lateral orbital wall can further be removed using the ronguer. The periorbita is then opened in a T-shaped configuration, to expose the orbital mass. Gentle dissection is carried out to separate the mass, and a cryoprobe helps in dissection. Hemostasis is ensured before closure. The lateral orbital wall is then replaced with the help of sutures within the preplaced holes, cyanoacrylate glue or with the use of microplates. The periosteum over the bone, orbicularis and skin are then closed in layers.

Approach to the Orbital Apex (Transcranial Orbitotomy)

The superior approach to the orbital apex is either by a transfrontal or a temporofrontal (panoramic) incision. A frontal bone flap is created by the neurosurgeon, following which the superior orbital rim and anterior orbital roof are opened. The frontal lobe is then elevated to expose the posterior orbital roof, which is opened to expose the optic canal. It is indicated for orbital apex tumors, decompression of the optic canal, debulking of sphenoid wing meningioma, and dissection at the superior orbital fissure. Orbital tumors can be excised by opening the periorbita (extradural approach), whereas orbitocranial tumors (such as optic nerve and sphenoid wing meningiomas) are explored by opening the periorbita and dura (intradural approach). After surgery, the bone flap is returned to its natural position.

Combined Approach

Lateral and Medial Orbitotomy

The transcaruncular medial orbitotomy can be combined with lateral orbitotomy, for large medial intraconal or extraconal lesions. The lateral orbitotomy in this case allows space for orbital contents to shift laterally ("access" orbitotomy), providing better exposure in the medial orbit.

Orbital Decompression for Thyroid Orbitopathy

A combined lateral and medial orbitotomy, as the procedure of choice, for orbital decompression to relieve optic neuropathy or decrease proptosis resulting from thyroid ophthalmopathy. A transcaruncular medial orbitotomy is performed for ethmoidectomy. A lateral orbitotomy helps burring away of the body of the sphenoid wing. This balanced two wall orbital decompression is less likely to result in postoperative diplopia compared to the standard technique of decompression of the orbital floor and medial wall.

Orbital surgery requires adequate clinical evaluation, orbital imaging and perioperative planning. CT scan and/or MRI are indispensable in accurate surgical planning. Numerous approaches to various orbital spaces are available. An

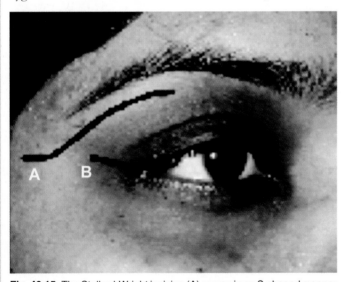

Fig. 40.15: The Stallard-Wright incision (A) curves in an S-shaped manner from the lateral half of the brow toward the lateral bony orbital rim. The Berke-Reese incision (B) is an extension of the lateral canthotomy incision and requires lateral canthal reconstruction during closure

adequate knowledge of orbital anatomy, surgical approaches and operating techniques results in better functional and cosmetic outcome.

COMPLICATIONS

Like any other surgical procedure, complications can occur during orbital surgery. Pressure packing and the use of bipolar cautery can usually control intraoperative hemorrhage. Perioperative intravenous antibiotics are given prophylactically following surgery to prevent orbital cellulitis. Ocular motility restriction due to muscle contusion usually settles in a few weeks unless its nerve supply is compromised. Damage to the optic nerve is the most serious complication, indicated by intraoperative pupillary dilatation. This may require intravenous methylprednisolone injections postoperatively. Acquired ptosis following orbitotomy procedure can be observed for spontaneous improvement for six months before surgical correction is undertaken.

Section

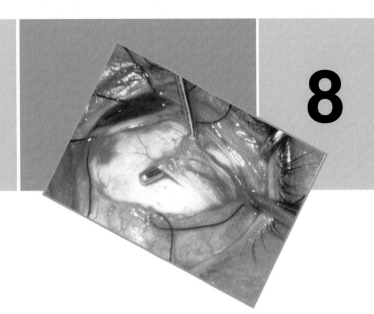

8

Strabismus

Strabismus

Kanwar Mohan

AMBLYOPIA

Amblyopia is a decrease in visual acuity in one or both eyes that results from an inability to use the eye or eyes for central fixation during the critical period of visual development. In human beings this critical period is thought to be from birth to approximately 6 years of age. A diagnosis of amblyopia is made when a patient has subnormal distance visual acuity despite refractive correction with spectacles or contact lenses and when no ophthalmoscopic organic cause can be detected to account for the decreased vision. Actually, even a difference of one Snellen line visual acuity between the two eyes can be considered amblyopia. However, for all practical purposes, a visual acuity difference of minimum two Snellen lines is diagnosed amblyopia by most of the ophthalmologists. The incidence of amblyopia ranges from 0.5 to 3.5% in preschool and school-age children, from 2.0 to 2.5% in the general population and from 4 to 5% in eye outpatient.

Types of Amblyopia

Strabismic Amblyopia

Strabismus accounts for 33 to 45% cases of amblyopia. If we consider the relative risk; strabismus patients are nearly 15 times more prone to become amblyopic than non-strabismus individuals. Strabismic amblyopia results from the suppression of the images in the deviating eye. Esotropia accounts for about 61%, whereas exotropia accounts for only 6% of the cases of strabismic amblyopia. Esotropes more often favor one eye for fixation compared to exotropes. Therefore, one can expect to find amblyopia far more often in esotropes than in exotropes. The higher prevalence of amblyopia in esotropes may also be related to the nasotemporal asymmetry of the retinocortical projections. In esotropia, the fovea of the deviating eye has to compete with the strong temporal hemifield of the fellow eye, whereas in exotropia, the fovea competes with the weaker contralateral nasal hemfield. Strabismic amblyopia does not occur in intermittent exotropia because there is fusion at one distance.

Any amblyopia associated with intermittent exotropia is either anisometropic or from some cause other than the strabismus. Amblyopia occurs only rarely in hypertropes because they usually manage to maintain fusion in some positions of gaze with an anomalous head posture.

The children with strabismic amblyopia present approximately 2.5 years earlier than those with anisometropic amblyopia. This is because strabismus is often observed by the parents and consequently advice is sought early, whereas, anisometropic amblyopia tends to go unnoticed because there is no accompanying sign. The appearance of amblyopia is more closely correlated with duration of strabismus than with the age of the child at the time the squint appeared.

Anisometropic Amblyopia

Anisometropia accounts for about 30% of the cases of amblyopia. Each 0.25 diopter difference between the refraction of the two eyes causes 0.5% difference in size between the two retinal images and a difference of 5% is probably the limit, which can be tolerated. Beyond this, the aniseikonia results in amblyopia in the more ametropic eye. Anisometropia of more than two to three diopters is often sufficient to cause amblyopia. In anisometropia, the foveal images in two eyes differ in size and clarity, which causes failure of fusion and a passive suppression of the blurred images, leading to amblyopia. The incidence of amblyopia is low in myopic anisometropia because the child can see near objects clearly thus preventing disuse. The depth of amblyopia has not been found to correlate with the degree of anisometropia. Stereoacuity is reduced in proportion to the depth of amblyopia (difference in visual acuity between both eyes) and anisometropic amblyopia with a difference of three or more Snellen lines is associated with reduced or absent stereoacuity.

Stimulus Deprivation Amblyopia

It is the least common but most damaging form of amblyopia that results from unilateral cataract, complete ptosis, corneal opacity and prolonged occlusion of the normal eye for the treatment of amblyopia. In unilateral stimulus deprivation, in addition to the decreased optical quality of the image, received by the fovea of the deprived eye, competition exists between this blurred image and the focused image received by the fovea of the healthy eye. Thus, form vision deprivation and abnormal binocular interaction are active amblyogenic factors. In bilateral stimulus deprivation, no such competitive situation is present and form vision deprivation is the only amblyogenic factor.

Isoametropic (Refractive) Amblyopia

Isoametropic amblyopia is bilateral and associated with approximately equally large hyperopia, myopic or astigmatic errors, or combinations of these. It occurs due to the effect of blurred retinal images.

Meridional Amblyopia

Meridional amblyopia occurs due to uncorrected astigmatism. It results from selected visual deprivation in a specific visual meridian.

Idiopathic Amblyopia

In some amblyopes no amblyogenic factor is detected. Clinically, such patients have foveal suppression of the amblyopic eye. It has been postulated that this may be due to some amblyogenic factor, such as transient anisometropia in infancy, which might have disappeared with advancing age.

Pathomechanism of Amblyopia

Abnormal binocular interaction and form vision deprivations are the two-amblyogenic factors in pathomechanism of amblyopia.

Types of Amblyopia	Abnormal Binocular Interaction	Form Vision Deprivation
Strabismic	+	−
Anisometropia	+	+
Stimulus Deprivation		
Unilateral	+	+
Bilateral	−	+
Isometropic	−	+
Meridional	+	+

Clinical Characteristics

Single letter visual acuity is better than linear acuity in amblyopic eye. This is due to crowding phenomenon because of contour interaction between the neighboring test optotypes. In the course of treatment of amblyopia, single letter acuity improves more rapidly than line acuity. Also greater the difference between the linear and single letter acuity, the poorer the prognosis. Visual acuity of amblyopic eye is better under scotopic conditions than under photopic conditions. Neutral density filter characteristically improves the visual acuity by one or two lines in patients with developmental amblyopia. This is due to scotopic conditions produced by neutral density filter.

The visual evoked response to pattern stimuli is usually abnormal in the amblyopic eye. In a small percentage of amblyopic eyes, the swinging light test is abnormal, suggesting an afferent pupillary defect. Increased central spatial summation, decreased central lateral inhibition, increased foveal cone receptive field size and dissociation between form and light senses have been demonstrated in amblyopic eyes.

Diagnosis of Amblyopia

In school-age children, the diagnosis of amblyopia is easy as one can record visual acuity on the Snellen's chart and detect any difference in visual acuities between both eyes. However, in infants and preschool-age children, Teller acuity cards can be used to assess vision but the correlation between Teller visual acuity and Snellen acuity is at present unreliable. Fixation preference test is a useful and reliable way of determining the presence or absence of amblyopia in the presence of strabismus in the infants and preschool groups. The presence of free alternation indicates equal visual acuity. The amblyopic patients will show fixation preference for the sound eye and stronger the fixation preference for the sound eye, poorer the visual acuity of the amblyopic eye.

If there is no manifest strabismus but amblyopia is suspected, the fixation pattern is studied after artificially creating a vertical strabismus with a 10-prism diopter (PD) prism held vertically in front of one eye. Wright and associates in a study evaluated the sensitivity of standard fixation preference testing and the 10 PD fixation test in diagnosing amblyopia. Standard fixation preference test showed 100% sensitivity for diagnosing amblyopia of three lines or more. All patients with three lines or more of amblyopia showed abnormal fixation pattern with standard fixation test, while 25% of the patents with equal vision showed abnormal fixation pattern, thus a false positive rate of 25%. Patients with tropia less than 10 PD gave 40% false positive response versus 8% in patients with tropia greater than 10 PD. The 10 PD fixation test showed only 1.5% false positive results in patients with tropia less than 10 PD. They concluded that standard fixation preference testing could be used to diagnose moderate to severe amblyopia in patients with tropias greater than 10 PD, while 10 PD fixation test should be used in patients with straight eyes or tropias less than 10 PD.

Treatment

The decision to treat unilateral amblyopia depends upon the age of the patient and the amount of difference in visual acuity or fixation preference between the two eyes. In children up to 6 years of age, a difference of even one line in visual acuity between the two eyes is sufficient to indicate the need for treatment. However, in children older than 6 years with only one line difference between the two eyes, the decision to treat amblyopia should be weighed against the likelihood of success and the time and financial effort involved. There is little hope of equalizing the visual acuity of a child over 6 years with this small a difference between the two eyes. The surgeon should not postpone strabismus surgery in such a child because of a prolonged attempt to improve the visual acuity of the amblyopic eye to 6/6. Similarly, in preschool-age children, a mild fixation preference is acceptable for strabismus surgery. However, in all other situations, the amblyopia should be treated prior to strabismus surgery. If amblyopia is not treated prior to surgery, sensory fusion will be defective and the fusion lock that holds the eyes straight after surgery will not be present and the eyes will gradually deviate again. Also the amblyopia treatment is very likely to be ignored and discontinued after strabismus surgery because the parents feel happy and relaxed with straight eyes of the child. Hence, amblyopia should be treated prior to strabismus surgery.

Occlusion Therapy

Occlusion therapy is by far the most commonly practiced method to treat amblyopia. Occlusion of the dominant eye (conventional occlusion) is the best method in the treatment of amblyopia regardless of the fixation pattern of the amblyopic eye. The following occlusion schedule is suggested:

Age up to 1 year: Three days of conventional occlusion followed by one day of inverse occlusion (occlusion of the amblyopic eye).

Ages >1−3 years: Four days of conventional occlusion followed by one day of inverse occlusion.

Ages 4−6 years: Six days of conventional occlusion followed by one day of inverse occlusion.

Age>6 years: Seven days of conventional occlusion without any inverse occlusion.

At no time both eyes are opened together. Patch should be applied as soon as the child wakes up and should be removed only after the child goes to sleep. Full-time occlusion (occlusion during all waking hours) is preferred over part-time occlusion (occlusion for few hours).

Type of Occluder

A skin patch is preferred over any occluder that attaches on the spectacles, such as Doyne's occluder, ground glass, etc., because the child can easily peep over the glasses, thus, nullifying the effect of occluder. We advise a patch made of 2-inch wide micropore adhesive tape. A small piece of paper is stuck in the center of the patch to ensure complete blockage of light and form and to allow free and comfortable movement of the eyelids underneath the patch (Fig. 41.1). Commercially available skin patches are costly. A patch made out of micropore tape is very economical and can be very easily prepared by the parents. Occlusive contact lenses are an alternative for those allergic to patch. However, they have a limited role because of difficulty in insertion and removal and the possibility of displacement.

Occlusion treatment is reinforced with near visual exercises, such as threading beads, tracing pictures, joining dots, hand video games, etc. These tasks put extra stress on the amblyopic eye and facilitate the recovery of vision.

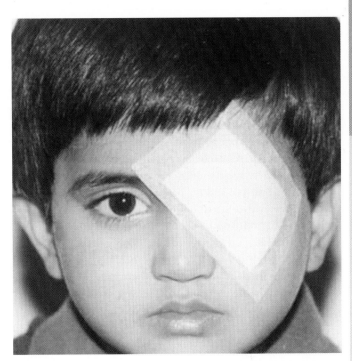

Fig. 41.1: Child wearing a patch made out of 2" wide micropore tape

Follow-up

After starting occlusion treatment, the child should be followed-up at an interval of one week per year of age, e.g. a 2-year should be followed-up at an interval of two weeks and a 4-year old child should be followed-up at an interval of four weeks. It is utmost important to record visual acuity using the same Snellen chart and under same illumination otherwise one would inappropriately record a better or worse visual acuity because an amblyopic eye sees better under scotopic conditions and poorer under photopic conditions. The fixation pattern of the amblyopic eye at each visit in preschool-age children is noted to assess any change in visual status. The child is never allowed to close his/her eye with his/her hand because the child may see with the supposedly closed eye through the chinks in between the fingers. Similarly, a child may memorize the letters in Snellen lines. So, one has to be careful in recording visual acuity in children. It is important that one should watch the child while he is reading the chart so that one can detect whether he is actually reading the chart or has memorized the letters.

When to Stop Full-time Occlusion?

Full-time occlusion is stopped only when vision in the amblyopic eye becomes equal to that of the dominant eye or if there has been no further improvement in vision despite at least 3 months of occlusion treatment sincerely or when fixation becomes alternating.

How to Maintain the Improved Vision?

When maximum visual improvement has been achieved by full-time occlusion, full-time occlusion is stopped and the improved visual acuity is commonly maintained by part-time occlusion of the dominant eye. The maintenance part-time occlusion is continued till the age of 8 or 9 years because it is around this age that the visual acuity becomes stable and the chances of recurrence of amblyopia are minimum.

Penalization

Penalization of the fixing eye by atropinization has a very limited role in the treatment of amblyopia. It can be used only to treat mild degree of amblyopia because despite atropinization, the visual acuity in the dominant eye may still be better than that of the amblyopic eye and the patient may still prefer to use the dominant eye. Also penalization produces a blurred stimulus, which may be more amblyogenic than no stimulus with total occlusion. Hence, the danger of occlusion amblyopia is probably greater with penalization. Therefore, penalization is not the preferred modality to treat amblyopia. However, it can be used to maintain the vision improved by occlusion treatment.

Pleoptics

Pleoptics, which involved dazzling of the retina around the fovea by an intense light hoping that the fovea would function better after turning off the light, has been discarded as a modality to treat amblyopia in most strabismus clinics because of a complex and time-consuming procedure.

CAM Vision Stimulator

CAM stands for Cambridge, England, where the apparatus was first studied. Here normal eye is occluded only for seven minutes during the treatment and the patient draws games on a transparent cover placed over slowly rotating, high contrast and sharp edged gratings. Though the initial studies reported promising results, subsequent studies found it much less effective than occlusion therapy. Hence, CAM vision stimulator is not preferred modality to treat amblyopia.

Pharmacological Agents

Some drugs like citicoline and levodopa have been recently tried to treat amblyopia. Citicoline has been found to improve visual acuity in both the sound and the amblyopic eye for at least six months after 15 days of treatment. Several investigators have reported the efficacy of levodopa in improving visual acuity in childhood amblyopia. Mohan and associates found an improvement in visual acuity in 74% of their patients treated with levodopa. They reported no side effects and found that at least 50% of their patients maintained visual acuity at 1-year follow-up.

Thus, attempts have been made towards a pharmacological treatment of amblyopia. Larger studies with longer patient follow-up are needed before these drugs are prescribed as a routine for the treatment of amblyopia.

Role of Patient Compliance

Patient compliance is the most important factor for the successful treatment of amblyopia. Occlusion treatment requires a lot of patience and entails repeated visits to the doctor. It needs a lot of cooperation from the child because an occlusive patch is psychologically disturbing and educationally disruptive. The parents should be explained the importance of patching. The teacher's cooperation can also be sought in motivating the child to wear a patch.

Prognosis

Amblyopia caused by stimulation deprivation due to cataract, corneal opacity etc. has the poorest prognosis. Strabismic amblyopia has better prognosis than anisometropic amblyopia. Amblyopia due to unilateral high hypermetropia has a poor prognosis than amblyopia due to unilateral high myopia. Older the patient age at the time of starting the treatment, poorer the prognosis. Occlusion treatment gives best results for up to 6 years of age. Patients older than 6 years have a slower improvement and require a longer treatment. We have observed visual improvement with occlusion treatment in patients up to 15 years of age. Hence, a trial of occlusion should be given even in older amblyopes, if the patient is willing to wear a patch.

To summarize, occlusion treatment is the most effective modality that has stood the test of time and till date no other modality has been able to replace it. An early detection and timely treatment of amblyopia by occlusion is utmost important to prevent a permanent visual loss due to amblyopia.

STRABISMUS IN CHILDHOOD

Esodeviations are the most common types of ocular misalignment, constituting over 50% of ocular deviations in the pediatric population. Esodeviations frequently seen in children include infantile esotropia, accommodative esotropia, partially accommodative esotropia and basic or nonaccommodative esotropia. Exodeviations commonly seen in children include infantile exotropia and intermittent exotropia. A vertical deviation, especially hypertropia, is frequently associated with horizontal deviation. A purely vertical deviation is rare in children. Whenever a child with ocular deviation is brought for consultation, the ophthalmologist should enquire from the parents the age at the onset of deviation, the type of deviation whether convergent or divergent or vertical, the mode of onset whether sudden or gradual, the course of deviation whether intermittent or constant, any inciting cause, such as illness, fatigue, fever, trauma, etc., birth history whether the child was born full-term or premature, history of birth asphyxia and whether the milestones of the child were normal or delayed.

Convergent Squint in a Child

When the parents bring a child with the history of inward turning of eye/eyes, the first thing the ophthalmologist should see is whether the child has a true esotropia or an appearance of esotropia called pseudoesotropia. Pseudoesotropia is caused by a flat broad nasal bridge or prominent medial epicanthal folds (Fig. 41.2). The observer sees less sclera nasally, which gives the

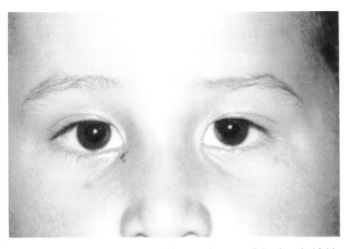

Fig. 41.2: Pseudoesotropia caused by prominent medial epicanthal folds

impression that the eye is turned in toward the nose, especially when the child looks to either side. Pseudoesotropia can be easily differentiated from a true esotropia by cover-uncover test, which will show no movement of either eye in the former and an outward movement of either eye in the latter. Costenbader found that out of 753 patients suspected by their parents to have esotropia, 47% had pseudoesotropia. It is important to differentiate between a true esotropia and a pseudoesotropia because a true esotropia requires a detailed work-up and management, whereas a pseudoesotropia requires no treatment but only an assurance that as the child grows, the bridge of nose will become prominent and the appearance of esotropia will disappear. However, true esotropia can develop later in children with pseudoesotropia and therefore, parents should be cautioned that reassessment is required, if the appearance does not improve.

After a diagnosis of true esotropia is established, it is important to differentiate whether the child has infantile esotropia or accommodative esotropia or acquired basic esotropia or a combination of accommodative and basic esotropia. Each of these types of esotropia has its characteristic clinical features, which help in differentiating it from others.

Infantile Esotropia

Infantile esotropia is characterized by:

- The onset of esotropia is before 6 months of age. As esotropia is very rarely present at birth, the term "congenital esotropia" used previously has now been mostly replaced by "infantile esotropia."

- The angle of deviation is usually in excess of 35 PD. About 50% of the patients have a deviation larger than 50 PD. The deviation is stable and approximately same at distance and near fixation. Since it is difficult to get an infant to fix at distance for the prism cover test, the exact measurement is generally impossible and the deviation at distance can be only approximated, by observing the patient.

- Mild to moderate hypermetropia is present in nearly 90% of the patients. Hypermetropia is rarely in excess of 2.0 D and glasses are seldom indicated. Those having higher amounts of hypermetropia (+ 4.0 D or more) tend to show a decrease in deviation with time and 10 to 20% of these patients will eventually develop an exotropia. Hence, one should follow a conservative approach rather than an early surgical treatment in such patients.

- Many patients show alternate fixation in primary position and cross-fixation on gazing to either side. In cross-fixation, when the patient looks to the right, the left eye will be adducted and used for fixation and abduction of the right eye appears restricted. When the patient looks to the left, the right eye will be adducted and used for fixation and abduction of the left eye appears restricted (Fig. 41.3). Thus, the child may falsely appear to have a bilateral sixth nerve paralysis. However, a bilateral sixth nerve paralysis can be easily ruled out by closing one eye of the child or by doll's head phenomenon, which will show normal abduction in both eyes.

- Developmental amblyopia develops in approximately 40% of the patients. It is generally accepted that amblyopia is unlikely to develop in patients who cross-fixate. However, Dickey, et al., found significant amblyopia in 50% of cross-fixators. They suggested that the point at which alternation of fixation occurs was a reliable means of detecting amblyopia. If there was equal visual acuity, alternation occurred at the mid-line with each eye. If there was amblyopia, the sound eye would continue to follow the target beyond midline into abduction before the poorer seeing eye pick-ups fixation.

- Dissociated vertical deviation (DVD) is present in 46 to 90% of patients with infantile esotropia. DVD is infrequent before the age of 2 years and may develop years after the satisfactory alignment of the esotropia. This possibility should be told to the parents. Hiles and associates found the onset of DVD greatest during the second year of life. Following the third year, it occurred at a mean rate of 10%

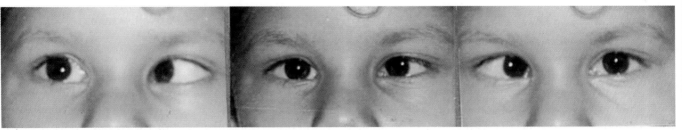

Fig. 41.3: Infantile esotropia with cross fixation. There is pseudorestriction of abduction in both eyes

per year. Early horizontal alignment did not decrease the incidence of DVD, suggesting that DVD is a time-related phenomenon.

- Overaction of one or both inferior oblique muscles is present in 78% of the patients and it is so marked that it occurs spontaneously without having the patient perform version movements. However, it is rarely detectable before the age of 1 year. Hiles and associates noted the onset of inferior oblique overaction to be most frequent during the second year of life with mean rate of 33% per year; the greatest occurrence was during years three and seven. It is likely that this represents more advanced stage of the disease.

- Approximately half of the cases with infantile esotropia have micronystagmus. It is usually latent nystagmus, which is predominantly horizontal jerk nystagmus elicited by occluding either eye. It is usually of small amplitude and patient commonly has a null point indicated by a head turn or tilt. Therefore, if a child with infantile esotropia has an abnormal head posture, look for latent nystagmus. Rotatory nystagmus can also occur but it is much less common than latent nystagmus.

- Infantile esotropes do not have any potential for central fusion. Inspite of perfect surgical alignment of their eyes, these patients achieve only peripheral fusion. They never achieve normal stereopsis. Though some stereoacuity is usually present after treatment, it is of low quality.

Accommodative Esotropia

When we accommodate, a certain amount of convergence is associated with it, which is called accommodative convergence. The relationship between accommodative convergence and accommodation is called AC/A ratio. The normal AC/A ratio is 3–5, which means that one diopter of accommodation is associated with 3–5 PD of accommodative convergence. When a patient makes excessive effort to accommodate, it will cause excessive accommodative convergence, resulting in esotropia, called accommodative esotropia.

Accommodative esotropia usually develops between 1 and 3 years of age. This is the age when children start to look for details. Although they do not read, they nevertheless look with great attention at near objects, toys, etc. This calls into play their accommodation and may precipitate an esotropia. It is known that 10% of accommodative esotropia occurs prior to age 1 year. It has also been reported that accommodation may reach the adult level by the fourth month of life and 15% of infantile esotropia patients have infantile accommodative esotropia. In these patients, the angle of esotropia is less than that in infantile esotropia and the other characteristics of infantile esotropia such as inferior oblique overaction, DVD and latent nystagmus are also less frequent. Probably 50% of such patients may achieve correction of esotropia by full correction of hypermetropia. It has been recommended that if hypermetropia is 2.25 D or more despite the deviation being constant in infantile

esotropia, accommodative esotropia should be suspected and full refraction should be prescribed. Accommodative esotropia also can start at a much later time (between seven and fifteen years of age). Usually, this is precipitated by some factor, such as physical or emotional trauma, illness, etc., responsible for breaking down the previously successful use of relative accommodation in a latent hypermetrope.

In accommodative esotropia, near deviation is greater than distance deviation by more than 10 PD. The hallmark of accommodative esotropia is a variable deviation. Therefore, when a variable esotropia is not found, accommodative esotropia must be suspected.

Initially, the deviation is intermittent and may cause intermittent diplopia. The child may react to diplopia by showing irritability and by closing one eye. However, within a few days, suppression develops and the child returns to her/his normal behavior and no longer closes one eye. After a longer time, anomalous retinal correspondence develops to protect the child from any further sensory symptoms. Ultimately, constant esotropia may replace intermittent esotropia and may lead to developmental amblyopia.

Accommodative esotropia is commonly of two types:
i. Refractive accommodative esotropia
ii. Nonrefractive accommodative esotropia (High AC/A accommodative esotropia).

Refractive Accommodative Esotropia

In refractive accommodative esotropia, usually there is a mild to moderate hypermetropia (2.0 to 6.0 PD). When a patient has uncorrected hypermetropia, there is image blur. The patient will try to clear the image blur by increasing accommodative effort which, in turn, will cause excessive accommodative convergence. If fusional divergence amplitude is insufficient to compensate for this overconvergence and in the presence of a normal AC/A ratio, esotropia will develop and this esotropia is refractive accommodative esotropia. The patient's fusional reserve may be depleted by illness, fatigue and emotions. Some patients with uncorrected hypermetropia prefer blurred vision over the constant effort to accommodate. So they remain orthophoric but develop ametropic amblyopia.

In refractive accommodative esotropia, esodeviation is larger at near than at distance fixation. As this type of esotropia is related to hypermetropia, a full correction of hypermetropia, determined by cycloplegic refraction, will make the eyes orthophoric.

Nonrefractive Accommodative Esotropia

In nonrefractive accommodative esotropia, the effort to accommodate elicits an abnormally high accommodative convergence response, i.e. there is an abnormally high AC/A ratio. A high AC/A ratio can be taken more seriously, if the cycloplegic refraction reveals only a small amount of hypermetropia or if it reveals myopia or emmetropia. Accommodative esotropia with relatively low refractive errors (up to 4 D) are more likely to have high AC/A ratio, whereas those with high refractive errors (over 4 D) are more likely to have normal AC/A ratio. In one series of high AC/A accommodative esotropia, the average refractive errors were + 2.25 D. This is 2.50 D less than the average refractive error of the patients with purely refractive accommodative esotropia. Infrequently, high hypermetropia does occur with a high AC/A ratio and when it does, the refractive accommodative esotropia adds on to the high AC/A ratio esotropia.

In high AC/A esotropia, the deviation is significantly greater at near than distance fixation. In fact, there may be no esotropia for distance fixation in some patients. It is unrelated to refractive error meaning thereby that the correction of refractive error has no effect on esotropia. Practically, nonrefractive accommodative esotropia is suspected when there is a significant esodeviation at near fixation with refractive error fully corrected and the diagnosis is confirmed by establishing the presence of a high AC/A ratio, measured with the lens gradient method.

Partially Accommodative Esotropia

Partially accommodative esotropia is the combination of accommodative and basic (nonaccommodative) esotropia. Here a residual esotropia exists despite full correction of a hypermetropic refractive error or prescription of bifocal lenses or miotics or both. It can occur in two clinical situations:

i. A child initially has infantile esotropia on which an accommodative element becomes superimposed as the child grows older, often accompanied by a larger hypermetropia than was first measured.

ii. A child initially has accommodative esotropia. After alignment of the eyes with glasses or bifocal lenses, a nonaccommodative element becomes superimposed. It may be due to hypertrophy or contracture of the medial rectus muscles, conjunctiva or Tenon's capsule.

In partially accommodative esotropia, the residual deviation, after full correction of hypermetropia or prescription of bifocal lenses, is same for near and distance fixation. This deviation is usually constant and is therefore, typically associated with the suppression, anomalous retinal correspondence and amblyopia.

Acquired Nonaccommodative or Basic Esotropia

It includes esotropia with onset after 6 months of age but usually limited to childhood. Characteristically, an accommodative factor is absent; the refractive error is insignificant and the near deviation is approximately equal to the distance deviation. At the onset, the angle of strabismus, generally is smaller than in patients with infantile esotropia, but the angle tends to increase to a magnitude of 30 to 70 PD. The parents frequently associate the deviation with injury, illness or emotions. It has been postulated that such patients have an excessive convergence tonus that is controlled initially by fusional divergence but is disrupted easily by exogenous factors.

Other Conditions Which May Be Present with Esotropia

Duane's retraction syndrome (DRS) Type 1: DRS Type 1 is characterized by abduction deficiency, normal or mildly restricted adduction and retraction of the globe with narrowing of the palpebral fissure on attempted adduction of the affected eye. There may be orthophoria or esotropia in primary position with face turn.

Nystagmus blockage syndrome (NBS): Nystagmus blockage syndrome is based on the fact that convergence dampens nystagmus. It is thought that the patient unconsciously converges the eyes so that nystagmus will be decreased, which, in turn, improves visual acuity. Nystagmus blockage syndrome occurs in 10 to 12% of patients with infantile esotropia. It is characterized by nystagmus that begins in early infancy and is associated with esotropia. In these patients both eyes may be simultaneously markedly esotropic. Any attempt to abduct either eye provokes manifest nystagmus. Sometimes the strabismus is variable and the eyes only become markedly esotropic when the child tries to look carefully at something. This syndrome may be confused with bilateral sixth nerve palsy. If nystagmus is present on attempted abduction, the diagnosis of nystagmus blockage syndrome associated with infantile esotropia is almost certain.

An additional feature of NBS is when you occlude the non-fixing eye, the fixing eye remains in the convergent position and the patient turns head in the direction of the uncovered fixing eye. For example, when the patient is fixing with the right eye and you occlude the left eye, the patient turns the face to the right. This abnormal head posture allows the uncovered eye to persist in an adducted position. One is often unable to get the child to abduct either eye even by using the doll's head phenomenon. Occlusion of one eye for several hours may encourage movement of the other eye past the midline.

Also when a base out prism is placed before the fixing eye in a child with NBS, the fellow eye will remain in adduction and esotropia will actually increase. This phenomenon does not occur in children with infantile esotropia.

Congenital sixth nerve palsy: Congenital sixth nerve palsy in an otherwise healthy child is rare. It usually causes esotropia in the primary position. The child will have a compensatory face turn toward the palsied eye to maintain binocular vision. There will be deficiency or absence of abduction on doll's head phenomenon.

Sensory esotropia: Poor vision in one eye in a child presents severe obstacle to binocular vision and may cause strabismus. Sidakaro and von Noorden observed esotropia and exotropia with almost equal frequency when the onset of visual impairment occurred at birth or between birth and five years of age. Ellsworth reported esotropia as the presenting sign in 11% of children with retinoblastoma.

Moebius syndrome: Moebius syndrome consists of congenital facial diplegia (bilateral facial palsy) of variable degree and a congenital bilateral paralysis of lateral gaze. Vertical and convergence eye movements are spared. Partial atrophy of tongue, paralysis of the soft palate and muscles of mastication may occur. Infantile esotropia has been found in 38% of the patients with Moebius syndrome. Therefore, the parents of a child with infantile esotropia should be questioned about any sucking or feeding problems and the child should be examined for any associated systemic abnormalities of Moebius syndrome.

Clinical Evaluation

Measurement of the deviation: The following points should be kept in mind while measuring deviation:

i. The deviation should be measured after correction of the refractive error, if any.

ii. The deviation should be measured for near and distance fixation in the primary position. Also measure the deviation in up and down position to detect any "A" and "V" pattern.

iii. As the prism and cover test gives most accurate measurement of the deviation, the deviation should preferably be measured by using prism and cover test. Since it is difficult to get an infant to fix at distance for the prism and cover test, record approximate deviation at distance. Krimsky or Modified Krimsky test is used to measure deviation only if the child is not at all cooperative for the prism and cover test. Hirschberg's method gives the least accurate assessment of deviation.

iv. An accommodative target is used for fixation at near. Near deviation should be measured with accommodation fully controlled. Children with accommodative esotropia may keep their eyes aligned at near fixation by accommodating only partially or not at all. Therefore, use of a fixation target that requires full accommodation to identify small details is necessary. Such a target is usually termed as accommodative target. Fixation light is not an accommodative target. Hence, measurement for near deviation is performed by asking the patient to fix on torchlight.

Assessment of visual acuity: It is extremely important to assess visual status in a child so that amblyopia can be detected and treated early. In infants and preschool age children, an approximate assessment of visual acuity can be done indirectly by observing the fixation pattern of the squinting eye. A child with unilateral squint is presumed to have a severe amblyopia, whereas a child with freely alternating squint is presumed to have equal vision in both eyes. In school-going children, visual acuity can be assessed on Snellen's chart.

Examination of extraocular movements: One should look specifically for any limitation of abduction and overaction of superior and inferior oblique muscles. If there is a limitation of abduction on version, see if it improves with duction. Limitation of abduction could be due to Duane's retraction syndrome, sixth nerve palsy, cross-fixation and medial rectus contracture due to long-standing esotropia.

Cycloplegic refraction: Ideally any child with convergent squint should have refraction under atropine cycloplegia. Atropine uncovers an average 0.34 D more hypermetropia than cyclopentolate and 0.8 D more hypermetropia than tropicamide. Atropine is the drug of choice for cycloplegic refraction in children, especially up to six years of age. So one should not hesitate in using atropine. Atropine eyedrops cause more systemic side effects. Therefore, it is safe to use atropine eye ointment twice a day for three days (a total of six applications). However, it has been found that even four applications of atropine eye ointment are sufficient to uncover total hypermetropia and six applications are really not necessary.

Measurement of fusional divergence amplitude: If possible fusional divergence amplitude should be measured for near and distance fixation.

Fundus examination: Every child presenting with strabismus should have fundus examination to rule out any fundus pathology, such as retinoblastoma, macular lesion and optic atrophy accounting for strabismus.

Treatment

Correction of the Refractive Error

Patient with infantile esotropia

An infant with a hypermetropia of +2.0 D or greater under cycloplegia should be prescribed glasses.

Patient with refractive accommodative esotropia

Any child up to 4 years of age with a refractive error greater than +1.50 D should be prescribed full cycloplegic retinoscopic findings (Figs 41.4A and B). However, in a child older than 4 years, the ophthalmologist should prescribe the minimum power lens that will provide both binocular single vision with esophoria and maximum visual acuity. The goal of the treatment is not orthophoria but esophagi because in isochoric state, the patient continues to exercise fusional divergence amplitude. A child may not be able to attain maximum visual acuity with full radioscopy refraction because of latent hypermetropia. If a small reduction in radioscopy findings improves visual acuity and also maintains alignment and binocular vision, this reduction can be made. If the patient becomes intermittently isotropic because of this reduction, the reduction has been too great. Therefore, the ophthalmologist must avoid enthusiastically decreasing the patient's hypermetropia correction in order to improve visual acuity. Most of the patients are able to adapt to full radioscopy glasses. However, an occasional patient may not accept the glasses. One can advise instillation of atropine eye ointment once every day for two weeks in such patients to get them to begin wearing their glasses.

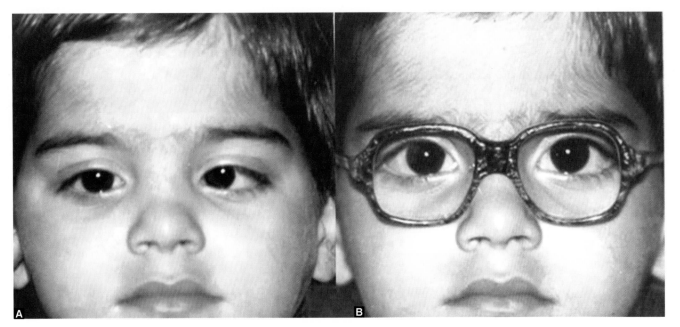

Figs 41.4A and B: Refractive accommodative esotropia: (A) Left esotropia without glasses (B) Eyes straight with glasses

All patients should be followed-up carefully. An infant should be seen monthly until it is certain that the glasses control the deviation. Once an infant is stabilized with the proper refractive correction, radioscopy should be repeated after every three months. For patients, aged 1–5 years, radioscopy should be repeated every six months and after that, yearly. If another one diopter of refractive error is found, a new prescription for glasses should be given.

Will the child have to use glasses for the rest of life?

This will depend upon the amount of hypermetropia present. Generally, children under the age of 3 years with hypermetropia spherical errors of less than 3.5 diopters have a good chance of getting rid of their glasses when they are visual adults, i.e. around age 8–9 years. There may be a decrease in the hypermetropia, as they get older. When hypermetropia exceeds 4 diopters or when there is a marked astigmatic refractive error, glasses will be necessary for clear vision, as well as for keeping the eyes correctly aligned. In these cases the parents should be told it is likely that some sort of optical correction will be necessary throughout the child's life.

Patients over 8 years of age whose refractive error is less than + 3.50 D and whose esotropia is fully controlled with glasses may be helped by orthoptic exercises. The aim of this treatment is to enable the patient to have straight eyes without glasses. The child must be highly motivated to give up wearing glasses. Treatment consists of ensuring that the child appreciates diplopia whenever an esotropia occurs. Teaching the child to relax accommodation without glasses, so that esotropia is eliminated and the child has blurred but single binocular vision, follows this. When the child can maintain this easily, exercises are aimed at establishing clear single binocular vision for distance without glasses and then later for near without glasses. Some children can begin to leave their glasses off and maintain clear binocular vision comfortably after six weeks, while others require several months to achieve this. Once control of the deviation has been established, the strength of the glasses may be reduced gradually and in some cases eliminated.

Swan reported that 38% of the 39 adult patients treated for refractive accommodative esotropia in childhood had not outgrown their hypermetropia and were still wearing glasses full-time. Their hypermetropia became maximum (median 5.7 diopters) by the age of 6, decreased in adolescence and then stabilized (median 4 diopters). Nearly all depended on relaxed accommodation to maintain alignment when they removed their glasses.

Deterioration of accommodative esotropia

It is widely recognized that accommodative esotropia although initially intermittent, tends to progress to a constant deviation if treatment is delayed. Constant esotropia can then lead to permanent loss of bifixation. Dickey and Scott reported that 13% of their patients with accommodative esotropia deteriorated over a follow-up period of 10 years. The prevalence of deterioration was 77% when the onset of esotropia was within the first year of age and 20% when the onset of esotropia was between one to two years. The rate of deterioration was extremely low when the onset of esotropia was after 24 months. Also there was an increasingly higher rate of deterioration, the longer the delay in starting antiaccommodative therapy.

It is known that the maintenance of bifixation (stereopsis of 50 arc seconds or better) is possible in accommodative esotropia patients, if the eyes are straightened during intermittent esotropia stage or shortly after the esodeviation becomes constant. Therefore, if deterioration of ocular alignment occurs, an early and aggressive intervention is necessary to prevent the loss of bifixation.

Patient with high AC/A accommodative esotropia

It is advisable to prescribe +3.0 D executive flat-topped bifocals with bifocal segment bisecting the pupil or touching the lower border of the pupil when the child looks straight ahead. (Figs 41.5A and B). If the full distance correction has been used, +3.0 D bifocal additions enable the patient to fix up to a distance of 33 cm without having to exert accommodation. Spectacle frames with adjustable nose pads are usually not satisfactory because the adjustment does not last long. Frames with a solid nose pad are more satisfactory for this purpose. If bifocals are indicated, it is desirable to prescribe them at the first visit, thus obviating the need to repurchase spectacles following the second visit.

Once bifocal glasses have been obtained, follow-up infants every three months, patients aged 2–5 years every six months and after age 5, yearly. At each follow-up visit, the patient undergoes retinoscopy and a difference of 1 D or more requires, prescribing new glasses.

By the time the child reaches age 5, an attempt should be made to reduce the power of bifocal segment gradually in decrements of 0.75–1.0 D. The aim is to maintain the patient's fusion while leaving him/her esophoric at near. By the time, the patient reaches the age of visual adulthood, i.e. 8 or 9 years, an attempt can be made to remove the bifocals. In a study on long term results of bifocal therapy for accommodative esotropia, Ludwig and associates found that although bifocals were successfully discontinued in a majority of patients at an average age of 9.5 years, a significant percentage still required long-term wear. The only factor that predicted long-term bifocal wear was a relatively high AC/A.

When bifocals are being withdrawn antisuppression exercises and exercises to increase fusional divergence amplitudes may be helpful in maintaining fusion. This is also a time when topical anticholinestrase preparations may be prescribed. Anticholinesterase eyedrops produce an accumulation of acetylcholine at myoneural synapses of the ciliary muscles, which results in a decrease in the nerve impulse required for accommodation. A reduction in accommodative effort then leads to a reduction in accommodative convergence. Phospholine iodide 0.03, 0.06, 0.125 percent solution is the most commonly used drug. It is important that anticholinestrase eyedrops should be stopped at least 6 weeks before succinylcholine, a depolarizing muscle relaxant, which can be used during general anesthesia otherwise fatal apnea can occur.

Treatment of amblyopia

Amblyopia should be treated before any surgery is planned for infantile esotropia or for nonaccommodative esotropia.

Role of Surgery

Surgery for infantile esotropia

The beneficial effect of accurate alignment by age 2 year in infantile esotropia is well established. There is only scanty clinical evidence that alignment before age 1 year, much less before age 6 months may yield a better quality of binocularity

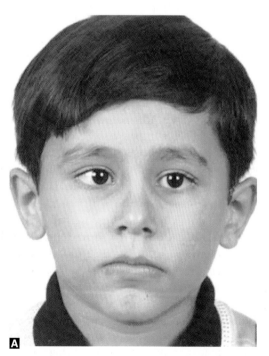
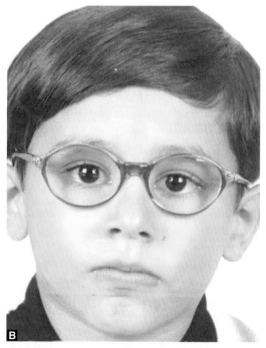

Figs 41.5A and B: High AC/A accommodative esotropia: (A) Right esotropia without glasses (B) Eyes straight with executive flat-topped bifocals bisecting the pupil

than alignment by age of 2 years. Surgery is not advised before 6 months of age. The best therapeutic result that can be expected is the development of peripheral fusion, which will allow a low grade of stereopsis. The advantage of obtaining peripheral fusion is that the eyes have some force other than mechanical alignment holding them together to produce a more stable alignment and cosmesis. Gross stereopsis may be some advantage in judging depth. To achieve this result, the deviation should be surgically reduced to 10 PD or less, which means that infantile esotropia is converted into monofixation syndrome. Approximately 50% of the patients, whose eyes have remained so aligned, will develop a monofixation syndrome and the remainder will end up without fusion or stereopsis. However, before surgery is considered, the diagnosis must be complete and the developmental amblyopia should have been treated. Once accurate measurements, equal fixation preference and a trial of spectacles for hypermetropia in excess of 2.75 D is achieved, there seems no practical reason for delay. Ing reported that the majority of infantile esotropes showed a significant increase in the quantity of the deviation while being followed. Therefore, any delay may actually necessitate greater amounts of surgical treatment.

The surgical treatment can be either unilateral recession of the medial rectus and resection of the lateral rectus or bilateral recessions of the medial rectus muscles. A relative indication for doing unilateral surgery is the developmental amblyopia. In the absence of developmental amblyopia, it appears to make little difference whether one does a unilateral or bilateral surgery. It is true that a recess-resect surgery is likely to produce some incomitance but this incomitance is usually insignificant because it occurs only in extreme positions of gaze. It has been found that a medial rectus recession of 5.5 mm is not necessarily the maximum that can be done. A 7 mm bimedial recession can be done for deviations exceeding 60 PD and it results in only a slight decrease in adduction.

Caputo and associates reported that a preferred alignment shortly after infantile esotropia surgery should be within 10 PD of esotropia because all of their patients who had consecutive exotropia (> 10 PD) were either orthophoric or exotropic (≤ 10 PD) six months after surgery.

Surgery for infantile esotropia associated with myopia

Only 5 to 11% of patients with infantile esotropia are myopic. Shauly and associates reported that surgical results of infantile esotropia were similarly favorable in controls and myopes between 2.00 to 5.0 D, whereas high myopes (greater than −8.0 D) had higher percentage of postoperative under corrections. They suggested that the conventional amount of recession or resection of muscles should be increased in high-myopic cases with infantile esotropia, because less effect is produced per millimeter of recession/resection initially; and in the long-term, the constant stimulus to accommodative convergence apparently causes recurrent esotropia.

Surgery for infantile esotropia associated with developmental delay

About 50% of children with cerebral palsy have congenital strabismus syndrome. It is particularly associated with those children who have hypertonicity and spasticity. They have a more variable surgical effect. Since these patients are likely to get less spastic and less hypertonic as they grow older, surgery should be delayed as long as possible. The only indication for surgery is when the patient is aware of being teased. Surgery, therefore, in these cases should be delayed until at least 5 or 6 years of age.

Pickering and associates reported that developmentally delayed children had an average 5.28 PD more effect per millimeter of surgery, compared to normal children. They suggested that bilateral medial rectus recessions in developmentally delayed children might be better postponed in some cases, deferred for smaller angles or decreased in amount.

Effect of surgery for infantile esotropia on infant development

There is evidence that early surgery for correction of infantile esotropia improves infant development. Rogers and associates reported an improvement in fine motor skills in 35% of such children. Visually directed reaching and grasping increased in 41% of children in their study. This increase in development appears related to enhanced depth perception.

Surgery for nonaccommodative component of partially accommodative esotropia

The nonaccommodative component of mixed esotropia is treated surgically just like basic esotropia and the amount of surgery should be based on the amount of residual esotropia, measured at distance with full hypermetropic correction. Wright and Bruce-Lyle reported that augmented surgery by increasing the amount of surgery provides better postoperative alignment and fusion than standard surgery in esotropia associated with hypermetropia more than 3.0 D. They recommended surgical recessions based on the average of the near deviation with correction and near deviation without correction.

Course of accommodative component after surgery for the non-accommodative portion of the mixed esotropia

Raab reported that the accommodative component after surgery for the nonaccommodative esotropia in mixed esotropia subsides during the first postoperative year in 30% of the patients and thereafter much more gradually so that it remains clinically important in about 50% of such patients for at least 6 years and in a substantial minority for several years, thereafter. Thus, the accommodative esotropia appears to behave the same in pure and in mixed forms.

Surgery for high AC/A ratio esotropia

There are several reports that described the success of a single medial rectus recession in patients with a high AC/A ratio. Procianoy and Justo reported alignment within 10 PD in 96%

of patients with high AC/A ratio and near esotropia of 15 to 35 PD following a 6 to 8 mm unilateral medial rectus recession. However, it must be remembered that surgery in high AC/A ratio esotropia is not the first modality for treatment and it is reserved only for cases that refuse to wear bifocals.

Surgery for nonaccommodative (basic) esotropia

Surgical therapy for basic esotropia is the same as for infantile esotropia. Chamberlain and Sheppard and associates reported the use of a unilateral medial rectus recession of 3.5 to 4.0 mm to treat esodeviations measuring less than 20 PD. A unilateral medial rectus recession of 6 or 6.5 mm can be performed for esotropia of 30 to 35 PD and one can achieve straight eyes or esotropia within 12 PD postoperatively in 80% of the patients.

Surgery for "a" or "v" pattern and dissociated vertical deviation

Surgery for vertical patterns should be done at the time of the bimedial recession or recession-resection surgery. The treatment of DVD is not recommended at an early age because it has a tendency to improve slightly as the patient grows old. The treatment of DVD should be left until the school age and even later if cosmesis is acceptable.

Divergent Squint in a Child

We usually see two types of divergent squint in children: infantile exotropia and intermittent exotropia, the latter being more common than the former.

Infantile Exotropia

Exotropia beginning during the first year of life in otherwise normal, healthy children is rare and occurs much less frequently than infantile esotropia. It may be associated with cerebral palsy or other neurological disease, which should be considered in their evaluation. Infantile exotropia has a number of clinical characteristics similar to infantile esotropia. It is characterized by a large angle (greater than 25 PD) and constant exotropia that begins during the first 6 months of life (Fig. 41.6). Usually the patient has alternate fixation and therefore, strabismic amblyopia is rare. If left untreated, it would most certainly provide the same barrier to the development of single binocular vision as infantile esotropia. Inferior oblique overaction, dissociated vertical deviation and latent nystagmus very often associated with infantile esotropia are also frequently seen in children with infantile exotropia.

Treatment: Treatment of infantile exotropia includes correction of refractive error, treatment of associated amblyopia, if any and an early surgery for alignment of eyes as in infantile esotropia. Hypermetropia in excess of 3 diopters or myopia in excess of 2 diopters requires spectacle correction before surgery. Either bilateral lateral rectus recession or unilateral recess-resect surgery may be performed. The aim of surgical treatment is to align the eyes within 10 PD of orthophoria by the age of 2 years.

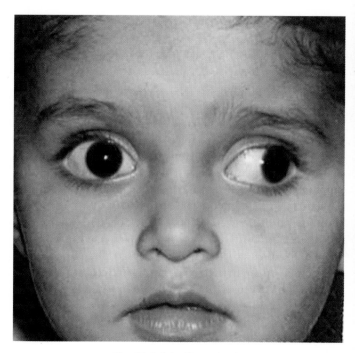

Fig. 41.6: Infantile exotropia

Intermittent Exotropia

Intermittent exotropia is a periodic divergence of the visual axes. The onset of intermittent exotropia is usually in childhood and sometimes in infancy.

Natural history

It generally begins as exophoria and the deviation usually becomes manifest first at distance when the fusional convergence amplitude at distance is exceeded. Later the deviation becomes manifest at near fixation.

The tropic phase of intermittent exotropia most commonly occurs under the conditions of fatigue, illness or visual inattention. The extent to which an exodeviation is controlled by fusion depends not only upon its size but also to a large extent on the general health, attention, alertness and level of anxiety of the patient. Considerable variation in the degree of fusional control from one examination to another is not a surprising finding. Therefore, repeated examinations at different times during the day are required to assess the condition thoroughly. The anxiety associated with impending operation releases extra energy, permitting the patient to keep his eyes aligned and the inexperienced surgeon may get confused. In 75% of the patients, the deviation progresses as revealed by an increase in duration and frequency of the tropic phase. Progression may be related to the decrease in tonic convergence that occurs as a child grows. A manifest deviation may ultimately appear at near. The deviation remains unchanged in 9% of the patients and improves in 16% of the patients without treatment.

When intermittent exotropia first develops in the visually immature child, transient diplopia occurs. However, very quickly suppression and later on anomalous retinal correspondence develops to protect the child from diplopia during the exotropic phase. During the exophoric phase, normal retinal correspondence is present. During the fusional phoric phase, stereopsis is normal or nearly normal. As the frequency and duration of tropic phase increases, some patients experience a decline in stereopsis even during the phoric stage.

Symptoms

Intermittent exotropia usually does not cause headache, asthenopic symptoms or reading problems unless there is also associated convergence insufficiency.

Monocular eye closure in bright sunlight: A patient with intermittent exotropia frequently closes one eye when outdoors in bright sunlight. No definite reason has so far been found for this. It has been thought that the bright sunlight dazzles the retina so that the fusion is interrupted and exophoria breaks into exotropia. At this stage, the diplopia occurs and the patient closes one eye to avoid diplopia. However, it is not certain because diplopia is not a frequent complaint. It has also been suggested that it may be due to decreased fusional convergence amplitude in bright sunlight. In a study by Wiggins and Gunter K von Noorden, it was found that binocular photophobia threshold was significantly lower in those reporting eye closure compared with those who did not. They suggested that monocular eye closure was a mechanism to reduce visual discomfort in bright light and are not related to the avoidance of diplopia. The bright light is the stimulus and eyelid closure the response and it is always the nondominant or deviated eye on which the reflex is expressed. This symptom may or may not improve after surgery. However, sunglasses give the patient relief and avoid the necessity of closing one eye.

Micropsia: Micropsia is a less well-known symptom of intermittent exotropia. These patients use accommodative convergence to control exodeviation at distance and convergence and accommodation are associated with objects appearing smaller.

Clinical Evaluation

Measuring the deviation

The following points should be kept in mind:
- The distance deviation should preferably be measured by asking the patient to fix at a target, placed at greater than 6 meter. This will allow the full deviation to be determined under natural viewing conditions.
- The deviation should always be measured with accommodation controlled by proper refractive correction.
- An accommodative target (a sufficiently small target) is used so that if the patient exerts accommodative convergence to maintain alignment of eyes, the target will appear blurred. Young patients may use voluntary convergence to overcome deviation at near fixation and in some cases the compensatory mechanism may extend to control distance deviation. Unless the target for distance forces the patient to relax accommodation and with it convergence, true deviation at distance may not be revealed. For example, in a

patient with visual acuity of 20/20, measure the angle when the patient reads 20/30 line on the chart. To recognize the letters in 20/30 line, the patient must relax accommodation. Whenever he invokes accommodation, the letters will appear blurred.

Based on the difference between the near and distance deviation, intermittent exotropia has been divided into the following types:

Basic type: The deviation is same for near and distance fixation.

Convergence insufficiency type: The near deviation is at least 15 PD (PD) greater than the distance deviation.

Divergence excess type: The distance deviation is at least 15 PD greater than the near deviation. It can be true divergence excess or pseudodivergence (simulated divergence) excess. To differentiate between these two, occlusion test should be done. In true divergence excess exotropia, there is an actual excessive divergence innervation and there will be no effect of occlusion on deviation, i.e. the distance deviation will still be at least 15 PD greater than near deviation. It is present in only 4% of the patients with divergence excess exotropia. In pseudodivergence excess, the near deviation is obscured by excessive convergence innervation and the distance deviation is at least 15 PD greater than the near deviation on routine testing. However, on occlusion of one eye for 30–45 minutes, the near deviation will be often equal or even greater than that at distance. Majority of the divergence excess exotropia patients have pseudodivergence excess.

Occlusion Test

Occlusion test should be done whenever intermittent exotropia is present only at distance or when the deviation at distance is at least 15 PD greater than that at near. The habitually deviating eye is occluded for at least 30–45 minutes and sometimes even for 24 hours. When the occluding patch is being removed, put the occluder in front of the other eye (Fig. 41.7). Opening of

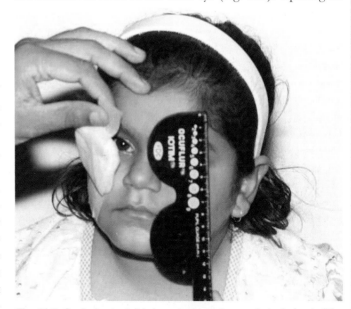

Fig. 41.7: Occlusion test: It is important to put an occluder in front of the other eye when removing the occluding pad

both eyes even for a moment may reinstate the active convergence mechanism by which the child controls the near deviation. Therefore, measure the near deviation with prism and alternate cover test without keeping both eyes open even for a few seconds.

The use of +3.00 D lenses in place of occlusion test to measure deviation at near is not recommended because the occlusion test removes binocular fusion stimuli, whereas +3.0 D lenses provide only an indication of AC/A ratio.

Lateral Incomitance

Lateral incomitance refers to exotropia in which deviation is at least 20% less to each side than that in the primary position for distance fixation. It has been shown that patients with lateral incomitance are more likely to have surgical overcorrection. Some authors have suggested that lateral incomitance must be 5—10 PD or more to be significant. The decrease in the deviation in lateral gaze is asymmetric in most cases. About 50% of the patients with lateral incomitance are known to have limitation of abduction. Moore found significant lateral gaze incomitance of 5 PD in 22% of his patients. However, Repka and Arnoldi reported a true incomitance greater than 5 PD in only 9% of the patients. They reported that significant lateral incomitance could be induced in every patient by improperly positioning the neutralizing prism. They recommended 300 of head turn and placement of the neutralizing prism over the adducting eye rather than on the abducting eye. This will fix the amount of abduction of the abducting eye at 300, an amount unlikely to encounter end gaze mechanical limitation. They also suggested that the neutralizing prism should be placed with its posterior surface perpendicular to the direction of the fixation target. Even a small rotation of prism from this correct position can yield significant artifactual lateral incomitance. Lateral incomitance can be ignored in children under the age of 8 years and it seems to disappear after surgery for the deviation in the primary position.

Vertical Deviation

Vertical deviations are present in 16 to 52% of patients with intermittent exotropia. It is present in most instances at distance fixation and not at near fixation. It is caused by overaction of the inferior oblique muscle in 1/3rd of the patients, whereas in 2/3rd of the patients no definite cause is found. Davies advised that in those cases in which no cause for the vertical component could be found, the distance hypertropia should be ignored as it usually disappears after the horizontal surgical procedure. "A" or "V" patterns and dissociated vertical deviation can also occur in intermittent exotropia and can also be encountered subsequently in patients operated for intermittent exotropia.

Sensory Adaptations

Routine sensory testing should be done before other dissociating tests, such as acuity testing or prism cover test. The patient with intermittent exotropia suppresses the deviating eye while the eye is tropic. Suppression is then switched off when the eyes are straight. In patients with divergence excess exotropia, a latent strabismus at near fixation often coexists with a manifest strabismus at distance fixation. Thus, normal binocular vision is constantly being reinforced and sensory adaptations are infrequent or when present, are only superficially established. Stereo acuity deteriorates concomitantly with loss of fusional control in patients with intermittent exotropia.

Refractive Errors

Most recent studies have shown that the distribution of refractive errors in exotropes resembles that in the non-strabismic population.

Treatment

Correction of refractive error: A cycloplegic refraction should be done. Myopic patients with exodeviation should be prescribed full correction. Children with exodeviation and hypermetropia less than 2.0 D are not given the correction. In older presbyopic patients, near prescription may cause deviation to become manifest. In such patients, the weakest possible aid for comfortable near vision is prescribed.

Use of minus lenses: The use of 2.00 to 4.00 D overcorrecting minus lenses, either in upper segment bifocals for divergence excess or in lower segment bifocals for convergence insufficiency have been tried to reduce exodeviation by stimulating accommodative convergence. This form of treatment often results in asthenopia and is not recommended. However, it can be used only as a temporary measure in patients with high AC/A ratio.

Base in prisms: Base in prisms can be used to enforce bifoveal stimulation. Only one half to one third of the deviation is prismatically corrected. However, image distortion by prisms makes compliance a problem.

Part-time occlusion: Part-time occlusion of the preferred eye for 3 to 5 hours a day is expected to convert manifest deviation into latent in about 40% of the patients by increasing the fusional convergence amplitude. If there is no improvement after four months, occlusion is discontinued.

Orthoptic exercise: Orthoptics should not be used as a substitute for surgery but rather as a supplement. It has not been proved that surgical results are functionally superior to those who have not received orthoptics or that surgery can be avoided altogether by using this form of treatment.

Surgical Treatment

Aim of treatment: The aim of treatment is to eradicate suppression and reduce or eliminate the exotropia. The only method that currently appears to be successful in eliminating suppression is to operate when the child is young, preferably under 4 years of age and prevent any recurrence of the exotropia that stimulates the suppression. Even an exotropia of as little as 5

PD can trigger suppression. One can seldom get reliable repeatable measurements before the age of 2 years and therefore, if possible, surgery should be postponed until then. Patients operated on before the age of 4 years have a better prognosis than those operated on at age 6 years or older when the suppression is more entrenched. The primary goal of the surgery is to provide the opportunity for normalization of binocular functions by restoring a favorable alignment. To attain this goal, one must correct the largest exotropic deviation measured.

Indications for Surgery

- Amount of deviation: If the surgery is indicated for functional reasons, the angle of deviation should be at least 15 PD for distance or near. From a cosmetic point of view, 15 PD exotropia is seldom significant and cosmetic surgery is usually not performed unless the deviation measures at least 20−25 PD.
- If exotropic phase is present at least 50% of the times.
- If the following signs of progression are present at the time of initial examination or develop when the patient is under observation:
  − Increase in size and frequency of deviation
  − Gradual loss of fusional control and deteriorating stereopsis
  − Development of suppression as evidenced by the absence of diplopia during the manifest phase of deviation.
  − Definite evidence of defective binocular single vision existing.
- If the patient has asthenopic symptoms.

Choice of Surgical Procedure

Most surgeons agree that bilateral lateral rectus recession should be performed for the true divergence excess exotropia and recession-resection on the nondominant eye for the convergence insufficiency type of exotropia. There is no general agreement regarding the choice of procedure for the basic and pseudodivergence excess type of intermittent exotropia. In these patients, it is surgeon's choice as bilateral lateral rectus recession and unilateral recession-resection provides equally good results. Surgeon should anticipate a few PD of overcorrection with recession-resection procedure and a 10−15 PD overcorrection with bilateral lateral rectus recession.

Many authors have reported good surgical success with unilateral lateral rectus recession 6−8 mm for intermittent exotropia up to 20 PD. Feretis and associates reported more satisfactory motor and functional results by performing 11.5 mm to 12 mm unilateral lateral rectus recession in patients with 14−16 PD intermittent exotropia. The overcorrection obtained by this method was 4−6 PD.

Where to Overcorrect?

Because of the tendency of an exodeviation to drift postoperatively, small overcorrection of 10 PD to 15 PD in immediate postoperative period is desirable in a visually mature patient (over age 4 years) as this tends to stabilize the functional results and thus, it stabilizes the eventual alignment of eyes. Children with intermittent exotropia have already developed single binocular vision and have the potential for normal stereopsis. If one overcorrects a visually immature child (below age 4 years), it will lead to monofixation syndrome, which may lead to amblyopia and loss of stereopsis.

Overcorrection is not predictable. In one series, where an overcorrection was attempted in every patient, only 37% were overcorrected postoperatively. In another series, where overcorrection was avoided, 40% were overcorrected.

Where to Undercorrect ?

In a visually immature child, a slight undercorrection should be attempted because there is a greater danger of monofixation syndrome in the slightly overcorrected esotropic condition than that in slightly undercorrected exotropic condition.

A patient with lateral incomitance has the risk of overcorrection. Therefore, one should avoid bilateral lateral rectus recession in these patients and also reduce the amount of surgery by 1 mm each in recession-resection procedure.

Results of Surgery

The postoperative status of 156 patients operated for intermittent exotropia revealed microexotropia in 32%, subnormal binocular vision in 50% and a complete sensory cure in only 17% of the patients. In another series, patients who were orthophoric or slightly esophoric at 33 cm and 6 meters were examined by asking the patient to fixate at a target at the end of 25 meter corridor, it was found that most of the patients had small constant exotropia. Hence, complete restoration of normal and stable binocular vision in patients with intermittent exotropia presents a major challenge.

Factors Affecting Surgical Results

The age of the patient at the onset of intermittent exotropia and at the time of surgery has not been found to affect the motor surgical outcome. Preoperative sensory changes also affect the surgical result. In a study by Lee associates, patients with diplopia had a surgical success rate of 92%, compared to 74% in those with suppression. They suggested that surgery should be performed before diplopia changes to suppression, which represents an abnormal sensory change in binocular vision.

In a recent study by Abroms and associates, it was found that patients with intermittent or constant exotropia had a significant greater chance of achieving superior sensory outcome (a stereoacuity better than 60 seconds of arc), if they were surgically aligned before 7 years of age or before 5 years of strabismus duration or with intermittent as compared with constant exotropia.

ADULT STRABISMUS

An adult presenting with strabismus may have its onset in childhood or later on. It can broadly be divided into the following groups:

i. Untreated childhood strabismus
ii. Residual strabismus
iii. Consecutive strabismus
iv. Sensory strabismus
v. Paralytic strabismus
vi. Restrictive strabismus.

Scott and associates classified adult strabismus into two groups. If the onset of strabismus was before the age of 9 years, it was termed as the before visual maturity (BVM) group and if the onset of strabismus was after the age of 9 years, it was termed as the after visual maturity (AVM) group. They found that the horizontal strabismus in adults usually had the onset before visual maturity and the paretic or restrictive strabismus usually had the onset after visual maturity. In a study of strabismus in patients over the age of 60 years, Magramm and Schlossman found that the strabismus was of adult onset in 71% and of childhood onset in 29% of the patients. Paralytic, restrictive and sensory factors were the main etiologies in the adult onset group. The number of esodeviations was equal to the number of exodeviations, whereas in childhood, esodeviations far outnumber the exodeviations. Strabismus following cataract surgery and retinal detachment surgery form a unique group in older patients presenting with strabismus.

Special Points in Clinical Presentation

Asthenopia

If an adult with strabismus reports symptoms of asthenopia, it is important to ask how long the symptoms have been present. If they have only been present a few months in-patient with childhood-onset strabismus, it is extremely unlikely that the asthenopic problems will have anything to do with strabismus. Similarly, if the patient has no fusion, it is generally safe to assume that asthenopic symptoms are unrelated to strabismus.

Adults with intermittent exotropia commonly present with visual symptoms, such as diplopia, headache and difficulty in near work and eye fatigue. Occasionally, they may say they are aware of trying to control the position of the eye and this annoys and tires them. This is because convergence mechanism becomes relatively less active as the patient grows old. Therefore, exophoria at near is more difficult to control. The patients having heavy demands for near work have more visual symptoms. This is in sharp contrast to children with intermittent exotropia where the visual problems are rare and they present mostly with squint or history of closing of one eye in sunlight. Diplopia is uncommon in childhood.

Symptomatic Alternation

Some patients who spontaneously alternate fixation and have no fusion will complain of an apparent jump in position of the object of regard, in the process of changing conscious fixation from one to the other eye. This may cause problems in driving, reading or playing ball games.

Special Points in Assessing Adults with Strabismus

- Every patient must be refracted.
- Measurement of the deviation should be performed in all positions of gaze at distance fixation with and without full optical correction in place. Also one should measure the deviation at near fixation with and without full optical correction in place. If a patient has no fusion and an amblyopic eye, only an uncorrected refractive error (especially hypermetropia) of the fixing eye may affect alignment. No matter what the uncorrected refractive error is in the deviating nonfixing eye, it is irrelevant to the alignment of the eyes. Therefore, there is no need not to prescribe refractive correction for such an eye.
- Once the strabismus has been measured with the prism and cover test, the accuracy of the measurement should be checked by using a prism until the patient first sees double. This will confirm the exact amount of strabismus present in that gaze position. These patients immediately experience diplopia once the deviation becomes overcorrected and the image of the fixation target crosses even one prism diopter over the retinal midline.
- A larger than normal binocular visual field is present in exotropia and a smaller binocular visual field in esotropia. The reduction in the binocular field of vision associated with the straightening of a large angle exotropia may be noticeable to the patient and should be explained before surgery. A bonus of straightening a marked esotropia without fusion is an expansion of the binocular visual field.
- If a patient has an exotropia in excess of 35 PD in the primary position, the eyes should be examined specifically in down gaze. If there is a marked increase in exotropia, it is almost always associated with overaction of the superior oblique muscles. It is thought that if the eyes have been markedly exotropic for many years, the superior oblique muscles take up the slack and are somewhat contracted, resulting in the increased exotropia in down gaze. These cases will require tenotomy of both superior oblique muscles. If attention is not directed to the overacting superior oblique muscles in such a situation, recurrence of the exotropia is very common.
- If one plans adjustable suture strabismus surgery, make a note in the chart whether the postoperative adjustment can be done without the patient's glasses or whether glasses make a difference to the deviation and must be worn for the adjustment.
- There is a high incidence of concomitant medical disorders in some of the older patients. This should be an important consideration in planning the type of anesthesia. Many of these patients may require local anesthesia in lieu of general anesthesia.

Surgery for Adult Strabismus

Compared with children, adults with strabismus make very demanding patients. They perceive even the tiniest cosmetic defect. They are actually aware of any sensory change, such as diplopia, that may be precipitated by altering the alignment of their eyes. Some even expect to acquire fusion despite having the congenital strabismus syndrome. Therefore, it is important to ask the patient the question "What are you hoping to achieve with treatment?" This usually clarifies the patient's expectation: cosmetic improvement, relief of diplopia or binocular vision with fusion and stereopsis. Three main reasons to correct adult strabismus have been listed:

i. Restoration of fusion and elimination of diplopia.
ii. Expansion of binocular visual fields in patients with esotropia.
iii. Improvement in psychosocial functioning.

Restoration of Binocular Fusion and Elimination of Diplopia

Adults with intermittent exotropia usually seek treatment for visual symptoms, including diplopia, headache and difficulty in near work and ocular fatigue. Major indication for strabismus surgery in patients older than 60 years is diplopia and asthenopia. The restoration of binocular fusion and elimination of diplopia is accepted as a reason to correct strabismus in adults.

It has been demonstrated that strabismus surgery in adults can produce both restoration of alignment and binocular function. Kushner found that 85% of adults with strabismus who were well aligned postoperatively demonstrated binocularity at six weeks postoperatively by the Bagolini's glasses test regardless of the type of deviation present preoperatively, the duration of strabismus, or the depth of amblyopia in the deviating eye. He stated that this was a functional improvement postoperatively as compared with preoperative levels. Morris and associates reported that with good alignment, sensory fusion could be obtained in cases of long standing strabismus in adults. They stated that the goal of strabismus surgery is to align the eyes as close to orthotropia as possible to allow fusion to develop. Scott and associates also found some degree of sensory fusion postoperatively in many of their patients with adult strabismus with onset before visual maturity and in 92% of their patients with onset of strabismus after visual maturity. Even 29% of their patients with infantile esotropia had some sensory fusion. These observations indicate that restoration of alignment, elimination of diplopia and sensory fusion are functional benefits that can be obtained through strabismus surgery in adults. Clearly, adult strabismus is more than just a cosmetic problem and treatment is worthwhile.

Expansion of Binocular Visual Fields in Patients with Esotropia

Wortham and Greenwald recorded preoperative and postoperative binocular visual fields in esotropic patients and concluded that there was an expansion of the binocular visual fields that was approximately equal to the change of the strabismus deviation. This expansion of the visual fields occurred irrespective of the present of amblyopia. Kushner also had a similar observation. Operating on adults with exotropia may produce a dissatisfied patient because of the loss of the supernormal visual field experienced by patients with exotropia and this must be explained to the patient.

Improvement in Psychosocial Functioning

Satterfield and associates studied the psychosocial aspects of strabismus in adults. Using the Hopkins Symptom Checklist, they found that adults with uncorrected strabismus had higher levels of distress than the normal population. Strabismus had an adverse effect on their livelihood by affecting their ability to obtain work, maintain a good self-image, maintain good interpersonal relationships and perform in school, work and sport activities throughout their lives. Clearly, the psychosocial aspects of strabismus should be a major factor in dealing with patients with strabismus. The correction of adult strabismus offers the opportunity for potential improvement in binocular fusion, expanded binocular visual fields and improved psychosocial functioning.

Postoperative Diplopia in Adult Strabismus

Scott and associates reported on the prevalence of diplopia preoperatively and postoperatively in adults with strabismus. They demonstrated that diplopia was not uncommon, either preoperatively or at some time in the postoperative period. Persistent diplopia in adults following strabismus surgery, however, was uncommon. They found that though 39% of the patients experienced diplopia sometime in the immediate postoperative period, only 1.4% of the patients had it at the last postoperative visit. They concluded that the fear of producing diplopia following strabismus surgery in adults is not well founded and the risk is very low.

Surgical Overcorrection for Intermittent Exotropia in Adults

It has been shown that adult patients with intermittent exotropia frequently have recurrence of 10 to 15 PD within a few months of surgery. This has resulted in some surgeons in advising a deliberate overcorrection in order to leave the patient with 10 PD of esotropia immediately after surgery. However, it leads to diplopia. Therefore, it is essential to warn patients before surgery about the inevitable occurrence of diplopia postoperatively, if they are esotropic. If esotropia does not resolve with the eye becoming slightly exotropic again, permanent diplopia will result. If esotropia persists, the patient has the option of base out stick-on Fresnel prisms while awaiting resolution. Spontaneous resolution is unlikely, if the esotropia has persisted unchanged for at least 3 months. These patients will require surgical correction of esotropia.

Stability of Strabismus Surgery in Adults

Although the alignment obtained by surgery in adults without fusion tends to be more stable than in children, it is important to inform the patient that although the eyes appear approximately straight immediately after surgery, the deviation may sometimes recur in as little as a few days to a few months. Conversely, the eyes may remain well aligned for the rest of the patient's life. There are no indicators that help to predict, which result will occur. Recurrence is particularly common after surgery for exotropia in patients without fusion.

Central Fusion Disruption

Adults can lose their ability to fuse and this gives rise to intractable diplopia. Loss of the motor ability to maintain sensory fusion occurs occasionally following severe head trauma. A similar type of fusion defect may occur following improvement of vision in cases of unilateral sensory deprivation due to cataract or severe corneal scarring. The longer the duration of the deprivation, the most likely this is to occur. Improving the vision in a previously sensorially deprived eye may make the patient aware of intractable diplopia, even if vision is restored to the same level as that of the unaffected eye. A patient with central fusion disruption is able to obtain momentary superimposition of the diplopic images. However, there is a complete inability to maintain fusion; the images typically bob-up and down as if the eyes are trying to avoid fusion.

Recovery is unfortunately rare. It is very difficult but not impossible to regain fusion in cases, resulting from unilateral sensory deprivation. The treatment involves providing the best possible visual acuity in such eye and then superimposing the images from each eye by adjustable strabismus surgery and prisms. However, patients in this situation still have functional limitations and occlusion of one eye may be necessary to enable the patient to function normally.

BOTULINUM TOXIN IN THE MANAGEMENT OF STRABISMUS

There are seven antigenically distinct forms of botulinum neurotoxin (type A to G) produced by the bacterium *Clostridium botulinum* that are among the most powerful neuroparalytic agents known. Botulinum toxin A is easily made in culture. Scott in 1978 introduced the use of botulinum toxin type A injection into the extraocular muscle as an effective alternative to conventional surgery for strabismus. Since then, it has been used in the management of various forms of strabismus.

Mechanism of Action

The botulinum neurotoxins acts primarily on the peripheral cholinergic synapses, where by inhibiting the release of the neurotransmitter acetylcholine, they cause the widespread muscular paralysis. It is now believed that at least three steps are involved in the inhibitory action of botulinum toxins. First step is a binding step whereby the toxin attaches rapidly to the presynaptic nerve membrane. Second step, is an internalization step in which toxin crosses the presynaptic membrane and the third step is, whereby toxin inhibits the release of neurotransmitter substance, acetylcholine.

Preparation of Type A Toxin

Cultures of *C. botulinum* are grown up under anerobic conditions. When the maximum yield of toxin has been attained usually after 72 hours, the toxin is harvested by centrifugation after acidifying the culture. The precipitated crude toxin is redissolved and purified by a series of procedures involving ammonium sulphate precipitation and ion-exchange chromatography. The potency of the purified toxin is assessed and an appropriate quantity of the purified toxin solution is added to a diluent containing lactose and human serum albumin. The diluent provides protection to the toxin during freeze-drying and also acts as a bulking agent for the freeze-dried product. Prior to freeze-drying, the diluted toxin is dispensed into vials and then it is freeze-dried. The freeze-dried toxin retains stability even when kept at 4°C for not less than 3 years.

Technique of Injection

Botulinum toxin is dissolved in sterile isotonic saline and is injected into the extraocular muscle with a specially constructed needle electrode used with an amplifier to provide auditory information to the surgeon regarding the electromyographic (EMG) response. The surgeon places the needle at the muscle insertion and advances it into the muscle under direct vision until a suitable EMG response is obtained. The injection consists of 0.05 to 0.15 ml of a suitable dilution of the toxin.

Topical anesthetic drops provide anesthesia. Children can be treated using a small dose of intravenous ketamine to provide temporary sedation but this agent frequently causes nightmares and hallucinations.

Onset and Duration of Action of Botulinum Toxin

Botulinum toxin produces a dose-related, temporary paralysis of the injected muscle, which comes on about three days after injection and the maximum effect is roughly seven days after injection. The effect lasts for about 8–12 weeks. The paralysis results in a temporary overcorrection of the ocular deviation. A considerable alignment change persists for years after the paralysis is gone. The tendency for the eyes to return toward the original deviation over a period of months or years can be easily managed by repeat injection of the toxin.

Side Effects

There have been no systemic side effects of botulinum chemodenervation. The toxin may spill over to the adjacent muscles and may result in transient vertical deviation. The levator muscle is very sensitive to botulinum toxin and ptosis is a common occurrence but it is entirely reversible. Only occasionally a permanent damage to the injected muscle may occur.

Uses of Botulinum Toxin in Squint Management

Sixth Nerve Palsy

In acute sixth nerve palsy, botulinum toxin injection into the medial rectus muscle temporarily relieves diplopia and prevents contracture of the medial rectus while the patient awaits recovery. In chronic sixth nerve palsy, a transposition procedure may be enhanced by botulinum injection into the medial rectus rather than recession. This reduces the risk of anterior segment ischemia.

Adult Strabismus

Botulinum toxin has been used to treat concomitant horizontal strabismus (primary, residual and consecutive), sensory strabismus, postretinal detachment surgery strabismus and dysthyroid ophthalmopathy in adults.

Childhood Strabismus

There is less literature on the use of botulinum toxin in childhood strabismus. This is partly because the electromyography guided injection technique requires a local anesthetic and is inapplicable under general anesthesia. The technique can be used with local anesthetic and intravenous ketamine in children, but ketamine frequently causes nightmares and hallucinations. Also, side effects of the botulinum toxin due to spread to other extraocular muscles and the levator are commoner in children because of the small orbit. Several authors have treated essential infantile esotropia with botulinum injection. Campos and associates reported that botulinum toxin could be effective in essential infantile esotropia when children are treated by age 7 months. Tejedor and Rodriguez compared reoperation and botulinum toxin injection, in the management of children who needed treatment after surgery for acquired esotropia. They reported that botulinum injection was as effective as reoperation in these children.

Nystagmus

Botulinum toxin A has been used to treat oscillopsia due to intractable nystagmus in multiple sclerosis.

Current Status of Botulinum Toxin in Strabismus Management

The role of botulinum toxin in strabismus management is clear in muscle paresis and other situations where binocular potential is good. However, more thoughtful and well-designed studies are needed to clearly define its role in other situations.

Surgical Treatment of Strabismus

Vinita Singh

Strabismus surgery is distinct, firstly because the movement of the tissue is the essential component of the final goal of the surgery and, secondly, because at present time and in the near future there is a small chance that further surgery may be necessary. It is therefore important to design the surgical technique so as to avoid excessive restrictions on the eye, minimally disturb the strength and leverage of muscles, preserve tissue planes, and maintain a record of preoperative details thus allowing necessary surgical reintervention to be easily accomplished.

Strabismus surgery is one of the frequent types of ophthalmic surgery. The variability in the surgical results, which is seemingly beyond the surgeon's control, is a cause of dilemma amongst most ophthalmologists. Some of this variability can rightly be attributed to unpredictable patient responses, but a substantial amount can be attributed to measurement and judgment errors and variations in the surgical technique. With advances in diagnostic methods, better understanding of different forms of strabismus, functional interplay between various muscle groups, availability of better and safer suture materials and needles, surgical procedures have changed remarkably specially with reference to the performance of bolder surgery and an attempt to correct large deviations and combined horizontal and vertical deviations with a one stage procedure. Use of adjustable sutures permits bolder and more accurate surgery in unpredictable situations.

AIMS OF STRABISMUS SURGERY

The aim of surgery for strabismus is to restore the alignment of the visual axes so as to facilitate binocular single vision. Strabismus surgery has primarily a "mechanical" effect, to alter the position of the globe in the orbit and to realign the visual axes. It has no direct "sensory" or "innervational" effects. These are secondary to binocular sensory adaptations of the eyes to the surgically created new stimulus situation, which is expected to restore comfortable binocular single vision and strengthen binocular functions. When functional recovery is

difficult or impossible then cosmetic reasons call for a surgical intervention.

In order to avoid postoperative frustration, the purpose and achievable realistic goal should be clearly defined prior to surgery. While a satisfactory cosmetic appearance can almost always be obtained with strabismus surgery, functional cures are more difficult and sometimes impossible. Complete functional cure implies freely mobile eyes with ability to maintain ocular alignment in all directions of gaze and have binocular single vision with fusion and stereopsis. Achievement of at least some degree of binocularity is an important part of the goal both functionally and cosmetically, for the ability of both eyes to work together stimulates them to remain aligned and hence ensures the stability of the surgical result.

Indications for Surgery

Surgical treatment is indicated in patients of squint to restore ocular alignment for:

i. Functional reasons in patients in whom the deviation precludes the development of binocular functions or interferes with comfortable binocular vision.

ii. Cosmetic reasons in patients in whom the deviation causes a cosmetic concern. Cosmetic blemish due to misaligned eyes can be a considerable social and emotional handicap, and strabismus surgery for cosmetic reasons alone is certainly justified.

iii. Correcting the compensatory head posture even in the absence of obvious strabismus, such as in paretic squints, retraction syndromes.

iv. Eliminating globe retraction in some cases of Duane's syndrome.

Patient Evaluation

When the need for surgery has been established, the evaluation of the patient is done for the following:

i. To define the fusion potential and the achievable realistic goal in terms of the stability of ocular alignment, binocularity and restoration of ocular motility. This should be clearly communicated to the patient and attendants, so as to avoid postoperative frustrations to both, the surgeon as well as the patient.

ii. To determine the most appropriate surgical approach. To alter the position of the eyes, the action of a muscle can be weakened, strengthened or modified by altering its position on the globe. These procedures may be performed singly or in combination. To determine the most appropriate surgical approach and muscle or muscles to be operated upon, it is necessary to carefully assess all the clinical findings and then decide the type and amount of operation on an individual basis rather than routinely applying one or the other procedure.

The following factors influence the above:

The age of onset, presentation and duration of squint: It is generally agreed that children with congenital strabismus should be treated as early as possible if there is to be any chance of gaining even limited binocular vision. When strabismus is acquired or intermittent, the chances of regaining at least some binocular vision with appropriate treatment are generally higher. The potential for the restoration of binocular vision decreases with the increased duration of strabismus. Untreated infants lose this potential quickly, whereas strabismic adults and older children retain at least some potential for binocular vision for many years.

Visual acuity: Uncorrected and corrected visual acuity should be evaluated for each eye separately, as well as binocularly. All attempts should be made to attain equal or near equal vision in both eyes. This is important for achieving predictable and stable surgical results. In the presence of intractable amblyopia the surgical results are unpredictable, for the eye may have a tendency to revert back to its original position, or the deviation may get over corrected. In such patients the aim is to have a cosmetically acceptable residual angle that is slightly convergent.

Binocular functions: Extraocular muscle surgery can only restore the alignment of the two eyes but the most important component of the neuromuscular apparatus that maintains this position is the binocular fusion faculty. If the estimate of the state of fusion faculty, called the fusion potential, is high then even an approximate surgical correction may be sufficient to achieve stable ocular alignment with binocular single vision. If on the other hand, the estimate of the fusion potential is low then the postoperative ocular alignment may be unpredictable and unstable.

The fixating eye: Preoperatively, wherever possible, an attempt should be made to make the patient able to alternate. If monocular surgery is planned in the absence of amblyopia then it is preferred to operate on the dominant eye, as this is the eye that governs the binocular motor reflexes.

Angle of strabismus: Although the degree of correction per millimeter of muscle surgery is variable, the amount and behavior of the preoperative angle of strabismus is an important deciding factor for the surgical approach and the amount of surgery. The deviation is measured for near and distance fixing each eye and in various directions of gaze. It is attempted to correct the deviation present when the preferred eye is used, as this is the eye that governs the innervations being sent to each eye. Medial rectus surgery is preferred if the near deviation is significantly more and lateral rectus surgery is considered when the distance deviation is more. A or V pattern with horizontal strabismus can be corrected by combining recess/resect surgery with up/down displacement, slant procedures or oblique muscle surgery. Surgery is aimed to correct the basic deviation, regardless of whether it is intermittent or constant.

Refraction: Any clinically significant refractive error is corrected and a period of several weeks is allowed for adaptation to the new optical correction before determining the amount of deviation that needs to be corrected surgically.

Ocular motility: A preoperative estimation of both uniocular (ductions) and binocular (versions) movements is necessary to plan the surgery so as to normalize the excursions of the eyes and as far as possible to symmetrize and restore ocular alignment in all directions of gaze.

Diplopia charting: Diplopia charting is helpful in identifying the areas of maximum diplopia, under or overacting muscles and deciding the most appropriate surgical procedure which would restore binocular single vision in maximum area of the practical binocular field.

Forced duction test: Forced duction test is performed to assess the passive movements. If it reveals mechanical restrictions, not anticipated preoperatively, the original surgical plan may have to be modified on the table at the time of surgery.

It is obvious from the above account that due to several variables affecting the surgical plan and outcome, we cannot have a blanket formula applicable to every patient. However, if surgery is planned on the basis of individual findings in each patient, and supported by appropriate preoperative and postoperative binocular training, then a high percentage of merely immediate satisfactory cosmetic realignments would change into lasting good results.

ANATOMICAL CONSIDERATIONS

Before discussing the surgical procedures it is necessary to consider some anatomical aspects that are important for the safety and success of extraocular muscle surgery. As ocular motility is an important outcome in strabismus surgery, it is essential to know and respect the structures that allow it. The movement of the eye within the orbit is brought about by six extraocular muscles, four recti and two obliques for each eye. In addition, an intricate fascial network, comprising of Tenon's capsule, intermuscular septum, and muscle capsule separates the globe from the orbital fat and provides smooth slippery surfaces for the free movement of the globe within the sub-Tenon's space. Scarring of any of these structures will result in restricted motility. Let us first study the location of the extraocular muscles on the globe and tissue planes that must be passed to reach them and restored during surgery so as to minimize complications and allow free ocular motility.

Extraocular Muscles

The four recti originate in the orbital apex at the annulus of Zinn (Fig. 42.1), then pass forward though the orbital fat and sub-Tenon's space and insert onto the sclera. The usual insertion width and limbus to insertion distance of the extraocular muscles are illustrated in Fig. 42.2.

The superior oblique is the longest and the thinnest extraocular muscle. It originates from the annulus of Zinn and then courses forward along the nasal orbital wall to reach the trochlea. It becomes tendinous approximately 10 mm behind the trochlea. After passing through the trochlear pulley it courses posteriorly and laterally to penetrate the Tenon's capsule about 3 mm nasal to the superior rectus. As it passes under the superior rectus it fans out on its way to its broad (7–15 mm) insertion onto the superior temporal quadrant posterior to the equator of the globe (Figs 42.2 and 42.3). The broad insertion gives the superior oblique its three functions, viz. incyclotorsion, depression and abduction. Hooking the compact superior oblique tendon in the sub-Tenon's space nasal to the superior rectus, prior to its fanning out will prevent the risk of the incomplete capture of the tendon.

The inferior oblique originates from the anterior nasal orbital floor just posterior to the orbital margin and passes posteriorly and laterally, penetrating the Tenon's at the lateral border of the inferior rectus. In the sub-Tenon's space it continues in the same direction around the globe (Fig. 42.4), passing under the lateral rectus to reach its insertion into the sclera

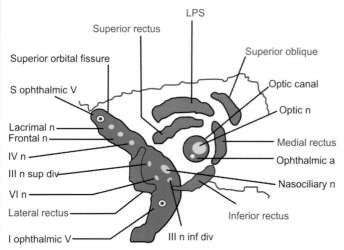

Fig. 42.1: Topographic arrangement of muscle origins in the annulus of Zinn (right orbit)

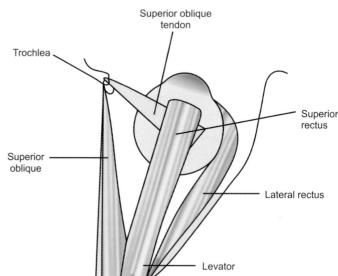

Fig. 42.3: Superior view of the right orbit

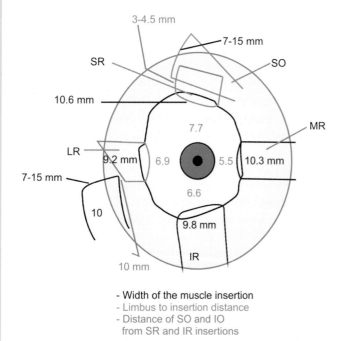

- Width of the muscle insertion
- Limbus to insertion distance
- Distance of SO and IO
  from SR and IR insertions

Fig. 42.2: Sites, shapes and average sizes of the insertions of extraocular muscles of the right eye

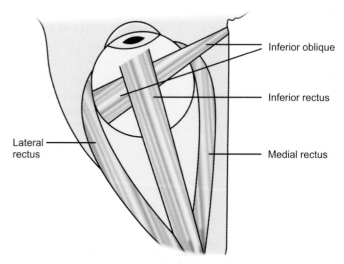

Fig. 42.4: Inferior view of the right orbit

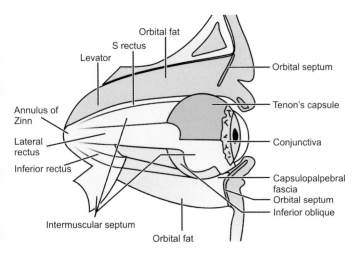

Orbital fat
S rectus
Levator
Orbital septum

Annulus of Zinn
Tenon's capsule

Lateral rectus
Conjunctiva

Inferior rectus
Capsulopalpebral fascia
Orbital septum
Inferior oblique

Intermuscular septum
Orbital fat

Fig. 42.5: Fascia covering the eye and extraocular muscles

just anterior to the macular area (Fig. 42.2). The posterior fibers are responsible for elevation and abduction and the anterior fibers for excyclotorsion.

Fascial Coverings

The fascial coverings around the globe and extraocular muscles comprise of the Tenon's capsule, intermuscular septum, muscle capsule and orbital fat (Fig. 42.5).

Tenon's Capsule

Tenon's capsule is a dense white avascular fascial layer of elastic connective tissue surrounding the eye and extraocular muscles in the anterior orbit, and the globe in the posterior orbit. The extraocular muscles originate outside the Tenon's capsule and penetrate it prior to the insertion onto the globe. The recti enter the Tenon's posterior to the equator while the obliques enter it anterior to the equator of the globe. The muscle capsule is attached to a sleeve of Tenon's capsule at its point of penetration, allowing the movement of the muscle through the Tenon's capsule. The inner surface of the Tenon's capsule is smooth and opposed to the sclera, posteriorly, and muscle capsule and intermuscular septum, anteriorly. Strabismus surgery is performed on the anterior portion of the muscle contained within the sub-Tenon's space.

Intermuscular Septum

The intermuscular septum is a sheet of thin transparent, avascular tissue extending from a muscle's capsule to the capsule of adjacent extraocular muscle. It lies between the anterior Tenon's capsule and the sclera and forms a fascial plane joining the extraocular muscles. Anteriorly it fuses with the Tenon's capsule about 3 mm from the limbus. This combined fascial plane then fuses with the conjunctiva about 1 mm from the limbus. This has important implications for the strabismus surgeon. While doing the forced duction test it is safer to grasp the conjunctiva near the limbus where a stronger structure exists. This minimizes the chance of conjunctival tear. An incision at the limbus, where these three structures are fused, will immediately expose the correct plane for hooking the muscle. Whereas in a posterior incision the conjunctiva, Tenon's and the intermuscular septum will have to be passed separately to reach the correct plane for extraocular muscle surgery.

Muscle Capsule

Surrounding each muscle and its tendon is an avascular connective tissue capsule. It provides a smooth surface to the extraocular muscle. Its inner surface is associated intimately with muscular blood vessels. Opening of the muscle capsule may result in hemorrhage in the surgical field; it would also leave an exposed muscle surface thus increasing the risk of adhesions.

There are attachments between the muscle capsules of the oblique and the rectus muscles as they cross. The medial rectus, the strongest extraocular muscle, has a relatively straight course, and has no direct capsular attachment to an oblique muscle. It is, therefore, at the greatest risk of slipping back into the posterior orbit through the Tenon's.

A potential space exists between the muscle and its capsule. It is, therefore, possible for a muscle to slip within its own capsule. Care must therefore be taken to pass the muscle suture through the entire thickness of the muscle substance rather than superficially where it may engage only the muscle capsule and subsequently result in the slippage of the muscle.

Check Ligaments

These are sheets of elastic connective tissue extending from the muscle to the overlying Tenon's. These are seen easily during surgery when the Tenon's capsule is retracted to expose a rectus muscle that has been hooked. These have to be severed to allow the free mobility of the muscle postoperatively in its altered position.

The Orbital Fat

The orbital fat and its framework of connective tissue, septa, provide a firm cushion to support the globe and yet allow it to move freely within the orbit. Anteriorly it comes forward to about 10 mm of the limbus. The Tenon's capsule separates it from the muscle capsule and the intermuscular septum. An inadvertent opening of the Tenon's more than 10 mm from the limbus will allow the orbital fat to herniate in the sub-Tenon's space, where it tends to incite an intense inflammatory reaction resulting in scaring and adhesions, causing the eye to be pulled in a deviated position with restricted motility. Subsequent surgery to restore the fascial planes is difficult and almost always unsuccessful.

Capsulopalpebral Fascia and Ligament of Lockwood

It originates from the terminal fibers and tendon of inferior rectus, runs forward and divides into two around the inferior oblique, fuses with the orbital septum prior to its insertion onto the tarsus of the lower lid (Fig. 42.6). It acts as a lower lid retractor. While operating on the inferior rectus, failure to sever

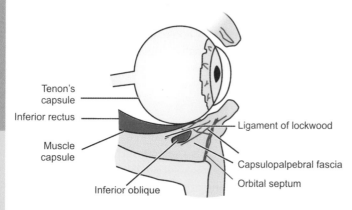

Fig. 42.6: The capsulopalpebral fascia

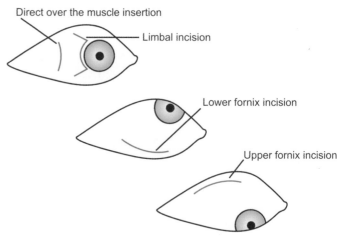

Fig. 42.7: Conjunctival incisions for extraocular muscle surgery

its attachments to the capsulopalpebral fascia will result in a change of the height of the lower lid leading to a change in the width of the palpebral aperture.

The blending of the sheaths of the inferior oblique and inferior rectus muscles and their extensions to the sheaths of medial and lateral rectus, tarsal plate of the lower lid and orbital septum forms a suspending hammock to support the eyeball and is termed suspensory ligament of Lockwood.

SURGICAL TECHNIQUES

Anesthesia

The extraocular muscles can usually be operated upon painlessly under local anesthesia. General anesthesia is required only for small children and apprehensive or nervous older children and adults. After topical anesthesia with four percent lidocaine, an equal mixture of two percent lidocaine with adrenaline and 0.5 percent Bupivacaine with hyaluronidase 25 IU/ml is infiltrated in the retro or peribulbar space. Facial block is usually not required.

Exposure of the Muscle

The eye is rotated in the direction opposite to the muscle to be operated, with the help of one or two-stay sutures at the limbus or conjunctival fixation forceps (Figs 42.7 and 42.8). The muscle insertion is approached through transconjunctival incisions at the limbus, directly near the muscle insertion or indirectly in the fornix (Fig. 42.7). Each has its advantages and disadvantages.

The limbal incision (Fig. 42.8 A), described by von Noorden, is the most popular due to certain inherent advantages. At the limbus the three tissue planes the conjunctiva, Tenon's and the intermuscular septum are fused into one, hence can be dealt by a single incision. No or minimal tissue dissection between the conjunctiva and the Tenon's is required, hence there is minimal tissue reaction postoperatively. Besides the limbal incision has the added advantage that the bare sclera closure or conjunctival recession can be performed. The surgical scar near the limbus is cosmetically more acceptable than the more posterior conjunctival incision placed directly over the site of muscle

insertion. This direct approach, described by Swan and Talbot, has the advantage of simplicity, in that it provides easier access and better exposure for posterior surgery and muscle displacement procedures and the disadvantage that, as the conjunctiva and Tenon's here are well defined separate layers, it requires the meticulous identification and restoration of tissue planes in order to prevent unwanted adhesions and a bad scar. The fornix incision described by Parks, has the advantage that it does not leave a scar visible in the palpebral aperture, causes least discomfort to the patient, allows three adjacent muscles to be approached through one incision, in fact all the six extraocular muscles can be tackled through two fornix incisions (the inferior rectus, lateral rectus, and inferior oblique through the lower temporal fornix and the superior rectus, medial rectus and superior oblique through the upper nasal fornix) and permits any necessary subsequent surgery to be comfortable, as it leaves no conjunctival or Tenon's scar directly over the muscle. It has the disadvantage of complexity as it requires the identification and meticulous dissection of tissue planes.

Recti

After the sub-Tenon's muscle plane has been reached (Fig. 42.8 B), the muscle along with its capsule is hooked (Fig. 42.8 C). A second hook is passed under the insertion from the other side to ensure that the complete muscle is engaged (Fig. 42.8 D). The insertion is cleared. The muscle is stretched on the hook and freed by severing its fascial connections as far back as the white condensation of the Tenon's appears. The check ligaments are already severed by dissection up to this point. Usually this point is 9–10 mm behind the muscle insertion. Dissection beyond this point may result in the herniation of the orbital fat. The muscle should be freed of its fascial connections without disturbing its capsule. While clearing the superior rectus muscle, care must be taken to avoid injury to the levator muscle and the superior oblique tendon and while clearing the inferior rectus, care must be taken to free it from the fascial connections and the capsulopalpebral fascia in order to maintain the level of the lower lid.

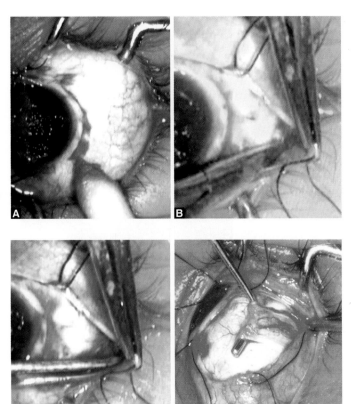

Figs 42.8A to D: Exposure of extraocular muscle limbal conjunctival incision (A). Conjunctiva and Tenon's reflected. (B). Muscle insertion is hooked below the Tenon's (C). Second hook is passed and muscle is cleared (D)

Once the muscle and its insertion has been isolated and cleared, the required surgical procedure can be performed.

Inferior Oblique (Figs 42.9A to H)

The inferior oblique muscle is captured in the inferotemporal quadrant through an incision at the limbus (Fig. 42.9A) or in bulbar conjunctiva and intermuscular septum 7–9 mm from the limbus. After exposure of the bare sclera in the lower temporal quadrant the lateral rectus muscle is hooked from the inferior side (Fig. 42.9B). This is now used to rotate the eye ball superonasally and also as a landmark for identifying the inferior oblique muscle. By blunt dissection under the tenons the inferior oblique belly is hooked under direct visualization avoiding injury to the nearby vortex vein. The lateral rectus hook is now released. Using a second hook, the whole width of the inferior oblique is cleared (Fig. 42.9C). The desired procedure is now performed taking care to include all fibers of the inferior oblique. Failure to do so may account for residual postoperative inferior oblique overaction.

Superior Oblique

The superior oblique tendon is hooked under direct visualization through a conjunctival incision in the superonasal quadrant. Blind sweeping should be avoided for fear of damage to the vortex vein. Like the inferior oblique muscle, care must be

taken to include all fibers in the procedure. Incomplete tenotomy or tenectomy is a common cause of undercorrection.

SURGICAL PROCEDURES

The horizontal recti are by far the most commonly operated extraocular muscles, the vertical recti and the oblique follow. The surgical procedures on extraocular muscles can be grouped as follows:
1. Weakening operations
2. Strengthening operations
3. Operations to modify the action of an extraocular muscle.

Weakening Operations

Since Dieffenbach introduced tenotomy to weaken the action of an extraocular muscle in 1839, great strides have been accomplished in the field of surgery on extraocular muscles. The unavoidable outcome of tenotomy was a large number of overcorrections with little to undo it. Except for unusual cases, tenotomies have been largely replaced by recessions.

Recession

The muscle insertion is secured by sutures to a predetermined location, on the sclera, behind its original insertion. Unlike free tenotomy this procedure permits the grading of the weakening effect, prevents the excessive retraction of the muscle and leaves the muscle in a position that it is available for any necessary subsequent surgery. The weakening effect of recession is due to the loss of contractile force caused by the shortening of the muscle, reduction in the arc of contact and the necessary disruption of some of the supporting structures during surgery (Figs 42.10 A to 42.11 J).

Recession of recti: The recession of the *medial rectus* should be restricted to a maximum of 6 mm. Larger recessions of 6–8 mm are often required on the *lateral rectus*. In adults with large exodeviations exceeding 70 PD as much as 10–12 mm, lateral rectus recession can be done with nil to minimal restriction of abduction postoperatively. Even though this places the insertion behind the anatomic equator there is sufficient arc of contact to allow the muscle to exert rotational force. To retain sufficient arc of contact and to ease the placement of sutures while performing large recessions hang-back and hemihang-back techniques of recession can be adopted.

Recessions of 5–6 mm can be safely performed on the *vertical recti*. Provided necessary precautions are taken and the amount of surgery is not excessive, the procedure is effective and free from complications. Due to close relationship between the superior rectus and levator of the upper lid and between the inferior rectus and capsulopalpebral fascia of the lower lid, great care must be taken in dissecting the muscles from all fascial connections.

Recession of inferior oblique: Inferior oblique myectomy was the procedure of choice for weakening of the inferior oblique till Parks in 1972 demonstrated the recession of the inferior

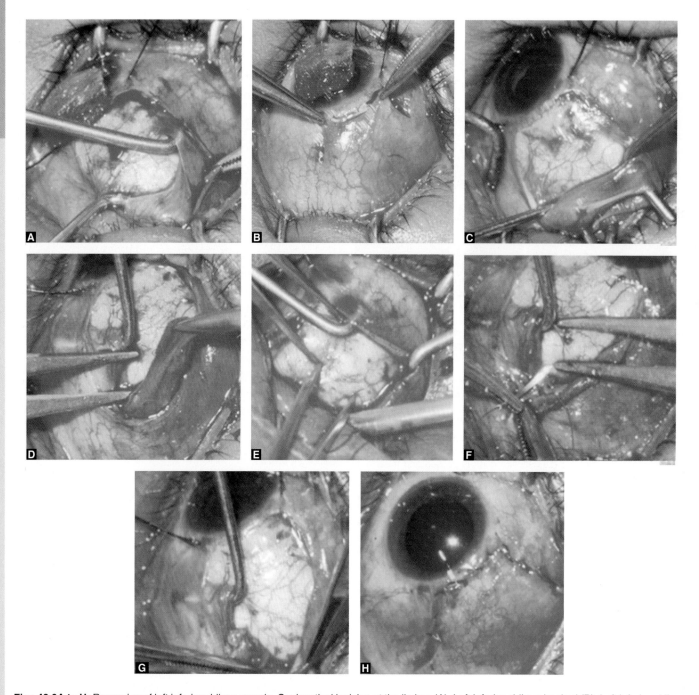

Figs 42.9A to H: Recession of left inferior oblique muscle. Conjunctival incision at the limbus (A). Left inferior oblique hooked (B). Left inferior oblique exposed (C). Left inferior oblique disinserted (D). The Fink point (E). The Park Schie point (F). Stitched at Park Schie point (G). Conjunctival incision closed (H)

oblique to be safe and effective (Fig. 42.12 A). Weakening of the inferior oblique can be achieved by recessing it to a point 3 mm inferior and 2 mm lateral to the lateral border of the inferior rectus insertion, the Scheie Park point (Figs 42.12 B and 42.9 F). The recession may be done to a point 8 mm infero-posterior (6 mm inferior and 6 mm posterior) to the lower border of the lateral rectus insertion, the Fink point (Fig. 42.9 E). The reduction in a hyperdeviation by the recession procedure is 8–12 PD. Selective weakening of its elevation action can be achieved by the anteroplacement of its insertion. Anterior displacement of the recessed inferior oblique has been found

to enhance its weakening effect. Elliot and Nankin report excellent results by placing the recessed inferior oblique just anterior to the temporal border inferior rectus insertion.

Recession of superior oblique: Though weakening the superior oblique by recession, has the theoretical advantage of providing a graded effect. It has the disadvantage that it changes the basic mechanics of its actions. It collapses its broad insertion and creates a new focal insertion anteriorly. At this new insertion the superior oblique no longer acts as a depressor. It is important to replace the tendon posterior to the equator, which is difficult. Postoperative limitation of depression has been observed with

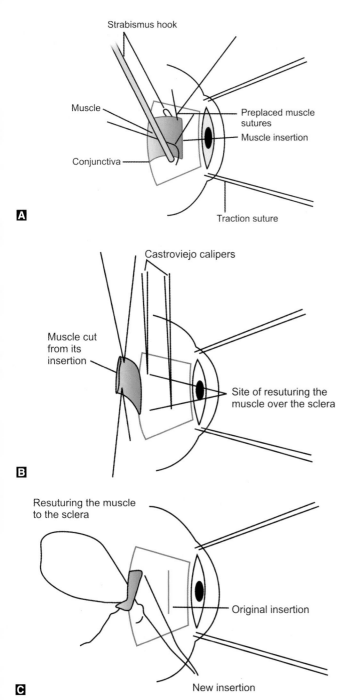

Figs 42.10A to C: Recession of the left medial rectus. The muscle is hooked and preplaced sutures passed at the insertion (A). The muscle is cut at the insertion and precalculated site for new insertion marked at the sclera (B). The muscle sutured at the new site behind the original insertion (C)

the recession of the superior oblique. Other procedures, such as tenotomy or tendon lengthening are therefore preferred for weakening the superior oblique.

Hang-back and hemihang-back recession: Both these techniques of recession weaken the action of an extraocular muscle. The muscle is recessed and suspended with the help of sutures in both procedures. In HB the sutures pass through the original

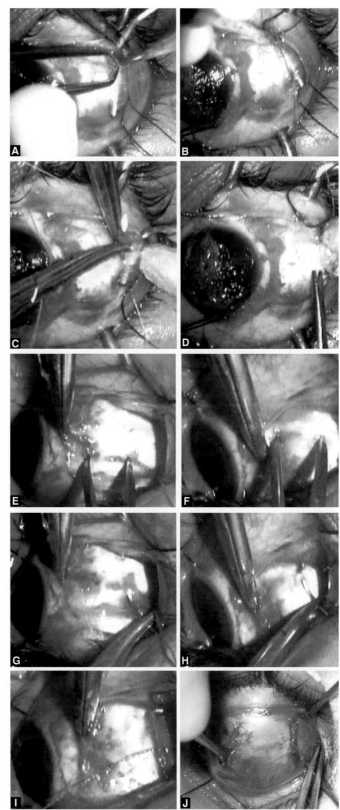

Figs 42.11A to J: Recession of a rectus muscle after the rectus muscle is hooked and cleared, the insertion is cauterised (A) and secured on two preplaced sutures (B and C). It is then cut at the insertion (D). Two marks are put at the sclera, one for the upper end and one for the lower end of the precalculated site for the recessed muscle insertion (E and F). The upper and lower borders of the cut insertion are then sutured to this new site (G and H). This is further strengthened by a central suture (I and J)

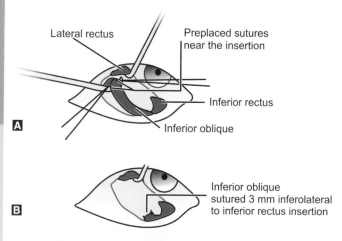

Figs 42.12A and B: Right inferior oblique recession

Marginal Myotomy

A marginal myotomy is performed by severing the muscle fibers at the upper and lower borders (Fig. 42.14). It effects the actual weakening of the muscle by reducing the number of contractile elements without changing its arc of contact. This procedure has been found highly effective in further reducing the action of an already maximally recessed rectus muscle or one that cannot be recessed. The reduction of the deviation by this procedure, on a rectus muscle, has been estimated to be about 10–16 PD. This procedure can be done on the superior and inferior oblique muscles also.

Tenotomy or Myectomy

Free tenotomy on *recti* is performed only in unusual cases, such as lateral rectus tenotomy in III nerve paralysis and inferior rectus tenotomy in thyroid myopathy.

Tenotomy is also performed as a weakening procedure on the oblique muscles in patients with cyclovertical paralysis, A/V patterns, or primary oblique muscle overaction.

Percutaneous myectomy of an inferior oblique muscle at its origin, first described in 1906 by Duane, has largely been abandoned. Myectomy or tenotomy of an inferior oblique muscle is usually performed through a conjunctival incision about 8 mm from the limbus, in the inferotemporal quadrant between its

insertion stump and in hemihang-back from the sclera posterior to the insertion, half way between the original insertion and the proposed site of recession (Figs 42.13A to D). 6–0 vicryl or ethibond sutures can be used. Both these procedures have the advantage that the arc of contact is minimally disturbed and the risk of scleral perforation is minimal as the posterior awkward suture placement is avoided. Larger recessions can therefore be safely performed without disturbing the ocular movements.

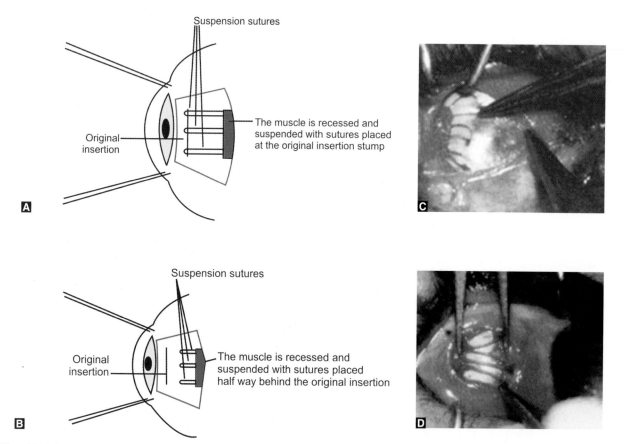

Figs 42.13: Hang-back recession of left lateral rectus (A). Hemihang-back recession of left lateral rectus (B). Hang-back recession of right lateral rectus (C). Hemihang-back recession of right lateral rectus (D)

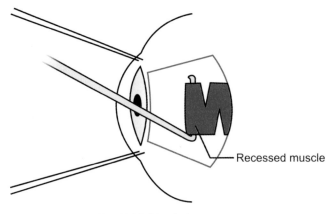

Fig. 42.14: Marginal myotomy

insertion and the inferior rectus insertion. Though the choice as to the best procedure for inferior oblique weakening is unclear, a recession of the inferior oblique is preferred in most cases, as this procedure permits the subsequent handling of the muscle if need arises. An overcorrection following the weakening of the inferior oblique is rare, but may occur if performed on a normally or minimally overacting muscle.

Tenotomy of the superior oblique muscle is usually performed, midway between the insertion and the trochlea where the tendon is compact, through a conjunctival incision in the upper nasal quadrant medial to the superior rectus insertion (Fig. 42.15). A weakening operation on an overacting superior oblique reduces hyperdeviation in its field of action. It is also effective in reducing incyclotropia and A-pattern. In patients of Brown's syndrome, forced duction test should be performed, after the tenotomy preoperatively, to confirm the complete release of the restriction.

Posterior Fixation Suture (Faden Operation)

Posterior fixation suture (Faden operation) or retroequatorial myopexy is performed by suturing a rectus muscle to the sclera behind the equator (Figs 42.16A to 42.17 C).

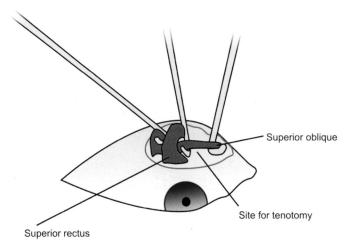

Fig. 42.15: Tenotomy of right superior oblique

In principle this decreases the leverage between the center of rotation and the line of pull by shortening the effective arc of contact in the direction of action of the muscle producing a selective weakening in the direction of primary action of the muscle without disturbing the ocular balance in other positions of gaze (Fig. 42.16 B). Because this procedure does not affect the primary ocular position, it must be combined with a recession where there is a need to correct the deviation in the primary position.

The posterior fixation suture has been successfully tried wherever a selective weakening, in the direction of action of the muscle, is required, such as a paretic strabismus on the yoke muscle, dissociated vertical deviations, nystagmus blockage syndrome, convergence excess type of esotropia and Duane's retraction syndrome.

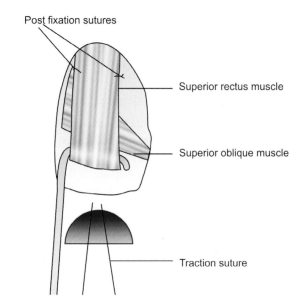

Fig. 42.16A: Posterior fixation suture of the right superior rectus

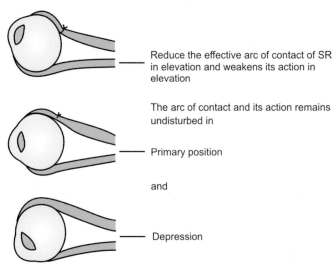

Fig. 42.16B: Posterior fixation suture of the SR muscle–Mechanism of action

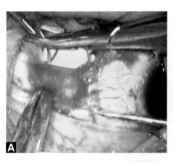
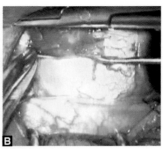
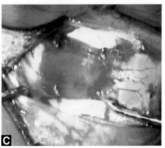

Figs 42.17A to C: Retroequatorial myopexy (Faden suture) of left medial rectus. Upper suture (A). Lower suture (B) and both sutures applied (C)

Botulinum Toxin to Weaken the Action of a Muscle

Weakening the action of an extraocular muscle by chemically denervating the motor nerve terminals is an accepted method of treatment in selected patients of strabismus. Botulinum toxin A (*Botox*) is injected transconjunctivally under local anesthesia, into the belly of the extraocular muscle about 2.5 mm from its insertion. This approximates the location of the motor end plate; here it inhibits the release of neurotransmitter acetylcholine leading to the functional denervation of the extraocular muscle. An electromyography needle connected to an audible EMG amplifier is helpful in guiding the injection needle.

Two nanograms of Botulinum toxin reconstituted in non-preserved saline in the dilution of 1–12 units/0.1 ml is the commonly used dose. The drug-induced weakness or paralysis of the extraocular muscle lasts for 2–8 weeks or more. This usually results in permanently changed ocular alignment as the injected muscle lengthens and its antagonist contracts. Extrajunctional acetylcholine receptors may develop in the atrophied muscle leading to the reinnervation, reversal and eventual recovery of the drug-induced paralysis. Repeat injections can be given when necessary.

A deviation of less than 35 PD can be corrected to within 10 PD or less in most of the patients. Overcorrections are rare. The results in esotropia are generally better than in exotropia. Botulinum toxin has been successfully used in selected patients of paralytic squints, postoperative adjustment of undercorrections or overcorrections, esotropia of less than 40 PD in poor surgical candidates, and in strabismus following retinal detachment surgery.

Strengthening Operations

The action of a muscle can be enhanced by shortening it, so that the tension and hence the pull caused by it increases. This

can be achieved in a controlled manner by resecting or plicating a precalculated length of the muscle or its tendon; it can also be achieved by advancing the muscle insertion. Excessive resection may mechanically restrict the movement of the globe in the opposite direction and, therefore must be avoided.

Resection Operation

A precalculated length of the muscle is resected and the cut end is stitched to the site of the original insertion (Figs 42.18 A to 42.19 I). When combined with a recession of the ipsilateral antagonist, it has a stabilizing effect on the result and enhances

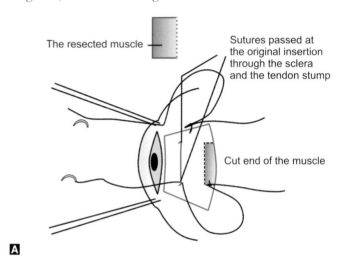

The resected muscle

Sutures passed at the original insertion through the sclera and the tendon stump

Cut end of the muscle

A

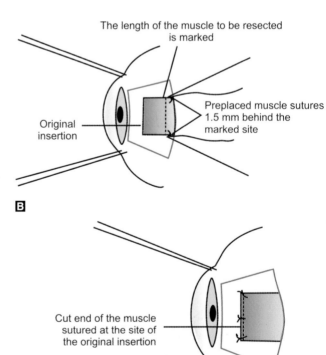

The length of the muscle to be resected is marked

Original insertion

Preplaced muscle sutures 1.5 mm behind the marked site

B

Cut end of the muscle sutured at the site of the original insertion

C

Figs 42.18A to C: Resection of left lateral rectus. Preplaced sutures are passed in the muscle behind the mark of the muscle to be resected (A). The muscle is resected and the sutures are passed at the original insertion (B). The cut end of the muscle is sutured at the original insertion (C)

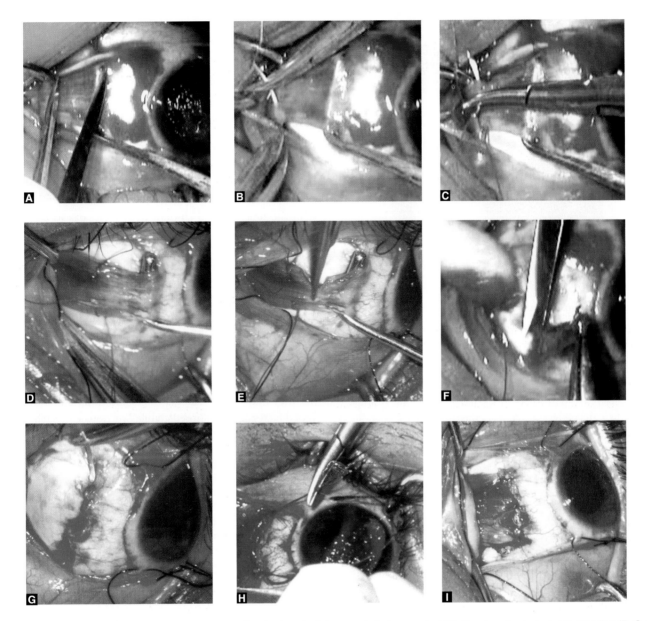

Figs 42.19A to I: Resection of rectus muscle. Measuring the length of the muscle to be resected (A). Preplaced sutures behind the line (B, C, D). The tendon is cut along the marked line (E). The tendon stump cut and removed. (F). The cut end brought to original insertion (G, H, I)

the amount of correction. Though it improves the action of the resected muscle, resection alone has little or no effect on the primary ocular position. Resection of one or both medial recti has therefore been successfully used for the treatment of the selected cases of primary convergence insufficiency.

Horizontal rectus muscles: The minimal amount of resection on the horizontal recti is 4 mm and the maximal amount is 7 mm on the medial rectus and 10 mm on the lateral rectus.

Vertical rectus muscles: Resection procedures can be performed on the vertical recti (Fig. 42.20) with precautions similar to that for recession techniques. The minimal and maximal amounts of resection are 4 mm and 6 mm respectively.

Inferior oblique muscle: Due to the proximity of its insertion to the fovea, resection procedure on the inferior oblique muscle

is technically difficult and risky. Besides, the procedure has been found to be ineffective in improving ocular motility in the field of action of this muscle; it is therefore not recommended. Alternatively, whenever the need for such a surgery is felt, weakening of the yoke muscle, i.e. the superior rectus of the other eye, has been found to be effective.

Superior oblique muscle: Shortening of the superior oblique tendon by plication is effective in improving the depression of the adducted eye and counteracting excyclotropia. It is preferable to do plication of the superior oblique tendon (tenoplication) through a transconjunctival route in the upper temporal quadrant (Fig. 42.21). The plication can be performed in the upper nasal quadrant also, but the risk of the capture of the tuck in the trochlea and the restriction of oblique elevation (acquired Brown's syndrome) postoperatively is higher. To prevent this,

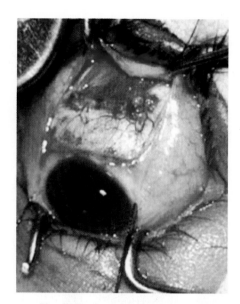

Fig. 42.20: Superior rectus resection

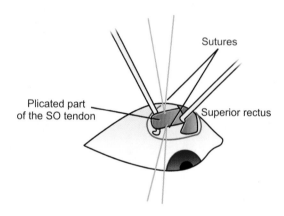

Fig. 42.21: Tenoplication of right superior oblique

the plication should be done near the nasal border of the superior rectus while using the upper nasal approach.

Selective strengthening of the intorsion action can be achieved by the selective plication of only the anterior fibers of the superior oblique tendon. This procedure was first described by Ito in 1964 and since then this name has been used to refer to any procedure involving only the anterior half of the superior oblique tendon.

Combined Weakening-Strengthening Operations

Weakening of a muscle combined with the strengthening of its antagonist in the same operative session adds greatly to the effectiveness of each procedure and postoperative stability of the ocular alignment. Resection alone is usually not enough for the treatment of manifest tropia. The corrective effect of a resection procedure on the ocular deviation seen in the immediate postoperative period gradually reduces during the next six weeks.

Adjustable Sutures

Adjustable sutures can be placed after recessing or resecting a muscle. Several techniques of placing adjustable sutures have been described. After suturing the muscle to the sclera, the sutures are brought forward and tied in a bow-tie fashion so that the effect of surgery can be modified in the immediate postoperative phase by pulling on or loosening the sutures, the former being simpler. It is therefore desirable to leave the muscle more posterior than finally desired so that any adjustment will involve tightening the sutures and advancing the muscle. To leave the suture loose for readjustment in a resection procedure, more than the precalculated amount of muscle, has to be resected. Adjustable sutures are, therefore, better used with a recession procedure.

An attempt to modify the result of surgery in the immediate postoperative phase implies that the immediate postoperative ocular position is predictive of the final outcome. This however, is not the case except for large undercorrections and overcorrections that often tend to persist. Moreover, the precise evaluation of ocular alignment and suture adjustment in the immediate postoperative phase is difficult and impractical in children. Their routine use is therefore not recommended, but they may be of value in adults and older children with an added factor for the unpredictability of outcome, such as previous operations, scarring, contracture or endocrine myopathy.

Operations to Modify the Action of an Extraocular Muscle (Muscle Transposition Operations)

The action of an extraocular muscle can be modified by shifting its insertion so that the direction of the pull caused by it is altered. The raising or lowering of horizontal rectus insertions and nasal or temporal transposition of vertical rectus insertions are performed in selected cases for the correction of A/V patterns, vertical deviations, and for enhancing the effect of horizontal corrections. The raising or lowering of a horizontal rectus insertion has a weakening effect on its horizontal action in up or down gaze, respectively, in favor of its vertical action in the direction of the shift. The amount of up or down displacement may vary from 5 mm to full tendon width (about 11 mm) in nonparalytic squints to transfer of a rectus insertion to the insertion of another muscle in paralytic squints. In nonparalytic squints, an up or down displacement of the horizontal recti has been found to be effective with no torsional effects or limitation of ocular motility.

Paralytic Strabismus

Muscle transpositions are effective in restoring some degrees of motility in the field of action of the paretic muscle, i.e. some restoration of elevation by the transposition of medial and lateral rectus insertions to that of superior rectus in elevator paralysis (Fig. 42.22 A) and the transposition of superior and inferior rectus insertions to the lateral rectus in VI nerve palsy.

To overcome the risk of anterior segment ischemia, while combining muscle transpositions with resection of the paralyzed muscle, partial tendon widths can be sutured to the paralyzed muscle (Figs 42.22 B and C). This is known as the Jensen's procedure.

In desperate situations of third nerve palsy, the tendon of the superior oblique can be used to aid adduction by transplanting it either to the medial border of the superior rectus or to the medial rectus after freeing it from the trochlear tunnel. The former procedure is simple but results in excessive intorsion, the latter requires extensive dissection.

These procedures should not be performed if there is limitation of passive movement and mechanical factors are responsible for the limitation of movement.

Correction of A/V Patterns

The muscle utilized for the correction of A/V patterns depends upon the overacting or underacting muscle responsible for the pattern of the deviation (Fig. 42.23). An exotropia is the one that is most troublesome to the patient. Even a small degree of

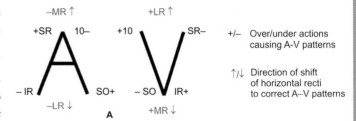

Fig. 42.23: Etiology and correction of A-V patterns

an exotropia may require treatment. The A/V patterns respond satisfactorily to weakening procedures on the overacting superior and inferior obliques respectively. The other muscles are utilized when obvious oblique overactions or underactions are not present.

For correction of A/V patterns, the insertion of a horizontal muscle is moved in the direction in which it is desirable to most decrease its horizontal action and in the direction opposite that in which one wishes its horizontal action to be more effective. An up displacement of the lateral rectus (Fig. 42.24) results in a relative decrease in its abduction action in the up gaze and a reduction of V-pattern, and a down displacement to a reduction of A-pattern. Similarly, an up displacement of the medial rectus results (Fig. 42.25) in a reduction of A-pattern and down displacement in a reduction of V-pattern. It helps to remember that to correct a vertical incomitance (A/V patterns), the medial recti have to be shifted toward the apex and the lateral recti have to be shifted toward the base of the A or V (Figs 42.23 and 42.26).

While doing recess/resect procedures on the horizontal recti, A-V patterns can be corrected by weakening or strengthening the upper and lower borders by different amounts and suturing the muscle in a slanting manner (Fig. 42.26). The direction of the slant depends upon the pattern of the deviation. The muscle insertion is made parallel to the limbs of the A or V (Figs 42.27 and 42.28).

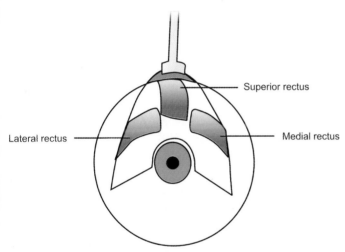

Fig. 42.22A: Up-transposition of medial and lateral rectus for elevator paralysis right eye

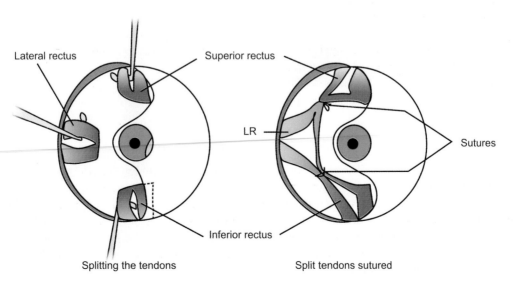

Figs 42.22B and C: Transposition of lateral halves of SR and IR to LR in right LR paralysis (Jensen's procedure)

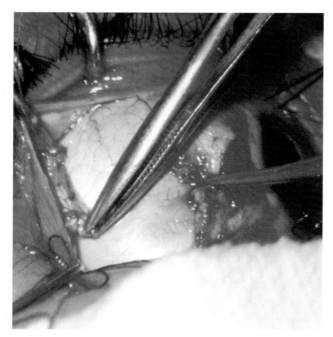

Fig. 42.24: Recession and updisplacement of right lateral rectus for V exotropia

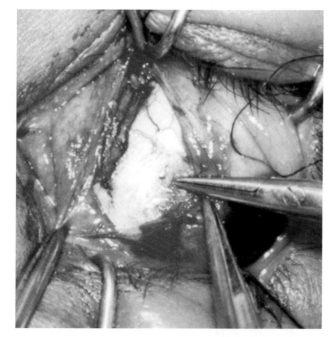

Fig. 42.25: Recession and updisplacement of left medial rectus for A esotropia

Anteroplacement of Obliques

The muscle insertion can be transposed so as to selectively alter the action of a muscle. Anteroplacement of the obliques selectively weakens their vertical action in favor of the torsional action. Sagittalization by the lateral and anterior advancement of only the anterior fibers of the superior oblique insertion (Fig. 42.29) enhances its torsional action without affecting its depression action. These procedures are not required very frequently but have proven to be of value in carefully selected patients.

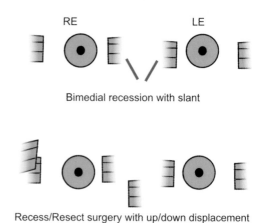

Bimedial recession with slant

Recess/Resect surgery with up/down displacement

Fig. 42.26: Correction of V esotropia

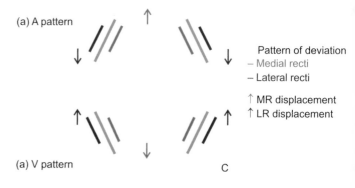

(a) A pattern

Pattern of deviation
– Medial recti
– Lateral recti

↑ MR displacement
↑ LR displacement

(a) V pattern   C

Fig. 42.27: The placement of slanting insertions for correction of A-V patterns.

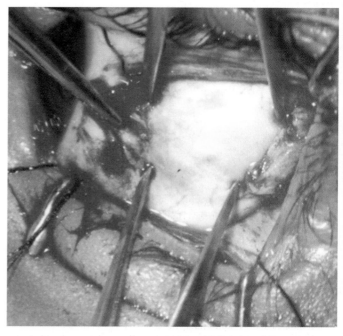

Fig. 42.28: Slanting recession of left lateral rectus for V exotropia

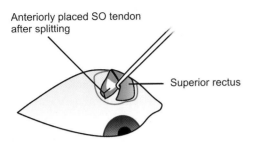

Anteriorly placed SO tendon after splitting

Superior rectus

Fig. 42.29: Anteroplacement of half of the right superior oblique tendon

Use of Plastic Materials

Plastic materials, such as supramid sheaths or tubes are used during strabismus surgery in selected cases for following purposes:

i. To prevent adhesions and preserve muscle functioning after the isolation of the muscle from scar tissue in reoperations.
ii. To add to the tendon length. 4–7 mm long strip of the silicone band is used as a sheath expander for elongating the superior oblique tendon in Brown's syndrome.

AMOUNT OF OPERATION

The surgical results depend upon several variables described earlier and on the surgical technique, manner in which the muscle is exposed, how thoroughly it is freed, how the muscle sheath is dealt with, placement of sutures and other factors. Each surgeon must therefore establish through experience the approximate effectiveness of his technique. In addition, a number of unknown mechanical and innervational factors remain, so that an identical surgical procedure on different patients may have different results; hence the surgical strategy has to be planned individually for each patient. Although the surgical result and its stability is dependent upon several variables and it is difficult to arrive at a mathematical formula, it is essential to have some guidelines as to what result to expect from a particular surgery, in order to be able to plan the surgery to be undertaken.

Surgery is planned with the aim of symmetrizing the action of the extraocular muscles rather than performing symmetrical surgery; hence ductions, versions, gaze incomitance, and deviation for near and distance fixation must be considered. The larger the deviation the greater will be the effect of same amount of surgery. In older children and adults, larger operations are required than in younger children with a comparable deviation. Recession is more effective than resection in reducing a deviation. A graded combination of resection with recession has an added mechanical advantage and a stabilizing effect on the surgical result. Due to the difference in the anatomical direction and the arc of contact of the horizontal recti, recession procedure is more effective when performed on the medial rectus and resection is more effective when performed on the lateral rectus. The result of surgery on the vertical recti is more predictable. The amount of correction also depends upon the strength and the thickness of the operated muscle. It is expected to get a correction of 3–5 PD and 3–4 PD per mm of recession of the medial and lateral rectus respectively, and 6 PD per mm recession of the vertical recti, 2–3 PD and 2–4 PD per mm of resection of the medial and lateral rectus respectively, and 4 PD per mm resection of the vertical rectus.

On the basis of clinical experience the following guidelines have been found to be useful.

Horizontal Deviations

The amount of correction usually obtained by the minimal and maximal amount of biomedial or bilateral recession is 15–20 PD and 30–40 PD respectively, being lesser by bilateral rectus recession. The amount of correction usually obtained by the minimal and maximal amount of recess/resect operation in one eye is 20–25 PD and 40–50 PD respectively, being lesser in exodeviation. In consideration with other individual variables, Table 42.1 is helpful in planning the surgery.

Cyclovertical Deviations

Small degrees (less than 8 PD) of hyper/hypotropia can be safely ignored while operating on large horizontal deviations. Comitant hypo or hyper deviations of 10–14 PD can be eliminated by raising or lowering the insertions of the horizontal recti while performing surgery for horizontal deviation. Adjustable

Table 42.1: Correction by horizontal muscle surgery

	Esodeviation		Exodeviation	
Surgery Deviation	MR rec	MR rec/LR res	LR rec	LR rec/MR res
< 30 PD	5-6 mm OE 4 mm BE	4 mm/5-6 mm OE	5-7 mm BE	5-7 mm/4-5 mm OE
30-45 PD	5 mm BE	5-6 mm/6-7 mm OE	8-10 mm BE	7-8 mm/5-6 mm OE
> 45-60 PD	6-7 mm BE	5-7 mm/8-10 mm OE	10-12 mm BE	8-10 mm 5-7 mm OE
> 60 PD	MR rec 5-6 mm BE+LR res 8-10 mm OE or MR rec 5 mm BE+LR res 7-8 mm BE		LR rec 8-12 mm BE + MR res 5-6 mm OE or LR rec 7-10 mm BE+MR res 5-6 mm BE	

- When 3 or 4 muscle surgery is planned, it is preferred to proceed in a stage wise manner, particularly in younger patients.
- The amount of surgery on the medial and lateral recti and which muscle to be tackled first is determined on the basis of near and distance deviations, gaze, and vertical incomitance, if any.
- When persistent esotropia is associated with conjunctival fibrosis then MR recession may have to be combined with conjunctival recession.
- If esodeviation is significantly more for near than for distance then biomedial recession may have to be combined with faden on the medial recti.
- For A-V patterns surgery may have to be modified as discussed in the text.
- OE: one eye; BE: Both eyes.

Table 42.2: Correction by vertical muscle surgery

Amount of hypertropia	Choice of surgery
15-20 PD	SR rec 4-6 mm OE or IO rec OE
20-30 PD	SR rec 4-6 mm + IR res 4-6 mm OE or SR rec 4-6 mm + IO rec OE
Alternating sursumduction	SR rec 5-7 mm OE/BE with faden if necessary.

- OE: one eye; BE: Both eyes.

sutures may be particularly helpful to eliminate troublesome diplopia in down gaze due to residual small tropias.

The results of surgery on the vertical recti (Table 42.2) are more predictable than on the horizontal recti.

Many methods for the surgical correction of dissociated vertical deviations have been tried, with no consensus as to the best approach. Large (7–12 mm) recessions of the superior rectus muscles with or without a faden procedure have been found to be effective. Large resections of the inferior rectus muscles and recess/resect procedures on the vertical rectus muscles have been tried with varying degrees of success.

Overacting oblique muscles are weakened by one of the appropriate procedures described earlier. Weakening procedures on the superior and inferior oblique muscles usually do not affect the horizontal alignment in primary position. The surgery to correct the oblique muscle overaction or underaction, usually takes care of the associated cyclodeviation also. In rare situations, when a cyclic deviation is symptomatic in the absence of a vertical or horizontal deviation, such as in cases of mild superior oblique paresis, selective torsional effect can be obtained by shifting only the anterior portion of the superior oblique insertion, the sagittalization or modified 'Harada-Ito' procedure.

PARALYTIC SQUINT

The aim of treatment in a case of paralytic squint is to restore comfortable binocular vision, without the necessity for the adoption of compensatory head posture, over as large an area of the central and lower part of the binocular visual field as possible, and to make the ocular movements of both eyes as symmetrical and equal as possible.

Surgical intervention is considered when the ocular deviation becomes stationary that is there is no regression or progression and the underlying disease causing the palsy is no longer active.

The secondary effects of a paralysis or paresis of an extraocular muscle are as follows:
i. Overaction of contralateral synergist (the yoke muscle) with its hypertrophy.
ii. Overaction of the ipsilateral (direct) antagonist due to unopposed action and secondary contracture.
iii. Inhibitional paresis of the antagonist of the overacting synergist in the other eye.

The aim of surgery is to restore and symmetrize ocular movements, to eliminate compensatory head posture, and

restore ocular alignment as far as possible. If a small residual deviation is unavoidable, then it is better that it be in the upper and not in the lower or central part of the visual field.

The surgery for paralytic squint is planned on the basis of secondary overactions and underactions; one or several of the following operations may have to be performed in a stepwise manner:
i. Recession of the overacting contralateral synergist, the yoke muscle.
ii. Recession of the overacting (or fibrotic) ipsilateral antagonist.
iii. Strengthening of the weak, palsied muscle by resection and/or transplanting tendons of adjacent muscles, i.e. the superior and inferior rectus to the palsied lateral rectus.

If there is no contracture of the ipsilateral antagonist then the yoke muscle is weakened first, whereas in the presence of a contracture the ipsilateral antagonist is weakened prior to tackling other muscles. The amount of correction depends upon the degree and duration of palsy and secondary effects on other extraocular muscles.

SPECIAL FORMS OF STRABISMUS

A special therapeutic challenge exists in certain special forms of strabismus. Some of these are Duane's retraction syndrome, superior oblique sheath syndrome, strabismus fixus, congential fibrosis syndrome, and thyroid myopathy. Apart from their individual features, each of them has considerable amount of restrictive element. The associated retraction and palpebral fissure width changes add to the cosmetic problem. Surgery usually fails to restore complete ocular motility and binocular single vision over the entire area of the binocular field; it is therefore indicated only when there is a significant deviation in the primary position, an uncomfortable compensatory head posture or significant globe retraction. The aim of surgery is to restore cosmetic appearance, ocular alignment and binocularity in primary gaze and as large area of visual field as possible and to eliminate compensatory head posture. The general principles for planning the surgery are similar. The clinical evaluation of the restriction is confirmed by a forced duction test and surgery is done primarily to release the restriction and then to restore the ocular alignment. Strengthening the antagonist of a fibrotic or a cocontracting muscle in an attempt to correct the ocular alignment, without releasing the restrictive element is unlikely to give a satisfactory result; on the other hand, it may aggravate the retraction and the cosmetic problem. For example, in Duane's retraction syndrome with limitation of abduction, limitation and retraction of the globe in adduction, a positive forced duction test for the lateral rectus, medial rectus resection on an exotropic eye is likely to enhance the retraction with no or minimal effect on the ocular alignment whereas a medial rectus recession on an esotropic eye may improve the ocular alignment without any undesirable effect on the retraction. A recession of both horizontal recti graded in accordance with the primary ocular position has been found to be effective in restoring the ocular alignment in primary position, eliminating compensatory head posture and minimizing globe retraction. It has also been found to be effective in controlling vertical leashes (vertical slipping of tight muscles) often associated with Duane's syndrome. Satisfactory results have been reported with posterior fixation sutures with or without the recession of the horizontal recti.

The indications and aims of surgery for superior oblique sheath syndrome are same as discussed above. Dissection and release of a tight superior oblique sheath has been found to have good but not lasting results. Superior oblique tenotomy with all its disadvantages has therefore, been advocated. This may lead to superior oblique paralysis in the long run, requiring subsequent surgery to weaken the contralateral inferior rectus. Recently, there are reports of satisfactory results with tendon lengthening procedures.

Suturing the Muscle to the Sclera

The muscle is restitched to the sclera at the desired site by means of the preplaced muscle sutures at the upper and lower borders of the cut edge. An additional suture is used to secure the center of the cut edge and restore the natural curve of the muscle insertion. While suturing the muscle at the desired site, a small 1.5–2 mm superficial bite in the sclera is all that is necessary and this avoids the danger of penetrating the globe. In a resection procedure, a bite only through fibers left at the original insertion stump is not enough and should include the superficial sclera as well.

Closure of the Wound

It is preferable to close the Tenon's capsule separately using minimal absorbable sutures (Figs 42.30 A and B). Separate closure of the Tenon's ensures the normal anatomical covering of the extraocular muscle and the sclera and prevents adhesions of the bulbar conjunctiva to these underlying structures.

Sometimes in a limbal incision, separate closure of the Tenon's may not be necessary. The conjunctiva should be closed accurately (Fig. 42.30 C) taking care to avoid leaving the exposed tags of Tenon's as these tend to form granulomas. The suture material for conjunctival closure is entirely the surgeon's choice. Absorbable sutures incite more tissue reaction than nonabsorbable silk sutures, but are preferred by some, particularly in small children, as they do not have to be removed. However, the tissue reaction with silk sutures is distinctly lesser and we do not find their removal a problem.

Irrespective of the exposure, suturing and closure techniques, it is important to obtain hemostasis to handle tissues with gentleness with regard for tissue planes. This adds to the postoperative patient comfort and success of the surgery.

POSTOPERATIVE CARE

Period of hospitalization after strabismus surgery depends upon the time that the effect of general anesthesia lasts. Most in town patients, operated under local anesthesia can leave the hospital the same day and out of town patients can leave the next day.

Postoperatively the patient is examined 24 hours, seven days and six weeks after surgery. Nonabsorbable conjunctival sutures are removed on the seventh postoperative day. Dressing is kept on the operated eye for 24 hours. It may be done for 48 hours in patients with bare sclera closure. Patching of both eyes has no benefit and is very distressing to the patient, hence should not be done.

Topical corticosteroids plus antibiotics are used for 2–4 weeks postoperatively. Systemic antibiotics are used for 3–5 days and antiinflammatory drugs are used as and where required.

Postoperatively the patient should wear the necessary refractive correction as soon as the dressing is removed. Minor adjustments in the spectacle power postoperatively may help the patient to exercise better binocular control and overcome

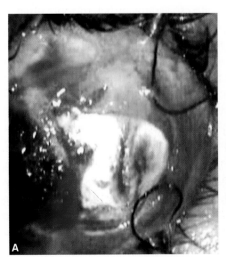
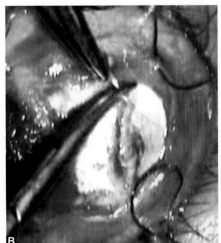
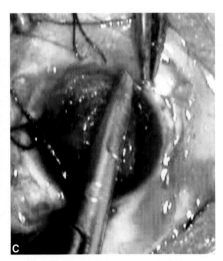

Figs 42.30A to C: Wound closure. Tenon's closure (A and B). Conjunctival closure (C)

small residual deviations. Wherever planned, postoperative orthoptics should be started as soon as the tissue reaction has subsided, this is frequently within two days and certainly within one week.

COMPLICATIONS

Preoperative

Preoperative complications during strabismus surgery are few and mostly can be prevented or satisfactorily dealt with if proper care and respect for tissue and tissue planes are exercised.

Excessive bleeding: Excessive bleeding is usually not a problem if appropriate surgical planes are identified. If bleeding is a repeated problem with a surgeon then careful self-reassessment of the technique is called for. Occasionally excessive bleeding may result from cutting a conjunctival vessel, attempting dissection between muscle fibers and muscles sheath or from accidentally cutting into the muscle during exposure. Sometimes the scleral muscle stump bleeds after the muscle has been cut. When it does occur, it can usually be managed satisfactorily by proper sponging and cautery. Control of bleeding is essential before continuing with the operation since hematoma and subsequent scarring will unfavorably influence the surgical result.

Scleral perforation: Scleral perforation is extremely rare with the use of modern, fine spatulated needles. Usually the size and shape of needles permit them to perforate the sclera without causing retinal holes. In case, it is suspected, the site should be examined carefully by thorough indirect ophthalmoscopy through dilated pupils.

Lost muscle: Muscle may be lost due to a broken suture or rarely by cutting it on the wrong side of the clamp. Usually it can be grasped and resutured. If it has slipped more posteriorly, then it can usually be grasped through the opening in the muscle sheath. While looking for a posteriorly slipped muscle, do not look back along the globe itself for that is not the natural direction of the muscle. It is headed toward the orbital apex which is directly posterior for the medial rectus, nasal for the lateral rectus, inferior for the superior rectus, and superior for the inferior rectus.

Blind grasping and suturing of unidentified tissue to the globe will result in unwanted restrictions of ocular motility and should not be done. If the muscle cannot be found then the globe should be fixed by traction, with scleral stay sutures, in the direction of action of the lost muscle, i.e. full adduction in case of a lost medial rectus. The eye should remain in this position for two weeks. If no function is observed after that time then the case should be dealt like any other paralytic squint. Resecting and suturing the Tenon's to the muscle stump has also been recommended in case of a lost muscle.

Oculocardiac reflex: It is a transient phenomenon that results from pulling on the muscle specially the medial rectus. It results in vagal stimulation leading to bradycardia. Usually the cardiac rhythm is restored immediately after the pull on the muscle is relaxed. It can be minimized or prevented by atropine injection and to some extent by retrobulbar block.

Anatomical variations in the extraocular muscles: These are rare. When found, the variation should be doubly confirmed with the known landmarks and carefully recorded by a photograph or sketches. If a muscle is found to be absent and the absence conforms to the ocular movements, the surgery is as for any paralytic squint. Most variations are iatrogenic, stemming from prior surgery. A good preoperative record of previous surgical procedures will prevent most surgical surprises.

Postoperative

Postoperative complications with strabismus surgery are few and trivial. The agony due to some of the unavoidable postoperative discomfort can usually be minimized with good patient communication regarding what he should expect in terms of redness, discharge, vision, diplopia and position of eyes.

Overcorrections and Undercorrections: Small overcorrections and undercorrections are not uncommon and are usually compensated for by a patient with a reasonable binocular potential. Large overcorrections and undercorrections cause serious concern to the patient and his relatives. A large deviation in the early postoperative phase with inability to bring the eye even to the midline suggests a slipped muscle and calls for an immediate exploration and resuturing of the muscle. Once the possibility of a slipped muscle is ruled out it is desirable to reassure the patient, wait and watch, continuing the appropriate conservative treatment with spectacles, prisms or alternate occlusion as and where indicated. In some of these patients there is a reduction in this untoward result; hence there is no need for immediate resurgery. Usually it is preferable to wait for at least six weeks before considering reoperation. While reoperating on overcorrections, an attempt to undo the previous surgery is not always the best option. Other muscles can be operated upon with equal or more ease and effectiveness.

Diplopia: Patients operated for comitant heterotropia often are troubled by postoperative diplopia, which occurs in response to the newly acquired position of the eyes. It may persist from a few days to weeks or even months. Its duration depends upon the patient's ability to ignore it and hence is more prolonged and troublesome in adults. It usually disappears with time. When the residual deviation is too small for resurgery, persistent troublesome diplopia can be relieved with prisms. Alternate occlusion often helps patients to learn alternate suppression.

Decreased muscle function: Minimal limitation of action of an operated extraocular muscle may appear in the immediate postoperative phase. This is probably due to the excessive handling of the muscle or splinting of the eye by the patient due to postoperative pain and inflammation. It usually recovers in a week or two. Severe limitation of movement on the other hand may indicate a slipped muscle, and calls for careful examination and necessary intervention.

Infection: Serious complications related to infections leading to endophthalmitis, orbital cellulitis or suture abscess have been reported but are extremely rare.

Allergic reactions: Mild to moderate allergic reactions to suture material are more common than infections and may present as ocular discomfort, conjunctival congestion, chemosis and swelling of lids during 6–8 weeks after surgery. Treatment with topical corticosteroids is usually enough. Localized granulomas may appear 2–4 weeks after surgery. Treatment is by topical corticosteroids. Occasionally, excision may become necessary.

Conjunctival cysts: Occasionally, small conjunctival cysts filled with clear fluid may form. These can usually be evacuated by a needle puncture.

Corneal Dellen: Corneal Dellen may appear as whitish elevated areas near the margin of the cornea specially when the limbal incision is used. They are due to interruption in the tear film. They can be prevented by the proper closure of the limbal wound and resection or recession of any excessive conjunctiva to prevent tissue elevation near the limbus. They can be relieved by a pad and bandage.

Anterior Segment Ischemia: Anterior segment ischemia is a very rare but serious complication. It occurs due to the disruption of blood supply to the anterior segment, as a result of injury to the anterior ciliary arteries when three or four recti are operated upon in one sitting. Adults are more susceptible than children.

Ischemia manifests within 24 hours of surgery as corneal edema, haze, Descemet's folds, mild keratic precipitates and cells in aqueous. Segmental iris atrophy, distorted pupil and cataract appear late. Treatment consists of intensive topical and systemic corticosteroids.

RESULTS

The aim of all strabismus surgery is the mechanical restoration of ocular alignment to facilitate and strengthen binocular vision. Full functional cure is difficult and sometimes impossible. Untreated infants lose the potential for binocular development rapidly; hence to achieve good or at least some degree of binocular vision in children with congenital strabismus surgical alignment should be aimed as early as possible preferably by the age of 18 months. When the strabismus is acquired or intermittent, chances of regaining binocular vision with appropriate ocular alignment are greatly increased. The potential for binocular restoration however, decreases with the duration of strabismus. Depending upon the multiple variables described earlier, the outcome of strabismus surgery may be one of the following:

I   a. Orthophoria or asymptomatic heterophoria with normal visual acuity in both eyes, stable ocular alignment, normal retinal correspondence, normal fusional amplitudes and normal stereopsis.

   b. Orthophoria or asymptomatic heterophoria with normal visual acuity in both eyes, stable ocular alignment, normal retinal correspondence, reduced fusional amplitudes and reduced stereopsis. These patients may need orthoptic exercises to strengthen the fusional amplitudes.

II. Stable ocular alignment with microtropia and mild amblyopia. These cases have small angle esotropia or exotropia (+/- 10pd), mild amblyopia, central, peri or parafoveolar fixation, ARC with reduced fusional amplitudes reduced or absent stereopsis. Treatment for amblyopia may be useful.

III. Cosmetically acceptable small angle esotropia or exotropia (+/- 20pd) with suppression or amblyopia, absent fusion and absent stereopsis. Some patients may have ARC and reduced fusional amplitudes. Prisms may be helpful in some patients to overcome suppression and strengthen fusional reflexes. The ocular alignment in these patients may not be stable.

IV. Cosmetically unacceptable residual or consecutive squint. These patients require resurgery and till that is done they need the usual care of uniocular and binocular vision by glasses, occlusion and prisms.

Due to the complexity of the sensory and motor neuromuscular apparatus of the eyes, the variability in results is unavoidable even in the most experienced and skillful hands, but it can be minimized by attention to detail in preoperative evaluation and surgical technique. Finally, the visibility of the result, in terms of cosmetic appearance and properly functioning eyes, is most gratifying to the patient and his relatives and gives a satisfaction akin to that achieved after successful cataract surgery. Fortunately, an unsatisfactory cosmetic appearance can usually be corrected with further surgery unless a disastrous step has been taken during the previous surgery.

Though some recent studies claim less variable results by incorporating axial length measurements in planning the amount of surgery, there is still a long way to go in the understanding of various factors, and the pursuit to improve functional results and minimize the variability of motor results after strabismus surgery continues.

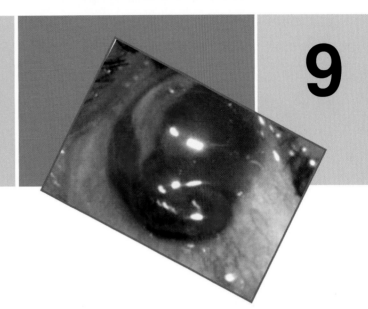
Trauma

43. Ocular Trauma

Ocular Trauma

S Natarajan, Kavita Rao, Arindam Chakravarti

INTRODUCTION

Ocular trauma is the most important preventable cause of blindness in all age groups. It is the cause of blindness or partial loss of vision in more than half a million people worldwide. The National Eye Institute Trauma System Registry (NETSR) report on penetrating eye injuries noted that 83% of the patients were men and the median age was 27 years, ranging from 1 to 92 years of age. Posterior segment trauma is the most common causes of severe visual loss after eye trauma.

Over the past few years, there is an improvement in the management of ocular trauma cases due to advancement in imaging techniques, instrumentation and observation systems. Vitreoretinal surgery for complications of ocular trauma has evolved greatly over the years due to a better understanding of the pathophysiology and pathoanatomy of vitreoretinal complications of eye trauma.

The NETSR has reported that 22% of 2,939 cases of penetrating eye injury were the result of assault, while 21% of the injuries occurred at the worksite. In the worksite related cases, the most common causes of injury were projectiles, sharp objects, blunt objects and blasts. However, prevention of injuries at workplace is often not very realistic. Thus, the efficient management of ocular trauma is of eminence. Ocular injuries have not received enough attention in India and the statistics on eye trauma are not yet available.

A study by Dandona and associates found that ocular trauma affected 1 in 25 people in the urban population and 1 in 167 was estimated to be blind in at least one eye due to trauma. The majority of trauma resulting in blindness occurred during childhood and young adulthood, usually while playing, was higher in males and in the lower socioeconomic group.

EVALUATION AND INITIAL MANAGEMENT

The goals of evaluation are to determine subsequent diagnostic and therapeutic decision and to be of prognostic significance. The following examination should orderly be:

- Recognition of emergency conditions—life threatening/ ocular emergencies (chemical injuries, central retinal arterial occlusion) in which case the treatment will continue along with evaluation.
- The recognition of complete extent of ocular involvement and its classification.
- Concurrent medical conditions.
- Ancillary tests.

OCULAR TRAUMA CLASSIFICATION SYSTEM

The Ocular Trauma Classification Group was organized to establish a system to classify categorically mechanical injuries of the eye. This system provides unambiguous definition for each term and has become the common international language of ocular trauma terminology improving the accuracy in both clinical practice and research (Table 43.1).

This classification system is based on four specific variables that have been shown to be prognostic of final visual outcome. These variables can clinically be assessed on initial ophthalmological examination or during initial surgical procedure. For open globe injuries in which an intraocular foreign body is not suspected, this classification system does not rely on more sophisticated testing, such as ultrasonography or computed tomography. Cases in which there is a high clinical suspicion of an intraocular foreign body that cannot be confirmed on clinical examination or in closed-globe injuries in which media opacity prohibits examination of intraocular structures ancillary testing including X-ray, computed tomography or ultrasonography is required to classify injuries.

The group established a classification system based on standard terminology and features of eye injuries at initial examination that have prognostic significance. The classification system established is limited to the mechanical injuries of the globe. Chemical, electrical and thermal ocular injuries are not included. The classification system has been subdivided for open and closed injuries of the globe because

Table 43.1: Definitions of ocular trauma

Terms	Definitions	Remarks
Eyewall	Sclera and cornea	Though technically the wall of the eye has three coats posterior to the limbus, for clinical purposes it is more feasible to restrict the term "eye wall" to the rigid structure of the sclera and cornea
Closed globe	The eye wall does not have a full thickness wound	Caused by partial thickness sharp (contusion) and superficial foreign body force (lamellar laceration), blunt force (contusion) and superficial foreign body
Open globe	The eye wall has a full thickness wound	The cornea and/or sclera sustained through and through injury
Rupture	Full thickness would be caused by a blunt object	The eye wall gives way under blunt force at its weakest point, which may or may not be at the impact site
Laceration	Full thickness corneal and/or scleral wound caused by a sharp object	The globe opening occurs at the site of impact
Penetrating injury	Single, full thickness wound of the eye wall, usually caused by a sharp object	No exit wound has occurred
Intraocular foreign body injury	The retained foreign object causes a single entrance wound	Technically a penetrating injury, but grouped separately because of different treatment and prognosis implications
Perforating injury	Two full thickness wounds (entrance and exit) of the eye wall usually caused by a missile.	The two wounds caused by the same agent.
Contusion	Closed-globe injury resulting from a blunt object; injury can occur at the site of impact or at a distant site secondary to changes in globe configuration or momentary intraocular pressure elevation.	No full thickness eye wall injury.
Lamellar laceration	Closed-globe injury of the eye wall or bulbar conjunctive usually caused by a sharp object; the wound occurs at the impact site.	Partial thickness defect of bulbar conjunctiva or eye wall.
Superficial foreign body	Closed-globe injury resulting from a projectile; the foreign body becomes lodged into the conjunctiva and/or eye wall but does not result in a full thickness eye wall defect.	The force of impact may be blunt/sharp or both.

the resultant pathological responses and treatment strategies are quite different depending on the integrity of the globe.

This classification system is based on four specific variables that have been shown to be prognostic of final visual outcome: type of injury; grade of injury; visual acuity at initial examination; presence of a relative afferent papillary defect in the involved eye and the zone of injury based on the location of the globe opening in open-globe injuries or the most posterior structure involved in closed globe injuries. The classification primarily is done at the time of initial examination. In cases requiring initial surgical repair, modification of the initial classification is done during surgery. Additionally, gained information would suggest alternative classification for the injury.

Type of Injury

The type of injury refers to the mechanism of injury. Classification of the type of injury is based primarily on the circumstances of the injury.

Grade of Injury

The grade of injury is based on visual acuity of the injured eye at initial examination. The testing is done for distance and near.

When possible, all testing is done with patients' corrective lenses with or without pinhole. Visual acuity of no light perception is confirmed with a bright light source while the fellow eye is completely occluded. Visual acuity is a physiologic variable limited by its subjective nature. Nevertheless, it has proven to be the strongest predictor of visual outcome in open-globe injuries.

Relative Afferent Pupillary Defect

Relative afferent pupillary defect grossly measures optic nerve and retinal functions. The testing utilizes swinging flash light test. If one pupil is mechanically or pharmacologically nonreactive or cannot be visualized because of media opacity, it can still be assessed by observing the consensual response in fellow eye.

Zone of Injury

The zone of injury is defined by the location of the most posterior full thickness aspect of the globe opening. Zone I injuries occur when the opening of the globe is isolated to the cornea or corneoscleral limbus. Zone II injuries are those that involve the anterior 5 mm of the sclera. Zone III injuries are those that extend the full thickness into the sclera more than 5 mm posterior to the corneoscleral limbus. In cases of multiple corneoscleral openings, the zone is defined as the most posterior opening. In case of intraocular foreign bodies, the zone is defined as the entry site, whereas in perforating injuries, the zone is defined as the most posterior defect, generally, at the exit site.

For closed-globe injuries, since no full thickness opening of the eye wall has occurred, the categories of intraocular foreign body, penetrating, perforating and rupture do not apply. Instead, closed-globe injury, involves blunt forces resulting in contusion injury, sharp forces resulting in lamellar-lacerating injury, or injuries that result in superficial foreign bodies. These foreign bodies become lodged in the bulbar conjunctiva, cornea or sclera, and are defined as superficial because they do not result in a full thickness defect in the eye wall. When a combination of injury types occur, then the mixed-injury category is more appropriate.

The zones in closed-globe injuries are based on the anteroposterior anatomic location of injury. However, because closed-globe injures do not involve full thickness wounds, these injuries are zoned according to the tissues injured.

Zone I

Zone I injuries are superficial injuries limited to the bulbar conjunctiva, sclera or cornea. These include corneal abrasions, traumatic conjunctival hemorrhages and intracorneal foreign bodies.

Zone II

Zone II injuries involve structures in the anterior segment up to and including the lens apparatus and include the lens, zonules and pars plicata.

Zone III

Zone III injuries are posterior injuries, involving the pars plana, choroids, retina, vitreous or optic nerve. When structures in more than one zone are involved, the zone of the most posterior involvement classifies the injuries.

Ancillary Testing

Over the past decade, diagnostic ancillary techniques have been found to be extremely useful in the initial management of ruptured globes. The imaging methods used are: plain X-ray orbit, ultrasonography, computed tomography (CT) scan, magnetic resonance imaging (MRI) and electophysiological tests. Plain X-ray and ultrasonography give sufficient information in most of the cases of a planned surgical approach.

Electrophysiological Tests

Both Electroretinogram (ERG) and visual evoked potential (VEP) have both been used as valuable prognostic indicators, especially in opaque media. Hirose and associates found that though a recordable ERG and VEP did not always indicate a good prognosis, a nonrecordable ERG tended to indicate a poor visual outcome. Others found the VEP to be the single best predictor of visual outcome. ERG also has a role in the assessment of metallosis bulbi.

X-ray

Though the role of X-ray has diminished due to more sophisticated modalities, it still remains a cost effective means of screening for foreign bodies and orbital integrity. The shape and number of foreign body can be determined and their localization has become more accurate using ultrasonography determined axial lengths.

Ultrasonography

B-scan and A-scan are useful to detect the effects of trauma on the anterior and posterior segment in opaque media. Immersion techniques are used to delineate anterior lesions such as hyphema, iridodialysis, lens integrity and position. Posteriorly the presence of vitreous hemorrhage, posterior vitreous detachment, retinal detachment, posterior segment scleral wounds, choroidal detachments and blood in the suprachoroidal space can be detected. It is useful in the evaluation of intraocular foreign body (IOFB), metallic and nonmetallic and their localization relative to the ocular coats. Contact ultrasound with sterile covers can be done in the operation theatre after repair of large lacerations (Fig. 43.1).

Computed Tomography

Computed Tomography (CT) scan of the orbit is a standard diagnostic and noninvasive technique used to locate intraocular foreign body, especially smaller than 1 mm size and less radiodense objects of slightly larger size. It is used to detect the size of orbital wall fractures and incarceration of orbital contents. It is a confirmatory technique for ruptured globe showing the presence of intraocular air bubbles. Signs of scleral rupture on CT include "Flat Tyre Sign", i.e. flattening of the posterior surface and evidence of scleral thickening. It is best to insist on the thinnest possible slices with overlapping cuts. The only drawback of CT in localization is seen one or more foreign bodies have a sufficient attenuation coefficient and volume to cause streak and Hounsfield artifacts.

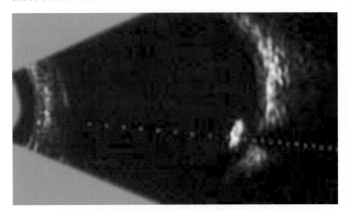

Fig. 43.1: B-scan ultrasonography shows retained intraocular metallic foreign body

Magnetic Resonance Imaging

This investigative technique provides superior tissue definition and resolution. However, it cannot be used in the suspicion of a ferromagnetic IOFB which could be dislodged and produce further damage to the eye. With its superior resolution, it helps in evaluation of occult scleral ruptures, large hemorrhagic choroidal detachments and dense vitreous hemorrhage. It can be used to detect radiolucent and wooden, plastic and glass IOFB. Inspite of the cortical bone being hypointense, the hyperintensity of the orbital fat allows orbital fractures to be well visualized.

ANTERIOR SEGMENT TRAUMA

Conjunctival Injury

Blunt Trauma

The conjunctiva is one component of the first line of ocular defense and is involved in many cases of blunt trauma to the eye and orbit. Common clinical findings are either bleeding or air under the conjunctiva. Although subconjunctival hemorrhage is alarming in appearance, timely management and reassurance of hematoma will initially spread and then, without treatment, gradually absorb over approximately 2 weeks.

Foreign Body

Single or multiple foreign bodies embedded in the conjunctiva and cornea is common in the setting of minor occupational accidents. Minor non-penetrating foreign bodies have irritative consequences and are potential indicators of a concurrent intraocular or intraorbital foreign body, which needs inspection of the entire globe for a perforating wound. Removal of foreign body embedded in the conjunctiva is done by sweeping with cotton tipped applicator or fine forceps with the aid of topical anesthesia. Many inert materials can remain indefinitely within the conjunctiva without adverse reaction.

Laceration

Conjunctival lacerations (Fig. 43.2) may occur in settings of injury and involving sharp projectiles, notably broken glass. Clinical signs may readily be evident upon external or slit lamp examination as a conjunctival surface defect with prolapse of Tenon's tissue or orbital fat or exposure of sclera. Careful inspection of the conjunctival defect can be done using topical anesthesia followed by dilated ophthalmology. Surgical repair is not needed for small conjunctival laceration unless the defect us greater than 1 cm. Careful inspection for underlying occult scleral lacerations is a must.

Corneal Injury (Closed Globe Injury)

Contusion

A direct, focal, concussive blow causes mechanical deformation injury to endothelium, causing severe intraocular damage.

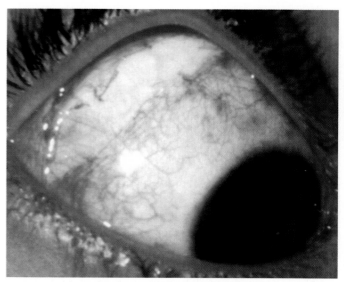

Fig. 43.2: Conjunctival laceration

Acute appearance of corneal edema is an alarming feature but visual improvement usually occurs within 3 months. Corneal rupture is an uncommon consequence of blunt trauma.

Foreign Body

Clinical signs of presence of foreign bodies are blurred vision, photophobia and foreign body sensation, which are evident through biomicroscopy. Foreign bodies present for more than 24 hours show associated stromal infiltration. A corneal foreign body is usually extracted using topical anesthesia at the slit lamp. Discrete, superficial foreign bodies are dislodged using a foreign body spud or disposable 25-gauge needle under magnification. More deeply embedded foreign bodies, most often noninfectious retained for several days, are difficult to extract but it should carefully be examined to determine possible perforation into the anterior chamber and may be allowed to remain or extrude spontaneously, while foreign bodies of large and more central warrant surgical removal. Following removal, the foreign body should be cultured to look for any potentially infectious infiltrate.

Abrasion

Superficial abrasions of the corneal epithelium are caused by direct or tangential impact from a foreign body most commonly from a fingernail, plant, paper, etc. which are microbial contaminated, leading to the possibility of secondary infection. The clinical diagnosis is usually evident upon biomicroscopic examination of the cornea, where an epithelial defect is most vividly appreciated with fluorescein or rose bengal stain.

Corneoscleral Tears

Lamellar corneal lacerations are detected by careful slit lamp evaluation (Fig. 43.3). In these cases, cornea is not perforated and anterior chamber is not entered. Intraocular pressure by applanation tonometry should be done only if laceration site can be avoided. Seidel test should be negative.

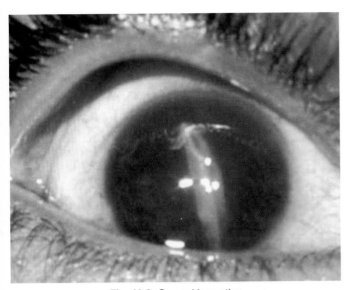

Fig. 43.3: Corneal laceration

Occasionally bandage soft contact lens is used with antibiotic eye drops along with cycloplegia. Re-evaluation should be done daily.

Subconjunctival Hemorrhage

There may be a history of eye injury with a sharp object. Slit lamp examination reveals subconjunctival hemorrhage, corneal laceration with or without prolapse of intraocular content (Fig. 43.4), shallow or deep anterior chamber compared with normal eye, hyphema. Once the diagnosis of full thickness corneoscleral tear is established, further examination should be avoided until the time of surgical repair to prevent extrusion of intraocular contents.

The following measures should be taken:
- Protect the eye with shield
- Keep patient nil orally
- Systemic antibiotics

Analgesic and antiemetics may be prescribed to prevent Valsalva effect. Surgical procedure, accurate wound closure, is important for watertight wound, thus maintaining anterior chamber, intraocular pressure postoperatively.

During the procedure, anterior chamber should be maintained by use of viscoelastics edges of the wound are realigned, but suturing may become difficult due to viscoelastic. Excess viscoelastic should be swabbed away.

Repair of the corneal component should be done first followed by scleral component. If corneal tear crosses limbus, then the repair should begin at limbus with 10-0 nylon suture followed by closure of remaining corneal tear. Vitreous, lens fragments, foreign body prolapsed in the wound should be excised. Care should be taken to avoid traction on vitreous. If uvea or retina protrudes, it should gently be reposited by sweeping the iris with spatula through paracentesis at limbus. Necrotic unhealthy uveal tissue should be excised. Vertical tears are closed first followed by shelved tears, as they tend to open up suturing.

Suturing Technique

10-0 nylon on spatula shaped cutting edge needle is used. Sutures with equal bites placed perpendicular to wound edge at depth of 75% to 90% of corneal stroma. Wound edges should firmly be approximated (Fig. 43.5).

Stellated Corneal Lacerations

Closure can be achieved with "X" sutures. In large perforations with extensive tissue loss, full thickness penetrating keratoplasty can be performed as primary procedure.

Scleral Tear Repair

Such an injury has to be repaired. Conjunctival peritomy is done to expose the wound. Prolapsed vitreous excised. Prolapsed non-necrotic uvea and retina reposited with spatula.

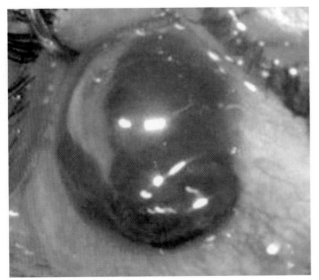

Fig. 43.4: Corneal laceration with iris prolapse

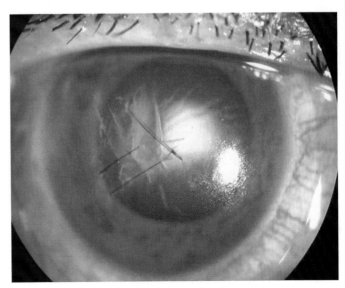

Fig. 43.5: Suturing technique

Scleral wound is closed with 7-0 vicryl. Exploration of the globe should always be done to trace the posterior extent of the tear. Scleral repair should be done as far posteriorly as possible. Necrotic tissue should be excised and prolapsed vitreous is excised with microvit. Prolapsed excised tissue should be sent for microbiological examination.

Subconjunctival broad-spectrum antibiotics are used at the end of the procedure. Intravitreal antibiotics, like vancomycin 1 mg and amikacin 200 µg, are given in cases of contaminated wounds involving vitreous. Postoperatively systemic antibiotics are added. Steroids are to be avoided, if infection is suspected.

Hyphema

Clot formation and integrity are maximum in 4–7 days. Rebleeding occurs in 3.5% to 38% of patients usually 2–5 days following trauma. Clot retraction is thought to be a key factor in rebleeding. Antifibrinolytic agent such as aminocaproic acid given as 50 mg/kg as a 5 days course is thought to reduce the risk of rebleeding. Fibronolytic agents to lyse the clot cause significant corneal toxicity. Tissue plasminogen activator (tPA) is affected in the clearance of hyphema, but may contribute to rebleeding if used within 48 hours of the initial bleed (Fig. 43.6).

The followings are the indications for surgical drainage:
- IOP > 59 mm Hg for 5 days or > 35 mm Hg for 7 days
- High IOP associated with corneal staining
- Total hyphema not resolving after 5 days.

Surgical Procedure

A bimanual approach with the hand held 20-gauge infusion cannula and a vitreous cutter is recommended as this allows a controlled removal with less risk of globe hypotony.

Angle Recession Glaucoma

The forceful expansion at the equator following blunt trauma may cause tissue separation, which can lead to both acute and long-term glaucoma. The injuries include acute and long-term glaucoma. The injuries include a tearing of the papillary margin, tear of the peripheral iris and a tear of the ciliary body itself. The typical tears occur into the face of the ciliary body between the scleral spur and the region of iris insertion between the circular and the longitudinal muscles. Gonioscopy reveals unevenness in the width of the ciliary body band and a width greater than one trabecular meshwork. If the muscle is torn from its attachment to the scleral spur, a cyclodialysis cleft is seen. Tears in the surface of the trabecular meshwork are seen as torn iris processes or a white prominent scleral spur.

Following injury, the intraocular pressure may be elevated in association with inflammatory cells, angle recession and hyphema. Use of topical steroids to reduce inflammation and trabecular scarring should continue for 6 weeks. If more than 180° of the angle is recessed, there is up to a 10% chance of subsequent development of chronic glaucoma. Standard glaucoma management should be followed.

Cyclodialysis on the other hand are associated with hypotony and require treatment in the form of laser photocoagulation, cryotherapy or direct suturing. The iridodialysis, if large, is repaired along with the reconstruction of the anterior chamber. It is essential in cases that may require silicone oil to prevent corneal touch. An artificial polymethylmethacrylate iris has been designed for patients with traumatic aniridia who require silicone oil injection.

Traumatic Cataract

Traumatic cataracts (Figs 43.7 and 43.8) are associated with inherent complications like corneal tears, iridodialysis, posterior capsular rent, anterior capsule tear and zonular dialysis. Majority of these patients are young in whom good visual outcome and early visual rehabilitation is a must. Modalities of management of traumatic cataracts are extracapsular surgery with intraocular lens and small incision cataract surgery. Of late, small incision cataract surgery and phacoemulsification has become more popular because of early visual rehabilitation.

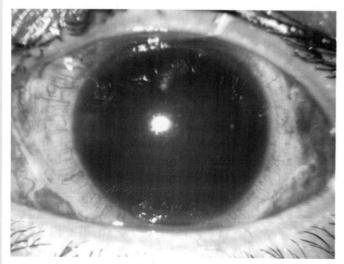

Fig. 43.6: Posttraumatic hyphema

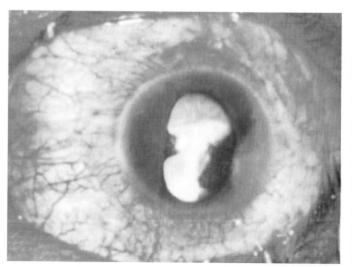

Fig. 43.7: Traumatic cataract

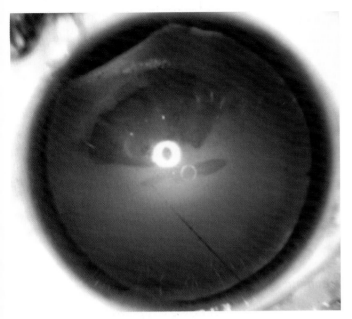

Fig. 43.8: Traumatic cataract with zonular dialysis

Preoperative anterior segment evaluation by slit lamp examination, tension applanation, gonioscopy and posterior segment evaluation should be done by indirect ophthalmoscopy and in cases where fundus examination is difficult due to opaque media; B-scan ultrasonography should be done.

General anesthesia is preferred to achieve good hypotony during surgery. But in conditions where it is not possible, local anesthesia can be given with extra precautions like 100 ml intravenous Mannitol given half an hour before surgery for good hypotony. Facial block should be given before retrobulbar block and ocular massage should be avoided. Surgical steps should be modified depending on the situation. Scleral tunnel of 6–6.5 mm is adequate. Capsulorhexis is preferred, as in cases with preexisting posterior capsule rents, intraocular lens can be placed over the anterior capsule rim. In cases with anterior capsule rupture, anterior capsulotomy should be completed by can-opener type capsulotomy or linear capsulotomy carefully removing the anterior capsule tags with Vannas scissors. Hydroprocedures, like hydrodissection, should be done in selected cases. In cases with penetrating injuries and anticipated posterior capsule rents, it is avoided or done with caution. Nucleus is prolapsed into the anterior chamber by wheeling with Sinsky's hook. Irrigation and aspiration of cortex is done by Simcoe cannula. In cases with posterior capsular rent, irrigation and aspiration in that area should be done last to avoid vitreous disturbance. Vitreous disturbance should be anticipated and managed meticulously by automated anterior vitrectomy. Salient features of small incision cataract surgery in traumatic cataract include less induced astigmatism due to small tunnel size: anterior chamber is well maintained due to valve effect of the tunnel; hence intraoperative manipulations like automated anterior vitrectomy can be done without further damaging the already compromised endothelium. Surgeon has to be

trained for this technique and facility for automated vitrectomy becomes crucial.

Postoperative Management

Postoperative management includes systemic antibiotics and analgesics. Commonest problem encountered postoperatively is iritis, which may be aggravation of preexisting iritis, which can successfully be controlled by antibiotic steroid eye drops. In cases with corneoscleral injuries, steroid eye drops should be avoided and can be replaced with nonsteroidal anti-inflammatory group of eye drops. Adequate postoperative mydriasis is helpful.

CLOSED GLOBE POSTERIOR SEGMENT TRAUMA

Mechanism of Contusion

Blunt trauma to ocular, periocular or cranial regions produce ocular damage by coup or contrecoup mechanisms. Coup injuries cause local trauma directly at the sight of injury. Contrecoup damage occurs at a site opposite to the site of impact. Anteroposterior compression of the eye results in a horizontal displacement of the eye fluids. The posterior segment structures are stretched and may tear. Damage occurs at tissue interfaces especially at the chorioretinal and scleral interface and hence retinal damage is common.

Traumatic Maculopathies

Commotio Retinae

Commotio Retinae was first described by Berlin in 1873. Blunt trauma to the anterior portion of the globe may produce commotio retinae anywhere in the posterior segment though typically occurring to the site of impact. It takes several minutes to hours to manifest. It is seen as a geographic pattern of gray-white cloudy opacification of the outer retina with ill-defined margins. If the entire posterior pole is involved, a pseudo-cherry-red spot is seen. Visual acuity drops when the macula is affected. Experimental model suggests that the visual outcome of an eye with commotio retinae is dependent on the number and location of damaged photoreceptors. Histopathological examination shows major alteration in the outer retina with edema in the outer plexiform, nuclear and photoreceptor layers. Fluorescein angiography shows blocked choroidal fluorescence, but there is no change in the retinal or choroidal vascular permeability. Retinal pigment epithelium alterations may be seen. The prognosis is usually good unless associated with other injuries. The lesion may resolve completely or there may be varying degrees of retinal pigment epithelium mottling, which in severe cases may appear to be a pseudoretinitis pigmentosa syndrome.

Purtscher's Retinopathy

Purtscher's retinopathy was first described by Purtscher in 1910 as a syndrome of sudden blindness in traumatized eyes associated with multiple areas of superficial retinal whitening located primarily in the posterior pole. In Purtscher's retinopathy, the setting is one of severe head trauma, or chest compression in the absence of direct trauma to the globe. The frequency of this condition is unknown. Other presenting features were scattered intraretinal hemorrhages and preretinal hemorrhages. In its classical form, Purtscher's retinopathy consists of marked generalized retinal edema, macular edema, multiple patches of peripapillary superficial retinal whitening, intraretinal hemorrhages and disc edema (Fig. 43.9). Purtscher called this condition angiopathia retinae traumatica and postulated that the white spots were lymphatic extravasations caused by a sudden increased in intracranial pressure related to head trauma. Traumatic retinal angiopathy has come to be known as Purtscher's retinopathy and the white patches are now recognized as cotton wool spots.

In the acute stages of Purtscher's retinopathy, the following fluorescein angiographic findings have been demonstrated: normal choroidal filling with some blockage of background choroidal fluorescence; impaired or occluded retinal capillary nonperfusion or leakage; late perivenous staining and/or partial vein obstruction and optic disc edema.

Choroidal Rupture

Indirect choroidal ruptures result from compressive injury to the posterior pole of the eye with horizontal expansion of the globe. The elastic retina and tough sclera resists rupture, but the relatively inelastic Bruch's membrane is prone to rupture along with overlying retinal pigment epithelium and underlying choriocapillaris. They are usually single, curvilinear, concentric and temporal to the disc, but may rarely be nasal, multiple and radial (Figs 43.10A and B). The rupture is obscured by overlying hemorrhage and, as the lesion resolves, a yellow-white scar is seen. Visual acuity is affected if the tear passes through the fovea and a variety of field defects may be seen. The fluorescein angiography helps to detect small ruptures and their location

in reference to the foveal center. Histopathological studies showed that bleeding follows choroidal rupture, fibrovascular tissue proliferation and retinal pigment epithelium hyperplasia. After stabilization, the patients need to be re-evaluated for secondary choroidal neovascularization.

Retinitis Sclopetaria

Retinitis sclopetaria, chorioretinitis sclopetaria and chorioretinitis proliferans are all names that have been applied to a distinct fundus picture that may follow high-velocity missile injury to the orbit by high-velocity missile, such as a BB pellet. It is attributable to shock waves produced in the orbit by the missile either directly adjacent to the path of the missile and the macula. Extent of ocular damage is determined by the missile's proximity to the globe, its velocity and its size.

Traumatic Macular Hole

Traumatic macular hole (Fig. 43.11) is found in association with postcontusion injuries: commotio retinae, subretinal hemorrhage and choroidal rupture, whiplash maculopathy and

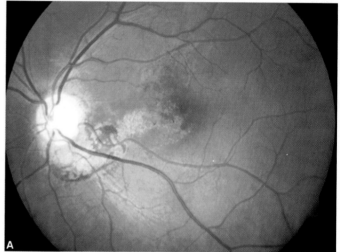

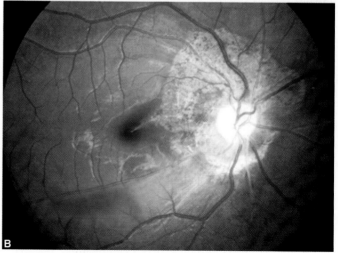

Figs 43.10A and B: Choroidal rupture

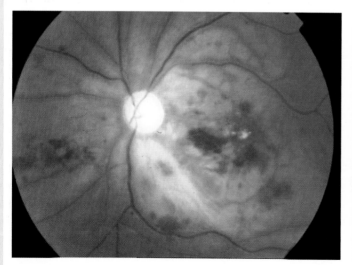

Fig. 43.9: Purtscher's retinopathy

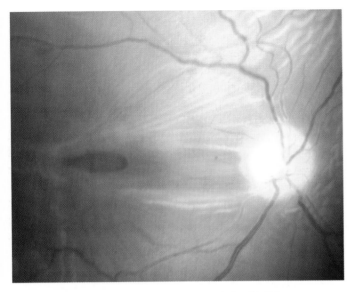

Fig. 43.11: Traumatic macular hole with RD

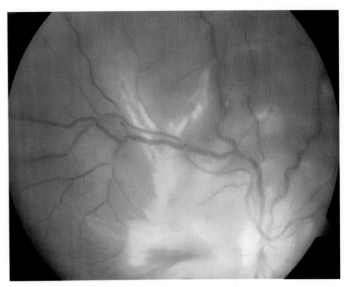

Fig. 43.12: Traumatic retinal detachment

cystoid macular edema. Postcontusion necrosis may result in cystoid macular edema and the development of cystic space that coalesce to produce a large cyst. Rupture of inner layer of a larger macular cyst may produce a lamellar hole. If both the inner and the outer walls of a macular cyst disappear, a full thickness hole may develop. Acute vitreofoveal traction, a partial or complete separation of the posterior vitreous phase from its adherence to the macula can create a macular hole. Differentiation of lamellar holes from full thickness macular holes is associated by biomicroscopic recognition of an intact outer retinal layer and the absence of any subretinal fluid in the lamellar hole. Optical coherence tomography (OCT) outlines the depth of the hole, surrounding retinal changes and the extent of vitreous traction. Visual acuity drops to 20/80−20/200 along with a central scotoma and metamorphopsia. The macular hole and its localized detachment may remain stationery, however, progressive detachment of the posterior pole and peripheral retina has been known to occur with a traumatic macular hole. Treatment consists of vitrectomy, air/fluid exchange with Brilliant Blue or Indocyanine green dye staining to peel the internal limiting membrane and C_3F_8 injection followed by postoperative prone positioning for 3 weeks. Postoperative OCTs are done to document macular hole closure.

Traumatic Retinal Tears and Detachment

Retinal tears due to trauma are the results of transmission of an external force to the globe with resultant distortion. Ocular contusion produces a forceful anteroposterior compression of the globe, with a resultant lateral expansion of the equatorial region and disinsertion or tearing of the retina. Two major mechanisms may lead to retinal tears after blunt trauma. The first results from changes in the shape of the globe with secondary tractional effects on the vitreous base. Other rare manifestations include vitreous base avulsion, retinal dialysis and giant retinal tears; all of these may be associated with retinal detachment. The second type of retinal tears result from fragmentation and necrosis of the retina at the site of direct trauma to the sclera.

Retinal tears associated with direct trauma are often associated with intraretinal hemorrhages and retinal edema; producing large, irregular retinal tears. Retinal tears not associated with retinal detachment caused by ocular contusion may be treated with cryopexy or photocoagulation. Retinal detachment requires scleral buckling or vitreoretinal surgery (Fig. 43.12).

Traumatic Endophthalmitis

Postoperative endophthalmitis is most frequently caused by gram-positive cocci, staphylococcus epidermis. Traumatic endophthalmitis is unique in having a high incidence of bacillus species, in particular B. cereus. The diagnosis of traumatic endophthalmitis depends on a high index of suspicion followed by the application of appropriate diagnostic procedures and culture techniques. The recognition of endophthalmitis following trauma may be obscured by the consequences of the trauma itself, such as pain, swelling, redness, media opacity and loss of vision (Fig. 43.13). The management of traumatic endophthalmitis includes three clinical settings: prophylaxis of endophthalmitis, initial management of suspected endophthalmitis (presumptive treatment) and subsequent management of culture-positive cases. The specific elements of management include intraocular antibiotics, vitrectomy and steroids. Intravitreal antifungals along with oral antifungals may be required in the setting of documented fungal endophthalmitis. But most of these patients need vitrectomy and prognosis is usually poor.

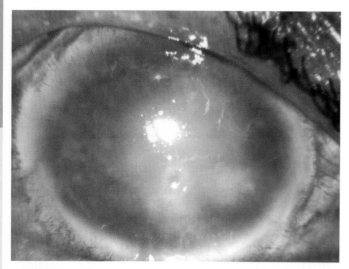

Fig. 43.13: Traumatic endophthalmitis

Open Globe Posterior Segment Trauma

The final insult is a result of the trauma as well as the effect of the reparative processes. The initial inflammatory reaction, as well as blood, is an important stimulus for significant cellular proliferation. Cells such as myofibroblasts proliferate along the scaffold of the vitreous gel and along the surface of the retina. Myofibroblasts subsequently contract resulting retinal detachment. Collagen deposition occurs on the surface of the detached retina and causes further immobilization. Pars plana lacerations appear to be associated with more damage than wounds more posteriorly perhaps due to the vitreoretinal relations in the area of the vitreous base and ora serrata. Penetrating injury through the retina itself rarely causes rhegmatogenous retinal detachment and the usual response is tractional detachment.

Vitrectomy and Penetrating Injury

Vitrectomy permits the removal of vitreous hemorrhage and other opacities and the scaffold on which the cells proliferate. The stimulus to intraocular inflammation is diminished limiting the formation of membranes and traction on the retina.

Timing of Vitrectomy

Immediate vitrectomy is done if there is an infectious endophthalmitis, risk of rapid toxic damage from IOFB and retinal detachment. In most cases, however, it is performed 4–14 days after injury to allow the media to clear up and a posterior vitreous detachment to occur thereby simplifying the surgery.

Indications

Major indications include non-clearing vitreous hemorrhage, vitreous hemorrhage with retinal detachment, IOFB, endophthalmitis, posterior perforations, giant retinal tears, macular holes, sympathetic ophthalmitis.

Basic Steps

A standard three-port vitrectomy is done avoiding sites of scleral rupture. Core vitrectomy done followed by posterior cortical removal, along with a meticulous anterior vitrectomy to remove anteroposterior traction. Areas of vitreoretinal adhesions are freed from the rest of the vitreous to relieve traction. Membranes and retinal adhesions are removed with forceps; traction bands and fibrovascular proliferation are cut after diathermy. Perfluorocarbon liquid is used to stabilize the retina. Endolaser is applied around areas of retinal breaks. Long-term tamponade is achieved with silicone oil or C_3F_8. Scleral buckle is required to support the vitreous base and retinal breaks.

Special Situations in Vitrectomy

Retinal Incarceration

After a complete vitrectomy, a circumferential relaxing retinotomy is made just posterior to the incarceration site followed by scleral buckling. For more posterior incarcerations relaxing retinotomies, circumscribing the incarceration site along with prolonged tamponade is required.

Subretinal Hemorrhage

Traumatic submacular hemorrhages and hemorrhagic retinal detachments may produce significant retinal damage if not managed timely. Han and associates described three indications for surgical management including retinal breaks elevated by hemorrhage, massive hemorrhagic retinal detachment involving the posterior pole and bullous detachment of the retina. A three-port pars plana vitrectomy followed by internal drainage through retinotomies is required. If the blood is liquefied, it is removed with a cannula. Clotted blood is removed with forceps or lysed by tPA injection.

Suprachoroidal Hemorrhage

Suprachoroidal hemorrhage needs surgical intervention in the presence of kissing choroidals, development of severe glaucoma, severe eye pain, macular involvement with anterior retinal displacement and associated retinal detachment. A pars plana vitrectomy with a temporary infusion cannula at the limbus is performed. Phakic eyes may require lensectomy. The drainage sclerotomy are radially made in the area of greatest hemorrhage at or just posterior to the insertion of the recti muscle. Upon entering the suprachoroidal space, the cyclodialysis spatula is used to facilitate removal of the hemorrhage. A limited anterior vitrectomy is performed with subsequent injection of perfluorocarbon liquid to push the suprachoroidal blood anteriorly, allowing the drainage from the sclerotomy sites.

Perforating (Double Penetrating Injury)

The initial treatment should be limited to the closure of the anterior wound. The posterior wounds often close spontaneously and vitreoretinal surgery should be deferred to 7–10 days after the injury. During vitrectomy, the vitreous incarceration should carefully be excised so as not to reopen the wound. Retinal incarceration is managed with relaxing retinotomies. Prolonged internal tamponade and scleral buckling are required.

Intraocular Foreign Body

Posterior segment IOFBs penetrating through sclera retains the highest momentum (Fig. 43.14). The incidence of IOFBs is in young males with an average age of 20–40 years. Ocular damage is caused by the IOFB due to the penetrating injury itself as well as associated microbial endophthalmitis, toxicity and other inflammatory reactions. The ocular reaction elicited depends on the size of the foreign body, the vascularity of the surrounding tissues and the chemical reactiveness of the foreign body. Reactive metallic foreign bodies can cause extensive damage known as metallosis bulbi following electrolytic dissociation. They need urgent removal by vitrectomy. Other indications for immediate surgical intervention are vegetative foreign bodies and endophthalmitis.

Inert foreign bodies, like glass, may be observed if they are not causing any complications like retinal detachment or vitreous hemorrhage.

Siderosis

Iron either pure or as an alloy is the most frequently seen metallic IOFB. Iron contamination of ocular tissue causes a characteristic clinical picture termed 'Siderosis'.

The iris assumes a brownish color pupil becomes mid dilated due to damage to the sphincter dilatory muscles and eventually nonreactive to light and accommodation. Iron deposits in the epithelial cells of the anterior capsule of the lens forming brownish dots. Pigmentary degeneration of the retina develops in the periphery, extending posteriorly causing concentric visual field loss. Retinal arterioles sclerose and fine pigmentary changes occur at the macula. Iron infiltration of the trabecular meshwork causes a type of open angle glaucoma. ERG is very sensitive diagnostic tool showing reduced b-wave amplitude, which is reversible.

Chalcosis

Copper or its alloys (e.g. bronze, brass, etc.) IOFBs are seen most commonly with wire injuries or shell explosives. Pure copper usually causes a severe acute inflammatory reaction. Copper alloys cause clinical findings similar to endogenous chalcosis due to hepatolenticular degeneration. These include a Kayser-Fleisher ring, sunflower anterior subcapsular cataract, metallic refractile particle in the anterior chamber, a greenish iris and a brilliant highly refractile deposit on the surface of the retina. Copper deposits on limiting membranes, whereas iron deposits intracellularly causing more extensive damage.

Management of Dislocated Crystalline Lens

A standard three-port vitrectomy is followed by lensectomy with the vitreous cutter if the nucleus is soft. For harder nuclei, ultrasonic fragmentation is done. The lens is first aspirated into the mid-vitreous cavity and then fragmented. This procedure can be facilitated, by floating the lens into the vitreous cavity by perfluorocarbon liquids. Sometimes, if the nucleus is hard, after doing vitrectomy, it can be manipulated into the anterior chamber with the help of MVR blade or microvit and then removed by corneal or scleral section. Scleral fixated intraocular lens implantation may be planned in the same sitting.

Rarely, the crystalline lens may be lodged in the subconjuctival space following trauma, a condition known as traumatic phacocele (Fig. 43.15). This condition requires surgical extraction of the lens by anterior approach with scleral fixated IOL implantation.

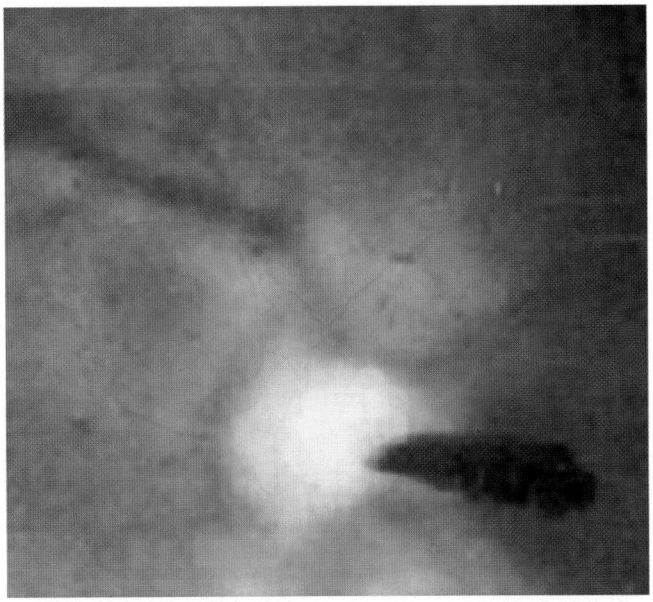

Fig. 43.14: Fundus photograph shows intraocular foreign body in front of the optic disc

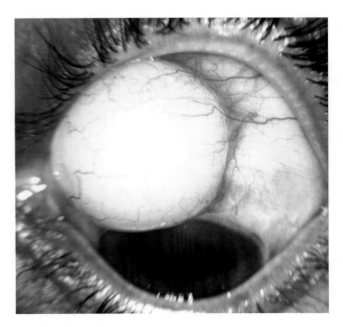

Fig. 43.15: Traumatic phacocele

Post traumatic Posterior Dislocation of Posterior Chamber Intraocular Lens

Blunt trauma may lead to posterior dislocation of the IOL in the vitreous (Fig. 43.16). Associated retinal breaks, retinal detachment or vitreous hemorrhage may be present. The condition is managed by standard three-port vitrectomy, the IOL is grasped with forceps and manipulated into the anterior chamber. It is removed either through a corneal section or scleral section. Some surgeons prefer to inject PFCL over the posterior pole to facilitate grasping the IOL without causing any iatrogenic breaks in the retina. SFIOL or PCIOL may be planned in the same sitting depending on the extent of capsular support present.

MANAGEMENT OF RETAINED INTRAOCULAR FOREIGN BODY

Diagnosis and Localization

The history and physical examination will be complemented by appropriate ancillary tests. A careful history is crucial in all cases of trauma. Special focus should be laid on the circumstances and possible mechanism of injury. If an IOFB is suspected, the ophthalmologist should attempt to determine the material, its likelihood of contamination and the force with which it struck the eye. Identification of entrance wounds, the path of a suspected foreign body and prompt fundus examination are the areas of prompt attention. Radiographs are perhaps the simplest and most readily available method of IOFB identification, but are of limited use. CT scanning has become the standard method of detection and location of IOFBs. Anteriorly located IOFBs may be discovered through CT scan. It will help in identification of metallic and nonmetallic IOFBs and composition of nonmetallic IOFBs. MRI is also used to identify and localize IOFBs, but magnetic IOFBs have been shown to move on exposure to the magnetic field. Ultrasound, particularly high-frequency ultrasound, is more effective than plain films in the detection of IOFBs.

Surgical Technique

Magnetic Extraction

External and internal electromagnets can be used to remove magnetic foreign bodies from the posterior segment via a direct or indirect approach. The direct approach refers to application of the electromagnet over the sclera directly adjacent to the IOFB. The IOFB should be located in the intraretinal or subretinal space or over the pars plana and the location must be accessible for scleral incision. The indirect refers to application of the electromagnet above the pars plana at a distance from the IOFB. This is done when the IOFB is located in the vitreous, over the retina without evidence of retinal penetration, or posteriorly (when a pan retinal or intraretinal location is inaccessible to extraction through adjacent sclera). This approach is used primarily for small, magnetic, intravitreal IOFBs. However, this system does not provide accurate foreign IOFB location.

Vitrectomy

Vitrectomy is used in cases of nonmagnetic, large, or subretinal IOFBs, eyes with opaque media, or more generally, whenever IOFBs cannot be removed by a magnet (Fig. 43.17). When the IOFB is poorly visualized due to cataract or vitreous hemorrhage, vitrectomy or lensectomy are necessary. If the IOFB is nonmagnetic, intraocular forceps or gentle aspiration with a soft-tipped instrument is used. Extension of the scleral port may be required to remove the foreign body. If the foreign body is too large, it has to be removed via a limbal wound. Injection of perfluorocarbon liquid has been suggested as a means to protect the macula during this maneuver. The visual prognosis depends largely on the site of impaction, with macular involvement portending a poorer visual prognosis.

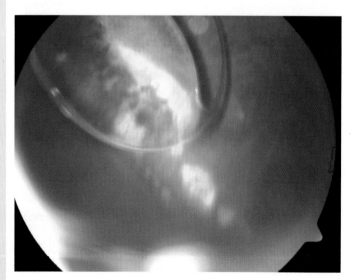

Fig. 43.16: Traumatic posterior dislocation of IOL

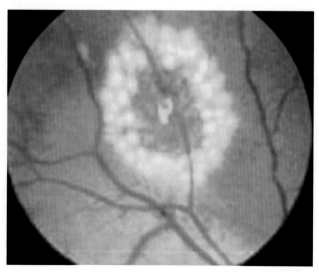

Fig. 43.17: Fundus photograph shows laser marks around the site of a foreign body removed following pars plana vitrectomy

Chemical Injuries of the Eye: Alkali and Acid Burns

Chemical injury are potentially devastating ocular surface injuries that may result in permanent unilateral or bilateral visual impairment. Severe ocular chemical injuries require rapid assessment and initiation of treatment. Alkali injuries are usually more severe than acid injuries, the latter tending to remain confined to the ocular surface and producing more superficial damage (Table 43.2).

Alkali Burns

The most common chemical causing alkali burns are ammonia (NH_3), lye (NaOH), potassium hydroxide (KOH, caustic potash), magnesium hydroxide [$Mg(OH)_2$] and lime [$Ca(OH)_2$]. When ammonia and lime are in direct contact with the eye, their lipid solubility results in extreme rapid penetration. Magnesium hydroxide may add to the thermal injury produced by fireworks. Lime is the most common cause of alkali injuries in the construction work place, but it penetrates poorly into the corneal stroma.

Though alkali differs in their ability to penetrate the eye, the mechanism by which the hydroxyl ion causes damage to the eye is the same for all alkaline substance. The cation determines the ability to penetrate the tissues. Alkalis are lipid soluble and are able to penetrate with or without cellular death. Deeper penetration causes changes in the trabecular meshwork, lens and ciliary body. Ciliary body involvement causes a change in the constituents of the aqueous humor. The pH increases and correlates with tissue damage. The ability to concentrate ascorbate decreases the aqueous levels.

Collagen loss in the form of stromal ulceration is the common occurrence and usually occurs after 2−3 weeks of injury. Several enzymes that may account for this process have been found in the cornea. These include glycosidases and proteases. Collagenolytic activity has been demonstrated early in the corneal epithelium but peaks at 14−21 days. Calcium and zinc ions are necessary for collagenase activity. The infiltrating polymorphonuclear leucocyte and fibroblasts may also play a role.

Corneal ulceration usually stops when the epithelium becomes intact or when the cornea becomes totally vascularized. The cornea in the reparative stages presents a picture typical of localized scorbutus. The ciliary body normally concentrates ascorbate in the aqueous humor. Ascorbate is necessary for the synthesis of nature collagen.

Acid Burns

The acids that are the most clinically important sources of chemical injuries are sulfuric acid (H_2SO_4), sulfurous acid (H_2SO_3), hydrofluoric acid (HF), hydrochloric acid (HCl), nitrous acid (HNO_3) and acetic acid (CH_3COOH).

Sulfuric acid is the most commonly encountered and a common industrial acid and a component of automobile battery acid. Sulfuric acid reacts with water in the precorneal tear film producing heat and charring of the corneal and conjunctival

Table 43.2: Therapy for chemical eye injury

I. Initiate primary therapy:

a. Irrigate—With water or sterile saline, if available, which is preferred as it is isotonic and sterile. For a minimum of 30 minutes, adequacy can be assessed by measuring the pH of the inferior cul-de-sac

b. Remove particular matter or dissolve with 0.01–0.05 M solution of EDTA

c. Debride devitalized tissue—Debatable

d. Initiate antimicrobial therapy

e. Mydriatic—Cycloplegic agent

f. Antiglaucoma medication—IOP is best determined by a pneumotonometer or an electronic tonometer. Carbonic anhydrase inhibitors are preferred over topical therapy

g. Corticosteroids—Topical preparations to decrease the number of inflammatory cells. They may be used during the first 10 days even if the epithelium is not intact. Thereafter, they are continued only if epithelial healing occurs

h. Topical collagenase inhibitors—10–20% N-acetyl cysteine (Mucomyst) every 2 hours. 0.5% suspension of Medroxy progesterone also inhibits production of collagenase

i. Subconjunctival heparin: 0.75 ml in cases with perilimbal ischemia may promote revascularization

j. Hydrophilic contact lens facilitates corneal epithelial regeneration and is left for 6–8 weeks

k. Scleral lenses and symblepheron rings

II. Promote epithelial wound healing (using one or more of the following):

a. Tear substitutes and lubricants

b. Punctal occlusion in severely dry eyes

c. Lid closure (taping, pressure patch, tarsorrhaphy)

d. Therapeutic soft contact lens

e. Fibrinonectin (investigational)

f. Epidermal growth factor (investigational)

g. Ocular surface (conjunctival or limbal) transplantation

h. Keratoepithelioplasty

III. Limit ulceration and support repair by:

a. Minimizing corticosteroid use after 10 days, unless re-epithelialization is complete

b. Use of one or more of the following:

- Progestational steroids (provera 1%)
- Ascorbate—Oral 2 gms per day or a topical 10% solution to be used only in ulcerative conditions.
- Citrate—Decreases availability of calcium required for collagenase activity
- Tissue adhesive (isobutyl cyanoacrylate) and soft contact lens
- Conjunctival flap
- Keratoplasty—Patch graft, lamellar keratoplasty, penetrating keratoplasty

IV. Avoid complications (using one or more of the following):

a. Antiglaucoma medications (inhibitors of aqueous production)

b. Cycloplegics

c. Lysis of conjunctival adhesions (glass rods)

d. Long-term anti-inflammatory therapy

e. Retinoic acid

f. Ocular surface transplantation prior to penetrating keratoplasty

epithelium. Sulfurous acid is formed from sulfur dioxide and water and commonly used as a fruit and vegetable preservative. When an injury occurs from a refrigerant, the severity is related to the penetration of the acid. Hydrofluoric acid is a weak inorganic acid that produces skin burns and severe ocular injury, mainly because of the toxicity of the fluoride ion. Hydrochloric acid produces severe ocular injury relatively infrequently and has unique feature of producing a yellow epithelial opacity.

Acid burns generally produce less severe injuries than alkalis because they have the ability to coagulate the epithelial surface forming a relative barrier to further penetration. The corneal stroma has a buffering capacity for solutions with a pH less than 4. The lesions produced are sharply demarcated and significant ischemia is not encountered.

Clinical Course and Evaluation

Roper-Hall (Ballen) classification of alkali burns is shown in Table 43.3. McCulley has divided the clinical course of chemical injuries into four phases (Figs 43.18A to 43.20):

Table 43.3: Roper-Hall (Ballen) classification of alkali burns

Grade 1	• Excellent prognosis • Corneal epithelial damage • No ischemia
Grade 2	• Good prognosis • Cornea hazy but details of iris seen • Ischemia affects less than one third of the limbus
Grade 3	• Guarded prognosis • Total loss of corneal epithelium • Stromal haze obscures iris details • Ischemia affects one third to one half of the limbus
Grade 4	• Poor prognosis • Cornea opaque • Obscuring view of iris or pupil • Ischemia affects more than one half of the limbus

1. *Immediate phase:* It is the first phase immediately after a chemical injury, where the detailed examination will be done after completion of copious irrigation. Proper examination should be carried out which can provide information regarding ultimate prognosis.

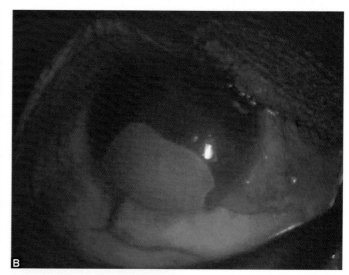

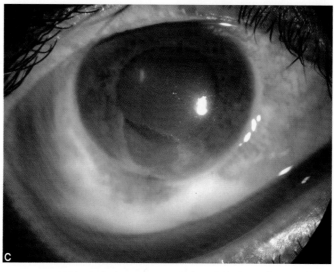

Figs 43.18 A to C: Various grades of chemical injury

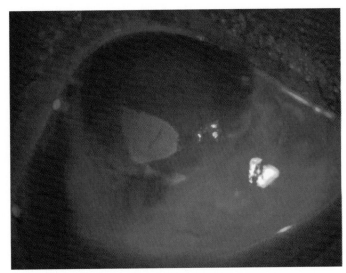

Fig. 43.19: Corneal epithelial defect with inferior conjunctivalization

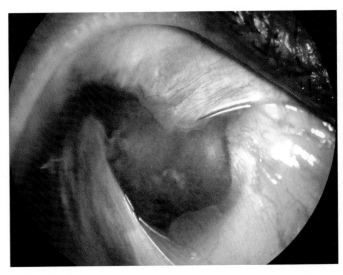

Fig. 43.20: Extensive symblepharon following chemical injury

2. *Acute phase:* This phase refers to the first week after injury, where re-epithelialization and keratocyte proliferation and migration occur concurrently with progressive ocular surface and intraocular inflammation. Clinical features include conjunctival and corneal epithelial defects, corneal edema, prelimbal ischemia and vascular thrombosis, fibrinous iritis, cataract and raised intraocular pressures.

3. *Early reparative phase:* This phase refers to 7–21 days after injury. The epithelium starts degenerating along with corneal neovascularization and invasion of inflammatory cells. In cases with severe endothelial damage, retrocorneal fibrous membranes develop. The iritis usually disappears. The dreaded complication of corneal ulceration occurs in this phase.

4. *Late reparative phase:* This phase refers to 21 days or more after injury. There may be progression of stromal ulceration and perforation may occur. There is progressive corneal vascularization and loss of corneal nerves. Tear film abnormalities result from a diffuse loss of goblet cells and scarring with loss of accessory lacrimal gland. The eyes may be glaucomatous though severe damage and fibrosis of the ciliary body results in hypotony and eventual phthisis bulbi. Cataract may develop conjunctival scarring results in symblepheron formation, trichiasis and entropion. The injured eyes can be classified into two groups. In first group, epithelialization has been completed or nearly completed and in second group, conjunctival re-epithelialization is required for all resurfacing and corneal re-epithelialization has proceeded poorly or not at all.

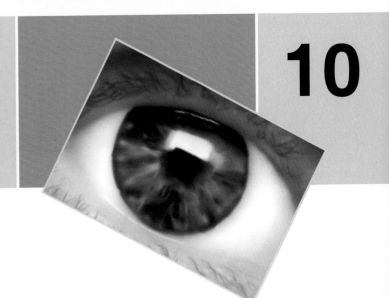

Section 10

Practice Management

Ophthalmology Practice Management

Sandeep Saxena, Puneet Saxena, Manoj K Tangri

A successful practice comes not only from excellent surgical skills and judgment, but also from good business management. Business management skills are generally more important in solo or small group practices because a health care professional is involved in the daily management of his or her office. However, in large group practices, business management knowledge and experience are important for every member of the practice because the business environment is frequently complex. Running a successful practice requires the following management philosophy to set the ground rules for running an orderly, efficient and ethical office:

* Dedication towards providing the highest quality of care to patients.
* Emphasis on the fact that patients are the most important assets.
* Importance of remembering patients' names and treating patients with courtesy.
* Fairness and insistence on the spirit and cooperation and teamwork among employees.

SETTING SPECIFIC GOALS FOR SUCCESS

Setting performance goals is vital to managing yourself and your practice. In doing so, you may have made a common mistake–confusing objectives with activities. Activities are not objectives. Activities are how you achieve the objectives, the outcome-based goals. An activity for an ophthalmology practice might be to research the needs of a certain target patient population. An outcome would be to increase the revenue, generate a specific number of employer contracts or exceed customer service expectations. Your first step in establishing goals and taking action should be to focus on outcomes not activities. Once you have that focus, you must choose from the following four measures for measuring success:

I. **Speed and time:** Many practices evaluate their performance by whether they can respond to patients within a reasonable time.
II. **Cost:** Cost is familiar to all practices. A laser vision correction center needs to monitor new patient acquisition costs.
III. **Specifications and expectations:** This concept applies to any performance challenge that demands adherence to one or more product specifications or customer expectations.
IV. **Positive yields:** This involves determining what positive impacts you are trying to accomplish. Many positive yields are familiar, such as revenue, profits and market share. Others are less familiar, such as the strength of comanagement relationships.

When you know how you will be measuring your progress, its time to set specific performance goals:

* **Specific goals:** The more tightly you define your goal, the more focused your actions will be.
* **Measurable goals:** Goals must be measurable, if the practice hopes to benefit from the tracking and feedback that is so critical for the performance.
* **Aggressive and achievable goals**: Set ambitious goals to push the practice beyond the comfort zone, but do not make the goals too far to reach.
* **Relevant goals:** The goals you set should pertain directly to your practice's performance challenges.
* **Time deadline for goals:** Without a time deadline, the practice has no built-in performance accountability.

The challenging business of change will become second nature as you learn to distinguish between outcomes and activities, thus, allowing you to focus in the end on performance. This outcomes-based management approach will transform your practice into a smoothly working instrument of sustainable performance cycles.

Making Resolutions

Making resolutions is easy. Making them stick is something else. Some simple and practical steps, which can help you to turn your resolutions into accomplishments, are the following:

Focus on Your Goal

A clear and measurable goal makes all the difference. Focus on what you want to create instead of the problem. This simple principle can be applied to resolutions involving your practice.

By being very specific about what you want, you further define your goal and create a clear picture of what you want to accomplish.

Determine Where You Are and Compare

Do not compare yourself to where you were last year or to what your competition is, unless that's where you want to be. When determining reality, opinions don't count. Back up your perceptions with real data. You cannot increase your referrals, if you do not know how many referrals you have now. Once you've clearly established where you are and where you want to be, you will soon train yourself to take only those actions that lead to your goal.

Involve Others

The bigger the picture you envision, the more you will have to involve others. Most of your resolutions will involve the participation of other members in one of following three roles. Mentors who will provide guidance, support people who will help in work and monitors who will hold you accountable. Each team member needs to have a clear grasp of current reality if they will be going to help you make progress towards your goal.

Stepping into the future, do not worry that the goal you are picturing is too big. Think of this new millennium as a clean slate. Carefully paint a picture of what you want your practice to look like next year. Then with the help from your team, make that picture a reality.

Successful Practice

Some of the most successful practices are that they are in charmed locations. Some surgeons work in markets so rural that staffing and facility costs are a fraction of what their urban counterparts pay. Only the most fortunate surgeons can work in easy markets. The following list can help assure control of your business affairs and ultimate commercial success, even in the most demanding markets:

Make Great Decisions

After making sure that your decision is ethical and legal, most decisions are based on their profitability. Gather the facts and let facts make your decision.

Make Collective Business Decisions

Engaging every individual likely to be impacted by your decision is good. Getting the opinion of people smarter or more experienced, than you are on the subject, is important. The sharpest clinical minds are often frustratingly dull when applied to business affairs.

Strive Daily to Increase Profitability

Large profits and quality gains are less common in mature practices. However, even the most developed and refined practice can make small, incremental improvements.

Leave Your Options Open

Think twice before abandoning patient services, closing an office or dismissing a key staff member. Take an introductory laser in situ keratomileusis course to stay current, even if you never plan to perform refractive surgery.

Remain Diversified

Sharply falling profitability in the present scenario is just the latest in along list of hard lessons. For safety, no single patient service and no single payer should represent more than a third of your cash flow.

Cultivate Better Relationships

Be balanced in your relationship building, including patients, staff, local institutions, vendors and fellow doctors. End each year with better relationships.

Be Disciplined

Most practices that get into trouble do so because their lead doctors are undisciplined in one way or another. They set performance standards for staff members that they are unwilling to keep themselves. In any area where you have a history of being poorly self-disciplined hire an outside source of discipline.

Work Harder and Smarter

The most financially successful surgeons are those who did exceptionally well because they simply worked harder than their peers did.

Seize Opportunity

The most successful people in business are rash and opportunistic. Have sufficient personal and business capital reserves on hand to be able to accept reasonable risks.

Review Every Major Business Decision

Using your current income statement as baseline, review the impact of adding a satellite office, a doctor or a practice service to your practice. Have the intellectual integrity to believe the numbers rather than relying on hunches. At the same time, trust your instinct. A bad feeling about a potential project should trump even the rosiest financial projections.

Office Planning and Procedures

Developing plans for office size and divisions is one of the most important decisions. With limited starting funds one will err in obtaining office space that is too small. Even if some space is left unused at the beginning, the cost of paying extra monthly rent will outweigh the cost of moving the office in the future because of inadequate office space. A minimum of 1,200 square feet should be obtained and 1,500 square feet is not excessive for a one-physician practice. The interior of the office should always be clean, organized and well maintained.

The efficiency, friendliness and convenience of routine office procedures are extremely important for the development of your successful practice. These procedures should ensure high quality patient care, as well as efficient utilization of resources. The patient's initial contact usually occurs by telephone. It cannot be overemphasized that the person who has first contact with a patient is extremely important in creating the patient's proper positive perception of your practice.

Strategic Practice Plan

Moving your practice forward requires more than good intentions. You really need to have a strategic plan, unless you care where your practice is going to end. Strategic planning is a process that helps a practice visualized and positioned itself for the future. The result of this process is a living document offering strategic alternatives for your practice's future success. A strategic plan is not static. It changes as your planning assumptions change. Strategic planning focuses on the big picture. It does not require a comprehensive, detailed financial budget projected years into the future. Generally, strategic plans should cover a three-year planning. Beyond that length of time, the value of strategic and tactical alternatives is greatly diminished because of the rapidly changing health care environment. To plan for your future effectively, the following questions have to be answered about your current status and future goals:

a. How you are performing as compared to your peers?
b. What do you do well?
c. What do you do poorly?
d. What are your competitors' strengths and weaknesses?
e. Will your practice be full service provider or specialty focused?
f. Whether your practice will emphasize quality or value?
g. Whether your practice will aim for niche or broad market penetration?
h. What threatens the future of your practice?
i. What opportunities exist for your practice?

Strategic planning process can be divided into following steps:

Situation Analysis

You must analyze your current situation by looking at the key factors that define where your practice stands. This information will give your planning process a reference point and enhance your ability to make meaningful decisions.

Practice history: Create a chart that shows how your practice has performed during the past three years. This review should compare income statements and important practice statistics and ratios, both over time and in comparison with industry benchmarks. The main purpose is to identify trends and problems and then determine the reason for them. Understanding historical trends helps in assessing strengths and weaknesses more accurately. This is essential if you want to make effective choices for the future.

Patient referral and demographic data: This is a key area of your review regarding patient sources and demographics. These are both important in understanding of patient dynamics and market share. Prepare a spreadsheet showing patient referral sources and analyze the data. It is important to know where your patients live and whether you have gained or lost patients from each area. Create a separate spreadsheet for each service you offer and you will need to explain the trends you uncover.

Productivity: Review your productivity during the three-year period, you are analyzing. This data should include the amount of billing and collections, as well as the number of patient visits and major surgeries performed. This information is important when you explore future options. This data may also shed light on overall practice trends.

Competition: Analyze your competitors. Obtain physician names, subspecialities and services. Obtain surgical market share information from your sources. Analyze their strengths and weaknesses. Their strengths might include: being first in the community, excellent reputation, quality outcomes, subspeciality/full service provider, prominent location, excellent positioning, good Website, ownership of an outpatient surgery center, a state-of-the-art facility and excellent referral relationships. Weaknesses might include poor patient skills and outcomes, inferior location, lack of Website or an inferior one, and limited or no specialty coverage.

Business structure: Analyze your current business structure. Share your strategic plan with your tax advisor before you implement your plan.

Future trends: The last step in your situation analysis is an analysis of other trends that will affect your practice in the future. These include:

- Population trends in your service area.
- Profitability trends.
- Technology trends.

Analysis of Your Practice's Strengths, Weaknesses, Opportunities and Threats

This analysis is the most important step performed in the planning effort. It is vital that you commit proper management resources to the effort. Create two charts for this analysis. The first should help you analyze your practice's strengths and weaknesses. List the different areas of your practice, which may include clinic efficiency, state-of-the-art equipment, services provided, information technology, quality of facility, location(s), marketing abilities, Web site, image, training, morale, employee skills, patient satisfaction, consultation hours, quality of care and patient education. The second chart should allow you to evaluate opportunities and threats. Your list of opportunities may include partner addition, satellite expansion, marketing opportunities, adding/deleting services, referral resource opportunities, mergers or acquisitions, staff addition, improving operational efficiencies, corporate structure, methods to increase market share and optometric networking opportunities. Your list of threats may include hospital and competitive developments, socioeconomic changes, workforce issues and governmental regulations. Your discussion concerning opportunities and threats is one of the most important parts of your strategic planning effort. Combating threats and taking advantages of opportunities is the essence of strategic planning.

Mission Statement

A mission statement is a declaration of a business purpose and core beliefs. It is the guiding light that keeps your practice moving in the right direction. Unfortunately, mission statement has been thought of as a corporate tool, of little relevance to the world of medicine. Few ophthalmologists take mission statement seriously. A mission statement can motivate staff, provide general guidelines for day-to-day operations, create an image you want to project and provide a philosophical guideline for every staff person to follow. This should include some comment about the services you provide, the markets you serve and the level of customer service you plan to offer. The mission statement should reflect your true feelings and philosophies. Credibility and trust within your practice will be severely damaged if your actions routinely contradict your mission statement.

Goal Setting

Goal setting starts by deciding what actions should be taken to minimize or eliminate threats to your practice and take advantage of opportunities. Use your situation analysis data to guide you.

Tactical Planning

Tactical steps define specific actions to be taken, due dates for those actions and responsible individuals. Without such details being specified, goals simply won't be accomplished. Part of the tactical planning should include periodic evaluation or reevaluation of the economic and political wisdom of each goal.

Implementation

Implementation of your tactical plan will require ability and commitment on the part of your staff. Long range planning frequently requires timing and goal modification because of unforeseen factors that arise. To make sure that your implementation stays on track, hold quarterly meetings to review progress and update tactics and goals. Strategic planning is important to the success of any business and ophthalmology practices are no exception.

Positioning the Practice

For marketing to be effective, your practice has to stand out from the crowd. Unless your practice is located in a rural area, you are probably one of a number of eye care options for prospective patients. You have to generate a public image that will set your practice apart from all the others and make patients think that you are the best person to care for their eyes. The most successful practices are those that generate a clear idea about who they are, what they stand for or what they do, in the minds of their patients. This is referred to as "positioning". The following steps will help you in positioning your practice:

Emphasize Specific Characteristic of Your Practice

It is much easier for patients to remember products that are specifically positioned. Patients will be most likely to remember you and your practice, if you can get them to identify you with one simple and clear idea.

Make Your Message Unique

It won't do you any good to position your practice as "high class", if other practices are in your area convey the same message. Choose a message no one else is using.

Make Your Message Relevant

Make sure the thing you emphasize about your practice gets right to the heart of what your patients want.

Convey Convincing Message

In addition to providing a clear image, provide convincing reasons that patients should come to you. Mention your impeccable success rate.

When determining your position, remember that being first is often preferable to being better. A leadership position does have its caveats. First and foremost, you must be willing to invest time and money to educate patients on the positioning you choose. Also, after you have educated patients on your practice's new position, another practice may try to squeeze in on your position. If this happens, remind your patients that you were there first. Telling your patients that you exist isn't sufficient. You have to make them remember you via a clear, distinct image. Position yourself for success.

Competitive Practice Analysis

Your competition is changing in today's dynamic health care arena. Your patients do have a choice. You need to be conscious of who your current competitors are and what they are up to. If you are not careful, other doctors in your market will make inroads into their territory. You need to know as much about your competitors as possible. Hence, you will know how to position yourself so prospective patients will choose your practice and your current patient will not be switching to another doctor.

A competitive analysis is a thought provoking and time-consuming way to check the climate of your marketplace and evaluate your position relative to other doctors who are available to your patients. For a competitive analysis the following questions need to be answered:

1. Who are your major competitors are and where are they located?
2. How are they perceived in the market place?

3. How does your practice rank in terms of size and practice strengths relative to your competitors?
4. What major services do your competitors offer right now and what might they offer in the near future?
5. What methods do they use to promote themselves?
6. Who are their patients?
7. What are their pricing strategies?
8. Does your practice have any features that differentiate it or give it an advantage over your competition?
9. What services of your competitors are superior or distinct?
10. What services of your competitors have distinct weaknesses?

While many of these questions can be answered relatively easily by you, some observational research will be required. When an ophthalmic practice determines that its product is superior, either in term of features, performance, supporting services or image, emphasizing that competitive advantage is a good way to attract patients. While checking out your competition, emphasizing your strong points in the market place can do a lot to draw patients to your door, but it won't compensate for problems within your own practice. So, take some time to make sure your own practice is in order and not lose all those new patients your competitive analysis will help you bring in.

Marketing

Medical schools have avoided teaching the topic of marketing, in the belief that it is "unprofessional". Marketing is not, as many physicians assume, advertising. It is learning what consumers need, producing a product that meets that need and then telling them that you have done so. Marketing and advertising are frequently confused. Advertising is a part of marketing that deals with selling services to a targeted segment of population. Typically, marketing deals with four major variables: price, product, position and promotion. Marketing improves instead of worsening the medical care, because it forces the physician to understand and satisfy the entire range of patients' wants and needs. With the increase in health care providers and the rising sophistication of buyers, ophthalmologists desperately need to understand marketing, for it quite probably will be one of the factors that separate the practices that succeed from those that fail.

Many of us assume that if we provide the highest quality of care we can, patients will come to us. In doing so we assume that the market wants what we want to provide. This is not necessarily true. Patients want high quality care. But how do they judge an abstract term like quality? We know that outcomes are important, also important are factors like location, consultation hours, fees and bedside manner. In the marketing field, when a provider concentrates on the product rather than the need, its called "marketing myopia". Your practice must do more than provide what you consider to be high quality care. You must determine the wants and needs of your target market and then deliver on those wants and needs more effectively and efficiently than your competitors do. Before making any business decisions, take the time to assess your market and its needs.

Determine what services are needed and how do the patients want those services delivered. The patient judges you not on your services, which are intangible, but on the tangible aspects of their encounters: the place, people and equipment. They generally want to see an office that is professional and up-to-date. The staff has to be friendly, courteous and skilled. The hours should be convenient. Communication with the patient should be thorough, personalized and easy to understand. You have to be believable, reliable and responsive. Also you should consider efficiency, productivity and positive patient outcomes.

Work to delight your patients. Patients who are happy with your service will return to your practice and tell friends and referring physicians too. If a patient does have a complaint, resolve it as quickly as possible.

Your staff is an extension of you. Staff members can truly make or break a practice. If they project a caring attitude or do their jobs well, your image will be enhanced and patients will be much more likely to return to your practice. Before involving staff in your marketing efforts, think of them as your internal market. Studies show that the top service organizations consider their employees as a separate market and work hard to make them happy.

Ophthalmologists must remain flexible to respond effectively to changing consumer tastes and needs in today's business environment. Always be attuned to ways to make the patient visit more enjoyable. Be sure to keep patients informed about new techniques, treatment and products. Present this news in a way that lets patient know that you embrace change that makes their lives better.

The most effective marketing for doctors is the kind that happens without formal advertising. The best referrals still come from current patients and colleagues. When a referral does come your way, send a note of thanks. Reach out to potential patients through activities that are important to them. Give your time through speaking or eye-health screenings. Take an educational approach. For really "hot" topics, such as refractive surgery/other newly developing techniques, consider organizing seminars for family physicians and allied health professionals. Have separate seminars for current patients and the general public. Invest in a comfortable, convenient location and some upscale refreshments. Give patients printed materials, which describe office policies, hours, products and services that are available. This information should be contained in an attractive office brochure that projects a very positive image. Prepare professional looking literature that describes common visual and eye conditions and the treatments available from your office. The better you communicate with your patients, the more satisfied they would feel.

Smart Marketing Plan

Marketing blunders can cripple a practice. In this competitive environment, you must have a carefully constructed marketing plan and budget to succeed. One of the most difficult decisions facing practice administration is how much to spend on marketing. If you allocate insufficient funds and resources to marketing, you run the risk of either losing your competitive position, or if your center is new, failing to establish a secure position in your market. The following critical steps are involved in developing an effective and smart marketing plan and budget:

- *Analyze your market:* You must recognize that each market is unique. Effective advertising depends not just on the reach, frequency and message, but also on what your competitors are doing to capture the market place. Similarly, markets are constantly changing. You may find that what has worked for you in the past may not continue to work in the future.

- *Identify your strengths:* Before you spend on a marketing campaign, it is imperative that you develop a clear understanding of exactly what it is you are offering to your patients. Identify those qualities or factors that differentiate your center from others in the market. The more your doctors and staff contribute to formulating the overall marketing message, the more they are going to internalize and believe in that message.

- *Review performance to date:* Before deciding where you want to go, take time to review where you have been. Analyze what percentage of your patients is generated through external advertising and other sources. Discern any positive or negative trends in the profile of your customer base.

- *Assess your target market:* Assess the demographics of your patients and identify your target market. Analyze whether you can find an opportunity to build business in a previously undeveloped segment of your market. Determine what can be done to penetrate this market.

- *Set quarterly goals:* Just as it is critical to involve your team in the formulation of your overall marketing strategy, it is equally important that your staff participate in setting quarterly goals. Identify opportunities for improvement and decide which resources can be allocated to achieve these goals.

- *Establish a budget:* Successful centers typically spend approximately 5 to 15% of their gross revenue on marketing. A start-up center will usually spend a higher percentage to establish its position in the market. Conversely, a well-established center may not have to spend as much on external advertising and can focus its effort on internal marketing to ensure a steady stream of word-of-mouth referrals.

- *Determine your marketing mix:* Depending on your quarterly goals, decide how much you want to spend on each of the following categories:
  1. *External advertising:* This includes the print media and direct mail.
  2. *Internal marketing:* This includes newsletters, patient satisfaction surveys and other methods of getting your message to your patients.

Its helpful to prepare a detailed spreadsheet based on your marketing mix. Based on your projected revenue for the quarter, you can allocate your marketing funds to every component in your marketing plan.

- *Establish proper infrastructure:* If your marketing efforts get the phones ringing, but you are not able to capitalize on those increased calls, your efforts will be wasted. It is important to anticipate this key question from your prospective patients: "Why should I choose your center?" Your staff should be able to handle that make-or-break question with assurance and conviction. Be sure to capture as many callers as possible.

- *Start marketing campaign:* Once you are satisfied that all your systems are in place, that all calls will be measured and tracked, that your staff is well trained and that your consultations can be scheduled fairly quickly, begin your marketing campaign.

- *Monitor and modify:* You can only manage what you can measure. Your practice involves a two-stage process:
  1. Conversion of callers to consultation
  2. Conversion of consultations to surgeries. Monitor your performance at each stage. If your consultation rate is low, concentrate and improve your staff's telephone skills. If your consultations are not resulting in surgeries, offer patients a better experience when they come in for your consultation. If your center is achieving a high conversion rate at both stages, but your marketing campaign has not produced the number of additional calls you had anticipated, do not hesitate to modify your campaign.

With any form of marketing, there is always an element of trial and error. It may take two or more attempts before finding the marketing mix and/or message that works best for your practice. The main key is to monitor the results of your marketing campaign and to be flexible enough to change the campaign when change is necessary.

Budgeting the Marketing Plan

One of the best hedges against an economic slump is making sure your practice has a solid foothold in the market place and getting that foothold is primarily a matter of effective marketing. There is no universal agreement about how to budget for marketing. Following three strategies help in determining the amount that is sufficient for marketing:

1. *Sales percentage:* This method bases your marketing budget on a percentage of last year's profits or next year's anticipated profits (or a combination of the two).
2. *Competitive parity:* This method involves determining which advertising vehicles and strategies are being used by practices that dominate your marketplace. Your budget is then determined in relation to the competition.
3. *Objective-driven:* A strategically planned and budgeted marketing campaign is only as good as the objectives it meets. This method requires the most work, but it also offers the most focused results.

A new practice requires a bigger marketing budget than an established practice. Once you get established, your marketing costs should level out. Following three considerations should be kept in mind:

1. *Cuts can backfire:* Practices that slash advertising budgets during periods of economic recession invariably end up losing market share when the economy rebounds.
2. *Plan ahead:* Whenever possible plan in advance. This proactive planning will enable you to secure the lowest rates and the best inventory.
3. *Track your results:* Tracking the success of your current marketing efforts is an integral part of deciding how much to spend on which parts of your marketing budget.

The big picture is that advertising your practice is not a community obligation, nor is it a vehicle to educate the population of your area. Advertising has to be done to earn revenue, to solidify your position in the market place so you can withstand economic fluctuations and to help you gain the resources necessary to improve your facility and provide better care. Marketing is not just a current expense, it is a long-term investment.

Price Issue

Pricing is affecting virtually every practicing ophthalmologist, at every price point. Three things influence price: the evolving technology, evolving patient demographic and the evolving market. During the past few years there has been an incredible explosion in the evolution and supply of technology. With this will come saturation of the supply of technology and falling prices. The demand for various surgeries has also changed, based on a changing patient. Factored into demand is market segmentation. In most communities, the market has segmented into discount, value and premium categories. Approximately 25% of the market is discount-oriented, compared with 50% in the value and 25% in the premium sectors. Thus, about 75% of the customers in most markets are not driven on price, but other factors.

You and your staff can respond to the areas you can influence, namely patient needs and marketing. Today's surgery patients are late adapters. Understanding what drives late adapters emotionally is the key to success. Most patients have concern about having surgery on their eyes. Patients want in-depth knowledge about the procedure. The key to successful marketing is creating and following a comprehensive, budgeted plan that includes patient communications (customer service, brochures and newsletters), public relations, community outreach and Internet marketing and advertising. While the plan should focus on strategies and tactics, it more needs to address how you will market your brand (i.e. the memorable identity that you want others to know you by). Keep your brand in front of patients and you will become a recognized entity. The following strategies will help you minimize the price issue and close sales:

- *Focus on one-to-one relationship with each patient:* The key to increased sales and patient satisfaction is delivering to each prospective patient's emotional needs. Take every opportunity to inform and educate at every stage. At the first opportunity, create a dialogue to understand patient's needs; ensure that your clinic environment is geared towards patient comfort; train your team to connect with the patient and not process patients and ensure that the customer-service standards you set for doctors and are geared toward patient care.

- *Focus on the surgeon:* There is no better way to get around the price issue than focusing your marketing messages and strategies around your surgeon. The ophthalmologist and his or her personality, expertise and experience separate every practice from its competition.

- *Focus on the referral base*: It is five times harder to get new patient than to keep an existing patient. Hence, any time, money and effort you direct toward your patient database will be worth it. Periodic newsletters are invaluable part of any patient communications program.

- *Focus on E-marketing:* In addition to using traditional strategies in marketing, you should focus on how to best use the power of the Internet. You need to give visitors—both patients and prospective patients—multiple opportunities to connect with you.

Market Share

As ophthalmology practices have developed, there has been the understandable scramble of providers jockeying for market advantage. Price reduction strategy occurs in every industry. Traditionally, price compression will surface in mature phase of a product or service's evolution. In the rush by many providers to gain market share, price compression decreases a good portion of industry's profitability. In time, financial fall out will reduce the number of low-price providers and the price will rise to a more reasonable long-term number. Not all providers have reduced prices. This means that the industry is experiencing price stratification. Low prices can differentiate providers, but high prices can do the same. However, when setting higher prices, it is important that the patient sees a clear advantage for choosing the higher price. This means they must perceive more value from a particular provider. This could be in the form of surgeon experience, brand awareness, reputation, celebrity endorsement or the latest technological advances. In marketing, introducing an advanced, revolutionary version of a product always has a perceived value to a patient. Building your entire brand around it is problematic. Do not build your market brand on technology alone, because it will eventually weaken your position. Conversely, the ability to become known for the latest advancements in technology over the long haul has tremendous value. When the next great advancement hits the market, the patient in your market would call your center first, because you have built a brand known for being the authority in your community. This is an excellent way to use technology to enhance your brand value. There are certain things, which you can do to capture enough market share to be successful. Do not try to be all things to all patients. You will gain market share by narrowing the scope of its target audience. Target marketing is most likely the future of success. You need to use this strategy more often to your advantage. Seeking help from experts in the field can help ensure your practice gets a fair share in your marketplace.

Patient Service

In the 21st century, time has come where you have to make patient service, the number-one priority. A well-run, profitable practice must know when patients arrive, how long it takes for them to be examined and advised and at what time they leave the clinic. The route to success is having a patient not get lost or overlooked in the system. A time routing sheet can be devised to help in finding areas of congestion and eliminating problems before they get out of hand. A time routing sheet should contain following items: patient name, chart number, time of arrival, time patient was brought to the examining room, time of examination and advice, time patient left office and miscellaneous notes. Using this system creates an accurate charting of patient flow and gives you a record of the amount of time a patient spends in clinic. Patients value their time and are adept at discerning what your practice is doing to improve their visits. Waiting is a major source of complaints for clinics. In today's world, medical professionals must find ways to better serve the patients. Exceptional customer service is what keeps people loyal.

Patient Care

Better patient care can be provided without cutting corners. Clinicians get maximum support from their team and latest equipment. You cannot do it alone. It takes a highly competent team working with the latest equipment. You cannot achieve the increase overnight. It takes planning and patience as you and your team refine the patient-care process. Clinical experience makes it possible. A new way to schedule patients is required. The patient visits can be divided into "longs" and "shorts". The long visits are complete or complex follow-up examinations. The short visits are postoperative check and quick follow up examinations. To keep the schedule going, you need to have great phone triage. Make sure your reception desk understands how to schedule patients, including emergencies. Along with regular appointments always schedule a few slots for emergencies. Divide some days between surgery and clinic. One option is to have clinic in the morning so that in case of any surgical delays, the clinic schedule is not disturbed. It is important to invest in newer equipment, which is faster and easier to operate. This kind of pace won't work unless the office is streamlined. Create customized forms to reduce time-spent writing. Ask your staff members to suggest changes that will improve efficiency. When hiring new staff, screen carefully. Good people once hired will learn quickly and try to serve patients well. An experienced and competent staff makes efficient practice possible. Don't try to operate in a vacuum. Visit other practices to see what they are doing to increase efficiency. Invite other practices to visit yours. Visitors often ask questions/make suggestions that may lead to further refinements.

Improving Referrals

Patients and doctors are the single most important source of new patients. Concentrate on efforts on developing and nurturing referral relationships with other physicians, allied health personnel and patients. Other physicians and allied health professionals will never refer to you unless they are aware of who you are and what you do. Once you know some referring doctors, stay in touch with them. Assume a profile in the local medical society and in the hospital staff. Meet and greet other doctors any chance you get. Always be available. Always agree to see patients who are referred to you. Always take other doctors' calls. Always share information with the referring doctor. No matter how inconvenient they are, referrals are an opportunity and not a burden. Always follow up immediately with the referring doctor by sending a brief letter describing the diagnosis and treatment plan. Follow up with the patient. Make a quick personal call or drop a letter to the patient asking how he or she is doing and repeat any instructions or advice. Just by your behavior, you can open doors or close them. If you feel other doctors respected and valued, they will return the favor in ongoing referrals that sustain your practice for years to come.

Benchmarking Ophthalmology Practice

Surviving in today's increasingly competitive marketplace necessitates setting appropriate fees, tracking economic factors (net income and market share) and carefully managing overhead. Knowing your practice's number is important. But seeing where your practice stands in relation to other successful practices can be even more valuable; it can help you pinpoint areas in which your practice may be in need of attention. For the majority of ophthalmic practices, the analysis and maintenance of their own economic health entails an annual benchmarking effort. More frequent analyses both facilitate the process and make the ophthalmic office far more efficient. Weekly business analysis (quick-keys review) will give you the ability to identify and correct negative conditions early, when they are relatively easy to address. The quick-keys review should take little time and cost. Like any proactive tool, its purpose is to prevent the extensive amounts of time, money and effort that a long-detected business problem can cost a practice (Table 44.1). The following comments will help in clarifying the meaning of some of the categories:

- *Net income and expenses:* Having too high a level of expenses is a common problem, particularly in areas of marketing, staffing and fees paid for surgical room assess.

- *Global fee structure:* The most successful refractive practices do not try to compete by lowering price. Instead, they sell their services on the basis of their skills and experience and the quality of care and follow up they offer.

- *Accounts receivable:* If your accountant uses the accural system, this number may be misleading; the accrual system allows some existing debt to be omitted from this number.

If your accountant uses the cash system, your accounts receivable figure should be representative of your true current situation.

- *Surgery room charges:* This figure will vary depending on volume.
- *Miscellaneous expenses:* Usually this covers for expenses, such as insurance/cleaning/depriciation/laundry.
- *Ratio of assets to liabilities:* Generally, anything higher than 5:1 should be considered excellent. However, a lower ratio may simply indicate a major recent purchase.
- *High-volume competitors:* To complete these calculations you will have to take into account the number of people living in your area.

Set your schedule for benchmarking. Select a day and time when you will routinely perform the review. Monday morning report alerts you about where you need to focus that week. Identify your fields. Choose the categories for analysis that represent the revenue and cost items most indicative of any business problems needing immediate attention. They are the same ones you focus on in your yearly study, such as revenue breakdown by service, major surgical volume, wages and overhead. As you track the figures weekly, you will be able to identify performance trends and areas in need of improvement, as well as any potential problems. You may well find that this analytical tool helps you to develop and introduce new business ideas into the practice. Program your system to collate the necessary information. For each item, have it provide the year-to-date figure for both the current and previous year, the difference between those figures and the percentage of that difference. Once established, your quick-keys program should

run automatically. Set time aside to review this data and report areas of concern. The first step in making things better is finding out where there is room for improvement.

Embracing Efficiency

If you are trying to set up a hospital-based system of total customer responsiveness then, specialize, create a niche and differentiate yourself. In order to achieve this, five value-added strategies must be followed.

I. *Top quality:* The first value-added strategy is to provide top quality, as perceived by the patient. In order to do this, you have to measure patient satisfaction, find where it is lacking and then set up plans to improve it.

II. *Superior service:* The second value-added strategy is to provide superior service and emphasize the intangibles. This means doing little things that make you special. Even if they are marginally better than the competition, the groundwork is done for success.

III. *Extraordinary responsiveness:* The third value-added strategy is to achieve extraordinary responsiveness. Concentrate on surgery room turnover, ease in booking cases and so forth. Try to get things faster and quicker than they have ever been done before.

IV. *International perspective:* The fourth value-added strategy is to be an internationalist. This means travelling around in the country and the world and keeping your eyes and ear open to what is going on elsewhere to see who is better, what systems work better and trying to copy these systems.

V. *Uniqueness:* The fifth value-added strategy is to create uniqueness. Strive to be as different and as special as possible. Dream of being the best and then make that dream come true. If you want to achieve excellence, you can get there today. As of this second, quit doing less than excellent work.

Adopting New Technology

Ophthalmologists today find themselves confronted with a continuous stream of appealing new high-tech equipment. Advanced technology can quickly grab your attention and some technologies may indeed prove to be welcome and profitable additions to your practice. But before you commit to any new technology, you need a plan to evaluate its potential for your specific situation. The following questions have to be answered:

1. Will the technology benefit the patients; which of them will benefit most?
2. What special training is required to perform the new procedure?
3. Who pays for the procedure and at what price?
4. What is the profile of the patient who will have this procedure?
5. How many patients routinely seen in practice qualify for the procedure?
6. How can more patients be attracted and at what cost?

Table 44.1: Retained earning and market share calculation

Items	Benchmark	Actual	Difference	Areas of concern
Net income (percentage of gross)	61–64%			
Expenses (percentage of gross)	36–39%			
Total fee				
Accounts receivable	10%			
Marketing budget	5% of revenue			
Ratio of assets to liabilities	5:1			
High-volume competitors in area				
Overhead				
Marketing	5%			
Travel and *CME	0.5%			
Legal and Accounting	0.5%			
Medical Supplies	2%			
Surgery Room Charges	8%			
Office Rent	4%			
Staff Salaries	9%			
Professional Fees	2%			
Miscellaneous Expenses	5–10%			
Total				

*CME: Continuing medical education

7. What is the "per use" cost of the technology?
8. What are the additional costs in facilities, equipment supplies and people?
9. Which competitors are likely to offer the service?
10. Will there be new competitors and what is their value proposition?
11. How does the new technology fit into my practice?

These questions can be answered both objectively and subjectively, with the overall conclusions helping to guide your decision to acquire any new technology.

Computers in Medical Practice

Computers have made many office tasks easier. Although expensive to purchase, maintain and service, use of computer may be worthwhile because it eases the workload of the office.

Computerizing medical records leads to reduced costs. Some systems even have the capability of using digital imaging systems for fluorescein angiograms, in which images are networked into the examining rooms. Computerized medical records improve documentation. As you will get more and more busy, it will become more difficult to document every detail of a complete eye examination. Legibility is another important aspect of documentation. It may also increase efficiency by standardizing the medical record format and making it easier to locate and pull charts. Certain items can now be scanned into the computerized record.

Impact of Information Technology

In recent years, there has been an exponential growth in information technology and its impact on ophthalmology practice. The Internet has revolutionized the speed of access to information. Numerous peer-reviewed journals are now available on the World Wide Web (www). Most freely accessible sites offer a table of contents with abstracts. Some journals are now being published, solely, on the Internet. It is essential for you to develop skills in tracking down the best available current literature. Literature searches are no longer just a research tool but have become an indispensable part of clinical practice. MEDLINE and EMBASE are the most popular and useful computerized databases. Modern information technology has opened a world of instant communication and vast tracts of easily accessible information for you. The earlier you embrace this technology and exploit it, the sooner you will be able to face the challenges.

Doing Business on the World Wide Web

A Web site is a great boost for a practice and is almost required today. In this Internet-dominated era, it has become commonplace for medical practices to set up Web sites accessible to patients and the public and to interact with their patients by e-mail or online. Physician-hosted Web sites can provide access to valuable sources of information, permit more convenient opportunities for physicians to communicate with their patients and to serve as an effective marketing tool for the group.

Proper management of an eye care practice requires constant attention to details in all areas of business. Unlike clinical problems, business issues often do not have only one or two correct answers, but several compromising options.

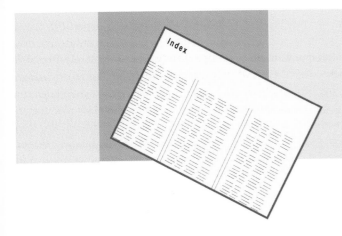

Index

Page number with (f) indicate figures and with (t) indicate tables.

Index

877